EIGHTH EDITION

Counseling Nursing Families

A Lactation Consultant's Guide

Judith Lauwers
BA, FILCA
IBCLC Retired

Kristina Chamberlain
CNM, ARNP, IBCLC, PMH-C

Rosann Edwards
RN, MScN, PhD, IBCLC

Jennie Wagner
EdD, RN, MSN, MBA, CNE, IBCLC

JONES & BARTLETT
LEARNING

LEAARC
In partnership

World Headquarters
Jones & Bartlett Learning
25 Mall Road
Burlington, MA 01803
978-443-5000
info@jblearning.com
www.jblearning.com

Jones & Bartlett Learning books and products are available through most bookstores and online booksellers. To contact Jones & Bartlett Learning directly, call 800-832-0034, fax 978-443-8000, or visit our website, www.jblearning.com.

Substantial discounts on bulk quantities of Jones & Bartlett Learning publications are available to corporations, professional associations, and other qualified organizations. For details and specific discount information, contact the special sales department at Jones & Bartlett Learning via the above contact information or send an email to specialsales@jblearning.com.

30314-8

Production Credits
Vice President, Innovative Learning and Assessment Solutions: Ada Woo
Senior Director, Content Production and Delivery: Christine Emerton
Director, Product: Melissa Kleeman Moy
Acquisitions Editor: Sophie Fleck Teague
Senior Outsourcing Specialist: Carol Brewer Guerrero
Content Coordinator: Samantha Gillespie
Content Management: MPS Limited
Manager, Intellectual Properties and Content Production: Kristen Rogers
Content Production Manager: Belinda Thresher
Senior Intellectual Property Specialist: Colleen Lamy
Senior Product Marketing Manager: Lindsay White
Director, Product Fulfillment: Aaron McKinzie
Purchasing Manager: Wendy Kilborn
Composition: S4Carlisle Publishing Services
Project Management: S4Carlisle Publishing Services
Cover Design: MPS Limited
Text Design: S4Carlisle Publishing Services
Intellectual Property Specialist: Faith Brosnan
Intellectual Property Specialist: Maria Leon Maimone
Cover Image (Title Page, Part Opener, Chapter Opener): © best_vector/Shutterstock
Printing and Binding: Sheridan Kentucky

Library of Congress Cataloging-in-Publication Data
Names: Lauwers, Judith, author. | Edwards, Rosann, 1975- author. | Chamberlain, Kristina, author. | Wagner, Jennie (Jennie M.), author.
Title: Counseling nursing families : a lactation consultant's guide / Judith Lauwers, Rosann Edwards, Kristina Chamberlain, Jennie Wagner.
Other titles: Counseling the nursing mother
Description: Eighth edition. | Burlington, MA : Jones & Bartlett Learning, [2027] | Preceded by: Counseling the nursing mother / Judith Lauwers, Anna Swisher. Seventh edition. [2021] | Includes bibliographical references and index.
Identifiers: LCCN 2024061652 | ISBN 9781284018271 (paperback)
Subjects: MESH: Breast Feeding | Counseling--methods | Infant Nutritional Physiological Phenomena | Lactation--physiology | BISAC: HEALTH & FITNESS / Breastfeeding
Classification: LCC RJ216 .L354 2025 | NLM WS 125 | DDC 649/.33--dc23/eng/20250715
LC record available at https://lccn.loc.gov/2024061652

6048

Printed in the United States of America
29 28 27 26 25 10 9 8 7 6 5 4 3 2 1

Brief Contents

Contents

Color Plate – See the color plate at the end of the book for full-color images.

Preface

Counseling Nursing Families (formerly titled *Counseling the Nursing Mother*) remains unique among lactation texts in its focus on counseling and communication skills. We hope you will gain an appreciation of the significance of counseling techniques and how your style and approach can enhance your interactions with families and thus your effectiveness. Topics are presented within a counseling framework, with practical suggestions and evidence-based information interwoven throughout the text. We hope the insights shared within these pages will assist you in applying knowledge and research to day-to-day clinical practice with an appreciation of counseling challenges and how to help families meet their needs.

Features for educators and students set this text apart from other lactation resources as an ideal text for lactation education. The text is written from a teaching perspective to help the reader grow professionally in the lactation field, with a focus on reaching out to the current generation of families. These features make this text an indispensable resource for lactation educators, students, and interns and provide helpful study tools for the certification exam.

- The comprehensive Glossary contains definitions of over 900 terms used in lactation practice.
- New *Conversation Starters with Parents* appear at the end of each chapter, with examples of open-ended questions to model counseling related to the chapter topics.
- Bulleted lists at the end of chapters identify significant takeaway messages for the information presented in the chapter.
- Full-color photographs identify clinical conditions, and scores of photographs, figures, and tables provide concise summaries and images of topics.

This eighth edition is newly titled *Counseling Nursing Families* to embrace the rich diversity of families, which include mothers and fathers as well as nonbinary and non-cisgender parents. It has been thoroughly reviewed and revised to reflect cultural diversity, equity, and inclusion. Parents are addressed in nongendered terms except where context requires reference to a specific gender. The adjective *breastfeeding* is replaced with *nursing* to acknowledge that parents breastfeed, chestfeed, and pump feed for their babies. The noun *breastfeeding* is replaced with *feeding* or *nursing* to reflect that human milk feeding is the natural form of infant feeding.

With LEAARC as the coauthor, content focuses on what a student, clinician, or counselor needs to know to help nursing families. Chapters are thoroughly updated to include new research regarding the science of lactation, clinical protocols, and counseling methods. Several topics were reorganized within chapters or moved to other chapters to improve flow.

Chapter Features

Chapter 1: Infant feeding practices, lactation recommendations, and global initiatives were updated. Discussions of wet nursing, informal milk sharing, HIV protocols, lactation rates and initiatives, Code violations, and Baby-Friendly designation were expanded.

Chapter 2: The chapter was newly titled "Interdisciplinary Lactation Care." Discussions of lactation consultant practice settings, peer counselor support, interdisciplinary collaboration, and the parent's role on the healthcare team were updated. The "Healthcare Team Approach" section, "Home Health Lactation Program" section, and financial considerations for practice settings section were removed.

Chapter 3: Discussions of cultural factors in lactation support, family dynamics, social behavior, sharing knowledge, and decision-making were updated. Health equity, disparities, inequalities, and systemic inequities were clarified and expanded. Discussions of cultural humility and cultural practices and support were expanded. A new section on microaggression was added. Discussions of intercultural and multilingual communication and the use of interpreters were expanded. Sections on motivational interviewing and working with lesbian, gay, bisexual, transgender/transsexual, queer/questioning, plus (LGBTQ+) families were moved to Chapters 5 and 21, respectively.

Chapter 4: Health consumerism, adult learning, self-confidence, and the role of humor were substantially revised. Discussions of caregiver confidence and guilt were updated. The section "Components of Communication" was moved to Chapter 5.

Chapter 5: The section on communication previously located in Chapter 4 was added, and the chapter was retitled "Communication and Counseling Skills." Discussions of counseling skills for information gathering, affirmation, and education were updated. New sections on trauma-informed care and adverse childhood experiences were added.

Chapter 6: The sections on anticipatory guidance, problem-solving, elements of consultations, and documentation were updated. The sections on consultation methods was updated and expanded to include email, texting, telehealth, and communication challenges during the pandemic.

Chapter 7: The sections on breast anatomy, growth, and function were updated. Discussions of nerve anatomy, techniques for addressing nipple inversion, and the importance of regular self-examination were revised. Discussion of the connection between oxytocin and bonding behavior and the discussion of modifying a syringe to evert a nipple were removed.

Chapter 8: The chapter was retitled "Nutrition in Pregnancy and Lactation." Discussions of basic nutrients, nutritional intake, weight loss, healthy food choices, nutrition guidelines, and standards were updated. The section "Practical Suggestions for Diet" was removed.

Chapter 9: Sections on maternal health, infant health, and properties of colostrum and human milk were extensively revised and updated. A figure on modulating microbiota was changed to a table. Discussion of nutritional components, immunological factors, and immunological and obesity protection of milk was updated. Tables with ranges for early milk intake and comparing human milk to that of other mammals were removed.

Chapter 10: Discussion of the prevalence of, need for, and selection of infant formula was updated, along with discussion of industry practices. The sections on the composition of infant formula and precautions and consequences of its use were updated and expanded.

Chapter 11: Discussions of medications, smoking, caffeine, and alcohol intake were updated. The section on illicit drugs was revised, and the section on opiates was reorganized. The table on the safety of medications was replaced. The section on environmental contaminants was reorganized and revised.

Chapter 12: Discussions of infant feeding choice and the influence of family and friends were extensively revised. A section on mental health factors was added. The section on preparing for nursing was updated, with revisions to the nipple correction discussion. The section on selecting a health-care provider was extensively revised. A section on online support groups and social media influencers was added.

Chapter 13: The sections on prenatal, birth, and postpartum practices were reviewed and updated. Discussions of elective cesarean delivery, labor induction, and postpartum rooming-in were substantially revised. The World Health Organization's Ten Steps for Successful Breastfeeding were updated to reflect current guidelines, including the addition of monitoring and collection of data regarding the feeding status of newborns. The figures on outcomes of labor intervention and the Ten Steps for Successful Breastfeeding appraisal tool were removed.

Chapter 14: The section on newborn assessment was reviewed and updated. Sections on colic and jaundice were revised to reflect current evidence and research. The concept of "purple crying" was introduced. New data and a table on racial/ethnic differences in sudden infant death syndrome (SIDS) rates were added. Discussion of the causes of excessive crying was extensively revised.

Chapter 15: Discussions of newborn feeding reflexes and nursing positions were updated. The sections on assisting with feedings, nursing multiples, and tandem nursing were extensively revised.

Chapter 16: Discussions of latching, sucking, and milk transfer were reorganized and updated. The sections on the physiology of infant sucking, nutritive and nonnutritive sucking, and use of pacifiers and bottles were extensively revised. Discussions of problems with latch and sucking were reviewed and updated, including the addition of current recommendations for the management and treatment of mastitis spectrum disorders.

Chapter 17: The sections on commitment to nursing, establishing milk production, and breast abscess were updated. Discussions on nipple pain and plugged duct (changed to *ductal narrowing*) were extensively revised. The section on mastitis was thoroughly revised, including up-to-date recommendations for the management and treatment of mastitis spectrum disorders. A table on causes of and treatments for plugged ducts was removed.

Chapter 18: The sections on infant growth and development, nursing in public, and traveling were updated. Teething and biting were moved to another section in the chapter. The sections on toddler nursing and weaning were extensively revised. Discussion of complementary feeding was updated based on current research and global recommendations.

Chapter 19: Discussions of recognizing sufficient milk production and risks for low production were revised. The section on increasing milk production was updated, with substantial revisions to the discussion of the use of domperidone. Discussion of infant growth concerns was updated, with revisions to the section on assessing and managing faltering growth (previously failure to thrive). The table on baby feeding requirements was removed.

Chapter 20: Discussions of acquiring the parental role, sexual adjustments, and contraception were updated. The section on postpartum depression was updated and expanded to include survivors of intimate partner violence and adverse childhood experiences. Discussion of the father's role was updated to reflect partners regardless of gender. Physical recovery after birth, preparing for a home birth, and details of baby training programs were removed.

Chapter 21: Discussions of opposition to nursing and low-income, single, and teen parents were updated. The section on grandparents was shortened. Discussion of family lifestyle was removed, and intimate partner violence was moved to Chapter 21. The section on LGBTQ+ families previously located in Chapter 3 was added.

Chapter 22: Discussions of nursing techniques and tools were updated. The sections on nipple eversion and use of a nipple shield, pacifier, and breast pump were extensively revised. Discussions of digital techniques and manual expression were updated. Discussions of human milk banking, informal milk sharing, and alternative feeding methods were updated.

Chapter 23: The section on infant jaundice was revised, and phototherapy recommendations were updated. Discussions of hypoglycemia, delayed nursing, resisting nursing, and preferring one side were updated. The sections on relactation, inducing lactation, and nursing during emergencies were substantially revised.

Chapter 24: Family-centered care and shared decision-making were emphasized for families of high-risk infants. The section on neonatal intensive care was substantially revised, including feeding protocols, discharge planning, and support at home. Discussion of preterm infants was updated, including feeding effectiveness, the importance of human milk, skin-to-skin care, transition to nursing, and care at home. Discussions of late-preterm infants, postterm infants, and infant demise were updated. The table on development of preterm infant feeding behavior was removed.

Chapter 25: The section on managing nursing through a separation was updated. The section on COVID-19 and nursing was updated with current recommendations and evidence. Discussion of the H1N1 virus was removed. Discussions of the Zika and Ebola viruses were moved to Chapter 26. The section on combining working and nursing was thoroughly updated. Discussion of formula company marketing to working parents was removed.

Chapter 26: The sections on autoimmune disorders, thyroid disorders, polycystic ovary syndrome (PCOS), phenylketonuria (PKU), and infectious disease were updated. Discussions of diabetes, obesity, milk insufficiency, cystic fibrosis, and disabilities were extensively revised. A section on Zika and Ebola viruses was added.

Chapter 27: Discussions of congenital anomalies, phenylketonuria, and galactosemia were updated. Discussions of phenylalanine-free formula, Down syndrome, and neurologic conditions were substantially revised. The sections on cleft defects, spina bifida, and hydrocephalus were updated. Discussion of caregiver compassion fatigue was added.

Chapter 28: Discussions of healthcare provider lactation knowledge and preparing for the lactation profession were updated. The section on simulation-based clinical education was expanded. Discussion of the newly formed International Board Certified Lactation Consultant (IBCLC) Commission and a section on expert witness testimony were added. Discussion of employment as an IBCLC was removed.

Chapter 29: The sections on types and structure of articles, critical reading, and application of findings were updated. Discussions of evidence-informed practice, case studies, longitudinal studies, and predatory practices were expanded. New sections were added on online studies and nomenclature. One practice article was removed.

Chapter 30: Discussions of leadership, creating change, and lactation promotion were updated. The assertiveness discussion was shortened, and discussion of the art of persuasion was removed. The table on personality types of Americans was removed. Discussion of healthcare provider education was moved to Chapter 2.

This eighth edition of *Counseling Nursing Families* is the final edition for Judith Lauwers, who has retired after coauthoring the previous seven editions. As the coauthor of this edition, LEAARC will continue in future editions to present ongoing learning, research findings, and counseling skills through the text's unique perspective. *Counseling Nursing Families* will continue to be an important resource for new generations of lactation consultants and other healthcare providers.

Judith Lauwers

Kristina Chamberlain

Rosann Edwards

Jennie Wagner

Acknowledgments

A text of this scope is the result of collaboration with scores of colleagues throughout the history of the lactation consultant profession and multidisciplinary support for nursing families. Our thanks and appreciation go to all who have enriched our understanding of the art and science of lactation. Their generosity and selfless sharing of resources and insights for this edition (*Counseling Nursing Families*) and previous editions (*Counseling the Nursing Mother*) help promote lactation consulting to new generations of professionals. We thank everyone who assisted in large and small measures with the previous seven editions of this text.

We appreciate the voices of the many colleagues who have raised awareness of equity, inclusion, and diversity in our profession. Their wisdom guided our approach to this *Eighth Edition*. We hope our contribution to the conversation will enrich readers' appreciation for cultural humility in their interactions with families and colleagues. We thank the many families from whom we have learned so much about the miraculous bonds of nursing and parenting. We also appreciate the families who generously gave their time for photos and for sharing their lactation journey.

Profound thanks to all the coauthors who helped guide previous editions of *Counseling the Nursing Mother*. The *First Edition* resulted from a shared vision by Candace Woessner and Judith Lauwers for a text to teach healthcare professionals and counselors the knowledge and skills to support nursing families. Candace continued to collaborate on the *Second Edition* and helped set the unique tone of a warm and nurturing approach to helping families. Debbie Shinksie kept the flame burning for the *Third Edition*, followed by Anna Swisher, who coauthored the past four editions. Thank you to all of you amazing women for your contributions to the lactation profession.

This *Eighth Edition* marks a collaboration between Judith Lauwers and the Lactation Education Accreditation and Approval Review Committee (LEAARC). Kristina Chamberlain, Rosann Edwards, and Jennie Wagner enthusiastically spearheaded LEAARC's role as coauthor and updated several chapters. Thank you to additional chapter contributors Cheryl Benn, Susan Fuchs, T'Errah Jessup, Elaine Webber, and Nadine Wodwaski. Thank you also to chapter reviewers Amy Black, Petra Colindres, Carolina Cardona-Lopez, Carrie Westmoreland Miller, and Julie Theriault.

Many thanks to Every Mother, Inc. for the addition of numerous photographs from the Breastfeeding Curriculum developed for the Women, Infants, and Children (WIC) program through the U.S. Department of Agriculture (USDA) Food and Nutrition Services. The program's emphasis on counseling skills also inspired the new Conversation Starters with Parents that were added at the end of each chapter.

We owe tremendous thanks to the talented team at Jones & Bartlett Learning, including Tina Chen, Product Manager; Carol Guerrero, Senior Outsourcing Specialist; Belinda Thresher, Content Production Manager; Veerakumar Thiagarajan, Project Manager; Maria Maimone and Faith Brosnan, Intellectual Property Specialists, as well as Karan Rana, Content Manager at MPS Limited, for shepherding us through the revision and production process with patience and grace.

We extend our deepest gratitude to our families for their support, encouragement, and inspiration throughout this journey. Their unwavering support has sparked and sustained our passion for nurturing babies and families of all backgrounds and sizes, reminding us of the profound impact that care and connection can have on future generations.

Contributors

Cheryl Benn, RM, IBCLC, DCur
Registered Midwife
Palmerston North, Manawatu, New Zealand

Susan Fuchs, MS, IBCLC
Drexel University
Philadelphia, Pennsylvania

T'Errah Jessup, MPH, IBCLC
Wildflower Lactation & Postpartum Care, LLC
Winston-Salem, North Carolina

Elaine Webber, DNP, PPCNP-BC, IBCLC
University of Detroit McAuley School of Nursing
Detroit, Michigan

Nadine Wodwaski, DNP, MSN-ed, CNS, RN
University of Detroit Mercy
Detroit, Michigan

Reviewers

Amy Black, IBCLC
Milk Matters Lactation
Lactation Education Resources
Woodbridge, Virginia

Carolina Cardona-Lopez, DMD, IBCLC
Doctor of Dental Medicine
Cesar, Valledupar, Columbia

Petra Colindres, MA, RDN, CD, IBCLC
Office of Superintendent of Public Instruction (OPSI)
Olympia, Washington

Beth Stuesse, MSN, RNC-IAP, RNC-OB, RNC-MNN, C-EFM, C-ONQS, CLC, CBS, CCE, CHBE
Clinical Assistant Professor of Nursing
Maryville University
St. Louis, Missouri

Julie Theriault, MA
University of North Carolina—Chapel Hill
Chapel Hill, North Carolina

Carrie Westmoreland Miller, PhD, RN, CHSE-A, IBCLC, FAAN
Montana State University
Bozeman, Montana

Learning Features for Students

In addition to serving as a resource for clinical practice, *Counseling Nursing Families* is designed to impart the specialized knowledge and skills needed to help nursing families. It is ideal as the first text for students preparing to practice as lactation consultants and for increasing skills in counseling and communication. Content is intentionally written in easy-to-read terminology so that students may learn basic information before advancing to more scientific texts. Several special features make this a meaningful resource for students.

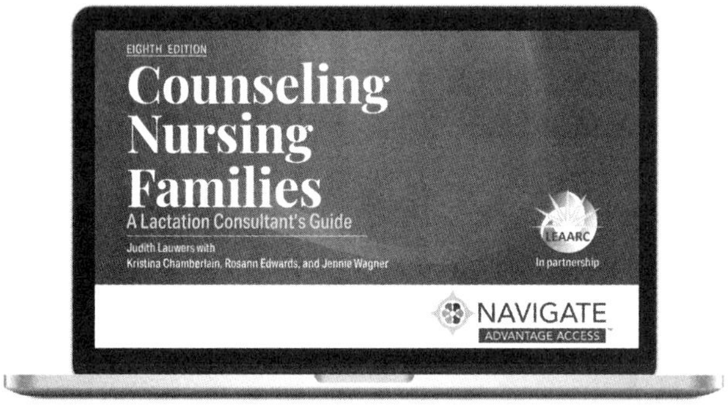

Key Terms	▪ Every chapter begins with a list of Key Terms to help the reader anticipate topics that will be presented in the chapter. The terms appear in bold within the chapter and their definitions appear in the Glossary.
Conversation Starters with Parents	▪ Following each chapter summary, sample open-ended questions to ask parents will guide the reader in approaching counseling related to the chapter topics.
What You Learned—At a Glance	▪ Every chapter ends with bulleted lists to identify significant takeaway messages. The lists serve as an overview of the chapter, a valuable study guide, and a quick reference when working with families.
Glossary	▪ An extensive Glossary appears at the end of the text. Definitions are provided for more than 900 entries, including all Key Terms in the text and other terminology used in lactation. The Glossary is a helpful study tool for students when completing classwork and preparing to take the certification exam. Practitioners may find this resource useful in practice as well.
Full-Color Clinical Photographs	▪ Full-color clinical photographs appear in both the printed text and the Navigate eBook. Students may refer to these when preparing to take the certification exam.

An image bank is available to qualified instructors.

We Value Your Feedback

Do you love this text? Spot an error you'd like to report? Follow this QR code to give us your observations and suggestions for improvement.

PART 1

Promotion and Support

CHAPTER 1

Lactation Advocacy in the Modern World

Lactation advocacy among caregivers and parents is much more complex than it may seem. The superiority of human milk over substitutes is well documented and widely acknowledged by the scientific, medical, and lay communities. It is not easy to understand why parents choose artificial feeding for their babies despite all the evidence in favor of human milk. Governments and institutions may fail to protect lactation. Caregivers may not recommend nursing to their clients or may not be able to answer questions or provide help when complications arise. Parents may receive contradictory messages from healthcare professionals, friends, relatives, or social media. Recognizing the dynamics of infant feeding practices and the political and sociological factors involved is essential to creating tangible and enduring change that will promote and protect nursing and optimize maternal and infant health.

KEY TERMS

1,000 Days
Baby-Friendly Community Initiative (BFCI)
Baby-Friendly Hospital Initiative (BFHI)
Breastfeeding Report Card
Centers for Disease Control and Prevention (CDC)
Complementary feeding
Cross-nursing
Exclusive nursing
Global Strategy for Infant and Young Child Feeding
Healthy People 2030
Innocenti Declaration
International Code of Marketing of Breast-milk Substitutes (the Code)
Malnutrition
Maternity Practices in Infant Nutrition and Care (mPINC)
Milk banking
Milk sharing
Mortality
Neo-BFHI
Office on Women's Health
Paradigm shift
Patient Protection and Affordable Care Act
Protecting, Promoting, and Supporting Breastfeeding
Ten Steps to Successful Breastfeeding
The Joint Commission
U.S. Department of Agriculture (USDA)
U.S. Surgeon General's Call to Action to Support Breastfeeding
United Nations Children's Fund (UNICEF)
Wet nursing
World Health Assembly (WHA)
World Health Organization (WHO)

Infant Feeding Practices Throughout History

Humans are one of over 4200 types of mammals, all of which feed their young with their species-specific milk (Webb, 2019). The biological norm for human babies is human milk. Historically, human babies have been fed human milk—either the milk of the baby's biological parent or the milk of another parent (**Figure 1-1**). Babies in colonial America typically were nursed through their second year.

Despite human milk being the norm for human babies, parents throughout history have made a conscious choice not to nurse their children. Wealthy or royal families often chose wet nurses or hand feeding (feeding with a bottle, cup, or other device) to prevent breast sagging, regain fertility quickly, or exhibit class status. Thus, human milk substitutes have been available for centuries. Only in recent history, however, have more infants in industrialized nations received substitutes rather than human milk (Papastavrou et al., 2015; Stevens et al., 2009). Globally, nursing is still the primary feeding method for infants.

Milk from Other Women

Wet nursing—the act of nursing a baby other than one's own—dates back as far as 2000 BC (Stevens et al., 2009). Before the advent of mass manufacturing of artificial milk, wet nurses provided the necessary nourishment when nursing was not possible or desired. Wet nurses predominantly faced economic hardship and relinquished nursing their own children (West & Knight, 2017). Awareness of the importance of human milk has increased the incidence of wet nursing in some parts of the world (Norsyamlina et al., 2021).

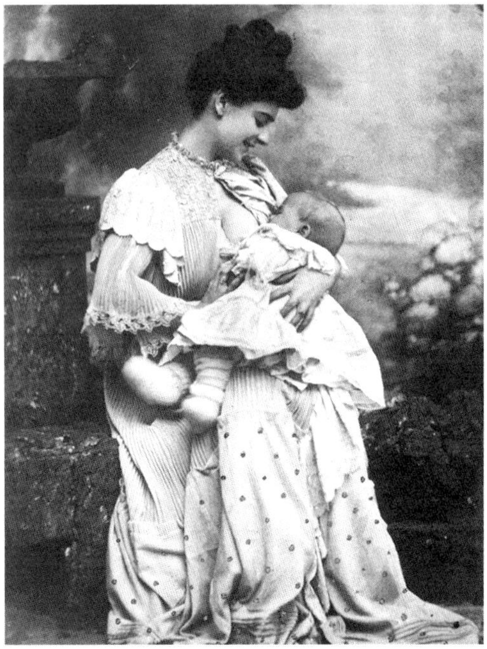

Figure 1-1 A baby nursing in the early 1900s.

Printed with permission of breastfeedingart.net

Cross-nursing has been practiced in many cultures. Cross-nursing is when parents in a family, community, or group nurse each other's children. Almost 30% of parents in a Brazilian study, mostly adolescents, reported practicing cross-nursing, predominantly with relatives or friends (von Seehausen et al., 2017).

Milk sharing is the provision of one parent's milk for another parent's child, sometimes at no cost and sometimes for sale. The practice is common in the United States among middle-income, college-educated women who self-identify as Caucasian/White (Kullman et al., 2022; Palmquist & Doehler, 2016). Donors and recipients typically share milk with family members, friends, and people they have met within their community or online. Informal milk sharing is typically facilitated through the internet and exchanged in person. For-profit milk sharing often requires shipping and risks contamination.

There is some concern about the lack of healthcare provider involvement in informal milk sharing and the safety of the milk compared with the screening and quality control provided by formal donor milk banks. Perceptions of risk are lower when social ties are familiar and trust is established (Palmquist & Doehler, 2016). Milk-sharing donors and recipients predominantly engage in positive safety practices that lower the risk of bacterial contamination of shared milk (Reyes-Foster et al., 2017). Safe practices include handwashing, sanitizing equipment, storing milk at room temperature for no longer than 8 hours and frozen for no longer than 6 months, defrosting milk in warm water or in the refrigerator, and transporting milk on ice. Donor screening and testing safety tips are available on the internet and Facebook.

Milk banking offers a safe alternative to parents who cannot nurse or who cannot produce enough milk. Availability is limited, and preterm or ill babies in intensive care units are the highest-priority recipients. A milk bank is a collection point where healthy nursing parents donate their milk. The first known human milk bank was established in 1909 in Vienna. The first one in the United States opened in 1911 in Boston. By the height of their popularity in the early 1980s, there were 23 milk banks in Canada and 30 in the United States. Since the isolation of human immunodeficiency virus (HIV) in human milk in the mid-1980s and the increase in the production of preterm formulas, the number of milk banks declined.

Research continues to demonstrate improved outcomes for infants given human milk. Furthermore, the risks of artificial formula are now widely recognized by the public and the medical community. The demand for expressed human milk is growing, and human milk banks offer the safest option. There are now human milk banks in over 60 countries, with some operating in low-income and middle-income countries (Haiden & Ziegler, 2016). There are over 200 milk banks operating in more than 20 countries throughout Europe (European Milk Bank Association [EMBA], 2023).There are 30 in North America (Human Milk Banking Association of North America [HMBANA], 2023). **Chapter 22** discusses milk banking and donor milk.

Advent of Human Milk Substitutes

During the 18th and 19th centuries, advances in medicine, science, and technology resulted in remarkable changes in infant feeding practices. Artificial milks emerged in the mid-19th century primarily to provide nutrition for infants in institutions. By the 1880s, newborns began to receive cow's milk in large numbers. Milk factories provided pasteurized cow's milk and home sterilizers to the public (Wolf, 2001). As technology made infant formula more available, parents increasingly turned to artificial feeding. This typically led to full weaning before the infant was 3 months old (Salmon, 1994).

Increased infant **morbidity** (illness) and **mortality** rates led healthcare providers to caution against the dangers of artificial feeding. In the same period, pediatricians emerged as a new subset of healthcare providers with infant feeding expertise to guide the selection of appropriate food for babies. The pediatrician provided a prescription based on a mathematical formula comprising the infant's age, weight, pallor, overall health, stool consistency, and any pertinent medical diagnoses (Wolf, 2020). Mass production of infant formula emerged by the 1920s, as it became clear that babies could receive a standard formula. Because pediatricians were no longer needed to prescribe a formula, pediatrics evolved into a profession of specialists in well-baby care and preventive medicine. Many in the pediatric profession continue to be heavily influenced by the infant formula industry through sponsorship of conferences, education, meetings, and other events (Nestle, 2013; Waterston & Yilmaz, 2016).

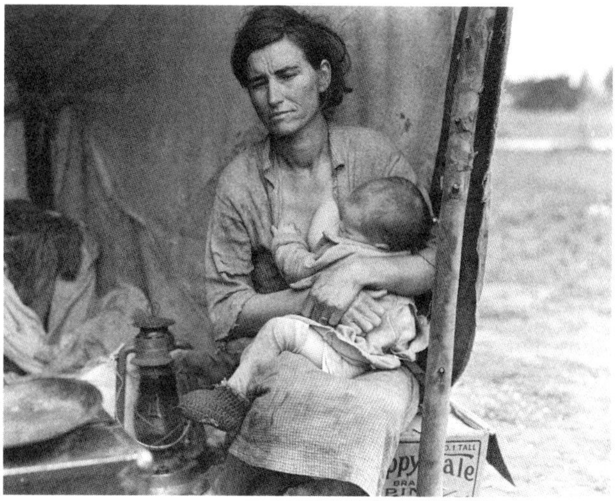

Figure 1-2 Nursing became associated with lower social status.

The feeding of human milk substitutes continued to increase in popularity in the 20th century with cow's milk products promoted as the modern way to nourish infants. As the popularity of artificial feeding grew, its attractiveness and accessibility became associated with higher-class, educated families. Nursing, in turn, became associated with lower social status, as depicted in **Figure 1-2** (Lange, 1936). The popularity of human milk substitutes eventually trickled down through all social strata until most babies throughout the industrialized world received a milk substitute from a bottle rather than nursing. Western society began to idealize the sexuality of the breast in men's magazines and mass media, an impression that continues to affect nursing rates (Grant et al., 2022).

The sexual objectification of the female body subverted women's biological function to nourish and nurture their babies. By 1971, lactation reached an all-time low in the United States, with only 24% of babies nursed at least once before hospital discharge (Ryan et al., 1991). A lost generation of nursing parents gave rise to peer support organizations and, later, the lactation consultant profession composed of allied health professionals skilled in assisting and supporting nursing families.

Separation of Parents and Babies

The Industrial Revolution had brought greater accessibility of human milk substitutes, providing women of all social strata new options for feeding their infants. Soldiers who returned home at the end of World War II found a new landscape in family life. Spouses who had entered the workforce in large numbers during the war enjoyed the freedom and challenge of working outside the home while still raising a family. Feeding practices that liberated them from their babies led to a cultural belief in many industrialized societies that artificial feeding was the norm and nursing was the exception. Around the same time, childcare experts promoted regimented feeding schedules, stressed the need to trust scientific development in infant feeding, gave poor lactation advice, and robbed parents of trusting their instincts.

Dramatic changes also took place in birth practices throughout the industrialized world. By the early part of the 20th century, medical advances and improved hygiene reduced birth mortality rates. Before that time, babies were traditionally born at home with family members and midwives providing strong and continuous support that facilitated labor and birth. Lactation was regarded as part of the birth process, with the baby beginning to nurse at the end stage of labor and birth.

As medical technology advanced, childbirth moved from the home to a clinical hospital environment. Control of birth shifted to medical staff, often compromising the family's personal needs. Today, birth in most industrialized nations typically occurs in a hospital, with the birthing dyad surrounded by technology and medical personnel. Birthing practices created a separation of the dyad, regimented infant care, and interference with initiating lactation (Davis-Floyd & Cheney, 2019). Parents had limited access to their babies during their critical first week of life, with babies brought to them on a strict schedule for brief feeding periods.

Lactation Revisited

Early in the 20th century, members of the medical community began to question the wisdom of feeding babies human milk substitutes. Healthcare professionals advocated for medical students to spend more time observing and studying lactation (Sedgwick & Fleishner, 1921). Researchers noted that the babies studied with IQs exceeding 130 were all nursed (Hoefer & Hardy, 1929). Professional articles on lactation and infant feeding began to appear in medical literature in the 1950s. Key among them was seminal research by Dr. Mavis Gunther (1955) and Dr. Niles Newton (Newton and Newton, 1950). Support groups for nursing families emerged in 1956 through grassroots efforts started by La Leche League International (LLLI) and other lactation support organizations (LLLI, 2023). Lactation was promoted as a healthy and natural method of infant feeding, a messages that continues to resonate today, as depicted in **Figure 1-3**.

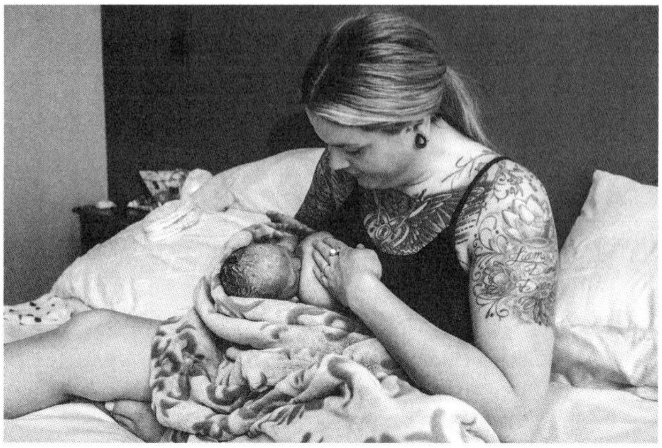

Figure 1-3 A modern-day baby nursing.
Printed with permission of Tiarra Doherty.

The movement back to nursing began among educated, upper-social-class families, the same as the trend toward artificial feeding had previously. Society refocused on asserting the needs and autonomy of the family and protecting the health of infants and children—a message that continues today (Feldman-Winter et al., 2022). The feminist movement of the 1960s prompted women to seek economic and social equity with men. Some committed to healthy living, with nursing being an intrinsic part of that lifestyle. However, some feminists considered nursing to be restrictive. The debate about feminist ideals generated by these two opposing viewpoints continues today. **Chapter 3** discusses feminism and lactation.

Lactation Recommendations

Lactation-friendly health care is the goal of global promotion, protection, and support of lactation. Such a climate empowers and enables parents to nurse. Optimal maternal and infant health and minimal cost to the family, community, and environment form the basis of these recommendations. The American Academy of Pediatrics (AAP), the **World Health Organization (WHO)**, and the American Academy of Family Physicians (AAFP) recommend that babies nurse exclusively for 6 months and continue nursing with appropriate complementary food for up to 2 years and beyond (AAFP, 2023; Meek & Noble, 2022; WHO, 2023). This recommendation, which had previously been nursing up to 1 year and beyond, was jointly updated in 2022 by the AAP, WHO, and AAFP. The change corresponds with the importance of nutrition during the "first 1000 days," the period from conception to 2 years of age (Schwarzenberg et al., 2018).

Exclusive nursing means that healthy infants receive no drinks or foods other than human milk, except for oral rehydration, vitamin and mineral drops, or medicines. To optimize the probability of exclusive nursing, infants should receive no pacifiers or artificial teats (nipples). They should feed in response to hunger cues, with no limits placed on frequency or length of feedings. Most infants who are nursed exclusively receive at least 8 to 12 feedings in 24 hours, including night feedings.

Lactation Initiation and Duration

Lactation rates differ significantly throughout the world. Variations in the definition of exclusive nursing from one country to another present a challenge when attempting to compile meaningful statistics. According to the **United Nations Children's Fund (UNICEF**, 2021**)**, 49% of infants nurse in the first hour of birth, 65% nurse exclusively for the first 2 days, and 62% continue nursing to 12–23 months. The WHO reports that 44% of infants aged 0–6 months worldwide nursed exclusively from 2015 to 2020 (WHO, 2021a). The WHO estimates that about 820,000 child lives could be directly saved every year with the promotion of optimal lactation, appropriate complementary feeding, and the provision of supplements in food-insecure populations (WHO, 2021b).

Lactation Rates in the United States

U.S. lactation initiation rates have risen slowly since the grassroots movement in the 1950s. The annual **Breastfeeding Report Card**, begun by the **Centers for Disease Control and Prevention (CDC)** in 2008, reports the rates of nursing infants in each U.S. state. Rates are affected by income, educational level, race/ethnicity, prevalence of obesity, and smoking (Anstey et al., 2017). Rates of exclusive nursing at 3 and 6 months remain low despite increases in initiation. Rates are higher in western and northeastern states and lower in the Southeast. The wide range of initiation rates among U.S. states demonstrates the need for geographic interventions.

The CDC reports that of infants born in 2019, 83% initiated lactation, 56% were still nursing at 6 months, and 36% continued through 12 months. Almost half were still exclusively nursing at 3 months (CDC, 2024). **Table 1-1** presents data for the 2022 CDC Breastfeeding Report Card. **Table 1-2** breaks down U.S. lactation rates by race/ethnicity (CDC, 2021). **Chapter 3** discusses lactation in the context of race and ethnicity.

Table 1-1 Breastfeeding Report Card

Key Breastfeeding Indicators	Rate
Infants who are ever breastfed	83.2%
Infants who are breastfed at 6 months	55.8%
Infants who are breastfed at 1 year	35.9%
Infants who are breastfed exclusively through 3 months	45.3%
Infants who are breastfed exclusively through 6 months	24.9%
Breastfed newborns who receive formula supplementation within the first 2 days of life	19.2%

Data from Breastfeeding Report Card. United States, 2022. Centers for Disease Control and Prevention. https://www.cdc.gov/breastfeeding/pdf/2022-breastfeeding-report-card-h.pdf

The Healthy People initiative establishes national objectives every decade and monitors progress toward improving the health of Americans. ***Healthy People 2030*** reduced the number of objectives in all areas from previous years to prioritize the most pressing public health issues (Office of Disease Prevention and Health Promotion [ODPHP], n.d.). The 2030 objectives for lactation are summarized in **Table 1-3** (ODPHP, n.d.).

Increasing Lactation Rates

Educating the public about the importance of lactation dates back to the late 19th century. Efforts focused defensively on the benefits of lactation, enumerating all the reasons why babies should be nursed. Public awareness then shifted to the hazards of *not* nursing and the reasons babies should not receive a human milk substitute. A classic IQ study illustrates this **paradigm shift** in the way society views infant feeding. The study reported that preterm infants receiving human milk have higher IQ levels than those receiving infant formula (Lucas et al., 1992). Because the biological norm is for an infant to receive human milk, infants who have nursed have normal IQs. Thus, infants who do not receive human milk have lower-than-normal IQs. Health outcomes from nursing are indisputable evidence of the risks of not nursing. This paradigm shift in perception and attitude promotes public recognition of the negative consequences of artificial feeding and helps parents make informed and healthy choices.

Table 1-2 Breastfeeding Rates by Race/Ethnicity in 2021

Race/Ethnicity	n	Any Breastfeeding			n	Exclusive Breastfeeding	
		Ever Breastfed	Breastfed at 6 Months	Breastfed at 12 Months		Exclusive Breastfeeding Through 3 Months	Exclusive Breastfeeding Through 6 Months
Hispanic	4528	83.4±2.1	56.1±2.6	37.0±2.5	4445	45.6±2.7	25.9±2.3
Non-Hispanic White	12735	86.2±1.0	63.4±1.4	42.5±1.4	12353	50.3±1.5	29.2±1.3
Non-Hispanic Black	2250	75.4±2.8	51.7±3.1	31.0±2.9	2202	39.0±3.0	24.4±2.7
Non-Hispanic Asian	1151	92.7±2.0	73.9±4.1	50.8±4.7	1102	46.0±4.7	30.2±4.3
Two or more races	1879	85.2±2.7	58.4±3.6	38.9±3.5	1836	43.2±3.6	23.2±2.9

Data Source: Rates of Any and Exclusive Breastfeeding by Sociodemographic Characteristic Among Children Born in 2021. Centers for Disease Control and Prevention. https://www.cdc.gov/breastfeeding/data/nis_data/data-files/2019/rates-any-exclusive-bf-socio-dem-2019.html

Table 1-3 *Healthy People 2030* Goals for Lactation

Number	Objective	Baseline (Year Measured) %
MICH-21	Increase the proportion of nursing infants who are breastfed	(2006 births)
MICH-21.1	Ever	74.0
MICH-21.2	At 6 months	43.5
MICH-21.3	At 1 year	35.9
MICH-21.4	Exclusively through 3 months	33.6
MICH-21.5	Exclusively through 6 months	14.1
MICH-22	Increase the proportion of employers that have worksite lactation support programs	25.0 (2009)
MICH-23	Reduce the proportion of breastfed newborns who receive formula supplementation within the first 2 days of life	24.2 (2006 births)
MICH-24	Increase the proportion of live births that occur in facilities that provide recommended care for lactating mothers and their babies	2.9 (2009)

MICH = Maternal, Infant, Child Health.
Data from U.S. Department of Health and Human Services. Office of Disease Prevention and Health Promotion. Healthy People 2030. Washington, DC. Available at https://odphp.health.gov/healthypeople/objectives-and-data/browse-objectives/infants

Global Lactation Initiatives

By the mid-1970s, health experts recognized the need for a global effort to stem the tide of negative health outcomes for children. The documentary film *Bottle Babies* (1975) brought the tragedy of illness and death from the unethical marketing practices of formula companies to the world's attention. A 1978 U.S. Senate hearing led by Senator Edward Kennedy provided the impetus for global action to monitor corporate practices in the marketing of infant formula. Spearheaded by the WHO, the **World Health Assembly**

(WHA), and UNICEF, several international initiatives provided a beacon for lactation promotion at all levels. These initiatives give healthcare professionals and administrators clear guidelines for the establishment of policies and practices that promote, protect, and support lactation.

International Code of Marketing of Breast-milk Substitutes

In 1981, the WHA adopted the **International Code of Marketing of Breast-milk Substitutes (the Code)** to promote safe and adequate infant nutrition. The aim of the Code is to protect and promote lactation while ensuring the appropriate marketing, distribution, and use of human milk substitutes. A main principle of the Code is that healthcare facilities should not promote human milk substitutes, feeding bottles, or teats. Subsequent WHA resolutions have clarified the Code's principles and closed loopholes.

The United States was the last country to sign the Code because of aggressive lobbying by the infant formula industry. Although the Code was affirmed by all WHO member states, it awaits enactment into legislation or enforceable regulations at the national level in many countries. Too few countries have robust measures in place, and very few countries include milk products labeled for use up to at least 36 months of age as designated products in their legislation. In addition to control of the marketing of human milk substitutes, there is a need to implement laws and policies to prevent inappropriate promotion of commercially produced complementary foods (Zehner et al., 2019). Aggressive marketing of these foods undermines appropriate **complementary feeding** of infants (Hadihardjono et al., 2019). **Chapter 10** discusses formula company marketing practices.

Countries with weak or nonexistent Code legislation are vulnerable to continued aggressive marketing by the formula industry (Soldavini & Tailie, 2017). In 2018, the WHA introduced a new resolution, supported by leading maternal and child health organizations, to limit marketing claims about human milk substitutes for infants and young children. The United States threatened the government of Ecuador with economic sanctions if Ecuador introduced the proposed resolution. The Russian Federation introduced the resolution instead, and other countries voted to support it (Jacobs, 2018; Wernick, 2018; WHO, 2018b).

Understanding the International Code

Table 1-4 highlights the main points of the Code, which calls for regulating the marketing and distribution of products represented to be suitable as a partial or total replacement for human milk. Any product that is promoted for children younger than 6 months of age has the effect of replacing human milk in a child's intake. The intent of the Code is to regulate the advertising and promotional techniques used to sell foods marketed or otherwise represented to replace human milk, as well as feeding bottles and artificial nipples (WHO, 2017). Manufacturers and distributors of products within the scope of the Code should disclose any contributions made to health workers, such as fellowships, study tours, research grants, or conferences.

Healthcare facilities that uphold the Code do not accept free or low-cost supplies of human milk substitutes. They purchase milk substitutes for wholesale price in the same way as other foods and medicines. They provide no promotional materials for human milk substitutes during pregnancy or in a birth facility. Artificial feeding is demonstrated only by health workers and only to families who need it. Human milk substitutes are kept out of public view. The facility accepts no sample gift packs with milk substitutes or related supplies. Health workers and their families accept no financial or material inducements to promote products within the scope of the Code.

Code Implementation and Compliance

Implementation and enforcement of the Code are inconsistent. As of April 2020, 136 (70%) of 194 WHO member states had enacted legal measures to implement it. Of these, 25 countries had measures substantially aligned with the Code, and 42 countries had measures that were moderately aligned. Less than half of the countries prohibited the donation of free or low-cost products or samples, or prohibited product information other than what is scientific and factual (WHO, 2020). The Cambodian government adopted the Code as the national standard with a pilot training system for implementation. The challenges and lessons Cambodia faced can guide Code monitoring and policy change in other countries (Hou et al., 2019). The current status of nation-specific Code enforcement is available from the WHO (2018). **Chapter 10** discusses Code compliance by formula manufacturers.

Table 1-4 The International Code of Marketing of Breast-milk Substitutes

Code Provision	Implications to Consider
Under the scope of the Code, items marketed or otherwise represented to be suitable as human milk substitutes can include foods and beverages such as the following: ■ Infant formula ■ Other milk products ■ Cereals ■ Vegetable, fruit, and other pureed preparations ■ Juices and baby teas ■ Follow-on milks ■ Bottled water	Whether or not a product is within this definition will depend on how it is promoted for infants. Any products that are marketed or represented as suitable substitutes for human milk will fall into this category. Because babies should receive only human milk for the first 6 months, any other food or drink promoted for use during this time will be a human milk substitute.
Regarding advertising and information, the Code recommends that: ■ Advertising of human milk substitutes, bottles, and teats to the public should not be permitted ■ Educational materials should explain the benefits of nursing, the health hazards associated with bottle feeding, the costs of using infant formula, and the difficulty of reversing the decision not to nurse ■ Product labels should clearly state the superiority of human milk, the need for the advice of a healthcare worker, and a warning about health hazards; and they should not show pictures of babies or other pictures or text idealizing the use of infant formula	Health workers, such as lactation consultants and peer counselors, need to press their legislators for measures that will implement the Code in full. This would protect parents from advertising in parent magazines and on television. It would also prevent direct company contact with parents through hotlines, internet sites, mailings, home-delivered supplies of formula, and baby clubs.
Regarding samples and supplies, the Code recommends that: ■ No free samples should be given to pregnant clients, parents, or their families ■ No free or low-cost supplies of human milk substitutes should be given to birthing facilities or any other part of the healthcare system	Under the Code, free or low-cost supplies can be distributed only outside of the healthcare system and must be continued for as long as the infant needs them. In the United States, this is usually for 1 year. Elsewhere, it is for at least 6 months. The healthcare system encompasses healthcare workers, including lactation consultants and peer counselors.
Regarding healthcare facilities and healthcare workers, the Code recommends that: ■ There should be no product displays, posters, or distribution of promotional materials ■ No gifts or samples should be given to healthcare workers ■ Product information for health professionals should be limited to what is factual and scientific	This provision also covers bottles that are provided and shown in advertisements by breast pump companies that are clearly feeding bottles, even when no teats are shown. Pens and pads of paper with the name of a formula company are examples of gifts.

Even in countries where the Code is written into law, many health workers and institutions breach the law despite being aware of it. A study of eight countries revealed that 64% of families with young children reported exposure to promotion of products covered under the Code in the previous 6 months. Almost 20% of families with an infant less than 6 months of age were advised by a healthcare provider to feed their child food or drink other than human milk. About 20% of providers had contact with a representative of a formula company in the previous 6 months to distribute promotional materials, samples, or free supplies (Lutter et al., 2022).

In many healthcare facilities, representatives from infant formula companies distribute free samples, gifts, and sponsorships to health staff. This occurs freely where healthcare authorities have no practical rules and regulations in place to implement the Code in their institutions. Concerns about formula contamination scandals have prompted many hospital systems in the United States to discontinue distributing formula bags. The Joint Commission requirement that hospitals log all formula lot numbers in case of recall has helped make this a corporate risk management decision, not a local decision.

There are systemic failings at all levels, including a lack of political will and a lack of formal and transparent governance structures (Forsyth, 2019). Monitoring and education are needed to better promote the elements of the Code, identify violations, and restrict access to families with inappropriate marketing messages. Legislation must be accompanied by effective information and training to ensure that healthcare providers and manufacturers comply with evidence-based practice. The WHO and UNICEF provide monitoring protocols, tools, and guidance to assist countries in strengthening monitoring and enforcement of the Code (WHO & UNICEF, 2017). Several actions can help colleagues and facilities adhere to the Code and develop an awareness of instances in which a facility violates it:

- Remove posters, videos, and leaflets that advertise products marketed or otherwise represented to be suitable as human milk substitutes.
- Do not use educational materials for parents that are produced by the pharmaceutical or formula industry, including smartphone apps for pregnancy and lactation.
- Remove videos on artificial feeding from the hospital's television channel and provide individual instruction only to parents who do not nurse.

Ten Steps to Successful Breastfeeding

Formula manufacturers ignored the Code throughout the 1980s. Few governments enacted legislation to enforce it. Artificial feeding increased and lactation rates declined. To improve lactation rates throughout the world, UNICEF and the WHO issued a 1989 joint statement entitled **Protecting, Promoting, and Supporting Breastfeeding**. The statement led to the formation of the **Ten Steps to Successful Breastfeeding** (WHO, 1989). The Ten Steps were updated in 2018 (**Figure 1-4**) based on 2017 WHO and UNICEF guidelines to help WHO member states and their partners, policymakers, government institutions, and organizations make evidence-informed decisions in implementing programs for infant and young child feeding (IYCF) (WHO & UNICEF, 2018).

In 1990, WHO and UNICEF reaffirmed their commitment to nursing with the **Innocenti Declaration** on the Protection, Promotion and Support of Breastfeeding. The declaration called for the establishment of national breastfeeding coordinators in all countries, universal use of the Ten Steps to Successful Breastfeeding by birth facilities, implementation of the Code, and legal protections for employed nursing parents.

Critical management procedures

1a. Comply fully with the International Code of Marketing of Breast-milk substitutes and relevant World Health Assembly resolutions.
1b. Have a written infant feeding policy that is routinely communicated to staff and parents.
1c. Establish ongoing monitoring and data-management systems.
2. Ensure that staff have sufficient knowledge, competence and skills to support breastfeeding.

Key clinical practices

3. Discuss the importance and management of breastfeeding with pregnant women and their families.
4. Facilitate immediate and uninterrupted skin-to-skin contact and support mothers to initiate breastfeeding as soon as possible after birth.
5. Support mothers to initiate and maintain breastfeeding and manage common difficulties.
6. Do not provide breastfed newborns any food or fluids other than breast milk, unless medically indicated.
7. Enable mothers and their infants to remain together and to practise rooming-in 24 hours a day.
8. Support mothers to recognize and respond to their infants' cues for feeding.
9. Counsel mothers on the use and risks of feeding bottles, teats and pacifiers.
10. Coordinate discharge so that parents and their infants have timely access to ongoing support and care.

Figure 1-4 Ten Steps to Successful Breastfeeding.

UNICEF. Ten Steps to Successful Breastfeeding. https://www.unicef.org/documents/baby-friendly-hospital-initiative

Baby-Friendly Hospital Initiative

In 1991, at a time when breastfeeding rates were historically low, UNICEF and WHO launched the **Baby-Friendly Hospital Initiative (BFHI)**. The goal of BFHI is to help birth facilities support initiation of nursing and transform their services through implementation of the Ten Steps to Successful Breastfeeding. The Baby-Friendly designation process is controlled by national authorities, using global criteria that can be applied in every country. The internationally defined term "Baby-Friendly" is used by facilities that satisfy the global criteria for the BFHI.

Health facilities worldwide are designated as Baby-Friendly, with the initiative being adopted more slowly in some countries than in others. Globally, only 10% of births occur in facilities that are designated as Baby-Friendly. In 2021, a total of 2,097,036 births took place in BFHI-accredited hospitals (Hernández-Aguilar, 2022). In 2023, there were more than 590 Baby-Friendly-designated hospitals and birthing centers in all 50 U.S. states, the District of Columbia, and the Commonwealth of Puerto Rico. In the United States, almost 10 million babies have been born in Baby-Friendly-designated facilities since the program began in 1996. Nearly 28% of U.S. births now occur in Baby-Friendly facilities (Baby-Friendly USA, 2023).

Improved feeding practices are significantly higher in Baby-Friendly hospitals as compared with those that are not designated as Baby-Friendly (Liberty, 2019; Patterson et al., 2018; Procaccini et al., 2018; Wouk, 2017). Cesarean birth rates are lower (Di Mario et al., 2013), and lactation rates are higher among special care infants (Parker et al., 2013). Attitudes of healthcare professionals and lactation-related care practices improve as well (Mäkelä et al., 2022; Pramono et al., 2021; Shing et al., 2022). BFHI-advocated practices have a positive effect on lactation knowledge and planned duration (Lubold, 2017; Munn et al., 2016), as well as on maternal and infant health. There is an increased likelihood that babies will nurse exclusively for the first 6 months (Ducharme-Smith et al., 2022; Hockamp et al., 2022) and will continue nursing for 2 years or beyond with appropriate complementary foods.

Although lactation rates are higher in Baby-Friendly facilities, it has been difficult to maintain or increase rates. There has been a decreasing trend since 2018. In 2022, the early-initiation rate was 65%, and the rate for exclusive nursing from birth to discharge was 55%. The rate for exclusive nursing at 6 months was 19%. During that same period, implementation of the Ten Steps did not improve globally (Hernández-Aguilar, 2022).

Achieving Baby-Friendly Designation

A Baby-Friendly designation means that a facility meets high global standards with at least 75% of babies exclusively nursing at discharge. The process for receiving Baby-Friendly recognition involves an internal self-assessment, an assessment by outside evaluators, and a presentation of the findings by UNICEF. The process varies by country because government officials make adaptations to complement their country's standards.

Meeting BFHI standards to achieve designation can be difficult for some hospitals (Bruney et al., 2020; Burnham et al., 2021). Both hospital and community factors influence attainment of BFHI designation. BFHI designation in the United States is more likely for teaching hospitals that are part of a health system that serves communities with higher birth totals (Tafili et al., 2022). Lack of uniformity in BFHI initiation and the perception of its benefits at all levels of the health system create challenges to achieving Baby-Friendly designation (Wieczorek et al., 2016). Lack of adequate protection and aggressive formula marketing continue to undermine investments in lactation promotion (Hernández-Cordero, 2022). Opposition from the healthcare establishment and the formula industry creates obstacles as well.

Lack of support from national and state authorities and low awareness or acceptance of the need for the initiative among government departments, healthcare systems, and parents also create obstacles (Pérez-Escamilla et al., 2023). Advocacy, political will, financing, research, and coordination are key to fostering an environment for lactation (Hernández-Cordero, 2022). Lack of political will or buy-in from senior managers is a significant barrier. Hospitals cite stringent criteria, excessive paperwork, insufficient technical assistance, and bureaucracy as challenges. The lack of Code implementation affects BFHI indirectly by discounting the importance of lactation.

Although potential costs may be cited as a deterrent by some facilities, the number of lactation-supportive practices a hospital has in place is not significantly associated with higher costs (Allen et al., 2014). Hospitals can purchase formula at the same average discount of about 90% off the retail price as for other items such as diapers and OB pads (Srinivas et al., 2015). Endorsements of hospital administrators and government policymakers, effective leadership in changing practice, staff training, controlling the marketing influence of formula companies, and integrating hospital and community health services all affect successful implementation of BFHI. Guidance is available for creating Baby-Friendly practices in hospitals, clinics, and healthcare provider offices; complementary feeding; care of HIV-positive parents; and community services (WHO & UNICEF, 2018).

Maintaining Baby-Friendly Designation

Maintaining BFHI designation is challenging. Most facilities lack monitoring systems to ensure that staff adhere to BFHI standards. Many countries cite the high costs of ongoing training to maintain staff skill levels because of staff turnover (Arslanian et al., 2022). To ensure sustainability, the WHO calls upon countries to fulfill nine key responsibilities through a national BFHI program (WHO, 2018a):

- Establish or strengthen a national breastfeeding coordination body.
- Integrate the Ten Steps into relevant national policy documents and professional standards of care.
- Ensure the competency of health professionals and managers in implementation of the Ten Steps.
- Utilize external assessment systems to regularly evaluate adherence to the Ten Steps.
- Develop and implement incentives for compliance and/or sanctions for noncompliance with the Ten Steps.
- Provide technical assistance to facilities that are making changes to adopt the Ten Steps.
- Monitor implementation of the initiative.
- Advocate for the BFHI to relevant audiences.
- Identify and allocate sufficient resources to ensure the ongoing funding of the initiative.

Global protection of lactation requires family-friendly employment policies, enforcement of the Code, and investment in workforce training for successful large-scale implementation and sustainability of the BFHI. Community-based counseling and avoiding conflicts of interest with infant formula companies are also key to protection. Although BFHI designation is not the only option for a successful lactation program, its structure can be a means to improve lactation policies.

Critical Review of BFHI

Critics have questioned BFHI recommendations on pacifier use, rooming-in, and skin-to-skin care (Gomez-Pomar & Blubaugh, 2018). BFHI has clarified that it recommends that healthy term infants may use pacifiers at infant nap or sleep time after lactation is well established (Baby-Friendly US, 2023). This aligns with the AAP guidelines to promote safe sleep. Negation of the importance of rooming-in was refuted by a later study showing that success with continual exclusive nursing in the postpartum period is dependent on full rooming-in (Wu, 2022). Although strong evidence exists in support of the benefits of skin-to-skin care, there are multiple reports of sudden unexpected postnatal collapse in the neonate (SUPC) that warrant caution (Bass et al., 2016; Davanzo et al., 2015; Feldman-Winter et al., 2016; Ferrarello & Carmichael, 2016; Lutz et al., 2016). Clinicians are encouraged to teach parents guidelines for safe pacifier use, skin-to-skin care, and rooming-in.

Concern about insufficient milk intake causing increased hospitalizations of newborns who nurse exclusively, along with the death of one infant, gave rise to the Fed Is Best Foundation. This advocacy group cites dangerous gaps in lactation management and education. Fed Is Best provides research, education, and resources for parents and health workers to practice safe infant feeding with human milk, formula, or a combination of both (Fed Is Best Foundation, 2024). The concerns addressed by the group underscore the importance of implementing all aspects of Baby-Friendly practices, including parent education, monitoring of infant intake, and supplementation when it is medically indicated.

Neo-BFHI

In 2009, professionals from Sweden, Norway, Denmark, Finland, and Canada met to expand the BFHI to neonatal care. The group recommended promoting BFHI as a facilitator of family-centered care and interdisciplinary staff education, with increased access to lactation consultants (Benoit & Semenic, 2014; Nyqvist et al., 2013). The **Neo-BFHI** core document was published in 2015 (Nyqvist et al., 2015). In 2020, the WHO/UNICEF published recommendations for nursing small, sick, and preterm newborns that align with the Neo-BFHI (WHO, 2022).

Neo-BFHI conforms to the Ten Steps to Successful Breastfeeding with three guiding principles, as described in **Table 1-5**. There is international readiness for expansion of Baby-Friendly standards to neonatal settings. By 2019, 36 countries had begun implementing the Neo-BFHI recommendations (Maastrup & Hajek, 2019). The initiative has produced improvements in attitudes and practices in neonatal units (Cabrera-Lafuente et al., 2022; Mäkelä et al., 2022). Lack of resources to support parental presence, barriers to milk expression, and a high rate of formula feeding may present challenges for some facilities (Abugov et al., 2021).

Baby-Friendly Community Initiative

The **Baby-Friendly Community Initiative (BFCI)** is an extension of step 10 of the Ten Steps to Successful Breastfeeding and the BFHI. BFCI provides continued lactation support to communities after discharge by creating a comprehensive support system at the community level through support groups. It addresses nutritional and developmental needs, including environmental sanitation, personal hygiene, and equity. The seven-point community initiative (presented in **Figure 1-5**) has been implemented in numerous countries around the world (Baerug et al., 2016; Kavle et al., 2019; Maingi, 2018;

Table 1-5 Neo-BFHI Core Principles and Standards

	Principle	Standards
Guiding principle 1	Staff attitudes toward the mother must focus on the individual mother and her situation.	■ Every mother is treated with sensitivity, empathy, and respect for her maternal role. ■ Mothers are supported in making informed decisions about milk production, lactation, and infant feeding. ■ Mothers receive focused, individualized support with respect to milk production, lactation, and infant feeding.
Guiding principle 2	The facility must provide family-centered care, supported by the environment.	■ Family-centered care is integrated into the organization and functioning of the neonatal ward. ■ The presence of the father in the neonatal ward is encouraged at all times because he is the mother's supporter and the infant's caregiver. ■ The care of infants admitted to the neonatal ward is transferred gradually by the staff to the parents, beginning as soon as possible after birth. ■ The neonatal ward provides practical support, such as a place to rest, sleep, and eat, that will enable mothers/parents to stay with their babies as long as they want. ■ The neonatal ward provides an individualized, developmentally supportive environment that is appropriate for the infants and the parents and that facilitates lactation.
Guiding principle 3	The healthcare system must ensure continuity of care from pregnancy to after the infant's discharge.	■ Care in regard to lactation support during each stage of healthcare delivery (prenatal care, the arrival of a "potentially" critical infant, the acute/critical care phase, the stable-improving phase, the transfer-discharge phase, and the follow-up or continuing care phrase) is consistent. ■ Information regarding the infants' medical management and families' preferences is shared among the relevant healthcare providers, institutions, and organizations involved in lactation support.

Reproduced from Nyqvist KH, et al. *Neo-BFHI: The Baby-friendly Hospital Initiative for Neonatal Wards. Core document with recommended standards and criteria.* Nordic and Quebec Working Group; 2015.

1. Have a written breastfeeding policy that is routinely communicated to all healthcare staff.
2. Train all staff involved in the care of mothers and babies in the skills necessary to implement the policy
3. Inform all pregnant women about the benefits and management of breastfeeding.
4. Support mothers to initiate and maintain breastfeeding.
5. Encourage exclusive and continued breastfeeding, with appropriately-timed introduction of complementary foods.
6. Provide a welcoming atmosphere for breastfeeding families.
7. Promote co-operation between healthcare staff, breastfeeding support groups, and the local community.

Figure 1-5 Baby-Friendly Community Initiative seven-point plan.

Kavle JA, et al. Baby-Friendly Community Initiative-From national guidelines to implementation: a multisectoral platform for improving infant and young child feeding practices and integrated health services. *Matern Child Nutr.* 2019 Jan;15 Suppl 1(Suppl 1):e12747.

Schmied et al., 2019; Walsh et al., 2023). Kenya developed the first national BFCI guidelines, which inform national- and subnational-level implementation. The initiative has increased the likelihood of exclusively nursing infants during the first 6 months of life (Kimani-Murage, 2021). BFCI is a promising platform to integrate into other sectors, such as early child development, agriculture, water, sanitation, and hygiene.

Global Strategy for Infant and Young Child Feeding

In 2003, in a bid to further strengthen world attention on infant feeding practices, the WHO and UNICEF collaborated to create the **Global Strategy for**

- Development of comprehensive national policies on infant and young child feeding
- Use of an evidence-based, integrated, comprehensive approach
- Consideration of the physical, social, economic, and cultural environment
- Healthcare support of exclusive breastfeeding for 6 months
- Supportive work environments to increase exclusive breastfeeding rates
- Support of breastfeeding with complementary foods for up to 2 years and beyond
- Provision of adequate, timely, safe complementary foods
- Guidance to families in exceptionally difficult circumstances
- Legislation and regulations to ensure adherence to the International Code of Marketing of Breastmilk Substitutes and subsequent World Health Assembly resolutions

Figure 1-6 Components of the Global Strategy for Infant and Young Child Feeding.

Data from World Health Organization (WHO). *Global Strategy for Infant and Young Child Feeding*. Geneva: World Health Organization; 2003.

Infant and Young Child Feeding (WHO, 2003). The Global Strategy builds on the Code, the Innocenti Declaration, and the BFHI. It places those initiatives in the overall context of national policies, programs on nutrition and child health, and several other declarations and conventions.

The Global Strategy addresses appropriate, evidence-based feeding practices for infants and young children that are essential for attaining and maintaining proper nutrition and health. It identifies essential interventions to ensure that children develop to their full potential, free from the adverse consequences of compromised nutritional status and preventable illness. The initiative charges governments, international organizations, and other concerned parties with ensuring that their collective action contributes to the attainment of these goals.

Major components of the Global Strategy are presented in **Figure 1-6**. The initiative reasserts exclusive nursing for the first 6 months of life and nursing with appropriate complementary foods for up to 2 years and beyond. It calls for employee support, culture-specific nutrition counseling, skilled support to parents and caregivers, and appropriate response to global emergencies. Specific strategies within the healthcare system include skilled counseling, implementation of the BFHI, routine nutrition intervention, and guidance in appropriate complementary feeding. IYCF practices increase the rates of early initiation of lactation and exclusive nursing at 3 and 6 months. Such practices also decrease diarrheal disease, stunting, wasting, and infant mortality (Lassi et al., 2020).

The Global Strategy urges implementation, monitoring, and reassessment of BFHI-designated facilities. It calls for expanding the BFHI to include clinics, health centers, and pediatric hospitals. It urges the adaptation of the BFHI to the feeding of infants and young children affected by HIV/AIDS. It urges that those responsible for emergency preparedness should be well trained to support appropriate feeding practices consistent with BFHI's universal principles. The initiative aims to reduce the consequences of childhood undernutrition, specifically diarrheal disease, measles, malaria, and lower respiratory infection. Low-cost, high-quality complementary foods for infants and young children in the developing world contribute to the eradication of infant and child **malnutrition**. Optimal nursing in the first year and complementary feeding practices can prevent about one-fourth of deaths in children under 36 months of age.

IYCF practices vary in communities because of differences in knowledge, culture, health service use, and other socioeconomic factors. Key facilitators include family support and government policies that are well aligned with global technical guidance. Family misperceptions of age-appropriate feeding, inadequate financing, and evidence gaps hamper efforts to adopt the recommended practices (Avula et al., 2017). An assessment of 84 countries revealed a lack of attention to policy in almost all areas (Gupta et al., 2019). Globally, monitoring of IYCF practices, data collection, budgeting, and preparedness and planning for appropriate and safe practices in emergencies is inadequate. Bottle feeding is prevalent, and Code violations are commonplace (Zakarija-Grković et al., 2020).

Infant formula companies are major players in the effort against the enforcement of IYCF legislation (Harris et al., 2017). Where food security is a concern, poverty reduction, rather than IYCF programs, is viewed as the solution. The U.S. initiative Alive & Thrive aims to reduce undernutrition and death caused by suboptimal IYCF practices. This organization is active in Bangladesh, Ethiopia, and Vietnam and has expanded its programs into Burkina Faso, India, Nigeria, and throughout the Southeast Asia region (Alive & Thrive, 2023).

A flexible, systematic, collaborative approach facilitates comprehensive IYCF programs. Training, strategic partnerships, and social media coordinated at the national level reach multiple audiences (Baker et al., 2018). Large-scale implementation of IYCF counseling in diverse environments is strengthened by training, supportive supervision and leadership, financing, incentives, partnerships, and monitoring

(Sanghvi et al., 2016). Face-to-face interventions, combined with social mobilization and relevant mass media, are effective in improving IYCF practices (Graziose et al., 2018; Osendarp & Roche, 2016). IYCF practices are especially crucial for infant and child survival during humanitarian crises (Prudhon et al., 2018; Shaker-Berbari et al., 2018).

1,000 Days Challenge

World leaders issued a **1,000 Days** challenge in 2010 to accelerate progress toward reducing hunger on a global scale. Key nonprofit organizations, including the Gates Foundation, partnered to form the 1,000 Days organization, named for the 1000 days between pregnancy and the child's second birthday. The challenge advocates globally for prenatal nutrition, exclusive nursing, and healthy complementary nutrition (1,000 Days, 2023).

Globally, malnutrition is responsible for 45% of all child deaths, stunting of 149 million children, and wasting of an additional 45.4 million children (UNICEF, 2023). Chronic deficiency in nutrition during the first 1000 days of a child's life, from conception to age 2, is among the main causes of stunting. Frequent infectious illnesses during this period also play a major role. Lack of human milk substantially elevates the risk of illness. The 1,000 Days challenge promotes targeted action and investment to improve nutrition (including exclusive nursing for 6 months and appropriate complementary foods) for nursing parents and children in this critical period.

U.S. Initiatives

Lactation promotion is reflected in several initiatives in the United States, including requirements from **The Joint Commission** and several government-based initiatives. To be successful, government initiatives need a long-term plan for sustaining the program and sound administrative and financial management. Staff and funds devoted exclusively to the promotion of programs will lead to the identification of key obstacles and strategies for overcoming them. Government-based programs depend on continued funding and support from one political administration to the next.

U.S. Department of Agriculture

The **U.S. Department of Agriculture** uses a social marketing approach to lactation education and support that is implemented at the state and local levels of the Special Supplemental Nutrition Program for Women, Infants, and Children (WIC). Percentages among families in WIC in 2019 were 74.7% initiation, 40.3% at 6 months, and 23.6% at 1 year (CDC, 2022). Exclusive nursing was 35.5% at 3 months and 17.8% at 6 months. The Six Steps to Achieve Breastfeeding Goals for WIC Clinics publication identifies the need for exclusive nursing to become the social norm and strongly recommends that WIC clinics adhere to the Code (National WIC Association, 2011).

Office on Women's Health

The **Office on Women's Health** in the U.S. Department of Health and Human Services (USDHHS) launched a National Breastfeeding Awareness Campaign in 2004, the first of its kind since 1911. The campaign encouraged exclusive nursing for 6 months, with a goal of increasing lactation rates to 75% (Merewood & Heinig, 2004). The Ad Council, a private, nonprofit organization, ran the campaign, titled Babies Were Born to Be Breastfed. Public service announcements spoke to the general market and targeted the Black community because of low lactation rates among that population. Lobbying efforts by the infant formula industry weakened the messages by removing significant content about health risks. The formula industry outspent the Ad Council, pouring $80 million into revising the campaign compared with the $30 million donated to it (Haynes, 2009).

The Office on Women's Health website provides employer solutions for supporting nursing employees (USDHHS, 2023). The searchable online resource provides businesses with tips and solutions used in a wide variety of industry settings. More than 200 employers in 22 industry sectors share solutions for creating space, time, and accommodations for expressing and storing milk or on-site infant care.

Centers for Disease Control and Prevention

About every 2 years, the CDC invites all hospitals across the country to complete the **Maternity Practices in Infant Nutrition and Care (mPINC)** survey. Survey questions focus on specific areas of hospital care that affect how babies are fed (CDC, 2023). The mPINC measures lactation-related practices against recommended standards at all intrapartum care facilities across the United States. It compares these practices by state, with each state's mPINC score representing the level of lactation support in its facilities. The survey measures the support of lactating hospital employees as well as patients.

Data from the mPINC survey are summarized in the CDC's Breastfeeding Report Card. The 2022 Breastfeeding Report Card for infants born in 2015 in the United States reported that 83.2% of infants initiated lactation, and 55.8% continued at 6 months. At 1 year, 35.9% were still nursing. The rate for exclusive nursing through 3 months was 45.3%, and the rate was 24.9% through 6 months. The CDC added new support indicators to the 2022 Breastfeeding Report Card to measure paid family and medical leave (PFML) and licensing regulations for childcare centers to support and encourage best practices. In 2022, the CDC and March of Dimes launched the National Network of Perinatal Quality Collaboratives (NNPQC) to support state-based perinatal quality collaboratives for improvements in maternal and infant health (CDC, 2022).

The Joint Commission

The Joint Commission accredits U.S. hospitals and is instrumental in improving the quality of care that patients receive. The organization instituted five perinatal care core measures in 2009 to stimulate and guide quality improvement efforts. Core Measure 5 requires that hospitals with 1100 or more births per year report the rate of exclusive human milk feedings during the newborn's entire hospitalization as a percentage of all full-term births, considering intention to nurse. In 2019, a sixth perinatal core measure was added for Unexpected Complications in Term Newborns (The Joint Commission, 2019). The PC-06 measure includes reporting of traumatic birth and neonatal jaundice to encourage policies that support nursing families and increase exclusive human milk feeding rates.

American Academy of Pediatrics

The AAP endorsed the Ten Steps to Successful Breastfeeding in 2009. Because of its stance on pacifier use to reduce the incidence of sudden unexplained infant death, the AAP did not support a categorical ban on pacifiers. However, they voiced strong support for the remaining tenets of the Ten Steps. This strengthened efforts within the U.S. healthcare system to institute practices that support lactation. The updated 2022 AAP Policy Statement: Breastfeeding and the Use of Human Milk encourages social and systemic changes, including inclusive language that reflects gender-diverse families (AAP, 2022).

Surgeon General's Call to Action to Support Breastfeeding

The 2011 U.S. Surgeon General, Dr. Regina Benjamin, issued the **U.S. Surgeon General's Call to Action to Support Breastfeeding**. It included 20 action areas that focused the country's attention on reducing barriers to lactation. At the time, lactation initiation rates were 75%, 43% were nursing at 6 months, and 22% were nursing at 12 months (USDHHS, 2011). The Call to Action helped to increase those rates to today's 83.2% initiation, 55.8% at 6 months, and 35.9% at 12 months (CDC, 2022). The Call to Action also called for ensured access to International Board Certified Lactation Consultants (USDHHS, 2011).

Patient Protection and Affordable Care Act

The U.S. 2010 **Patient Protection and Affordable Care Act** contains several elements of lactation support. The healthcare law requires employers to provide reasonable break time and a place for pumping that ensures privacy without intrusion from coworkers and the public for employees who are not exempt from overtime to express milk. It requires most health insurance plans to provide lactation support, counseling, and equipment (including breast pumps) during pregnancy and throughout lactation. If state laws provide greater protection, employers must comply with those state laws (U.S. Department of Labor, Wage and Hour Division [USDLWHD], 2010).

The 2023 Providing Urgent Maternal Protections Act (PUMP Act) closed some loopholes in the 2010 provision. It extends similar pumping breaks and private space to certain salaried workers who were not previously covered. This includes teachers, registered nurses, farmworkers, truck and taxi drivers, home care workers, and managers. Employees can sue for monetary remedy if their rights are violated. They must be compensated if they are not completely relieved from their work duties during a pumping break (USDLWHD, 2023).

Grassroots Initiatives

Grassroots promotion efforts also target nursing families. Reaching Our Sisters Everywhere (ROSE) focuses on reducing lactation disparities among Black communities across the United States. The organization seeks to strengthen the health of babies and families through mentoring, training, support groups, education, legislation, health policies, and social marketing (ROSE, 2023). MomsRising, an online multicultural organization, educates the public on critical issues facing families and mobilizes grassroots actions. MomsRising reaches out to local, state, and national leaders; amplifies national dialogue; lobbies at state capitols and on Capitol Hill; and helps hold corporations accountable (MomsRising, 2023).

Summary

Infant feeding practices have evolved throughout history with parents who chose not to nurse using wet nurses or artificial infant formula to feed their babies. Concerns about infant health and morbidity led to a resurgence of nursing with many parents embracing the idea of nursing their babies. For the most part, healthcare providers share the conviction that nursing is the optimal method for infant nutrition. Despite this intellectual agreement, nursing families need support and advice in societies dominated by artificial feeding messages; sometimes-hostile societal attitudes; and aggressive, unethical formula industry marketing. Numerous global and country-specific initiatives underscore the importance of human milk and strengthen promotion efforts around the world.

What You Learned—At a Glance

Conversation Starters with Parents

- How many babies have you observed nursing?
- What might prevent you from exclusively nursing your baby for 6 months?
- What exposure have you had to formula feeding?
- How supportive of nursing is your hospital?

Historical Infant Feeding Practices

- There is a rich history of wet nursing and sharing of human milk.
- There is a cultural belief in many countries that human milk substitutes are the norm.
- The field of pediatrics emerged with the need for infant feeding experts to guide the selection of human milk substitutes and continues to be heavily influenced by the infant formula industry.
- Around 1920, the medical community began to question the wisdom of feeding babies human milk substitutes because of poor health outcomes.

Nursing Recommendations and Rates

- Babies should nurse exclusively for the first 6 months and for 2 years or longer.
- There are great disparities in infant feeding practices among and within countries.
- Racial disparities affect lactation rates.

Global Lactation Initiatives

- 1981: WHO adopted the International Code of Marketing of Breast-milk Substitutes to promote safe infant nutrition.
- 1989: After countries ignored the Code, UNICEF and WHO issued a joint statement that led to the Ten Steps to Successful Breastfeeding.
- 1991: UNICEF and WHO launched the BFHI to promote practices to support lactation in birth facilities.
- 2003: WHO and UNICEF created the Global Strategy for IYCF to strengthen world attention on infant feeding practices.
- 2010: World leaders issued a 1,000 Days challenge to accelerate progress toward reducing hunger and malnutrition globally.
- 2018: WHO and UNICEF revised BFHI implementation guidelines and the Ten Steps to Successful Breastfeeding.

Lactation Initiatives in the United States

- 1997: Department of Agriculture launched "Loving Support Makes Breastfeeding Work" to increase lactation initiation and duration in WIC.
- 2004: The Office on Women's Health launched a National Breastfeeding Awareness Campaign with public service announcements.
- 2007: The CDC began the biannual mPINC survey to measure lactation-related practices.
- 2009: The Joint Commission instituted five perinatal core measures to assess hospital practices, adding a sixth one in 2019.

- 2009: The AAP endorsed the Ten Steps to Successful Breastfeeding.
- 2010: The Patient Protection and Affordable Care Act included several elements of lactation support.
- 2011: The Surgeon General issued a Call to Action to Support Breastfeeding.
- 2014: The Office on Women's Health launched an interactive website to showcase employer solutions for supporting employees.
- 2014: Grassroots promotion focused on the lactation needs of Black people and underserved families.

References

1,000 Days. 2023. https://www.thousanddays.org

Abugov H, et al. Barriers and facilitators to breastfeeding support practices in a neonatal intensive care unit in Colombia. *Invest Educ Enferm.* 2021;39(1):e11.

American Academy of Family Physicians. Family physicians supporting breastfeeding. 2023. https://www.aafp.org/about/policies/all/breastfeeding-position-paper.html

American Academy of Pediatrics. The AAP policy statement: breastfeeding and the use of human milk. *Pediatrics.* 2022;150(1):e2022057988. https://www.aap.org/en/patient-care/breastfeeding/policies-on-breastfeeding/

Anstey EH, et al. Racial and geographic differences in breastfeeding—United States, 2011–2015. *MMWR Morb Mortal Wkly Rep.* 2017;66:723–727.

Arslanian KJ, et al. How much does it cost to implement the Baby-Friendly Hospital Initiative training step in the United States and Mexico? *PLoS One.* 2022;17(9):e0273179.

Avula R, et al. Scaling-up interventions to improve infant and young child feeding in India: what will it take? *Matern Child Nutr.* 2017;13(suppl 2).

Baby-Friendly USA. Baby-friendly facilities in the U.S. 2023. https://www.babyfriendlyusa.org/about/

Baerug A, et al. Effectiveness of Baby-Friendly community health services on exclusive breastfeeding and maternal satisfaction: a pragmatic trial. *Matern Child Nutr.* 2016;12(3):428–439.

Baker P, et al. What drives political commitment for nutrition? A review and framework synthesis to inform the United Nations Decade of Action on Nutrition. *BMJ Glob Health.* 2018;3(1):e000485.

Bass JL, et al. Unintended consequences of current breastfeeding initiatives. *JAMA Pediatr.* 2016;170:923–924.

Benoit B, Semenic S. Barriers and facilitators to implementing the Baby-Friendly Hospital Initiative in neonatal intensive care units. *J Obstet Gynecol Neonatal Nurs.* 2014;43(5):614–624.

Bottle Babies. Directed by Peter Krieg, Kenya. 1975. Distributed by Unifilm, 419 Park Avenue South, New York, NY 10016.

Bruney T, et al. Achieving Baby-Friendly designation at a large metropolitan center. *Am J Perinatol.* 2020;37(04):430–435.

Burnham L, et al. Perspectives of nurses in Mississippi on implementation of the Baby-Friendly Hospital Initiative. *J Obstet Gynecol Neonatal Nurs.* 2021;50(4):392–401.

Cabrera-Lafuente M, et al. Breastfeeding practices in neonatal wards in Spain. Neo-BFHI international survey. *An Pediatr (Engl Ed).* 2022;96(4):300–308.

Centers for Disease Control and Prevention. Breastfeeding report card United States 2022. 2022. https://www.cdc.gov/breastfeeding/pdf/2022-breastfeeding-report-card-h.pdf

Centers for Disease Control and Prevention. Maternity Practices in Infant Nutrition and Care Survey (mPINC). 2023. http://www.cdc.gov/breastfeeding/data/mpinc/

Centers for Disease Control and Prevention. NIS-Child data results. November 4, 2024. https://www.cdc.gov/breastfeeding-data/survey/results.html

Davanzo R, et al. Making the first days of life safer: preventing sudden unexpected postnatal collapse while promoting breastfeeding. *J Hum Lact.* 2015;31:47–52.

Davis-Floyd R, Cheyney M. *Birth in Eight Cultures.* Long Grove, IL: Wavelength Press; 2019.

Di Mario S, et al. Baby-friendly hospitals and cesarean section rate: a survey of Italian hospitals. *Breastfeed Med.* 2013;8(4):388–393.

Ducharme-Smith K, et al. Exposure to baby-friendly hospital practices and breastfeeding outcomes of WIC participants in Maryland. *J Hum Lact.* 2022;38(1):78–88.

European Milk Bank Association. 2023. https://europeanmilkbanking.com/

Fed Is Best Foundation. 2024. https://fedisbest.org

Feldman-Winter L, Goldsmith JP; Committee on Fetus and Newborn, Task Force on Sudden Infant Death Syndrome. Safe sleep and skin-to-skin care in the neonatal period for healthy term newborns. *Pediatrics.* 2016;138:e20161889.

Feldman-Winter L, et al. Academy of Breastfeeding Medicine position statement: breastfeeding as a basic human right. *Breastfeed Med.* 2022;17(8):633–634.

Ferrarello D, Carmichael T. Sudden unexpected postnatal collapse of the newborn. *Nurs Women's Health.* 2016;20:268–275.

Forsyth S. Formula milk studies couldn't exist without industry. *BMJ.* 2019;364:l367.

Gomez-Pomar E, Blubaugh R. The Baby Friendly Hospital Initiative and the Ten Steps for Successful Breastfeeding. A critical review of the literature. *J Perinatol.* 2018;38:623–632.

Grant A, et al. Views and experience of breastfeeding in public: a qualitative systematic review. *Matern Child Nutr.* 2022;18(4):e13407.

Graziose MM, et al. Systematic review of the design, implementation and effectiveness of mass media and nutrition education interventions for infant and young child feeding. *Public Health Nutr.* 2018;21(2):273–287.

Gunther M. Instinct and the nursing couple. *Lancet.* 1955;265(6864):575–578.

Gupta A, et al. The world breastfeeding trends initiative: implementation of the global strategy for infant and young child feeding in 84 countries. *J Public Health Policy.* 2019;40(1):35–65.

Hadihardjono DN, et al. Promotions of breastmilk substitutes, commercial complementary foods and commercial snack products commonly fed to young children are frequently found in points-of-sale in Bandung City, Indonesia. *Matern Child Nutr*. 2019;5(suppl 4):e12808.

Haiden N, Ziegler EE. Human milk banking. *Ann Nutr Metab*. 2016;69:8–15.

Harris J, et al. Changes in the policy environment for infant and young child feeding in Vietnam, Bangladesh, and Ethiopia, and the role of targeted advocacy. *BMC Public Health*. 2017;17(suppl 2):492.

Haynes S. Evaluation of the National Breastfeeding Awareness Campaign: implications for the WIC campaign. 2009. http://www.nationalacademies.org/hmd/~/media/Files /Activity%20 Files/Nutrition/USDABreastfeeding/09 _Haynes_Suzanne.pdf

Hernández-Aguilar MT. BFHI network news brief. *J Hum Lact*. 2022;38(4);792–796.

Hernández-Cordero S, et al. Countries' experiences scaling up national breastfeeding, protection, promotion and support programmes: comparative case studies analysis. *Matern Child Nutr*. 2022;18(S3):e13358. https://doi.org/10.1111/mcn.13358

Hockamp N, et al. The role of breastfeeding promotion in German hospitals for exclusive breastfeeding duration. *Matern Child Nutr*. 2022;18(2):e13326.

Hoefer C, Hardy M. Later development of breast fed and artificially fed infants. *JAMA*. 1929;92(8):615–620.

Hou K, et al. Pilot implementation of a monitoring and enforcement system for the International Code of Marketing of Breast-Milk Substitutes in Cambodia. *Matern Child Nutr*. 2019;15(suppl 4):e12795.

Human Milk Banking Association of North America. 2023. https://www.hmbana.org/welcome2.html

Jacobs A. Opposition to breast-feeding resolution by U.S. stuns world health officials. *New York Times*. July 8, 2018. https://www.nytimes.com/2018/07/08/health/world-health-breastfeeding-ecuador-trump.html

Kavle J, et al. Baby-friendly community initiative—from national guidelines to implementation: a multisectoral platform for improving infant and young child feeding practices and integrated health services. *Matern Child Nutr*. 2019;15(S1):e12747.

Kimani-Murage EW, et al. Effectiveness of the baby-friendly community initiative on exclusive breastfeeding in Kenya. *Matern Child Nutr*. 2021;17(3):e13142.

Kullman KC, et al. Human milk sharing in the United States: a scoping review. *Breastfeed Med*. 2022;17(9):723–735.

La Leche League, International. A brief history of La Leche League, International. 2023. https://llli.org/about/history/

Lange D. Nipomo, Calif. March 1936. Migrant agricultural worker's family. Seven hungry children. Mother aged 32. Library of Congress Prints and Photographs Division, Washington, DC 20540. hdl.loc.gov/loc.pnp/pp.print

Lassi ZS, et al. Impact of infant and young child feeding (IYCF) nutrition interventions on breastfeeding practices, growth and mortality in low- and middle-income countries: systematic review. *Nutrients*. 2020;12(3):722.

Liberty AL, et al. A geospatial analysis of the impact of the Baby-Friendly Hospital Initiative on breastfeeding initiation in North Carolina. *J Hum Lact*. 2019;35(1):114–126.

Lubold AM. The effect of family policies and public health initiatives on breastfeeding initiation among 18 high-income countries: a qualitative comparative analysis research design. *Int Breastfeed J*. 2017;12:34.

Lucas A, et al. Breast milk and subsequent intelligence quotient in children born preterm. *Lancet*. 1992;339(8788):261–264.

Lutter CK, et al. Violations of the International Code of Marketing of Breast-Milk Substitutes: a multi-country analysis. *BMC Public Health*. 2022;22(1):2336.

Lutz TL, et al. Sudden unexplained early neonatal death or collapse: a national surveillance study. *Pediatr Res*. 2016;80:493–498.

Maastrup R, Haiek L. Compliance with the "Baby-friendly Hospital Initiative for neonatal wards" in 36 countries. *Matern Child Nutr*. 2019;15(2):e12690.

Maingi M, et al. Effectiveness of Baby Friendly Community Initiative (BFCI) on complementary feeding in Koibatek, Kenya: a randomized control study. *BMC Public Health*. 2018;18(1):600.

Mäkelä H, et al. Healthcare professionals' breastfeeding attitudes and hospital practices during delivery and in neonatal intensive care units: pre and post implementing the Baby-Friendly Hospital Initiative. *J Hum Lact*. 2022;38(3):537–547.

Meek JY, Noble L. Technical report: breastfeeding and the use of human milk. *Pediatrics*. 2022;150(1):e2022057989. https://doi.org/10.1542/peds.2022-057989

Merewood A, Heinig J. Efforts to promote breastfeeding in the United States: development of a national breastfeeding awareness campaign. *J Hum Lact*. 2004;20(2):140–145.

MomsRising. 2023. https://www.momsrising.org

Munn AC, et al. The impact in the United States of the Baby-Friendly Hospital Initiative on early infant health and breastfeeding outcomes. *Breastfeed Med*. 2016;11:222–230.

Nestle M. *Food Politics: How the Food Industry Influences Nutrition and Health*. Berkeley, CA: University of California Press; 2013.

Newton N, Newton M. Relationship of ability to breast feed and maternal attitudes toward breast feeding. *Pediatrics*. 1950;5(5):869–875.

Norsyamlina CAR, et al. A cross-sectional study on the practice of wet nursing among Muslim mothers. *BMC Pregnancy Childbirth*. 2021;21(1):68.

Nyqvist KH, et al. Expansion of the Baby-Friendly Hospital Initiative Ten Steps to Successful Breastfeeding into neonatal intensive care: expert group recommendations. *J Hum Lact*. 2013;29(3):300–309.

Nyqvist KH, et al. *Neo-BFHI: The Baby-Friendly Hospital Initiative for Neonatal Wards. Core Document with Recommended Standards and Criteria*. Nordic and Quebec Working Group; 2015.

Office of Disease Prevention and Health Promotion. (n.d.). Infants overview and objectives. *Healthy People 2030*. U.S. Department of Health and Human Services. https://health.gov/healthypeople/objectives-and-data/browse-objectives/infants

Osendarp SJ, Roche ML. Behavioral change strategies for improving complementary feeding and breastfeeding. *World Rev Nutr Diet*. 2016;115:184–192.

Palmquist A, Doehler K. Human milk sharing practices in the U.S. *Matern Child Nutr*. 2016;12(2):278–290.

Papastavrou M, et al. Breastfeeding in the course of history. *J Pediatr Neonatal Care*. 2015;2(6):00096.

Parker M, et al. 10 years after Baby-Friendly designation: breastfeeding rates continue to increase in a US neonatal intensive care unit. *J Hum Lact*. 2013;29(3):354–358.

Patterson JA, et al. The effect of Baby-Friendly status on exclusive breastfeeding in U.S. hospitals. *Matern Child Nutr*. 2018;14(3):e12589.

Pérez-Escamilla R, et al. Breastfeeding: crucially important, but increasingly challenged in a market-driven world. *Lancet*. 2023;401(10375):472–485.

Pramono A, et al. Social value of maintaining baby-friendly hospital initiative accreditation in Australia: case study. *Int J Equity Health*. 2021;20(1):22.

Procaccini D, et al. Baby-Friendly practices minimize newborn infants weight loss. *Breastfeed Med*. 2018;13(3):189–194.

Prudhon C, et al. Informing infant and young child feeding programming in humanitarian emergencies: an evidence map of reviews including low and middle income countries. *Matern Child Nutr.* 2018;14(1):e12457.

Reaching Our Sisters Everywhere, Inc. 2023. https://www.breastfeedingrose.org

Reyes-Foster BM, et al. Human milk handling and storage practices among peer milk-sharing mothers. *J Hum Lact*. 2017;33(1):173–180.

Ryan AS, et al. Recent declines in breast-feeding in the United States, 1984 through 1989. *Pediatrics*. 1991;88(4):719–727.

Salmon M. The cultural significance of breastfeeding and infant care in early modern England and America. *Soc Hist*. 1994;28:247–269.

Sanghvi T, et al. Achieving behaviour change at scale: Alive & Thrive's infant and young child feeding programme in Bangladesh. *Matern Child Nutr.* 2016;12(suppl 1):141–154.

Schmied V, et al. Place of sanctuary: an appreciative inquiry approach to discovering how communities support breastfeeding and parenting. *Int Breastfeed J*. 2019;14:25.

Schwarzenberg SJ, Georgieff MK; Committee on Nutrition. Advocacy for improving nutrition in the first 1000 days to support childhood development and adult health. *Pediatrics*. 2018;141(2):e20173716.

Sedgwick JP, Fleishner EC. Breastfeeding in the reduction of infant mortality. *Am J Public Health*. 1921;11:153–157.

Shaker-Berbari L, et al. Infant and young child feeding in emergencies: organisational policies and activities during the refugee crisis in Lebanon. *Matern Child Nutr.* 2018;14(3):e12576.

Shing J, et al. The influence of the Baby-Friendly Hospital Initiative and maternity care practices on breastfeeding outcomes. *J Hum Lact*. 2022;38(4);700–710.

Smith P, et al. (eds.). *Beyond Health, Beyond Choice: Breastfeeding Constraints and Realities (Critical Issues in Health and Medicine)*. New Brunswick, NJ: Rutgers University Press; 2012.

Soldavini J, Taillie LS. Recommendations for adopting the International Code of Marketing of Breast-Milk Substitutes into U.S. policy. *J Hum Lact*. 2017;33(3):582-587.

Srinivas GL, et al. Eradicating reliance on free artificial milk. *J Hum Lact*. 2015;31(1):53–56.

Stevens E, et al. A history of infant feeding. *J Perinat Educ*. 2009;18(2):32–39.

Tafili A, et al. Association of hospital and community factors on the attainment of Baby-Friendly designation: a breastfeeding health promotion. *Matern Child Nutr.* 2022;18(3):e13388.

The Joint Commission. National Hospital inpatient quality measures: perinatal care core measure sets. 2019. https://manual.jointcommission.org/releases/TJC2018B/MIF0393.html

United Nations Children's Fund. Infant and young child feeding. September 2021. https://data.unicef.org/topic/nutrition/infant-and-young-child-feeding/

United Nations Children's Fund. UNICEF Annual Report 2023. https://www.unicef.org/reports/unicef-annual-report-2023

U.S. Department of Health and Human Services, Office of the Surgeon General. *The Surgeon General's Call to Action to Support Breastfeeding*. Washington, DC: Office of the Surgeon General; 2011. https://www.surgeongeneral.gov

U.S. Department of Health and Human Services, Office on Women's Health. Supporting nursing moms at work. 2023. https://www.womenshealth.gov/supporting-nursing-moms-work/resources#2

U.S. Department of Labor, Wage and Hour Division. Section 7(r) of the Fair Labor Standards Act—Break Time for Nursing Mothers Provision. 2010. https://www.dol.gov/agencies/whd/nursing-mothers/law

U.S. Department of Labor, Wage and Hour Division. FLSA protections to pump at work. 2023. https://www.dol.gov/agencies/whd/pump-at-work

von Seehausen MP, et al. Factors associated with cross-nursing. *Cien Saude Colet*. 2017;22(5):1673–1682.

Walsh A, et al. Improving breastfeeding support through the implementation of the Baby-Friendly Hospital and Community Initiatives: a scoping review. *Int Breastfeed J*. 2023;18(1):22.

Waterston T, Yilmaz G. Sponsorship of paediatricians/paediatric societies by the Baby Feeding Industry—a position paper by the International Society for Social Paediatrics and Child Health. *Child Care Health Dev*. 2016;42(2):149–152.

Webb A. *Mammalogy: Adaptation, Diversity and Ecology*. Forest Hills, NY: Callisto Reference; 2019.

Wernick A. Why did the US try to block a UN resolution encouraging breastfeeding? Living on Earth. August 12, 2018. https://www.pri.org/stories/2018-08-12/why-did-us-try-block-un-resolution-encouraging-breastfeeding

West E, Knight RJ. Mothers' milk: slavery, wetnursing, and black and white women in the Antebellum South. *J South Hist*. 2017;83(1):37–68.

Wieczorek CC, et al. The struggle for inter-professional teamwork and collaboration in maternity care: Austrian health professionals' perspectives on the implementation of the Baby-Friendly Hospital Initiative. *BMC Health Serv Res*. 2016;16:91.

Wolf JH. *Don't Kill Your Baby: Public Health and the Decline of Breastfeeding in the Nineteenth and Twentieth Centuries*. Columbus, OH: Ohio State University Press; 2001.

Wolf JH. Historical research: the origin of "formula": state of the science, 1890s. *J Hum Lact*. 2020;36(3):410–413.

World Health Organization. *Protecting, Promoting, and Supporting Breastfeeding: A Joint WHO/UNICEF Statement*. Geneva, Switzerland: World Health Organization; 1989.

World Health Organization. *Global Strategy for Infant and Young Child Feeding*. Geneva, Switzerland: World Health Organization; 2003.

World Health Organization. *Guidance on Ending the Inappropriate Promotion of Foods for Infants and Young Children: Implementation Manual*. Geneva, Switzerland: World Health Organization; 2017. https://www.who.int/nutrition/publications/infantfeeding/manual -ending-inappropriate-promotion-food/en/

World Health Organization. Implementation guidance: protecting, promoting and supporting breastfeeding in facilities providing maternity and newborn services: the revised Baby-Friendly Hospital Initiative. 2018a. https://www.who.int/publications/i/item/9789241513807

World Health Organization. *Marketing of Breast-Milk Substitutes: National Implementation of the International Code, Status Report 2018*. Geneva, Switzerland: World Health Organization; 2018b.

World Health Organization. *Marketing of Breast Milk Substitutes: National Implementation of the International Code, Status Report 2020*. Geneva, Switzerland: World Health Organization; 2020. https://www.who.int/publications/i/item/9789240006010

World Health Organization. Infant and young child feeding. June 9, 2021a. https://www.who.int/news-room/fact-sheets/detail/infant-and-young-child-feeding

World Health Organization. Infant and young child feeding. February 2021b. https://www.who.int/news-room /fact-sheets /detail/infant-and-young-child-feeding

World Health Organization. WHO recommendations for care of the preterm or low-birth-weight infant. 2022. https://apps.who .int/iris/bitstream/handle/10665/363697/9789240058262 -eng.pdf

World Health Organization. Breastfeeding recommendations. 2023. https://www.who.int/health-topics/breastfeeding#tab=tab_2

World Health Organization, United Nations Children's Fund. *NetCode Toolkit. Monitoring the Marketing of Breast-Milk Substitutes: Protocol for Ongoing Monitoring Systems*. Geneva, Switzerland: WHO; 2017.

World Health Organization, United Nations Children's Fund. *Implementation Guidance: Protecting, Promoting and Supporting Breastfeeding in Facilities Providing Maternity and Newborn Services—the Revised Baby-Friendly Hospital Initiative*. Geneva, Switzerland: WHO; 2018. https://www.who.int/publications/i /item/9789241513807

Wouk K, et al. Systematic review of evidence for Baby-Friendly Hospital Initiative step 3: prenatal breastfeeding education. *J Hum Lact*. 2017;33(1):50–82.

Wu HL, et al. Rooming-in and breastfeeding duration in first-time mothers in a modern postpartum care center. *Int J Environ Res Public Health*. 2022;19(18):11790.

Zakarija-Grković I, et al. Are our babies off to a healthy start? The state of implementation of the Global Strategy for Infant and Young Child Feeding in Europe. *Int Breastfeed J*. 2020; 15(1):51.

Zehner E, et al. Marketing and infant and young child feeding in rapidly evolving food environments. *Matern Child Nutr*. 2019;15(S4):e12810.

CHAPTER 2

Interdisciplinary Lactation Care

Lactation care is an integral part of maternal and infant health. Lactation consultants, healthcare providers, educators, and parents all have an important roles on the lactation care team. Families need all members of their healthcare team to provide consistent care, support, and advice to help them achieve their lactation goals. Lactation assistance is most effective when caregivers work collaboratively with each other and with families. This includes any healthcare worker whose profession touches families during pregnancy, birth, or early childrearing. Lactation consultants and peer counselors are important members of the healthcare team whose primary focus is lactation.

KEY TERMS

Code of Professional Conduct
Commission on Accreditation of Allied Health Education Programs (CAAHEP)
Core Curriculum for Interdisciplinary Lactation Care
International Board Certified Lactation Consultant (IBCLC)
International Board of Lactation Consultant Examiners (IBLCE)
International Classification of Diseases (ICD-11) codes
International Lactation Consultant Association (ILCA)
Lactation Education Accreditation and Approval Review Committee (LEAARC)
Scope of Practice
Standards of Practice
Superbill
Third-party reimbursement
Warmline

Lactation Consulting Profession

New parents in earlier generations turned to elders in their families for advice and support in all areas of infant care, including lactation. In today's world, parents initiating lactation in a culture with decades dominated by artificial feeding often have no experienced family members or friends to help them. The lactation consultant profession emerged in 1985 to provide caregivers and families specialized knowledge and skills in lactation management and support.

The professional lactation consultant (**Figure 2-1**) is the primary member of the healthcare team to advocate for the nursing dyad. This advocacy extends to the nursing couple as well as to the infant as a separate individual. Lactation consultants use specialized knowledge and skills while working at the baby's pace. Because their primary focus is lactation, they may suggest alternative plans for lactation care as they collaborate with the rest of the healthcare team.

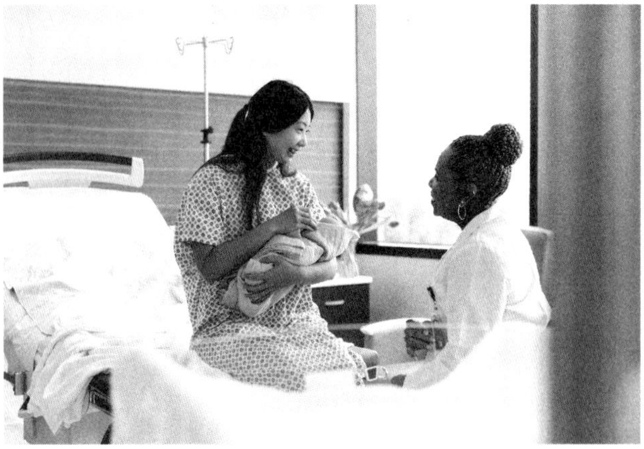

Figure 2-1 Lactation consultant on staff in the hospital.

The service that lactation consultants provide builds on the relationship between parents and their healthcare providers. Enlightened providers will change non-evidence-based practices through the sharing of clinical data and positive feedback from families. Lactation consultants can help facilitate this communication between parents and their healthcare providers to improve the support families receive. Provider support and guidance increase rates of exclusive nursing at 6 months and continued nursing at 12 months (Yourkavitch & Hall Smith, 2022).

Individuals enter the lactation consultant profession from a variety of backgrounds. Because of their professional education and experience, it is a natural progression for healthcare providers working in maternal/child health to expand their services to include lactation consulting. Many nutritionists and dietitians move into lactation support because of their understanding of the importance of human milk to lifelong health. Some lactation consultants begin their careers as peer counselors and then acquire the advanced education, skills, and credentials to work professionally as part of the healthcare team. Others enter lactation consulting from unrelated fields after nursing their own children and developing a desire to help parents with lactation.

Growth of the Profession

Interest in a specialized field began in the early 1980s with the advent of professional education for lactation management through various private programs. Several professional texts on lactation management emerged. Some were directed to the medical profession, and others, such as this text, were directed to the practical aspects of working with families. In 1984, then U.S. Surgeon General C. Everett Koop identified professional education as one of six core areas to be addressed in the lactation field. The following year, a pioneering group of leaders solidified the new lactation consultant profession with the creation of a certification board and a professional association. The education pillar of the profession followed later in 2008.

The **International Board of Lactation Consultant Examiners (IBLCE)** emerged in 1985 to develop and administer a professional certification examination. The exam measures the knowledge and skills necessary for safe and effective practice as a lactation consultant. It is administered in multiple languages and in countries across all major continents. A candidate for certification who meets education requirements and completes the examination can become an **International Board Certified Lactation Consultant (IBCLC)**. The IBCLC credential requires recertification every 5 years. Information about current requirements is available at the IBLCE website at https://www.iblce.org.

The **International Lactation Consultant Association (ILCA)** was formed in 1985 as the professional association for lactation consultants. ILCA's vision is "world health transformed through breastfeeding and skilled lactation care." The association's mission is to "advance the IBCLC profession worldwide through leadership, advocacy, professional development, and research" (ILCA, 2024). ILCA publishes the *Journal of Human Lactation* (*JHL*), a peer-reviewed scientific quarterly journal. The association also hosts an annual international conference and an extensive website with professional resources. Their Global Partner Program links organizations at the international, national, regional, and local levels.

The **Lactation Education Accreditation and Approval Review Committee (LEAARC)** was formed in 2008 to establish standards in lactation consultant education. LEAARC's mission is to "advance the global development of lactation education, appraise compliance with established standards, and provide ongoing educator support" (LEAARC, 2024a). Their vision is "global access to consistent foundational and continuing professional lactation education" (LEAARC, 2024a). In its role as a Committee on Accreditation for the **Commission on Accreditation of Allied Health Education Programs (CAAHEP)**, LEAARC reviews and recommends lactation programs in postsecondary institutions for accreditation (CAAHEP, 2024). LEAARC also provides formal recognition to didactic courses and clinical instruction for nonacademic lactation offerings.

Several documents guide the lactation consulting profession, including a **Code of Professional Conduct** (IBLCE, 2022), a **Scope of Practice** (IBLCE, 2018b), **Standards of Practice** (ILCA, 2013), and Clinical Competencies for the Practice of IBCLCs (IBLCE, 2018a). The profession's **Core Curriculum for Interdisciplinary Lactation Care** promotes consistency in evidence-informed lactation education and clinician practice (LEAARC, 2024b).

Diversifying the Lactation Consultant Profession

In 2014, the IBLCE, ILCA, and LEAARC held a summit to shed light on the need to diversify the lactation consultant profession to include underrepresented groups (ILCA, 2014). Summit participants identified several areas where improvement is needed. In the United States, where the majority of IBCLCs reside, African American, Hispanic, and Native American communities are underrepresented in the profession. Worldwide, the profession also needs to engage males, young adults, and lay counselors, along with members of the lesbian, gay, bisexual, transgender/transsexual, queer/questioning, questioning plus (LGBTQ+) community. Implicit bias training and application of critical race theory can help lactation organizations and employers better understand the historical context of lactation and move toward greater diversity within the field (Broomfield-Massey & Noor, 2018; Thomas, 2018).

Reaching Our Sisters Everywhere (ROSE) seeks to strengthen the health of Black babies and families across the United States (ROSE, 2023). The National Association of Professional and Peer Lactation Supporters of Color (NAPPLSC) was formed in 2015 to cultivate a community of diverse professional and peer lactation supporters in the United States (NAPPLSC, 2023). The organization partnered with the Carolina Global Breastfeeding Institute (CGBI) to implement the Reclaiming, Improving and Sustaining Equity (RISE) Lactation Training Model. RISE assists in establishing accredited lactation consultant education programs to increase the representation of people of color as IBCLCs in vulnerable communities (CGBI, 2023).

Practicing as a Lactation Consultant

Lactation consultants work in hospitals, healthcare provider offices, public health clinics, home health care, and private practice. A lactation consultant's background and experience may dictate their practice setting. In many cases, hospitals, healthcare provider offices, and home healthcare agencies require that the lactation consultant possess additional licensure as a registered nurse. Health clinics may employ a lactation consultant who is also a registered dietitian or nutritionist. Employers that provide lactation support to their workers are a growing practice venue for lactation consultants. Healthcare education and background may not be required for providing employee support. Experienced lactation consultants may establish a private practice in their community, a setting that requires extensive experience with a great variety of nursing dyads.

Any of these practice settings will need space that provides privacy, and an area for office work and lactation equipment and supplies. Easy access to necessary equipment and resources will increase efficiency in consultations, recordkeeping, and report. Some lactation consultants provide lactation devices during consultations. A large practice may offer breast pump rentals and retail sales of breast pumps, pump kits, replacement parts, adapters, power packs, and feeding devices. **Table 2-1** describes these and other possible resources for equipping a lactation consultant practice.

Practicing in a Hospital

Most lactation consultants work in hospitals, guiding and supporting families as they integrate their new baby into their lives. Hospital-based lactation consultants have the potential to greatly influence parents' self-confidence and competence as they begin nursing. The role of a hospital-based lactation consultant varies with the size of the facility and the resources available for lactation services. A robust program in a hospital with many births may employ a team of lactation consultants who provide both inpatient and outpatient services. A smaller hospital with fewer births may employ one lactation consultant for inpatient care on a part-time or full-time basis. Some hospitals may relegate lactation support to a staff nurse or provide no lactation support at all. The growing trend to outsource allied health caregivers in the United States also applies to lactation consultants. Some hospitals contract for lactation services in the same way as they contract with nutritionists, dietitians, respiratory therapists, and other specialties. Regardless of the hospital's size and lactation services, there are certain universal aspects to the role of a hospital-based lactation consultant.

Table 2-1 Resources for Lactation Consultant Practice

Office	■ Desk, chair, and filing cabinet ■ Computer and printer ■ Reference library
Communication	■ Dedicated cell phone or telephone line ■ HIPAA-compliant email and text access ■ Business website or blog
Consultations	■ Comfortable chair or couch with arms where parents can nurse, preferably one that can be wiped clean ■ Footstool to place in front of the chair to teach positioning ■ Pillows of various shapes and sizes (with removable cases to ensure safe hygiene practices) to help parents with comfortable positioning ■ Toys that can be cleaned to keep toddlers busy during the consultation
Infant assessment	■ Changing table where the baby can be laid securely for examination ■ Calibrated digital scales for pre- and post-feeding weights ■ Paper products or linens to use on the changing table and scale
Lactation devices	■ Breast pumps for rental and/or purchase and their accessories or sources where parents can obtain them
Disposable supplies	■ Medicine droppers ■ Small cups for cup feeding ■ Nipple shields ■ Nursing supplementers ■ Small amounts of formula to feed babies who need calories ■ Olive oil to improve the vacuum of the breast pump flange

HIPAA = Health Insurance Portability and Accountability Act.

Providing Skilled Lactation Care

One of the most important aspects of lactation care in the hospital is ensuring that someone who is skilled in lactation assessment observes at least one feeding for every nursing dyad before discharge. A lactation consultant is not always able to visit all parents on a given day. In some hospitals, the lactation consultant may visit only the dyads referred to them by nursing staff for special help, based on acuity levels (Mannel, 2011). Therefore, staff nurses provide much of the ongoing teaching and support as parents learn how to nurse during their hospital stay.

Lactation consultants need to ensure that staff members have the necessary instruction and guidance to provide consistent, skilled care. In-service training and appropriate lactation policies, procedures, care plans, and discharge instructions will ensure consistency. Hospital staff skilled in basic lactation care and handling common postpartum challenges will permit lactation consultants to respond to referrals for more complex situations. **Chapter 13** discusses a lactation consultant's role in postpartum lactation care.

Working with Peer Counselors

Some hospitals employ both lactation consultants and peer counselors to enhance the support they provide to nursing families. Lactation consultants work closely with peer counselors, who provide an important adjunct service to lactation care in the hospital. Counselors typically visit all nursing parents to provide basic information and support. They refer parents who experience problems to the lactation consultant for more skilled assistance and support. This model works well in hospitals with high numbers of nursing parents and a limited number of lactation consultants.

A Healthy Start program in one large city in the United States collaborated with a local hospital to provide multilevel lactation promotion. The program provides a safety net for low-income families and racial/ethnic groups from pregnancy through the postpartum period. Peer counselors conduct weekday rounds alongside the hospital's part-time lactation consultant. They educate parents on reasons to nurse, safe sleep, well visits, and positioning. They also inform parents about referrals for breast pumps, low-income assistance, and behavioral health. Counselor support continues for 6 months postpartum (Leruth et al., 2017).

Lactation Staffing Levels

Even motivated, experienced nursing parents may encounter early challenges that require skilled support. Sufficient lactation consultant coverage would ensure that every nursing parent receives a lactation visit before discharge. As discussed earlier, a hospital may provide 24-hour lactation coverage, have coverage during the workweek or for one shift, or outsource lactation services to contractors.

Table 2-2 Recommended Lactation Consultant Staffing in a Community Hospital

Mannel and Mannel (2006) ratio 1:783 nursing couplets

Category	*FTE Ratio*	*Calculations*	*Number*	*FTEs*
Number of nursing dyads		1000 × 85%	850	
Inpatient dyad	1:783	850 ÷ 783		1.1
Outpatient dyad	1:1292	850 ÷ 1292		0.7
Telephone follow-up	1:3915	850 × 2 1700 ÷ 3915	1700	0.4
Education	0.1:1000	1 × 0.1	1	0.1
Research	0.1–0.2			0.1
Program development/administration	0.1:1000	1 × 0.1	1	0.2
Total FTEs				2.6

FTE = full-time equivalent (40 hours per week.

Lactation consultants care for high-acuity nursing parents, educate other healthcare providers, and may administer complex lactation services. Almost one-third of a lactation consultant's time can be spent in indirect clinical activities, such as education, research, program development, and administration (Mannel & Mannel, 2006). Administrative tasks may include policies, procedures, documentation, staffing, personnel management, parent information, statistics, quality assurance, and hospital leadership. These nonclinical responsibilities must be factored into calculating accurate staffing needs to provide optimal lactation care.

A study by Mannel and Mannel (2006) calculated that a community hospital with 1500 deliveries and an 85% lactation rate would require about 2.5 full-time employees (FTEs) for the care of healthy, full-term newborns. This level of coverage permits three inpatient clinical consultations of approximately 30 minutes each for every nursing dyad, along with a follow-up phone call, as described in **Table 2-2**. The recommended number of FTEs increases with special care infants and postdischarge visits. Clinical time spent with each dyad in the neonatal intensive care unit would be about 5.5 hours, compared with 2.2 hours for healthy, full-term infants.

Practicing in Public Health

Public health clinics offer several avenues of employment for lactation consultants. Many clinics provide one-on-one counseling, classes, and postpartum support groups. Lactation consultants counsel parents or supervise and train counselors to provide that service. They provide information to agencies that deliver prenatal, labor and delivery, postpartum, pediatric, or daycare services. They participate in local, state or province, and national workshops, consortiums, and committees. Nutrition assistance programs are often part of a clinic's services.

Public health clinics encounter diverse lifestyles, with services that are sensitive to families' cultural and socioeconomic values. Many families relocate frequently, making ongoing contact challenging. Lifestyles and priorities among clinic families may differ from those of clinic staff. Focusing on parents' love and concern for their children helps to establish common ground for meaningful communication and assistance.

Nutrition Assistance Programs

In the United States, the Special Supplemental Food Program for Women, Infants, and Children (WIC) provides nutritious foods and services to nursing families with children up to 5 years of age. WIC serves 53% of all infants born in the United States (U.S. Department of Agriculture [USDA], 2023). Eligibility requires an annual income at or below 185% of the U.S. Poverty Income Guidelines (USDA, 2022b).

In Canada, the Canada Prenatal Nutrition Program (CPNP) provides similar services to over 45,000 pregnant people, parents, and caregivers across Canada (Public Health Agency of Canada, 2021). A distinguishing feature of the Canadian program is that it provides no free formula except as a compassionate response to a family that has run out of formula and cannot afford to purchase more.

Lactation Promotion in WIC

A glimpse into how the U.S. WIC program operates provides insight into similar public health programs throughout the world. WIC encourages exclusive nursing, provides anticipatory guidance, and helps create and advocate for a supportive environment that will help families carry out their feeding intentions. WIC provides prenatal classes, support lines, electronic messaging, mobile apps, and health professional training. Nursing participants receive supplies to help support their nursing. They may participate in WIC longer than non-nursing participants and receive support through peer counselors. A lactation consultant working in WIC often trains and supervises peer counselors, who reflect the community they serve. Cultural issues are discussed in **Chapter 21**.

WIC participants who exclusively nurse receive an enhanced food package to align with their higher calorie needs. WIC updates its food packages at least every 10 years to reflect nutrition science, public health concerns, and cultural eating patterns. The food packages were last changed in 2024. Food packages that reward lactation increase rates of exclusive nursing (Rasmussen et al., 2017).

In 2020, WIC produced a comprehensive, competency-based Breastfeeding Curriculum through a cooperative agreement with Every Mother, Inc. to train all levels of WIC staff in state and local WIC agencies. Through a tiered approach, the program trains support staff, peer counselors, Competent Professional Authorities and other health professionals, and WIC Designated Breastfeeding Experts. The training standardizes education throughout the agency to provide consistent care for WIC clients.

Lactation initiation and exclusivity rates are lower among WIC participants compared with all children born in the United States. In 2019, 74.7% of infants were ever nursed compared with 83.9% in the non-WIC population (Centers for Disease Control and Prevention [CDC], 2022). Socioeconomic characteristics common among the WIC population may contribute to these lower lactation rates. The WIC population includes twice as many Black and Hispanic/Latino families as the overall U.S. population. About 70% of WIC participants live below the poverty threshold compared with 10.5% of the general U.S. population (USDA, 2022b). **Chapter 3** provides further discussion of these vulnerable populations.

Working in a Healthcare Provider Practice

Working in an obstetric, pediatric, or family practice group offers an opportunity to care for families through many stages of lactation. Most of the care is preventive, with infants who are healthy and normal as well as those who require special care. Lactation consultants may work specific hours in the provider's office or on-call from home. The office may contact the lactation consultant or refer parents directly, with client load dependent on the provider's number of clients. Coverage will need to be arranged when the lactation consultant is unavailable to ensure that parents receive the help they need.

Lactation Services in a Healthcare Provider Practice

Having a lactation consultant on staff provides great marketing potential for a healthcare provider practice. Lactation consultants free up the time providers would otherwise spend helping parents with lactation. The expertise lactation consultants bring to the practice helps inform providers and staff of new research and practices. Shared appointments with the primary care provider and lactation consultant can provide consistent support and guidance. Parents benefit from the immediate face-to-face knowledge and support from the lactation consultant. Some pediatricians are IBCLC certified.

A lactation consultant may divide their time between pediatric and obstetrical practices. Lactation classes and support groups are natural extensions of services to parents in obstetric and pediatric practices. Prenatal contact provides an opportunity to help in the feeding decision, dispel misconceptions, explore lactation history and goals, and perform breast assessments in preparation for lactation. Contacting the hospital in the morning to determine which expectant parents need a visit will help in planning rounds.

Lactation consultants in these community settings guide parents through the early weeks of lactation, providing essential follow-up after hospital discharge. The practice may offer a 24-hour telephone **warmline** for parents to leave a voice message or email support via a secure electronic platform. It may also offer services through telemedicine, discussed further in **Chapter 6**.

Practicing in Home Health Care

Home visiting programs are an effective strategy to support families with young children. They increase lactation initiation, duration, and exclusivity (Arbour, 2019; Mersky et al., 2021; Pádua et al., 2022). Agencies differ in their services and policies for eligibility and the duration of the visits. Programs are designed to provide information, referrals, and parenting support to reduce child maltreatment, improve maternal and child health, and improve early school readiness (Health Resources and Services Administration, 2023). A home care agency with a lactation consultant on staff can provide lactation follow-up after hospital discharge. Hospitals customarily contract with managed care companies to provide home care services. Home health services begin with discharge planning and continue through home visits and community referrals.

A home environment is less structured than a hospital room, requiring flexibility in the way care is provided. Helping parents lower their expectations about showering, dressing, or cleaning the house for a visitor encourages them to get the rest they need. Social amenities and emotional support may be substantially different from what occurs in a hospital setting. Family dynamics may be quite different, with the partner, siblings, and grandparents often present. This provides insight into the parent's support system and opportunities to educate family members. Obtaining permission before discussing personal matters will ensure privacy. This section describes a possible progression of home visits by a lactation consultant.

A first home visit may start with asking about the birth experience to identify potential problems with lactation, such as the possibility of a sleepy baby because of birth interventions. Talking about the birth and any disappointments may help parents gain perspective and move on to other parenting elements, such as lactation. The lactation consultant assess the dyad, observe and assess feedings, learn how feeding is going, and build the parent's self-confidence. Anticipatory guidance will help avoid potential complications, such as nipple pain, engorgement, or low milk production.

A second visit typically occurs around day 5 or 6 after childbirth. The parent may be more rested, relaxed, and confident. Discussion can focus on long-term issues, such as managing feedings after returning to work and accessing community support. The visit typically includes another complete assessment of the dyad, including a breast exam and observation of a feeding. At least six or more wet diapers and three or more stools in 24 hours would be expected. Full-term infants who nurse exclusively typically lose about 6–7% of their birth weight by day 3 (Bertini et al., 2015; Flaherman et al., 2015). If weight has not rebounded by day 5 or 6, close follow-up is warranted. A 10% weight loss in the first 3–5 days is excessive and requires supplementation (Dewey et al., 2003; Miyoshi et al., 2020).

Working in Private Practice

A seasoned IBCLC with extensive experience assisting a wide variety of nursing families may consider opening a private practice. Private practice lactation consultants are dependent on referrals to maintain and expand their client base. Establishing a large system of referrals from contacts with other lactation consultants, hospitals, caregivers, and previous clients can take several years. An additional medical credential beyond IBCLC designation (e.g., nurse, nurse practitioner, physician, dietitian, or midwife) can enhance referrals. These licensed credentials also make it more likely that insurance companies will provide reimbursement. However, nonlicensed IBCLCs can be reimbursed by insurance in some situations.

Private practice allows lactation consultants to arrange their schedules around family functions and other responsibilities. Working part time in a hospital helps maintain peer relationships while also helping clients in the early postpartum period. Involvement in community coalitions and other professional groups provides additional networking opportunities. The keys to success include sound business practices, time to care for clients, reliable documentation, and marketing the practice.

Business Structure

Consulting with an accountant or tax attorney before opening a private practice can help avoid potential tax and business pitfalls associated with running a business. A small business course from a local community college may help those with no business background. Books, seminars, and internet resources also provide information on how to start a small business and run a home office. The Internal Revenue Service (IRS) provides webinars and extensive information on U.S. federal tax requirements on its website (IRS, 2024). Being self-employed may provide tax benefits, which an accountant can help identify.

Office Location

A private practice may be managed in an office in the community, at home or through home visits. If in the home, a local zoning board can identify any restrictions on home businesses, signs, parking, or supplies. Client visits may require additional coverage on homeowner's insurance. Removing personal items and clutter from the consultation room creates a professional environment. Framed professional awards and certificates of academic and community achievement will enhance credibility. An office in a commercial building requires rent, insurance, utilities, business signage, and maintenance. It needs to be located where clients will feel comfortable, with outdoor lighting for evening appointments, security, snow removal, and adequate parking. Many commercial offices offer secretarial services for small businesses, including copying, faxing, phone, and virtual voice-mail systems. If visits are in parents' homes, calling or texting before the visit avoids miscommunication about the date or time and is an opportunity to confirm the address. A cell phone will provide security, and the global positioning system (GPS) can help locate the home.

Regardless of setting, consultations require a location that ensures privacy and is not within hearing distance of others in the home or adjacent offices. This protects parents' privacy so that they can discuss sensitive issues. Bathroom facilities, safe and easy access to and from the office, and convenient parking are also needed. Intake forms, such as informed consent, history, and privacy notices, can be made available online through a secure server service. Clients can complete forms and pay online, or they can pay through an electronic tablet or notebook at the appointment, using secure platform applications designed specifically for lactation consultants. An integrated credit card reader for payments and emailing receipts to clients facilitates a paperless practice. If paper documentation is preferred, several client charts can be prepared on a clipboard so that they are ready to give to parents at the beginning of the visit. Insurance and healthcare providers expect electronic communication, so any paper documentation will need to be scanned and sent via secure (encrypted) electronic communication, including fax or email.

Marketing the Practice

A sound marketing strategy will guide the success of a private practice. Networking with other lactation consultants through social media, email, and conferences can provide insights into effective marketing strategies. Clients will come primarily from professional referrals, referrals from past clients, and marketing through the internet and places in the community. Many successful private practices use social media and websites that offer lactation information and describe their services. Including links to other lactation and parenting sites will increase online traffic. Mobile apps such as LatchMe (2024) provide an advertising opportunity. In addition, ILCA's Find a Lactation Consultant directory lists IBCLCs who are also ILCA members (https://www.ilca.org). Press releases and interviews through local news outlets and other media will further increase exposure.

Many routine aspects of private practice provide marketing opportunities. Meeting with healthcare providers at their offices to confer about clients and provide staff education enhances relationships. Connecting with hospitals, clinics, birthing centers, and childbirth educators will acquaint them with the practice. Sending a well-crafted report to providers after client visits demonstrates the lactation consultant's professionalism and expertise. Some circumstances may warrant enclosing a copy of relevant research articles as well. All this increases the likelihood that a provider will refer parents to the practice. Of course, satisfied clients are the best sources of referrals. Attention to meeting their needs will reap marketing benefits as they recommend the practice to friends and family and return for help with future babies.

Third-Party Reimbursement

If a private practice does not have in-network provider status with a parent's insurance carrier, the parent will need to pay their fee directly to the practice and send the receipt to their insurance company for reimbursement. An internet search for lactation **superbills** will identify forms designed specifically for **third-party reimbursement** of lactation consulting services. Some insurance companies require their own insurance reimbursement forms rather than a superbill. Information about coding, coverage of lactation care and services, and filing of claims is available for members from USLCA (2023).

In the United States, the Patient Privacy and Affordable Care Act requires that insurance providers cover the rental of an electric breast pump or the purchase of a consumer breast pump. Care plans should describe the type of pump (manual or electric), length of rental coverage, and when it is needed (before or after the baby's birth). Some insurance plans require preauthorization from the healthcare provider. **Figure 2-2** illustrates a sample referral letter for a breast pump rental that can accompany the

[Date]

To insurance carrier for: [client's name]
Name of policyholder:
Policy number:

The following explanation of medical need is provided in order to expedite insurance coverage for the rental of an electric breast pump.

[Name of parent] delivered the high-risk infant [name of baby] on [date]. The child is too immature or ill to nurse. However, it is well established that human milk provides optimal infant nutrition for the first 6 months of life. Thus, the parent of a preterm or high-risk newborn is encouraged to pump in order to provide milk for the baby and to maintain lactation until the baby can nurse.

The double electric breast pump is the most efficient, effective, and physiologic means of simulating the sucking action of a normal infant. Inexpensive manual, battery-operated, or small electric breast pumps are an adjunct to milk expression for occasional use when a large electric pump is unavailable. A piston-type electric breast pump is essential for the maintenance of adequate milk production when a child is unable to nurse. Such pumps cost approximately $1400 and thus are far more economical to rent.

The electric pump will be necessary until the baby is able to take all required nutrition by nursing. An electric breast pump is not a convenience for the parent; rather it is a medical necessity in the best interest of the child's health.

Sincerely,

[Healthcare Provider]

Figure 2-2 Healthcare provider letter for insurance coverage for rental of a breast pump.

reimbursement form. A dated copy of the provider's prescription could also be attached (a sample is provided in **Figure 2-3**). In the United States, this would include **International Classification of Diseases (ICD-11) codes** from the Centers for Medicare & Medicaid Services (CMS). Some codes may apply only if a healthcare provider is present for the consultation.

Client Services

Private practice lactation consultants need to be available to clients at established times and arrange coverage when away from the practice. Coverage by a reliable person who shares a compatible philosophy and approach to lactation will ensure that clients receive consistent help. The use of a cell phone, voice mail, or electronic messaging will ensure that parents can reach the practice and leave messages after hours. The lactation consultant is legally required to respond if a client leaves a message.

It is best practice to require that a new client sign a consent form before the first consultation. The form can include consent for future visits as well as permission for photographs for teaching purposes. A standard assessment form will ensure that essential information is collected and consistent. Preparing a report to the client's healthcare providers immediately after the client visit will ensure accurate reporting. Discussion of documenting feeding assessments and writing provider reports is presented in **Chapter 6**.

Record retention requirements are available from a state, province, or country agency. Materials to retain include client records, appointment books, call logs, financial records, and receipts. Records retained on a computer should be saved frequently through a secure online (cloud) backup service. In the United States, a free Health Insurance Portability and Accountability Act (HIPAA) security risk assessment tool is available from the U.S. Department of Health and Human Services (USDHHS, 2023). **Chapter 28** discusses documentation as it relates to legal liability.

Topic	Information to include
Consultation	Consult [lactation consultant's name] for evaluation, assessment, and treatment of [diagnosis and ICD-11 code].
Breast pump rental	Use of hospital-grade electric breast pump to obtain milk to feed to the baby. Classified as durable medical equipment.
Breast pump rental	Use of electric breast pump for treatment of [diagnosis and ICD-11 code].
Infant feeding supplies	Use of a [name of device] to ensure the baby's adequate caloric intake.

Figure 2-3 Examples of information to include on a prescription.

Interdisciplinary Healthcare Team

A team approach in health care includes a variety of professionals and advocates performing specialized functions designed to meet the physical, emotional, and psychological needs of clients. Interdisciplinary care encourages collaboration among relevant healthcare professions to capitalize on collective knowledge and skills. This interprofessional collaboration increases client and staff satisfaction, safety, quality, cost containment, and value (Institute of Medicine, 2015). Interdisciplinary teamwork (depicted in **Figure 2-4**) is characterized by common goals, complementary skills, shared decision-making, and shared accountability for outcomes. Team members foster trust and mutual respect for the roles of the various professional disciplines. Humility, listening, and

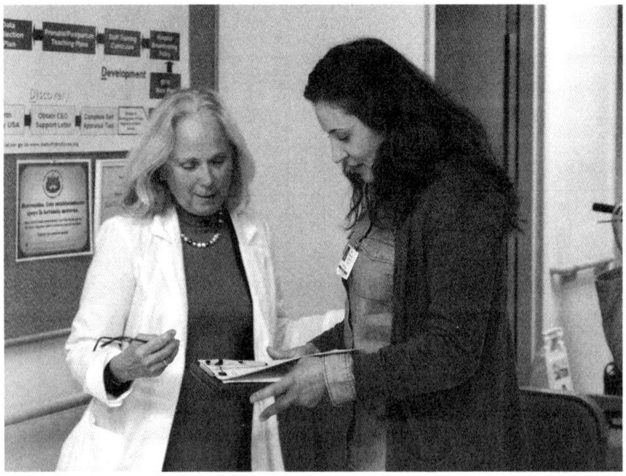

Figure 2-4 Healthcare team members conferring about a client.

Photo by Every Mother, Inc. and Regina Maria Roig-Romero.

learning from each other help to build trust and open communication (Sangaleti et al., 2017).

The course of pregnancy, birth, postpartum, and early child care brings families into contact with an array of healthcare professionals. Interdisciplinary care is especially important in lactation, with a team of caregivers meeting the needs of parents and infants from pregnancy through weaning (Reeves et al., 2018). Education and support from healthcare providers communicating positive views on lactation to new parents is a proven effective intervention (Gavine et al., 2022).

A collaborative approach requires that healthcare professionals understand and respect the credentials, scope of practice, and functions of each member of the team. Working together requires trust; open communication; and valuing the knowledge, skills, and insights everyone brings to the team. Interdisciplinary competency in knowledge, attitude, and working with others in the community helps healthcare providers meet the needs of nursing families. Integrating interprofessional competencies in curricula of various disciplines, as well as in-service training, can facilitate effective interprofessional collaboration (Vaseghi et al., 2022).

Primary disciplines relevant to interdisciplinary lactation care include lactation consulting, obstetrics, midwifery, pediatrics, nursing, neonatal intensive care, and dietetics. A lactation healthcare team may include lactation consultants, physicians, midwives, nurses, nurse practitioners, physician assistants, dietitians, pharmacists, childbirth educators, doulas, and **peer counselors**. Nurses and midwives are especially crucial because they can often spend more time educating parents than do other healthcare providers. Doula-led lactation education and support are shown to improve outcomes for diverse women from underserved areas (Louis-Jacques, 2022). If feeding complications occur, additional specialists may include physical therapists, occupational therapists, chiropractors, dentists, pharmacists, social workers, speech-language pathologists, and surgeons.

Knowledge Gaps on the Healthcare Team

There is a significant lactation knowledge deficit in all areas of health care (Meek, 2020). Lactation education in university health science, nursing, and medical programs may be lacking or inconsistent (Chuisano & Anderson, 2020). Medical schools may focus on biochemistry and medical issues related to lactation rather than practical management and support. Pediatric, obstetric, and family planning residents receive insufficient lactation education during their training (Feldman-Winter et al., 2017; Meek, 2020; Rodriguez & Shattuck, 2017). Lactation knowledge and skills are reportedly inconsistent among multidisciplinary pediatric healthcare professionals, particularly when it comes to complex clinical scenarios (Hookway & Brown, 2023).

Midwifery training lacks in-depth knowledge of lactation physiology and management (Altwalbeh, 2021). Nursing education does not always prepare students with the necessary knowledge, skills, and attitudes to help with lactation (Holtzman & Usherwood, 2018; Wallenborn et al., 2018; Webber & Serowoky, 2017). Nurses report feeling a low level of preparedness for practice in the first few years after graduation. New graduates must navigate the complex process of honing clinical skills while learning the organization's culture (Schmitt & Schiffman, 2019). Lactation education varies for pediatric nurse practitioners, who increasingly provide more pediatric and family health care. Although curricula promote lactation, programs vary in the amount of education and range of clinical opportunities for students (Brzezinski et al., 2018; Chuisano & Anderson, 2020). Pharmacists frequently interact with nursing parents regarding medication safety, yet their training may lack lactation content (Byerley et al., 2022; Harahsheh et al., 2024).

Parents are more likely to continue nursing when they receive consistent encouragement from their clinicians (American Academy of Pediatrics [AAP], 2022; McFadden et al., 2017). Healthcare providers rely on their background and training when educating and advising their clients. However, many of them lack the lactation knowledge, counseling skills, and professional education and training needed to help families (Blitman et al., 2022; Fahey et al., 2021; Mulcahy et al., 2022). Providers may rely on their own lactation experience or those of family members and clients to inform their practice (Garner et al., 2016). Negative or problematic experiences may bias the information and advice they give to clients. Providers who have had positive lactation experiences are more likely to promote lactation among their clients and staff (Eren et al., 2018; Sattari et al., 2016). **Chapter 28** discusses ways to fill the gap in lactation knowledge.

Support from the Healthcare Team

New parents flourish when they are supported and validated in their decisions. Healthcare providers exert tremendous influence over their clients. They are an important resource, especially for nursing families in rural and remote areas with limited resources (Dumphy et al., 2016; Goodman et al., 2016; Grubesic & Durbin, 2017). Providers' attitudes and cultures affect their level of lactation promotion and support (Garner et al., 2016; Radzyminski & Callister, 2015). Supportive providers who talk with their clients about lactation from a sound knowledge base can positively influence initiation and continuation. Some healthcare providers specialize in lactation support. The Academy of Breastfeeding Medicine provides a helpful protocol for lactation supportive practices in a healthcare provider's office (ABM, 2013).

A lack of adequate knowledge and skills may affect a healthcare provider's comfort level in promoting and supporting lactation (Baerg et al., 2021). Apparent nonsupport can result from reluctance to pressure parents or make them feel guilty about their choice to not nurse. An ambivalent approach transmits a message that infant formula is equally healthy and fails to promote human milk as optimal infant nutrition. Conveying the importance of lactation is no different than with other health choices, such as immunizations, preventive care, car-seat use, dental checkups, or avoidance of cigarette smoking and drugs of abuse. The issues of guilt are explored further in **Chapter 4**.

Peer Counselor Support

Many families have no access to experienced family members and friends to support them and teach them how to nurse. Peer counselors with experience nursing their babies can fill this gap and provide a supportive culture. Counselors of the same ethnicity as the community they serve can promote equity and enhance parents' ability to relate to them as role models (Rhodes et al., 2021). Research continues to document the value of peer support in increasing parents' confidence (Chang et al., 2022), initiation and duration rates (Martinez et al., 2020; Pyles et al., 2021; Ware, 2021), and exclusive nursing rates (Gavine et al., 2022; Keenan-Devlin et al., 2021; Saniel et al., 2021; Short et al., 2022).

Role of the Peer Counselor

Validation and support are valuable aspects of peer counselor services. Parents tend to deal with personal stresses by talking about them with others who share or understand their situation. Researchers have identified increased levels of self-esteem, confidence, empowerment, and satisfaction among nursing parents who receive peer support (Burns et al., 2020; Hopper & Skirton, 2016; Robinson et al., 2016).

Peer counselors receive training in counseling and lactation care. They offer anticipatory guidance to help parents learn what to expect, avoid potential problems, and resolve issues before they become unmanageable. They present options to parents and encourage them to participate actively in decisions about their babies' care. They typically emphasize limited separation of the nursing dyad, exclusive nursing for at least 6 months, and baby-led weaning. Helping parents manage a return to work or school and addressing variations in feeding styles that require compromise reflect counselors' flexibility and acceptance.

Community-Based Peer Support Groups

Step 10 of the Ten Steps to Successful Breastfeeding calls for ensuring that parents have timely access to ongoing support and care after hospital discharge. Peer support groups reinforce parents' traditional patterns of seeking and receiving advice from relatives and friends. Many parents who leave the hospital nursing fail to continue because they lack the necessary support and information to do so. Support groups educate parents about their options, help them make informed choices, and increase their self-confidence. In addition to counseling, they may provide written materials, regular group meetings, and special programs. Some groups provide help through internet websites, social forums, podcasts, and blogs.

Effective support groups accommodate the style and needs of the families and communities they serve. Regular community-based peer support group

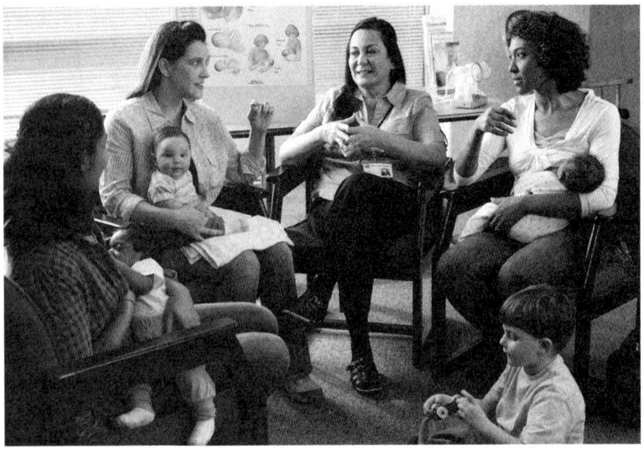

Figure 2-5 Breastfeeding support group.

Courtesy of U.S. Department of Agriculture's Food and Nutrition Service.

meetings held at a time and location convenient to families in their community will ensure accessibility. Meetings encourage friendly and informal discussion and participation through questions, demonstrations, and small-group discussions. Networking with others in the group provides an outlet for parents who lack contact with other nursing families. Parents benefit from the mutual sharing of experiences and the opportunity to be with other nursing parents and babies. Counselors offer support to new parents, helping them gain a feeling of self-reliance and reassurance. This social support and encouragement influence lactation continuation (Lee et al., 2019; Nabulsi et al., 2019; van Dellen et al., 2019). Meetings offer a valuable counseling opportunity as well (**Figure 2-5**).

Working with Peer Counselors

Establishing relationships with peer counselors and other support people in the community will enhance the effectiveness of lactation consultants in any area of practice. A collaborative working relationship between lactation consultants and peer counselors contributes to continuity in lactation care and support and promotes the continuation of lactation (Lee et al., 2019).

Many lactation consultants offer volunteer time to peer support groups. The value of building relationships and goodwill in the community makes this a worthwhile service and presents a unified program of support to families. **Table 2-3** presents possible services to a peer support group. Developing a peer support group, training group leaders, and being available as a resource is a worthy venture. Other ways to actively reach out include speaking at childbirth classes and clinics, sharing information with professionals, and speaking to high school health classes.

Table 2-3 Lactation Consultant Services to a Breastfeeding Support Group

Reciprocal referral system	■ Lactation consultants refer parents to the support group for continuing support. ■ The support group refers parents to lactation consultants when a situation requires a greater level of expertise. ■ A greater number of parents receive the necessary support and information.
Counselor training	■ Train counselors in counseling skills and lactation information to ensure that they provide quality counseling and accurate information. ■ Ensure that support and education are consistent with the lactation consultant's philosophy and approach. ■ Provide continuing education in the form of study nights, seminars, and workshops. ■ Be available as an adviser and to answer questions from counselors. ■ Review written materials for counselors and parents.
Assisting with support group activities	■ Speak at parent or counselor meetings. ■ Help organize outreach programs managed by the group. ■ Encourage community programs that address both parents and the medical community.
Liaison	■ Assist as a liaison between the support group and the medical community. ■ Maintain two-way communication when parents have problems, keeping healthcare providers and the support group informed.

Online Lactation Support

In an age when most adults own smartphones and regularly use apps and the internet, it is understandable that new parents increasingly seek lactation information and support online. They reach out to the internet for coping with difficulties, anticipatory guidance, and information on milk production. Parents who feel isolated and lack professional or family support may be drawn to online support. Online support normalizes lactation and offers shared experiences. It is reassuring, empathetic, and easily available (Moon & Woo, 2021; Morse & Brown, 2022; Regan & Brown, 2019). For some parents, knowing that information and guidance are a click away may provide the support they need.

Social media support promotes positive long-term lactation by increasing confidence, knowledge, and attitudes (Robinson et al., 2019a; Wilson, 2020). Many parents attribute their continued nursing to the online support they received (Black et al., 2020; Blackmore et al., 2022; Morse & Brown, 2021). Positive imagery of African Americans and shared online experiences improve confidence with nursing in public and prolonged duration (Robinson et al., 2019a, 2019b). Experiences of online support for some parents may include judgment for using formula, polarizing debates, and unhelpful information with no administrative oversight (Regan & Brown, 2019).

Many parents join online support groups that provide 24-hour access where they can post messages and wait for responses. They find support groups, such as those through Facebook, to be a convenient and preferred source for accessing lactation information and support. Australia and the United Kingdom host countrywide Facebook groups where parents receive immediate information and support from a trusted community (Australian Breastfeeding Association [ABA], 2023; The Breastfeeding Network [UK], 2023).

The Parent's Role on the Healthcare Team

Parents' active participation in their care is integral to the functioning of the healthcare team. Being validated and empowered in their parenting strengthens their role as equal members of their babies' and their own healthcare teams. Sharing the positive features of lactation with their providers helps modify or change provider attitudes, opinions, and practices. Busy healthcare providers may not recall all the details of a situation. Parents can summarize plans that were previously discussed and work with their provider on how to adapt the plans to the present situation.

A parent's assertiveness and clear communication with their healthcare providers and lactation consultants will reinforce their role as equal members of the team. Focusing on problems could cause providers to prescribe unnecessary practices for what they perceive to be a concern. For example, mentioning that the baby is fussy may result in the healthcare provider prescribing a formula supplement because of a concern about low milk production. The parent may simply have general questions about caring for a fussy baby and may not have considered a correlation between nursing and the baby's fussiness. Clear communication will avoid misunderstandings and unnecessary interventions.

Learning About Lactation

Ideally, lactation education begins before or during pregnancy and continues throughout the postpartum period. A combination of prenatal and postpartum education and support improves lactation initiation and continuation rates (Gavine et al., 2022). Parents learn about lactation through reading, prenatal and postpartum classes, personal assistance, and exploring the internet. They benefit from help in sorting through all the available information and deciding what will work for them and their baby. Lactation consultants serve as facilitators to gently guide them, using scientific knowledge and practical experience to nurture and protect lactation. Parents benefit most from a program that provides a range of services, such as those described in Table 2-3.

A lactation consultant's primary role with parents is to teach practical information about lactation, point out options, and offer useful suggestions. Learning why a certain technique works the way it does and the reasons behind suggestions will help parents understand them, relate to them, and adapt them to their situation. Learning in this manner will provide the tools to handle future similar circumstances and to grow in self-confidence. (Adult learning is discussed in **Chapter 4**.) Lactation research is dynamic and extensive. Remaining current with relevant literature and practices will ensure appropriate advice. **Figure 2-6** describes points for educating parents.

- Communicate clearly and simply.
- Offer the least complicated explanation in lay terms.
- Relate information in a friendly and low-key manner, neither overwhelming parents nor making them appear uninformed.
- Relate only information that is current, correct, and evidence based–not opinion or one person's experience.
- If information conflicts with information obtained from another source, check the source for accuracy and try to help resolve the conflict.
- If unable to answer a question, tell the parent you will research it and follow up later.

Figure 2-6 Tips for educating parents.

Information and advice parents receive must be obtained from a reliable source. Anything beyond the lactation consultant's scope of practice must be presented in a manner of educating, not prescribing treatment. This is not the case for those who have prescriptive authority, such as a physician, nurse practitioner, or physician assistant. Information on prescription drugs changes frequently based on current research, making it challenging to have the most up-to-date information when talking with parents. One authoritative source on medications and lactation is the current edition of *Hale's Medications and Mothers' Milk* (Hale & Krutsch, 2024). Parents can share this information with their baby's healthcare provider, who should be their ultimate adviser.

Managing Conflicting Advice

Lactation consultants are instrumental in promoting health consumerism and encouraging parents to assume an active role in their family's health care. At times, a lactation consultant's advice may conflict with advice from other healthcare providers. The disparity does not necessarily indicate that one side is incorrect. Rather, it illustrates the variety of opinions in obstetrics and pediatrics. Acknowledging any confusion caused by conflicting information will help parents resolve it and develop a plan that works for them.

When a conflict occurs, urging parents to make their own choices will help them work toward suitable solutions. The lactation consultant might communicate directly with the provider or share information with parents that they can discuss with their provider. Suggesting ways that parents can interact with their healthcare providers will strengthen their skills and confidence. Polite assertiveness, a positive attitude, and a willingness to work with their providers to resolve a conflict will strengthen their position. **Chapter 4** further discusses health consumerism and informed consent.

Summary

Parents who receive support from a strong healthcare team are empowered to participate in decision-making as informed health consumers. Lactation consultants are part of an interdisciplinary healthcare team that provides consistent care to parents and infants as they establish lactation. Whether the practice setting is a hospital, clinic, healthcare provider practice, home health care, private practice, or a corporation, a commitment to nursing families is the driving force behind all lactation support. Peer counselors have valuable roles in supporting parents. Lactation consultants can help coordinate this support by maintaining a reciprocal relationship with community support groups. Assertiveness and clear communication reinforce parents as equal members of the healthcare team.

What You Learned–At a Glance

Conversation Starters with Parents

- What do you know about lactation consultants?
- What services for nursing families are available in your hospital?
- What support for nursing families is available in your community?
- How supportive are your healthcare providers with nursing?

The Lactation Consultant Profession

- The lactation consultant profession emerged in 1985 to provide caregivers with specialized knowledge and skills.
- The IBLCE administers the certification examination for IBCLCs.
- ILCA is the international professional association for lactation consultants.
- LEAARC promotes standardization and excellence in lactation education.

Lactation Consultants in Hospital Practice

- Visit nursing parents.
- Teach parents and staff.
- Provide equipment and supplies for parents.
- Maintain hospital-based lactation programs.

Lactation Consultants in Public Health Programs

- Serve low-income families.
- Counsel families with cultural, socioeconomic, and lifestyle differences.
- Teach classes and facilitate support groups.
- Teach and supervise peer counselors.

Lactation Consultants in a Healthcare Provider Practice

- Care for parents with a full range of lactation experiences.
- Have client loads that depend on the provider's client load.
- Teach classes and facilitate support groups.
- Provide services during pregnancy.
- Visit parents in the hospital.
- Provide follow-up and support.

Lactation Consultants in Home Health

- Follow up with nursing parents after discharge.
- Assess the nursing parent, baby, and feeding.
- Provide anticipatory guidance on long-term issues.

Lactation Consultants in Private Practice

- Have extensive experience with dyads and situations.
- Manage a business and lactation equipment.
- Market the practice and establish a referral base.
- Bill for services and facilitate reimbursement.
- Provide office or home visits and follow-up.
- Document consultations, send healthcare provider reports, and retain records.

Members of the Lactation Team

- Inadequate lactation education in medical and nursing schools results in knowledge gaps among healthcare providers.
- Healthcare providers need to be proactive in protecting and promoting lactation.
- Connecting parents with peer support ensures continuing assistance and support.
- Peer support increases lactation initiation, exclusivity, and duration.
- Assertiveness and clear communication reinforce parents as equal members of the healthcare team.
- Parents benefit from help in sorting through information from social media.
- Anything beyond the lactation consultant's scope of practice must be presented as educating, not prescribing treatment.

References

Academy of Breastfeeding Medicine; Grawey AE, et al. ABM clinical protocol #14: breastfeeding-friendly physician's office: optimizing care for infants and children, revised 2013. *Breastfeed Med.* 2013;8:237–242.

Altwalbeh D. Breastfeeding knowledge and attitudes among midwifery diploma students in Jordan: a descriptive study. *Int J Community Based Nurs Midwifery*. 2021;9(4):325–335.

American Academy of Pediatrics. The AAP policy statement: breastfeeding and the use of human milk. *Pediatrics.* 2022;150(1):e2022057988. https://www.aap.org/en/patient-care/breastfeeding/policies-on-breastfeeding/

Arbour M, et al. National quality improvement initiative in home visiting services improves breastfeeding initiation and duration. *Acad Pediatr.* 2019;19(2):236–244.

Australian Breastfeeding Association. 2023. https://www.facebook.com/ozbreastfeeding/

Baerg K, et al. Learning needs of family physicians, pediatricians, and obstetricians to support breastfeeding and inform physician education. *Can Med Educ J.* 2021;29;12(6):55–61.

Bertini G, et al. Physiological weight loss chart helps to identify high-risk infants who need breastfeeding support. *Acta Paediatr.* 2015;104(10):1024–1027.

Black R, et al. Women's experience of social media breastfeeding support and its impact on extended breastfeeding success: a social cognitive perspective. *Br J Health Psychol.* 2020;25(3):754–771.

Blackmore A, et al. The effectiveness of virtual lactation support: a systematic review and meta-analysis. *J Hum Lact.* 2022;38(3):452–465.

Blitman E, et al. Breastfeeding mothers' experiences with community physicians in Israel: a qualitative study. *Int Breastfeed J.* 2022;17(1):62.

Broomfield-Massey K, Noor S. Consider the context: commentary on "'You Know if You Quit, That's Failure, Right?': Barriers to Professional Lactation Certification" by Erin V. Thomas. *J Hum Lact.* 2018;34(3):471–477.

Brzezinski L, et al. Pediatric nurse practitioner barriers to supporting breastfeeding by mothers and infants. *J Perinat Educ.* 2018;27(4):207–219.

Burns ES, et al. Breastfeeding support at an Australian Breastfeeding Association drop-in service: a descriptive survey. *Int Breastfeed J.* 2020;30;15(1):101.

Byerley EM, et al. Breastfeeding and the pharmacist's role in maternal medication management: identifying barriers and the need for continuing education. *J Pediatr Pharmacol Ther.* 2022;27(2):102–108.

Carolina Global Breastfeeding Institute. RISE (Reclaiming, Improving, and Sustaining Equity) lactation training model. 2023. https://sph.unc.edu/cgbi/rise-lactation-training-model-reclaiming-improving-and-sustaining-equity-2/

Centers for Disease Control and Prevention. Breastfeeding report card United States 2022. 2022. https://www.cdc.gov/breastfeeding/pdf/2022-breastfeeding-report-card-h.pdf

Centers for Disease Control and Prevention. Facts: nationwide breastfeeding goals. 2020. https://www.cdc.gov/breastfeeding/data/nis_data/data-files/2019/rates-any-exclusive-bf-socio-dem-2019.html

Centers for Disease Control and Prevention. NIS-Child data results. November 4, 2024. https://www.cdc.gov/breastfeeding-data/survey/results.html

Chang YS, et al. Views and experiences of women, peer supporters and healthcare professionals on breastfeeding peer support: a systematic review of qualitative studies. *Midwifery*. 2022;108:103299.

Chuisano SA, Anderson OS. Assessing application-based breastfeeding education for physicians and nurses: a scoping review. *J Hum Lact*. 2020;36(4):699–709.

Commission on Accreditation of Allied Health Education Programs. 2024. https://www.caahep.org

Dewey KG, et al. Risk factors for suboptimal infant breastfeeding behavior, delayed onset of lactation, and excess neonatal weight loss. *Pediatrics*. 2003;112(3 Pt 1):607–619.

Dumphy D, et al. A breastfeeding quality improvement project in rural primary care. *J Hum Lact*. 2016;32(4):633–641.

Eren T, et al. Breastfeeding experiences of female physicians and the impact of the law change on breastfeeding. *Turk Pediatri Ars*. 2018;53(4):238–244.

Fahey N, et al. Knowledge of breastfeeding and kangaroo mother care practices among general practitioners in rural western India. *Food Nutr Bull*. 2021;42(3):460–463.

Feldman-Winter L, et al. National trends in pediatricians' practices and attitudes about breastfeeding: 1995 to 2014. *Pediatrics*. 2017;140:1229.

Flaherman VJ, et al. Early weight loss nomograms for exclusively breastfed newborns. *Pediatrics*. 2015;135(1):e16–23.

Garner CD, et al. Discontinuity of breastfeeding care: "there's no captain of the ship". *Breastfeed Med*. 2016;11(1):32–39.

Gavine A, et al. Support for healthy breastfeeding mothers with healthy term babies. *Cochrane Database Syst Rev*. 2022;10(10):CD001141.

Goodman LR, et al. Breastfeeding barriers and support in a rural setting. *MCN Am J Matern Child Nurs*. 2016;41(2):98–103.

Grubesic TH, Durbin KM. Breastfeeding support: a geographic perspective on access and equity. *J Hum Lact*. 2017;33(4):770–780.

Hale T, Krutsch K. *Hale's Medications & Mothers' Milk 2025-2026: A Manual of Lactational Pharmacology*. 21st ed. New York, NY: Springer Publishing Company; 2024.

Harahsheh MM, et al. Community pharmacists' current practice and educational needs in breastfeeding support in Jordan: a cross-sectional study. *J Hum Lact*. 2024;40(1):132–142.

Health Resources and Services Administration. Maternal, infant, and early childhood home visiting program. 2023. https://mchb.hrsa.gov/programs/homevisiting/

Holtzman O, Usherwood T. Australian general practitioners' knowledge, attitudes and practices towards breastfeeding. *PLoS One*. 2018;13(2):e0191854.

Hookway L, Brown A. The lactation skill gaps of multidisciplinary paediatric healthcare professionals in the United Kingdom. *J Hum Nutr Diet*. 2023;36(3):848–863.

Hopper H, Skirton H. Factors influencing the sustainability of volunteer peer support for breast-feeding mothers within a hospital environment: an exploratory qualitative study. *Midwifery*. 2016;32:58–65.

Institute of Medicine. *Measuring the Impact of Interprofessional Education on Collaborative Practice and Patient Outcomes*. Washington, DC: National Academies Press; 2015.

Internal Revenue Service. Small business and self-employed tax center. 2024. https://www.irs.gov/Businesses/Small-Businesses-&-Self-Employed

International Board of Lactation Consultant Examiners. Clinical competencies for the practice of IBCLCs. 2018a. https://iblce.org/wp-content/uploads/2018/12/clinical -competencies-2018.pdf

International Board of Lactation Consultant Examiners. Scope of practice for IBCLCs. 2018b. https://iblce.org/wp-content/uploads/2018/12/scope-of-practice-2018.pdf

International Board of Lactation Consultant Examiners. Code of professional conduct. 2022. https://iblce.org/wp-content/uploads/2022/08/2022_August_17_Code-of-Professional-Conduct_FINAL.pdf

International Lactation Consultant Association. Standards of practice for international board certified lactation consultants. 2013. https://ilca.org/wp-content/uploads/2021/05/Standards-of-Practice-for-International-Board-Certified-Lactation-Consultants-newlogo.pdf

International Lactation Consultant Association. *2014 Lactation Summit Design Team, Summary Report of the 2014 Lactation Summit: Addressing Inequities Within the Lactation Profession*. Raleigh, NC: International Lactation Consultant Association; 2014. https://ilca.org/wp-content/uploads/2020/06/Summary-Report_2014LactationSummit-FINAL1.pdf

International Lactation Consultant Association. 2024. https://ilca.org/about/

Keenan-Devlin LS, et al. Clinically integrated breastfeeding peer counseling and breastfeeding outcomes. *J Perinatol*. 2021;41(8):2095–2103.

Lactation Education Accreditation and Approval Review Committee. 2024a. https://leaarc.org/about.html

Lactation Education Accreditation and Approval Review Committee; Campbell SH, et al. (eds.). *Core Curriculum for Interdisciplinary Lactation Care*. Burlington, MA: Jones & Bartlett Learning; 2024b.

LatchMe. Breastfeeding app. 2024. https://www.latchmd.com/

Lee YH, et al. Effects of education and support groups organized by IBCLCs in early postpartum on breastfeeding. *Midwifery*. 2019;75:5–11.

Leruth C, et al. A multilevel approach to breastfeeding promotion: using healthy start to deliver individual support and drive collective impact. *Matern Child Health J*. 2017;21(Suppl 1): 4–10.

Louis-Jacques AF, et al. Doula perspectives on lactation education and breastfeeding support for diverse, low-income women: a field report. *Ecol Food Nutr*. 2022;61(5):638–648.

Mannel R. Defining lactation acuity to improve patient safety and outcomes. *J Hum Lact*. 2011;27(2):163–170.

Mannel R, Mannel RS. Staffing for hospital lactation programs: recommendations from a tertiary care teaching hospital. *J Hum Lact*. 2006;22(4):409–417.

Martinez NG, et al. "Real-world" effect of a peer counselor on breastfeeding outcomes in an urban prenatal clinic in the United States. *BMC Pregnancy Childbirth*. 2020;20(1):671.

McFadden A, et al. Support for healthy breastfeeding mothers with healthy term babies. *Cochrane Database Syst Rev*. 2017;2:CD001141.

Meek JY, et al. Landscape analysis of breastfeeding-related physician education in the United States. *Breastfeed Med*. 2020;15(6):401–411.

Mersky JP, et al. Home visiting effects on breastfeeding and bed-sharing in a low-income sample. *Health Educ Behav*. 2021; 48(4):488–495.

Miyoshi Y, et al. Determinants of excessive weight loss in breastfed full-term newborns at a baby-friendly hospital: a retrospective cohort study. *Int Breastfeed J*. 2020;15(1):19.

Moon H, Woo K. An integrative review on mothers' experiences of online breastfeeding peer support: Motivations, attributes and effects. *Matern Child Nutr*. 2021;17(3):e13200.

Morse H, Brown A. Accessing local support online: mothers' experiences of local breastfeeding support Facebook groups. *Matern Child Nutr*. 2021;17(4):e13227.

Morse H, Brown A. The benefits, challenges and impacts of accessing social media group support for breastfeeding: a systematic review. *Matern Child Nutr*. 2022;18(4):e13399.

Mulcahy H, et al. Breastfeeding skills training for health care professionals: a systematic review. *Heliyon*. 2022;8(11):e11747.

Nabulsi M, et al. A multi-component intervention to support breastfeeding in Lebanon: a randomized clinical trial. *PLoS One*. 2019;14(6):e0218467.

National Association of Professional and Peer Lactation Supporters of Color. Accessed May 3, 2023. https://www.facebook.com/NAPPLSC/

Pádua AR, et al. An intervention program based on regular home visits for improving maternal breastfeeding self-efficacy: a pilot study in Portugal. *Matern Child Health J*. 2022;26(3):575–586.

Public Health Agency of Canada. Canada prenatal nutrition program. 2021. https://www.phac-aspc.gc.ca/hp-ps/dca-dea/prog-ini/cpnp-pcnp/

Pyles TEH, et al. Breastfeeding sisters that are receiving support: community-based peer support program created for and by women of color. *Breastfeed Med*. 2021;16(2):165–170.

Radzyminski S, Callister LC. Health professionals' attitudes and beliefs about breastfeeding. *J Perinat Educ*. 2015;24(2):102–109.

Rasmussen KM, et al. New opportunities for breastfeeding promotion and support in WIC: review of WIC food packages, improving balance and choice. *J Nutr Educ Behav*. 2017;49(7 suppl 2):S197.e1–S201.e1.

Reaching Our Sisters Everywhere, Inc. 2023. https://www.breastfeedingrose.org

Reeves S, et al. Teamwork, collaboration, coordination, and networking: why we need to distinguish between different types of interprofessional practice. *J Interprof Care*. 2018;32(1):1–3.

Regan S, Brown A. Experiences of online breastfeeding support: Support and reassurance versus judgement and misinformation. *Matern Child Nutr*. 2019:15(4):e12874.

Rhodes EC, et al. Promoting equity in breastfeeding through peer counseling: the US Breastfeeding Heritage and Pride program. *Int J Equity Health*. 2021;20(1):128.

Robinson A, et al. Facebook support for breastfeeding mothers: a comparison to offline support and associations with breastfeeding outcomes. *Digital Health*. 2019a;5:2055207619853397.

Robinson A, et al. It takes an e-village: supporting African American mothers in sustaining breastfeeding through Facebook communities. *J Hum Lact*. 2019b;33(3):486–499.

Robinson K, et al. Reactions of low-income African American women to breastfeeding peer counselors. *J Obstet Gynecol Neonatal Nurs*. 2016;45(1):62–70.

Rodriguez Lien E, Shattuck K. Breastfeeding education and support services provided to family medicine and obstetrics-gynecology residents. *Breastfeed Med*. 2017;12(9):548–553.

Sangaleti C, et al. Experiences and shared meaning of teamwork and interprofessional collaboration among health care professionals in primary health care settings: a systematic review. *JBI Database System Rev Implement Rep*. 2017;15(11):2723–2788.

Saniel OP, et al. Effectiveness of peer counseling and membership in breastfeeding support groups in promoting optimal breastfeeding behaviors in the Philippines. *Int Breastfeed J*. 2021;16(1):53.

Sattari M, et al. Infant-feeding intentions and practices of internal medicine physicians. *Breastfeed Med*. 2016;11:173–179.

Schmitt CA, Schiffman R. Perceived needs and coping resources of newly hired nurses. *SAGE Open Med*. 2019;7:2050312119833216.

Short VL, et al. Feasibility, acceptability, and preliminary impact of an mHealth supported breastfeeding peer counselor intervention in rural India. *Int J Gynaecol Obstet*. 2022;156(1):48–54.

The Breastfeeding Network (UK). 2023. https://www.facebook.com/TheBreastfeedingNetworkUK/

Thomas EV. "You know if you quit, that's failure, right?": barriers to professional lactation certification. *J Hum Lact*. 2018;34(3):454–466.

United States Lactation Consultant Association. Position paper—professional lactation support staffing in the hospital setting. *Clin Lact*. 2021;12(3).

United States Lactation Consultant Association. 2023. https://uslca.org/inside-uslca/committees/licensure/

U.S. Department of Agriculture, Food and Nutrition Services. Women, Infants and Children: 2022–2023 WIC Income Eligibility Guidelines. 2022b. https://www.fns.usda.gov/wic/ieg-2022-2023

U.S. Department of Agriculture, Food and Nutrition Service. What's in your WIC food package: what your WIC food package offers if you're breastfeeding. 2023. https://wicbreastfeeding.fns.usda.gov/whats-your-wic-food-package

U.S. Department of Health and Human Services. HHS releases security risk assessment tool to help providers with HIPAA compliance. 2023. https://www.hhs.gov/hipaa/for-professionals/security/index.html

van Dellen SA, et al. The effect of a breastfeeding support programme on breastfeeding duration and exclusivity: a quasi-experiment. *BMC Public Health*. 2019;19(1):993.

Vaseghi F, et al. Interprofessional collaboration competencies in the health system: a systematic review. *Iran J Nurs Midwifery Res*. 2022;27(6):496–504.

Wallenborn JT, et al. The impact of the professional qualifications of the prenatal care provider on breastfeeding duration. *Breastfeed Med*. 2018;13(2):106–111.

Ware JL, et al. African American breastfeeding peer support: all moms empowered to nurse. *Breastfeed Med*. 2021;16(2):156–164.

Webber E, Serowoky M. Breastfeeding curricular content of family nurse practitioner programs. *J Pediatr Health Care*. 2017;31(2):189–195.

Wilson JC. Using social media for breastfeeding support. *Nurs Womens Health*. 2020;24(5):332–343.

Yourkavitch J, Hall Smith P. Women's status, breastfeeding support, and breastfeeding practices in the United States. *PLoS One*. 2022;17(9):e0275021.

CHAPTER 3

Sociological Perspective on Lactation Support

The norms and perceptions of society strongly influence lactation promotion and support. Sociology examines the history, development, organization, and problems of people living together as social groups. It is a scientific study of social behavior; thought; and how we depend on, interact with, influence, and are influenced by others. This chapter explores lactation support from a sociological perspective, including insights into the needs of nursing families and the most effective strategies to help them reach their goals. Understanding the characteristics of acculturation into a dominant culture; bias; and the impact of racial, ethnic, and health disparities will help you honor the beliefs, customs, and values of families. Awareness of social thinking and social behavior will help you understand parents' perceptions and how they process information and media messages.

KEY TERMS

Acculturation
Conformity
Cultural humility
Culture
Demographics
Dominant culture
Empowerment
Evidence-based practice
Evidence-informed practice
Health disparities
Health equity
Health inequities
Implicit bias
Institutional bias
Liminality
Microaggression
Motivational interviewing
Myers-Briggs Type Indicators
Primary group
Secondary groups
Sensory input
Social determinants
Social marketing
Structural bias
Systemic bias
Technology-mediated support
Vulnerable population

Cultural Factors in Lactation Support

The commonality of people who share a culture, territory, and identity binds them together through relationships and interactions. The pattern of these relationships forms the social structure of a society. We each hold a particular position within society that influences the aspects of the culture we will experience. **Culture** involves all that we learn and transmit across generations. It includes the ideas, values, and practices that allow us to carry out our collective lives in relative order and harmony. Culture defines the foods we eat, the clothes we wear, the language we speak, the values and beliefs we hold, and the practices we follow.

Liminality describes a transitional stage that exists between a previous cultural norm and a return to that norm. Lactation is a transition period that occurs after pregnancy and birth and before weaning, when the nonpregnant, nonlactating status resumes. Liminal states become culturally unacceptable when the duration and the ending are not defined (Dowling & Pontin, 2017). For example, cultural pressure to wean intensifies as families continue nursing beyond their culture's accepted normal period.

Dominant Culture

A **dominant culture** consists of the specific behaviors, rituals, values, and social customs that have been established as a societal norm. Although numerous subcultures exist along with the dominant culture, members of the dominant culture have a significant presence in communication, education, law, government, and business. Thus, the dominant culture holds the balance of power and can impose its values and norms on subcultures, including vulnerable populations.

Subcultures

Subcultures within a culture vary by social class, ethnicity, race, religion, gender identity, lifestyle, goals, and interests. The identity of a subculture may revolve around its ethnic heritage, economic circumstances, or geographic region. A subculture often has a distinctive language and form of communication. We tend to evaluate others' customs, practices, and behaviors in light of our own subculture and experience. We need to understand and respect each cultural practice in terms of its place in the larger cultural context. Social values correspond to each individual subculture. We cannot dismiss the worth of practices within a subculture merely based on what we consider to be "right" and "wrong." For example, it may be easy to dismiss certain dietary or infant care practices as unimportant if they do not reflect best practice. For families in that culture, however, practices may carry deep meaning or reflect family tradition. Those practices may therefore contribute positively to their overall parenting identity. We need to approach and assess each person and cultural influence individually and with acceptance and a willingness to understand.

Some cultures promote beneficial practices such as carrying a baby close, unrestricted nursing, and long-term lactation. If a parent believes that pinning a band around the baby's abdomen will prevent an umbilical hernia, such a practice is not harmful to the baby and does not need to change. On the other hand, the custom of restricting consumption of fresh fruit for several weeks postpartum may affect nutritional status. There is a belief in some cultures that colostrum is harmful to the baby. This can result in delayed lactation until the colostrum changes to mature milk. Sensitive guidance regarding these practices can help to preserve the baby's health and the establishment of lactation.

Acculturation

Families who leave their native country have several characteristics in common when they work toward becoming part of a new culture. They share a sense of loss of their own culture, an environment in which they developed a set of beliefs and attitudes that are central to their lives. People's degree of **acculturation** (integration into a new culture) depends on how firmly they cling to traditional values. Members of succeeding generations replace old values with new ones as cultural differences become more diffuse. Factors that influence behavior are age, educational and social exposure, the intent to return to their country of origin, economic status, contact with older relatives, and the part of the country in which they reside. The lower classes tend to hold on to traditional values, whereas the middle and upper classes are more likely to incorporate new practices into their value system.

Families exhibit a wide range of value systems, family support, and interest in lactation. Members of some subcultures may desire to adapt to the dominant culture. Those who wish to integrate into Western culture may be influenced by mass media and perceive artificial infant milk to be the desired method of infant feeding. Even though lactation is the norm in their native culture, families may choose to formula feed to fit into their new surroundings.

Health Equity

Health equity is the opportunity for all people to attain their full health potential. Achieving health equity requires valuing everyone equally and removing obstacles to health for families among a **vulnerable population**. Vulnerability can result from poverty; ethnic, racial, or gender discrimination; or lack of access to good jobs with fair pay, quality education and health care, adequate housing, and safe environments. Equitable access to health care is crucial to achieving health equity.

Vulnerability can affect lactation in several ways. Housing insecurity is a significant risk factor for lower rates of exclusive nursing (Reno et al., 2022). Immigrants often live in communities with food insecurity (Miller et al., 2018; Walsemann et al., 2017). Low income increases the risk of poor mental health for parents (Bates et al., 2021). Early introduction of complementary foods is common among low-income families (Hornsby et al., 2021).

Prenatal enrollment in the Special Supplemental Nutrition Program for Women, Infants, and Children (WIC) increases the odds of feeding infants in response to hunger and satiety cues (Hudak & Benjamin-Neelon, 2021). Nursing support can encourage addicted parents to stop drug or alcohol use and can empower their parental caregiving (Schroeder et al., 2019). Delaying or preventing parent–infant separation after birth would assist incarcerated parents with lactation (Wouk et al., 2022).

Health Disparities

Health disparities occur when there are differences in health outcomes between segments of the population based on **social determinants** (Crear-Perry et al. 2021). Social determinants are conditions in the environment in which people are born, live, learn, work, play, worship, and age (Healthy People 2030, 2025). Determinants of health disparities may be socioeconomic, demographic, environmental, or geographic. Poverty, education status, race and ethnicity, gender, insurance status, and other factors influence the development of illness, the ability to obtain and use health care, and health outcomes. Systemic and structural social determinants such as racism, classism, and gender oppression contribute to inequities in health care access and outcomes.

The attitudes and behaviors of healthcare providers can contribute to health disparities (FitzGerald & Hurst, 2017; Hall et al., 2015). Addressing the needs of families within their varying sociocultural contexts may improve lactation rates (Bueno-Gutiérrez et al., 2021). Adverse social determinants of health regarding education, employment, food, neighborhood, and housing contribute to ongoing disparities in lactation (Standish & Parker, 2022). *Healthy People 2030* recognizes the effect of social determinants on health outcomes. Eliminating disproportionate morbidity and mortality among families of color is a health imperative (Asiodu et al., 2021; Crear-Perry et al., 2021; Hamed et al., 2022). The *Healthy People 2030* website provides tools and resources to examine data demographically by race and ethnicity (Healthy People 2030).

Health Inequities

Health inequities are measures of health for population groups or social classes associated with attributes such as income, education, race, and ethnicity. Inequity often results from gaps in access or inadequate care for disadvantaged groups. Health inequities are associated with social disadvantage and are pervasive around the globe. People with higher incomes often live longer and have better health and a better quality of life. Disadvantaged populations face inequitable access to quality health care and inequities in housing, education, environment, and social capital. During the COVID pandemic, nursing duration appeared to be affected more by inequities in health insurance than by education (McCloskey, 2023).

Racial and ethnic disparities are associated with a lack of health equity and children's health. Minority ethnic groups and indigenous populations are at increased risk for obesity (Isong et al., 2018; Min et al., 2018), poorer cardiovascular health (Pool et al., 2017), poorer vitamin D status (O'Callaghan & Kiely, 2018), and lower longevity (Wu et al., 2017). Inequity in maternal, newborn, and child health is associated with socioeconomic disparities (Gadson et al., 2017; Howell & Zeitlin, 2017; Kavle & Landry, 2018). There is evidence that epigenetic changes caused by multigenerational trauma and discrimination in historically subjugated groups may continue to negatively affect health outcomes in these groups (Conching & Thayer, 2019; Lehrner & Yehuda, 2018).

Racial and Ethnic Disparities in Lactation

Nursing families are affected by health disparities (Temple Newhook et al., 2017; Venu et al., 2017). Large racial and ethnic disparities exist in lactation rates for both Black and Latino families at national, state, and territorial levels. Because racial and ethnic groups vary geographically, efforts tailored to address each region's specific disparities are needed (Chiang et al., 2021). Systemic barriers in health care related to access, quality, support, and resources hinder lactation for Black people across generations (Stevens-Watkins et al., 2022). Lactation rates in the United States are lowest among African Americans and families living in rural areas (Antsey et al., 2017; Jones et al., 2015; Louis-Jacques et al., 2017).

The gap in lactation initiation between Black and White people in the United States is narrowing. However, there are large differences in exclusivity, duration, and the ability of parents to follow through on their intentions (Hemingway et al., 2021; Morrow et al., 2021). Black people disproportionately experience insufficient education and support, lack of knowledge about lactation, and concerns about navigating nursing and employment (Beauregard et al., 2019). Lack of encouragement and incomplete or incorrect information by healthcare providers may contribute to the lower lactation rates among African Americans (Asiodu et al., 2017), who are more likely to receive advice on formula feeding.

Interventions for Disparities

Protective interventions can reduce inequalities and inequities in lactation promotion and support among high-risk populations (**Figure 3-1**). A Black-focused model of lactation care for prenatal and postpartum practitioners can address lactation disparities in the Black community by increasing standardization and accountability (Gorbunova et al., 2023). Tapping into the strengths of African Americans who nurse the longest and tailoring interventions to that population may help increase lactation rates among low-income African Americans (Barbosa et al., 2017; Gross et al., 2017).

Strengthening support by family and social networks and engaging childcare centers and religious bodies in lactation promotion could help mitigate some of the disparities (Gyamfi et al., 2021). Enforcing the International Code of Marketing of Breast-Milk Substitutes may also help address inequalities and inequities in lactation (Zehner et al., 2019). Teaching healthcare providers about cultural and economic barriers to lactation can ensure appropriate education for nursing families. Helping hospitals that serve high-risk populations work toward Baby-Friendly Hospital practices will improve the health of families in their care. Reaching out to employers of low-wage staff can expand worksite lactation support to low-income families. Promoting culturally sensitive peer counseling in the community, as with WIC in the United States and the Canada Prenatal Nutrition Program, will ensure continuity of care for low-income families.

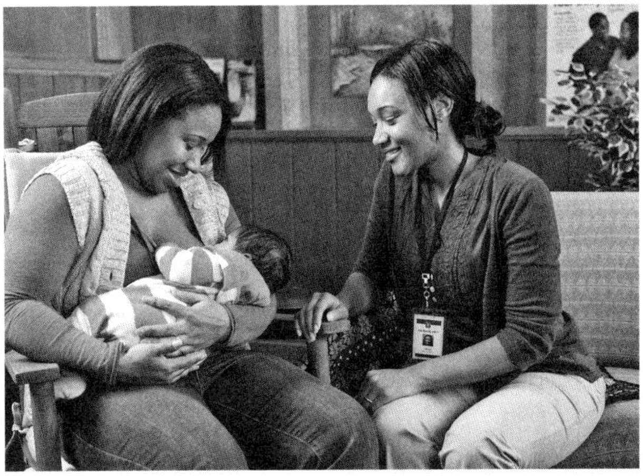

Figure 3-1 People of color need support to nurse.

Courtesy of U.S. Department of Agriculture's Food and Nutrition Service.

A 2022 White House Blueprint for Addressing the Maternal Health Crisis in the United States calls for improvements in lactation support by reducing systemic inequities that create disparities in access to health care. The initiative notes that Black people are three times more likely to die from pregnancy-related complications compared with White individuals. Native Americans are more than twice as likely to die from pregnancy-related complications compared with White individuals. Those who live in rural America are about 60% more likely to die (The White House, 2022).

Awareness of inequities is a necessary first step toward changing behavior. Targeted educational campaigns increase awareness of health disparities. Health equity can be improved through community-based programs that provide pregnancy and postnatal care, including home visits. The effectiveness of educational and public health efforts to reduce lactation disparities may be enhanced if support is tailored to acknowledge cultural differences and address factors that make formula feeding expected within their communities.

Cultural Humility

Because countries are increasingly diverse, healthcare professionals need to provide care that transcends cultural and language boundaries. Approaching families with **cultural humility** helps you understand and value the cultural norms, values, language, customs, beliefs, and healing traditions that shape a family's approach to health and illness. Recognizing cultural and historical factors that influence attitudes toward seeking help from healthcare providers will increase access to help when it is needed. This awareness will work toward eliminating long-standing disparities in the health status of people of diverse racial, ethnic, and cultural backgrounds.

Cultural humility occurs within the context of diversity and a power imbalance. It includes ethnic and racial differences and differences in sexual preference, social status, interprofessional roles, and healthcare provider–client relationships. Cultural humility in health care shifts the balance of power from the clinician to the client. It is an ongoing process of mutual respect, self-exploration, and self-critique and involves a willingness to honor the beliefs, customs, and values of others and accept them for who they are. This is distinctly different from a cultural competence approach, which implies that we can become competent in completely understanding the lived experiences of others. Cultural competence implies an end product of attaining understanding, whereas cultural humility is a lifelong process of developing new habits (Cassidy, 2024; Robinson et al., 2021).

Cultural humility requires continuous and humble learning and recognition of the various forms of bias. **Structural bias** is perpetuated through a society's cultural values that are ingrained in daily life. **Systemic bias** is prejudice, bigotry, or unfairness directed toward individuals of an oppressed or marginalized group. **Institutional bias** occurs when policies and practices within an organization discriminate against groups of people. **Implicit bias** is an involuntary personal thought process that results in unconscious favoritism toward or prejudice against people of a particular ethnicity, gender, or social group. Left unchecked, these biases can contribute to the inequitable treatment of others, which then perpetuates health inequities. Gender-inclusive language and cultural humility will help in achieving health equity and creating a supportive environment.

Implicit Bias

Implicit bias is influenced by media, literature, teachers, family, peers, and other sources of information. Unconscious bias is one of the greatest impediments to effective communication. It can cause us to interpret the behaviors, values, and beliefs of others through the lens of our own beliefs and experiences (Clohisy et al., 2017). Common areas where unconscious bias contributes to health disparities are gender, race, and ethnicity (Payne & Hannay, 2021; Saluja & Bryant, 2021).

Healthcare providers have a responsibility to root out inequities in the healthcare system and manage their implicit bias (Gopal et al., 2021; Vela et al., 2022). Educators recognize the need to better equip the members of the healthcare workforce to recognize their unconscious bias and learn cultural humility. Medical school coursework helps students use self-reflection to recognize the impact of their cultural background and learn to overcome unconscious biases (White et al., 2018). Simulations using scenarios with clients of diverse backgrounds help students recognize their implicit bias and develop cultural knowledge, awareness, and sensitivity to avoid cultural misunderstandings (Bahreman & Swoboda, 2016). Promoting self-awareness and introspection will help healthcare providers embrace cultural humility in their interactions with clients and colleagues.

Microaggression

Implicit biases can manifest in the form of **microaggressions**. A microaggression is subtle behavior directed at a member of a marginalized group that has a negative, derogatory effect (Hook et al., 2016). People are often well intentioned, and they do not aim to offend anyone. However, unconsciously, they may act differently and unintentionally infer that the person who receives the microaggression is not fully accepted or valued. The person who displays the microaggression may want to consciously promote equality, but instead, they minimize the existence of discrimination and deny personal bias.

Microaggressions may be verbal or nonverbal and may be conscious or unconscious. They may imply that the dominant culture is normal and that the minority culture is atypical. They may stereotype members of an underrepresented group or express disapproval of or discomfort with them. Reflecting on the connotations a remark or action might have can help us be more conscious of microaggressions and avoid them.

Family Dynamics

Understanding a community's **demographics** and cultural practices will assist you in framing your interactions. In many Western cultures, the individual is the basic social entity and the building block of social relations and institutions. In other cultures, the family is the dominant unit, and decision-making is the responsibility of the family rather than an individual member. Decisions may be made by the eldest male or other male figure in the family group. Extended family members often provide a support system for raising children. Taking cues from families helps you respond appropriately and show your interest in and respect for their culture. Because certain ways of touching the baby or referring to the baby may be taboo in that culture, always ask permission when you wish to touch the baby. If you are unsure about a cultural practice, do not hesitate to ask. Most families are receptive to explaining cultural practices to people who are sincerely interested.

Learning about families' beliefs and adapting suggestions to meet their needs will help you approach parents with cultural humility. Cultural taboos and beliefs taught by elders influence pregnancy, childbirth, and postpartum practices throughout the world (Modjadji et al., 2023; Nandagire et al., 2019; Withers et al., 2018). Cultural beliefs form our view of reality. A family's cultural convictions may be more important than science-based practices. To counsel effectively, take care not to interfere with family dynamics. Providing clear, accurate information and working within the family framework in a climate of acceptance can strengthen extended family support. Handouts and websites in the family's native language may help allay concerns. Computer-based lactation education holds promise, especially for families living in rural areas (Abbass-Dick et al., 2017; Grassley et al., 2017).

Visiting parents in their homes can help you obtain a more complete picture of their physical and emotional environment. Some families might be reluctant to invite strangers into their homes or may feel embarrassed by their living arrangements. However, they may respond to a friendly and sincere interest in their welfare. Learn the cultural customs of greeting and inclusion of others before you visit. For example, it is customary in many cultures to remove one's shoes when entering the home. If you observe shoes at the front door, remove yours as well. Americans tend to be very businesslike and consider it unprofessional to mix "business" with socializing. However, offers of drinks or food are important rituals in some cultures, and it can be considered rude to refuse.

Cultural Differences in Health Practices

Values and priorities vary greatly among families of different cultural backgrounds. Cultural beliefs may create health and illness behaviors that vary significantly from your own. Understanding these differences will avoid alienating parents with recommendations that are irrelevant or ignored. Culture affects the way parents regard health and the measures they take to prevent or treat illness. Some regard healthcare providers and the scientific community with great respect. Others place more faith in self-care or folk medicine. Others have deep-seated mistrust of the medical community, based on historical medical mistreatment (Fontanarosa & Bauchner, 2018). Some parents may adopt cultural practices that align with evidence-based recommendations and dismiss or postpone those that contradict recommendations (MacMillan Uribe et al., 2022). Parents are more likely to follow your suggestions when they fully understand the reasons behind your advice.

Intercultural experiences provide an opportunity for personal and professional growth, enabling you to view yourself and others more objectively. Learning about a family's culture and unique beliefs will help you clarify your own beliefs. You can become more aware of how your own convictions, customs, and prejudices affect how you counsel parents from cultures different from your own. Accept families where they are, and work to put your beliefs aside while providing care. Inappropriate advice can upset or confuse parents and cause friction with other family members. You risk your credibility and rapport if you discredit beliefs families have held their entire lives. Do not try to change culturally based practices unless they are detrimental to safety or health. It is the parents' responsibility to accept or reject the information you give them.

Organizations such as EthnoMed (2024) and National Center for Cultural Competence (NCCC, 2024) provide online resources for culturally sensitive and appropriate care. EthnoMed offers translated materials specifically for health care, including caring for refugee and recent-immigrant families. The NCCC offers healthcare provider assessments and distance-learning modules.

Cultural Practices with Lactation

The practice of lactation is based mostly on the habits, standards, and behaviors in a particular society. To counsel parents from another culture effectively, learn the values and cultural practices that can influence the nursing of their babies. Views on breast function, milk quality, and traditional practices underlie acceptance or nonacceptance of lactation (Daglas & Antoniou, 2012). If a parent discards their colostrum because of a belief that it is valueless or undesirable, you can explain the medical value of colostrum in their language and geared to their culture while realizing that their cultural beliefs may predominate. Likewise, parents may bottle-feed to avoid conflicting with cultural norms in their community.

Some cultures have taboos on prenatal or postpartum food (Lokossou et al., 2021; Zhou et al., 2022). The concept of "hot" and "cold" forces being "good" and "bad" for new parents is common in Asian culture. Some traditions discourage consuming cold foods and beverages for several weeks or months. Hot teas and soups will help ensure fluid requirements are met. When culturally important foods were provided in one study, lactation initiation rates soared from 16.7% in the hospital to 66.7% by 3 months after the intervention (Galvin et al., 2008). Some cultural beliefs place limitations on postpartum activity that an uninformed caregiver may interpret as a lack of compliance. By recognizing this, you can educate extended family and encourage their involvement in postpartum care.

Many cultures promote prelacteal feeds (El-Gilany & Abdel-Hady, 2014; Gul et al., 2014; Raheem et al., 2014). Some follow practices related to religious beliefs (Rehayem et al., 2020). Some favor artificial feeding or mixed feeding (Odeniyi et al., 2020). The practice of *los dos* (both) may be common, that is, combining nursing with formula. Some cultures promote early complementary foods (Goldbort et al., 2021; Yalçin et al., 2022; Zhang et al., 2020).

Prenatal education and outreach with culturally tailored interventions may help change practices. Parents from that culture who nursed their children can aid your promotion efforts and help you learn beliefs and child-rearing practices that dominate in their culture. Experienced parents can also help you understand effective measures for supporting and educating new families.

Immigrant families who have high lactation initiation and long duration rates in their native country tend to continue initially in their new country. Their practices may be compromised by their degree of acculturation. Lactation rates and duration can decrease for children who are born after the families immigrate (Dennis et al., 2019; Joseph et al., 2019; Kanatoula et al., 2019). Lack of knowledge and misinformation are barriers to lactation for immigrant populations. An inability to communicate in English and a lack of effective transportation create obstacles to accessing prenatal and postpartum health programs and services. Anticipatory guidance and education are important for these families, including how they can nurse when returning to work or school.

Language and Communication

A sensitive understanding of a family's culture and language is essential to establishing effective communication. Communities throughout the world are composed of multiple languages and literacy levels. Literacy—a set of reading, writing, basic math, speech, and comprehension skills—is needed to function in society. Literacy skills enable people to better develop their knowledge and achieve personal goals. Literacy is considered a social determinant of health and is associated with a range of health outcomes. Limited language proficiency, low literacy, and low health literacy of clients are common communication challenges in healthcare (The Joint Commission, 2018).

Health Literacy

Literacy skills are especially important when navigating health care and working with healthcare professionals. Health literacy is the degree to which individuals can find, understand, and use information and services to inform their healthcare decisions and actions. It is influenced by the language we speak and our ability to communicate clearly and listen carefully. Our age, socioeconomic status, cultural background, past experiences, cognitive abilities, and mental health affect how we communicate, understand, and respond to health information (U.S. Department of Health and Human Services [USDHHS], 2010).

People of all ages, races, incomes, and education levels are affected by limited health literacy. The effect is more common in socially disadvantaged populations and can lead to health disparities (Schillinger, 2020). Clients with limited health literacy experience difficulties with self-management, including adherence, communication, and knowledge (van der Gaag et al., 2022). A high literacy level is associated with exclusive nursing (Stafford et al., 2021) and duration (Vila-Candel et al., 2021). In a multicenter study, the health literacy levels of about half the participants were low or inadequate (Valero-Chillerón et al., 2022). At 6 months postpartum, one-third of participants were still exclusively nursing.

Individuals with basic health literacy skills can generally respond well to education that is directed to clearly defined goals and specific circumstances, such as prevention activities and behavioral change. Advanced health literacy skills enable individuals to derive meaning from different forms of communication, apply new information to changing circumstances, and discriminate between different sources of information. Individuals with advanced health literacy can respond to education that is more interactive and accessible through structured communication channels such as mobile apps and interactive websites.

To engage effectively, clinicians need to tailor communication with clients to their level of health literacy. This includes using plain language that is culturally appropriate and in the client's preferred language. Shared decision-making and empowerment can improve health literacy and promote autonomy and greater control over healthcare decisions (Nutbeam & Lloyd, 2021).

Intercultural Communication

Cultural humility and appropriate verbal and nonverbal skills are the foundation of effective intercultural communication (Tuohy, 2019). If a parent speaks another language, determine their level of proficiency in speaking the dominant language or whether they require language interpretation. Consider any specific cultural aspects that might affect communication and ways to respond to and accommodate their specific communication needs. Watch for nonverbal cues and messages through facial and body expressions. For example, a nod of the head accompanied by a bland or puzzled look can indicate confusion. To ensure that parents understand your instructions, you can ask that they repeat the instructions or repeat what you demonstrated. You can also demonstrate a technique and summarize the important points at the end of your conversation.

Understanding the nuances of body language is important to intercultural communication. The meaning of body language is not universal. Direct eye contact is often expected in Western cultures, whereas it is regarded as aggressive or confrontational in some Asian cultures. Certain hand gestures may have a positive meaning or be considered rude or obscene. Touch can convey support and empathy or may be unacceptable in some cultures. In some cultures, nodding and smiling do not denote understanding and you cannot assume that a parent comprehends what you are saying because of these gestures.

Multilingual Communication

Cultural barriers can seem greater when accompanied by a language difference. Language barriers may interfere with communicating effectively with parents. Poor communication contributes to inequalities and can negatively affect the ability to provide appropriate, timely, and effective care (Ali & Watson, 2018; Pérez-Stable & El-Toukhy, 2018). Communication errors can occur when either the healthcare provider or the client is speaking a second language (Renata et al., 2015). It is important to speak slowly and clearly and provide simple explanations.

Maximizing communication is especially important when discussing a feeding problem. Parents with limited English proficiency may be able to speak and understand English well enough to communicate about lactation in general. However, when experiencing a problem, they may need to converse in their native language to be understood and to comprehend your advice.

As society's multilingual character continues to grow, medical communication in multiple languages is gaining attention. Effectively communicating with clients involves understanding the community's linguistic practices and explaining health concepts in the client's language (Ortega & Prada, 2020). If you are not multilingual, you can learn common phrases used in lactation in the languages of families in your community (a Spanish glossary appears in the Appendix). Many communities offer classes in conversational medical terminology. The use of translation technologies such as Google Translate, Skype Translator, or multilingual healthcare apps are other alternatives. There are cautions about limitations, such as accuracy, when using technology-based translation (Panayiotou et al., 2019).

Use of Interpreters

When available, a trained professional language interpreter or informal bilingual healthcare staff or family member on site is an effective choice (Chen et al., 2017). Remote interpreting services may also be available through communication technologies such as Skype, telephone, or video link (Dowbor et al., 2015). Professional interpreters help provide linguistically appropriate health care (Luan Erfe et al., 2017). Language interpreters available through secure remote teleconferencing services provide enhanced communication in a face-to-face encounter. When there is no interpreter to assist you, a colleague or a parent's bilingual friend or relative may be able to assist. Parents may be more receptive to sharing intimate information with a same-sex interpreter.

Try to ensure that the language interpreter is communicating accurately and not adding opinions or values that differ from what you want to convey. When interpreters are used, training all staff on how to work with them will optimize communication (The Joint Commission, 2018). Including professional interpreters as part of the interprofessional healthcare team will enable them to be more proficient in lactation jargon and in the variety of cultural differences in the community (Krystallidou et al., 2021).

Bilingual Aids

Parents who have difficulty reading English will likely not benefit from lengthy print articles or books. Brief pamphlets with simple themes and illustrations written at an appropriate reading level are a better alternative. Providing demonstrations with visual aids such as dolls, lactation devices, or video clips (preferably in the parent's language) will be effective. Teaching tools and lactation information are available online in many languages. Sources include the World Health Organization (https://www.who.int), the United Kingdom's National Health Service (https://www.who.intwww.nhs.uk), and the U.S. National Library of Medicine (https://www.who.intwww.nlm.nih.gov/medlineplus). Local social services may be helpful as well.

Social Behavior

Heredity and environment contribute to the development of the person we become. Social situations influence our thinking, how we perceive ourselves and others, and how we form impressions of others. Perceptions and social norms govern all social behavior, even though much of the time, we are unaware of these influences. Through social interaction, we develop an identity, a set of beliefs, and a range of skills that will allow us to participate in society.

Personality

Social behavior is influenced by the specific qualities, attributes, traits, and mannerisms that distinguish one person from another. Although personality is largely consistent and firmly grounded, our specific needs, motives, attitudes, or reactions can influence a change in behavior. We may even alter our personality as part of a gradual maturing process or in response to major life events. Childbirth and parenting are two life events that modify personality. Having a child enables parents to embrace unconditional love and learn selflessness as they tend to their child's needs.

All of us regard ourselves as having certain traits, habits, relationships, and ways of behaving. This self-image influences our attitudes and behavior with others and the way we act in different situations. Self-image is an outgrowth of our background and experience. It is influenced by how we see ourselves, how we would like to perceive ourselves, how we believe others perceive us, and how we would like others to perceive us. Sometimes, self-image can conflict with societal or personal expectations. A parent, for example, may feel pressured by their partner or peer group to nurse but personally does not want to do it. They may consider nursing, but internally, they recoil from the physicality of lactation. This may result from social conditioning or even from a history of physical or sexual abuse or domestic violence.

Recognizing parents' personality characteristics, as well as your own, will provide insight into how to approach them. For example, if you are introverted, extroverts may respond to your quiet assurance as calming, or they may become irritated if you equivocate or appear hesitant. Direct statements of fact and care plans phrased in terms of "results" may be better received by extroverts. If you are extroverted, you can take your cues from introverted parents to avoid appearing overbearing, insensitive, or "bossy." More reserved parents might respond best to suggestions and being asked for their opinion. Personality tests identify personality types and show how individuals obtain and process information and how they make decisions. Many are based on the **Myers-Briggs Type Indicators** personality inventory, presented in **Table 3-1** (Myers & Briggs Foundation, 2024).

Table 3-1 Personality Types and Behavior

	Thinking	Feeling
Sensing	*Sensing-Thinking*	*Sensing-Feeling*
	Rational in decision-making	Practical and pragmatic
	Driven by logic rather than values	Driven by values rather than logic
	Practical and pragmatic	Makes decisions based on subjectivity
	Expends considerable effort to search for information	Likely to consider others when making a decision
	Avoids risk	Shares risks with others
	Identifies with material objects	Aware of how material objects influence others
	Makes decisions for the short term	Makes decisions for the short term
Intuitive	*Intuiting-Thinking*	*Intuiting-Feeling*
	Takes a broad view of personal situation	Takes a broad view of personal situation
	Relies on imagination, yet uses logic to approach decisions	Imagines a wide range of options in making a decision Highly people oriented and likely to consider views of others
	Imagines a wider range of options in making a decision	Makes decisions based on subjectivity
	Willing to take a risk	Seeks risk
	Makes decisions for the long term	Makes decisions for an indefinite period of time

Myers & Briggs Foundation. Myers-Briggs Type Indicators personality inventory. 2024. http://www.myersbriggs.org/

Ethics

Morals and ethics greatly influence social behavior. Moral customs may change with each new generation. Ethical values, on the other hand, are enduring and may or may not coincide with what is currently and locally considered to be moral. An ethical culture creates a humane environment that treats others as unique individuals, values their worth, treats them with respect, and elicits the best from everyone. Our ethical values influence how we behave and how we treat others and create conditions for them to thrive, both individually and collectively. It is impossible to practice ethical habits all the time. Ethical living in its fullest sense is an aspiration we can only approach. Our challenge is to integrate our internal personal needs and external social needs, determine right from wrong, and make ethical decisions (Beauchamp & Childress, 2019).

Figure 3-2 illustrates strategies for managing ethical dilemmas, which include building trust, empowering parents through support and information, and ensuring appropriate follow-up (Noel-Weiss et al., 2012). The International Board of Lactation Consultation Examiners (IBLCE) Code of Professional Conduct guides an International Board Certified Lactation Consultant's (IBCLC's) behavior (IBLCE, 2022). Ethical issues relevant to the lactation profession are discussed further in **Chapter 28**.

Attitude

Social behavior is influenced by attitude. The mores and cultural norms of society, personal experience, family, and friends all influence the attitudes we develop. Our early childhood, family background, educational level, and subculture all contribute to differences in our attitudes and behavior. Generally, the more information we have about something, the more likely we are to form attitudes about it, either positive or negative. Understanding how attitude affects parents' behavior will help in finding ways to effectively counsel them. Keeping your message simple, evidence based, and succinct increases the likelihood of acceptance.

A positive attitude and mindfulness are associated with nursing intention (Grano et al., 2022; Hulsbosch et al., 2021; Hulsbosch et al., 2023). Being mindful means paying full attention to experiences with a curious, open, and accepting attitude. Self-control and openness affect lactation self-efficacy positively, whereas neuroticism and anxiety affect lactation self-efficacy negatively (Corby et al., 2021; Menekse et al., 2021). Positive emotions, conscientiousness, agreeableness, extraversion, and openness are positive predictors of exclusive nursing (Padashian et al., 2021; Verbeek et al., 2019).

Understanding attitudes among adolescents and young adults is important to lactation promotion efforts. Social influence and exposure to lactation as a cultural norm are important predictors of positive attitudes about nursing among adolescents (Swanson et al., 2017) and university students (Hamade et al., 2014; Jefferson, 2017). Secondary school education on lactation, which could influence attitudes at a

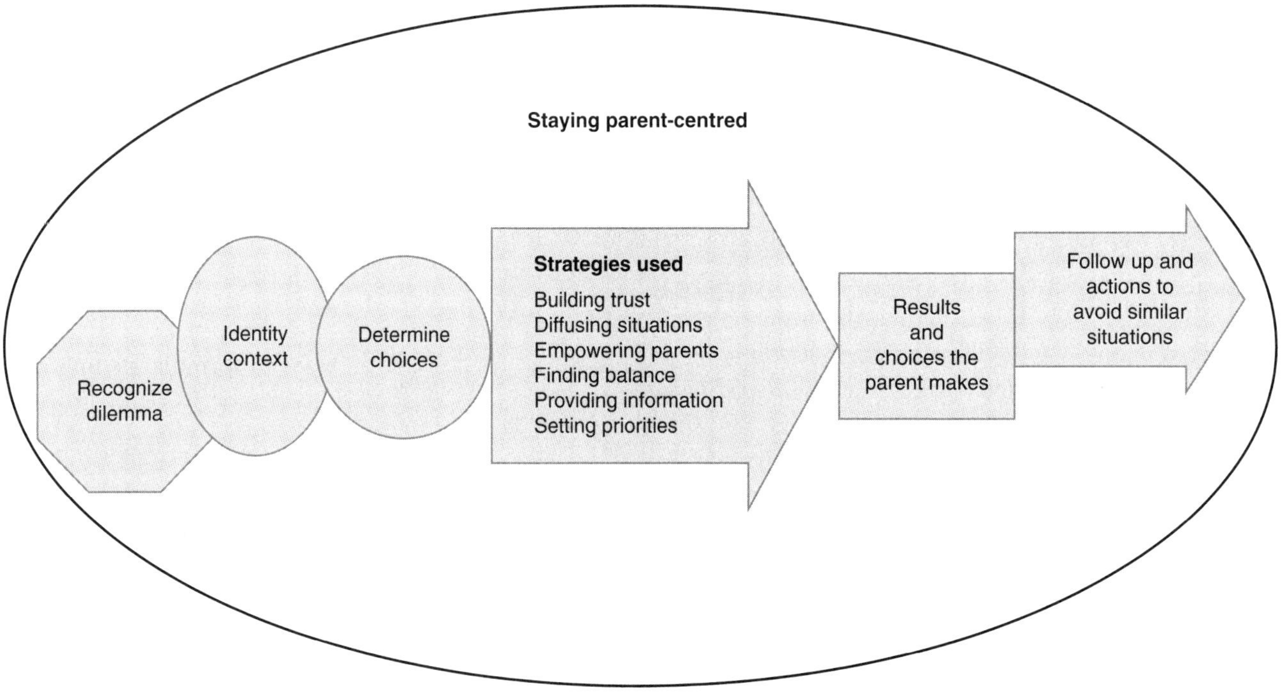

Figure 3-2 Managing ethical dilemmas.

Reproduced from Noel-Weiss J, et al. Exploring how IBCLCs manage ethical dilemmas: a qualitative study. BMC Med Ethics. July 23, 2012;13:18. http://www.ncbi.nlm.nih.gov/pmc/articles/PMC3467169/. "Figure 1. Conceptualization of the Steps in Managing an Ethical Dilemma."

young age, varies widely (Čatipović et al., 2018; Singletary et al., 2017). Education tailored to adolescents and university students can positively affect future intentions to nurse (Ben Natan et al., 2018; Reyes et al., 2019; Yang et al., 2019).

Healthcare provider attitudes can have a major influence on the choices their clients make and the attitudes their clients form. Many healthcare professionals were trained in an era when scheduled formula feeding was the norm. Many of them artificially fed their children. Even healthcare professionals having children today frequently formula feed. The belief that formula is "just as good" as human milk may guide their attitudes and actions. Formula manufacturers promote this belief through aggressive marketing targeted specifically at the healthcare community.

Perception

We receive an almost infinite number of stimuli daily through sight, hearing, sound, taste, and touch. This **sensory input** produces our perception of the world. Our perception and what we expect to see are influenced by our expectations, motives, and learning, which are all based on our previous experiences. What we expect to perceive often strongly influences what we do perceive and how we attribute causes to behavior. For example, differences exist among ethnic groups in the perception of and reaction to lactation barriers (Fischer & Olson, 2014). Some parents may describe their baby's feeding behaviors as "He's being lazy; he's just using me as a pacifier; he doesn't want to nurse." Informing them about normal infant behavior, instinctive needs, and feeding patterns may help alter parents' perceptions of their baby's behaviors.

We can often perceive brief stimuli without being consciously aware of them. Such subliminal perception can result from a brief visual presentation, from embedded or hidden imagery or words, or from spoken messages that are accelerated and at low volume. Subliminal messages predominate most commercial advertising and motivate people to behave in a certain way without being aware of what motivated it. Infant formula manufacturers spend millions of dollars on advertising to ensure that the image of a baby bottle or their logo connotes quintessential babyhood. They often portray optimal eye contact and a wide smile for a parent feeding a bottle to their baby versus eyes averted with minimal facial expression for a nursing parent. The influence of subliminal messaging makes it especially important to avoid materials produced by formula companies.

Predicting Behavior

Understanding people's attitudes provides insight into how to predict their behavior. Intention is the best predictor of behavior. Attitude occurs along a scale that ranges from positive to negative intentions (Schiffman et al., 2019). We are primarily influenced by people who are significant and important in our lives—family, friends, and coworkers. When faced with a decision, we may first consider how we believe they would respond. Thus, new parents often consider significant people in their lives when deciding how to feed their baby. **Chapter 12** discusses influences on the decision to nurse.

Attitude Changes

Although attitudes are relatively enduring, they are easier to change than core beliefs and values. Recognizing the circumstances that caused an attitude can help interpret it correctly. Attitudes can change because of personal experience and exposure to new sources of information. A healthcare provider, for example, who experienced severe jaundice with a previous client may treat jaundice more aggressively than established guidelines and quickly recommend formula supplementation. The provider may be influenced to change recommendations after learning more about best practices relative to lactation.

Personality plays a pivotal role in how quickly attitudes are likely to change, as well as what may trigger the change. Individuals who crave learning are likely to form positive attitudes in response to messages that are rich in information. Others will respond more readily to messages and impressions that appeal to their emotions. Thus, parents who intend to nurse for a short time may change to long-term lactation after witnessing their baby enjoying nursing and when they are more skilled with it. Healthcare providers who learn about the improved health outcomes of infants who nurse may change previous less favorable attitudes. Negative outcomes of formula feeding and learning about the risks of not nursing can change the beliefs and attitudes of both parents and healthcare providers.

Motivation

Motivation is a driving force behind behavior. All behavior is goal oriented, and all goals derive from some form of need. Learning new information motivates us to choose a behavior that helps fulfill a goal or need. Self-motivation is the ability to find enthusiasm, interest, and passion for a particular goal and

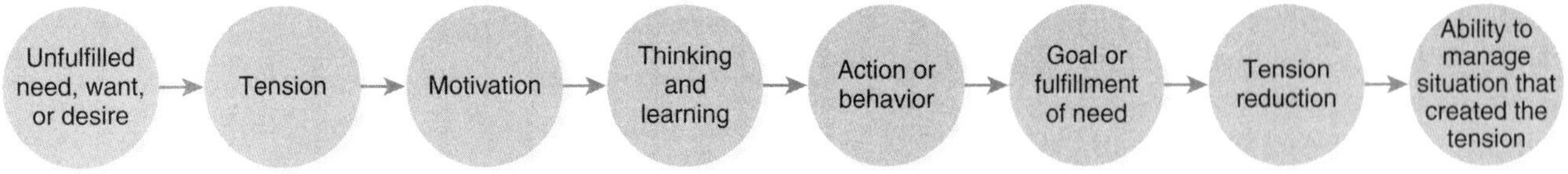

Figure 3-3 Path of motivation.

use them as the driving force to achieve it. Reaching the goal reduces tension and enables us to manage the situation that triggered the need to act. **Figure 3-3** illustrates this path.

Self-regulated motivation predicts positive outcomes for lactation intent and postpartum hospital outcomes (Akgün & Taştekin, 2020; Martin et al., 2022). It increases the rate of exclusivity at 6 weeks and any nursing at 12 weeks postpartum (Lau et al., 2022). Self-motivated parents may initiate lactation because of their beliefs and emotions despite being discouraged by others. However, discouragement by healthcare providers may decrease the motivation to nurse in others. This underscores a need for evidence-based birth practices and education of providers and the public to support lactation (Fabiyi et al., 2021).

The goals we select to pursue depend on our needs, personal experiences and interactions, cultural norms and values, self-image, and physical and social environment. Approach behavior directs our actions toward a positive goal. Avoidance behavior directs our actions against a negative outcome. Babies exhibit approach and avoidance behaviors that communicate their needs to parents and other caregivers. Refer to **Chapter 14** for more information about infant behavior.

Parents oriented toward approach behavior are more likely to nurse, to nurse longer, and to continue nursing when they experience initial difficulties (Scharfe, 2012). A parent who nurses because of the health benefits to the baby will persevere through challenges to achieve the desired goal of a healthy baby. A parent who has internalized stories about potential lactation difficulties may choose not to nurse to avoid that potential outcome. Educating parents to avoid or minimize lactation difficulties will help them set positive goals and make healthy choices for their babies.

Our motivations and goals change from childhood to old age as each season of life unfolds. The encouragement you offer parents to sequence such seasons may be a refreshing "new" thought as they merge parenthood with a career. By understanding this cultural dynamic, you can tailor your approach and sensitively help parents meet their needs and reach their feeding goals. **Motivational interviewing** is an effective technique in the counseling process, as discussed in **Chapter 5**.

Relationships

Relationships form the basis of our behavior with others. They are forged through work-related contacts, social interactions, and our involvement with groups and organizations. Childhood lays the foundation for adolescent and adult functioning. Many social psychologists believe a child's first relationship determines the way they approach and interact with other people (Ainsworth et al., 1978; Bowlby, 1976, 1982). The first 2 years of life are vital in determining personality, social behavior, and the ability to form relationships. Experiences during this critical time can set the stage for the way we approach future social situations. A parent who is securely attached to their infant prefers nursing over bottle feeding and initiates feedings more often than an unattached parent (Linde et al., 2020). Infant bonding is discussed in **Chapter 13**.

Group Behavior

We all belong to a variety of groups, both formal and informal. Groups influence how we communicate and interact with one another, how we perform tasks, and how we achieve goals. We gain our initial experiences through family, considered a **primary group** because it is there that we form close, personal, and enduring relationships. We mature in **secondary groups** through school, work, and religion, as well as through social and recreational activities. Relationships in these secondary groups focus on activities and are relatively impersonal.

Group participation addresses many social needs, such as needs for approval, a sense of belonging, and friendship. Members of peer groups in similar life stages, such as reading or study groups, play groups, or neighborhood associations, can form long-term friendships as they move through adult life stages together. Lactation and the lactation profession have produced peer support groups, a professional association (International Lactation Consultant Association), and many regional parent and professional organizations.

The strong beliefs and mutual commitment among the members of these secondary groups create a familial relationship like that of a primary group.

Power and Empowerment

Empowerment means to give authority or power. Power establishes controls within relationships, with the level of power largely dictated by the relationship. Healthcare professionals possess expert power derived from their specialized body of knowledge and extensive training. Health consumers, who typically are under the care of several healthcare providers, acquire increased levels of knowledge and power to control their outcomes. A goal of this text is to empower healthcare professionals in promoting lactation and empowering families in their feeding decisions and management.

Healthcare providers and consumers alike have and use power in their relationships with one another. With wide access to medical information through the internet and other resources, today's consumers are better informed and more demanding than ever before. As a result, the social distance between the consumer and the healthcare provider is narrowing. Client rights, health-related support groups, alternative therapies, and complementary practices are all balancing forces that permeate the healthcare arena. Consumers are transforming themselves from nonexperts to experts through easy information access. The center of power is shifting, and the face of healthcare has been forever altered because of social and scientific developments.

There is a strong correlation between perceived control and nursing duration. When healthcare providers relinquish coercive power and help parents take more control over their health needs and the prevention of problems, parents are empowered to gain mastery over their lives. This approach helps develop an awareness of the root causes of problems and a readiness to find solutions. True empowerment occurs when healthcare providers transform how they relate to clients. Respect, safety, holistic care, partnership, concern for general well-being, valuing relationships, and social connectedness are factors leading to parents' empowerment.

Feminism and Lactation

Empowerment of women is a cornerstone of feminist theory, which regards social expectations and roles as potentially oppressive to women. Issues concerning reproductive rights and sexuality are a critical source of ambivalence within feminism (Ignjatović & Buturović, 2018). There is an inherent tension in feminism's respect for autonomy while valuing women's roles in nurturing and nursing their babies (Smith, 2018).

Because lactation requires time with and access to the baby, some feminists consider it to be a gender difference that compromises a woman's autonomy and stands in the way of liberation. They suggest that lactation promotion reinforces power inequity and creates maternal guilt related to infant feeding. Recognizing women's needs and balancing infant feeding discussions on the health importance of human milk with the lived experiences of nursing can optimize maternal voice and autonomy and help reduce guilt (Benoit et al., 2016).

A feminist health approach to lactation advocacy regards it as incorporating women's needs as biological and reproductive social beings. It views lactation as part of natural parenting in the context of women's "identity work" (Faircloth, 2017). Unregulated online milk sharing may be viewed by some as a feminist act that contributes to demedicalizing the provision of human milk and making it communally available (Palmquist, 2015).

A health-activist approach would create the social and economic conditions that make lactation possible, successful, and valued for all women. A key to this effort is understanding the complex, multifactorial barriers facing underrepresented populations (Eni et al., 2014; Spencer et al., 2015). Feminist health activism includes removing economic and ethnic barriers to lactation, improving support from healthcare professionals, and improving home–work balance.

Knowledge and Culture

The culture and times in which we live influence our body of knowledge. Societal values, beliefs, and accepted wisdom often challenge the authenticity of scientific knowledge. The human condition changes continually in response to social influence and science, making it difficult to predict human behavior and social trends. The ubiquity of computer technology and the internet has created profound social change and links individuals collectively in an online, global society.

Evidence-Based Care

An evolution in scientific thought gave rise to the pursuit of **evidence-based practice**. In an evidence-based society, scientific validation sways medical practices. However, scientists do not always

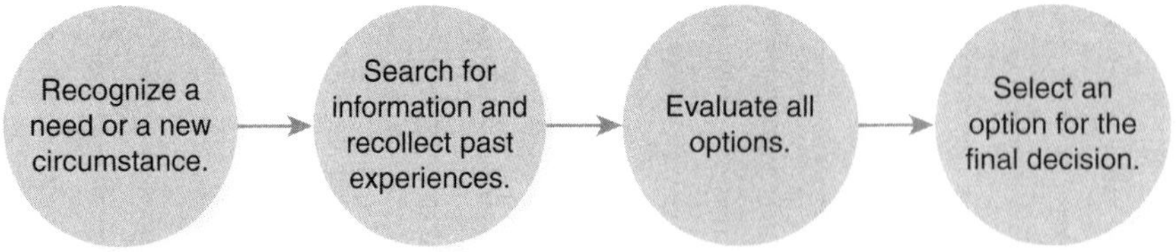

Figure 3-4 Decision-making process.

agree on how to approach research. One scientist may attempt to establish constant truths, whereas another scientist may attempt to disprove apparent truths. Sometimes, researchers accept conclusions from their predecessors and address only certain puzzles that are inherent in those conclusions. Those conclusions form the paradigm within which most healthcare professionals operate until evidence accumulates that repudiates accepted practice and thinking.

The public generally relies on the media's interpretations of research results rather than attempting to decipher the original research. Sound bites of information in the media about a particular study may cast lactation in a negative light. Careful examination of the actual research may reveal that the conclusions support lactation. Tools for critical thinking and discernment are discussed in **Chapter 29**.

Evidence-Informed Practice

An evidence-based approach can discount caring, intuition, and other "nonscientific" variables. **Evidence-informed practice** values the clinician's knowledge and experience along with clinical intuition and reasoning skills as critical factors in providing care. It values clients' cultures, previous experiences, and preferences to create an individualized care plan. Much of lactation care is experiential, based on anecdotal reports. For example, the use of cabbage for engorgement was rediscovered from century-old practices that had been lost in a bottle-feeding culture (Rosier, 1988). Although modern research does not validate the effectiveness of this practice, anecdotal experience reveals it to be useful. Likewise, lactation consultants often observe trends among their clients that influence their care regimens. It is important that we balance such intuitive practices with evidence-based options.

Decision-Making

We continually make decisions concerning every aspect of daily life. Decision-making begins when we recognize a need or new circumstance, search for information, recall past experiences, and evaluate alternatives. We judge the information against each alternative, select from among the alternatives, and make a final decision. Motivation, perception, learning, personality, and attitudes influence our decisions. Generally, we make decisions without stopping to think about what is involved in the process. **Figure 3-4** illustrates the decision-making process.

Personal knowledge and a flexible environment are the best predictors of clients' satisfaction with their healthcare decisions (Osorio Galeano et al., 2023). Parents may seek guidance online or from family or friends as they encounter issues such as teething, when to feed the baby, nursing in public, and a myriad of parenting decisions. For a complicated issue such as frenotomy or a trial of labor after a cesarean section, they will collaborate with their caregivers (Chang et al., 2022; Ray et al., 2020).

Shared decision-making between caregivers and parents will help parents navigate decisions for complex feeding issues. Involving them in the decision-making process respects their right to be involved in their healthcare decisions. Parents will thus feel empowered to make healthcare decisions that reflect their preferences, which increases compliance. This leads to increased satisfaction and self-efficacy and better health outcomes (Jiang et al., 2021).

Influencing Decisions

Influencing another person's decision-making begins with an appeal to their needs and interests. Sometimes, objective, factual appeals are an effective method of persuasion. At other times, emotional appeals are more effective. In general, more educated audiences respond better to factual appeals, and less educated people respond more to emotional appeals. However, culturally mediated parenting practices such as "baby training" may shape parents' responsiveness to infant hunger cues. This is evidenced by highly educated parents who embrace scheduled, restrictive feeding programs despite abundant medical information supporting cue-based feeding (Little et al., 2018).

Individuals who are highly involved in decision-making are more likely to evaluate the pros and cons

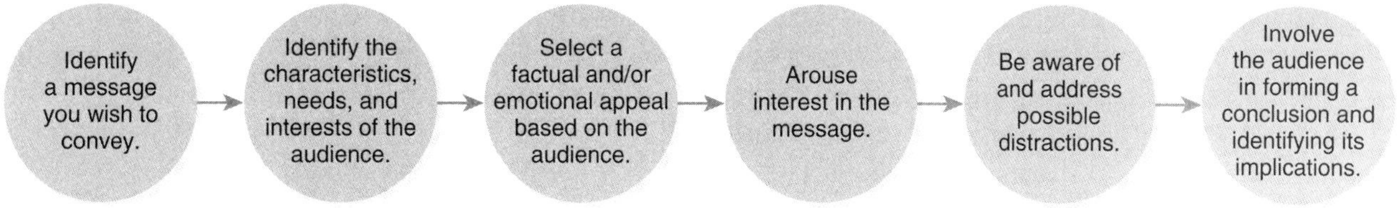

Figure 3-5 Influencing a person's decision-making.

of a message. Making a message memorable and persuasive begins by arousing interest in it and giving the other person a reason to listen. Asking questions generates involvement and helps to identify the points of interest that will be most effective. Interest will ripen into desire only after we remove the lingering doubts from the other person's mind. Recognizing this relationship, many lactation consultants increase participation in prenatal classes by asking parents to voice their questions at the start of the class. If no one volunteers, several "ice-breaker" questions proposed rhetorically can draw out discussion.

It is important to be aware of any distractions that may impede someone's ability to receive and retain the key points of a message. A message will not get through if individuals are engrossed in their thoughts or are emotionally unavailable. The use of humor attracts attention, increases comprehension, and enhances appreciation of a message. Lactation-related humor, such as cartoons or anecdotes, can enliven a class and diffuse embarrassment. **Figure 3-5** illustrates the process of influencing a person's decision-making. **Chapter 4** discusses humor as a communication tool.

Social pressure and a need to conform to a social norm can influence decision-making. **Conformity** involves acceptance of a change based on attitude and behavior in accordance with social norms. For example, a parent whose family and friends support nursing will be more likely to make that infant feeding decision. Likewise, if the climate of acceptance leans toward bottle feeding, a parent may feel pressured toward that choice. The support of one person can have a considerable effect on another to comply with or to resist social pressure. Thus, caregiver support for lactation may influence a parent to resist social pressure to bottle-feed.

Compliance occurs when we change our behavior or attitude but do not accept a change completely. For example, a parent may nurse only because they are told that it is best for them and their baby. The degree to which we comply may depend in part on our self-esteem and knowledge. Building influence through education and support may increase confidence and lead to true acceptance.

Social Media

On average, 60% of the global population uses social media. There were 4.9 billion social media users in the world as of March 2023 (Ruby, 2023). The prevalence of receiving information from social media influences how we make decisions. Accessing information on social media can lead to a shift in the power balance and increase decision-making quality. It empowers parents to follow healthcare provider recommendations and to be responsible for their own lives. It can enhance well-being and improve self-management and self-control (Smailhodzic et al., 2016).

Technology-mediated-support is increasingly used by healthcare providers to engage with clients online through telephone conversations, text chats, videoconferencing, and other social media tools and applications. Pairing of health care with social media can be successful with the right balance between digital and traditional health care (Farsi, 2021). The use of social media by clients and healthcare professionals can increase confidence in their relationships, increase knowledge about treatment options, and promote active communication during consultations. Providers need to ensure that their comments are objective, professional, and within their scope of practice.

Social media is a dominant form of communication during pregnancy and early parenting. Expectant and new parents use a variety of social media platforms to seek information and give and receive support (Frey et al., 2022; Morse & Brown, 2022). They turn to online sources for information (65%), esteem support (18%), and emotional support (10%) (Wagg et al., 2019). They increasingly seek information and support using Facebook, apps, websites, online videos, podcasts, and email (Galvão et al., 2021). Parents respond favorably to the anonymity and nonjudgment offered online (Rathbone & Prescott, 2019). They value social media support groups in normalizing lactation and helping them achieve their goals (Black et al., 2020; Wilson, 2020). Racial and ethnic minority groups often seek health information on YouTube for their children, offering opportunities to disseminate culturally relevant messages (Lama et al., 2022).

Social network sites facilitate communication and connections among health professionals in clinical practice, professional networks, and education (Chan & Leung, 2018; Vukušić Rukavina et al., 2021). Public health communication strategies, such as lactation promotion, depend on influencer attitudes and beliefs (Moukarzel et al., 2021). Users can disseminate false information quickly (Venegas-Vera et al., 2020). Information shared by interested citizens rather than professionals may be inaccurate or taken out of context (Moukarzel et al, 2020). This can unintentionally spread misinformation and non-evidence-based practices. Due diligence can assess the credibility of the information obtained and its source (Farsi et al., 2022).

Social Marketing

Marketing is a potentially powerful technology for bringing about socially desirable behaviors. This concept gave rise to the field of **social marketing**. The principles of social marketing can apply to a diverse set of social challenges. Social marketers analyze, plan, execute, and evaluate programs designed to influence human behavior. The premise of social marketing is to help individuals consider and choose a strategy that fits their readiness for action and their resources. The Centers for Disease Control and Prevention (CDC) provides marketing tips on health communication through a Health Communication Gateway (CDC, 2024).

Product, price, place, and promotion—the "four Ps" of marketing—are the primary variables that determine people's likelihood of changing their behavior. Designing programs that reflect what consumers truly want and that influence positive behavior change requires careful analysis of these marketing factors and how they interact.

- *Product*, within the context of social marketing, is a commodity, service, or health practice (e.g., lactation).
- *Price* involves the barriers or costs associated with adopting a behavior (e.g., acceptance of the choice to nurse by family and friends).
- *Place* encompasses either the location where the product or services can be accessed or the channels of communication and distribution points for the messages (e.g., lactation consultants, healthcare providers, peer counselors, and health facilities).
- *Promotion* constitutes messages that are memorable and persuasive (e.g., anticipatory guidance and education about lactation or subliminal messages about formula feeding).

The cultural norms of society have a powerful influence over health behavior decisions such as infant feeding method. Exposure to lactation and increasing positive attitudes and beliefs are important as a focus for public campaigns (Vari et al., 2013). The WIC food assistance program in the United States uses a national promotion campaign to increase initiation and duration rates of nursing among WIC participants, increase public awareness of the importance of lactation, and improve the environment of support for nursing families. Lactation campaigns on college campuses influence students' and employees' attitudes, subjective norms, intentions, knowledge, and awareness (Dinour & Bai, 2022). National campaigns lead to policy improvements in maternity benefits and workforce development.

Summary

Culture defines the values and beliefs we hold and the practices we follow. Openness and flexibility enhance interactions with people from other cultures. Taking cues from families shows interest in and respect for their culture. Poverty, education status, race and ethnicity, gender, and insurance status inhibit equitable access to healthcare and lead to inequities in health.

Motivation, perception, learning, personality, and attitudes all come together to influence the decision-making process. Healthcare providers and consumers have and use power in their relationships with one another. The social distance between consumers and healthcare practitioners is narrowing because of wider access to health information through social media. Societal values, beliefs, and accepted wisdom often challenge the authenticity of scientific knowledge. Evidence-informed care values the clinician's knowledge and experience along with clinical intuition and reasoning skills.

What You Learned–At a Glance

Conversation Starters with Parents

- How do cultural traditions affect your infant feeding plans?
- How might your lifestyle affect your infant feeding plans?
- What is your perception of nursing?
- What influenced your infant feeding decision?

Culture

- The degree to which families merge into a new culture depends on how firmly they cling to traditional values.
- Caregivers need to respect differences in values, beliefs, and practices.
- Vulnerable populations face inequitable access to quality health care.
- Awareness of inequities and implicit bias is the first step toward changing behavior.
- Learning community characteristics enhances sensitivity to cultural beliefs.
- Parents benefit from networking with other parents.

Cultural Humility

- Adapt counseling to income level, educational level, lifestyle, and support system.
- Accept health and illness behaviors that do not compromise lactation or safety.
- Learn customs and body language to help you respond appropriately.
- Learn phrases in common languages within the community you serve.
- Teach with internet and mobile app tools, visual aids, and return demonstrations.
- Enlist help from others in the culture to promote lactation.

Social Behavior

- Lactation may go against a perceived cultural norm.
- Exclusively nursing parents tend to have higher self-concept and self-satisfaction.
- IBCLCs are guided by the IBLCE Code of Professional Conduct.
- IBCLCs are expected to support the International Code of Marketing of Breast-Milk Substitutes and subsequent resolutions.
- Ethical practice requires integrating internal personal needs and external social needs.
- Empowering parents helps them take control of their health and validates their choices.
- Some feminists believe lactation compromises autonomy; others find it empowering.

Knowledge and Decision-Making

- A balanced approach combines evidence-based practice with evidence-informed practices.
- Empowering parents helps them to make informed choices and to be accountable.
- Addressing the needs and interests of parents and colleagues influences decision-making.
- Parents receive myriad—and mixed—messages from the media.
- The use of humor increases a message's acceptance and persuasiveness.

References

Abbass-Dick J, et al. The development and piloting of an eHealth breastfeeding resource targeting fathers and partners as co-parents. *Midwifery*. 2017;50:139–147.

Ainsworth M, et al. *Patterns of Attachment: A Psychological Study of the Strange Situation*. Hillsdale, NJ: Erlbaum; 1978.

Akgün P, Taştekin A. The effect of information-motivation-behavioral skills on breastfeeding success: a hypothetical model. *J Transcult Nurs*. 2020;31(4):378–386.

Ali PA, Watson R. Language barriers and their impact on provision of care to patients with limited English proficiency: nurses' perspectives. *J Clin Nurs*. 2018;27:5–6.

Antsey EH, et al. Racial and geographic differences in breastfeeding—United States, 2011–2015. *MMWR Morb Mortal Wkly Rep*. 2017;66(27):723–727.

Asiodu IV, et al. Achieving breastfeeding equity and justice in Black communities: past, present, and future. *Breastfeed Med*. 2021;16(6):447–451.

Asiodu IV, et al. Infant feeding decision-making and the influences of social support persons among first-time African American mothers. *Matern Child Health J*. 2017;21(4): 863–872.

Bahreman NT, Swoboda SM. Honoring diversity: developing culturally competent communication skills through simulation. *J Nurs Educ*. 2016;55(2):105–108.

Barbosa CE, et al. Factors distinguishing positive deviance among low-income African American women: a qualitative study on infant feeding. *J Hum Lact*. 2017;33(2):368–378.

Bates RA, et al. Co-occurring risk and protective factors and regulatory behavior of infants living in low-income homes. *Infant Behav Dev*. 2021;64:101598.

Beauchamp TL, Childress JF. *Principles of Biomedical Ethics*. 8th ed. New York, NY: Oxford University Press; 2019.

Beauregard JL, et al. Racial disparities in breastfeeding initiation and duration among U.S. infants born in 2015. *MMWR Morb Mortal Wkly Rep*. 2019;68(34):745–748.

Ben Natan M, et al. Breastfeeding knowledge, attitudes, intentions, and perception of support from educational institutions among nursing students and students from other faculties: a descriptive cross-sectional study. *Nurse Educ Today*. 2018;68:66–70.

Benoit B, et al. Infant feeding and maternal guilt: the application of a feminist phenomenological framework to guide

clinician practices in breast feeding promotion. *Midwifery*. 2016;34:58–65.
Black R, et al. Women's experience of social media breastfeeding support and its impact on extended breastfeeding success: a social cognitive perspective. *Br J Health Psychol*. 2020;25(3):754–771.
Bowlby J. Separation: anxiety and anger. In: *Attachment and Loss*. Vol 2. New York: Basic Books; 1976.
Bowlby J. Attachment. In *Attachment and Loss*. Vol 1, 2nd ed. New York: Basic Books; 1982.
Bueno-Gutiérrez D, et al. Breastfeeding counseling based on formative research at primary healthcare services in Mexico. *Int J Equity Health*. 2021;20(1):173.
Cassidy TM. Culture, cultural competence, and clinical care. *J Hum Lact*. 2024;40(2):216–220.
Čatipović M, et al. Breastfeeding intention and knowledge in secondary-school students. *Acta Clin Croat*. 2018;57(4): 658–668.
Centers for Disease Control and Prevention. Gateway to health communication. 2024. http://www.cdc.gov/healthcommunication/index.html
Chan WS, Leung AY. Use of social network sites for communication among health professionals: systematic review. *J Med Internet Res*. 2018;20(3):e117.
Chang WH, et al. Trial of labor after cesarean section. *Taiwan J Obstet Gynecol*. 2022;61(5):739–740.
Chen X, et al. Machine or human? Evaluating the quality of a language translation mobile app for diabetes education material. *JMIR Diabetes*. 2017;2(1):e13.
Chiang KV, et al. Racial and ethnic disparities in breastfeeding initiation—United States, 2019. *MMWR Morb Mortal Wkly Rep*. 2021;70(21):769–774.
Clohisy DR, et al. Leadership, communication, and negotiation across a diverse workforce: an AOA critical issues symposium. *J Bone Joint Surg Am*. 2017;99(12):e60.
Conching AKS, Thayer Z. Biological pathways for historical trauma to affect health: a conceptual model focusing on epigenetic modifications. *Soc Sci Med*. 2019;230:74–82.
Corby K, et al. Investigating predictors of prenatal breastfeeding self-efficacy. *Can J Nurs Res*. 2021;53(1):56–63.
Crear-Perry J, et al. Social and structural determinants of health inequities in maternal health. *J Womens Health (Larchmt)*. 2021;30(2):230–235.
Daglas M, Antoniou E. Cultural views and practices related to breastfeeding. *Health Sci J*. 2012;6:2.
Dennis CL, et al. Breastfeeding rates in immigrant and non-immigrant women: a systematic review and meta-analysis. *Matern Child Nutr*. 2019;15(3):e12809.
Dinour LM, Bai Y. Impact of Milk on the Move breastfeeding support campaign on students' and employees' attitudes, subjective norms, intention, knowledge, and awareness. *J Am Coll Health*. 2022;72(5):1599–1608.
Dowbor T, et al. Shrinking the language accessibility gap: a mixed methods evaluation of telephone interpretation services in a large, diverse urban health care system. *Int J Equity Health*. 2015;14:83.
Dowling S, Pontin D. Using liminality to understand mothers' experiences of long-term breastfeeding: "Betwixt and between," and "matter out of place." *Health (London)*. 2017;21(1): 57–75.
El-Gilany AH, Abdel-Hady DM. Newborn first feed and prelacteal feeds in Mansoura, Egypt. *Biomed Res Int*. 2014;2014:258470.
Eni R, et al. At the edges of embodiment: determinants of breastfeeding for First Nations women. *Breastfeed Med*. 2014;9(4): 203–214.
EthnoMed. 2024. http://www.ethnomed.org
Fabiyi CA, et al. Association between breastfeeding discouragement and breastfeeding behaviors. *J Obstet Gynecol Neonatal Nurs*. 2021;50(5):568–582.
Faircloth C. "Natural" breastfeeding in comparative perspective: feminism, morality, and adaptive accountability. *Ethnos*. 2017;82(1):19–43.
Farsi D. Social media and health care, part I: literature review of social media use by health care providers. *J Med Internet Res*. 2021;23(4):e23205.
Farsi D, et al. Social media and health care (part II): narrative review of social media use by patients. *J Med Internet Res*. 2022;24(1):e30379.
Fischer TP, Olson BH. A qualitative study to understand cultural factors affecting a mother's decision to breast or formula feed. *J Hum Lact*. 2014;30(2):209–216.
FitzGerald C, Hurst S. Implicit bias in healthcare professionals: a systematic review. *BMC Med Ethics*. 2017;18(1):19.
Fontanarosa PB, Bauchner H. Race, ancestry, and medical research. *JAMA*. 2018;320(15):1539–1540.
Frey E, et al. Parents' use of social media as a health information source for their children: a scoping review. *Acad Pediatr*. 2022;22(4):526–539.
Gadson A, et al. Exploring the social determinants of racial/ethnic disparities in prenatal care utilization and maternal outcome. *Semin Perinatol*. 2017;41(5):308–317.
Galvão DMPG, et al. Use of new technologies and promotion of breastfeeding: integrative literature review. *Rev Paul Pediatr*. 2021;40:e2020234.
Galvin S, et al. Practical intervention to increase breastfeeding initiation among Cambodian women in the US. *Matern Child Health J*. 2008;12(4):545–547.
Goldbort J, et al. Breastfeeding but not exclusively: exploration of Chinese American mothers' infant feeding practices. *J Hum Lact*. 2021;37(2):380–389.
Gopal DP, et al. Implicit bias in healthcare: clinical practice, research and decision making. *Future Healthc J*. 2021;8(1): 40–48.
Gorbunova T, et al. Could education be the best galactagogue? Development and content validation of provider and patient checklists to promote lactation among Black parents. *J Hum Lact*. 2023;39(3):500–504.
Grano C, et al. Predicting intention and maintenance of breastfeeding up to 2-years after birth in primiparous and multiparous women. *Psychol Health*. 2022;10:1–17.
Grassley JS, et al. Game-based online antenatal breastfeeding education: a pilot. *Appl Nurs Res*. 2017;33:93–95.
Gross T, et al. Long-term breastfeeding in African American mothers. *J Hum Lact*. 2017;33(1):128–139.
Gul S, et al. Newborn care knowledge and practices among mothers attending pediatric outpatient clinic of a hospital in Karachi, Pakistan. *Int J Health Sci (Qassim)*. 2014;8(2): 167–175.
Gyamfi A, et al. Black/African American breastfeeding experience: cultural, sociological, and health dimensions through an equity lens. *Breastfeed Med*. 2021;16(2):103–111.
Hall WJ, et al. Implicit racial/ethnic bias among health care professionals and its influence on health care outcomes: a systematic review. *Am J Public Health*. 2015;105(12):e60–e76.

Hamade H, et al. Breastfeeding knowledge, attitude, perceived behavior, and intention among female undergraduate university students in the Middle East: the case of Lebanon and Syria. *Food Nutr Bull.* 2014;35(2):179–190.

Hamed S, et al. Racism in healthcare: a scoping review. *BMC Public Health.* 2022;16;22(1):988.

Healthy People 2030. Healthy People 2030: building a healthier future for all. January 16, 2025.

Healthy People 2030 | odphp.healthhttps://odphp.health.gov/healthypeople.gov

Hemingway S, et al. Racial disparities in sustaining breastfeeding in a Baby-Friendly designated southeastern United States hospital: an opportunity to investigate systemic racism. *Breastfeed Med.* 2021;16(2):150–155.

Hook JN, et al. Cultural humility and racial microaggressions in counseling. *J Couns Psychol.* 2016;63(3):269–277.

Hornsby PP, et al. Timing of introduction of complementary foods and beverages to infants of low-income women. *Breastfeed Med.* 2021;16(7):547–552.

Howell EA, Zeitlin J. Quality of care and disparities in obstetrics. *Obstet Gynecol Clin North Am.* 2017;44(1):13–25.

Hudak KM, Benjamin-Neelon SE. Timing of WIC enrollment and responsive feeding among low-income women in the US. *Int J Environ Res Public Health.* 2021;18(14):7695.

Hulsbosch LP, et al. Breastfeeding intention and trait mindfulness during pregnancy. *Midwifery.* 2021;101:103064.

Hulsbosch LP, et al. Breastfeeding continuation is associated with trait mindfulness but not with trajectories of postpartum depressive symptoms. *Midwifery.* 2023;124:103770.

Ignjatović S, Buturović Ž. Breastfeeding divisions in ethics and politics of feminism. *J Sociol Soc Psychol Soc Anthropol.* 2018;60(1):84–95.

International Board of Lactation Consultant Examiners. *Code of Professional Conduct: International Board Certified Lactation Consultants.* Falls Church, VA: International Board of Lactation Consultant Examiners; 2022. https://iblce.org/wp-content/uploads/2022/08/2022_August_17_Code-of-Professional--Conduct_FINAL.pdf

Isong IA, et al. Racial and ethnic disparities in early childhood obesity. *Pediatrics.* 2018;141(1):e20170865.

Jefferson UT. Breastfeeding exposure, attitudes, and intentions of African American and Caucasian college students. *J Hum Lact.* 2017;33(1):149–156.

Jiang N, et al. Significance of patient participation in nursing care. *Altern Ther Health Med.* 2021;27(5):115–119.

Jones KM, et al. Racial and ethnic disparities in breastfeeding. *Breastfeed Med.* 2015;10(4):186–196.

Joseph J, et al. Postpartum breastfeeding experiences in the traditional-biomedical crossroads: a qualitative study using drawing with Vietnamese and Myanmarese refugee women in Australia. *J Adv Nurs.* 2019;75(11):2855–2866.

Kanatoula DD, et al. How does the degree of acculturation influence the intention to breastfeed, breastfeeding frequency, and breastfeeding duration in migrant women? A review of the publications from 2014–2018. *Z Geburtshilfe Neonatol.* 2019;223(5):271–279.

Kavle JA, Landry M. Addressing barriers to maternal nutrition in low- and middle-income countries: a review of the evidence and programme implications. *Matern Child Nutr.* 2018;14(1):e12508.

Krystallidou D, et al. Multilingual healthcare communication: stumbling blocks, solutions, recommendations. *Patient Educ Couns.* 2021;104(3):512–516.

Lama Y, et al. General and health-related social media use among adults with children in the household: findings from a national survey in the United States. *Patient Educ Couns.* 2022;105(3):647–653.

Lau CYK, et al. The effect of maternal self-regulated motivation on breastfeeding continuation. *Matern Child Health J.* 2022;26(2):441–448.

Lehrner A, Yehuda R. Cultural trauma and epigenetic inheritance. *Dev Psychopathol.* 2018;30(5):1763–1777.

Linde K, et al. The association between breastfeeding and attachment: a systematic review. *Midwifery.* 2020;81:102592.

Little EE, et al. Mother-infant physical contact predicts responsive feeding among U.S. breastfeeding mothers. *Nutrients.* 2018;10(9):1251.

Lokossou YUA, et al. Socio-cultural beliefs influence feeding practices of mothers and their children in Grand Popo, Benin. *J Health Popul Nutr.* 2021;40(1):33.

Louis-Jacques A, et al. Racial and ethnic disparities in U.S. breastfeeding and implications for maternal and child health outcomes. *Semin Perinatol.* 2017;41(5):299–307.

Luan Erfe BM, et al. Professional medical interpreters influence the quality of acute ischemic stroke care for patients who speak languages other than English. *J Am Heart Assoc.* 2017;6(9):e006175.

MacMillan Uribe AL, et al. Cultural influences on infant and toddler feeding among low-income Latinx mothers. *Matern Child Nutr.* 2022;18(4):e13342.

Martin H, et al. Breastfeeding motivation predicts infant feeding intention and outcomes: evaluation of a novel adaptation of the treatment self-regulation questionnaire. *J Hum Lact.* 2022;38(2):236–247.

McCloskey K, et al. Breastfeeding disparities during the COVID-19 pandemic: race/ethnicity, age, education, and insurance payor. *J Hum Lact.* 2023;39(4):615–624.

Menekse D, et al. An investigation of the relationship between mother's personality traits, breastfeeding self-efficacy, and perception of insufficient milk supply. *Health Care Women Int.* 2021;42(4–6):925–941.

Miller DP, et al. Longitudinal trajectories of food insecurity among children of immigrants. *J Immigr Minor Health.* 2018;20(1):194–202.

Min J, et al. Ethnic disparities in childhood BMI trajectories and obesity and potential causes among 29,250 US children: findings from the Early Childhood Longitudinal Study-Birth and Kindergarten Cohorts. *Int J Obes (Lond).* 2018;42(9):1661–1670.

Modjadji P, et al. Beliefs and norms influencing initiation and sustenance of exclusive breastfeeding: experiences of mothers in primary health care facilities in Ermelo, South Africa. *Int J Environ Res Public Health.* 2023;20(2):1513.

Morrow AL, et al. Breastfeeding disparities and their mediators in an urban birth cohort of Black and White mothers. *Breastfeed Med.* 2021;16(6):452–462.

Morse H, Brown A. The benefits, challenges and impacts of accessing social media group support for breastfeeding: A systematic review. *Matern Child Nutr.* 2022;18(4):e13399.

Moukarzel S, et al. Diffusing science through social networks: the case of breastfeeding communication on Twitter. *PLoS One.* 2020;15(8):e0237471.

Moukarzel S, et al. Breastfeeding communication strategies, challenges and opportunities in the twitter-verse: perspectives of influencers and social network analysis. *Int J Environ Res Public Health.* 2021;18(12):6181.

Myers & Briggs Foundation. 2024. http://www.myersbriggs.org/
Nandagire WH, et al. Exploring cultural beliefs and practices associated with weaning of children aged 0-12 months by mothers attending services at Maternal Child Health Clinic Kalisizo Hospital, Uganda. *Pan Afr Med J.* 2019;34:47.
National Center for Cultural Competence. Georgetown University. 2024. https://nccc.georgetown.edu/
Noel-Weiss J, et al. Exploring how IBCLCs manage ethical dilemmas: a qualitative study. *BMC Med Ethics.* 2012;13:18.
Nutbeam D, Lloyd JE. Understanding and responding to health literacy as a social determinant of health. *Annu Rev Public Health.* 2021;42:159–173.
O'Callaghan K, Kiely ME. Ethnic disparities in the dietary requirement for vitamin D during pregnancy: considerations for nutrition policy and research. *Proc Nutr Soc.* 2018;77(2):164–173.
Odeniyi AO, et al. Breastfeeding beliefs and experiences of African immigrant mothers in high-income countries: a systematic review. *Matern Child Nutr.* 2020;16(3):e12970.
Ortega P, Prada J. Words matter: translanguaging in medical communication skills training. *Perspect Med Educ.* 2020;9(4):251–255.
Osorio Galeano SP, et al. Preparing parents for discharge from the neonatal unit, the transition, and care of their preterm children at home. *Invest Educ Enferm.* 2023;41(1):e04.
Padashian F, et al. Examining exclusive breastfeeding in Iranian mothers using the five-factor model of personality traits. *J Taibah Univ Med Sci.* 2021;17(1):51–56.
Palmquist A. Demedicalizing breastmilk: the discourses, practices, and identities of informal milk sharing. In: Cassidy T, El-Tom A, eds. *Ethnographies of Breastfeeding: Cultural Contexts and Confrontations.* London: Bloomsbury Academic; 2015.
Panayiotou A, et al. Language translation apps in health care settings: expert opinion. *JMIR.* 2019;7(4):e11316.
Payne BK, Hannay JW. Implicit bias reflects systemic racism. *Trends Cogn Sci.* 2021;25(11):927–936.
Pérez-Stable EJ, El-Toukhy S. Communicating with diverse patients: how patient and clinician factors affect disparities. *Patient Educ Couns.* 2018;101(12):2186–2194.
Pool LR, et al. Trends in racial/ethnic disparities in cardiovascular health among US adults from 1999–2012. *J Am Heart Assoc.* 2017;6(9):e006027.
Raheem RA, et al. Determinants of the introduction of prelacteal feeds in the Maldives. *Breastfeed Med.* November 2014;9(9):473–478.
Ramoo S, et al. Breastfeeding practices in a hospital-based study of Vietnamese women. *Breastfeed Med.* 2014;9(9):479–485.
Rathbone A, Prescott J. "I feel like a neurotic mother at times"—a mixed methods study exploring online health information seeking behaviour in new parents. *Mhealth.* 2019;5:14.
Ray S, et al. Speaking in tongues: what parents really think about tongue-tie surgery for their infants. *Clin Pediatr (Phila).* 2020;59(3):236–244.
Rehayem A, et al. Infant feeding beliefs and practices of Arabic mothers in Australia. *Women Birth.* 2020;33(4):e391–e399.
Renata FI, et al. Overcoming language barriers in healthcare: a protocol for investigating safe and effective communication when patients or clinicians use a second language. *BMC Health Serv Res.* 2015;15:371.
Reno R, et al. Housing insecurity, housing conditions, and breastfeeding behaviors for Medicaid-eligible families in urban settings. *J Hum Lact.* 2022;38(4):760–770.
Reyes C, et al. Investigating the effectiveness of school-based breastfeeding education on breastfeeding knowledge, attitudes and intentions of adolescent females. *Midwifery.* 2019;70:64–70.
Robinson D, et al. The 5 Rs of cultural humility: a conceptual model for health care leaders. *Am J Med.* 2021;134(2):161–163.
Rosier W. Cool cabbage compresses. *Breastfeed Rev.* 1988; 1(12):28–31.
Ruby D. Social media users in the world [2023 demographics]. March 20, 2023. https://www.demandsage.com/social-media-users/#:~:text=There%20are%204.9%20billion%20social%20media%20users%20in,penetration%20rate%20is%2059.4%25%20as%20of%20January%202023
Saluja B, Bryant Z. How implicit bias contributes to racial disparities in maternal morbidity and mortality in the United States. *J Womens Health (Larchmt).* 2021;30(2):270-273.
Scharfe E. Maternal attachment representations and initiation and duration of breastfeeding. *J Hum Lact.* 2012;28:218–225.
Schiffman LG, et al. *Consumer Behavior.* 12th ed. New York: Pearson Education, Inc.; 2019.
Schillinger D. The intersections between social determinants of health, health literacy, and health disparities. *Stud Health Technol Inform.* 2020;269:22–41.
Schroeder D, et al. Rediscovering empowerment with breastfeeding in an urban First Nation's population. *BMC Pregnancy Childbirth.* 2019;19(1):509.
Singletary N, et al. Stakeholder views of breastfeeding education in schools: a systematic mixed studies review of the literature. *Int Breastfeed J.* 2017;12:14.
Smailhodzic E, et al. Social media use in healthcare: a systematic review of effects on patients and on their relationship with healthcare professionals. *BMC Health Serv Res.* 2016;16(1):442.
Smith PH. Social justice at the core of breastfeeding protection, promotion and support: a conceptualization. *J Hum Lact.* 2018;34(2):220–225.
Spencer B, et al. African American women's breastfeeding experiences: cultural, personal, and political voices. *Qual Health Res.* 2015;25(7):974–987.
Stafford JD, et al. Health literacy and associated outcomes in the postpartum period at Grady Memorial Hospital. *Matern Child Health J.* 2021;25(4):599–605.
Standish KR, Parker MG. Social determinants of breastfeeding in the United States. *Clin Ther.* 2022;44(2):186–192.
Stevens-Watkins D, et al. Social health care determinants of breastfeeding Black women: a multigenerational study. *Breastfeed Med.* 2022;17(8):666–672.
Swanson V, et al. "Both parents should care for babies": a cross-sectional, cross-cultural comparison of adolescents' breastfeeding intentions, and the influence of shared-parenting beliefs. *BMC Pregnancy Childbirth.* 2017;17(1):204.
Temple Newhook J, et al. Poverty and breastfeeding: comparing determinants of early breastfeeding cessation incidence in socioeconomically marginalized and privileged populations in the FiNaL study. *Health Equity.* 2017;1(1):96–102.
The Joint Commission. Communicating clearly and effectively to patients: how to overcome common communication challenges in health care. 2018. https://store.jointcommissioninternational.org/assets/3/7/jci-wp-communicating-clearly-final_(1).pdf
The White House. June 2022. White House blueprint for addressing the maternal health crisis. https://bidenwhitehouse.archives.gov/briefing-room/statements-releases/2024/07/10/the-white-house-blueprint-for-addressing-the-maternal-health-crisis-two-years-of-progress/

Tuohy D. Effective intercultural communication in nursing. *Nurs Stand.* 2019;34(2):45–50.

U.S. Department of Health and Human Services, Office of Disease Prevention and Health Promotion. National action plan to improve health literacy. 2010. https://health.gov/sites/default/files/2019-09/Health_Literacy_Action_Plan.pdf

Valero-Chillerón MJ, et al. Influence of health literacy on maintenance of exclusive breastfeeding at 6 months postpartum: a multicentre study. *Int J Environ Res Public Health.* 2022;19(9):5411.

van der Gaag M, et al. The importance of health literacy for self-management: a scoping review of reviews. *Chronic Illn.* 2022;18(2):234–254.

Vari P, et al. Community breastfeeding attitudes and beliefs. *Health Care Women Int.* 2013;34(7):592–606.

Vela MB, et al. Eliminating explicit and implicit biases in health care: evidence and research needs. *Annu Rev Public Health.* 2022;43:477–501.

Venegas-Vera AV, et al. Positive and negative impact of social media in the COVID-19 era. *Rev Cardiovasc Med.* 2020;21(4):561–564.

Venu I, et al. The breastfeeding paradox: relevance for household food insecurity. *Paediatr Child Health.* 2017;22(4):180–183.

Verbeek T, et al. Personality traits predict meeting the WHO recommendation of 6 months' breastfeeding: a prospective general population cohort study. *Adv Neonatal Care.* 2019;19(2):118–126.

Vila-Candel R, et al. Health literacy of pregnant women and duration of breastfeeding maintenance: a feasibility study. *J Adv Nurs.* 2021;77(2):703–714.

Vukušić Rukavina T, et al. Dangers and benefits of social media on e-professionalism of health care professionals: scoping review. *J Med Internet Res.* 2021;23(11):e25770.

Wagg AJ, et al. Online social support group use by breastfeeding mothers: a content analysis. *Heliyon.* 2019;5(3):e01245.

Walsemann KM, et al. Trends in food insecurity among California residents from 2001 to 2011: inequities at the intersection of immigration status and ethnicity. *Prev Med.* 2017;105:142–148.

White AA, et al. Self-awareness and cultural identity as an effort to reduce bias in medicine. *J Racial Ethn Health Disparities.* 2018;5(1):34–49.

Wilson JC. Using social media for breastfeeding support. *Nurs Womens Health.* 2020;24(5):332–343.

Withers M, et al. Traditional beliefs and practices in pregnancy, childbirth and postpartum: a review of the evidence from Asian countries. *Midwifery.* 2018;56:158–170.

Wouk K, et al. Lactation support for people who are incarcerated: a systematic review. *Breastfeed Med.* 2022;17(11):891–925.

Wu Y, et al. Life expectancies in Hawai'i: a multi-ethnic analysis of 2010 life tables. *Hawaii J Med Public Health.* 2017;76(1):9–14.

Yalçin SS, et al. Breastfeeding practices among Syrian refugees in Turkey. *Int Breastfeed J.* 2022;17(1):10.

Yang SF, et al. Breastfeeding knowledge and attitudes of baccalaureate nursing students in Taiwan: a cohort study. *Women Birth.* 2019;32(3):e334–e340.

Zehner E, et al. Marketing and infant and young child feeding in rapidly evolving food environments. *Matern Child Nutr.* 2019;15(S4):e12810.

Zhang X, et al. Cultural influences on complementary feeding beliefs amongst new Chinese immigrant mothers in England: a mixed methods study. *Int J Environ Res Public Health.* 2020;17(15):5468.

Zhou Q, et al. Breastfeeding practices 2008–2009 among Chinese mothers living in Ireland: a mixed methods study. *BMC Pregnancy Childbirth.* 2020;20(1):51.

CHAPTER 4

Empowering Parents to Nurse

Empowering parents to nurse is the role of every member of their healthcare team. Empowerment is a process that allows a person to gain the knowledge, skill sets, and attitudes needed to cope with new life circumstances. The focus of empowerment is on reducing the need for assistance and making parents more self-sufficient. For nursing parents, this includes encouraging and developing the skills required for problem-solving when difficulties arise.

People who demonstrate a sincere belief in nursing as the natural way to nourish an infant are the most effective in empowering lactation. This requires moving beyond a theoretical belief in lactation to instilling practices that promote and support nursing. Some healthcare providers may be reluctant to promote lactation for fear that they will create guilt in parents who choose not to nurse. Projecting ambivalence about lactation sends mixed messages and creates personal doubts. Providers who enthusiastically embrace lactation serve as powerful motivators and role models for both families and the healthcare community. An empowering partnership between providers and parents increases parents' confidence and self-esteem. This in turn fosters their independence, growth, and self-efficacy, as well as a positive learning environment. A positive learning climate actively involves learners in problem-solving and decision-making. Interactions laced with humor increase teaching effectiveness and help learners gain perspective during challenging times.

KEY TERMS

Consumer responsibilities	Health consumerism	Learning style
Consumer rights	Informed consent	Mixed message
Empowerment	Learning climate	Self-efficacy

Health Consumerism

Health care is a consumer-oriented system of preserving mental and physical well-being. **Health consumerism** positions clients as the primary decision-makers of their health care. A decision-making partnership between parents and their caregivers empowers families to accept responsibility for managing their health and the health of their children. Parents and their caregivers form a team that embraces parental involvement in shared decision-making which is the foundation of client-centered care. It leads to empowerment and promotes autonomy and greater control over healthcare decisions (Nutbeam & Lloyd, 2021).

As parents learn about lactation, they more clearly understand their options and develop the necessary skills to meet their lactation goals. They grow in self-confidence and self-esteem and mature as both individuals and caregivers for their children. The knowledge parents gain helps them understand how to manage feedings and enables them to make informed decisions about their care (Bahrambeygi et al., 2023).

The process of education is a joint venture to determine what parents need to make the best decisions for themselves and their babies. This philosophy of responsible and knowledgeable self-care forms the basis of the counseling approach promoted throughout this text.

Consumer Rights and Responsibilities

Consumers and healthcare providers share a two-way relationship of rights and responsibilities. Parents have a right to information that will enable them to grow as informed health consumers. Caregivers have a responsibility to inform consumers of healthy practices and the consequences of their actions. Parents have certain responsibilities as active health consumers. The **consumer rights** and **consumer responsibilities** for parents as active health consumers are summarized in **Table 4-1**. Hospitals typically have a client bill of rights as well. Constructive communication between caregivers and consumers is essential for effective, positive interactions. Clients who communicate their desires to healthcare providers are able to form healthy and mutually respectful working relationships. **Figure 4-1** provides suggestions to share with parents who wish to become better-informed healthcare consumers.

Table 4-1 Parents' Rights and Responsibilities

Parents have the right to:

- Understand what they are giving consent to
- Receive information concerning a drug or treatment before its administration
- Know about alternative treatment methods
- Accept or refuse treatment or advice without pressure
- Know whether a procedure is medically indicated or elective
- Have access to their complete medical records
- Seek medical opinions
- Be kept informed of the most current information
- Be treated as an equal partner in their health care
- Have their questions answered completely and courteously
- Be treated with respect
- Receive the best care possible, with a focus on prevention
- Make decisions regarding their treatment and that of their child
- Care for themselves and their child to the maximum extent of their ability

Parents have the responsibility to:

- Learn what is available and make informed choices
- Find caregivers who support their goals
- Be attentive to their caregivers with an open mind
- Indicate their preferences courteously
- Carry through on care plans
- Learn the approximate cost of a procedure in advance
- State why they change caregivers, if it occurs

Informed Consent

Informed consent protects client rights and autonomy. It indicates that a healthcare provider explains an intervention to clients before they agree to it. With informed consent, clients accept responsibility for becoming knowledgeable and actively involved in their healthcare decisions. Clients can sign a consent form either declining or requesting procedures (e.g., declining circumcision or vaccinations or giving consent to the use of blood products in emergencies). Consent forms can also educate consumers about unwise practices (e.g., the use of pacifiers or formula for a nonmedical reason). Signed consent forms protect both clients and healthcare providers. The client

- Acquire a medical vocabulary, subscribe to health electronic newsletters and magazines, access consumer-oriented medical references, research legitimate internet medical sites, and use the public library.
- Attend courses for nonprofessionals, such as classes in first aid or home health care. Check local high schools, colleges, online classes, or civic organizations for such programs.
- Enlist the services of caregivers and hospitals that welcome and encourage patients to become actively informed.
- Select an independent prepared childbirth class that provides information on alternatives, enhances your understanding, and encourages active participation in medical decisions.
- Learn to recognize early symptoms of illness, and investigate appropriate methods of treatment before contacting the caregiver. This preparation will enable you to have an informed and concrete discussion of the situation with the caregiver.
- If you are unfamiliar with a medical term or do not understand what was told to you, ask to have the point clarified and explained in simpler terms.
- Discuss alternatives with your caregiver, and ask why one course of treatment was chosen over another.
- If the situation warrants, seek a second (and even third) opinion. As a healthcare consumer, this is your right and your responsibility.
- Learn the cost of a recommended treatment, as well as the costs of alternative treatments.
- If you are uncomfortable or dissatisfied with your caregiver's advice, you are not legally required to comply with it in most cases. However, you must be aware of the medical risks. You have the right to make your own choices. Even if it seems to the caregiver that you have made a wrong choice, the ultimate consequences and responsibilities are yours.

Figure 4-1 Becoming an active healthcare consumer.

being actively involved in their care reduces the risk of medical liability in the event of an unfavorable outcome.

Helping Parents Become Informed Health Consumers

To be informed consumers, parents need to learn about lactation from trusted sources to help them select options that best suit their needs and goals. This requires that all members of their healthcare team are knowledgeable about best practices in lactation management. It also requires that parents can reach out to their healthcare professionals throughout lactation when questions or problems arise. Parents who seek health-related information from online sources will benefit from guidance on how to critically appraise internet sources and how to locate the highest-quality information (Jaks et al., 2019).

There is a wide range of understanding and comfort related to rights and responsibilities in health care. For example, an educated, professional couple will likely seek information regarding their health care. On the other hand, low-income, minority, teenage, or single parents are among the most vulnerable to patronizing attitudes of medical caregivers and may have a more difficult time finding appropriate and accessible health care.

Lactation consultants are viewed as knowledgeable members of the family's healthcare team who advocate for both parents and babies. At times, lactation consultant advice may differ from that of another caregiver on the parent's healthcare team. It is important to be tactful and respectful of the family's relationships with their caregivers. There may also be times when a parent chooses a course of action that is not considered best practice. After receiving the information they need to make informed decisions, parents need appropriate care that respects their choices.

Caregiver advice that commonly creates conflict involves practices that compromise the recommendation of exclusive nursing for 6 months. Questions or comments from parents may inadvertently cause a healthcare provider to recommend formula supplementation or early complementary foods. Hearing concerns about insufficient milk or frequent feedings may prompt such recommendations in a sincere attempt to solve what is perceived as a problem. Parents need to frame concerns in self-assured ways that avoid misunderstandings. Informed parents will have the confidence to determine what is best for them and their baby. Likewise, healthcare providers are more likely to work in collaboration with confident, informed parents.

Optimizing Learning

Learning is newly acquired knowledge that combines with experience to serve as feedback and influence future behavior in similar situations. Learning for humans ranges from the simplest, almost reflexive responses to abstract concepts and complex problem-solving. When confronted with a problem, we sometimes see the solution instantly. More often, however, we search for and evaluate information to help us make the best decision. Problem-solving enables us to gain some control over our environment and is pivotal to producing the desired response. Educating parents to be active participants in their problem-solving is empowering and increases their sense of control. Self-directed learning places responsibility on the learner to set goals, assess progress, identify resources, and seek feedback (Charokar & Dulloo, 2022; Robinson & Persky, 2020).

The four major elements of all learning theories are motivation, cues, response, and reinforcement. Motivation, discussed in **Chapter 3**, stems from a wish to satisfy an unmet personal need or goal. The greater the motivation, the more actively we engage in learning. Cues are the stimuli that give direction to our motives and guide our actions toward the desired outcome. Previous learning and reinforcement of past responses determine how we respond to those cues.

Reinforcement increases the likelihood of a specific future response as a result of new cues or stimuli. Such repetition increases the strength of the association and slows the process of forgetting. For example, learning how to position a new baby for feeding and practicing with help from a skilled caregiver help to hone a parent's lactation technique. Self-confidence increases with each successive feeding as the parent becomes more skilled at recognizing and responding to the baby's hunger cues.

Receiving and Storing Information

The human mind processes information similar to how a computer processes data. How the brain forms images and processes information depends on cognitive ability and the complexity of the information. **Figure 4-2** illustrates the processing of sensory input, using an example of showing a parent how to position the baby for feeding. Understanding this process is relevant for parents learning how to nurse their babies as well as for professionals learning the field of lactation and the skills for helping parents.

Sensory input is received: Parent is shown how to position the baby for feeding.
Input collects in the SENSORY STORE, where it is stored for 1–2 seconds.

When It Works	Why It Works	When Things Go Wrong
Input is ***processed*** within 1–2 seconds. ⇩ Input transfers to the ***short-term store*** and is retained for 30 seconds. ⇩	Parent is alert. It is a teachable moment. Parent is motivated. Process is described and demonstrated with a doll while parent begins to nurse.	Input is not processed in time. ⇨ Information is lost immediately. **Why It Went Wrong** Parent is tired or in pain. Parent lacks motivation. Parent is distracted.
Input is ***rehearsed*** within 30 seconds. ⇩	Parent practices nursing. Parent receives assistance and support in the early days.	Input is not rehearsed in time. ⇨ Information is not retained. **Why It Went Wrong** Parent doesn't do a return demonstration. No one visits to reinforce the process. Parent forgets important features.
Less than 5–6 items of input are received and rehearsed. ⇩ Input is ***encoded***. ⇩ Input transfers within 10 seconds to ***long-term store***, where 2–3 items are retained for days, weeks, or years. ⇩ ***Activation*** of input takes place to: ◆ Organize with new links. ◆ Expand network of relationships. ◆ Motivate search for more information. ⇩	Parent receives printed and verbal instructions about what to expect in the first week: frequency, duration, feeding cues, number of stools and voids. ***RESULT FOR PARENT*** ⬇ Parent has a solid grasp of basic management. Parent is ready to focus on additional factors for the next several weeks and months. Parent applies what was learned to new situations.	More than 5–6 items of input are received and rehearsed within 30 seconds. ⇨ Information overload. Information is not retained. Confusion takes place. Less effective choices. Poor decision making. **Why It Went Wrong** Parent receives 2 pages of printed and verbal instructions that include: Frequency, duration, feeding cues, number of stools and voids, what to eat, various positions for holding the baby at feedings, how to end a feeding, how to soothe a fussy baby, what to do about leaking, how to treat sore nipples and engorgement, when to start supplements, how and when to wean, how to express milk, how to manage lactation and returning to work, how to increase milk production, and how to nurse in public.
Recoding of input takes place to: ◆ Accommodate more information. ◆ Interpret and elaborate. ◆ Match frame of reference. ◆ Match prior knowledge. ◆ Activate long-term memory. ⇩	Parent continues to learn more about lactation at each stage of the baby's development and responds appropriately.	Does not match frame of reference or prior knowledge. ⇨ Retention and recall are hampered. Retrieval system fails. Forgetting takes place.
Retrieval of information.	Parent feels confident about their lactation knowledge and management techniques. Parent applies what they know when they nurse subsequent babies.	***RESULT FOR PARENT*** ⬇ Parent doesn't know how to feed on cue; starts early supplements and solids. Parent doesn't get a good latch; gets sore nipples. Parent weans early. Parent doesn't nurse subsequent babies.

Figure 4-2 Pathway for sensory input for lactation management.

The degree to which we form mental images, which depends on the frequency of input, influences our recall. When we perceive an image, it is temporarily stored in a series of memory "storehouses" in the brain. The image remains there for 1 or 2 seconds and is lost immediately unless it is processed and transferred to short-term memory. Short-term memory can accommodate only four or five items. Information is lost in approximately 30 seconds unless it is mentally repeated (rehearsed). Information we rehearse is transferred to long-term memory within 2 to 10 seconds, where it can remain for days, weeks, or even years.

Retention and Recall

How we retain information depends on the degree to which we repeat it or relate it to other knowledge or experience. Rehearsal enables us to hold information in short-term storage long enough for encoding to take place. When we encode information, we select a word or visual image to represent what we perceive. Both verbal and visual images are important in forming an overall mental image. Verbal images take less time to learn than visual images. Thus, combining verbal and visual images in one-on-one lactation assistance produces better retention than just viewing an online video.

Information can be lost when short-term storage receives a large amount of input at the same time. Offering too much information and too many suggestions will make it difficult for parents to encode and store the information. This overload can cause confusion and lead to poor decision-making. Parents receive an overwhelming amount of information on all aspects of care during the immediate postpartum period. Locating lactation information can be challenging for new parents, much less processing it!

When input reaches long-term storage, it is constantly organized and reorganized as new links are forged between chunks of information. As we gain more knowledge, we expand the network of relationships between data and may search for additional information. We relate new data to old data, thereby making the retained information more meaningful. The data we already encoded may be re-encoded to include larger amounts of information.

When we fail to retrieve information, forgetting occurs. It is often difficult for parents to recall specific instructions early in lactation. Reinforcing verbal instruction with written materials and other visual aids helps provide the necessary support they need at this time of change and confusion. The use of multimedia increases long-term retention and transfer of learning (Abdulrahaman et al., 2020; Hsu et al., 2022; Tang et al., 2018).

Involvement and Relevance

The way we process information depends on how relevant it is to us and our level of involvement. We are more willing to spend the effort required to process a message when it is personally relevant. We seek information, weigh it carefully, and evaluate its merits. When we are highly involved in or have a strong opinion about an issue, we may interpret something as being more positive than it actually is if it agrees with our opinion (Schiffman & Wisenblit, 2019). Individuals who have no strong opinion or stance will be more receptive to arguments both for and against an issue, or they may take no position at all. Visual cues and repetition can help reinforce messages for parents who may be having difficulty processing information or making decisions.

As illustrated in **Figure 4-3**, the human brain is often characterized in terms of a duality, with the left and right brains serving complementary functions (Corballis, 2019). The left brain is considered to be the highly active and verbal side of the brain that focuses on rational and realistic cognition. The right brain is considered to be more passive and focuses on emotions, symbolism, impulses, and intuition. The right and left hemispheres of the brain work together to process information. Greater learning and recall occur when there is both verbal and visual input.

Adult Learning

People attach more meaning to what they learn from experience than to what they learn passively. Adult learning uses teaching methods that meet the needs of adult learners. It empowers parents and engages them in actively learning rather than being passively taught. Simply informing adult learners what to do does not actively engage them in their learning or in shared

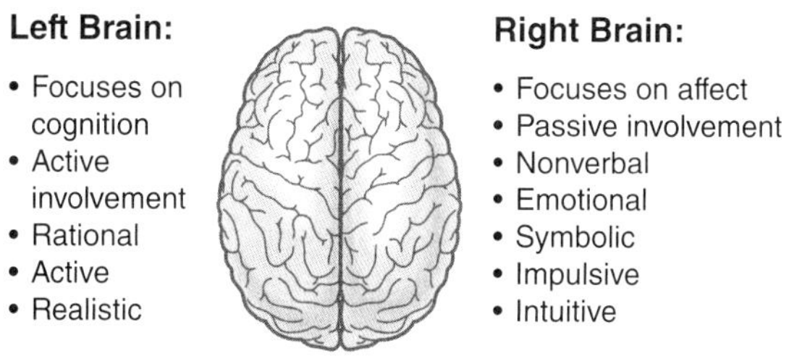

Figure 4-3 Split-brain theory.

decision-making. An adult's needs as a learner are different from those of adolescents. Mature learners bring with them an accumulation of life experiences, knowledge, and a belief system gained over their lifetime. Adults are generally practical, autonomous, self-directed, and goal oriented. They need to be free to direct themselves and assume responsibility for their decisions and actions.

The key to self-directed learning is that learners have the primary responsibility for planning, carrying out, and evaluating their own learning (Zénon et al., 2019). Although adults have a deep psychological need to be generally self-directing, they will benefit from help when learning new skills or going through life or role transitions. The role of a facilitator of adult learners is to guide their learning and help them reach their goals rather than merely supplying them with information. Through an adult learning approach, facilitators form a problem-solving team with parents to explore options and guide their decisions on what will work for them.

Readiness to Learn

Information must be relevant to have value for the adult learner. Adults generally become ready to learn when they have a need to cope with real-life tasks and problems. Drawing on previous knowledge and experience that is relevant and that adds value can help them connect to their learning. Approach adults as equals in life experience, respecting their knowledge and encouraging them to voice their opinions freely and engage in learning.

Adults are generally willing to engage in learning experiences before, after, and during a life-changing event (Hutchinson, 2019). They want to be able to apply the knowledge and skills they gain today to living more effectively tomorrow. The goal of any learning is to transfer new understanding and skills to a new setting. This involves using the behavior that was learned and refraining from other practices that were learned to be unhelpful. This transference is most likely to occur when the degree of learning is high and when learners can associate new information with something they already know. For example, acquiring the necessary skills and learning how to interpret and respond to infant cues in the early days of lactation sets the stage for effective management and continued growth.

Learning Climate

Effective body language and counseling techniques can create a **learning climate** that is relaxed, trusting, mutually respectful, informal, warm, collaborative, and supportive. Establishing rapport and a friendly, open atmosphere helps motivate learners. It is natural for learners to be anxious or nervous when faced with a new learning situation. High stress is a barrier to learning, and people learn best under low to moderate stress. Learners will respond positively to a rich, responsive, risk-free environment where they can practice and master new skills without judgment, have sufficient time for reflection, and receive positive reinforcement. Parents will learn best with a low degree of difficulty that avoids information overload. An effective learning climate is tailored to their developmental readiness and sequenced to their pace. Stimulating as many senses as possible and with positive reinforcement facilitates learning.

Adult Learning Techniques

Assessing parents' needs and their readiness to learn will help identify the most effective approach for each situation. Within a relaxed, trusting, collaborative, and mutually respectful learning environment, caregivers and parents can engage in shared decision-making. This approach enhances problem-solving skills and self-reliance. It encourages self-direction, risk-taking, active participation in setting goals, and ownership of the care plan and the outcome. Presenting parents with choices and asking what will work for them encourages self-direction as they practice techniques. Urging them to evaluate their learning affirms that they understand what they learned and that they know what will work best for their situation. Their competence and confidence will increase and foster greater self-esteem and independence.

Generational Differences

Generational differences can affect how adults engage in learning. While adults and adolescents respond to a learning experience in much the same way, their expectations may be greater in some areas. In addition, the dynamics of interactions with adults are quite different from those with adolescents. This is largely because of the way adults interact and the way they assess a facilitator's credibility. The healthcare team will interact with multiple generations of parents and their families:

- Baby boomer grandparents (born 1946–1964)
- Generation X older parents (born 1965–1980)
- Generation Y, or millennials (born 1981–1996)
- Generation Z, or iGen (born 1997–2010)
- Generation Alpha (born after 2010)

Although much is written about commonalities among generations of learners, generalities should not negate the individuality of learners (Schnapp et al., 2022).

However, recognizing common preferences for learning modes is helpful in planning approaches to educating parents, most of whom are young adults. Expectations and learning styles for young adults are different from those of previous generations (Eckleberry-Hunt et al., 2018; Shorey et al., 2021). Young adults were raised in a world of interactive media, the internet, and digital messaging technologies. They seamlessly and simultaneously use resources such as Facebook, online support groups, and mobile apps. Young adults value the use of technology, teamwork, and interactive learning (Rogers & Cohen, 2020). They want a learning environment in which they can make decisions; work at their own pace; and receive direction, feedback, and support (DiMattio & Hudacek, 2020). They prefer online tutorials or videos, interactive gaming, and virtual learning environments (Vizcaya-Moreno & Pérez-Cañaveras, 2020).

Learning Styles

Lifelong learning results from stimulation of all senses—visual, auditory, and kinesthetic. Thus, adults learn primarily through what they see, what they hear, and what they engage in physically. Some people use one sense more than others to learn or recall information. Those with dominance in the left brain generally learn better from verbal instruction and respond well to analytical and logical information. Right-brain learners tend to respond more readily to images, symbols, intuition, and emotion.

Although learners may have a preferred **learning style**, research reports no evidence that we learn better with our preferred learning style (Boland & Amonoo, 2021; Childs-Kean et al., 2020; Nancekivell et al., 2021; Yfanti & Doukakis, 2021). A single approach to teaching does not work for every learner, and most prefer a combination of modes. Engaging multiple learning styles can help visual, auditory, and kinesthetic learning to take place and contributes to better learning (Boland & Amonoo, 2021; Nancekivell et al., 2021). Multisensory education enhances learning and is more effective than one modality alone. Lectures alone have intrinsic deficiencies as a teaching method. The use of information technology and multimedia can reduce or eliminate some of these deficiencies. **Table 4-2** describes the three learning

Table 4-2 Basing Teaching on Learning Style

Learning Style	Traits	Ways to Reach Parents
Visual learners	▪ Prefer written instructions ▪ Learn best with visual aids, such as photographs, diagrams, and illustrations ▪ Respond well to carefully organized learning materials ▪ May study by reading notes and organizing them in an outline	▪ Well-organized and interesting visual materials presented in a variety of formats ▪ Handouts that are visually appealing and easy to read ▪ Variety of technologies, such as computers, videos, and live demonstrations
Auditory learners	▪ Extremely good at remembering what they say and what others say ▪ Learn best through verbal repetition and by repeating things aloud ▪ Enjoy discussing ideas and express their interest and enthusiasm verbally ▪ Are easily distracted by either too much or too little noise ▪ Can find it difficult to work quietly for long periods	▪ Rephrase points in several ways ▪ Write down key points before verbally presenting them to help avoid confusion ▪ Vary voice speed, volume, and pitch to increase interest ▪ Incorporate sounds, music, and other oral technologies
Kinesthetic learners	▪ Need to be physically involved in what they are learning ▪ Enjoy handling learning materials and respond well to hands-on activities ▪ Often take notes to keep busy, although they rarely use them ▪ Typically have good motor coordination ▪ Can remember how to do something after doing it once	▪ Allow them to move around the room ▪ Provide lots of tactile activities where they can handle and practice with items ▪ Encourage them to write down important points ▪ Ask for return demonstrations ▪ Incorporate multimedia, such as computers and video cameras, to engage them actively

Table 4-3 Levels of Learning

Result	Level	Feature	Examples for Teaching Parents
Tell me and I may remember. OR I hear and I forget.	Auditory – Lowest level	Conveys information verbally	▪ Information that does not require visual or interactive reinforcement ▪ A discussion of contraception, nutrition, or medications ▪ Reinforce the message with printed and online materials to help them recall what they were told
Show me and I may remember. OR I see and I remember.	Visual – Middle level	Adds visual reinforcement to verbal instruction	▪ Demonstrate positioning the baby for feeding with a doll ▪ Chart or computer animation of breast anatomy and changes ▪ Demonstrate manual expression with a cloth breast ▪ Demonstrate use of a breast pump or other device ▪ Show a cloth breast, video clips, and photographs with discussions of engorgement, mastitis, nipple pain, and thrush
Involve me and I may master. OR I do and I understand.	Kinesthetic – Highest level	Actively engages the learner in the learning process	▪ Demonstrate positioning with a doll while the parent initiates a feeding ▪ Demonstrate manual expression or breast pump use while the parent practices the technique

styles and shows how learners can be reached based on their style.

Levels of Learning

Involving parents as active participants in their learning will heighten their ability to acquire new knowledge and perform new skills well. Auditory learning conveys information verbally. Visual learning adds visual reinforcement to verbal instruction. Kinesthetic learning actively engages the learner in the learning process. Each of these three levels of learning, as described in **Table 4-3**, builds on the previous level.

There will be times in interactions when verbal instructions are sufficient and appropriate. Visual demonstrations added to the instructions will enhance the teaching, as in **Figure 4-4**. Online videos and other visual resources can teach many aspects of lactation, including positioning and hand expression. Having parents interact with their learning by practicing along with a demonstration will enhance their learning (**Figure 4-5**). This active participation also provides visual reinforcement to the caregiver of the parents' level of understanding and mastery of the technique.

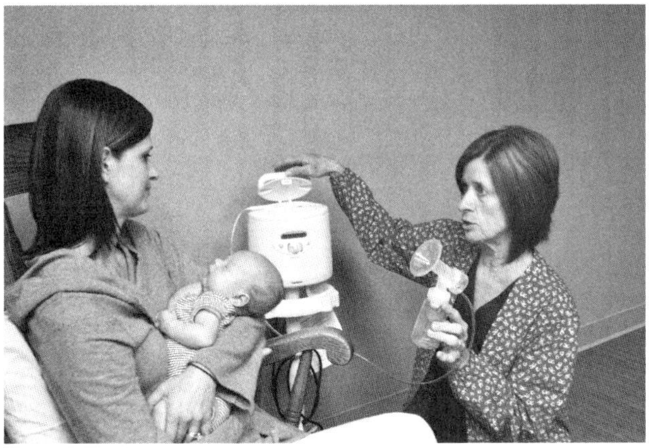

Figure 4-4 Demonstrating use of a breast pump.

Printed with permission of Anna Swisher.

Personalizing Learning

The rich background of experiences, capabilities, resources, and beliefs that parents bring to nursing make their needs different from those of other parents. Every parent and baby are a unique dyad. Relating to parents individually and on a personal level strengthens relationships and enhances caregiver effectiveness. Some parents will appear confident

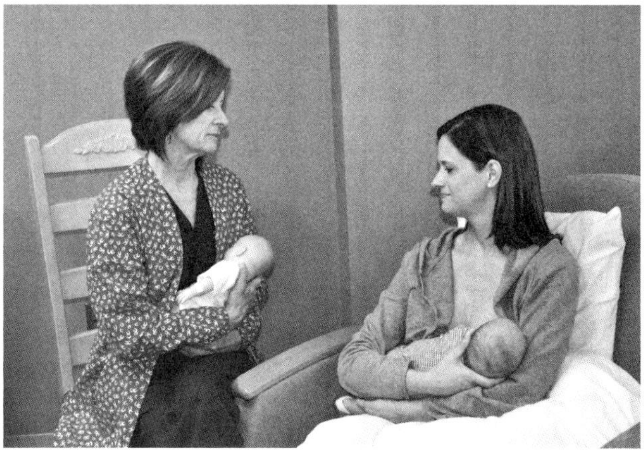

Figure 4-5 Demonstrating positioning with a return demonstration.

Printed with permission of Anna Swisher.

and knowledgeable. Others will have a greater need for increasing their self-esteem and confidence. Personalized education increases self-efficacy, reduces anxiety, and fosters a sense of self confidence (Brockway et al., 2017). Cultural and familial histories are important considerations as well (Thomson et al., 2020). Using the parent's and baby's names will personalize the exchange. Adapting to the family's language style, imagery, intensity, and sense of humor will help caregivers relate appropriately and sensitively.

Tailoring teaching and problem-solving to each dyad will help avoid appearing to have a rigid agenda. This individualized approach facilitates collaborative decision-making and client care. Capitalizing on parents' strengths and building on their capabilities will be especially helpful for parents who appear anxious or nervous when faced with a learning situation. When they learn a technique or overcome an obstacle, praise them for their accomplishment. Find something to praise about the baby as well. For example, "See how your baby looks at you!" or "Look at how your baby responds to your voice!" Because each parent and baby will learn at their own speed, it is important to keep pace with them. Be alert to signs of frustration or confusion and be prepared to slow down if it seems parents are not absorbing the teaching.

Respecting Parents' Autonomy

Parents have a great need to be autonomous and self-directed as they settle in with their babies. The very nature of a hospital environment results in a loss of a certain amount of control. Respecting parents' autonomy and self-direction will help them feel in greater control. Any intervention should have a valid reason for a caregiver becoming actively involved. Observing a parent's nursing technique may confirm that no help is needed. When assistance is appropriate, first teach techniques such as positioning and latch without touching the parent or baby. This hands-off approach actively involves parents in the learning process and contributes to their personal growth.

The "biological nurturing" approach to feedings respects an infant's innate ability to self-feed. Placing the baby skin to skin on the parent's stomach taps into a newborn's natural reflex to crawl up the parent's body, find the nipple, latch on, and begin to nurse. This hands-off approach allows caregivers to minimize interventions and ensure the parent's dignity and comfort (Colson, 2019). Some babies and parents will need a higher level of intervention, including hands-on help (Douglas & Keogh, 2017). When hands-on help is requested or required, always ask the parent permission to handle their baby and their body.

Facilitating Learning

Childbirth and lactation are life-changing events, optimal times for building on parents' willingness to learn. Asking pointed questions about the experience they bring to this life event (**Figure 4-6**) will engage them in determining their learning needs. A combination of teaching methods will help reach families in a wide variety of life circumstances with varied learning styles, needs, and knowledge levels. Methods include printed and verbal instructions, visual aids, and multimedia (computer, video clips, podcasts, online learning), as well as interactive learning, such as demonstrations, and verbal feedback. Personal stories enhanced with graphics and electronic content also engage learners. Parents respond favorably to receiving information in this way rather than through traditional medical information sheets.

- Is this their first baby, or are they an experienced parent?
- What exposure have they had to lactation?
- Do they have relatives or friends who nursed?
- Have they nursed before? If so, what was their experience like?
- What have they read or heard about lactation?
- What are their support system and resources?
- Do they have someone to help with caring for the baby or with nursing?
- How soon will they return to work or school?

Figure 4-6 Questions to assess a parent's learning needs.

Time for Practice

Observing a feeding session, as depicted in **Figure 4-7**, will help assess a parent's technique. If adjustments are needed, demonstrating the technique with a doll and asking for a return demonstration will avoid entering their space and touching the baby. **Figures 4-8** and **4-9** illustrate how to make the necessary adjustments to get a good latch and have the parent follow. Avoid physically placing the baby in position to nurse. Rather, talk the parent through the technique and remain available to help if needed as the feeding continues. This is a powerful approach that reinforces learning and allows time for reflection without judgment.

Transferring Learning to Home

Numerous teachable moments occur throughout a postpartum hospital stay. Optimal learning occurs when it takes place at a time when parents are most ready to learn. If a parent appears tired, distracted, or otherwise unable to focus, it is better to return later. When parents are stressed, discouraged, or uncertain, it is difficult to concentrate on learning or problem-solving until they work through their concerns. When they are receptive, help them talk through these emotional issues before attempting any new learning. Sequencing instruction to teachable moments will maximize the parent's ability to learn and to process and retain what was learned. When time allows, dividing learning into several visits will avoid offering too much information at one time.

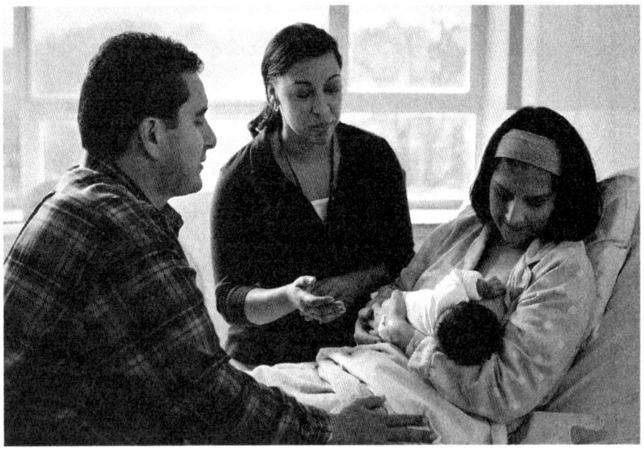

Figure 4-7 Observing a feeding.

Courtesy of the U.S. Department of Agriculture's Food and Nutrition Service.

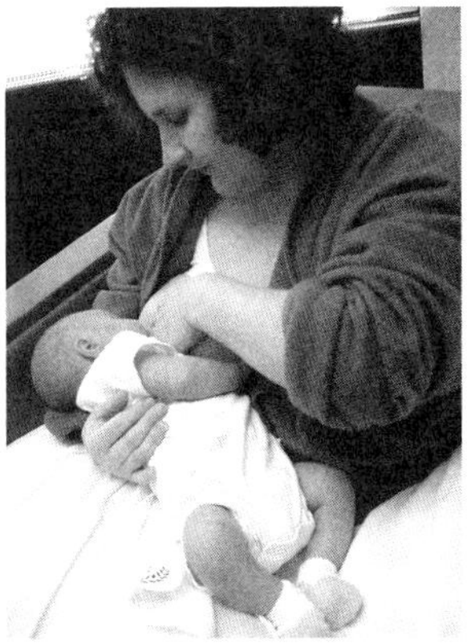

Figure 4-8 Positioning help is needed.

Printed with permission of Anna Swisher.

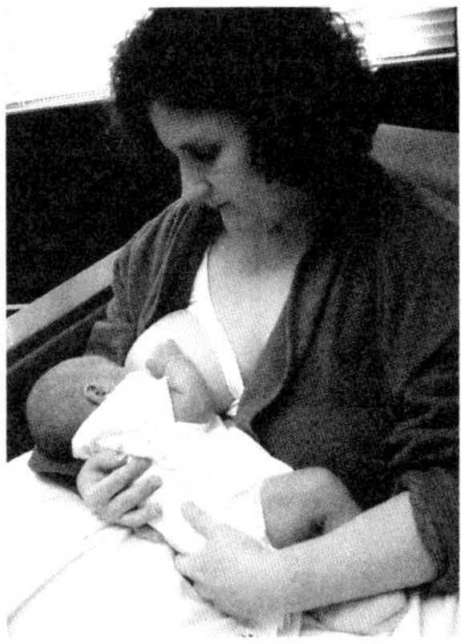

Figure 4-9 After positioning help.

Printed with permission of Anna Swisher.

- Will a return to work separate the parent and baby for regular periods?
- Are they a single parent?
- Are they a teen parent?
- Do they live with extended family?
- Do they have an active social life?
- Do they have demanding work responsibilities?

Figure 4-10 Questions to explore lifestyle concerns.

Parents appreciate help in accommodating lactation to their lifestyles. They will need to transfer what they learn about lactation in the hospital to their daily lives. The degree to which they learn and retain new skills in the early postpartum period will determine whether they can put them into practice at home. **Figure 4-10** provides questions to consider regarding lifestyle circumstances that may create challenges. Considering these lifestyle factors will help determine the best approach and most effective learning opportunities to help lactation fit into their daily lives.

Caregiver Confidence in Lactation

Healthcare professionals who promote lactation with confidence demonstrate that it is the best form of infant feeding and provide tangible encouragement and support. This in turn increases parents' self-confidence and empowers them to reach their feeding goals. Self-confident people inspire confidence in others. When caregivers approach parents with confidence in lactation and a belief in parents' ability to nurse, they help strengthen parents' confidence in their decisions and capabilities. Although most health workers agree with the evidence that nursing is superior to artificial feeding, fewer actively promote lactation with conviction. Some may be reluctant to take a strong stance on nursing after having fed their own babies formula. They may have had problems with nursing or had other personal experiences that diminished their perception of nursing.

Ambivalence and Mixed Messages

An approach laced with ambivalence and **mixed messages** fails to support families in making informed feeding decisions for their babies. A noncommittal attitude by health workers unwittingly promotes unhealthful practices by implying that artificial feeding is a choice equal to nursing. When parents fail to learn the important differences between the two feeding methods, they cannot make an informed choice about feeding their infant. Mixed messages compromise self-confidence and risk parents' second-guessing the wisdom of their decisions.

Caregivers need to avoid the implication that two equal infant feeding alternatives exist and that one is as good as the other. Asking, "Are you going to nurse or bottle-feed?" conveys a neutral stance and fails to inform parents about the health risks of formula to babies and the health risks to parents from not nursing. Unless an alternative is equally healthy and an equally good choice, questions should not imply endorsement or equality of the less healthy choice. Asking, "What questions do you have about nursing?" or "How can I help you with your feeding goals?" underscores the health imperative implicit in lactation. This messaging conveys the expectation that parents will nurse unless they respond otherwise.

If an expectant parent says they do not plan to nurse, a respectful and open-ended response might be, "I want to know how best to support you in your feeding choice. How did you decide on this option?" A sincere and supportive open-ended question can encourage parents to explore their motives, ask questions, and consider their choice. Even well-educated expectant parents may not recognize the importance of lactation to the health of both baby and parent. Exploring the factors behind the decision to formula feed will help dispel misunderstandings or allay fears. Helping parents become informed consumers empowers them to make healthy choices.

Obligation for Informed Choice

Consumer rights and caregiver responsibilities are significant elements in informed choice. Parents have a right to the information necessary to make an informed infant feeding choice. Caregivers have a responsibility to inform parents of their options so that they can make responsible decisions. All members of the healthcare team are responsible for educating families appropriately and helping them feel confident in nursing. Teaching should begin during antenatal care and continue throughout lactation. Caregivers should address parents' knowledge, health beliefs, and feeding intentions. They should also share evidence-based health information about the normalcy of nursing and the risks of artificial baby milk.

Guilt Related to Lactation

There are many forms of potential guilt associated with lactation. The fear of provoking guilt inhibits many caregivers from promoting lactation to their families. Parents who choose not to nurse may feel guilty because they worry they may not be doing what is best for their baby. Parents who wean early may feel guilt from not continuing to provide protection to their baby for the recommended time. Caregivers may feel guilty about the way they managed lactation in the past as new research changes best practice.

Caregiver Guilt in Promoting Lactation

Some caregivers may be reluctant to assertively promote lactation to their clients because of a fear that they will create guilt in parents who choose not to nurse. They may also worry about causing guilt in parents who choose to nurse and fail (Harrison et al., 2018). The rationale behind these fears fails to recognize the importance of nursing to the health of babies and parents. Withholding information to avoid making parents feel guilty denies a parent's right to make an informed feeding decision.

Guilt does not prevent caregivers from promoting healthy practices they know to be important. For example, when they advocate the use an infant car seat, they do not worry about offending parents who place their baby in danger by not using a car seat. Guilt is not a concern when informing parents about the need for immunizations or advising against cigarette smoking, illicit drugs, or alcohol. Guilt is not a consideration in recommending healthy diets, exercise, good hygiene, and dental care. Promoting lactation should be equally free of worry about causing parents to feel guilty if they choose a less healthy alternative. Healthcare providers who embrace lactation will be as assertive about promoting that health choice as they are with any other health practice.

Guilt from Not Nursing

Parents who do not nurse experience a loss at a conscious or subconscious level, regardless of whether the choice is by decision or imposed (Caes et al., 2021; Constantinou et al., 2021; Jackson et al., 2021). Withholding information about the superiority of human milk does not contribute to a trusting relationship with parents. Even worse, it can produce parental guilt if a child is diagnosed in later life with an illness for which human milk affords protection. As parents research their child's condition, they may learn that not nursing increased these risks. In addition to feeling guilty, the parents may then also regard the caregiver unfavorably for not helping them make an informed decision.

There are other considerable consequences of failing to promote lactation to parents who elect to formula feed. The cost of infant formula and feeding devices can strain family finances. Babies fed formula have higher rates of illness, sudden infant death, emotional neglect, and child abuse. They are at a greater risk for developing obesity, allergies, and asthma, among other health issues. The incidence of learning deficiencies is higher in children who are not nursed. IQ levels are lower as well. In addition, the potential for contamination of artificial baby milk places an infant's health at unnecessary risk. These realities are discussed in **Chapters 1** and **10** in more detail.

Guilt from Nursing Disappointment

A parent who tries to nurse and fails may feel guilt from the failure (McIntyre et al., 2018). Nursing parents assume a risk of having adequate milk production for their baby. Low milk production that requires supplementation can trigger feelings of guilt and anxiety. Perhaps a parent failed to receive the necessary caregiver support and encouragement to master lactation management techniques. Unsatisfying nursing experiences can create a sense of personal failure and abandonment. For some parents, the risk of failure may be more painful than the guilt of not nursing. Health providers can help avoid this by providing appropriate education and assistance and by creating safe and nonjudgmental spaces for parents to communicate through their disappointments.

Guilt from Past Actions

Some healthcare providers experience guilt when they consider the implications of their past actions. The lactation field continues to evolve in its recommended practices. That is the essence of evidence-based practice. As we learn more about lactation care and the consequences of past management, we change the way we practice. Past practices may have included unnecessary formula supplementation, frequent use of pacifiers, strict rules about frequency and length of feedings, arbitrary use of nipple shields, or sending families home with formula "gift packs." Caregivers may have presented lactation as complicated and reliant on a variety of gadgets and special techniques. Perhaps they formula-fed their own children and deal with the same guilt others experience from not nursing. They need to recognize that their past practices were based on what was considered appropriate at the time. Best practice evolves in the light of new information. Healthcare providers will continue to learn and change their practice based on research and new evidence.

Guilt as a Catalyst for Change

Guilt has the potential to motivate behavior change and can serve a positive purpose. By definition, guilt is "the act or state of having done a wrong or committed an offense." Parents who feel guilty about their choice not to nurse, to supplement with formula, or to wean early most likely believe that they are failing to do what is best for their baby. Their guilt can lead to personal growth and motivate them to change a particular behavior or action on behalf of their children. Caregiver guilt can be a catalyst for practicing evidence-based care, resulting in assertive advocacy of lactation and remaining current in best practices.

Parents' Self-Confidence

Self-confidence, a belief in our personal worth and our likelihood of succeeding, is an essential component of our daily lives. Self-confidence is especially important when facing a new life experience, such as childbirth or lactation. The degree to which parents trust their bodies and their capabilities affects their level of self-confidence. Some parents continue to nurse despite extraordinary difficulties, whereas others give up when they encounter the slightest problem. How we empower parents to trust their instincts and their babies may significantly affect their nursing satisfaction and duration. Self-confidence, image, and other emotional factors in self-perceptions are significant determinants of lactation outcome (Wouk et al., 2020).

Having a realistic picture of what to expect in childbirth and in the early days and weeks of lactation can be a pivotal factor in parents' self-confidence. Idealistic expectations can lead to emotional distress when the actual experience fails to meet expectations. This distress may be further compounded by feelings of guilt and inadequacy if premature weaning occurs. Clinicians have a responsibility to accurately reflect the reality of lactation and to support parents when they experience difficulties (Marshall et al., 2019).

Self-Efficacy

Belief in our abilities determines how we feel, think, behave, and motivate ourselves. Self-confidence is a combination of self-esteem and general **self-efficacy**, which is a belief in our ability to perform specific tasks. The most effective way of creating a strong sense of confidence in a new skill or role is through mastery of the necessary skills. Acquiring self-efficacy begins with setting a goal and making a commitment to achieve it. Individuals with high self-efficacy—those who believe they can perform well—are more likely to persist longer despite obstacles and challenges as they strive to attain their goals. They approach difficult tasks as challenges to be mastered and maintain a strong commitment. Validating parents for their capabilities leads to them making a greater effort to reach their goals (Albanese et al., 2019; Joulaie et al., 2019).

Providing lactation education to parents, supporting them in their attempts at mastery, and praising their accomplishments help empower them to attain high levels of personal self-efficacy with nursing. Their self-efficacy will increase as they learn and hone their lactation management skills. Parents who intend to formula-feed report poorer self-efficacy about lactation (Grant et al., 2019), whereas those who intend to nurse have higher levels of lactation knowledge (Suárez-Cotelo et al., 2019). Mastering lactation can increase a parent's belief in their abilities and their feelings of competence. Interventions aimed at improving self-efficacy with lactation are intended to result in longer and more exclusive nursing.

The early weeks of lactation are a pivotal time for establishing confidence with feeding practices. Immediate skin-to-skin contact after birth enhances nursing self-efficacy (Karimi et al., 2019). Many parents view nursing as the one thing they can control in their immediate postpartum environment. Increased self-efficacy lowers anxiety and can result in greater nursing intensity and exclusivity (Asimaki et al., 2022; Melo et al., 2021; Shipp, 2022). A perception that lactation hinders independence and self-identity (life apart from being a parent) may influence nursing duration and exposure to formula feeding (Bartle & Harvey, 2017). Helping parents feel in control of nursing can shift the perception that lactation hinders their independence and will help them transition more smoothly to the parental role.

Support, especially in-person contacts, is an essential component of improving lactation outcomes and reducing the isolation experienced by many new parents. Lactation promotion targeting the whole family increases parents' motivation and self-efficacy (Aghababaei et al., 2022; Wu et al., 2021). Peer support promotes self-efficacy, well-being, and **empowerment**. Civilian military wives report increased self-efficacy resulting from a sense of community and supportive lactation consultants and other healthcare facilitators (Ringo & Gephart, 2022). Support from parents' social networks promotes stronger self-efficacy in, duration of, and confidence in public nursing (Maleki-Saghooni et al., 2019; Robinson et al., 2019).

Low self-efficacy in the early postpartum period can risk early cessation of lactation. Many factors can make it difficult for new parents to have the needed knowledge for nursing. For example, there is a correlation between prenatal education and increased nursing duration (Kehinde et al., 2023). Therefore, parents of late-preterm and early-term infants may not have benefited from prenatal education. This may explain why these parents exhibit less exclusivity and lower self-efficacy and satisfaction with nursing (Ahmed & Rojjanasrirat, 2021). Achieving a positive and rewarding lactation experience helps produce feelings of power and accomplishment. Help and support beyond hospital discharge to increase self-efficacy and confidence can improve nursing duration and exclusivity. Timely follow-up, information, and support in the early weeks at home facilitate acquiring a sense of control that helps extend lactation.

Helping Increase Confidence

Confidence is a strong predictor of nursing duration and exclusivity (Fan et al., 2022; Khresheh &

Ahmad, 2018; Muelbert & Giugliani, 2018; Rocha et al., 2018). Prenatal education about nursing is an important factor in establishing parental commitment and increases parents' confidence that they can overcome later challenges. Parents with a high intention to nurse are less likely to supplement with formula. Increasing a parent's confidence in their ability to nurse increases the likelihood that they will initiate nursing exclusively, and nurse for longer.

Helping parents set feeding goals that fit with their unique needs and wants and providing the necessary education and support may enhance their self-perception and empower them to reach their goals. A combination of prenatal and postnatal peer support increases confidence and self-efficacy in nursing (Houghtaling et al., 2017). Telephone and virtual support can also provide reassurance, boost confidence, and increase the determination to continue (Harris-Luna & Badr, 2018).

Self-confidence and the quality of parent–infant relationships are strengthened when parents receive prenatal, postpartum, and ongoing support. This combination of education, support, and networking with other parents helps empower nursing families. A positive nursing experience can have a tremendous positive impact on a healthy taking on of the parental role. Peer, online, telephone, electronic, and person-to-person support help to create the safe community new parents need in acquiring their parental roles. A positive self-image and confidence in parenting are more likely to lead to positive parent–child attachments.

Parents who lack confidence have difficulty establishing positive parent–child attachments. Depressed parents may negatively affect the health and development of their children (Ali, 2018). Anxiety and depression are also associated with shorter nursing exclusivity and duration (Ngo et al., 2019; Vieira et al., 2018). Providing support for coping with the pressures linked to early parenting will encourage longer nursing duration. Strategies for managing stress include increasing lactation knowledge, staying relaxed, using positive self-talk, challenging unhelpful beliefs, learning problem-solving skills, reaching out to other new parents, and joining a community new-parents group.

Trusting Parents and Babies

Caregivers who demonstrate confidence in the capabilities of parents and babies build on parents' self-confidence and encourage them to engage in self-direction. Such empowerment requires caregivers to trust that parents and babies can assume control. Newborns have amazing capabilities from the moment of birth. Teaching parents how to read and respond to infant language, and refraining from interfering, allows babies to communicate effectively to have their needs met.

Likewise, believing in parents' abilities can help facilitate their growth. Parents who feel in control and have their successes acknowledged learn to trust themselves and their babies. They feel more independent, self-reliant, and confident. Consequently, they find it easier to adjust to taking responsibility for their learning. They develop problem-solving skills, accept the consequences of their decisions and actions, and control their outcomes.

Relinquishing Control

Trusting in the capabilities of parents and babies enables caregivers to relinquish much of the control that is traditionally associated with health care. New parents need the opportunity to use their inner resources to become self-sufficient. A parent who feels controlled may not recognize ways to help themselves. If they become dependent on others they may lose sight of their strengths, expecting others to solve their problems. They may also blame those same people if their problems persist. Caregivers can guide parents with their expertise while providing the knowledge and skills they need to follow their instinctive ability to nurse.

An expectant parent's privacy and autonomy are invaded the moment they pass through a hospital door. They are placed in a dependent role during labor, throughout delivery, and after they give birth. Hospital and healthcare provider policies often impose unnecessary controls and practices, with others making decisions about their care. The loss of control many parents experience during childbirth and postpartum care can undermine their confidence and sense of personal efficacy. Many parents choose to birth with midwives at birthing centers or choose a home birth to maintain greater control regarding their care and that of their infants (Yuill et al., 2020).

Minimizing Interventions

Lactation policies should model self-reliance and parental decision-making from the very beginning. Avoiding unnecessary interference and ensuring that any intervention has a clear and specific purpose will help parents reestablish some of their control. Parents are often told to hold their breast during a feeding, wear a bra with good support, avoid certain foods, feed on a schedule, use both sides at a feeding, or use only one side at a feeding. Such arbitrary rules are counterproductive to the goal of empowering parents to trust their instincts and their baby. Minimizing unnecessary interventions places control with babies and parents—where it belongs.

The Empowering Nature of Humor

Humor has a direct effect on mental and physical health and is important in all aspects of our lives. It is a way of life, an attitude. Humor can be an indirect form of healthcare communication between caregivers and clients. It can help to establish relationships, reduce tension and anxiety, release anger in a socially acceptable way, avoid or deny painful feelings, and facilitate learning (Hardy, 2020; Osincup, 2020; Proyer & Rodden, 2020). Personalities and levels of receptiveness will determine when humor is appropriate. Easterners are generally less likely to use humor as a coping strategy in comparison with their Western counterparts (Jiang et al., 2019). Extroverted people tend to have a greater appreciation for humor. Mild forms of humor can help even reticent parents relax and release oxytocin.

Humor in Health Care

Humor, as a component of health care, is a humanistic approach that conveys acceptance, respect, caring, and a genuine interest in helping. Humor evolves naturally in a relaxed climate of support and acceptance. Such an atmosphere enhances parents' self-concept and helps them remain tolerant and understanding of themselves and their baby. Parents who lack self-confidence, who are anxious about their ability to nurse, or who have little support from family or friends may find it difficult to find enjoyment. The warmth and caring transmitted to parents will help them use humor to relieve the stresses of learning how to be a parent and how to nurse. **Figure 4-11** illustrates how humor can help parents deal with the stress, tension, and frustration that are common in the early days of lactation.

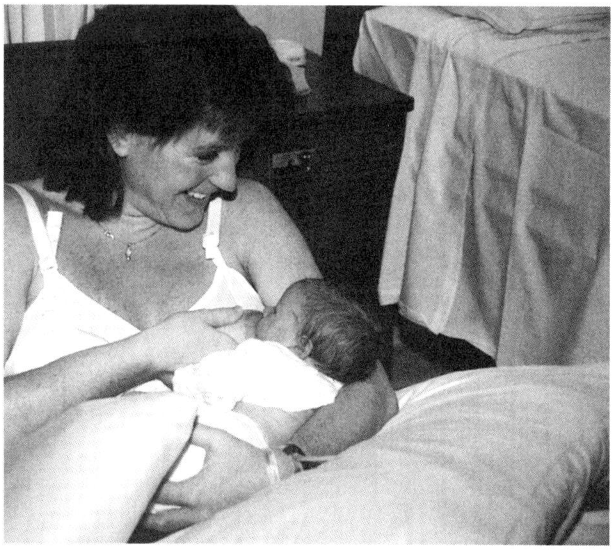

Figure 4-11 Parent laughing while beginning to nurse.

Printed with permission of Judith Lauwers.

Humor blended with a relaxed atmosphere and appropriate timing and style can help establish trust and enhance interactions with receptive parents. The use of humor can help parents gain perspective and recognize that a situation may not be as serious as it may seem. With a positive outlook, they are more likely to meet new challenges with enthusiasm and optimism. Parents will be better able to laugh at themselves and shake off missteps as they and their baby learn to respond to each other. Humor can be considered a form of preventive medicine. It increases self-confidence, improves parents' frame of mind and perspective, and helps them enjoy their baby.

Traditionally, healthcare providers have intentionally avoided humor in their interactions with clients. Incorporating humor into clinical interactions may be challenging for caregivers who take themselves too seriously. Health professionals can be so intent on becoming better in their profession that they fail to enjoy themselves in the process. Learning to laugh at ourselves helps us take ourselves more lightly and can reduce power imbalances with clients. Learning to enjoy life and its challenges will help us keep perspective and humanize our work with families. Humor can come through in the form of a warm and friendly approach, a smile, or a light touch. Such pleasantries are a valuable component in lactation care.

Health Benefits of Humor

Humor causes biochemical changes in the body that are enormously healing and therapeutic. Norman Cousins (1979) wrote about humor therapy that helped him recover from a life-threatening disease that produced intense pain and paralysis. Ten minutes of watching comedy films and reading humorous literature produced genuine laughter that had an anesthetic effect and gave him at least 2 hours of pain-free sleep. Gradually, he recovered and went on to research the symbiotic role of humor and wellness.

Therapeutic humor in health care promotes health and wellness by stimulating a playful discovery, expression, or appreciation of the absurdity or incongruity of life's situations (Osincup, 2020). Humor facilitates healing or coping, whether physical, emotional, cognitive, social, or spiritual. Humor therapy decreases agitation and increases well-being (Gonot-Schoupinsky & Garip, 2018; van der Wal & Kok, 2019; Yoshikawa et al., 2018). Individuals with advanced illnesses highly value humor. Humorous interactions with healthcare providers can be acceptable and appropriate despite the severity of illness (Pinna et al., 2018).

Medical experts know that negative emotions can create organic changes such as headaches and ulcers. It makes sense, therefore, that positive emotions can produce positive biochemical changes in the body as well. Laughter produces positive effects in most of the body's major physiologic systems (Hayashi et al., 2016; Lapierre et al., 2019; Law et al., 2018). It speeds heart rate, lowers blood pressure, accelerates breathing, and increases oxygen consumption. It can stimulate muscles and relax muscle tension, thereby reducing pain and anxiety. Laughter stimulates the cardiovascular system, the sympathetic nervous system, and the production of catecholamines and endorphins, thereby boosting the immune system. Following this arousal state, respiration, heart rate, and muscle tension return to below-normal levels.

Humor Enhances Learning

Humor increases the amount of adrenaline in the brain, stimulating alertness and memory and enhancing learning and creativity. Laughter incorporated into learning can help ensure that parents learn a lesson well. Shared laughter is energizing and increases the ability to take risks. Parents will be more comfortable and will therefore be more receptive to advice and feel more welcome to ask questions and offer input.

Humor and laughter increase productivity and contribute to learning enjoyment, interest, motivation, and creativity. Integrating humor with learning promotes critical thinking and emotional intelligence. A humorous approach stimulates divergent thinking and increases a willingness to look at a situation in a new way. This strategy frees the flow of ideas to consider new alternatives and solutions. Humor stimulates both the right and the left hemispheres of the brain at the same time and enables the brain to work at its fullest capacity. When the right and left brains are integrated and functioning simultaneously, the capacity for learning is at its highest level.

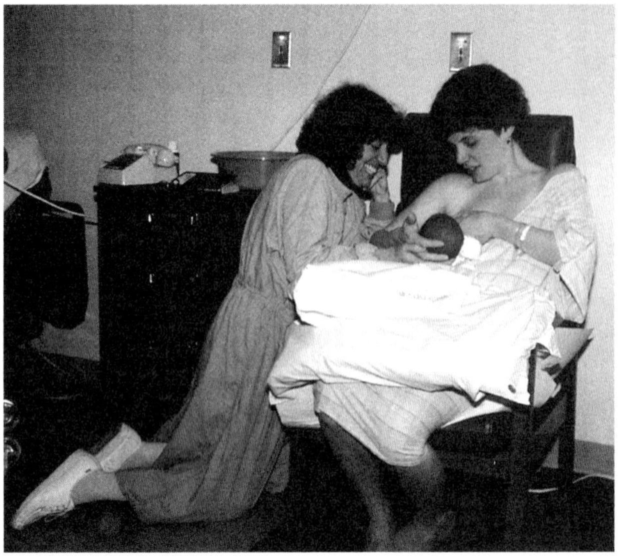

Figure 4-12 Using effective body language and humor.

Printed with permission of Judith Lauwers.

Humor in Lactation Support

Lactation support presents many opportunities for infusing teaching with humor. Parents are more likely to remember what they learn with the use of humorous imagery and stories laced with humor. Amusing terminology or a play on words can help when teaching lactation techniques. Keeping a humor diary can capture light moments with parents and could also be used for professional self-reflection. When used appropriately, humor enhances interactions and enriches the lives of families and colleagues (**Figure 4-12**).

It is important to recognize that not every situation calls for the use of humor. Parents in crisis may not respond favorably to a caregiver's attempts at humor. Assessing how receptive parents would be to lightening the mood with humor can indicate whether humor would be helpful or a hindrance to helping a client achieve their goals.

Summary

A caregiver's commitment, beliefs, attitude, and approach affect parents' ability to reach their feeding goals. Demonstrating a sincere belief in the importance of lactation increases parents' self-image and confidence. Teaching lactation to parents and providing opportunities for them to practice and repeat the techniques will help them master the necessary skills. Developing partnerships with parents to explore options in problem-solving helps them grow as active, informed, and responsible health consumers. New parents will continue to grow in a climate that relinquishes medical control, limits interventions, and trusts in their abilities and the abilities of their babies. A personalized approach with every parent—one that assesses their needs as adult learners, capitalizes on their strengths, and praises their accomplishments—helps lead to long-term satisfaction. Humor can help establish an optimal learning climate and develop rapport with parents.

What You Learned–At a Glance

Conversation Starters with Parents

- How involved are you in your healthcare decisions?
- How do you prefer to learn new information and skills?
- How confident do you feel in your ability to nurse your baby?
- How do you respond to health professionals using humor in your interactions?

Health Consumerism

- Members of the healthcare team are key players in helping parents become informed health consumers.
- Forming a partnership with parents empowers them to make decisions and accept responsibility for their actions.
- Control and power should be placed with the parents and baby, not with the caregiver.
- Reducing unnecessary medical interventions protects the rights of parents and babies.

Learning

- Reinforcing verbal instruction with visual aids, including demonstrations (and return demonstrations), internet resources, mobile apps, and written materials enhances learning.
- Offering too much information at one time can overwhelm parents and make it difficult for them to encode and store the information.
- An effective learning climate is relaxed, trusting, mutually respectful, informal, warm, collaborative, and supportive.
- An individualized approach recognizes learning needs and readiness and keeps pace with parents and babies.
- Actively involving the learner heightens learning and retention.
- Self-directed learning places responsibility on learners to plan, carry out, and evaluate their learning.

Confidence

- Assuming that parents will nurse their newborns unless they say otherwise promotes lactation as the normal and healthy feeding method.
- A neutral approach to infant feeding fails to teach parents about the health risks of not nursing.
- Past actions that were considered appropriate at the time are not a reason for caregiver guilt.
- Guilt can lead to personal growth and informed decision-making.
- People who have high self-efficacy persist longer to attain their goals.
- Parents with low nursing self-efficacy may be at risk for early weaning.
- The appropriate use of humor in interactions helps to reduce stress and enhances learning.

References

Abdulrahaman MD, et al. Multimedia tools in the teaching and learning processes: a systematic review. *Heliyon*. 2020;6(11): e05312.

Aghababaei S, et al. Promoting maternal self efficacy and paternal attitudes towards breastfeeding: a randomized controlled trial. *Glob Health Promot*. 2022; 29(4):17579759221091194.

Ahmed AH, Rojjanasrirat W. Breastfeeding outcomes, self-efficacy, and satisfaction among low-income women with late-preterm, early-term, and full-term infants. *J Obstet Gynecol Neonatal Nurs*. 2021;50(5):583–596.

Albanese I, et al. Achieving results-oriented goals through patient partnership. *J Gen Intern Med*. 2019;34(7):1072–1073.

Ali E. Women's experiences with postpartum anxiety disorders: a narrative literature review. *Int J Women's Health*. 2018;10:237–249.

Asimaki E, et al. Main biopsychosocial factors influencing breastfeeding: a systematic review. *Maedica (Bucur)*. 2022;17(4): 955–962.

Association for Applied and Therapeutic Humor. What is therapeutic humor? 2023. https://www.aath.org

Bahrambeygi F, et al. Hospital health literacy conceptual explanation: a qualitative content analysis based on experts and population perspectives. *J Edu Health Promot*. 2023;12:31.

Bartle NC, Harvey K. Explaining infant feeding: the role of previous personal and vicarious experience on attitudes, subjective norms, self-efficacy, and breastfeeding outcomes. *Br J Health Psychol*. 2017;22(4):763–785.

Boland RJ, Amonoo HL. Types of learners. *Psychiatr Clin North Am*. 2021;44(2):141–148.

Brockway M, et al. Interventions to improve breastfeeding self-efficacy and resultant breastfeeding rates: a systematic review and meta-analysis. *J Hum Lact*. 2017;33(3):486–499.

Caes L, et al. Exploring women's perceptions of pain when breastfeeding using online forums. *Int Breastfeed J*. 2021;16(1):84.

Charokar K, Dulloo P. Self-directed learning theory to practice: a footstep towards the path of being a life-long learner. *J Adv Med Educ Prof*. 2022;10(3):135–144.

Childs-Kean L, et al. Use of learning style frameworks in health science education. *Am J Pharm Educ*. 2020;84(7):ajpe7885.

Colson S. *Biological Nurturing: Instinctual Breastfeeding*. 2nd ed. Amarillo, TX: Praeclarus Press; 2019.

Constantinou G, et al. Reviewing the experiences of maternal guilt—the "motherhood myth" influence. *Health Care Women Int*. 2021;42(4–6):852–876.

Corballis MC. Evolution of cerebral asymmetry. *Prog Brain Res*. 2019;250:153–178.

Cousins N. *Anatomy of an Illness*. New York: Norton; 1979.

DiMattio MJK, Hudacek SS. Educating generation Z: psychosocial dimensions of the clinical learning environment that predict student satisfaction. *Nurse Educ Pract*. 2020;49:102901.

Douglas P, Keogh R. Gestalt breastfeeding: helping mothers and infants optimize positional stability and intraoral breast tissue volume for effective, pain-free milk transfer. *J Hum Lact*. 2017;33(3):509–518.

Eckleberry-Hunt J, et al. Is medical education ready for generation Z? *J Grad Med Educ*. 2018;10(4):378–381.

Fan HSL, et al. The association between breastfeeding self-efficacy and mode of infant feeding. *Breastfeed Med*. 2022;17(8):687–697.

Gonot-Schoupinsky FN, Garip G. Laughter and humour interventions for well-being in older adults: a systematic review and intervention classification. *Complement Ther Med*. 2018;38:85–91.

Grant A, et al. Understanding health behaviour in pregnancy and infant feeding intentions in low-income women from the UK through qualitative visual methods and application to the COM-B (Capability, Opportunity, Motivation-Behaviour) model. *BMC Pregnancy Childbirth*. 2019;19(1):56.

Hardy C. Humor and sympathy in medical practice. *Med Health Care Philos*. 2020;23(2):179–190.

Harris-Luna ML, Badr LK. Pragmatic trial to evaluate the effect of a promotora telephone intervention on the duration of breastfeeding. *J Obstet Gynecol Neonatal Nurs*. 2018;47(6):738–748.

Harrison M, et al. Navigating motherhood and maternal transitional infant feeding: learnings for health professionals. *Appetite*. 2018;121:228–236.

Hayashi K, et al. Laughter is the best medicine? a cross-sectional study of cardiovascular disease among older Japanese adults. *J Epidemiol*. 2016;26(10):546–552.

Houghtaling B, et al. Likelihood of breastfeeding within the USDA's food and nutrition service special supplemental nutrition program for Women, Infants, and Children population. *J Hum Lact*. 2017;33(1):83–97.

Hsu YM, et al. Effectiveness of multimedia-based learning on the improvement of knowledge, attitude, and behavioral intention toward COVID-19 prevention among nurse aides in Taiwan: a parallel-interventional study. *Healthcare (Basel)*. 2022;10(7):1206.

Hutchinson E. *Dimensions of Human Behavior: The Changing Life Course*. 6th ed. Thousand Oaks, CA: SAGE Publications, Inc.; 2019.

Jackson L, et al. Guilt, shame, and postpartum infant feeding outcomes: A systematic review. *Matern Child Nutr*. 2021;17(3): e13141.

Jaks R, et al. Parental digital health information seeking behavior in Switzerland: a cross-sectional study. *BMC Public Health*. 2019;19(1):225.

Jiang T, et al. Cultural differences in humor perception, usage, and implications. *Front Psychol*. 2019;10:123.

Joulaie M, et al. Maternal perception of self-efficacy and involvement in young children with prelingual hearing loss. *Indian J Otolaryngol Head Neck Surg*. 2019;71(1):48–53.

Karimi FZ, et al. The effect of mother-infant skin-to-skin contact immediately after birth on exclusive breastfeeding: a systematic review and meta-analysis. *J Turk Ger Gynecol Assoc*. 2019;21(1):46–56.

Kehinde J, et al. The effectiveness of prenatal breastfeeding education on breastfeeding uptake postpartum: a systematic review. *Midwifery*. 2023;118:103579.

Khresheh RM, Ahmad NM. Breastfeeding self-efficacy among pregnant women in Saudi Arabia. *Saudi Med J*. 2018;39(11):1116–1122.

Lapierre SS, et al. Effects of mirthful laughter on pain tolerance: a randomized controlled investigation. *J Bodyw Mov Ther*. 2019;23(4):733–738.

Law MM, et al. A comparison of the cardiovascular effects of simulated and spontaneous laughter. *Complement Ther Med*. 2018;37:103–109.

Maleki-Saghooni N, et al. Investigation of the relationship between social support and breastfeeding self-efficacy in primiparous breastfeeding mothers. *J Matern Fetal Neonatal Med*. 2019;24:1–6.

Marshall NE, et al. Impact of maternal obesity and breastfeeding intention on lactation intensity and duration. *Matern Child Nutr*. 2019;15(2):e12732.

McIntyre L, et al. Breast is best . . . except when it's not. *J Hum Lact*. 2018;34(3):575–580.

Melo LCO, et al. Anxiety and its influence on maternal breastfeeding self-efficacy. *Rev Lat Am Enfermagem*. 2021;29:e3485.

Muelbert M, Giugliani ERJ. Factors associated with the maintenance of breastfeeding for 6, 12, and 24 months in adolescent mothers. *BMC Public Health*. 2018;18(1):675.

Nancekivell SE, et al. A slippery myth: how learning style beliefs shape reasoning about multimodal instruction and related scientific evidence. *Cogn Sci*. 2021;45(10):e13047.

Ngo LTH, et al. Breastfeeding self-efficacy and related factors in postpartum Vietnamese women. *Midwifery*. 2019;70:84–91.

Nutbeam D, Lloyd JE. Understanding and responding to health literacy as a social determinant of health. *Annu Rev Public Health*. 2021;42:159–173.

Osincup P. How to use humor in clinical settings. *AMA J Ethics.* 2020;22(7):e588–595. https://journalofethics.ama-assn.org/article/how-use-humor-clinical-settings/2020-07

Pinna MÁC, et al. The use of humor in palliative care: a systematic literature review. *Am J Hosp Palliat Care.* 2018;35(10):1342–1354.

Proyer RT, Rodden FA. Virtuous humor in health care. *AMA J Ethics.* 2020;22(7):e615–618.

Ringo N, Gephart SM. Exploring greater rates of breastfeeding among civilian military wives. *Nurs Womens Health.* 2022;26(1):10–20.

Robinson A, et al. It takes an e-village: supporting African American mothers in sustaining breastfeeding through Facebook communities. *J Hum Lact.* 2019;35(3):569–582.

Robinson JD, Persky AM. Developing self-directed learners. *Am J Pharm Educ.* 2020;84(3):847512.

Rocha IS, et al. Influence of maternal confidence on exclusive breastfeeding until six months of age: a systematic review. *Cien Saude Colet.* 2018;23(11):3609–3619.

Rogers LS, Cohen MS. Medical education in pediatric and congenital heart disease: a focus on generational learning and technology in education. *Prog Pediatr Cardiol.* 2020;59:101305.

Schiffman L, Wisenblit J. *Consumer Behavior. What's New in Marketing.* 12th ed. Upper Saddle River, NJ: Pearson Education; 2019.

Schnapp BH, et al. Avocado toasted: mythbusting "millennials," "generation Z," and generational theory. *AEM Educ Train.* 2022;6(3):e10757.

Shipp GM, et al. Breastfeeding self-efficacy as a predictor of breastfeeding intensity among African American women in the Mama Bear Feasibility Trial. *Breastfeed Med.* 2022;17(5):453–458.

Shorey S, et al. Learning styles, preferences and needs of generation Z healthcare students: scoping review. *Nurse Educ Pract.* 2021;57:103247.

Suárez-Cotelo MDC, et al. Breastfeeding knowledge and relation to prevalence. *Rev Esc Enferm USP.* 2019;53:e03433.

Tang B, et al. Online lectures in undergraduate medical education: scoping review. *JMIR Med Educ.* 2018;4(1):e11.

Thomson G, et al. Exploring the use and experience of an infant feeding genogram to facilitate an assets-based approach to support infant feeding. *BMC Pregnancy Childbirth.* 2020;20(1):569.

van der Wal CN, Kok RN. Laughter-inducing therapies: systematic review and meta-analysis. *Soc Sci Med.* 2019;232:473–488.

Vieira ES, et al. Breastfeeding self-efficacy and postpartum depression: a cohort study. *Rev Lat Am Enfermagem.* 2018;26:e3035.

Vizcaya-Moreno MF, Pérez-Cañaveras RM. Social media used and teaching methods preferred by generation Z students in the nursing clinical learning environment: a cross-sectional research study. *Int J Environ Res Public Health.* 2020;17(21):8267.

Wouk K, et al. Positive emotions during infant feeding and breastfeeding outcomes. *J Hum Lact.* 2020;36(1):157–167.

Wu W, et al. Factors influencing breastfeeding practices in China: a meta-aggregation of qualitative studies. *Matern Child Nutr.* 2021;17(4):e13251.

Yfanti A, Doukakis S. Debunking the neuromyth of learning style. *Adv Exp Med Biol.* 2021;1338:145–153.

Yoshikawa Y, et al. Beneficial effect of laughter therapy on physiological and psychological function in elders. *Nurs Open.* 2018;6(1):93–99.

Yuill C, et al. Women's experiences of decision-making and informed choice about pregnancy and birth care: a systematic review and meta-synthesis of qualitative research. *BMC Pregnancy Childbirth.* 2020;20(1):343.

Zénon A, et al. An information-theoretic perspective on the costs of cognition. *Neuropsychologia.* 2019;123:5–18.

CHAPTER 5

Communication and Counseling Skills

Communication is a complex process that needs practice to be used effectively. Clinical communication is calculated, deliberate, purposeful, and focused. It is intended to collect information, to assess and modify behavior, to educate, to collaborate, and to provide emotional support. A clinician who cannot communicate well limits the quality of their care despite having excellent clinical understanding and technical ability. Skilled communication is central to building therapeutic relationships and positive client–clinician interactions.

Counseling is the most basic element in the helping process. Helping with lactation goes far beyond book knowledge, research, scientific principles, and clinical practice. In the absence of effective counseling skills, the knowledge and wisdom may be misunderstood or not absorbed. Members of the healthcare team have a responsibility to acquire the skills and techniques that will maximize their effectiveness in helping families.

KEY TERMS

Active listening
Affirmation
Attending
Attentive listening
Body language
Empathetic listening
Motivational interviewing (MI)
Open-ended question
Passive listening
Pretending
Probes
Reflective listening
Selective listening
Self-efficacy
Trauma-informed care
Vicarious trauma
Voice tone

Communication

Communication is a core clinical skill in health care (International Board of Lactation Consultant Examiners [IBLCE], 2023; White & Preda, 2022). It is influenced by culture, perceptions, values, relationships, context, and the content of a message. Interpersonal skills are key to communicating effectively and building relationships. Clear, accurate communication reduces confusion, frustration, and misinterpretation. Body language, tone of voice, and the words that are spoken determine how the message is received. Nonverbal language makes a far greater impression than the content of a message. Appearing rushed, speaking quickly, or failing to establish eye contact can hinder communication. Being aware of body language and other components of how you communicate will help you be more effective in your interactions.

Communicating over the telephone relies on voice tone and the spoken message without the advantage of conveying body language. Texting, tweeting, online support, and social media rely entirely on the written word, creating even greater challenges for effective communication. The absence of both body language and voice tone makes written messages pivotal. When any of the three components is inaccessible, even greater attention to the available component(s) is important.

The Importance of the Spoken Word

The words we use account for less than 10% of the message that is received (Fast, 2014). Because nonverbal elements of communication eclipse the spoken message, it is especially important that what we say creates the effect we want. Some words or phrases can unintentionally create doubt, send mixed messages, compromise self-confidence, or be offensive. They can create a negative impression or imply that a parent is doing something incorrectly. **Table 5-1** illustrates examples of phrases that send unintended messages. Attention to the words we use can avoid unintentionally offending parents and undermining their confidence.

Table 5-1 Phrases That Send Mixed Messages

What Is Said	What the Parent May Hear
You need your rest. I'll take your baby to the nursery for you.	■ You can't get enough rest if you keep your baby with you. ■ It doesn't matter if you skip a feeding. ■ We can give the baby a bottle of formula. ■ Formula is just as good as your milk.
Are you going to try to nurse?	■ You might not be able to nurse. ■ A lot of parents try and fail. ■ You can try, but don't be surprised if it doesn't work.
Do you have any milk yet?	■ You might not have enough milk for your baby. ■ We might need to give your baby a bottle. ■ You should have more milk by now. ■ Some parents never make enough milk.

The Use of "But"

The word *but* is often used to join two thoughts. However, doing so negates the first half of what is said and alters the intended message. Parent who is told, "You're holding your baby in a good position, but if you bring your baby in closer, you'll get a better latch" may think, "I'm not holding my baby right. I feel so dumb!" As soon as they hear the word *but*, they forget the first part of the statement. Although the intent was to help the parent learn how to achieve a better latch, the phrasing undermined their self-confidence.

A simple way to connect two thoughts without sending a negative message is to replace the word *but* with *and*. For example, "You have a good start positioning, and if you bring your baby in closer, you will get an even better latch." Another way to rephrase it is, "That's a great start. Now, if you bring your baby in closer, the latch will be even deeper." Improving technique without the suggestion that something is incorrect preserves parents' self-confidence and increases their growth.

The Use of "Should"

The word *should* is often used to convey a recommendation. However, saying it to parents risks sounding judgmental and implies your expectations or that they are doing something incorrectly. Eliminating the word *should* avoids sending a judgmental message or undermining parents' confidence. When teaching parents about feeding frequency, for example, instead of saying, "You should feed your baby whenever they demonstrate a hunger cue," you could say, "When you watch for hunger cues, you will know when to feed your baby." Both examples convey the same concept. However, the first one suggests what is correct and appropriate. The second one focuses on the parents' instincts and preserves their self-confidence.

Negative Imagery

Some phrases related to childbirth and lactation, such as *incompetent cervix*, *failure to progress*, *insufficient milk production*, and *growth faltering* can create negative images. Even words intended to be positive can suggest the possibility of something negative. For example, to indicate a desire to help parents succeed at nursing raises the possibility that they may not succeed. Using the term *inadequate milk production* when talking to a parent may create worry that milk production might be inadequate. Rephrasing such messages can send a more positive impression. For example, this response can refer to parents producing enough milk to meet their baby's needs.

Gender-Neutral Language

The way we use language can significantly affect those around us. Language can make people feel respected, or it can make them feel excluded. Using gender-neutral language demonstrates respect for people of all backgrounds, genders, and beliefs. Gender-neutral, also called *gender-inclusive*, language avoids reference to a particular sex or gender. For example, using the singular *they* instead of saying *he or she* is inclusive for males, females, and nonbinary individuals. Nonbinary or non-cisgender individuals may use pronouns such as *him* and *her*, or they may prefer the use of *they* and *their* as singular pronouns (Duckett & Ruud, 2019). Although it can feel awkward or forced when beginning to use gender-neutral language, repeated use can help it become a part of everyday communication.

Being aware of gendered language commonly used in our everyday lives can sensitize us to finding nongendered substitutes. For example, using the term *Latinx* instead of *Latino* or *Latina* when referring to people of Latin American descent avoids assigning gender. Replacing the terms *mother* and *father* with *parent* includes all parents regardless of gender. *Spouse/partner* can replace *husband/wife*. We can say *police officer* instead of *policeman/policewoman*, and we can say *everyone* instead of *ladies and gentlemen*. Sensitivity to our language will help avoid inadvertently offending others. Gender-affirming and inclusive care can positively affect parents' experiences. This sensitivity to language should guide professional writing and dissemination of research as well (Dodgson & Bamberger, 2021).

There is debate among healthcare providers, researchers, supporters, and parents themselves about the use of gender-neutral language in pregnancy, birth, lactation, and newborn care. Some assert that women have unique experiences, needs, and rights in relation to pregnancy, birth, and lactation that are not shared with others. They argue that terms such as *parents* and *families* as replacements for *mothers* diminishes women and can inappropriately include males and other family members (Gribble et al., 2022).

Avoid Undermining Confidence

Words are powerful and can be either empowering or discouraging. **Figures 5-1** and **5-2** share some real-life examples of interactions between parents and healthcare providers. Reflect on these parents' experiences and to the caregiver responses. Consider how to incorporate empowering approaches into working with families.

My first unsupportive comment came from a healthcare provider whom I work with and very much love and respect. She is both intelligent and down-to-earth. We were discussing my plan to practice baby-led weaning and how I was still nursing my then 13-month-old. She said, "Why are you still nursing? You know there is no benefit after 6 months, right?" That comment immediately broke my heart and made me question everything I believed about breastfeeding and my own instincts. It was a comment that shook me to the core. ~MK

In the hospital a required lactation consultant came to my room about an hour after birth. We were already skin to skin and my son already had nursed successfully. She grabbed my breast and was pushing it toward my son. I had to ask her to leave because I didn't find it helpful. ~JR

My last daughter Sophia had 4 solid months nursing, but when I started taking classes again I decided to use formula along with breastfeeding. Sophia could not hold down formula, and my production went down. Sophia was admitted into the children's hospital. They would not let me nurse her, which was devastating as a nursing parent. I argued my point that nursing would not hurt her and would only benefit her. They finally said I could nurse her. ~SA

When total parenteral nutrition was discontinued, one neonatologist called to tell me that they would be watching Calvin very carefully now that he was on "just breastmilk." If Calvin didn't gain enough weight on "just your milk," he wanted to introduce formula. I couldn't believe it. Not only had Calvin gained weight consistently, but due to his prematurity and damage to his bowel, the chance of necrotizing enterocolitis, a devastating intestinal infection, was something like 20 percent higher if they gave him formula! ~FW

Figure 5-1 Discouraging comments.

During every shift I would pump for my baby 2–3 times to maintain my production. It was a long walk to the "pumping room," and usually, at least once, I would run into one of our cleaning staff. This older woman was foreign and spoke with a thick Romanian accent. She used to tell me, "Good for you! Breastmilk is best!" and "That's one lucky baby!" ~MK

When my husband and I got pregnant we were absolutely clueless. At the time, I was on WIC and that was by far the biggest help. My breastfeeding counselor there gave me so much information. She was very honest, and that was the best thing I needed. She was my biggest help. ~JR

I'll never forget when he was up to 1-ounce bottle feedings. I tentatively asked when I could breastfeed. The nurse just looked at me and said, "Now." I cried, I was so happy! ~FW

Figure 5-2 Empowering comments.

Voice Tone

It is important that your **voice tone** matches your intended message. Voice tone is responsible for up to 38% of the message that is received (Fast, 2014). Thus, the voice tone you use during teaching and counseling has a dramatic effect on how parents interpret the messages they receive. Manner of speech can create a warm, friendly, even humorous atmosphere. Moderation in volume, rate of speech, and pitch contribute to an effective voice tone.

Moderating voice volume, rate, and pitch will have a positive effect on how your message is received. A moderate volume is not too loud and not too soft. Speaking too quickly can give the impression of being rushed and create an anxious or nervous feeling. Remembering to stop and breathe can avoid running out of breath and seeming rushed. Speaking too slowly can become irritating and create impatience. Often, our voices tend to get higher in pitch when we are irritated or excited. Consciously trying to maintain a moderate pitch will help control volume.

Body Language

Body language accounts for 52% of how a message is received (Fast, 2014). Body language encompasses all body movements, including smiling, eye contact, posture, space, and touch. It ranges from deliberate to unconscious gestures. A particular form of body language may apply to cultural practices. You can capitalize on using appropriate nonverbal messages to convey a sense of self-worth and empowerment. In addition, observing parents' body language will reveal whether they appear to be stressed or in pain (**Figure 5-3**). **Figure 5-4** presents factors to consider for identifying signs of stress or pain in parents. Women are typically better at recognizing emotions and express themselves more easily than men (Prentice et al., 2022).

Eye Contact

Our eyes are the most powerful of all body parts in transmitting information. Eye contact conveys a desire to interact and communicate. It creates a warm, caring, and inviting climate. Generally, maintaining eye contact at least 85% of the time is most effective in interactions. Blinking or looking away and back again can avoid too much intensity or the appearance of staring.

Failing to establish and maintain eye contact carries the risk of appearing too busy or distracted to fully engage. Eyes that are focused on documenting or otherwise averted, as in **Figure 5-5**, create a

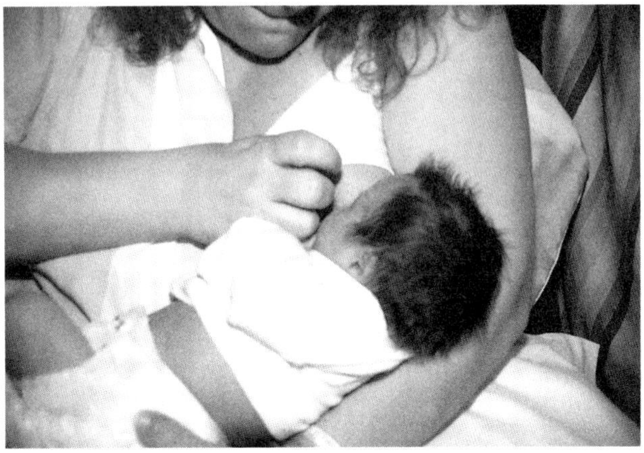

Figure 5-3 This parent's clenched hand conveys tension.

Printed with permission of Judith Lauwers.

- Do they welcome eye contact or avert their eyes?
- Do they sound confident or stressed and anxious?
- Is their facial expression animated or listless?
- Do they appear comfortable being touched, or do they move away?
- Do they sit or stand with an erect posture or does their body sag?
- Do they have an air of self-assurance, or do they seem passive and unsure?
- Do they appear relaxed or do they shift their body and fidget?
- Are their shoulders relaxed or are they hunched and tense while nursing?
- Are their feet relaxed or do their toes curl when the baby is feeding?

Figure 5-4 Reading body language for signs of stress or pain.

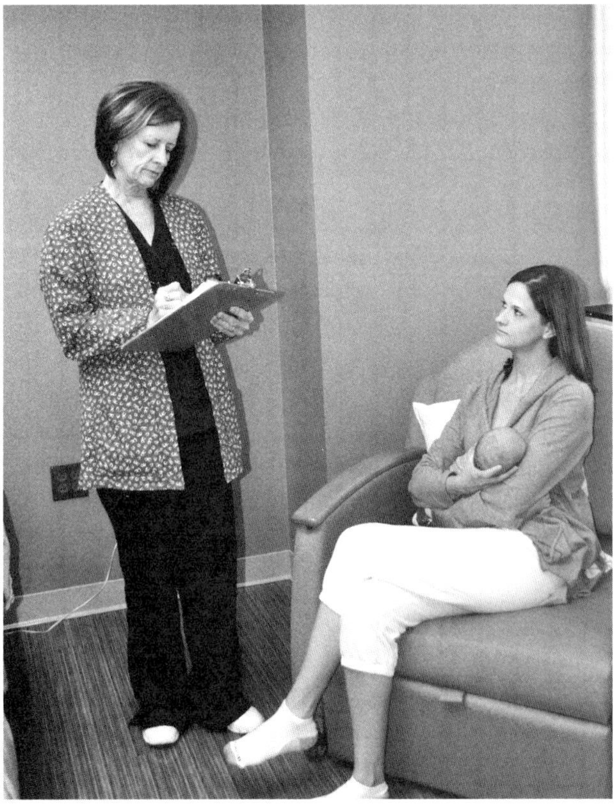

Figure 5-5 Caregiver exhibiting poor eye contact.

Printed with permission of Anna Swisher.

barrier that interferes with a meaningful exchange. Consciously engaging in eye contact enhances interactions. A study in telecommunication rated communication skills with the healthcare provider looking directly at the camera compared with looking at the computer screen (Helou et al., 2022). Looking at the camera was perceived as making eye contact and providing empathy and support. **Chapter 6** discusses teleconsultations.

Facial Expression

Presenting yourself with a calm, relaxed smile will put parents at ease. A pleasant facial expression creates a warm and inviting atmosphere. It is almost impossible not to return a smile, so when we smile, we elicit a smile in return. The warmth of a smile comes through even when speaking over the telephone.

We can tell a lot about what a person is thinking by the look on their face. The ability to understand facial expressions is an important part of nonverbal communication. Words do not always match emotions, and the face conveys what a person is feeling. Being observant of a parent's facial expression can alert you to underlying issues.

Body Posture and Position

Body posture is a key element of nonverbal communication. The way we stand and sit influences how others perceive us. Posture suggests our confidence level, our engagement with our surroundings, and our power status. Crossed arms or legs can convey disinterest and emotional distance. Adopting an open, relaxed, and comfortable body posture creates a warm and inviting climate that conveys an interest to communicate on a meaningful level. Sitting or standing squarely with both feet flat on the floor and arms resting in an open posture can achieve this. Leaning forward further conveys an interest in interacting.

Where we position our body when interacting with others affects their comfort and the effectiveness of the interaction. We all have a sense of personal space, the amount of space we need around us to feel comfortable. Being too close may invade another person's comfort zone and cause them to feel uneasy or awkward. Being too far away, as in **Figure 5-6**, can convey being too busy or disinterested in engaging meaningfully. A comfortable position—not too far away and not too close—will achieve the desired impression.

Another aspect of body position to be aware of is altitude. When two people interact, the height that each person assumes in relation to the other can create a perception of or an actual power imbalance in the relationship. People who want to appear superior to the other person use such posturing to their advantage. A caregiver looming over a parent, as in **Figure 5-7**, can cause the parent to feel intimidated and less in control. Placing parents at an equal or greater height establishes them as having the greatest importance. It leads to greater self-confidence and self-reliance, which is empowering. Sitting in a chair or kneeling on the floor create an atmosphere of working together as equals.

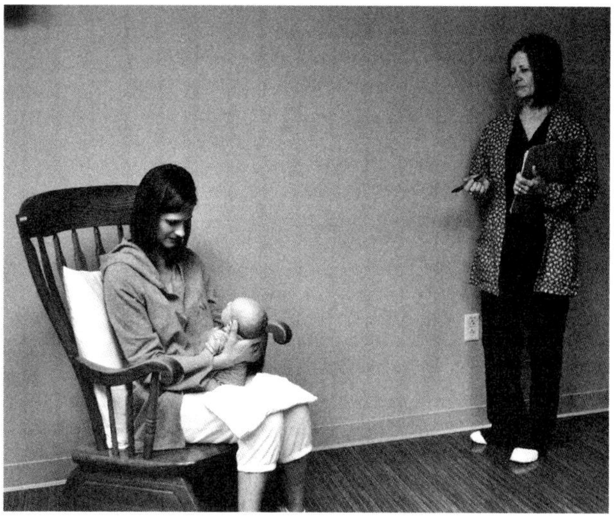

Figure 5-6 Caregiver too far away to engage in meaningful dialogue.

Touch

Touch is a powerful form of social support that communicates empathy and can be reassuring and calming. The touch of a hand, or an arm placed around someone's shoulder, can convey warmth, caring, and encouragement. Such a touch must come at the appropriate moment and within the appropriate context. Some people are uncomfortable touching or being touched by others. Be judicious in the use of any posture that involves body contact and be watchful for comfort cues.

Ask permission and explain the purpose before conducting a physical assessment or touching the parent, as in **Figure 5-8**. Also ask permission before invading a parent's space to hold the baby. When examining the baby's mouth or using another form of physical assessment, explain the purpose and ask permission. Seek opportunities to encourage parents to share control. When possible, perform

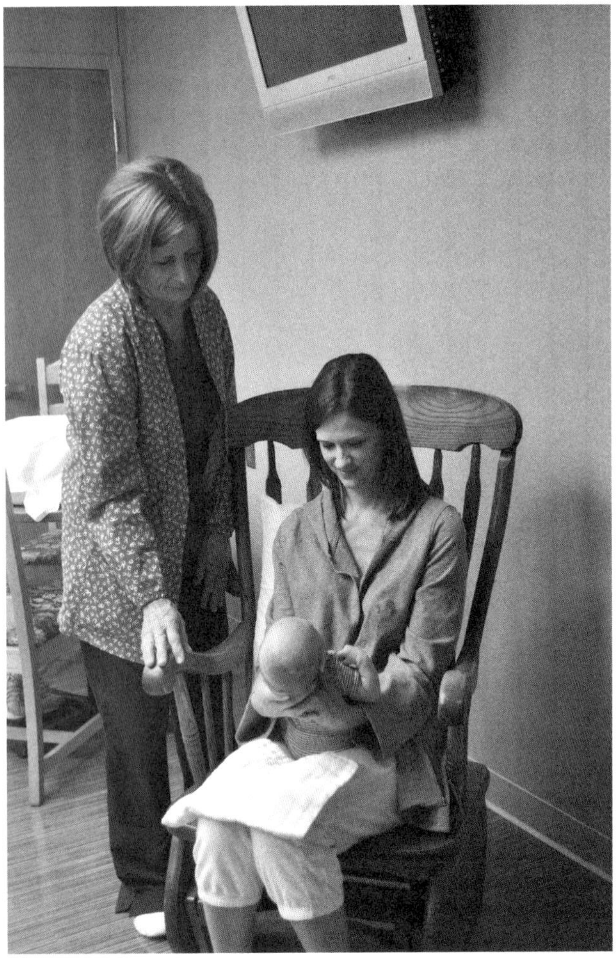

Figure 5-7 Caregiver positioned too high.

Printed with permission of Anna Swisher.

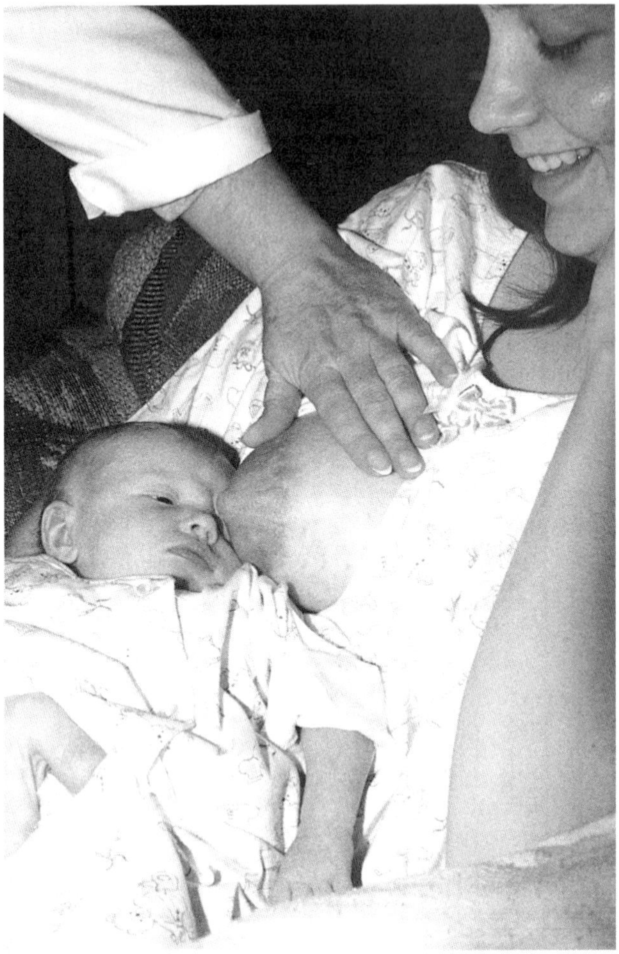

Figure 5-8 Ask permission before doing a physical assessment.

Printed with permission of Anna Swisher.

assessments with the parent holding the baby. When weighing the baby, the parent can move the baby on and off the scale. If the baby has a void or stool, the parent can change the diaper. Small steps like these convey respect for the parents' role and reinforce the concept that the baby belongs to them, not to the caregiver.

Cultural Differences

The messages conveyed by body language are not universal. Smiling, eye contact, personal space, touching, and posture can vary greatly from one culture to another. In some cultures, direct eye contact is considered rude. In Western culture, shaking the head up and down indicates agreement, and shaking it from side to side indicates a negative response. In other societies, side-to-side gestures mean yes, and nodding up and down means no. Some cultures are more comfortable with proximity and touch than others. Learning the cultural nuances among parents in your care will help in adopting and interpreting body language appropriately.

Personalize Your Approach

Effective counseling techniques will enable you to personalize your approach and give parents the support they need to develop confidence in their parenting and lactation. Talking through a situation helps parents relieve emotional stress, express themselves, learn, and participate in their outcomes. This increases their self-confidence and self-awareness, which leads to personal growth. Parents are then able to take responsibility for their choices and develop self-sufficiency.

Parents' satisfaction with their nursing outcomes can depend in part on the caregiver's perception of their needs, the use of counseling skills, and the caregiver's personality traits. Positive regard and respect acknowledge parents' individuality and worth without judgment, encouraging them to be open and authentic. Maintaining flexibility will help ensure use of the full range of skills to respond to parents appropriately at different stages in the counseling process. Counseling skills will help affirm and empower parents and avoid portraying lactation as problematic (Gallegos et al., 2018).

Participant-Focused Counseling

Participant-focused counseling will enable you to build rapport with parents and tailor education to their individual needs. Active listening skills will help you actively engage and hear how to help parents work lactation into their lives. Shared decision-making with parents leads to setting realistic goals that can lead to changing behavior. A key element in participant-focused counseling is parents developing trusting, personal relationships with their caregivers. Determining parents' concerns will help build positive connections and target information that is meaningful and relevant. Customized care helps parents reach their feeding goals and can reduce inequities (Furman et al., 2023).

Using the names of parents and babies helps personalize the exchange and enhances the helping relationship. It is especially important to use the baby's name with a parent who continually refers to "the baby." Not using the baby's name could indicate a parent's difficulty bonding with the baby. Your use of the baby's name will help model bonding for parents.

When addressing parents, ask them what they prefer to be called. Some parents may appreciate the formality of using their last name while others prefer to be called by their first name or nickname. It is also respectful to verify the correct pronunciation of names. Most people appreciate your taking the time to learn how to say their names correctly. Recognizing that many couples have different last names, verify the correct last names of support persons. Also ask if they have preferred pronouns.

Trauma-Informed Care

An approach to healthcare, known as **trauma-informed care** (TIC), considers an individual's experiences and how trauma may impact their lives. Trauma is prevalent among all races, ethnicities, ages, and socioeconomic backgrounds. It can result from abuse, violence, neglect, loss, war, or natural disaster. Trauma is more common in low-income populations and related to substance abuse, military life, homelessness, and gender orientation (National Child Traumatic Stress Network [NCTSN], 2023). Indigenous people experience multigenerational and historic trauma resulting from discrimination and forced relocation and cultural assimilation (Gameon & Skewes, 2020). Stressors from the 2020 global COVID-19 pandemic raised concerns about collective trauma and far-reaching harm to the mental health of parents and infants (Choi et al., 2020).

Childhood trauma and toxic stress have a cumulative effect that influences lifelong health and behavior. Adverse childhood experiences (ACEs) affect the survivor's physical, psychological, and social development and well-being into adulthood. ACEs include, but are not limited to, violence; neglect; discrimination; poverty; and emotional, sexual, and physical abuse. Home life may have involved divorce, substance abuse, domestic violence, incarceration, psychiatric disorder or depression, instability, or homelessness.

The prevalence of ACEs varies geographically. In one U.S. study, 61% of adults reported at least one ACE, and 16% reported four or more (Merrick, 2019). In a study of South African adolescents, 77% reported at least one ACE, and 21% reported four or more (Manyema & Richter, 2019). In one state in India, 91% of the youth experienced at least one ACE, and about 50% experienced three or more (Damodaran & Varghese, 2019).

TIC assumes that that any given person is more likely than not to have a history of trauma and acknowledges the role trauma has in their lives. It acknowledges the high prevalence of trauma, addresses the consequences of trauma, and facilitates healing. TIC provides a complete picture of a parent's life situation, both past and present. It enables caregivers to recognize how trauma may affect parents to better support them. Fellow staff and colleagues may also be trauma survivors and can be triggered by exposure to a parent's traumatic experiences, commonly known as *secondary trauma* or **vicarious trauma** (Isobel & Thomas, 2022; Kim et al., 2022).

Using a TIC approach enables you to recognize signs of past trauma exposure. It helps avoid unintentionally inflicting further trauma or triggering a reminder of past experiences. TIC ensures that parents feel safe, supported, and understood. Components of TIC include the following:

- Establish physical and emotional safety. Knock before entering a room. Introduce yourself and your role in every interaction. Protect parents' privacy and respect their boundaries. Ask permission before any physical touch, including handling the baby. If you need to observe a feeding, allow clothing to be shifted rather than removed. Use open and nonthreatening body positioning.

- Build trust and transparency. Be punctual, consistent, supportive, and nonjudgmental in your interactions. Provide anticipatory guidance and client-centered care that seeks input from parents and encourages them to ask questions. Give evidence-based explanations about what will be done, how, and why it is necessary. Ask permission before taking action.
- Offer peer support. If the parent is receptive, provide support resources from other trauma survivors for shared experiences and fostering relationships.
- Ensure collaboration, shared decision-making, and mutual support. Create opportunities for parents to build a sense of control and empowerment as active members of their care team. Provide options and tailor care to their specific situation, needs, goals and desires.
- Approach parents with cultural humility and seek to understand their beliefs and core values. Be sensitive to racial, ethnic, historical, and cultural backgrounds and gender identity. Recognize your own privilege and its impact on your perception of trauma responses.

TIC requires a multilevel commitment in policies, practices, workplace culture, and daily interactions (Fleishman et al., 2019). Pregnancy and the postpartum period are vulnerable, emotional times for parents. It is common for them to feel unskilled and uncertain in learning how to meet their baby's needs. These feelings can be amplified for trauma survivors. A trauma-informed approach helps survivors feel safe, supported, empowered, and understood. It helps them make positive, conscious choices in coping and healing as they transition to parenthood. **Chapter 20** discusses trauma survivors.

Step by Step Counseling Techniques

Counseling techniques help you create meaningful dialogue to enhance your helping role. The order in which you use these techniques can affect your effectiveness and the outcome of your interactions. You will want to first gather sufficient information and insights to understand the situation. Then provide **affirmation** and validation to begin to build rapport and help them feel comfortable and confident. After you have gathered information and provided affirmation, you are ready to educate and provide resources to help parents with their lactation management.

The variety of counseling techniques that are presented here can form your personal counseling "toolbox." Assess each contact and use the skills relevant to the situation. Practicing the techniques will determine which ones are compatible with your personality and approach. Use those that feel comfortable and that help you establish effective and supportive relationships with parents.

Step 1: Information Gathering

Information gathering enables you to assess parents' knowledge and understanding of how to manage their lactation. Counseling skills used during information gathering will encourage parents to open up as they explore their motivations, strengths, internal resources, and goals. When time is at a premium, it may be tempting to jump into problem-solving. This is especially endemic in hospital or other clinic settings where productivity is measured in numbers of encounters. A rush to problem-solve runs the risk of missing important clues about parents' needs. Counseling skills for sensitively and efficiently gathering information and insights will help you understand their feelings, goals, and other factors that influence their actions. Use of these skills helps parents feel safe sharing their ideas and concerns openly and helps you discern their needs more clearly.

The aim of counseling is for parents to become skillful and self-sufficient and able to make sound decisions about their nursing. By encouraging them to talk, reflecting their ideas, and clarifying their concerns, you help them understand their situation and identify knowledge gaps. Listening skills will enable you to gather information while providing the opportunity for parents to hear themselves and sort out their feelings and concerns. At times, you will need to direct the conversation to focus on specific points. Facilitating the conversation in this way helps parents recognize and clearly define their situation.

Listening

Listening as a counseling skill goes beyond everyday listening. It is a consciously active process of responding to total messages and perceiving with your ears, eyes, and imagination. It means being silent much of the time and encouraging parents to talk. You put your thoughts and interests aside and give yourself fully to listening. You avoid the temptation to interrupt and listen attentively to what parents say as well as what they do *not* say.

Everyday listening usually takes place at one of four levels. The lowest level of listening is ignoring. No doubt, most adults have experienced this level of listening with a child or pet! The next level is **pretending**, where the listener is trying to be polite but is not giving full attention to the speaker. It describes the noncommittal response you might receive if you interrupt someone who is deeply engrossed in texting, reading, or watching a movie. The third level is **selective listening**, in which the listener hears only certain parts of what is said. This can occur when you focus so much on how you plan to respond that you fail to listen carefully. The fourth level of customary listening is **attentive listening**, in which the listener is fully engaged and actively focuses on the words and the message.

Skilled Listening

Skilled listening requires time and patience. It often means waiting until parents develop an understanding of their feelings and concerns. Failure to help is often a result of snap judgments and not allowing time for parents to collect their thoughts so that you can learn the whole story. For example, if you ask how everything is going, the response may be, "Fine." Several minutes later, after you and the parent have talked about increases in the frequency of feedings at various stages in the baby's growth, their response may be, "Oh, no wonder my baby is nursing constantly!"

Encouraging parents to keep talking will help you gain insights into concerns they may have. Often, parents are not sure how they feel and need more time to talk and to feel at ease before communicating on a meaningful level. When there are mixed feelings or several concerns, you will need time and ample conversation before you uncover feelings and concerns. Listening skills that reinforce what parents say will clarify their statements, show acceptance, and encourage them to arrive at solutions. Effective listening conveys that you care about them enough to give them your total attention. Three listening skills that can help you gain this insight are attending, reflective listening, and empathetic listening.

Attending

Attending is a **passive listening** skill that confirms you are listening without asking questions or making comments. Examples include "Yes," "I see," "I can appreciate that," "Oh," "Mmmmm," and "Really." Attending is a valuable listening skill that encourages parents to continue talking freely. It has a strong reinforcing effect that helps them assume responsibility for the course of the discussion. Attending minimizes the tendency to intervene unnecessarily. Silence is another effective attending technique. Pausing in the conversation and waiting for parents to fill the silence encourages them to take a more active role. Attending includes visual observation and the use of eye contact, posture, gestures, and listening in a noninterfering manner.

The absence of any type of attending behavior, whether verbal or nonverbal, could discourage parents from pursuing a topic or cause them to feel that you are not interested in what they have to say. Your use of eye contact and other nonverbal behavior sends strong messages. If you avoid eye contact, cross your arms or legs, focus on charting, or seem otherwise unapproachable, you risk sending a message of indifference. It is difficult to alter such a negative impression with any verbal attempt to show interest. Direct eye contact; sitting at the parent's level; leaning forward with a natural, relaxed posture; calm gestures; and a pleasant, engaged facial expression transmit a positive nonverbal message and show that you are genuinely interested.

Reflective Listening

Reflective listening, also called **active listening**, helps establish a supportive climate as you gather information from parents. A reflective listening response accepts what the parent feels and encourages them to relax and respond openly. It is a warm, sincere, and considerate way of communicating that most people appreciate. Reflecting back what you believe parents mean shows acceptance of their viewpoints and feelings and encourages further discussion. It is validating and conveys that you are trying to understand how they feel and that you are interested in what they are saying. It also lets parents know whether you received their message completely and correctly.

Paraphrasing what was said encourages parents to respond and explain their situation further. It provides an opportunity for them to find solutions in an atmosphere in which they can grow and accept information. This example of reflective listening shows acceptance:

Parent: I'm not sure I can nurse much longer. My nipples are so sore that nursing is really unpleasant!

Response: It's no fun to feed Nolan when it hurts. We talked about how enjoyable nursing is, and this isn't fun at all. [This expresses understanding and validates the concern.]

Reflective listening can clarify a message by helping parents hear what they said and think about it. Your response may involve some interpretation. Their reaction to your response lets you know whether you understood correctly and focuses the conversation. Reflective listening is particularly useful when parents have only vague or as-yet-unspoken thoughts on a situation. It also helps with parents who are anxious or discouraged and not sure what their concern is or how they feel about it. You cannot offer suggestions until parents are ready to accept them. That will occur only after their situation and feelings are clear. Listening and encouraging parents to continue talking are crucial steps in defining their concerns. This example illustrates clarification with reflective listening:

Parent: Molly is 4 months old now and always looks around the room instead of nursing. I guess she's ready to wean.

Response: You're wondering if Molly is ready to wean. [The response will indicate whether to pursue a discussion about weaning or perhaps ways to minimize distraction.]

Instead of explaining right away that a 4-month-old infant does not usually self-wean and is probably just distracted, you first accept the parent's feelings, making no judgment. Later, after further discussion, you can offer information about developmental stages. Reflective listening helps parents feel comfortable sharing personal feelings after having talked for a while and developing trust. This example illustrates correcting an impression:

Parent: My nipples hurt.

Response: Your nipples are sore when you feed Ryan. [This includes interpretation that the soreness occurs during a feeding.]

Parent: Not just when I nurse, but after I wash them, too. [This is a correction, a clarifying message.]

Reflective listening serves as an important means of developing trust, encouraging a response, and clarifying what was said. You now have more information to help you in problem-solving—namely, washing the nipples after a feeding.

Empathetic Listening

As part of the counseling process, **empathetic listening** goes beyond merely reflecting words to understanding emotionally and intellectually. It is a deeper form of reflective listening and is the highest and most effective level of listening. Empathy is an element of compassionate care. Compassion flows from empathy and demonstrates sensitivity, kindness, and warmth. Empathetic care from healthcare providers is associated with positive outcomes including lowered rates of hospitalization and better control of chronic diseases (Hojat et al., 2018).

Empathetic listening requires that you listen with your ears, eyes, and heart, tuning in to the feeling, meaning, and behavior that are conveyed. It integrates your right brain and left brain so that you sense and feel what is being said. When you reflect a message back, you rephrase both the content and the feeling of what was said. With the use of this skill you deliver compassionate care and help parents work through their feelings as well as their thoughts. When you reflect what they seem to be saying, in your words, you help them hear the emotions they expressed. This example illustrates a compassionate, empathetic listening response:

Parent: I don't know whether I should nurse Juliette when we first arrive home from the hospital. Reese, our 2-year-old, is very clingy. I'm afraid nursing Juliette might make Reese jealous and even clingier.

Response: You're afraid that seeing you nurse Juliette will make Reese more demanding.

Hearing this repeated back with your interpretation will help clarify whether the message came through as intended. The parent's response may be, "Yes, Reese already needs a lot of attention. I'm not sure what will happen if I spend so much time nursing Juliette." If you misinterpreted the comment, the response may be, "No, I'm concerned that Reese may want to begin nursing again." This response will help you determine the direction to take.

Empathetic listening helps you gain information that will clarify a situation, which in turn makes it

Scenario	Possible meanings
A parent says, "I think I'll have to give my baby a bottle in the evening so that partner can do something for the baby."	• Parent wants to give a bottle. • Partner wants to give a bottle. • Partner feels left out. • Parent wants partner to be more active in child care. • Parent wants baby to sleep through the night. • Partner thinks the baby needs more nourishment. • Parent is thinking of weaning. • Baby is fussy and parent thinks milk production is too low. • Partner wants to help as the much as possible.
A parent says, "My mother-in-law is here helping me these first 2 weeks, but she bottle-fed."	• Mother-in-law does not support nursing. • Mother-in-law thinks baby isn't getting enough nourishment. • Mother-in-law is helpful around the house but does not support nursing. • Parent is embarrassed nursing in front of the mother-in-law. • Mother-in-law envies parent for being able to nurse. • Mother-in law wants to learn about lactation. • Mother-in-law is not familiar with differences between bottle feeding and lactation. • Mother-in-law does not know how to support the parent's nursing.
A parent says, "I have to wean to go to a wedding."	• The wedding is a convenient excuse to wean. • Parent does not want to nurse baby at wedding. • Partner wants parent to wean. • Parent doesn't realize she can miss a feed. • Parent doesn't know how to collect and freeze milk. • Parent is not comfortable nursing in public. • Parent wants more freedom. • Parent cannot wear her favorite dress because of breast size. • Parent's favorite outfit will not accommodate nursing in public.
A parent says, "I don't know how long I'll be able to nurse. My sister had to wean at 10 days because her milk dried up."	• Parent is worried that their milk may dry up. • Sister is unsupportive of nursing. • Parent does not know about growth spurts. • Parent is worried about the baby getting enough milk. • Parent is not getting enough encouragement to nurse. • Parent fears she may make sister look like a failure. • Parent has a ready excuse if anything goes wrong. • Parent is not sure how long they want to nurse.

Figure 5-9 Possible meanings from a parent's statements.

less likely that you will misinterpret the meaning. **Figure 5-9** contains a list of possible meanings for several statements. If you misinterpret the initial statement, your explanation or suggestions might be inappropriate and unhelpful. The wide range of possible meanings reinforces the importance of clarifying the intent. When using empathetic listening, keep your feedback statements tentative. You cannot be certain you know exactly what parents are feeling. Be mindful of your tone of voice and avoid sounding like a mind reader.

At times you may find it difficult to think of words to express feelings. The list of "feeling words" in **Figure 5-10** may help expand your vocabulary in reflecting your interpretation of emotions. Be specific in your responses. Try to avoid use of the general word *upset*, which can communicate that you do not really understand the emotion being expressed. When you receive a "feeling" message, think to yourself, "What emotion is the parent expressing?" and think of a word to describe that emotion. Empathetic listening responses become more spontaneous when you concentrate on identifying the emotion.

Probing

Probing is a technique for gathering information. **Probes** encourage parents to give more information and better define their situation. They help focus on specific concerns and direct the conversation to pinpoint issues and feelings that need to be addressed. Probing statements or questions will help you clarify and interpret a message.

Words that reflect "upset"	Words that reflect "happy"
angry	accepted
anxious	appreciated
defeated	better
difficult	capable
disappointed	comfortable
discouraged	competent
disrespected	confident
doubtful	empowered
embarrassed	encouraged
feel like giving up	enjoy
frightened	excited
guilty	glad
hate, hated	good
hopeless	grateful
hurt great	happy
inadequate	love, loved
left out	pleased
miserable	proud
put down	reassured
rejected	relieved
sad	respected
stupid	satisfied
unhappy	validated
unloved	wonderful
worried	

Figure 5-10 Words that reflect feelings.

Asking Open-Ended Questions

Asking **open-ended questions** is a useful skill for gathering information. It is the most direct way to learn what you need to know. An open-ended question cannot be answered with a simple yes or no. Questions requiring only a yes/no response include those that begin with words such as *are*, *is*, *do*, and *does*. Such closed questions elicit minimal responses and tend to shut down the conversation. In contrast, open-ended questions require more informative responses. They are the same questions a good reporter asks: *who*, *what*, *when*, *where*, *why*, *how*, *how much*, and *how often*.

For example, the likely answer to the question, "Are you eating well?" is yes, which provides no helpful information. Asking, "What did you eat today?" or "What do you usually eat for breakfast?" will elicit a response with more information about the parent's diet and eating patterns. This provides an opportunity for nutrition guidance if needed.

If you suspect a baby needs more frequent feedings, a response to, "Does Samantha nurse often enough?" may offer no insight into her feeding pattern. Asking, "How many times does Samantha nurse in 24 hours?" will help you learn more about feeding frequency so that you can provide appropriate assistance. You could also ask, "How many soiled and wet diapers has Samantha had over the past 24 hours?" As with many counseling skills, asking open-ended questions becomes easier and more natural with practice.

Use questioning wisely. Posing too many questions in sequence may seem like interrogating and cause parents to feel threatened or irritated. Continually asking questions can also interfere with encouraging shared decision-making. Parents may expect that they can describe symptoms and complaints and rely on you to provide solutions. You can discourage this pattern by using other skills to encourage parents to talk in a conversational style rather than answering a series of questions. Your goal is to encourage parents to talk freely and participate in finding solutions. Balancing open-ended questions with other counseling skills promotes **self-efficacy** and builds self-confidence and independence.

Clarifying

Clarifying will help gather enough information to understand a message clearly and avoid miscommunication. One way to clarify a point is to admit confusion about the parent's meaning and restate what you heard. You may also clarify what was said with reflective listening. Here are some examples of clarifying responses:

- "You feel that . . ."
- "It seems like . . ."
- "Let me see if I understand what you said . . ."
- "So you're saying you don't think you can nurse."

Interpreting

Like reflective listening, the skill of interpreting clarifies what is said, shows acceptance, and encourages a response. An interpreting response contains more of your thoughts and impressions than simple rephrasing and provides an analysis of what was said. An interpreting response may begin with "So you're saying that . . ." or "It sounds like you are saying . . ." or "That must mean . . ." Drawing together several statements and adding tentative conclusions is a way to interpret what was said.

When using interpreting, allow opportunity for parents to process what you have said and correct you if they believe you misinterpreted their message. The goal of this skill is for parents to interpret events in their lives and perceive their situation in

Scenario	Possible meanings
Parent of a 4-week-old infant: "I can't get anything done during the day because I'm nursing all the time." [Frustrated]	• You feel your housework is getting away from you. [Interpreting] • You're surprised a newborn needs so much time. [Reflective listening] • You wish you had more time to do other things. [Interpreting] • You seem to be nursing all day. [Reflective listening]
Parent of a 2-month-old infant: "Johnny is still waking up 2 times during the night, and I feel like a zombie most days." [Yawning]	• You're wondering if you'll ever get a good night's sleep. [Interpreting] • You feel tired because your sleep is interrupted. [Reflective listening] • It seems as if this will go on forever. [Interpreting] • You're wishing Johnny would sleep longer at night. [Reflective listening]
Parent of a 2-month-old infant: "My healthcare provider said Jimmy was doing very well, but that it was time to start cereal twice a day." [Confused]	• You're wondering if Jimmy needs solid foods at this time. [Reflective listening] • You don't feel Jimmy needs solid foods yet. [Interpreting] • You're wondering why your healthcare provider suggested cereal at this time. [Reflective listening]
Parent of a 1-year-old child: "Tommy and I enjoyed nursing so much, and now all of a sudden he would rather do other things than nurse." [Disappointed]	• You seem to miss the daytime feedings. [Interpreting] • Nursing times were such happy and warm times for you and Tommy. [Reflective listening] • Tommy seems to prefer toys and other activities. [Reflective listening]
Pregnant woman: "I want to nurse but I'm not interested in classes. Natural childbirth is horrible." [Fearful]	• You don't want to go through that. [Reflective listening] • You think natural childbirth is painful. [Interpreting] • It sounds as though you've heard about some unpleasant experiences. [Interpreting] • Natural childbirth is not what you want. [Reflective listening]

Figure 5-11 Distinguishing between interpreting and active listening.

new ways. You can use this skill to listen and respond empathetically.

Figure 5-11 presents examples that distinguish between interpreting and reflective listening. Interpreting encompasses empathetic listening to analyze a conversation and help parents gain perspective. Use this skill with discretion to avoid causing annoyance or offense from your interpretations. Reserve interpreting for times when you have a clear impression of what is said to help sort out feelings.

Redirecting

The goal of redirecting is to pursue a more meaningful dialogue that increases understanding for both of you. Redirecting is useful when parents seem to ramble or change direction to an unrelated topic. Typically, parents raise several topics during a conversation. When you believe they have touched on their main concerns, you can focus the conversation by pursuing an aspect you believe could be useful.

You may focus the conversation by repeating a particular point or reviewing several points. For example, you might concentrate on issues such as how the parent feels and how the baby has been acting. Redirecting is especially helpful in bringing talkative parents back to the important points that will help them. Examples of phrasing are "Tell me more about . . ." and "Can we talk about [topic] again?" With focusing, you sort through the various issues to identify topics you need to explore further. This example illustrates a need to focus the conversation:

Parent: Hi, Alicia. I really liked the book you recommended. I just wish my partner had been willing to read it. I gave it to my neighbor. She's going to have a baby next month.

Response: You say you would like your partner to learn more about nursing?

Parent: I sure do. Adam is worried about what our two kids will think when they see me nursing now that they're getting older. Our daughter, Lillian, is in nursery school and only knows about bottles. Our son, Eden, is in third grade. Eden plays Little League and is pretty good.

Response: Let's get back to your partner. Adam is afraid of how Lillian and Eden will react when they see you feeding the new baby?

In this example, the parent referred to their partner's attitude twice, and it was the first personal topic that was mentioned. Often, the first statement will provide a clue about parents' concerns, as will the number of times they mention a topic. After you have refocused the conversation, the parent's response will indicate the topic to pursue. With practice, this skill will become almost second nature.

Motivational Interviewing

Motivational interviewing (MI) engages parents by asking targeted questions to explore their motivations, strengths, internal resources, and goals. MI can reveal inner motivations and resolve uncertain feelings. Expressing empathy, being flexible with resistance, and promoting autonomy are aspects of this approach. The nonconfrontational, nonjudgmental approach of MI helps parents explore and resolve ambivalence while feeling supported.

MI is a widely accepted evidence-based approach to changing behavior (Gregory et al., 2022). Understanding what motivates people to change can help them find the internal motivation to take on healthy practices. The goal of a motivational interview is to use internal motivation instead of persuasion. It is a person-centered, goal-oriented approach to counseling that draws out a person's reasons for change rather than just giving them information about the desired behavior. MI can help parents identify discrepancies between their current behavior and their goals or values so that they can make the changes necessary to reach their goals (Tooley & Kolahi, 2022).

Parents who are influenced the most by other people may benefit from this counseling approach. MI may be especially effective with parents at high risk for formula feeding or for premature weaning. Selective reinforcement of statements made by the parents can strengthen their motivation for change (Bischof et al., 2021). The use of MI helps staff feel better prepared to promote lactation and give accurate information (Defoor & Darby, 2020). It enhances self-efficacy in nursing exclusivity and continuation (Naroee et al., 2020). An example of MI appears in **Figure 5-12**.

Step 2: Affirmation

A classic principle in any helping profession is that people don't care how much you *know* until they know how much you *care*. Affirmation conveys a sense of security, a climate of acceptance, and a genuine interest in parents' well-being. It reduces anxiety and validates parents' feelings, emotions, and concerns. When parents feel validated, in a calm and supportive atmosphere, they are better able to take in information and join in problem-solving. In contrast, if their emotions and frustrations are high, they may not be receptive to learning or addressing solutions. It is important to address a parent's emotional needs before beginning teaching and problem-solving.

Affirmation skills will help to lower pressure and stress and encourage parents to verbalize their feelings. Affirmation validates their concerns, shows acceptance, and praises their actions or attempts. These skills help you listen attentively and be alert to what parents are *not* saying. Parents who appear self-assured may have internal anxieties that reveal themselves through their body language or comments. Affirmation skills will help you build connections and rapport with parents that will help them process information. Demonstrating a sincere interest in parents and their concerns; showing enthusiasm for the things they are happy about; and conveying acceptance of them, their situation, and their decisions are all ways of providing affirmation.

Influencing parents in a positive way is a form of affirmation that can encourage them to continue to seek help and work toward solutions. New parents are often unsure of themselves. If the reality of caring for a baby does not match their expectations, they may become discouraged or susceptible to poor advice. Heartening words from you will counteract these negative factors to give them reassurance, build hope, and identify their strengths.

Reassuring

Reassuring is an affirmation skill that gives parents perspective and lets them know that many babies act like their baby. Babies have fussy periods, do not sleep through the night, do not nap when you want them to, feed frequently, and so on. Offering reassurance can help parents recognize that their situation is normal. You can gently let them know that it is okay to feel the way they do, and that their situation will improve as their baby grows.

Because this skill is easy to use, there may be a tendency to overuse it. Reassurance efforts sometimes come across as insincere sympathy or avoidance of

Alicia is 7 months' pregnant and is talking with a lactation consultant about how to feed the new baby.	
Speaker	**Dialogue**
Alicia	My first baby was formula fed and was sick a lot of the time. It would be great if my new baby is healthier. I've heard that if I nurse my baby won't be sick as much.
Consultant	Your first child was sick, and you are thinking nursing might make your new baby healthier. [*Reflective listening*]
Alicia	Yes, that's what I've read on the internet and heard in the news.
Consultant	It's great you're learning about lactation, Alicia. [*Affirmation*] You're right that nursing can help your baby to be healthy. Infection-fighting cells in human milk attack germs in the baby's body. Your milk will be like medicine for your baby.
Alicia	Yes, that's what I had heard. My older child had to have ear tubes inserted a few months ago because of so many ear infections. I'd love to avoid that with my new baby.
Consultant	It sounds like keeping your baby healthy is very important to you. Your baby will be lucky to have you as a parent. [*Affirmation*]
Alicia	It *is* important to me. I have a friend who formula fed and then nursed the second baby and said it made a big difference.
Consultant	You're thinking that if you nurse your new baby you might notice the same thing as your friend did. [*Reflective listening*]
Alicia	I hope so!
Consultant	It's great that you want to increase the chance of better health this time. [*Affirmation*] If you nurse, how do you think it will make you feel? [*Identifying internal motivation*]
Alicia	I would feel proud that what I'm doing is making my baby healthy.
Consultant	What an amazing way to start life with your new baby! [*Affirmation*] It sounds like you think nursing might be important for you and your baby. [*Reflective listening*] How confident do you feel about nursing? [*Open question*]
Alicia	I definitely want to, but I don't even know where to start
Consultant	Most parents feel uncertain the first time they nurse. [*Affirmation*] On a scale of 1 to 10, with 10 being VERY confident, how confident do you feel about being able to nurse? [*Open question*].
Alicia	I guess about a 3.
Consultant	That's a start! It sounds like you know nursing is good, you want to do it, but you're not feeling confident about it. [*Reflective listening*]
Alicia	Right.
Consultant	You didn't rate yourself at 1 so that shows you're motivated to give your baby a healthy start. [*Affirmation*] What could help increase your confidence that you can nurse? [*Probe*]
Alicia	I'd like to learn as much as I can about lactation. If I know more about it, I'll be able to know if it's something I can do.
Consultant	I'm happy to help with that. The hospital where you plan to deliver has a monthly prenatal class where you can meet with parents who are nursing for the first time. You can also attend the hospital postpartum support group to meet with other who are nursing. And I can give you some written materials and recommend other good resources on lactation. What do you think you would like to do? [*Open question*]
Alicia	I definitely want to go to the prenatal class, and written materials will help too. I didn't know I could go to a support group while I'm still pregnant. I'd love to talk with nursing parents and see babies nurse.
Consultant	So, what I heard is that your first baby did not nurse and was sick a lot. You want to nurse your new baby and would feel more confident if you could learn more. [*Summarizing*] Here are the materials we talked about. What do you plan to do to increase your confidence? [*Open question*]
Alicia	I'll read this material you gave me, and I'd like to buy a book on nursing. I'll also register for the prenatal class and try to make it to a support group meeting. [*Summarizing*]
Consultant	It sounds like you have a great plan, Alicia. I think you will do a great job. [*Affirmation*]
Alicia	Thanks so much. I'm getting excited about this now. Thanks for helping me talk it out.

Figure 5-12 Motivational interviewing.

This scenario was adapted in part from the U.S. Department of Agriculture, Food and Nutrition Services, WIC Breastfeeding Curriculum. The content of this publication does not necessarily reflect the view or policies of the U.S. Department of Agriculture, nor does mention of trade names, commercial products, or organizations imply endorsement by the U.S. Government.

discussing a parent's concern. Be careful not to give the impression that you are minimizing the importance of a parent's feelings or concerns. Keeping in mind that your goal is to build their confidence will help you decide when reassuring is appropriate. The following examples demonstrate reassuring responses:

- "Even though nursing in front of relatives can be difficult, it gets easier the more you do it."
- "You are really going through a rough period. The first 2 weeks with your baby are the most challenging. It will get easier as you and your baby become more experienced."

Building Hope

Hope is an antidote to discouragement and a source of relief from tension and unmet expectations. Building hope shows parents they are not alone. It gives those who are experiencing a bad time the feeling that the future may bring relief. Parents with long-term conditions, such as persistent nipple pain, a fussy baby, an unsupportive family, or a return to work can benefit from your use of this technique.

Building hope can begin by encouraging parents to discuss their feelings. Help them observe how their feelings relate to their present situation and how appropriate action can change their circumstances. Encouraging active participation helps them feel better so that they can function effectively. Here are some examples of responses that build hope:

- "You're discouraged that your baby wakes so many times during the night. Nursing more frequently during the day might encourage longer sleep periods at night."
- "Now that you've returned to work, you seem to feel like you are not giving your baby enough attention. Maybe you could set aside the first hour when you get home for just nursing and being together."

Identifying Strengths

Identifying strengths is a form of praise that helps parents focus on their positive qualities. It counteracts negative factors such as fatigue, a crying infant, or the inability to meet preconceived expectations. Reminding parents how well they handled a situation or how they can take advantage of a natural ability can encourage them to continue to find solutions. Reviewing past experiences that helped parents learn and grow can help them realize that they can handle their present challenges. It encourages them to develop and rely on their resources and is a step in the direction of self-efficacy. Discussing how parents resolved past problems is the essence of this technique.

Recalling peak moments with parents, such as their baby's first smile, a sibling's helpfulness, or an enjoyable evening with other new parents, can help them perceive their parenting experience as positive. Parents will recognize that they, their baby, and their family are special and that more memorable experiences will occur in the future. In the following examples, the responses identify strengths:

- "You handled that well."
- "You are already advocating for your child."
- "You seem really tuned in to your baby's needs."
- "You're the only one who can do that for your baby."

Use of Information-Gathering and Affirmation Skills

As stated earlier, gathering sufficient information and affirming parents need to occur before attempting to share information and seek solutions. Your counseling skills will help you select responses that are appropriate to each situation. **Table 5-2** illustrates

Table 5-2 Effective Use of Information-Gathering and Affirmation Skills

Expectant parent Kiara says, "I'm afraid that nursing might make my child too dependent."		
Listening Responses	Attending Active listening Empathetic listening	Hmmm, you do . . . You're worried that nursing will make your child too dependent. You want your baby to grow into an independent child, and you're not sure that nursing will make that possible.
Facilitating responses	Clarifying Interpreting Asking open-ended questions Redirecting	What do you mean by "too dependent"? You believe the dependency associated with nursing will keep your child from exploring the world. In what ways do you think nursing will make your child too dependent? Let's get back to your concerns about . . . (This would be used later if it becomes necessary to focus on Kiara's primary concern—dependence, or feelings of inadequacy as a prospective parent, or other concern.)
Affirmation responses	Reassuring Building hope Identifying strengths	Being a parent can be confusing. Many parents who bottle-feed also wonder how the attention they give their baby relates to later independence. You know, research has shown that given more attention and physical contact in the early years grow up to be more independent. It's great that you are concerned about your baby's independence, Kiara. How do you feel you can encourage your child to become independent?

Table 5-3 Helpful and Unhelpful Responses

Parent's Statement	Unhelpful Responses	Helpful Responses
I'm afraid nursing might make my child too dependent.	No, it makes a child more independent. (disagreeing) You need to read a book on parenting. (ordering) I really wanted to talk to you about . . . (changing the topic)	You're unsure how nursing will fit into your family. (reflective) You wonder how long your baby will want to nurse. (interpreting)
My labor wasn't what I expected.	Your baby is healthy; that's what matters. (minimizing) At least it's all behind you. (dismissive)	You're disappointed with the way it turned out. (reflective) It didn't go the way you hoped. (validating)
I'm not sure what to do when the nurse brings my baby to me.	Just hold your baby close to your nipple and your baby will figure it out. (dismissive) The lactation consultant will be here soon. (dismissive)	You're not sure what to do first when you hold your baby. (reflective) You're feeling a bit overwhelmed. (expanding)
I wish my healthcare provider would spend more time with me.	Healthcare providers have busy schedules. (dismissive) I can get you the healthcare provider's telephone number. (presumes)	You have some unanswered questions. (clarifying) What questions can I answer for you? (eliciting)
I have to go back to work in 6 weeks.	At least you can nurse until then. (minimizing) A lot of parents combine nursing and working. (fixing)	You're not sure you want to leave your baby. (clarifying) You're wondering how you can manage it. (reflective)
My healthcare provider says I have to give my baby formula.	Your healthcare provider knows best. (patronizing) A little formula won't hurt your baby. (minimizing)	You don't want to give your baby formula. (clarifying) You don't understand why your baby needs formula. (eliciting)
My baby cries all the time.	It's fine to let babies cry themselves to sleep. (unhelpful, fixing) It will get better. (minimizing)	You're worried you may not have enough milk. (clarifying) You're worried your baby doesn't want to nurse. (clarifying)

how the information-gathering and affirmation skills presented in this section may be used in responding to a parent's statement. **Table 5-3** presents examples of helpful and unhelpful statements in response to a parent's statement.

Step 3: Education

After you have gathered sufficient information and impressions and built rapport through affirmation, you are ready to begin educating and sharing resources with parents. When parents can identify their situation accurately, they can work with you to explore the options open to them. Education can range from stating simple facts about nutrition to educating parents on how their milk is produced. It may involve correcting parents' perceptions or lactation management. After working with parents to help them understand their situation, you can summarize the discussion and work with them toward solutions. **Chapter 6** discusses problem-solving.

Informing

Informing involves educating and explaining how something functions and why. Providing information and anticipatory guidance at the appropriate times helps parents grow and provides them with necessary resources to handle new challenges as they arise. Parents learn about lactation at prenatal and postpartum classes; at support group meetings; on the internet; and from caregivers, friends, and relatives. With such an array of information sources, they must sift through what is credible and recommended. To ensure that they obtain the best and most accurate information, you can educate them and suggest appropriate resources for self-learning. Following up with discussions of parents' questions and ideas enhances the impact of what they learn and inspires them to educate themselves further.

Explaining why things happen the way they do often makes basic facts more meaningful and relevant. For example, stating, "The more frequently you nurse, the more milk you will produce" may not convince a parent to feed more frequently. By comparison, explaining how nipple stimulation and milk removal increase hormone production, which in turn increases milk production, may help them better understand this process. Parents who develop a deeper understanding are more likely to institute practices that are compatible with their new knowledge.

Before giving information to parents, allow them enough time to explore their concerns and determine what they need to know. Ask yourself, "What information is needed, and is this the best time to provide it?" Determining the appropriate time for educating parents—the teachable moment—can be critical to their ability to accept and process the information. Much of the teaching you provide will occur organically as you help parents get started with nursing. When you observe a baby demonstrating feeding cues, for example, you can point out that this is the baby's way of showing hunger. As the baby begins to nurse, you can talk through positioning and the nuances behind various positions and latch.

Adults are more likely to remember information when it is learned through many senses. Hearing, seeing, and experiencing information in multiple ways will help reinforce new skills and information. Demonstrating techniques and asking parents to do a return demonstration will enhance their learning and help them become comfortable with managing their feedings. The use of breast models, dolls, and other tools will enrich your teaching and engage parents in their learning. In teaching hand expression, for example, you can demonstrate the technique on a breast model and ask for a return demonstration on the breast model or breast. You can then progress to the parent expressing milk as you talk through any needed adjustments. Adult learning is discussed in **Chapter 4**.

Correcting a Misconception or Mismanagement

Sometimes, you may need to correct parents' perceptions or correct the way they are managing feedings. For example, a parent may believe they must wean when their baby's teeth begin to erupt. You might start with an active listening statement such as, "You're worried it will hurt when Matthew has teeth." You can then continue with, "You will find that Matthew's tongue covers the bottom teeth during sucking." With this two-fold response, you have corrected the misconception and, at the same time, provided affirmation by accepting the parent's concern.

When correcting a misconception or mismanagement, using a warm and friendly tone of voice will provide information without making parents feel foolish or uninformed. Rather than saying, "You should . . ." or "I think . . . ," you can say, "You may want to . . ." or "You may find that when you . . ." or "What do you think about . . . ?" or "How would that work?" These types of responses help preserve parents' self-confidence while you educate them. The following example demonstrates a response to tactfully clear up a misconception:

Parent: Isn't it great that you don't get your period while you're nursing?

Response: That's true for some parents, Lisa. It doesn't always happen that way. There's a lot of variation among individuals. When you are lactating . . . [You can then explain the effect of lactation on menstruation and ovulation. Lisa had the general idea and just needed some clarification.]

Summarizing

Parents will benefit from a summary of their care plan that is concise and easy to understand so that they are certain of what to try. Summarizing reviews the highlights of what was discussed and reinforces important aspects. This skill is especially helpful after a lengthy conversation. When possible, urge parents to do the summarizing to confirm their understanding and help them assume responsibility for the care plan. You may say, for example, "From what we discussed, which things will you try to increase your milk production?" The following example illustrates a summarizing response:

Response: Amanda, you said you're having trouble expressing your milk at work. We talked about finding a more private place to pump, playing some soothing music, and trying to schedule a longer break so that you don't feel so rushed. You have an information sheet to take home with tips for working and nursing, along with links for online working parent support groups. How does that work for you?

Counseling Scenario

The counseling skills you use as you gather information will help clarify a parent's message and concerns and provide emotional support and validation. These skills produce essential information and impressions before you move on to educating and problem-solving. Your continued use of reflective listening, empathetic listening, and open-ended questions while you educate parents will establish a comfortable flow to the exchange. The counseling scenario in **Table 5-4** demonstrates the flow of information gathering, affirmation, and education as the parent, Linda, and the lactation consultant, Devyn, work toward problem-solving. Problem-solving and follow-up are discussed in **Chapter 6**.

Table 5-4 Scenario Using All Counseling Skills

Parent	Consultant Response	Comments
(Sounding weary and discouraged) I'm so tired. My baby has been getting up three times a night for the last 3 nights.	You really sound discouraged, Linda.	Devyn uses active listening to provide emotional support and personalizes the exchange by using Linda's name.
Yeah. I thought we were really getting somewhere with sleeping through the night last week. And now Michael acts starved at night.	It seems to you like Michael is backsliding.	Devyn continues to give emotional support through active listening and personalizes the exchange by using Michael's name.
I'll say—and just when my sister and my sister's three kids have come for a week's visit.	Mmmm. That's a lot of company.	Devyn uses an attending response and forms a hunch that Linda is too active, leading to a decrease in milk production. Linda did not say anything about activities with the sister. Devyn cannot assume immediately that Linda is too tired or that Michael isn't getting enough milk. Devyn needs to wait for Linda's response to know if this hunch is correct.
It is a lot of people, but my sister is very helpful; she's doing most of the cooking and keeping my house in better shape than I do!	That's great for you, Linda. So, your sister is more help than work for you.	Devyn learns that the first hunch was incorrect. The use of active listening encourages Linda to give more information.
Definitely.	Let's get back to what Michael is like during the day.	Devyn redirects the discussion back to the baby and uses Michael's name to personalize the exchange. Devyn seeks hidden factors that will help identify the problem.
Michael wakes up around 8:00 a.m. and eats, eats again around 10:30 and then naps, eats again at 1:00 and 3:00, then takes another nap until about 6:00. For the past couple of days, Michael fusses and eats a couple of times during the evening and goes to bed about 10:00.	Let's see, Linda, that's about six feedings during the day, so nine feedings in 24 hours. How does each feeding go?	Devyn uses Linda's name again to personalize the exchange. Devyn summarizes what was said and asks an open-ended question to gain more information.
Well, Michael fools around a lot, eating, looking around, and watching my sister's kids.	You know, Linda, this is the age when babies are easily distracted by people and motion and noise.	Devyn uses Linda's name and then responds with interpreting and educating to test whether these distractions are the cause of the problem.

(continues)

Table 5-4 Scenario Using All Counseling Skills *(continued)*

Parent	Consultant Response	Comments
Michael is definitely distracted. Every time someone comes near, Michael stops nursing and looks at them.	It's hard for Michael to pay attention to eating with so many people around.	Devyn uses Michael's name in an active listening response to voice an alternative hunch.
That's right.	So, you're saying that Michael is distracted a lot during the day and seems especially hungry at night.	Devyn uses Michael's name in an interpreting response to test the hunch.
Do you think Michael might be making up for not getting enough milk during the day?	That seems to be a possibility.	Devyn uses an attending response to encourage Linda to provide additional information that might shed more light on the situation.
That makes sense. When we were alone for a feeding yesterday, Michael ate for a long time and took an exceptionally long nap.	Michael seemed to sleep better after nursing with no distractions.	Devyn received confirmation that the hunch was correct and uses an interpreting response.
Yeah.	Linda, perhaps it might help if you nurse Michael in a quieter place during the day.	Devyn uses Linda's and Michael's names and suggests an alternative action.
I could go into the living room. The kids pretty much stay in the family room, and my sister and I could talk quietly.	Good idea. You might also try waking Michael sooner from the long afternoon nap and add an extra feeding in the afternoon.	Devyn uses Michael's name and suggests an alternative action. Linda has accepted the first suggestion and is trying to adapt it to the situation. Devyn can document this as the beginning of a plan of action.
Well, I could, but that would interfere with my making supper after my sister leaves. I really like that quiet time to make supper, and I hate to work on supper in the morning.	It wouldn't work for you. Okay, so you're going to try to nurse in a quieter place, to see if Michael is satisfied during the day and sleeps better at night.	Devyn realizes Linda does not like the second suggestion and uses active listening as a graceful way to withdraw the rejected suggestion. By not pushing it, Devyn shows support and validates Linda's right to decide how to handle the situation. Devyn uses Michael's name while summarizing what they have discussed and arriving at a plan of action. Although this example limits the plan to one option, there likely would be more suggestions in a real-life situation.
Yes.	Great, Linda! Please give me a call next week to let me how this has worked. Feel free to call me before then if you need to.	Devyn uses Linda's name and arranges follow-up.

Summary

Communication skills and counseling skills are essential for healthcare providers who work in a helping role. The ability of caregivers to communicate well determines the quality of care they provide. Being aware of body language and other components of communication and using effective counseling techniques will provide parents with the support and teaching to develop confidence in their parenting and lactation. Approaching parents in a warm, caring manner will show deep, genuine concern and empathy to help them take positive action in dealing with their situation. The communication and counseling skills presented in this chapter will help you gather information and insights, provide emotional support and affirmation, and provide education that will lead to problem-solving. Using counseling skills that are appropriate to each situation will help you develop and continue to improve your interactions with parents.

What You Learned—At a Glance

Conversation Starters with Parents

- How comfortable are you with personal space and touch?
- How has previous trauma affected you in your adult life?
- How confident do you feel with nursing?
- How do you respond when you feel overloaded with information?

Communication

- Communication is 10% spoken or written word, 38% voice tone, and 52% body language.
- Negative terminology can undermine self-confidence and send a judgmental message.
- Body language is powerful in engaging and empowering parents.
- There are cultural differences in body language, personal space, and being touched.
- Reading parents' body language will help determine their comfort and receptiveness.

Participant-Focused Counseling

- Participant-focused counseling builds rapport and targets education to individual needs.
- Caregivers' personalities affect their rapport with parents.
- Effective counseling requires gathering sufficient information and providing affirmation before teaching.

Trauma-Informed Care (TIC)

- Trauma is prevalent among all races, ethnicities, ages, and socioeconomic backgrounds.
- ACEs affect physical, psychological, and social development and well-being into adulthood.
- TIC assumes that all individuals are more likely than not to have a history of trauma.
- TIC ensures safety, builds trust, and offers support.
- TIC is sensitive to gender identity and to racial, ethnic, historical, and cultural background.

Information Gathering

- Listening skills facilitate gathering information and insights and help parents hear themselves to sort out their feelings and concerns.
- Effective listening involves verbal and nonverbal messages, perceiving with the ears, eyes, and imagination.
- Active listening gathers information, clarifies messages, shows acceptance, and encourages responses.
- Empathetic listening reveals emotions and supports parents as they work through their feelings.
- Clarifying, open-ended questions, reflecting, and redirecting help obtain more information, define the situation, and focus on specific concerns.

Affirmation

- Affirmation builds rapport and focuses on parents' feelings.
- Reassuring, building hope, and identifying strengths can positively influence outcomes.
- Caregivers need to gain parents' trust and clarify their situation before engaging in teaching.

Education

- Receiving timely information, anticipatory guidance, and resources enables parents to handle new challenges as they arise.
- Limiting the number of suggestions in a single counseling session will avoid overwhelming parents.
- Correcting misconceptions or mismanagement needs to be done with sensitivity and respect.
- Having parents summarize the conversation encourages self-direction and self-efficacy.

References

Bischof G, et al. Motivational interviewing: an evidence-based approach for use in medical practice. *Dtsch Arztebl Int.* 2021;118(7):109–115.

Choi KR, et al. Promotion of maternal–infant mental health and trauma-informed care during the COVID-19 pandemic. *JOGNN.* 2020;49:409–415.

Damodaran D, Varghese K. The unveiled Indian picture of adverse childhood experiences: socio-demographic correlates among youth in Kerala. *Int Soc Sci Rev.* 2019;6:1248–1257.

DeFoor M, Darby W. "Motivate to lactate": utilizing motivational interviewing to improve breastfeeding rates. *J Perinat Educ.* 2020;1;29(1):9–15.

Dodgson JE, Bamberger ET. Sex and gender inclusiveness in lactation research. *J Hum Lact.* 2021;37(2):237–241.

Duckett LJ, Ruud M. Affirming language use when providing health care for and writing about childbearing families who identify as LGBTQI. *J Hum Lact.* 2019;35(2):227–232.

Fast J. *Body Language: How Our Movements and Posture Reveal Our Secret Selves.* New York: Open Road Integrated Media; 2014.

Fleishman J, et al. Trauma-informed nursing practice. *Online J Issues Nurs.* May 31, 2019. https://doi.org/10.3912/OJIN.Vol24No02Man03

Furman L, et al. Understanding breastfeeding barriers at an urban pediatric practice. *J Racial Ethn Health Disparities.* 2023;10(2):581–592.

Gallegos D, et al. Can a phone call make a difference? Breastfeeding self-efficacy and nurse responses to mother's calls for help. *J Child Health Care.* 2018;22(3):433–446.

Gameon JA, Skewes MC. A systematic review of trauma interventions in native communities. *Am J Community Psychol.* 2020;65(1–2):223–241.

Gregory EF, et al. Motivational interviewing to promote interconception health: a scoping review of evidence from clinical trials. *Patient Educ Couns.* 2022;105(11):3204–3212.

Gribble KD, et al. Effective communication about pregnancy, birth, lactation, breastfeeding and newborn care: the importance of sexed language. *Front Glob Womens Health.* 2022;3:818856.

Helou S, et al. Physician communication skills in telemedicine: the role of eye contact. *Stud Health Technol Inform.* 2022; 290:849–853.

Hojat M, et al. The Jefferson Scale of Empathy: a nationwide study of measurement properties, underlying components, latent variable structure, and national norms in medical students. *Adv Health Sci Educ Theory Pract.* 2018;23(5):899–920.

International Board of Lactation Consultant Examiners. IBCLC detailed content outline. May 1, 2023. https://ibclc-commission.org/wp-content/uploads/2023/05/2023_IBCLC_Detailed_Content_Outline_FINAL.pdf

Isobel S, Thomas M. Vicarious trauma and nursing: an integrative review. *Int J Ment Health Nurs.* 2022;31(2):247–259.

Kim J, et al. A scoping review of vicarious trauma interventions for service providers working with people who have experienced traumatic events. *Trauma Violence Abuse.* 2022;23(5):1437–1460.

Manyema M, Richter LM. Adverse childhood experiences: prevalence and associated factors among South African young adults. *Heliyon.* 2019;5(12):e03003.

Merrick MT, et al. Vital signs: estimated proportion of adult health problems attributable to adverse childhood experiences and implications for prevention—25 states, 2015–2017. *MMWR Morb Mortal Wkly Rep.* 2019;68:999–1005.

Naroee H, et al. The effect of motivational interviewing on self-efficacy and continuation of exclusive breastfeeding rates: a quasi-experimental study. *Breastfeed Med.* 2020;15(8):522–527.

National Child Traumatic Stress Network. Populations at risk. Retrieved February 2, 2023. https://www.nctsn.org/what-is-childtrauma/populations-at-risk

Prentice F, et al. Gender differences in interoceptive accuracy and emotional ability: an explanation for incompatible findings. *Neurosci Biobehav Rev.* 2022;141:104808.

Tooley EM, Kolahi A. Motivating behavioral change. *Med Clin North Am.* 2022;106(4):627–639.

White SJ, Preda V. Communication as a clinical skill: a challenge in the delivery of safe and effective patient care. *Aust Health Rev.* 2022;46(1):62–63.

CHAPTER 6

Client Consultations

Parents have more positive lactation outcomes when they receive consistent encouragement, help, and guidance at appropriate times. A preventive approach is a time-saving method that is far more effective than crisis management. Some situations are more suited to counseling by phone, text, online, or email, whereas others require an in-person **assessment**. Sometimes, a situation has advanced by the time contact occurs, requiring more intense problem-solving. Collaborating with parents will help them recognize possible causes of problems and practical actions to resolve them. Use of counseling skills, as presented in **Chapter 5,** will help determine the situation and gain insights into what caused it. This chapter continues the helping process through a systematic approach to problem-solving, consultations, and documentation for working toward a solution.

KEY TERMS

Alternative hunches
Anticipatory guidance
Assessment
Bristol Breastfeeding Assessment Tool (BBAT)
Care plan
Electronic communication
Electronic health record
Electronic medical record
History
Hunch
Infant Breastfeeding Assessment Tool (IBFAT)
LATCH
Mother–Baby Assessment
SMART goals

Anticipatory Guidance

Anticipatory guidance is a proactive counseling technique that is used in individual consultations, support groups, and lactation programs throughout the world. All areas of the medical community engage in anticipatory guidance through preventive medicine. Well-baby checkups, dental exams, Pap smears, and routine eye exams are all examples of preventive care. Modern medicine clearly recognizes the benefits of early detection. Providing anticipatory guidance for lactation to new parents is helpful for all caregivers who work with families. Anticipatory guidance reduces stress, helps prevent negative outcomes, and empowers parents to sustain lactation in spite of challenges (Hsu et al., 2018; Jackson et al., 2021). It helps establish a foundation of knowledge that leads to optimal lactation practices. This investment of time and energy pays off in fewer problems and more positive outcomes. An enjoyable experience for parents, with less time spent on problem-solving, makes this a parent-friendly and time-saving approach.

Contact at key times can diminish or avoid problems. When parents receive practical information and support before significant milestones occur, they can anticipate impending changes and identify their needs. Anticipatory guidance prepares parents who feel uncertain about nursing by helping them know what to expect and increasing their confidence in meeting each new milestone (Kuliukas et al., 2019). The anticipatory guidance that clinicians provide helps reduce unmet needs and empowers parents along each step and different aspects of the parenting journey (Dosman et al., 2019; Garg et al., 2018; Ismail et al., 2018; Williams et al., 2019).

The Timing of Anticipatory Guidance

Anticipatory guidance needs to occur at a teachable moment, a time of optimal attention and capacity for learning when retention of information is highest and when decision-making takes place. The infant feeding decision usually occurs before the baby's birth, often even before pregnancy, as discussed in **Chapter 12**. Thus, early exposure to lactation information will help expectant parents make their infant feeding decisions.

Early education about the biological imperative of human milk for babies can help adolescents form healthy perceptions of sexuality and parenthood. Adolescents are receptive to learning about lactation during their secondary school years (Reyes et al., 2019). Adolescence is an ideal time for correcting misconceptions, promoting positive attitudes, and establishing a sound knowledge base (Čatipović et al., 2018). When adolescents reach adulthood, reinforcement of early concepts will further guide them in making sound decisions.

It is easier to address specific needs after establishing a comfortable relationship with parents. A climate characterized by acceptance, flexibility, and cooperation sets the stage for a positive nursing experience. Making contact during pregnancy helps build rapport and trust, which in turn increases the likelihood of accepting advice. After a program of comprehensive prenatal education, valuable time postpartum can be spent reinforcing and reviewing issues presented earlier.

The Need for Anticipatory Guidance

Nursing parents often lack role models, an experienced support person, practical and timely information, and the self-confidence to anticipate their babies' needs. The only source of information for some parents may be a brief discussion at a childbirth or postpartum class—or formula company misinformation. Many learn through websites or blogs replete with formula advertising and personal, non-evidence-based opinions. At a time when parents' energies and concentration are centered on their infant's birth and their changing role, retention of lactation information may be minimal at best. Parents may combine half-remembered instructions with incorrect information from well-meaning friends and relatives.

Some caregivers fail to support parents adequately through lactation challenges. Some may allow passionate advocacy to override awareness of how difficult it may be for a parent to implement their advice. A knowledgeable and sensitive caregiver is key to parents' ability to meet their feeding goals. Lactation consultants and peer counselors bridge the gap in teaching lactation management and providing emotional support (Broom et al., 2022; Thomson & Crossland, 2019).

Anticipatory guidance provided one step at a time can save parents and infants from potential feeding difficulties. Timely guidance can teach and inform parents well in advance of critical periods. Their preparedness and self-confidence will often be enough to prevent problems. Any problems that do occur will likely be of shorter duration and with less chance of recurrence.

Outreach Counseling

Lactation education needs to be viewed in the larger context of a preventive approach to health care, in much the same way that dental checkups help prevent cavities. Parents who receive continuing support and information prenatally and throughout lactation become prepared for what will unfold at each stage. Prevention counseling provides the anticipatory guidance parents need for increasing their self-efficacy and meeting the challenges of parenting with confidence.

Initiation and duration rates are higher when there is consistent encouragement, help, and guidance prenatally, during the hospital stay, and postpartum (Cordell & Elverson, 2021; Huang et al., 2019). Parents who receive necessary information and support have significantly longer lactation with fewer problems. Prenatal support is more effective than support given only after delivery. Support both before and after delivery produces the best results. Anticipatory guidance and concrete information are especially crucial for continuing to nurse after returning to work or school (Spatz, 2018, 2019). Lack of information is a key factor in premature weaning (Hamze et al., 2019). Refer to **Chapter 18** for further discussion on weaning.

When a caregiver's work setting does not allow extended outreach, a hotline, warmline, or electronic communication may be a practical method for reaching out to parents. Some parents may not desire frequent contact. Sensitivity to their cues will establish an opportunity for them to gracefully make their wishes known. For parents who prefer to manage their lactation privately, the most effective approach may be to let them know how to initiate contact.

Support Groups

Referring parents to breastfeeding support groups can provide the anticipatory guidance and lactation assistance they need. Community support groups are available through hospitals; La Leche League; Women, Infants, and Children (WIC); Breastfeeding USA; the Black Mothers' Breastfeeding Association (BMBFA); and similar organizations throughout the world. Online support groups are available on Facebook, Instagram, and Reddit.

Support groups typically provide the services of peer counselors, who are important partners in the parents' support team. They provide much of the prenatal and postpartum support and education new parents receive. Peer counselors typically communicate with families through phone, texts, email, and social media. Ideally, contact begins several weeks or months before delivery, and it may continue through weaning. Many support groups also host meetings for parents to attend. Lactation consultants can be instrumental in helping support groups to establish effective outreach to families in the community. **Chapter 2** discusses support groups.

Prenatal Contact

Reaching families during pregnancy can lay the groundwork for optimal lactation practices. Outreach counseling encourages expectant parents to educate themselves about lactation through online sources, reading, attending meetings or classes, observing babies nursing, and voicing their questions and concerns. The use of listening skills will help identify their feeding goals, the extent of their knowledge, and their need for support. Allowing ample opportunity to ask questions will ensure that their questions and concerns are addressed. Ensuring that they know how to contact you—whether by phone, text, or other electronic communication—and the best times to reach you will encourage them to reach out when they begin nursing.

Continuing Regular Contact

Parents benefit from frequent contact in the early weeks of nursing to ensure they understand the principles of managing feedings and minimizing challenges. **Table 6-1** presents guidelines for deciding how often to contact parents and what to discuss at each stage. The information parents learn through these contacts can help them learn the following:

- How to respond to hunger cues
- How to know when their baby has an effective latch
- How to ensure ample milk production
- How to respond to the baby's periods of increased hunger (growth spurts)
- Typical nursing patterns for babies of different ages
- How to trust themselves and their baby

Use of counseling skills will help determine when confidence and knowledge will sustain parents. As they learn more about their baby and managing feedings, the frequency of contacts can gradually diminish unless they experience problems. Initiating contact at times when the potential for problems typically occurs will give parents the support and advice they need. Detailed records and thorough evaluations of each contact will help determine appropriate follow-up. Your judgment and intuition, along with open communication and rapport with parents, will help you and the parents decide when contact can end.

Problem-Solving

An important element of counseling is helping parents minimize problems and find solutions when they arise. After receiving relevant support and gaining an understanding of a situation, parents will be better able to take positive action in dealing with their concerns. Problem-solving begins with gathering information and sorting through the facts to help parents clarify their situation. Obtaining sufficient information and impressions helps avoid jumping in with irrelevant or unnecessary problem-solving. This kind of troubleshooting often involves using intuition to develop a hypothesis, or **hunch**. Hunches will help focus your clinical reasoning and identify suggestions that will be most helpful to the circumstances.

Determining the Problem

Problems can occur even when parents practice sound feeding management. Helping them recognize possible causes and practical actions will lead to finding ways to resolve them. Sometimes, parents need to take immediate action to reduce their physical discomfort before investigating the causes of a problem. If they do not receive comfort measures early in the contact, they may be unable to hear or accept information. The comfort measures parents need may not necessarily

Table 6-1 Anticipatory Guidance Milestones

During pregnancy	Expectant parents will benefit from one or two contacts during their pregnancy. You can recommend books and videos, urge them to begin acquainting themselves with lactation, and invite them to attend a support group meeting. This is an opportune time to begin building rapport and discussing their expectations and preparation for childbirth.
When the baby is born	If you have contact with expectant parents during pregnancy, you can ask them to let you know when they deliver. You can ask if they would like you to visit them if there is no lactation consultant support in the hospital. If you are unable to visit in person, you can ask if they would welcome a telephone call or text. Encourage them to talk about their labor and delivery. You may be the only person who shows an interest in helping them verbalize any disappointments or concerns regarding their birth. Ask how they feel and how the baby is doing. Ask their baby's name and start referring to the baby by name. Be sure they know when the next contact will be and who will initiate it.
Just home from the hospital	Parents often benefit from being contacted within 2–3 days after they return home, and more frequently if they have problems. Try not to overwhelm them with too much information. Possible issues to explore are as follows: ■ How they feel and level of fatigue ■ Number of feedings, voids, and stools in 24 hours ■ Positioning the baby during feedings ■ How to know the baby is getting enough milk ■ How to avoid problems such as nipple pain and engorgement
Baby 1 week old	Contact at this time can review the following: ■ Feeding frequency typically increases at approximately 10 days old. ■ Breast size will decline in response to increased feedings. ■ Milk production depends on supply and demand. ■ Continuing to respond to the baby's hunger cues ■ Typical feeding patterns at this age
Before baby's 2-week checkup	Help parents understand what the baby's healthcare provider will be looking for at the first checkup. Discuss normal weight patterns and feeding patterns. Help them form questions to ask during the visit. Call again after the checkup to ask about weight gain and any recommendations that were made. Help them integrate the healthcare provider's suggestions into their feedings and clarify any possible misunderstandings.
Baby 6 weeks old	Remind parents that their baby may go through a hunger spurt in response to the parent returning to a more active lifestyle. Caution them that the increased feedings may be prolonged if their activity level results in missed feedings. Discuss the possible effects of oral contraceptives on lactation.
After the first month	Parents will benefit from continued contact as the need arises. Some parents welcome routine contact all the way through weaning. Others may prefer to reach out when they have questions or need help.

be related to nursing. For example, a parent may be in pain from a cesarean incision, gas from a medical procedure, or perineum tearing or stitching. They may have a backache from labor or from an epidural. Simple measures such as pillows, fresh water, and cold or hot packs may increase their physical comfort to allow for more effective problem-solving.

At times, parents may have waited a long time before initiating contact, or they may have received unhelpful, inappropriate, or contradictory advice. As a result, they might lack confidence in their feeding ability. Sometimes, a problem may have advanced to the point that the only recourse is to assist in weaning and provide emotional support. When this happens, reflective listening can validate the grief parents may feel. Recalling the positive aspects of nursing their baby may provide hope that feedings can follow a more rewarding course for a subsequent baby.

Critical Thinking

No single universal solution is appropriate for every feeding problem. Critical thinking skills will provide the judgment, knowledge, and intuition to form reflective judgments to problem-solve. Feeding problems are often complex, with multiple causes and no specific "right" solution. It is important to define all aspects of a situation clearly before looking for solutions. This may include the parent's medical history, labor complications and birth experience, breast assessment, feeding history, and milk expression. It may also include the baby's medical history, health status and temperament, prenatal concerns, and any postpartum complications. A feeding assessment will identify any issues with positioning, latch, and milk transfer.

Clinical reasoning is a complex process of identifying and prioritizing clinical data to develop a hypothesis and a **care plan** to confirm or refute that hypothesis (Richards et al., 2020). The critical thinking process requires clarifying the purpose and context, analyzing the sources of information, evaluating the arguments, making inferences and creating conclusions, and monitoring the results. Core critical thinking skills are described in **Table 6-2**.

Table 6-2 Core Critical Thinking Skills

Skill	Description
Interpretation	■ Clarify the problem and what caused it. ■ Determine if you understand the problem sufficiently. ■ Consider different viewpoints and arguments. ■ Decode the significance of data.
Analysis	■ Examine ideas and information from reliable sources. ■ Identify arguments and assumptions. ■ Make connections between ideas. ■ Systematically consider all aspects of the problem. ■ Consider each element in its wider context.
Evaluation	■ Assess the claim's credibility, strengths, and limitations. ■ Assess the quality of arguments that were made using inductive or deductive reasoning. ■ Evaluate how the quality of one source or argument compares with other sources. ■ Determine what contribution the argument makes to knowledge and clinical practice. ■ Consider your overall assessment of the source or argument. ■ Determine what claims need further investigation.
Inference	■ Consider relevant information needed to draw logical conclusions. ■ Conjecture alternatives. ■ Draw logically valid or justified conclusions.
Explanation	■ Present the results. ■ Justify your reasoning in terms of the considerations upon which the results are based. ■ Present reasons in the form of cogent arguments.
Self-regulation or self-correction	■ Analyze and evaluate your personal judgments and conclusions. ■ Question, confirm, validate, or correct your reasoning or results.

Data from APA Report: Expert Consensus Statement on Critical Thinking. (ERIC ED 315 423) and What is critical thinking? Monash University. https://www.monash.edu/learnhq/enhance-your-thinking/critical-thinking/what-is-critical-thinking.

Shared Decision-Making

Engaging parents in decision-making is pivotal to client-centered care (Tonelli & Sullivan, 2019). Shared decision-making is a process of collaborative deliberation that respects clients' autonomy and engagement, with both the caregiver and the care receiver sharing information (Elwyn, 2021). Caregivers provide options based on expertise and describe the risks and benefits of each option in detail. Clients share their comprehension of the options, their values, and their preferences. This collaborative approach reduces the patronizing element frequently encountered in health care (Fibuch & Ahmed, 2017; Street et al., 2017). It allows clients time to ask questions, consider the information, and process any uncertainties.

Parents' understanding will come more readily when they are equal partners in problem-solving. Providing emotional support, patiently listening, and encouraging parents to communicate openly validates their perception of a problem and encourages their participation in working toward a solution. This empathetic approach helps reduce anxiety and enables parents to be more patient and objective as they engage in joint problem-solving. They will be better able to help develop a plan that produces the best results and decreases the likelihood of recurrences. Working with parents to define their problems and explore possible actions helps them develop confidence and skills and assume responsibility for meeting future challenges.

Goal Setting

Setting the goals for problem-solving is an important part of shared decision-making. A formal approach to goal setting will help plan a path with a clear focus and increase the chances of achieving the goal. Goal setting with **SMART goals** is one method for creating and evaluating clinical goals. SMART stands for Specific, Measurable, Achievable, Realistic, and Time-based (Mind Tools, 2024). A specific goal has a much greater chance of being accomplished than a general goal. Measurable, concrete criteria will enable tracking of progress toward the attainment of the goal. A goal that is attainable and realistic will increase parents' willingness to work toward it. There must also be parameters for measuring progress toward achieving the goal. **Table 6-3** presents possible SMART goals for nursing parents.

Working Toward a Solution

The process of working toward a solution begins with forming a hunch and defining the problem. This may at times resemble peeling back the layers of an onion as you dig deeper into possible hidden factors related to the situation. Continuing to explore the circumstances will eliminate unrelated causes and lead to testing the hunch. Parents' feedback will determine any need to explore alternative hunches and look for other possible causes. After defining the problem, you and the parents can examine possible options for resolving it. Involving parents in developing a plan in this way increases the likelihood that they will follow it.

Table 6-3 SMART Goals for Nursing Parents

SMART Goal	Questions to Ask
Specific	What needs to be accomplished? What actions need to occur? What information or resources are needed?
Measurable	What will determine that the goal is accomplished?
Achievable	What will determine if the parent can achieve the goal?
Realistic	Is the goal realistic and within reach for this parent? Will the parent commit to achieving the goal?
Time-based	When will achievement of the goal be evaluated?

Step 1: Form a Hunch

Determining how parents view a situation, what they think caused it, and how they have tried to resolve it will help in forming a hunch about the cause and considering a possible solution. Forming a hunch is more of an unconscious reflex than a carefully reasoned analysis. Concentrating on a preliminary hunch helps focus observations and reduces aimless thinking. Continuing to use counseling skills to gather more information and impressions will further clarify and define the situation.

Step 2: Look for Hidden Factors

In many cases, hidden factors may contribute to a feeding problem. Infants who nurse frequently at night may sleep for long periods during the day. Parents who worry that their milk is not rich enough may have expressed milk and noticed the typical thin, watery appearance of their milk. Or they may no longer feel the sensation of copious milk production, and their baby is not gaining weight. Encouraging parents to talk and listening attentively to their needs and concerns will help identify any hidden factors.

Step 3: Test Your Hunch

Counseling responses such as "From what you're describing . . ." or "Let me see if I understand . . ." or "You seem to be. . ." can test your hunch. This helps parents hear what they are telling you so that they can provide further clarification if necessary. When parents complain that "It hurts when I nurse," for example, explore whether they are feeling the sensation when the milk lets down, the tugging sensation of sucking, or pain throughout a feeding. Pain thresholds vary considerably from person to person. You can quantify the perception of pain by asking, "What is your pain level on a scale of 0 to 10, with 0 being no pain and 10 being the worst pain ever?" The parent's response will help clarify the level of discomfort.

Step 4: Explore Alternative Hunches

The insights you gain in testing your initial hunch may lead to pursuing other hunches to resolve a problem. Exploring **alternative hunches** will further clarify the situation. Sometimes, a problem may remain ill-defined throughout several contacts, perhaps over several weeks. At such times, it may be necessary to develop a trial plan that addresses the most obvious symptoms or concerns. When parents recognize which actions are most effective, they can begin to narrow down the cause of a problem. Networking with colleagues and healthcare team members may help with your analysis. Difficulty in determining a problem's cause and solution can be frustrating for both caregivers and parents. Acknowledge this frustration and offer support and encouragement as you and parents continue to work through the problem together.

Step 5: Develop a Care Plan

Creating a care plan, with parents deciding on specific actions they will take, helps them develop self-efficacy and take responsibility for decision-making. Parents often need this kind of reinforcement, especially when they doubt their parenting abilities in other areas. They may ask, "When do I pick up my baby?" or "How warmly should I dress my baby?" or "Am I doing this right?" Empowering parents through counseling and shared decision-making will help them gain the confidence necessary to find the answers to these questions. Developing a care plan and follow-up are discussed later in this chapter.

Consultation Methods

Some consultations require an in-person visit for assessment and interaction. Voice and electronic communication methods, as discussed in **Chapter 2**, are appropriate for a good deal of follow-up that occurs after hospital discharge or a clinic or office visit. It is important to establish parameters when using voice or electronic communication. Telephone, texting, and email services carry an implied contract to respond in a timely manner. Make sure parents know how soon they can expect a response. Also, establish the types of issues you can address without visiting with them in person. Make sure parents fully understand any fees associated with an in-person consultation. Keeping a log of all communication with parents is an important component of client documentation.

Telephone Support

Telephone support for nursing families is a mainstay of peer counseling and hospital follow-up. Timely follow-up increases lactation initiation and duration (Chaves et al., 2019; Forster et al., 2019; Olson et al., 2019). Many lactation issues do not require in-person visits. For parents who voice concern that their baby is fussy or not sleeping through the night, for example, reviewing their feeding practices can ensure that they are nursing frequently enough. A concern about engorgement may be solved with adjustments in feeding routine. A telephone call can

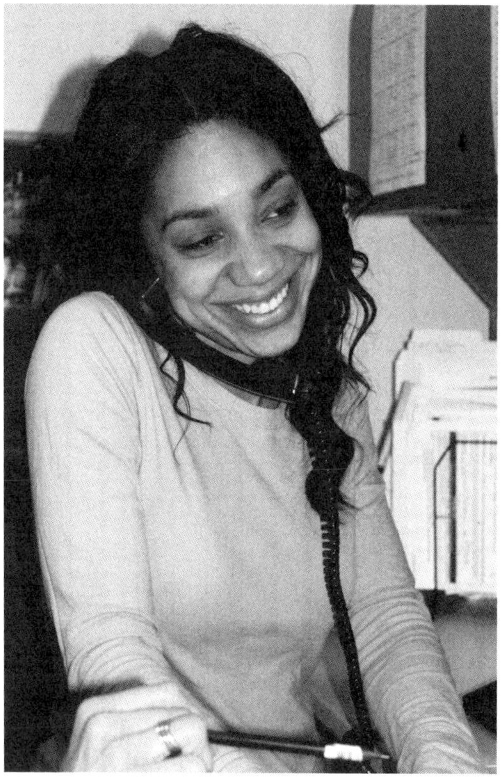

Figure 6-1 Smiling on the phone conveys warmth.
Photo by Every Mother, Inc.

provide the needed information, along with vocal reassurance and support.

Telephone support can be of great value in disadvantaged areas, perhaps because of the potential for greater social barriers (Thorpe et al., 2018). Families in low-income, inner-city, and rural areas with few resources often receive inadequate support after they leave the hospital. A lactation support line can help overcome this potential obstacle. Parents in underserved areas are unlikely to initiate calls for help with feeding, in part because they may undervalue nursing and their own needs (Hunt & Thomson, 2017).

Initiating telephone contact in a reassuring communication style can increase a parent's confidence. During face-to-face contacts, body language is a great indicator of how a message is received. Telephone contact lacks such visual cues and relies on voice tone and spoken words to relay messages. A smile and soothing voice tone will convey warmth and sincerity and enhance the exchange (**Figure 6-1**). Components of communication are discussed in **Chapter 4.**

Electronic Support

Electronic communication is increasingly replacing face-to-face contact. It is especially useful for factual questions, such as how to express milk or how to accommodate a return to work or school. Advances in technology allow a shift in the delivery of lactation support from traditional in-person care to virtual delivery. Lactation consultants, peer counselors, primary care providers and other caregivers use electronic communication to inform, reassure, encourage, and support nursing parents. These forms of communication offer a cost-effective, timely way to provide information and support, and to reinforce teaching (Mohamad Pilus et al., 2022; Sevda & Sevil, 2023).

Virtual care through smartphone applications, text messaging, and the internet can increase exclusive nursing (Blackmore et al., 2022). A lactation smartphone app is shown to increase lactation knowledge, attitude, and self-efficacy (Saucedo Baza et al., 2023; Seyyedi et al., 2021). Teaching modules with video clips downloaded to a personal tablet computer for parents with babies in the special care nursery resulted in increased attachment to their infants, greater perceived support, and increased exclusive nursing (Fu et al., 2021).

Texting

The use of texting for lactation support is very effective. Parents who receive regular text-based education and support nurse exclusively for longer periods and are more likely to meet their feeding goals (Bender et al., 2022; Harari et al., 2018; Unger et al., 2018). Because the length of text messages is limited to 160 characters, abbreviations help to keep messages brief. Providing a list of terms that are typically used will ensure that parents understand them. Reviewing the text before it is sent will ensure that it is clear and conveys the intended tone. It is important that message communication platforms are secure and protect client privacy. The use of texting for communication of routine healthcare issues is increasing, requiring improvements in the privacy and security of this medium.

Email

Some clinicians provide lactation support through email messages to clients. It is important to keep copies of all electronic correspondence to and from clients as part of their documentation. When emails are downloaded from the server to a hard drive, keeping backup copies online or on a storage device will protect the data over the long term.

Use of a secure, encrypted web-based (cloud) server for email communication protects client privacy. Clients are rightfully concerned about the potential for an **electronic health record** (EHR) to result in breached privacy and misuse of health data. Loss and theft of private health information are growing concerns, especially with the widespread use of EHRs and large data-security breaches (Chernyshev et al., 2018). Caregivers should inform parents of privacy issues and include a disclaimer at the bottom of any electronic transmission. **Figure 6-2** shows examples of such disclaimers. Chapter 28 discusses of confidentiality and privacy issues.

> NOTE: The information contained in this document may be confidential. If you have received this information in error, please contact me at [put your contact information here].
>
> NOTE: The information contained in this electronic mail may be privileged and confidential and protected from disclosure. If the reader of this message is not the intended recipient, or an employee or agent responsible for delivering this message to the intended recipient, you are hereby notified that any dissemination, distribution, or copying of this communication is strictly prohibited. If you have received this communication in error, please notify the sender immediately at [put your contact information here].

Figure 6-2 Electronic communication disclaimers.

Social Media

Many parents seek lactation information and support online through health-related websites and social networking groups. Receiving peer support on social media may positively influence norms and confidence in nursing, help overcome challenges, and extend nursing duration (Robinson et al., 2019). There is wide variability in information quality, website usability, and compliance with standards of medical internet publishing (Stokes-Parish, 2022; Zhang & Kim, 2022). Parents need to be discriminating in the advice they find online. Despite the ubiquity of the internet, it does not appear that online support will replace traditional methods of lactation support and education anytime soon (McFadden et al., 2017).

Telehealth

The use of telehealth, (illustrated in **Figure 6-3**) also called *telemedicine*, surged rapidly during the COVID pandemic and continues to be popular. Two-way electronic audiovisual technology offers clients and providers access to quality care when in-person care is not possible (Manocchia, 2020). Telehealth platforms are often encrypted and secure. One limitation is the availability of telehealth technology access and e-health literacy in resource-limited settings and low- and middle-income countries (Beheshti et al., 2022; Doraiswamy et al., 2020).

During the pandemic, almost half of U.S. hospitals provided virtual lactation consultations (Perrine et al., 2020). Remote consultations via teleconferencing

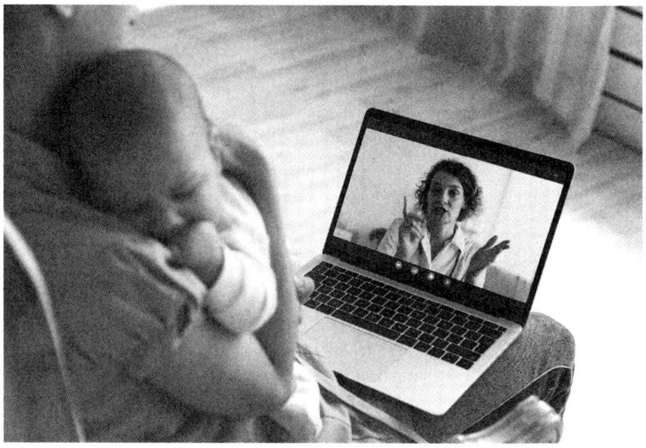

Figure 6-3 Telehealth expands outreach to clients.

have grown in popularity for both primary care and allied healthcare providers. Some pediatric groups provide remote lactation teleconference consultations. A growing number of lactation consultants provide remote consultations through videoconferencing. Telehealth can accommodate lactation issues that do not require in-person clinical assessment.

Telelactation interventions are well received by parents and healthcare providers (Bogulski et al., 2023; Chua et al., 2022). Telelactation is shown to increase nursing rates, duration, knowledge, and self-efficacy (Hubschman-Shahar, 2022). Remote access is especially helpful for families living in remote areas with no access to in-person lactation services (Demirci et al., 2019; Kapinos et al., 2019).

In-Person Visits

Many situations in lactation require that nursing parents and babies be present in person. If telephone or electronic communication causes concern or fails to provide sufficient insight, an in-person visit will be needed. Parents who seem shy or have difficulty expressing concerns may also need face-to-face interaction. Parents who acquire breast pumps from a pharmacy, business, or insurance company need assessment for properly fitting flanges. Parents who are using any device will need instruction and assistance in its use. In addition, the need for a device is often accompanied by a problem for which an in-person visit would provide insight into problem-solving.

Clinical Assessment

Clinical issues that require a physical assessment and evaluation are the most common reasons for in-person visits. A breast assessment, assessment of an infant's suck, or observation of a feeding provides insight into how to help with nipple pain or with difficulties caused by latch or positioning. Severe engorgement requires assessment to gain further insight into the cause and treatment. Concern about infant weight gain requires an infant assessment, observation of a feeding, and assessment of milk transfer, and possibly prefeeding and postfeeding weights. For legal protection, as well as for the baby's safety, it is advisable to insist on a consultation or referral to a healthcare provider for any concerns with an infant's weight.

Challenges with Face Masks

The advent of COVID brought challenges with the wearing of masks during in-person visits. A face mask creates a physical barrier to effective communication. It degrades hearing and interferes with lip reading, both of which can impede comprehension and engagement (Marler & Ditton, 2021). Interference with hearing and accurately interpreting what is being said obstructs clear two-way communication. Encouraging dialogue and providing time for questions and answers can help compensate for this communication deficit.

Face masks also interfere with reading facial expressions to interpret emotions and understanding. Smiles convey empathy, warmth, and genuineness in interactions. Frowns can convey confusion or lack of comprehension. The absence of these verbal cues affects the dynamics of the interaction and can impede parents' self-efficacy and sense of validation. Active listening and verbal affirmation of thoughts and feelings may help overcome the inability to observe facial expressions.

Communication recommendations when wearing face masks include the following:

- Minimize noise and distractions.
- If possible, show a picture of yourself without the mask.
- Encourage questions.
- Verbally recognize the challenges associated with mask wearing.
- Give verbal feedback to portray emotion (e.g., "I'm smiling back at you" or "I really empathize with the way you are feeling").
- Use culturally appropriate gestures and body language to express sentiment and indicate understanding (e.g., hand gestures such as thumbs-up and thumbs-down to clarify whether information has been adequately understood).
- Use flashcards, whiteboards, notepads, and information sheets to present or reinforce information.
- Use videos with specific clinical relevance.
- Safeguard confidentiality if voices are raised to compensate for mask wearing.

Elements of a Consultation

Lactation consultations may occur in hospitals, clinics, caregiver offices, pharmacies, or parents' homes. A personal introduction and using the parents' and baby's names will establish a supportive tone. Eye contact, a pleasant facial expression, and an approachable posture will transmit an interest to engage with parents in a meaningful way. The use of counseling skills will help gather information and insights while taking a history and performing assessments.

A consultation will include recording the reason for the visit, parent and infant histories and assessments, and any problems that are revealed. Impressions gained through observing a feeding, the physical assessments, and information obtained throughout the consultation will provide insights into any issues to address. Shared problem-solving can then lead to developing a care plan and determining any follow-up needed.

Obtaining Consent

Many elements of a lactation consultation involve interactions that require consent. A signed consent form protects both caregivers and clients. Consent may be implied in many healthcare settings. In a hospital or a medical group, for example, clients sign consent for all care provided within that setting. Explicit consent is advised even in those settings if a lactation visit includes clinical photos or the use of devices and techniques. In private practice, it is good practice to obtain signed consent *before* initiating a consultation. If a parent refuses to sign a consent form or crosses out significant parts, such as reporting to primary caregivers, it is risky to continue with the consultation. **Chapter 28** discusses informed consent.

A lactation consent should encompass all areas in which you will work with the dyad during the current and subsequent visits. This may include the following:

- Breast assessment
- Infant assessment, including oral structure and sucking
- Feeding assessment and assistance
- Use of devices and techniques related to infant caloric intake and feeding management
- Release of information to the insurance carrier
- Reports to and consultation with primary caregivers
- Use of information for educational purposes, including photographs
- Payment and rental or sale of any equipment if parents pay directly for the consultation

Privacy of Healthcare Information

Protection of health information is in place in countries throughout the world. The European Union (EU) Charter of Fundamental Rights stipulates that EU citizens have the right to protection of their personal data. The U.S. Health Insurance Portability and Accountability Act (HIPAA) requires that healthcare practitioners obtain signed consents for all clients to safeguard the privacy of their health information and prohibit its use or disclosure unless authorized by the client. Becoming knowledgeable about provisions for protection of client health information in a caregiver's geopolitical region can ensure compliance.

Speaking quietly and avoiding the use of parents' and infants' names in public areas will avoid incidental disclosures of client health information. Locked file cabinets and strong computer passwords provide additional safeguards. If parents participate in research, deleting identifiers at the earliest opportunity will protect their private and confidential information from improper use. Most country privacy provisions permit disclosure of a client's healthcare information to legally authorized public health authorities to prevent or control disease, injury, disability, or suspected child neglect or abuse.

Taking a History

Caring for a nursing dyad requires a complete **history** of both parent and baby. Using a standard history form will help avoid omitting essential questions. A history is part of the official health record and needs to be complete. If you exclude an item on the history form, leaving it blank could suggest it was overlooked. Inserting *NA* ("not applicable") in the space will indicate that it is not pertinent to the history.

Eliciting Information for History

Counseling skills will help gather information and impressions while recording pertinent information in the history form. Periods of silence, as well as verbal and nonverbal cues, will encourage parents to talk. Listen to what parents say as well as *how* they say it, observing their body language to reveal what they may *not* be saying. Open-ended questions can elicit detailed information for identifying issues to explore. For example, asking, "How many times does your baby nurse in 24 hours?" rather than "How frequently does your baby nurse?" quantifies the number of feedings. If the parent reports pain, ask them to score the pain on a scale of 1–10 to help determine the level of pain. Asking how many days or hours the pain is experienced quantifies the response rather than descriptions like "for a while" or "all the time."

Paraphrasing and summarizing the topics discussed during the history taking will help focus on important issues. Ask parents how they perceive a problem and when it began. Provide feedback and offer emotional support throughout the history taking. Build on the information parents provide to flesh out anything you do not fully understand. Be as specific as possible and try to record what parents say accurately and objectively, without interpretation.

Items to Include in a History

Medical histories vary in depth and focus. Relevant elements of a lactation history include the following:

- Previous lactation experience—including milk production, duration, problems, and parent's perception
- Past and current medications—including contraceptives, insulin, thyroid medication, and any herbs, vitamins, or food supplements taken regularly
- Current diet—including the amount and type of fluids consumed daily
- Previous surgeries—including laparoscopy, gallbladder or gastric bypass, and any accidents, hospitalizations, or disorders that could affect lactation
- Pregnancy, labor, and birth experiences with this baby—including complications, length of labor and any medications or intervention, and type of delivery and any intervention
- Postpartum experience—including timing of first feeding, rooming in, skin-to-skin care, supplementation, and any complications
- How current nursing is going—including feeding frequency and duration, milk expression, and supplementation
- Baby's gestational age, weight gain, sleeping, crying, and behavior
- Stooling and voiding frequency and any change in pattern
- Any current lactation problems, what parents have tried, and the results of their efforts

Performing Assessments

Physical assessments of the parent and baby will provide insight into factors that may affect nursing. Asking permission before examining the baby or parent will help preserve parents' sense of control in the consultation process. Visual assessment of the parent's breasts and nipples, noting any scarring or abnormalities, will identify potential problems. The infant's physical assessment should include signs of hydration, caloric status, and general health. In a hospital setting, the infant assessment also includes reviewing information charted by staff, particularly the baby's daily weight, intake, and output. **Chapter 14** discusses infant assessment in more detail.

Feeding Assessment

A feeding assessment will confirm a parent's technique and self-confidence as well as the baby's ability to latch and suck for effective milk transfer. Before beginning the assessment, ensure the parent's privacy and help them find a comfortable position for the feeding. Explaining that the purpose is to observe what the baby does during the feeding focuses the assessment on the baby rather than on the parent. This will be less threatening and intimidating and avoids the impression of the parent being judged.

Allowing the feeding to proceed at the baby's pace without any suggestions or interventions will provide a clear picture of what is going on. The feeding assessment should focus on the parent's and baby's positioning, the latch, the baby's sucking pattern, evidence of milk transfer, and the appearance and condition of the breasts and nipples at the end of the feeding. If there are concerns with infant weight gain, a full feeding assessment with prefeeding and postfeeding weights may be needed. **Chapter 19** discusses infant weight.

The time spent during the feeding assessment can be used to gain further impressions. Observing the dynamics of the feeding and interactions between parents and their babies will reveal their body language, temperaments, behavior, and emotional states. Casual conversation using counseling skills can uncover details of parents' support network, cultural beliefs and practices, and their economic and employment status. Parents can define their feeding goals and what they have done to prepare for nursing. Capitalizing on the time spent during the feeding assessment will help provide clarity in identifying the parent's needs.

Developing a Care Plan

After completing physical and feeding assessments, a clear idea should emerge of whether a problem exists and what actions are needed. If a parent describes nipple pain, for example, the discomfort may cause the baby to not receive sufficient calories. The goal would thus be to decrease the nipple pain while also providing sufficient calories to the baby. From these

- Ensure the baby receives adequate nourishment, including possible use of supplements.
- Support milk production, including possible milk expression.
- Describe elements of the problem.
- Identify factors that will help solve the problem and prevent its recurrence.
- Summarize the actions to be taken.
- Indicate criteria for follow-up, including time frame and targets.

Figure 6-4 Elements of a lactation care plan.

general goals, a specific care plan can lead to nursing without pain while transferring milk effectively.

Elements of a Care Plan

Having a standard format for a care plan will help ensure inclusion of all essential information. Elements of a care plan are depicted in **Figure 6-4**. Parents will need to understand what caused the situation and how they can avoid its recurrence. The care plan will describe the problem, options for solving it, and plans for follow-up. Depending on the nature of the problem, the plan may include a feeding plan for the baby along with measures for pain relief and maintaining or increasing milk production.

To eliminate confusion and overload and learn whether a particular action is helpful, it is best to develop a plan with only two or three actions for solving a problem. The way parents respond to information and suggestions provides important clues as to whether they feel that what is proposed will help. When parents like a suggestion and adapt it to their situation, they are more likely to try it. If they seem noncommittal or reply with "Yes, but . . . ," they may be indicating that they do not believe the suggestion will work or that they will likely not try that option. Gathering further information will continue to define possible solutions.

In a hospital setting, providing instructions before hospital discharge is essential to facilitating nursing at home. When nursing is going well at discharge, a diary of the baby's feedings, voids, and stools, along with instructions regarding what is normal and where to get help, may suffice. If there are problems or concerns, parents will need a written care plan based on the assessment of the dyad.

Summarizing and Follow-Up

Asking parents to summarize their care plan will confirm that they understand what was discussed and can integrate it. Including the partner in the consultation and discussion of the care plan will empower them as a couple. This further empowers the nursing parent and increases their self-confidence and self-reliance.

The care plan should indicate a time limit on the actions the parent will take and arrange for follow-up. You might say, "So, you will try [specified action] for 2 days and will contact me on Thursday to let me know how it worked. In the meantime, please contact me if it gets worse or if something else develops." Follow-up will help you learn if the plan worked and if additional suggestions are needed. Follow-up is discussed in a later section.

Online Resources for Care Plans

A variety of online resources and smartphone lactation applications can assist in creating care plans. Apps designed for clinicians include common symptoms, weight loss and feeding amount calculators, and forms (Sidhu et al., 2019; Wang et al., 2018). The Newt app calculates weight loss, and indicates whether the birth was vaginal or cesarean and whether the infant is nursed or artificially fed (Newt Newborn Weight Tool, 2019). LactMed, an internet resource from the National Library of Medicine, describes parent and infant medications and drug levels, possible side effects, and alternative drugs to consider (U.S. National Library of Medicine, 2019).

Parents can log feedings, voids, stools, growth rates, and other information with online apps. Many apps enable users to send information to their healthcare provider. Parents should be aware of the extensive data mining apps utilize, through which developers increasingly personalize information based on the tracked data. Some parents may value the personal advice sourced from their tracked behavioral and contextual data (Otte et al., 2019), whereas others may not like the intrusiveness.

Reporting to Caregivers

As a part of the lactation healthcare team, it is good practice to send reports to caregivers for both the parent and the baby within 24 hours of consulting with a client. When there are immediate concerns, it may be necessary to contact the healthcare provider directly to discuss them. A brief report may suffice after providing a breast pump or other device or assisting a client via phone or email. Regular communication is especially important for an independent, community-based lactation consultant who has infrequent contact with other members of the team. Educating the team through such reports increases the likelihood of referrals and continuity of care.

1. Date of the client's appointment.
2. Names and addresses of parent's physician and baby's physician.
3. Regarding: Parent's and baby's names and baby's date of birth.
4. Dear Dr....,
5. Parent appointment was at your request, was self-referred, was referred by (include name if possible).
6. If you called the provider's office to give a verbal report or sent a written report, you can mention this in your letter.
7. Because of... (reason for referral).
8. Brief description of the parent's history (general health, conception, pregnancy, and birth).
9. Assessment of breasts and nipples.
10. Brief description of the baby's history (birth, Apgar scores, in-hospital feeding, current feedings, output, weights, behavior, etc.).
11. Assessment and present status of the baby (muscle tone, activity, skin turgor, oral cavity, behavior, weight, and so on).
12. Assessment of the feeding (include feeding weights, if possible).
13. Your assessment of the situation.
14. Suggestions you gave to the parent and the action plan that was developed.
15. Arrangements for follow-up with the parent.
16. If the patient was referred to you, thank the provider for allowing you to participate in the care of their client. If the client self-referred, you may comment about working with the provider with this couple ("It was a pleasure...").
17. Sincerely yours,... (your name, credentials, address, telephone number, fax number, email address, and website).

Figure 6-5 Elements of a healthcare provider report.

Creating a healthcare provider report using computer software ensures a professional appearance and provides a permanent record. Proofreading the document carefully, using the spell-check feature, and consulting an online medical dictionary will further ensure a professional report. The report should provide pertinent contact information, such as name, credentials, address, telephone number, fax number, email address, and website. Reports that are sent electronically need to include privacy notices to help protect client confidentiality. **Figure 6-5** identifies elements to include in a healthcare provider report. **Table 6-4** describes a consultation scenario from obtaining consent through writing a follow-up report.

Providing Follow-Up

Following up with parents after a consultation indicates a genuine concern in helping them. It helps confirm whether the care plan worked, increases parents' competence and self-confidence, and protects the health of infants. With limited teaching time before hospital discharge, follow-up ensures that nursing gets off to a good start. Some hospitals provide outpatient visits on a fee-for-service or billable basis. In these cases, family cost is a consideration when scheduling follow-up because insurance companies may restrict the number of visits. Some hospitals provide outpatient visits at no additional cost to the client. Some make follow-up telephone calls or send secure electronic messaging after discharge.

When follow-up services are not provided, parents will need referrals to community services and support groups; online resources; and places to obtain lactation devices, receive continued support, and network with other nursing families. If a particular work setting does not allow for frequent contact with families, peer counselors in a community support group are a valuable resource for follow-up contacts. Low-income parents can be referred to public health clinic services such as WIC in the United States. These referrals to community-based support ensure that new parents have adequate resources after they leave your care.

Arranging Subsequent Contact

A parent's level of need and the urgency of a situation will determine the nature and timing of follow-up. Parents who have difficulty at every feeding or who lack confidence may benefit from frequent contact until the situation improves. Less critical or short-term situations may accommodate less frequent contact. For example, a parent who is discouraged while pumping milk for a preterm hospitalized infant might benefit from daily contact for a while. In comparison, a parent with a nonsupportive or interfering family member might prefer less frequent contact.

Clarify who will initiate each contact and whether it will be by telephone, text or other electronic communication, or a scheduled visit. If parents are asked to initiate contact and they do not, you can reach out several times, documenting each attempt and any message you leave. Electronic communications minimize missed calls and enable you to document that you provided follow-up. If follow-up is critical, such as in the case of an infant who is failing to thrive, it would be prudent to notify the baby's healthcare provider when a parent does not follow up as requested.

Contact parents anytime you gain important new information, need to correct information you gave them, or need to gather more information to help resolve a problem. Parents appreciate such concern about their welfare and that of their baby. Be sensitive to signals from parents that they no longer feel the

Table 6-4 Consultation Scenario

Situation: Jasmine says, "My son Tyrell just had his 2-week checkup. My healthcare provider is concerned because Tyrell is still just under birth weight. They said I may need to supplement with formula, and I am so upset. I wanted to nurse exclusively, and now I don't know what to do."	
Convey emotional support	"I can understand that it's upsetting, Jasmine, that your healthcare provider recommended supplementing with formula."
Obtain consent	Ask Jasmine to sign and date a consent form before proceeding with the consultation.
Gather information through parent and infant history and assessment	■ Number of feedings in 24 hours ■ Pattern of sleeping and nursing ■ Feeding cues and Jasmine's response to them ■ Audible swallowing during feedings ■ How feedings end ■ Tyrell's behavior during and after feedings ■ Number of voids and stools in 24 hours ■ What Jasmine knows about lactation ■ Whether supplements were prescribed or mentioned as a possibility if immediate measures do not increase weight ■ Tyrell's general appearance, hydration status, birth weight, hospital discharge weight, and present weight ■ Pre- and postfeed weights ■ Condition of Jasmine's breasts and nipples ■ Latch, positioning, and milk transfer ■ Hunch: Jasmine is unfamiliar with normal feeding cues, and Tyrell is not nursing frequently enough for adequate milk intake and weight gain.
Develop a workable plan	■ If Tyrell transfers milk well, nurse 10 or more times in 24 hours around the clock. ■ Teach feeding cues, baby-led feeding, and how to watch and listen for audible swallows. ■ Teach how to compress breast tissue to enhance milk transfer. ■ Identify sources of support and suggest household help through this time.
Follow-up	■ Call the next day to evaluate how changes in nursing routine are going. ■ Do a weight check in 2 days. Perform another prefeed/postfeed assessment if needed.
Healthcare provider's report	If Jasmine is unsure about the healthcare provider's exact request regarding supplements, call the provider's office to clarify. Send a report within 24 hours outlining the care plan.

need for continued follow-up. Always make sure they understand that they may contact you before the next prearranged contact.

Researching Outside Sources

Follow-up can help determine whether additional resources, such as online resources or specialists, will help resolve a situation. This may involve reaching out to colleagues, especially if a situation is beyond the assistance you typically provide to families. Many lactation consultants work alone, and colleagues are a valuable source of professional support. A situation may become clearer after receiving further input and a fresh outlook. A colleague may, for example, identify additional information to obtain. Online resources such as social network groups for lactation professionals, medical search engines, and lactation science websites are available as well. It is important to seek help whenever a situation cannot be resolved with available resources.

Evaluating the Consultation

Evaluating the results of a care plan is an essential element of problem-solving. Follow-up will indicate whether the plan was useful and whether further support or assistance is needed. If a plan does not resolve a problem, the situation may be more complicated than first thought and may require another assessment. It is important to determine whether parents adhered to the care plan. Perhaps they were overwhelmed by too many suggestions or were unable or failed to follow through with the plan. Perhaps family members interfered with their attempts. Perhaps the care plan was too rigid, and other alternatives might work better. Remaining flexible, networking with colleagues, attending educational offerings, and reading current research will help identify effective treatment options.

Assessing Counseling Effectiveness

Self-evaluation is a valuable element in follow-up that assesses the appropriateness of support, education, and problem-solving. **Figure 6-6** identifies a series of questions to evaluate counseling effectiveness (Isselman et al., 1993). The questions in **Figure 6-7** assess the progression of the consultation. The degree of affirmative responses to these questions will help identify improvements that are needed.

Self-evaluation is especially important when a situation remains unresolved. Such self-reflection helps caregivers learn from their failures and plan for further contact to work toward a solution. It is through failures and mistakes that we learn and grow. Bear in mind that you cannot always "fix" a lactation problem. Parents own their problems, as well as the responsibility for resolving them. At times, a situation may indicate an underlying issue or need that is beyond your scope to resolve. It may be helpful to discuss a less-than-positive outcome with a colleague.

1. My confidence in my counseling skills has increased over the past 6 months.
2. I have identified the counseling style in which I am most comfortable and effective.
3. I am able to adapt my counseling style to meet the needs of parents.
4. I now use more attending and listening skills in my counseling sessions.
5. I can now recognize when a parent is not listening during the counseling process.
6. I am better able to acknowledge my feelings that arise during the counseling process.
7. I am better able to acknowledge parents' feelings during the counseling process.
8. I have altered the way I conduct counseling session based on the recognition of my own or parents' feelings.
9. I evaluate the environment before beginning the counseling session.
10. I take steps to correct the environment before beginning the counseling session.
11. I have requested changes in my work site environment that will enhance the counseling process.
12. I need further instruction, encouragement, or evaluation to enhance my counseling skills.

Figure 6-6 Questions to evaluate the counseling process.

Element	Questions
Affirmation and support	• What support did I give? • Did the parent seem relaxed and talkative? • If not, what skills can I use to encourage parents to talk freely? • In what other ways could I have supported the parent?
Information gathering	• Did I gather enough information so that we both understood the problem? • If not, what further information do I need?
Education	• Did I give appropriate information? • Did the parent understand it? • If not, what further information do I need to provide?
Shared decision making	• Did we form a partnership for problem solving? • Did I empower the parent to be self-sufficient in problem solving?
Developing a plan	• Did we make the plan together? • Is the plan workable? • Did the parent seem satisfied with the plan? • If not, what alternative actions could I suggest? • How will I know if the plan worked?
Follow-up	• What follow-up did we arrange? • Who will initiate follow-up?
Documentation	• Did I document the contact adequately? • How were notes from previous contacts helpful? • How can I improve my method of documentation?
Satisfaction	• Did the parent seem satisfied with the contact? • Am I satisfied in my helping role with this parent? • If not, what can I do to improve?

Figure 6-7 Questions to evaluate a consultation.

Documentation

Standard documentation will ensure that consent, assessments, recommendations, care plans, evaluations of treatments, and follow-up are all recorded. In the United States, The Joint Commission accredits hospitals through stringent guidelines for charting, including acceptable and nonacceptable abbreviations and acronyms (The Joint Commission, 2019). Caregivers need to be familiar with documentation requirements in the work setting and hospital accreditation systems in their geopolitical region.

Charting provides valuable information about the parent and baby that will enable other care providers to refer to what was done and what was effective. Abbreviations should be avoided unless they are understood by everyone who might review the records. Documentation of care may also serve as evidence in legal proceedings and should be maintained in a secure location. **Figure 6-8** identifies elements to document.

Digital Documentation

The medical charts maintained for parents and babies in a hospital, clinic, or healthcare provider practice include much of the information needed for a lactation consultation. Most healthcare facilities rely on electronic charting for a seamless **electronic medical record** (EMR). The EMR contains all standard medical and clnical data, including the parent's medications and any pregnancy or birth complications. The baby's information will include gestational age, weight, and types and amounts of feedings. Reading these charts before a consultation will reveal the parent's and baby's histories. Any information relevant to lactation that is not already included can be added after the consultation.

- Parent's and infant's medical histories
- Birth experience
- Postpartum issues
- Lactation goals
- Consent for care
- Presenting problem
- Parent's assessment
- Infant's assessment
- Feeding documentation
- Evaluation
- Care plan and recommendations

Figure 6-8 Elements of lactation documentation.

Facilities also maintain an Electronic Health Record (EHR), which is a comprehensive history designed to share information from all providers involved in a client's care. It can be created, managed, and consulted by authorized providers and staff from multiple organizations (HealthIT.gov, 2023). EHRs enable clients' health records to move with them across providers, hospitals, and regions. There is a rapid push for electronic documentation of health records in industrialized nations.

Documenting a Feeding

Use of a standard method for documenting feedings will help in evaluating the essential elements of the feeding process. Someone knowledgeable in lactation management should observe and document at least one feeding every 8 hours during the immediate postpartum period. The Joint Commission Perinatal Care measure PC-05 in the U.S. requires documentation of exclusive human milk feeding during the newborn's entire hospitalization (The Joint Commission, 2014). In a busy hospital setting, a method that is simple and uncomplicated will ensure recording of complete and useful information about every nursing dyad. Teaching parents to chart much of their feeding information enables them to become self-sufficient and self-assured in their nursing.

There are many methods for charting observations of feedings. Regardless of method, it is important to avoid using terms such as *good*, *fair*, or *poor* to evaluate a feeding. When used alone, these terms provide very little useful information to another person who reviews the chart. Likewise, simply recording the duration of a feeding gives no indication of its quality. Many hospitals use standard lactation scoring forms, such as the ones described here. The use of such forms is usually included in a hospital's policies and procedures and may require working with the facility's administration to make any changes.

Breastfeed Observation Aid

Figure 6-9 illustrates a form created by the United Nations Children's Fund (UNICEF) and the World Health Organization (WHO) in their manual for training maternity staff throughout the world (UNICEF & WHO, 2009). The main categories to evaluate are observing the parent and baby, the breasts, the baby's position and attachment, and sucking. After observing a feeding, the clinician checks off (in the left column) the signs that feeding is going well. The right column identifies signs of possible difficulty. This method helps staff recognize when help is needed. The intent

BREASTFEED OBSERVATION AID

Parent's name____________________ Date____________

Baby's name____________________ Baby's age____________

Signs that nursing is going well:	**Signs of possible difficulty:**
GENERAL	
Parent:	*Parent:*
☐ Looks healthy	☐ Looks ill or depressed
☐ Relaxed and comfortable	☐ Looks tense and uncomfortable
☐ Signs of bonding with baby	☐ No mother/baby eye contact
Baby:	*Baby:*
☐ Looks healthy	☐ Looks sleepy or ill
☐ Calm and relaxed	☐ Is restless or crying
☐ Reaches or roots for breast if hungry	☐ Does not reach or root
BREASTS	
☐ Appear healthy	☐ Appear red, swollen, or sore
☐ No pain or discomfort	☐ Pain reported
☐ Well supported with fingers away from nipple	☐ Fingers touch areola
☐ Nipples protractile	☐ Nipples flat, not protractile
BABY'S POSITION	
☐ Baby's head and body in line	☐ Baby's neck and head twisted to feed
☐ Baby held close to parent's body	☐ Baby not held close
☐ Baby's whole body supported	☐ Baby supported by head and neck only
☐ Baby's nose faces nipple	☐ Baby's lower lip, chin faces nipple
BABY'S ATTACHMENT	
☐ More areola seen above baby's top lip	☐ More areola seen below bottom lip
☐ Baby's mouth open wide	☐ Baby's mouth not open wide
☐ Lower lip turned outwards	☐ Lips pointing forward or turned in
☐ Baby's chin touches breast	☐ Baby's chin not touching breast
SUCKING	
☐ Slow, deep sucks with pauses	☐ Rapid shallow sucks
☐ Cheeks round when sucking	☐ Cheeks pulled in when sucking
☐ Baby detaches when finished	☐ Parent detaches baby
☐ Signs of oxytocin reflex	☐ No signs of oxytocin reflex

Figure 6-9 United Nations Children's Fund (UNICEF) Breastfeed Observation Form.

of the checklist is to have the elements become ingrained in the clinician's memory so that noting the essential points becomes second nature when observing feedings.

Charting Lactation

Several tools are available for charting the progress of lactation, with scores assigned for the various elements. These tools are effective in assessing and charting lactation (Dolgun et al., 2018; Kuhnly & Chapman, 2018). **Table 6-5** describes the features of several lactation assessment tools that are commonly used. Copies of the tools can be found online. The tools vary in what they evaluate, with most of them focusing on both the parent and infant and assessing latch, sucking, swallowing and milk transfer, and positioning at feedings. The Infant Breastfeeding Assessment Tool (IBFAT) focuses primarily on the infant and does not assess position, latch, or swallow.

Table 6-5 Lactation Assessment Tools

Tool	Features
Infant Breastfeeding Assessment Tool (IBFAT) Matthews (1993)	■ Assigns a score of 0, 1, 2, or 3 to the following factors: • Infant state • Level of stimulation required to coax the infant to nurse • Rooting response • Time lapsed from initial attempt until the infant latches • Sucking pattern • How the parent feels about the feeding
Mother-Baby Assessment Mulford (1992)	■ Modeled after the 10-point Apgar system, with 2 points possible for each step ■ Assesses the following factors: • Signaling: agreement that a feeding will take place • Positioning: placement of the parent's and baby's bodies in relation to each other • Fixing: point at which the baby latches and begins to suck • Milk transfer: when sucking releases milk and the baby consumes the milk • Ending: outcome of the feeding session
LATCH Jensen et al. (1994)	■ Assesses the following factors: • Latch: baby's ability to latch • Audible swallowing: as a determinant of milk intake • Type of nipple: shape, size, and texture • Comfort of nipple and possible need for adjustment • Hold: able to achieve and maintain an effective latch ■ May be calculated online through MDApp at https://www.mdapp.co/latch-score-calculator-373/
Bristol Breastfeeding Assessment Tool (BBAT) Ingram et al. (2015)	■ Assigns a score of 0, 1, or 2 that rates the parent's need for help with the following: • Positioning: placement of the parent's and baby's bodies; parent's confidence • Attachment: rooting, wide mouth, quick latch, baby stays latched • Sucking: effective pattern, baby ends feed • Swallowing: audible, regular soft swallowing, no clicking

Summary

Anticipatory guidance helps parents achieve positive lactation outcomes and is ultimately less time-consuming for healthcare staff. The most effective method of lactation support focuses on early contact and follow-up so that problems can be prevented or minimized. The nature of a situation determines whether it requires a face-to-face visit or can be handled through telephone or electronic contact. A consultation should begin with establishing a receptive climate and then obtaining consent, gathering information through parent and infant histories, completing a parent and infant physical assessment, and observing a feeding. Problem-solving begins with sharing information, offering suggestions, and working with parents to develop a care plan, which includes follow-up to evaluate progress. All necessary documentation should be recorded appropriately, with a written report submitted to the caregiver as appropriate.

What You Learned–At a Glance

Conversation Starters with Parents

- What concerns you about nursing?
- How well prepared do you feel for nursing?
- How do you prefer to receive information and support for nursing?
- How comfortable are you with telehealth?

Anticipatory Guidance

- Anticipatory guidance is best given when retention is high and decision-making can occur.
- Initial learning before delivery allows postpartum teaching to focus on reinforcement.
- Lack of information is a key factor in premature weaning.

- A hotline, warmline, or electronic communication encourages parents to reach out.
- Many new parents need frequent contact during the early weeks of nursing.

Problem-Solving

- Sufficient information and impressions are needed before intervention or problem-solving.
- A nonassertive approach encourages parents to actively engage in problem-solving.
- Critical thinking and analysis skills help with judgments and defining solutions.
- Hidden factors that contribute to a problem need to be explored before acting on a hunch.
- Being open to new information will help in forming and exploring hunches.

Consultations

- A consultation may be in-person or via electronic communication.
- Obtaining consent and taking a history are the first steps in a consultation.
- Private healthcare information is confidential and must be protected by law.
- Feeding assessments should move at the baby's pace with no intervention unless necessary.
- Teaching can occur during the feeding assessment.
- Engaging parents in care plans ensures they understand and are committed to the plan.
- It is good practice to send a report to caregivers after a lactation consultation.

Follow-Up

- Follow-up confirms whether the care plan worked, increases parents' competence and self-confidence, and protects the health of infants.
- The parent's level of need determines the nature and timing of follow-up.
- Follow-up may be via electronic communication or an in-person visit.
- Referral to community-based support provides parents with needed resources.
- Follow-up includes researching additional resources and sources of professional support.
- Parents need to know how to reach out for follow-up contact.

Documentation

- Standard documentation includes a record of consent, assessments, recommendations, care plans, evaluations, and follow-up.
- Most healthcare facilities use electronic charting.
- Documentation needs to sufficiently record the quality of feedings.
- Teaching parents to chart their feedings increases their self-efficacy and confidence.

References

Beheshti L, et al. Telehealth in primary health care: a scoping review of the literature. *Perspect Health Inf Manag.* 2022;19(1):1n.

Bender W, et al. Text message-based breastfeeding support compared with usual care: a randomized controlled trial. *Obstet Gynecol.* 2022;140(5):853–860.

Blackmore A, et al. The effectiveness of virtual lactation support: a systematic review and meta-analysis. *J Hum Lact.* 2022;38(3):452–465.

Bogulski CA, et al. A comparison of audio-only and audio-visual tele-lactation consultation services: a mixed methods approach. *J Hum Lact.* 2023;39(1):93–106.

Broom M, et al. Impact of introducing a lactation consultant into a neonatal unit. *J Paediatr Child Health.* 2022;58(4):636–640.

Čatipović M, et al. Breastfeeding intention and knowledge in secondary-school students. *Acta Clin Croat.* 2018;57(4):658–668.

Chaves AFL, et al. Telephone intervention in the promotion of self-efficacy, duration and exclusivity of breastfeeding: randomized controlled trial. *Rev Lat Am Enfermagem.* 2019;27:e3140.

Chernyshev M, et al. Healthcare data breaches: implications for digital forensic readiness. *J Med Syst.* 2018;43(1):7.

Chua CMS, et al. Use of telelactation interventions to improve breastfeeding outcomes among parents: a mixed-studies systematic review. *Women Birth.* 2022;S1871-5192(22)00113-5.

Cordell A, Elverson C. Interventions to improve breastfeeding outcomes from six weeks to six months: a systematic review. *West J Nurs Res.* 2021;43(6):583–596.

Demirci J, et al. Telelactation via mobile app: perspectives of rural mothers, their care providers, and lactation consultants. *Telemed J E Health.* 2019;25(9):853–858.

Dolgun G, et al. Reliability and validity of the Bristol Breastfeeding Assessment Tool in the Turkish population. *Midwifery.* 2018;57:47–53.

Doraiswamy S, et al. Use of telehealth during the COVID-19 pandemic: scoping review. *J Med Internet Res.* 2020;22(12):e24087.

Dosman CF, et al. Anticipatory guidance for behaviour concerns: school age children. *Paediatr Child Health.* 2019; 24(2):e78–e87.

Elwyn G. Shared decision making: what is the work? *Patient Educ Couns.* 2021;104(7):1591–1595.

Fibuch E, Ahmed A. Bringing value strengthen bonds with your patients. *Physician Leadersh J.* 2017;4(3):50–53.

Forster DA, et al. Proactive peer (parent-to-parent) breastfeeding support by telephone (Ringing Up About Breastfeeding Early [RUBY]): a multicentre, unblinded, randomized controlled trial. *EClinicalMedicine.* 2019;8:20–28.

Fu ML, et al. Evaluation of an e-learning breastfeeding program for postpartum parents of moderately high-risk newborn infants admitted to the special care nursery. *J Perinat Neonatal Nurs.* 2021;35(2):177–187.

Garg P, et al. A case study of well child care visits at general practices in a region of disadvantage in Sydney. *PLoS One.* 2018;13(10):e0205235.

Hamze L, et al. Knowledge and attitudes towards breastfeeding practices: a cross-sectional survey of postnatal mothers in China. *Midwifery.* 2019;74:68–75.

Harari N, et al. Feasibility and acceptability of a text message intervention used as an adjunct tool by WIC breastfeeding peer counsellors: the LATCH pilot. *Matern Child Nutr.* 2018;14 (1):e12488.

HealthIT.gov. What is an electronic medical record? 2023. https://www.healthit.gov/providers-professionals/electronic-medical-records-emr.

Hsu HC, et al. Effects of pediatric anticipatory guidance on parents of young children. *West J Nurs Res.* 2018;40(3):305–326.

Huang P, et al. Individualized intervention to improve rates of exclusive breastfeeding: a randomised controlled trial. *Medicine (Baltimore).* 2019;98(47):e17822.

Hubschman-Shahar LE. Lactation telehealth in primary care: a systematic review. *Breastfeed Med.* 2022;17(1):6–21.

Hunt L, Thomson G. Pressure and judgement within a dichotomous landscape of infant feeding: a grounded theory study to explore why breastfeeding women do not access peer support provision. *Matern Child Nutr.* 2017;13(2):e12279.

Ingram J, et al. The development of a new breastfeeding assessment tool and the relationship with breastfeeding self-efficacy. *Midwifery.* 2015;31:132–137.

Ismail A, et al. The impact of anticipatory guidance on early childhood caries: a quasi-experimental study. *BMC Oral Health.* 2018;18(1):126.

Isselman M, et al. A nutrition counseling workshop: integrating counseling psychology into nutrition practice. *J Am Diet Assoc.* 1993;93:324–326.

Jackson KT, et al. A guide to anticipatory guidance for breastfeeding-related pain: a concept analysis. *Nurs Forum.* 2021;56(3): 752–757.

Jensen D, et al. LATCH: a breastfeeding charting system and documentation tool. *J Obstet Gynecol Neonatal Nurs.* 1994;23: 27–32.

Kapinos K, et al. The use of and experiences with telelactation among rural breastfeeding mothers: secondary analysis of a randomized controlled trial. *J Med Internet Res.* 2019;21(9):e13967.

Kuhnly JE, Chapman DJ. Qualitative analysis of registered nurses' perceptions of lactation assessment tools: why and how they are completed. *J Hum Lact.* 2018;34(1):32–39.

Kuliukas L, et al. Process evaluation of a peer-led antenatal breastfeeding class for fathers: perceptions of facilitators and participants. *BMC Pregnancy Childbirth.* 2019;19(1):48.

Manocchia A. Telehealth: enhancing care through technology. *R I Med J (2013).* 2020;103(1):18–20.

Marler H, Ditton A. "I'm smiling back at you": Exploring the impact of mask wearing on communication in healthcare. *Int J Lang Commun Disord.* 2021;56(1):205–214.

Matthews MK. Assessments and suggested interventions to assist newborn breastfeeding behavior. *J Hum Lact.* 1993;9(4):243–248.

McFadden A, et al. Support for healthy breastfeeding parents with healthy term babies. *Cochrane Database Syst Rev.* 2017;2:CD001141.

Mind Tools. SMART goals: how to make your goals achievable. 2024. https://www.mindtools.com/a4wo118/smart-goals

Mohamad Pilus F, et al. Effect of face-to-face and WhatsApp communication of a theory-based health education intervention on breastfeeding self-efficacy (SeBF intervention): cluster randomized controlled field trial. *JMIR Mhealth Uhealth.* 2022;10(9):e31996.

Mulford C. The Mother–Baby Assessment (MBA): an Apgar score for breastfeeding. *J Hum Lact.* 1992;8:79–82.

Newt Newborn Weight Tool. Penn State Hersey Medical Center. 2019. https://www.newbornweight.org

Olson T, et al. Going home with baby: innovative and comprehensive support for new parents. *Prim Health Care Res Dev.* 2019;20:e18.

Otte RA, et al. Tracker-based personal advice to support the baby's healthy development in a novel parenting app: data-driven innovation. *JMIR Mhealth Uhealth.* 2019;7(7):e12666.

Perrine CG, et al. Implementation of hospital practices supportive of breastfeeding in the context of COVID-19—United States, July 15–August 20, 2020. *MMWR Morb Mortal Wkly Rep.* 2020;69(47):1767–1770.

Reyes C, et al. Investigating the effectiveness of school-based breastfeeding education on breastfeeding knowledge, attitudes and intentions of adolescent females. *Midwifery.* 2019;70:64–70.

Richards JB, et al. Teaching clinical reasoning and critical thinking: from cognitive theory to practical application. *Chest.* 2020;158(4):1617–1628.

Robinson A, et al. It takes an e-village: supporting African American parents in sustaining breastfeeding through Facebook communities. *J Hum Lact.* 2019;35(3):569–582.

Saucedo Baza A, et al. A technological approach to improved breastfeeding rates and self-efficacy: a randomized controlled pilot study. *J Hum Lact.* 2023;39(4):679–687.

Sevda KÖ, Sevil İ. Continuous lactation support provided through the WhatsApp messaging application: a randomized controlled trial. *J Hum Lact.* 2023;39(4):666–678.

Seyyedi N, et al. Effectiveness of a smartphone-based educational intervention to improve breastfeeding. *Int Breastfeed J.* 2021;16(1):70.

Sidhu S, et al. Features and educational content related to milk production in breastfeeding apps: content analysis informed by social cognitive theory. *JMIR Pediatr Parent.* 2019;2(1):e12364.

Spatz DL. Helping mothers reach personal breastfeeding goals. *Nurs Clin North Am.* 2018;53(2):253–261.

Spatz DL. Protecting breastfeeding for adolescents who return to school. *MCN Am J Matern Child Nurs.* 2019;44(4):236.

Stokes-Parish J. Navigating the credibility of web-based information during the COVID-19 pandemic: using mnemonics to empower the public to spot red flags in health information on the internet. *J Med Internet Res.* 2022;24(6):e38269.

Street RL, et al. Engaging patients in the uptake, understanding, and use of evidence: addressing barriers and facilitators of successful engagement. *Patient Educ Couns.* 2017;100(1):4.

The Joint Commission. Specifications manual for Joint Commission national quality core measures. 2014. http://manual.jointcommission.org/releases/TJC2014A/

The Joint Commission. The official "do not use" list of abbreviations. Updated October 1, 2019. https://www.jointcommission.org

Thomson G, Crossland N. Using the behaviour change wheel to explore infant feeding peer support provision; insights from a North West UK evaluation. *Int Breastfeed J.* 2019;14:41.

Thorpe K, et al. Can a call make a difference? Measured change in women's breastfeeding self-efficacy across call interactions on a telephone helpline. *Matern Child Health J.* 2018;22(12):1761–1770.

Tonelli MR, Sullivan MD. Person-centred shared decision making. *J Eval Clin Pract.* 2019;25(6):1057–1062.

Unger JA, et al. Short message service communication improves exclusive breastfeeding and early postpartum contraception in a low- to middle-income country setting: a randomised trial. *BJOG.* 2018;125(12):1620–1629.

United Nations Children's Fund, World Health Organization. Baby-Friendly Hospital Initiative training materials. 2009. https://www.unicef.org/nutrition/index_24850.html

U.S. National Library of Medicine. LactMed App. Toxnet Toxicology Data Network. 2019. https://www.nlm.nih.gov /toxnet /Accessing_LactMed_Content_from_NCBI_Bookshelf.html

Wang C, et al. A Breastfeed-promoting mobile app intervention: usability and usefulness study. *JMIR Mhealth Uhealth.* 2018;6(1):e27.

Williams RC, et al. Relationships matter: how clinicians can support positive parenting in the early years. *Paediatr Child Health.* 2019;24(5):340–357.

Zhang Y, Kim Y. Consumers' evaluation of web-based health information quality: meta-analysis. *J Med Internet Res.* 2022;24(4):e36463.

PART 2

The Science of Lactation

CHAPTER 7

Lactation Anatomy and Physiology

The mammary gland is a marvelously complex organ that has ensured the survival of the human race. We nurse our babies, following our biological imperative as mammals. Historically, parents have instinctively nurtured their young, confident in their natural abilities to produce milk. It is only in recent decades that the study of the anatomy and physiology of the human breast has been a major interest to researchers. Scientists study every detail externally and internally. The growth of functioning breast tissue, milk synthesis (production), milk ejection, and types of nipples all receive intense scrutiny. Knowledge of lactation function has increased dramatically in recent years. Advances in molecular and genetic research have improved technologies such as ultrasound, magnetic resonance, and computer imaging to provide new insights. Heightened public awareness of breast cancer and its prevention has increased scientific interest. Staying current on the ever-changing understanding of this amazing organ is important for your clinical practice.

KEY TERMS

Acinus
Adrenal hormones
Alveoli
Amastia
Amazia
Areola
Athelia
Atrophy
Autocrine control
Autonomic nerves
Axilla
Bactericidal
Blood and lymph systems
Capillaries
Colostrum
Connective tissue
Cooper's ligaments
Dermis
Duct system
Ductal narrowing
Ductule
Dysphoric milk ejection reflex
Edema
Epidermal growth factor
Epidermis
Epithelium
Estrogen
Evert
Exocrine gland
Fatty tissue
Feedback inhibitor of lactation (FIL)
Fibroblast growth factor
Fibrocystic breast
Fistula
Flat nipple
Foremilk
Galactocele
Galactopoiesis
Glandular tissue
Gonadotropins
Hindmilk
Hydatid disease
Hypopituitarism
Hypoplasia
Hypothalamus
Inhibited letdown
Innervation
Insufficient glandular tissue
Insulin-like growth factor
Intercostal nerves
Intraductal papilloma
Inverted nipple
Involution
Keratin
Lactiferous sinus
Lactocyte
Lactogenesis
Lactogenesis I
Lactogenesis II
Lactogenesis III
Lactose
Letdown
Lobule
Lymph
Lymph nodes
Lymphatic system
Lysozyme
Malignancy
Mammary gland
Mammary ridge
Mammogenesis
Mature milk
Milk ejection reflex
Milk synthesis
Milk-producing tissue

Milk-transporting tissue
Montgomery glands
Myoepithelial cells
Nerves
Nipple pores
Nipple preference
Nipple shield
Normal fullness
Oxytocin
Paget's disease
Parenchyma
Pinch test
Pitocin
Pituitary
Placenta
Placental retention
Polymastia
Polythelia
Progesterone
Prolactin
Prolactin inhibitory factor (PIF)
Sebaceous
Secretory activation
Secretory differentiation
Sheehan's syndrome
Sphincter
Supernumerary nipple (accessory nipple)
Tail of Spence
Thelarche
Transforming growth factor β
Transitional milk
Trophic
Witch's milk

Anatomy of the Breast

The **mammary gland** is part of the body's intricate system of reproduction. Although it is called a gland, the breast is actually an organ. The human breast is an **exocrine gland** that functions and develops independently to extract material from the blood and convert it into milk (Alekseev, 2021). Variations in size and shape are especially evident during lactation, when breasts enlarge to accommodate **milk synthesis**. The rate of flow and the quantity of milk produced during lactation reveal their uniqueness. The nipple, **areola**, and **Montgomery glands** are located within the surface layer of the breast. Knowledge of skin, supportive tissue, **milk-producing tissue**, and **milk-transporting tissue** enables you to help parents understand normal changes that occur during pregnancy and throughout lactation. Awareness of markers for potential lactation problems is important for working with lactating families.

Skin

Most human contact with the environment comes through the skin. Skin, the body's largest organ, acts as a defensive covering for deeper tissue. It is flexible and elastic to allow for changes in tissue size. It acts as a screen against the damaging effects of light and performs respiratory and excretory functions—it breathes and perspires. The skin is composed of distinct cellular layers and contains hair, **sebaceous** glands, and sweat glands. Dead cells lie on the surface and living cells reside underneath. The **epidermis**, **dermis**, and hypodermis make up the major layers within the skin (de Szalay & Wertz, 2023).

Skin Layers

New cell growth in the germinating layer of the skin continually pushes dead cells out toward the surface. As the cells travel through the transitional layer, they undergo changes that cement them firmly together. This process creates a tough, hard, waterproof barrier against bacterial invasion. The outer skin layer, the epidermis, protects the inner layer, the dermis, from abrasion and water evaporation.

The epidermis is the outer layer of live epithelial cells. It covers and protects deeper skin layers from drying out and from bacterial invasion. Over the course of their life, skin cells progress through the epidermis, from their initial growth in the germinating layer to their loss of fluid in the transitional layer and on to the surface layer of dead skin, called **keratin** (**Figure 7-1**).

The dermis, which is composed of connective tissue, is the inner layer of the skin lying below the epidermis. It contains nerve endings, **capillaries** (small blood vessels), hair follicles, lymph channels, and other cells. Muscle cells are located under this layer, except around the areola and nipple, where the two intermingle. The deepest skin layer, the hypodermis or subcutaneous layer, binds the dermis to the underlying muscle. Areolar, elastic, and fat connective tissues reside here, as well as blood vessels and nerve endings (Grant, 2023).

Nipple

The nipple extends and becomes firmer when stimulated. This enables the baby to latch for nursing. The nipple is flexible and able to mold and elongate to conform to the baby's mouth during feeding. Nipple tissue is similar to the tissue in human lips, stretching easily and healing quickly. When the baby sucks,

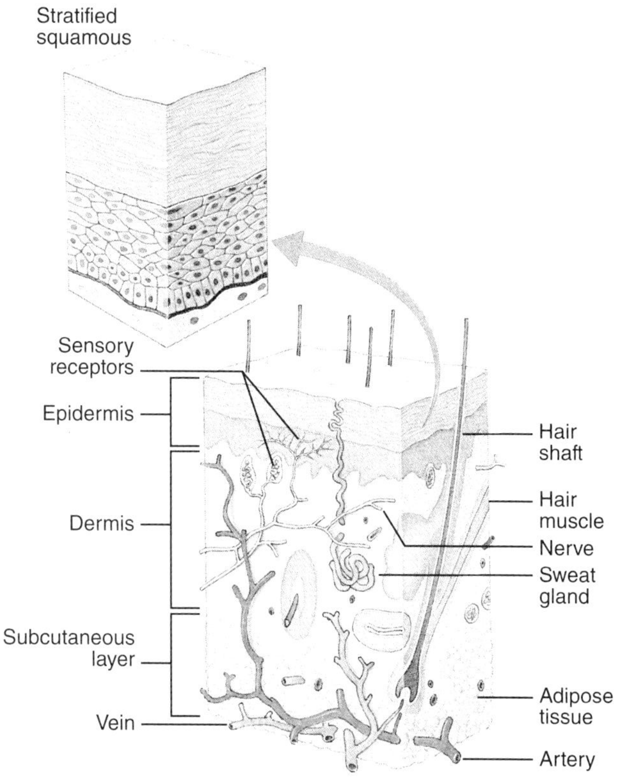

Figure 7-1 Skin layers.

sensory nerve endings in the nipple send a signal to the brain to trigger milk release via **oxytocin**.

The nipple is composed primarily of circular smooth muscle fibers that function as a closing mechanism for the milk ducts (Alekseev, 2021). **Ductule** openings, commonly called **nipple pores**, are located at the end of the nipple and enable the baby to receive the milk (**Color Plate 1**). The nipple has an average of 9 exiting ducts, spanning 4 to 18 (Geddes et al., 2021). Lawrence and Lawrence (2021) describe multiple ducts sharing a few common openings. They describe the diameter and position of the duct as being unrelated to whether it terminates close to the nipple or passes deeper into the tissue. This great variance in patent openings may explain why some parents lactate more successfully after breast surgery than others.

During the last trimester of pregnancy, changes within the ducts sometimes lead to a bloody nipple discharge. This phenomenon occurs when **epithelium** spurs that extend into the ducts are traumatized, resulting in bleeding. This type of bleeding does not affect lactation, and often stops when nursing begins. Known as "rusty pipe" syndrome because of the color of the blood, this condition typically resolves spontaneously (Mohamad et al., 2021). Usually, bleeding is associated with benign causes, such as an intraductal papilloma, a benign growth in the duct.

When a parent experiences a bloody nipple discharge, clarify how often it occurs. If they report bleeding more than once, you need to rule out trauma to the nipple from an ineffective latch or nipple compression during feedings. If there is no apparent reason for the bleeding, refer them to their primary healthcare provider or a breast specialist. Although the rate of carcinoma related to nipple discharge is low, **malignancy** should always be ruled out (Mohamad et al., 2021). Breast cancer is the most common cancer detected during pregnancy during lactation, and within the first year postpartum (Fazeli et al., 2023). About 1 in every 3000 pregnant individuals has breast cancer.

Areola

The areola is the dark circular area surrounding the nipple. Its size and color vary greatly. During puberty, menstruation, and pregnancy, the areola enlarges and becomes darker in color. There is little subcutaneous fat under the areola. The underlying ducts are superficial and easily compressed (Alekseev, 2021).

To achieve an effective latch, the baby's mouth needs to enclose a sizable portion of the areolar tissue. This enables the baby's tongue to compress a large amount of tissue against the palate to facilitate milk release. Some areolae are so large in diameter that the baby does not take the entire areola in their mouth. A guide for parents should be for the baby to take in areolar tissue well behind the nipple, usually at least an inch in diameter.

Montgomery Glands

The Montgomery glands, also called *Montgomery's tubercles*, are sebaceous glands located around the areola. They have a "pimply" appearance and secrete an oily substance that serves as a lubricant and a protective agent for the nipple. Montgomery gland secretions allow the skin to breathe and remain pliable. They are rudimentary mammary glands and may secrete a small amount of milk (Kantha, 2023).

Washing the nipples with any substance other than a gentle, unscented soap and plain water could remove this natural lubrication, dry out the skin, and reduce the scent. Use of creams or oils on the nipples is not usually necessary, and arbitrary use may reduce the amount of air reaching the tissue. Creams may also introduce a scent or taste that the baby dislikes or does not recognize.

Breast Anomalies

Polymastia, also referred to as *accessory breasts*, is the most common breast anomaly. It occurs most frequently in the axillae, although it can occur anywhere along the milk line (del Pilar Bérniz Laborda & Olivas-Menayo, 2023). The swelling of the accessory breast tissue during pregnancy and lactogenesis II can be uncomfortable. **Athelia**, a rare condition, is the complete absence of the nipple-areolar complex, although there is underlying tissue. Athelia is associated with genetic conditions and syndromes, including Poland's syndrome (Troupis & Markopoulos, 2023). **Amastia** is another rare condition where breast tissue and the nipple-areolar complex do not develop. Unilateral amastia is associated with pectoral muscle absence, as in the case of Poland's syndrome. Bilateral amastia is usually associated with other congenital anomalies. Amastia differs from **amazia**, which is the presence of the nipple-areolar complex with no underlying glandular tissue (Adekeye et al., 2023).

Supportive and Sustaining Tissue

Other tissues that are vital to lactation lie under the skin and between parts of the milk-producing and milk-transporting tissues. Connective tissues support the breast, and subcutaneous fatty tissues give it shape. **Nerves** provide a triggering mechanism for milk synthesis and release. The **blood and lymph systems** supply nutrients for milk, filter out bacteria, and remove dead cell parts.

Nerves

Innervation is the distribution of nerve fibers or nerve impulses. There is extensive **innervation** of the nipple and areola complex, involving both **autonomic nerves** and sensory nerves. Sensory nerve fibers innervate the smooth muscles in the nipples and blood vessels from the third, fourth, fifth, and sixth **intercostal nerves**. Most sensation to the nipple and areola comes from the fourth intercostal nerve (del Pilar Bérniz Laborda & Olivas-Menayo, 2023). Autonomic nerves can function independently with no outside influence. Sensory nerves in the breast trigger lactation (**Figure 7-2**). Intercostal nerves are located in the spaces between two ribs.

The nipple is believed to be more sensitive than the areola (Haider, 2023). The higher density of the nipple may possibly explain this difference. When the baby grasps a sufficient amount of tissue and sucks

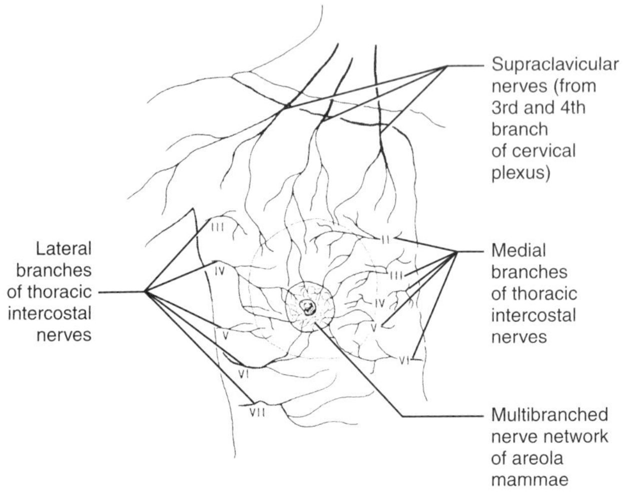

Figure 7-2 Innervation of the mammary gland.

Printed with permission of the International Lactation Consultant Association.

vigorously, it stimulates the deeper nerves and triggers oxytocin release and milk **letdown**. By comparison, a weak or tired baby or one who sucks on the nipple alone may not provide adequate stimulation to the deeper nerves. Ultimately, this lack of stimulation can result in less effective letdown and lower milk production. Studies suggest that parents with small breasts appear to have more sensitive nipple-areolar complexes than those with larger breasts (Bland et al., 2023).

Fatty Tissue

Fatty tissue holds all the structures within the breasts in place and, along with **glandular tissue** determines breast size. Fat cells are located throughout most of the tissue, between lobuli (plural of **lobule**) and milk ducts, and under the skin. There is very little fat immediately beneath the areola and nipple, an area dominated by muscular tissue and duct branching (**Color Plate 1**).

Large and small breasts are equally functional for nursing. Fatty tissues do not contribute to milk synthesis or transport. Therefore, size or the amount of fat has little impact on the quality or quantity of the milk. Some parents have large breasts with mostly fatty tissue and sparse alveolar growth (Alekseev, 2021). Others have smaller breasts with ample alveolar lobes and little subcutaneous fat.

Connective Tissue

Fibrous **connective tissue** supports and contains the fatty tissue and the tissues that produce and transport milk. Fibrous bands called **Cooper's ligaments** provide a framework to support the tissue. These ligaments attach the breast to the overlying skin and the underlying fibrous tissue enclosing the muscles.

Fibrous tissue holds the segments together and supports the ducts as they fill with milk.

Sagging breasts and protruding abdomens are associated with pregnancy, not lactation. Parents who do not nurse their infants experience the same effects. There is no research to support the notion that sagging can be lessened by the wearing of a good support bra during pregnancy and lactation. Caution parents to avoid tight bras or ones with an underwire or other stiff part that presses against milk ducts. The repeated pressure from these bras could contribute to **ductal narrowing**, previously referred to as *plugged ducts*.

Blood and Lymph Systems

The bloodstream provides the proteins, fats, carbohydrates, and other substances needed for lactation. Fluids containing these nutrients pass through the capillaries to the tissue spaces, where they are absorbed. Capillaries are small blood vessels that link the arteries and veins. The body has amazing control over the amount of blood that flows into tissue, maintaining circulation at a level that meets the needs of each tissue. When needs increase during menstruation and pregnancy, blood flow increases to this area to support tissue building. Later, when frequent sucking signals a need to increase milk production, more blood becomes available to provide the nutrients to make milk.

The **lymphatic system**—a complex network of capillaries, thin vessels, valves, ducts, nodes, and organs—functions like the bloodstream in reverse. **Lymph** is a thin, clear, slightly yellow fluid consisting of approximately 95% water. It contains a few red blood cells and variable numbers of white blood cells. The lymphatic system absorbs excess blood fluids from the tissue spaces and eventually returns them to the heart (**Figure 7-3**).

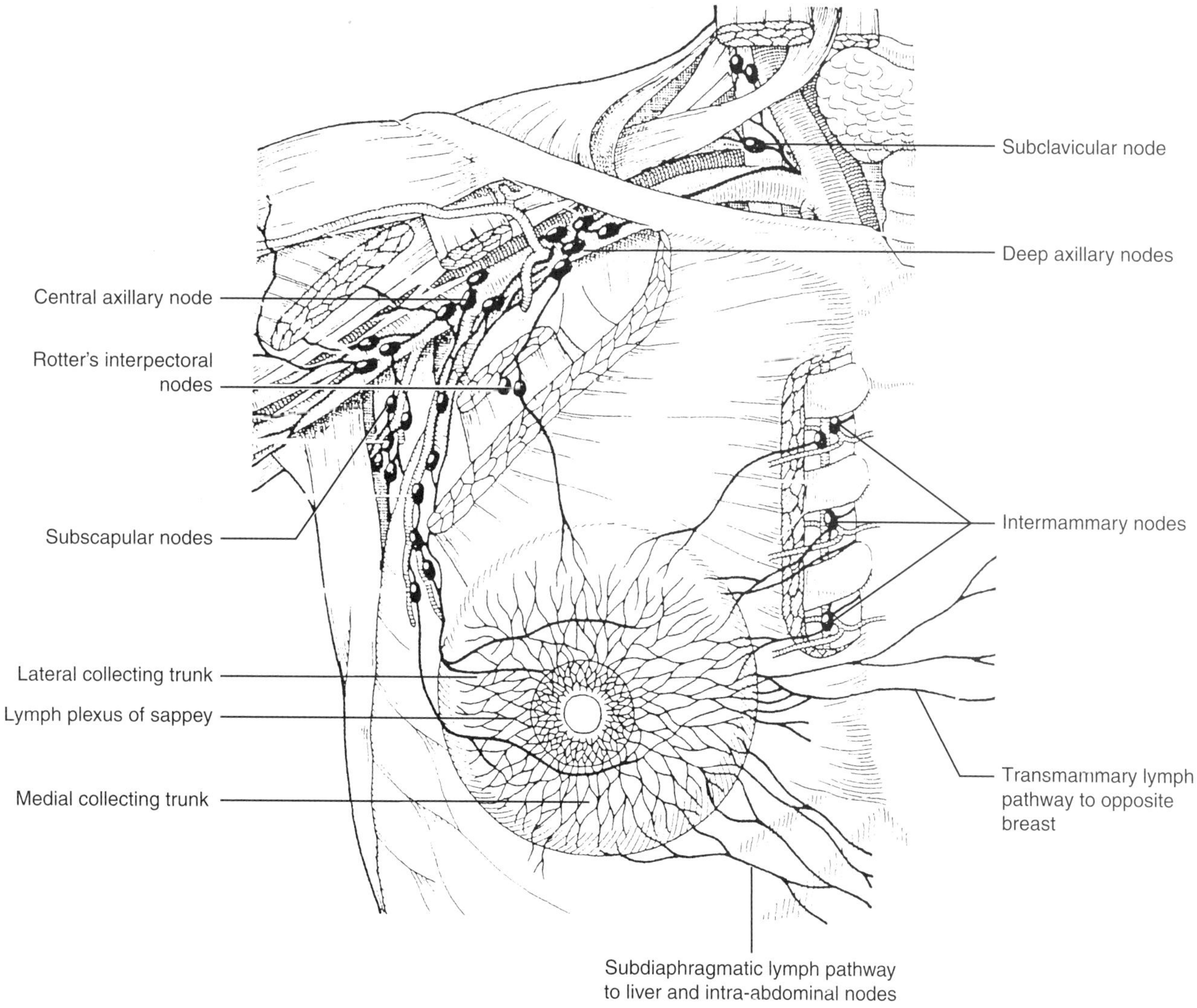

Figure 7-3 Lymphatic system of the breast.

Lymph nodes function as filters in the lymph vessels to trap bacteria and remove dead cell parts. Each node is a potential dam that arrests the spread of infection. At times, lymph nodes may swell and be painful. Most of the lymph fluid flows into the nodes in the armpit, where it traps bacteria that might otherwise travel up the ducts from the nipple or bloodstream. The swelling of a lymph node in the armpit could suggest that an infection is present in the breast, arm, or hand.

During engorgement, increased pressure from milk decreases blood and lymph flow. This can cause fluids to accumulate in the tissues, referred to as **edema**. With the lymphatic system at a standstill, the risk of local infection increases. When this occurs, bacteria and cell particles cannot be removed adequately, leading to poor drainage of the ducts and **alveoli**.

Generally, bacteria multiply faster in stagnant fluids than in moving fluids. Milk stasis provides a medium for bacterial growth. Poor drainage can lead to mastitis, an inflammation characterized by pain, swelling, redness, and fever. A parent with mastitis must remove milk as effectively as possible to reduce pressure. This can be accomplished by feeding the baby more frequently and thoroughly or by expressing milk. **Chapter 17** discusses engorgement and mastitis.

Glandular Tissue

Glandular tissue produces and transports the milk. The **parenchyma**—functional parts of the organ—are composed of many smaller individual glands, or lobuli. This highly efficient glandular tissue takes raw materials from the blood and creates essential nutrients for the baby. The lobuli consist of many milk-producing alveoli. The lobuli connect to a system of ducts, providing a passageway for the milk to flow.

Milk-Producing Tissue

Milk production occurs in small individual glands called *alveoli*. (The singular form is *alveolus*; also called **acinus**.) Alveoli group together to form lobuli, which are often compared visually to a cluster of grapes. The distribution of lobuli varies widely. Computer image research suggests that fewer lobes are present than previously believed, probably 7 to 10 per side (Haider, 2023; Puerta-Alcalde et al., 2023). The **tail of Spence** denotes the tissue that extends into the **axilla**, or armpit.

Alveoli consist of epithelial cells (**lactocytes**) encased in a dense, basketlike meshwork of smooth muscle, known as **myoepithelial cells**. Numerous capillaries surround the alveoli and transfer nutrient-rich blood, from which the alveoli make milk. Through this same system, the alveoli receive the hormones oxytocin and **prolactin**, which signal them to release and produce more milk.

Like other smooth muscle cells in the body, such as those in the uterine wall and nipple, myoepithelial cells contract when exposed to oxytocin released during sucking. The contraction of these cells in the alveoli results in a squeezing effect on the lobule, which forces milk down the ducts. **Color Plate 2** depicts alveoli filled with milk, and **Color Plate 3** depicts the interior of a milk-filled alveolus and its surrounding myoepithelial cells. **Color Plate 4** illustrates the constriction of the myoepithelial cells that forces milk from the alveolus into the duct.

Myoepithelial cells multiply and greatly increase in size during pregnancy and lactation. They decrease in size and number when nursing ends. From the time the alveoli begin to proliferate during pregnancy, alveolar cells constantly wear out and are replenished. The replenishment cycle continues throughout lactation.

Milk-Transporting Tissue

Milk flows through a system of mammary ductules, secondary ducts, and nipple pores, as illustrated in **Color Plate 1**. Formation of the **duct system** begins with a few small basic ducts in childhood. These ducts sprout and branch during puberty, forming tissue buds for the future development of alveoli and lobuli. With each ovulation, the ducts grow lengthwise as alveoli and lobuli develop.

During the first 4 to 5 months of pregnancy, sprouting and growth of ducts and alveolar development intensify. In the second half of pregnancy, the ducts and alveolar tissues become more specialized in preparation for their milk-related functions. There is great variance in duct systems.

During lactation, an intricate ductal system transports milk through the nipple pores. Each duct widens as milk passes through and then collapses when milk flow ceases. The duct system is much more random and intricate than presented historically in the literature. Sensitive imaging and three-dimensional computer design technologies have greatly increased our understanding of the lactating breast (Geddes et al., 2021).

Milk transfer to the infant relies on an intact duct system. Breast surgery or other interference with the milk-transporting system can compromise the ability to transfer milk to the infant. Assessment should include careful observation for scars. Surgery that severs milk ducts and nerves in the periareolar region has the greatest potential for compromising milk production and transfer. Reduction surgery may sever many milk ducts and nerves by removing the areola and milk-producing tissue and then reattaching the areola. Sometimes the nipple is shortened or reshaped (Faulkner et al., 2023). **Chapter 19** and **Chapter 26** discuss problems with milk transfer and long-term health conditions.

Earlier texts described the ducts beneath the areola as **lactiferous sinuses**. This understanding evolved from cadaver work by Sir Astley Cooper in 1840, where hot wax was injected into the breast of a lactating cadaver at the time of death. Scientists now hypothesize that the injection of the hot wax distended the cadaver's ducts, which led to the belief that lactiferous sinuses were larger than the rest of the ductule framework (Gnanavel et al., 2023). Modern real-time ultrasound computer imaging reveals a temporary dilation of the ducts during letdown as milk passes through the ducts. The ducts then collapse until the next surge of milk (Geddes et al., 2021). Unused milk flows backward through the ducts, which explains how bacteria can be introduced, sometimes causing mastitis.

Insufficient Glandular Tissue

Some parents have very small, poorly developed mammary tissue, a condition called **hypoplasia**. Unlike small but normally developed breasts, hypoplastic breasts are widely spaced (more than 1½ inches apart), tubular, frequently asymmetrical, and thin. These are all markers for **insufficient glandular tissue** (Jin et al., 2024). Some cases of insufficient glandular tissue may be less severe forms of amazia, described previously. **Color Plates 5 to 8** illustrate four common types of breasts. Type 4 illustrates hypoplasia.

If a parent is not producing enough milk, explore the possibility of underlying hormonal problems or insufficient glandular tissue. If they have tried all means of increasing milk production and cannot meet the baby's caloric needs, the baby will need donor milk or formula supplementation, until complementary foods begin. **Figure 7-4** presents signs of possible glandular insufficiency.

- Abnormal development of at least one breast
- Breast asymmetry, tubular breast shape
- Intramammary distance greater than 1.5 inches
- Disproportionately large or bulbous areolae
- Absence of typical breast changes that occur during pregnancy

Figure 7-4 Signs of possible glandular insufficiency.

Data from Marianne Neifert et al. (1990).

Molecular research investigates why some parents are unable to lactate successfully. Studies on the complex interplay of hormones, proteins, receptors, and cell differentiation in lactation are increasing (Hannan et al., 2023; Jin et al., 2024). One day, genetic therapies may be able to target insufficient milk production and help parents achieve full lactation.

Mammary Growth and Development

From the onset of puberty and throughout pregnancy, the mammary gland is in a stage of **mammogenesis**, when it develops into a functioning state. During pregnancy, it enters into **lactogenesis**, when milk synthesis and secretion are established. **Secretory differentiation** is commonly called **lactogenesis I**. **Secretory activation**, also called **lactogenesis II**, signifies copious milk secretion. With the establishment of **mature milk** and throughout lactation, the breast is in a state of **galactopoiesis**, also referred to as **lactogenesis III**. **Involution** occurs at the end of lactation, with the breast slowly returning to a near-prepregnant state. **Figures 7-5** and **7-6** compare breast appearance before and during pregnancy.

Fetal Stage

The beginnings of mammary development are noticeable in the fetus at 5 weeks of life. At this time, two **mammary ridges** (also called *milk lines*) are detectable, extending from the armpits to the inner thighs. Because the milk lines appear before genitalia, breasts develop in all babies regardless of gender. The lower parts of the milk lines disappear after several weeks. By 20 to 32 weeks, the upper parts develop and form milk ducts. The ducts form openings in the nipples that are depressed below the surface of the skin. Just before birth, the nipples push outward and become level with the skin. In some cases, this step fails, resulting in a partially or completely **inverted nipple**.

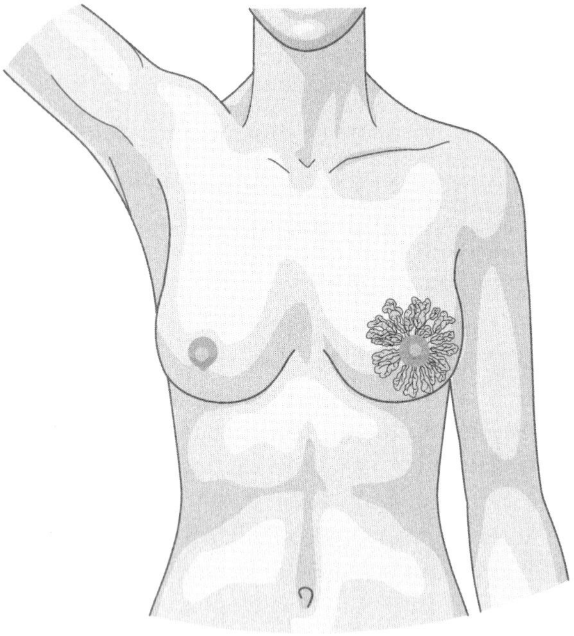

Figure 7-5 Breast before pregnancy.

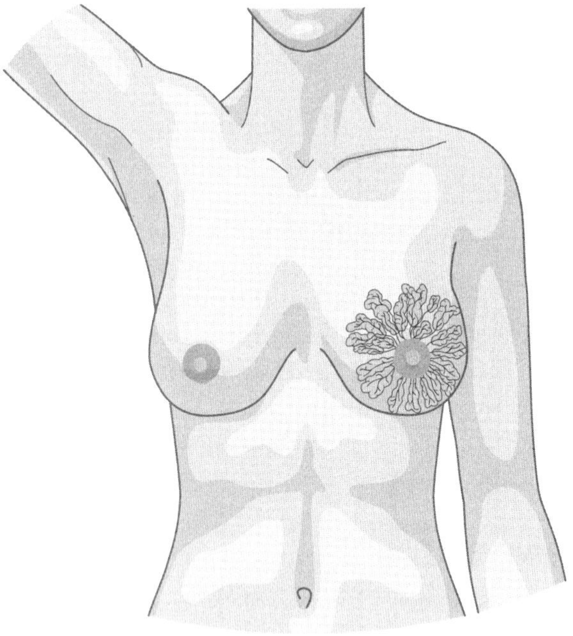

Figure 7-6 Breast during pregnancy.

Sometimes, the lower ends of the milk lines fail to regress, and the baby is born with **polythelia**, a condition in which there are one or more **supernumerary nipples** along this line. These nipples are sometimes called *accessory nipples*.

Some newborns secrete a colostrum-like fluid, referred to as "**witch's milk.**" This fluid consists primarily of shed epithelial cells and results from the transfer of hormones through the **placenta**. Babies born before term typically do not have this secretion. Left alone, the discharge disappears in about 20 days.

Puberty

Before the onset of puberty, the mammary gland is composed primarily of dense fibrous stroma and scattered ducts lined with epithelium. The majority of functional tissue development occurs during puberty and pregnancy, which are periods of increased hormonal activity. During puberty, **gonadotropins** produced by the **pituitary** raise **estrogen** levels. This maturation process, called **thelarche**, leads to increased fat deposits, new duct formation (by branching and elongation), and the appearance of lobular units. Estrogen, **progesterone**, **adrenal hormones**, and pituitary hormones control the growth and cell division process. Insulin, thyroid, and local growth hormones are also thought to have **trophic** effects, which means stimulating the activity of another gland (Haider, 2023; Hannan et al., 2023). Although structural growth is apparent during puberty, only a small amount of alveolar development occurs at this time. Slight development of functional tissue occurs during ovulatory cycles.

Because the mammary gland covers the bony rib cage, it grows outward. The skin that covers and contains it expands as it grows. The result is an evenly rounded organ with a protruding nipple. With the onset of menstruation, the body's hormonal balance is altered by the increased production of estrogen, which promotes the growth of ducts and the connective tissue between them. A thick layer of fat deposits under the skin to form the firm and enlarged adolescent breast. The areola and the nipple grow and take on a deeper color during puberty (and again in pregnancy).

The initial major changes in functional tissue are typically completed approximately 12 to 18 months after the first menstrual cycle. The formation of fibrous connective tissue and the laying down of fat continue to increase breast size during each adolescent menstrual cycle. The mammary gland is relatively inactive between puberty and pregnancy. Around 12 to 16 days before the onset of each menses, the ovaries release an egg, and estrogen levels increase. The reproduction of ductule tissue and the formation of alveolar cells begin to prepare for pregnancy. However, this proliferation is not significant in terms of size.

The fullness experienced when menses begins is attributable to the increased blood supply and excessive fluid retained in the tissues. After the end of each menstrual cycle, tissue growth regresses, and glandular cells degenerate. Fluid loss from the tissues returns the breast to its previous size. Regression of tissue growth is incomplete, and the ovulatory cycle slightly enhances mammary growth for parents younger than approximately 30–35 years of age. In terms of overall preparation for lactation, growth during pregnancy is far more significant than gains that occur during menstrual cycles.

Pregnancy

With the onset of pregnancy, the breast continues to develop into a functioning state. Hormonal changes cause a spectacular phase of growth and proliferation. During the first trimester of pregnancy (conception to 3 months), estrogen and progesterone levels cause the duct system to multiply. The skin begins to respond to internal enlargement, with an increase in the circumference of the nipple and areola. Increased pigmentation or darkening may accentuate this growth.

Montgomery glands, which often go unnoticed before pregnancy, enlarge or elongate. They may become noticeable by the first missed menstrual period, alerting the experienced parent to an early sign of pregnancy. The area takes on a rough, pimply appearance, which is most noticeable when the skin is cool. The Montgomery glands begin to secrete an oily substance to protect the nipple and areolar skin. This protective secretion continues throughout pregnancy and lactation.

The duct system continues to develop throughout the second trimester (4–6 months). Alveoli begin to appear as a result of placental prolactin (**Color Plate 1**). By the end of the second trimester, the blood supply and body fluids (lymph) that support alveolar growth and the multiplying number of alveoli increase the weight of the breast. **Colostrum** production is established, triggering the beginning of lactation.

General breast development continues throughout the third trimester (7–9 months). Stretch marks may appear as evidence of stress on the skin. The nipple and areola continue to darken and enlarge. The color may lighten somewhat when birth occurs and toward the end of lactation. This process is repeated with each succeeding pregnancy. The change in color and size often appears more pronounced in younger parents whose breasts are not fully mature when pregnancy occurs. Anecdotally, darkening of the nipple-areolar complex seems to be more pronounced in darker-skinned parents than in fair-skinned persons.

Lactogenesis

Lactogenesis is the three-stage maturation of alveolar cells to produce and secrete milk. Each stage of lactogenesis has a specific function in establishing milk synthesis and secretion:

- Stage I lactogenesis (secretory differentiation) starts at the beginning of the third trimester of pregnancy. Epithelial cells are converted to a secretory state. Plasma concentrations of **lactose**, total proteins, and immunoglobulin increase. Sodium and chloride decrease. Substances needed for milk synthesis are drawn from the bloodstream.
- Stage II lactogenesis (secretory activation) occurs at 2 to 5 days postpartum. It is referred to as the time when the colostral phase ends and **transitional milk** is produced. Blood flow increases, and copious milk secretion begins.
- Stage III lactogenesis (galactopoiesis) marks the establishment and maintenance of mature milk production. It occurs 8 to 10 days postpartum and is maintained by frequent milk removal, either by the infant nursing or by milk expression.

Awareness of factors that influence milk synthesis will enable you to explain to parents how frequent nursing increases milk production. Recognizing the factors that initiate milk ejection and the function of hormones in the letdown process will help you identify problems with milk release and assist parents in working out solutions.

Involution

Lactogenesis is followed by a period of involution, a normal process marked by decreasing breast size—**atrophy**—and a slow return to a near-prepregnant state. This is called *postlactational involution* and is distinct from the involution that occurs with menopause. Menopausal involution results in atrophy from reduced ovarian function (Hannan et al., 2023). Postlactational involution proceeds gradually in child-led weaning. Abrupt weaning results in rapid epithelial cell death and marked involution in a matter of days or weeks. Research suggests that brief lactation and/or rapid weaning may increase breast cancer risk. The mechanisms involved in gradual lactational involution may help prevent aberrant cell growth (Davis, 2017). After multiple pregnancies and extended nursing, some parents experience severe involution, in which fat deposits do not recur when the ducts regress (**Figure 7-7**). Loss of fat and shape can also occur without nursing. In the event of another pregnancy, alveoli regenerate, and lactation resumes.

Some parents have augmentation or other cosmetic breast surgery, including "lifts" after they wean. A parent may ask about the impact of surgical procedures on subsequent nursing. Referral to the research

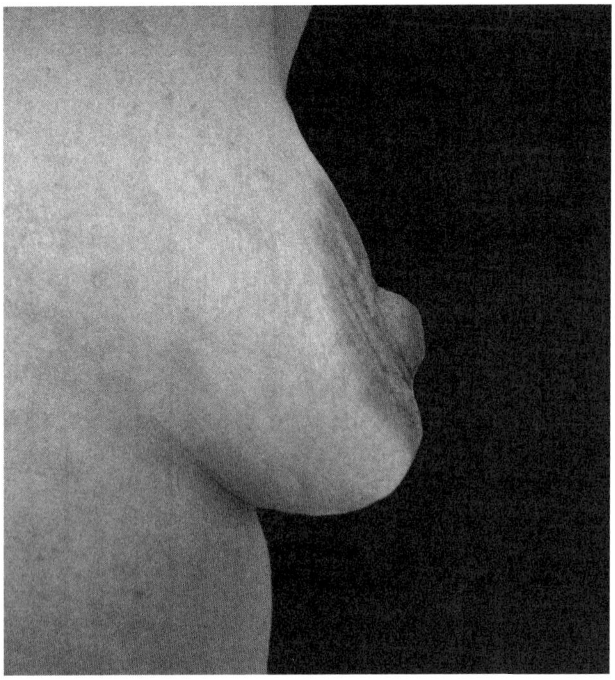

Figure 7-7 Involuted breast that has atrophied.
Printed with permission of Anna Swisher.

literature, to a lactation-savvy surgeon, and to bona fide online resources such as one from the CDC (https://www.cdc.gov/breastfeeding-special-circumstances/hcp/illnesses-conditions/breast-surgery.html) to help make an informed decision.

Hormonal Impact on Lactation

Hormones are chemical products of the endocrine glands that regulate the functions of specific organs or tissues. A comprehensive understanding of lactation hormones and their function will help you identify problems with milk synthesis and ongoing production. Lactation hormones affect letdown, milk production, functioning tissue, and other aspects of a parent's physiology. The growth, maturation, and function of the breast are a result of stimulation by four major hormones—estrogen, progesterone, prolactin, and oxytocin. Growth factor hormones are also involved, including **epidermal growth factor (ErbB)**, **insulin-like growth factors**, **fibroblast growth factor (FGF)** (Otuneye & Audu, 2023), and **transforming growth factor β** (TGF β) (Hannan et al., 2023).

Estrogen

Estrogen is produced in the ovaries, adrenal glands, and placenta. It stimulates growth of the uterus, vagina, and other reproductive organs. Estrogen is responsible for the development of secondary sex characteristics, such as the distinctive female skeleton, body contour, and mammary glands. This hormone causes the growth of mammary ducts and connective tissue between the ducts.

Progesterone

Progesterone is produced in the ovaries and placenta. In Latin the term means "for gestation." Along with estrogen, progesterone works to maintain the reproductive tract and menstrual cycle. This hormone is essential for the maintenance of pregnancy and aids in the development of the milk-secreting cells. Progesterone inhibits prolactin's effects during pregnancy. A retained placenta or placental fragment following delivery and its accompanying progesterone can impair stage II lactogenesis.

Prolactin

Prolactin is the hormone that promotes milk synthesis. It is produced in the placenta and in the anterior pituitary gland in the brain. In Latin the term means "for lactation." Anterior pituitary prolactin stimulates alveolar growth during pregnancy. Prolactin levels increase gradually during pregnancy and reach a peak of 20 times the normal value near term. The inhibitory effect of progesterone and estrogen during pregnancy prevents full lactation at that time. However, many individuals (especially multiparous parents) begin leaking colostrum by the second or third trimester.

Prolactin levels in the blood increase soon after sucking begins. Prolactin signals an increase in milk synthesis. It also serves as a natural tranquilizer and stimulates feelings of restlessness and yearning for the baby. This physiologically conditioned response stimulates positive interaction with the baby. Thus, prolactin is often credited with inducing bonding behavior.

Parents can keep prolactin levels high by ensuring an effective latch and avoiding the use of artificial nipples or pacifiers that may cause **nipple preference** or reduced nursing opportunities. They can provide unlimited access to nursing, at least every 1 to 3 hours in the early weeks and for as long as the baby wants at a feeding. Nursing during the night, when prolactin release in response to sucking is greatest, will help to keep prolactin levels high as well.

Oxytocin

Oxytocin is produced in the **hypothalamus** and travels through nerve fibers to the posterior pituitary, where it is stored. The infant's sucking stimulates nerve endings in the nipple. Nerve impulses then race through the hypothalamic region to the posterior pituitary and release oxytocin. Oxytocin is transported through the bloodstream to the breasts. The presence of oxytocin contracts the muscle layer, or myoepithelial cell, around each milk-producing cell. This response is called the **milk ejection reflex**, or *letdown*. In response, milk flows down the ducts and out through the nipple pores.

Parents will notice the beginning of milk ejection when the baby's sucking rhythm changes from rapid nonnutritive sucking (about 2 sucks per second) to regular deep, slow nutritive sucking (about 1 suck per second). Some parents may initially need several minutes of stimulus to produce a high enough level of oxytocin to induce letdown.

Pitocin is a synthetic exogenous form of oxytocin, often used to induce or augment labor. Synthetic oxytocin differs from endogenous oxytocin. The use of synthetic oxytocin during labor has been associated with delayed onset and reduced duration of nursing.

Hormonal Imbalances

Because hormones regulate the lactation process, a disturbance in hormone levels could potentially affect milk production and release. Pituitary, thyroid, and adrenal imbalances can all alter hormone levels, as can certain medications. This imbalance may cause either too little or too much milk production, release of milk at inappropriate times, or the inability to release milk at all. Lactation problems accompanied by a vague feeling of physical discomfort or a history of previous thyroid problems or menstrual irregularities may indicate a hormone imbalance. **Placental retention** can inhibit lactation by causing hormones to remain at pregnancy levels. The absence of fullness and changes in secretions can indicate the retention of placental fragments.

Parents who had difficulty conceiving or who became pregnant with the aid of reproductive technologies are at a higher risk for hormone imbalance and, consequently, milk insufficiency. Infertility treatment typically manipulates hormonal levels and, thus, can cause hormone-related lactation problems.

A parent who fits the profile for hormone problems needs a referral to a caregiver for a thorough hormonal screening to rule out hormone imbalance as a cause. The screening includes measurement of progesterone, thyroid function, prolactin, and testosterone levels. Chapter 26 discusses hormonal issues, such as pituitary and thyroid dysfunction and polycystic ovarian (or ovary) syndrome (PCOS), in more detail.

Sheehan's syndrome is a form of shock that can result from severe postpartum hemorrhage and hypotension. The condition is also referred to as **hypopituitarism** syndrome, *postpartum hypopituitarism*, and *postpartum pituitary insufficiency*. In this condition, blood pressure drops so low that blood fails to circulate to the pituitary gland. This causes some or all cells in the gland to stop functioning permanently. Colostrum production may have begun before going into shock. Because of the malfunctioning pituitary gland, however, the breasts will remain soft after delivery, and milk production may not occur. The damage to the pituitary gland is usually irreversible and may permanently rule out the prospect of nursing.

Milk Synthesis

Milk synthesis is the process of producing milk. Delivery of the placenta causes estrogen and progesterone levels to drop sharply and prolactin production in the anterior pituitary to increase dramatically. This combination of events signals the alveoli to secrete milk. Colostrum, the initial milk produced, gives way to transitional milk. This is followed by increased milk production and fullness, beginning between the second and fifth days postpartum. Initial milk production typically produces **normal fullness**. Parents who do not understand this normal physiological response (fullness) may mistake it for engorgement.

Colostrum Production

Alveoli begin producing colostrum in the fourth month of pregnancy. At first, only small amounts are released into the center of the lobuli. As pregnancy advances, colostrum production continues to fill the alveoli. Some colostrum may leak out through the cell pores. Protruding portions of the alveoli may break away into the lobule, causing colostrum to leak during the later months of pregnancy.

Colostrum appears as a semitransparent, thick, and sticky liquid ranging in color from clear to deep yellow, even orange. It contains water, minerals, fat droplets, lymphocytes, and similar cells. Cast-off alveolar cells in the colostrum offer a unique combination of nutrients designed to meet the nutritional and immunologic needs of the newborn. Colostrum acts as a natural lubricant and, because of its **lysozyme** content, is **bactericidal** (destroys bacteria).

Role of Hormones

When estrogen and progesterone levels drop at delivery, the high prolactin levels stimulate milk production. Prolactin receptor sites on the walls of the lactocytes in the alveoli allow prolactin to move into the lactocytes and stimulate milk synthesis. Prolactin levels increase again 10-fold in response to sucking. Prolactin levels are three to five times higher after 3 months postpartum than the levels typically found during menstruation. The amount of prolactin released is directly proportional to the degree of nipple stimulation (Jin et al., 2024). Continued nursing increases the frequency of this hormone.

Autocrine Control

Milk synthesis does not rely entirely on endocrine (i.e., hormonal) control. Over time, milk production becomes dependent on the frequency and degree of drainage. Thus, milk production changes from endocrine control to **autocrine control** (i.e., local control). It is believed that frequent milk removal in the early weeks increases the number and sensitivity of prolactin receptor sites, thus increasing milk synthesis. Prolactin receptors and frequent feedings are necessary for long-term milk production.

Autocrine control in lactation comprises local control within the breast. The control agent is a secretory product (in this case, milk) that influences the cell's activity. This relationship suggests that milk remaining after a feeding inhibits the production of more milk. Proteins inhibiting milk synthesis build up when time lapses, signaling the brain to slow the rate of synthesis (Hannan et al., 2023). These proteins have been previously called the **feedback inhibitor of lactation (FIL)**. Through this process, the parent produces only what the baby needs, thus and protecting energy expenditure during lactation. Autocrine control explains why parents can nurse with one side exclusively through the course of lactation and involute totally on the other side.

Prolactin Inhibitory Factors

Prolactin inhibitory factors (PIFs) prevent the release of prolactin at times when the baby is not nursing (Hannan et al., 2023). They are produced by neuroendocrine neurons, including dopamine, somatostatin, and γ-aminobutyric acid. Sucking deactivates PIFs, thereby allowing prolactin release. Feeding frequency and nipple stimulation significantly affect the level of prolactin that is released. In the absence of effective and frequent sucking to remove milk, prolactin release decreases, and autocrine inhibition begins. For this reason, it is important to encourage frequent feedings and ensure an effective latch that facilitates milk transfer.

Milk Ejection Reflex (Letdown)

Milk ejection, also referred to as *letdown*, is a reflex triggered by various stimuli when the baby sucks. Contact between the baby's tongue and the nipple stimulates nerve endings to send a message to the hypothalamus. The message goes to the anterior pituitary, which lowers levels of PIF and triggers prolactin release. As sucking continues, the posterior pituitary gland secretes oxytocin, contracting the smooth muscles around the alveoli and the uterus. This contraction forces milk down through the ducts to the nipple openings (**Figure 7-8**).

Milk ejection is bilateral—that is, it occurs at the same time on both sides. Sphincters at the end of the ducts prevent milk from flowing freely from the nonsucked side, however. A **sphincter** is a circular band of muscle fibers that narrows a passage or closes a natural opening in the body.

The baby obtains the milk through negative pressure generated by sucking. Initially, letdown causes active expulsion of milk through pressure within the ducts. This lasts for a very short time, and then the flow subsides. Positive pressure continues, and milk flow will continue with effective sucking. The free flow of milk provided by letdown is essential to move

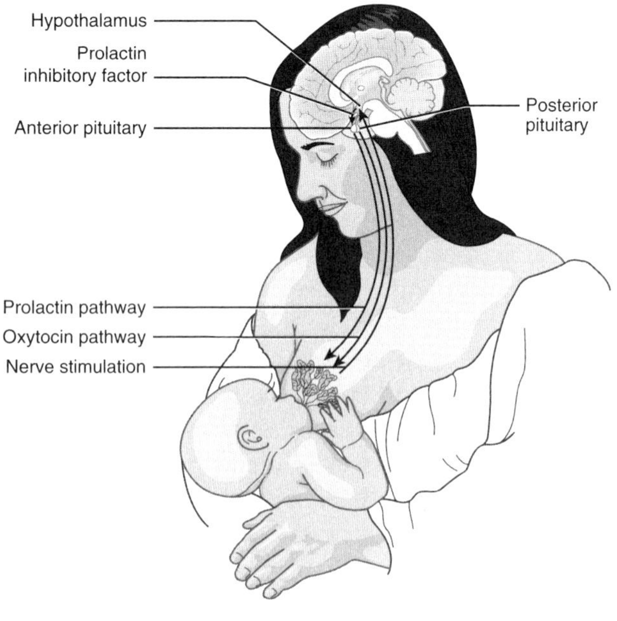

Figure 7-8 Hormone pathways during sucking.

fat globules down through the ducts. High-definition ultrasound shows that milk that is not removed flows back into the ducts (Geddes et al., 2021; Neville et al., 2023). When milk flow is interrupted in this manner, engorgement can develop, which may lead to ductal narrowing or mastitis.

Signs of Letdown

Several letdowns occur in a single feeding. Letdown may cause a tingling or tightening sensation as a result of alveoli contracting and forcing milk through the duct system. The initial letdown is usually the most noticeable because of the large volume of milk moved at that time. In the first few days postpartum, uterine contractions often accompany letdown owing to oxytocin's contraction of the involuting uterus.

Some parents do not notice the letdown reflex consistently in the first days and weeks of lactation. This is especially the case for parents who are nursing for the first time. Some may notice that milk drips from one side while the baby is nursing on the other side. Because letdown occurs bilaterally, this leaking is a sign that milk has let down in both breasts. Parents may also experience increased thirst or sleepiness. An awareness of letdown diminishes as the dyad becomes more experienced in nursing.

Parents can observe signs in their infant that indicate that their milk is letting down. Swallowing is more pronounced as the baby receives milk. Some babies may gulp or gag from the sudden rush of milk. In addition, parents can monitor the number of the baby's voids and stools for signs of milk transfer. By day 3, the baby should have three or more bowel movements and three or more wet diapers per day. By day 4, daily output should increase to four bowel movements and five wet diapers (Centers for Disease Control and Prevention [CDC], 2023). From the end of the first week of life through the first 6 weeks, six or more wet diapers and three to five stools per day indicate effective letdown and milk transfer.

A Functioning Letdown

A functioning letdown reflex is a necessary element in lactation. In its absence, the infant fails to receive an adequate amount of milk. Letdown enables the baby to receive most of the fat content in the milk, which tends to adhere to the duct lining. As letdown occurs, it forces this creamy **hindmilk** down into the ducts. The infant then receives more fatty milk after letdown as the feeding progresses. It is important that the duration of a feeding on each side is long enough for the baby to receive sufficient calories. Limiting nursing time on one side to switch to the other side could result in a large volume of **foremilk**, which contains fewer calories. In lactation, 50% of the calories come from the fat content.

Fat content correlates inversely with the amount of time between feedings (Tekin-Guler et al., 2023). The percentage of fat is higher when feedings are frequent, thereby minimizing differences between hindmilk and foremilk. The fat content of the foremilk can be higher than the fat content of the hindmilk, depending on the degree of fullness. The emptier the breast, the higher the fat content. These subtle differences have led to some practitioners ceasing to use the terms *foremilk* and *hindmilk*. However, given that the fat content toward the end of the feeding is higher than the fat content at the start of the feeding and because of the ubiquity of these terms, this text continues to use them, with the understanding that the percentage of fat varies from feeding to feeding, based on frequency. Restricting the number of feedings or limiting feeding duration can reduce fat intake. Every baby's nursing pattern is unique. It is advisable to allow the baby to finish nursing on one side rather than switching arbitrarily to the other side.

Inhibited Letdown

Letdown can fail to occur when nipple stimulation is weak, such as when the baby is not latching effectively. Fatigue, anxiety, fear, or pain can also inhibit letdown. Parents new to nursing often feel overtired because of lack of rest or overexertion is common. Some may feel tense and pressured by work, family commitments, or unsupportive family and friends. There may also be discomfort after childbirth or resulting surgery. Any of these circumstances could inhibit the secretion of oxytocin and release adrenaline. This, in turn, can negate the effects of oxytocin on the myoepithelial cells, thus inhibiting letdown.

If you suspect an **inhibited letdown**, a consultation will allow you to discuss possible emotional factors and ways to cope with stressors. You can also build the parent's confidence in the ability to nourish their baby by explaining that their body is able to sustain the baby now, just as it did during pregnancy. Suggestions for conditioning letdown in the next section will also help.

Conditioning Letdown

Relaxation techniques will help parents ease tension both physically and mentally during the early weeks of nursing, as described in **Chapter 15**. The less tension a parent experiences, the more likely they are to let down milk consistently during feedings. Nursing in a quiet location and a comfortable position can help ensure that letdown becomes a firmly established part of feedings. Such a pattern will condition parents psychologically for their milk ejection reflex to function. These conditioning techniques are especially helpful when parents are expressing milk because of being separated from their baby during feedings. Milk ejection can be triggered by picking up the baby, hearing a baby cry, turning on the pump, looking at the baby's picture, or thinking about the baby.

A small subset of parents experience a phenomenon with letdown called **dysphoric milk ejection reflex** (D-MER). This dysphoria, or experience of negative emotions, occurs a few moments before to a few moments after letdown. It is a physiological response caused by hormones and is different from postpartum depression (Liu et al., 2023; Nguyen et al., 2024; Ureño et al., 2019). Sensations include sadness, irritability, panic, agitation, and tearfulness. The feelings usually subside after a few minutes, although some parents feel these sensations throughout the feeding. It appears that oxytocin upregulates the stress response instead of downregulating it (Frawley & McGuinness, 2023; Uvnas-Moberg & Kendall-Tackett, 2018). An online resource, https://D-MER.org, provides information and support for parents experiencing D-MER and for practitioners caring for them.

Variations in Breast Structure and Function

The ability to produce and release milk depends in part on the physical condition of the breasts. A wide variety of sizes and nipple shapes can accommodate nursing. Only a few variations in structure create challenges. Parents can overcome differences in structure such as nipple inversion. Other circumstances, such as surgery that severed milk ducts, may make it necessary to supplement nursing with additional nutrition. In most circumstances, size and shape do not indicate how much milk can be produced.

Examining the Breasts

If a difficulty arises that you suspect may be related to the nipples or breasts, an examination is appropriate. A systematic exam can reveal the presence or absence of glandular tissue necessary for milk production. Some parents associate breast examination with illness or cancer prevention. Thus, make sure they understand the purpose of your examination. Use this opportunity to teach them about milk production and techniques that will help, such as breast massage, compression, and hand expression.

Before beginning a breast exam, ensure privacy to help the parent feel comfortable. Be aware of any customs of modesty that may make the parent uncomfortable. Ask permission and explain your purpose before you begin the exam. If written consent is required, be sure the parent has read and signed a consent form granting you permission to examine the dyad.

History

Normal breast changes during pregnancy include increased growth and tenderness, darkening of the areolae, and increased Montgomery gland prominence or "bumpiness." Ask parents open-ended questions, such as "What changes did you notice in your breasts during your pregnancy?" Use reflective listening to clarify what they say to you. Explore closely if they report no changes prenatally and ask if there were changes in bra size. If bra size increased from a B cup to a D cup, there is probably sufficient functioning tissue. Describing typical changes will help parents recollect how their breasts changed. Often, their partner is observant about breast growth and can help clarify changes that occurred.

Ask about any previous surgery or damage to the chest area. This may include surgical reduction or augmentation, cardiac surgery, central line placement, or any other procedure that could affect function. Even an automobile accident in which the seat belt placed severe pressure on the chest could damage tissue, as could sports or childhood injuries.

Assessment

Examining both breasts at the same time will enable you to observe their symmetry. Note the skin's elasticity; the presence of normal glandular growth; prominent veining; and any engorgement, lumps, swelling, or redness. Look for evidence of surgery that may have altered or severed some ducts (**Color Plate 9**).

Note nipple size and shape and the size of the areolae. Be sensitive and respectful when discussing the shape and size of nipples. If the message parents hear seems negative, they may not overcome that impression to reach their nursing goals. Reinforce with them that small and large breasts alike typically produce sufficient milk.

Gentle nipple compression will help assess the ability of the nipple to **evert** (protrude) for an effective latch. How a nipple reacts with compression indicates what is happening inside the infant's mouth during nursing. A nipple that retracts is considered short shanked and could cause nipple damage.

Differences in Nipples

Nipples are unique in shape, size, and the degree to which they evert. Nipple size varies greatly, ranging from 7 to 40 mm (Ventura et al., 2021). Nipple length ranges from 5 to 20 mm, with an average of 9.5 mm. These nipple differences could potentially affect nursing. Efficient milk transfer depends on a baby's ability to latch, form the tissue into a conical shape, and stretch it forward and then upward against the hard palate (roof of the mouth). A nipple that everts on stimulation aids the baby in finding and centering on the nipple. It also facilitates sufficient tissue to be drawn into the baby's mouth. A **pinch test**, as described in **Chapter 22**, can help test the ability of the nipples to evert.

Many differences exist in types of nipples. Variations include bifurcated nipples; dimpled nipples; extremely long nipples; and thick, "meaty" nipples that are not truly inverted but may be difficult for the baby to grasp. **Table 7-1** depicts nipples classified into five types according to how they appear before and after stimulation. Stimulation such as touch, cold, or gentle compression can reveal whether true inversion is present. The nipple in **Color Plate 10** appears normal and inverts, or retracts inward, when stimulated (**Color Plate 11**). The nipple in **Color Plate 12** appears dimpled—yet after pumping to release the adhesions, it everts.

Inverted Nipples

Nipples that do not evert are referred to as *inverted nipples*. Some parents believe they have inverted nipples, but if the nipple everts with stimulation, it is not truly inverted. The degree of nipple inversion typically decreases with each subsequent pregnancy. For some individuals the skin's increased elasticity during pregnancy decreases the extent of inversion.

Inverted nipples typically begin to respond to correction techniques during the last trimester of pregnancy. There is a theoretical possibility that nipple stimulation could result in preterm labor. Because of this concern, expectant parents should check with their caregiver before beginning any technique that involves nipple stimulation.

Inverted nipples are a factor in suboptimal infant feeding behavior. With a good match of the breast and baby's mouth, the baby takes in a large portion of the tissue and forms it into a cone-shaped teat. An infant typically takes in enough tissue to reach back almost to the juncture of the hard and soft palates (LeFort et al., 2021). When the tissue does not stretch to accommodate this pattern, the baby has difficulty maintaining suction. Milk transfer, therefore, often depends more on the pliability of the tissue to form a tight seal and maintain negative pressure than on the configuration of the nipple. Clinicians may try a variety of techniques to help evert nipples that are difficult for a baby to grasp. Some methods are more effective than others.

Devices to Evert Nipples

Some parents purchase breast shells and everting devices without consulting their caregiver or a lactation specialist to confirm that they need them. Like many aspects of lactation, interventions work well for some parents and are intimidating or overwhelming to others. Presenting information that informs, empowers, and yet does not overwhelm parents is a part of your counseling role. Approach each encounter with sensitivity and share prenatal guidance accordingly.

Breast shells have been promoted historically for improving nipple protrusion prenatally. However, a study concluded that neither the use of breast shells nor the practice of manually pulling the nipple to break adhesions before birth had a significant impact on nipple elongation (Kaya et al., 2024). Furthermore, prenatal nipple assessments can potentially undermine an expectant parent's confidence and commitment to nurse. Wearing shells between feedings has been suggested to improve nipple eversion by gently placing pressure on the skin, thereby stretching and pushing the nipple forward.

Some parents form the nipple by hand or with the application of ice or suction from a breast pump just before a feeding. Commercial devices such as LatchAssist, Supple Cups, Nipplette, and Evert-It also help elongate the nipple. **Chapter 22** provides detailed information about these devices and interventions. When using any eversion technique, it is important not to increase the suction to painful levels and to minimize the frequency of their use in order to avoid nipple damage.

A **nipple shield** is often used as a potential solution to inversion (**Color Plate 13**) and as a transitional tool for nursing (Kaya et al., 2024). Nipple shields are readily available in stores and online, resulting in parents purchasing them without guidance.

Table 7-1 Five Basic Types of Nipples

	At rest	Stimulated
Common nipple The majority of parents have what is referred to as a *common nipple*. It protrudes slightly when at rest and becomes erect and more graspable when stimulated. A baby has no trouble finding and latching onto this nipple to pull in a large amount of tissue and stretch it to the roof of the mouth.	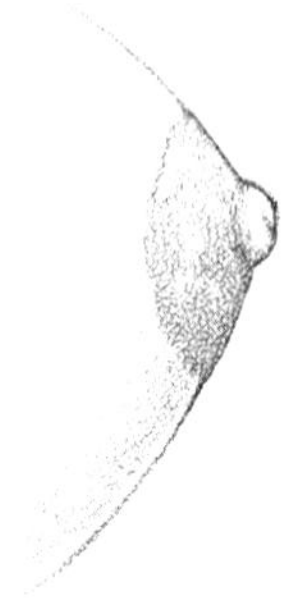	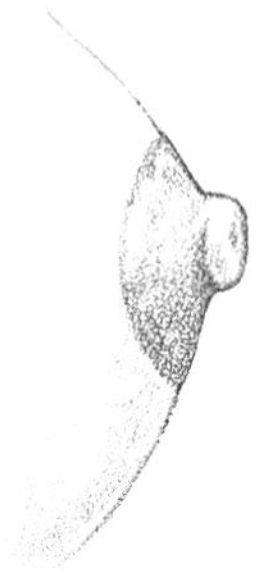
Flat nipple A **flat nipple** has a very short shank that makes it less easy for the baby to find and latch onto. In response to stimulation, this nipple remains essentially unchanged. Slight movement inward or outward may occur, but it is not enough to aid the baby in latching. This nipple may benefit from the use of nipple eversion techniques to increase protractility.	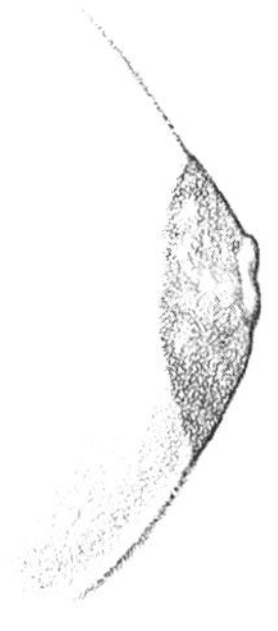	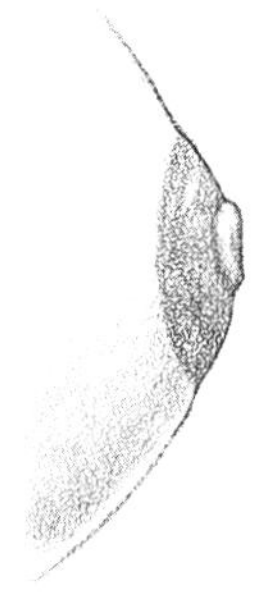
Inverted-appearing nipple An inverted-appearing nipple may appear inverted but becomes erect after stimulation. This nipple needs no correction and presents no problems with latch.	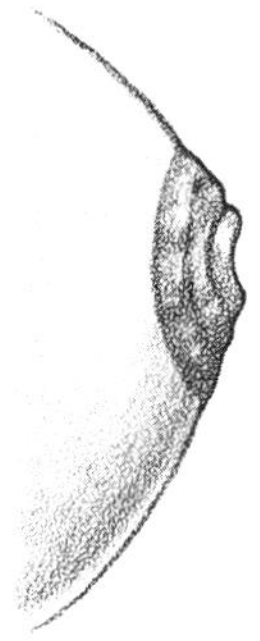	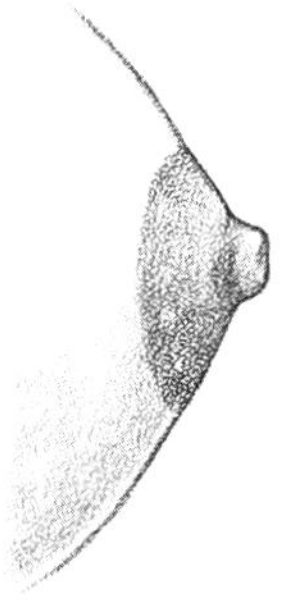
Retracted nipple A retracted nipple is the most common type of inverted nipple. Initially, this nipple appears to evert. However, on stimulation, it retracts, making latch difficult. This nipple responds well to techniques to increase nipple protrusion.	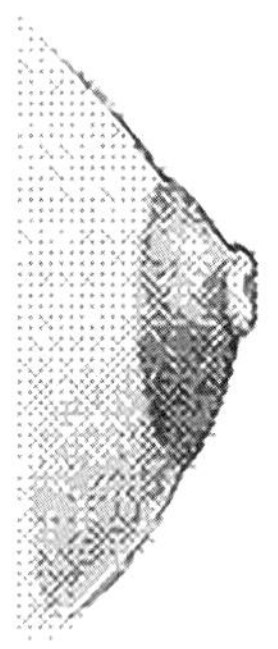	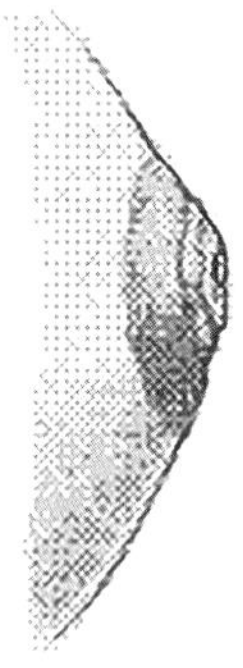
Inverted nipple A truly inverted nipple is retracted both at rest and when stimulated. Such a nipple is more difficult for the baby to latch onto. All techniques used to enhance protractility can be used to improve latch. Even if the nipple remains retracted, the baby may be able to latch if the parent helps sandwich the breast for the baby's mouth. Sometimes, milk expression will be required until the inverted tissue stretches and everts.	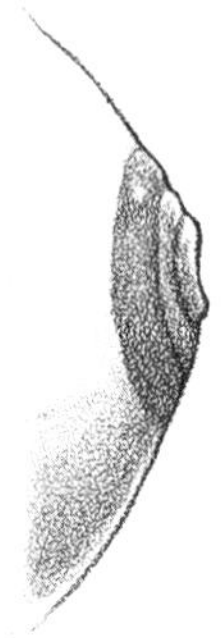	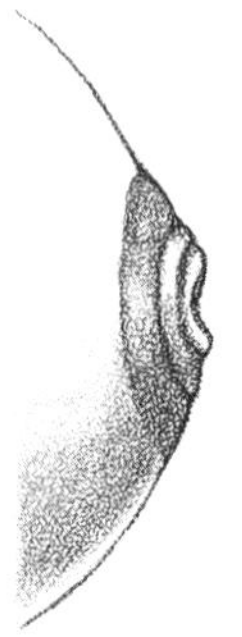

Selection must be based on correct size and material (e.g., silicon, not rubber or latex). There is a risk of infant preference for the artificial nipple, tissue damage, inadequate sucking stimulation, incorrect shield placement during feeding, and inadequate milk transfer. Optimally, a lactation consultant would monitor that a nipple shield is used appropriately. Chapter 22 discusses nipple shield use in more detail.

Surgical Correction of Inverted Nipples

Some parents opt for surgical "correction" of inverted nipples, primarily for aesthetic reasons but also to facilitate nursing (Feng et al., 2019; Kaya et al., 2024). Any breast surgery has the potential to affect lactation negatively, especially when it occurs in the periareolar area. A surgical procedure using two triangular areolar dermal flaps has proven successful for nipple inversion with no infection, hematoma, or nipple necrosis (Kim & Wee, 2023). It is important to ask parents whether they have had any breast procedure because they may not consider certain nipple inversion "correction" techniques to be surgery per se.

Lumps in the Breast

The general population usually associates lumps in the breast with cancer. However, many lumps associated with lactation are not a health risk. The normal state of a lactating breast is lumpy because of the enlarged milk-filled alveoli distributed throughout the tissue. Other lumps can occur from ductal narrowing or mastitis (discussed in **Chapter 17**). These conditions are usually temporary, with the associated lumps disappearing after alleviating their cause.

If a lump fails to move downward and begin to break up, consider a cause unrelated to lactation, and refer the parent to a caregiver who can identify the cause of the lump. Lumps associated with **fibrocystic breasts** change with the menstrual cycle, shrinking and becoming less noticeable after menstruation. Other types of cysts may also be present, as described next.

Galactocele

A **galactocele** is a benign cyst usually believed to be caused by a milk duct obstruction. It contains a thick, creamy collection of milk products and is compatible with lactation. Rarely, the material can be crystallized and chalky (Costas et al., 2023; Jaseem Hassan et al., 2018). Breast surgery, prolactin increases in pregnancy, and oral contraceptive use may contribute to the formation of a galactocele (Amaral et al., 2023; Gada & Bakhshi, 2024).

A galactocele sometimes oozes from the nipple when the cyst is compressed. Galactoceles can be aspirated, and some are removed surgically to prevent them from refilling. They can also resolve spontaneously, without the need for surgery. If surgery is required, nursing does not usually need to be interrupted.

During lactation, a hydatid cyst may be mistaken for a galactocele. **Hydatid disease** is a parasitic infection caused by tapeworm larva. It can be transmitted from animals to humans and occurs frequently in sheep-raising communities. It usually presents in the liver and lungs but can occur in the breast. Treatment requires antiparasitic medication and sometimes even surgery (Mesfin et al., 2023).

Intraductal Papilloma

An **intraductal papilloma** is a benign, nontender tumor within a milk duct. Intraductal papillomas are the second most frequent cause of a bloody breast discharge. They are usually associated with a spontaneous bloody discharge from one breast. Nursing may continue while serious disease is being ruled out. The discharge may stop, or a surgeon may remove the involved duct.

Malignancy

Breast cancer during pregnancy and lactation is relatively rare (about 3%). However, breast cancers found during pregnancy, lactation, or within a year after birth are typically more advanced and more aggressive with a poorer prognosis (Fazeli et al., 2023). Breast cancer rates during pregnancy and early postpartum are expected to increase with advanced childbearing age. As discussed earlier in this chapter, rapid weaning can also be a cause.

An infant's rejection of a breast may be a marker for malignancy (Portnow et al., 2023). Be careful not to confuse such rejection with the common occurrence of temporary refusal, as discussed in **Chapter 23**. Therefore, a lump in conjunction with an infant refusing to nurse needs to be referred to a specialist to rule out cancer. Nursing can continue if a biopsy is performed on a lump. In many cases, lumps are benign, and nursing is not interrupted. There is a small risk that a milk **fistula** (abnormal opening) may result from a biopsy, which can cause milk to leak from the incision site.

Researchers have identified significant changes in the milk proteins of cancerous breasts compared with noncancerous breasts. Analytical techniques may soon provide nursing parents with better options for early detection of breast cancer risk or disease (Aslebagh et al., 2019; Kondracka et al., 2023). Treatments for cancer, including chemotherapy and radiation, are not compatible with nursing. **Chapter 18** discusses unavoidable weaning and counseling in these difficult situations.

Paget's disease is a rare form of breast cancer that is usually unilateral (**Color Plate 37**). Almost half of all clients with mammary Paget's disease have a palpable lump at the time of diagnosis. Frequently, timely diagnosis is delayed when both the clinician and parent assume that the symptoms are a dermatological condition (Mariano et al., 2023). Encourage such parents to visit a breast specialist if unusual skin symptoms involving the nipple or areola fail to resolve quickly. Magnetic resonance imaging (MRI), sonography, and ductoscopic techniques have improved diagnosis and treatment (Babu et al., 2018; Mariano et al., 2023; Ogata et al., 2018). Markers for Paget's disease include the following:

- Itching, tingling, or redness in the nipple and/or areola
- Flaking, crusty, or thickened skin resembling eczema on or around the nipple
- A flattened nipple
- Yellowish or bloody discharge from the nipple

Regular Self-Examination

Breast self-examination (BSE) will help individuals become familiar with their breasts and comfortable handling them for lactation. BSE at various intervals will help identify changes over time and aid in the early detection of breast lumps. BSE can increase awareness, identification of danger signs, and timely intervention (National Breast Cancer Foundation, 2024; Polishwala et al., 2023).

Summary

The breast is an intricate system of sensory nerves, connective and fatty tissues, and milk-producing and transporting glands. Puberty triggers the development of functional breast tissue. Hormonal changes during pregnancy produce most of the growth toward lactogenesis. The areola undergoes changes in size and color, and the Montgomery glands become more pronounced. The breast experiences lactogenesis throughout pregnancy, transforming it into a state characterized by milk production and secretion.

Estrogen, progesterone, prolactin, and oxytocin hormones play crucial roles in milk production and release. Insulin, thyroid, and growth factor hormones are also involved. Blood carries proteins, fats, sugar, and other substances needed for lactation. The breast, in turn, takes these raw materials from the blood to create nutrients for the infant. This nutrition travels through a system of lobuli and ducts to the nipple, where it is discharged through several nipple pores. Surgery that damages the nerves or severs the milk ducts may compromise the ability to lactate fully.

What You Learned—At a Glance

Conversation Starters with Parents

- What are you doing to preserve the health of your breasts?
- What can you do to ensure that your milk production satisfies your baby?
- What changes did you notice in your breasts during your pregnancy?
- What changes do you notice in your breasts during and after a feeding?

Breast Anatomy

- Preserving the keratin layer and Montgomery gland lubrication will help avoid skin damage.
- When the baby sucks, sensory nerve endings in the nipple signal the brain to trigger milk release via oxytocin.
- The baby's latch needs to take in some areolar tissue.

Supportive and Sustaining Tissue

- There is extensive innervation in the nipple and areola complex.
- A deep latch and vigorous suck will stimulate the nerves.
- Breast size correlates to the amount of fatty tissue and does not predict milk production capacity.
- Breast sagging results from pregnancy, not lactation.
- Pressure from engorgement decreases blood and lymph flow, causes edema, leads to poor milk drainage, and risks mastitis.

Glandular Tissue

- Increased estrogen during menstruation produces growth of ducts and connective tissue.
- Sucking stimulates milk production and increases blood flow to provide nutrients to make milk.
- Raw materials from blood create nutrients in the alveoli.
- Myoepithelial cells surround the alveoli, contract when sucking releases oxytocin, and force milk down the ducts to the nipple.
- Widely spaced, tubular, asymmetric, and thin breasts are markers for insufficient glandular tissue.
- In the absence of pregnancy and lactation, tissue growth regresses, and glandular cells degenerate.

Mammary Growth and Development

- Functional tissue development during pregnancy is far more significant than gains during menstrual cycles.
- In the first trimester of pregnancy, the duct system multiplies, the skin stretches, nipple size and areola increase, the areola darkens, and the Montgomery glands become noticeable.
- Stage I lactogenesis (secretory differentiation) occurs at the beginning of the third trimester of pregnancy, when the breast begins to gather nutrients for milk synthesis.
- Stage II lactogenesis (secretory activation) occurs around the second to fifth day postpartum, when transitional milk is produced and copious milk secretion begins.
- Stage III lactogenesis (galactopoiesis) occurs about 8 to 10 days postpartum, when mature milk production is established.
- Lactogenesis is followed by a period of involution, when the breast returns to a nearly prepregnancy state and milk production ceases.

Hormonal Impact on Lactation

- Estrogen stimulates growth of the uterus, vagina, and other reproductive organs.
- Progesterone inhibits prolactin's effects during pregnancy.
- Prolactin stimulates alveolar growth and milk synthesis and induces bonding behavior.
- High prolactin levels can be maintained with unlimited, effective sucking and nursing at night.
- Oxytocin releases in response to sucking and contracts the myoepithelial cells (milk ejection reflex).
- Pituitary, thyroid, and adrenal imbalances can affect milk production and release.
- Sheehan's syndrome (hypopituitarism) can cause irreversible damage to milk-producing cells.

Milk Synthesis and Ejection

- Colostrum is established by the end of the second trimester.
- Delivery of the placenta causes estrogen and progesterone levels to drop sharply and prolactin to increase dramatically.
- Sucking inhibits the production of PIF, thereby allowing prolactin release to occur.
- Autocrine control inhibits milk production when milk remains in the breast.
- Letdown moves fat globules down through the ducts (hindmilk).
- Letdown can be inhibited by fatigue, anxiety, fear, or pain.
- Relaxation can help condition letdown.
- Frequent feedings, an effective latch, and ample milk transfer milk removal in the absence of effective and frequent sucking help protect milk production.

Variations in Breast Structure and Function

- Breast symmetry can be observed by examining both breasts at the same time.
- Truly inverted nipples are rare.
- An inverted nipple can be drawn out by sucking, an everter, breast pump, or nipple shield.
- The normal lactating breast is lumpy because of the enlarged, milk-filled alveoli.
- A galactocele may resolve spontaneously or may be compressed, aspirated, or removed surgically.
- An intraductal papilloma may produce a bloody discharge.
- Breast rejection may occur when malignancy is present.
- Paget's disease produces scaly, itchy nipples and areolae and sometimes bloody discharge.
- Breast surgery may damage functional tissue and require close monitoring for milk intake.

References

Adekeye A, et al. Pediatric and adolescent breast conditions: a review. *J Pediatr Adolesc Gynecol*. 2023;36(1):5–13.

Alekseev NP. *Physiology of Human Female Lactation*. Cham, Switzerland: Springer International Publishing. 2021.

Amaral RS, et al. Galactorrhea after breast augmentation: case report and literature review. *Rev Bras Cir Plást*. 2023;38:e0736.

Aslebagh R, et al. Combinatorial electrophoresis and mass spectrometry-based proteomics in breast milk for breast cancer biomarker discovery. *Adv Exp Med Biol*. 2019; 1140:451–467.

Babu B, et al. Bilateral mammary Paget disease in a young adult female. *Radiol Case Rep*. 2018;13(3):586–591.

Bland KI, et al. *The Breast: Comprehensive Management of Benign and Malignant Diseases*. St. Louis: Elsevier Health Sciences; 2023.

Centers of Disease Control and Prevention. Infant and toddler nutrition. 2023. https://www.cdc.gov/nutrition/infantandtoddler nutrition/faqs.html

Costas T, et al. Mammary tissue changes during pregnancy and breastfeeding. In: Gomes-Ferreira M, Olivas-Menayo J, eds. *Post-Maternity Body Changes: Obstetric Fundamentals and Surgical Reshaping*. Cham, Switzerland: Springer International Publishing; 2023:247–261.

Davis FM. The ins and outs of calcium signalling in lactation and involution: implications for breast cancer treatment. *Pharmacol Res*. 2017;116:100–104.

de Szalay S, Wertz PW. Protective barriers provided by the epidermis. *Int J Mol Sci*. 2023;24(4):3145.

del Pilar Bérniz Laborda C, Olivas-Menayo J. Nipple-areola complex restoration after breastfeeding. In: Gomes-Ferreira M, Olivas-Menayo J, eds. *Post-Maternity Body Changes: Obstetric Fundamentals and Surgical Reshaping*. Cham, Switzerland: Springer International Publishing; 2023:329–341.

Faulkner HR, et al. Safe reproducible breast reduction. *Plast Reconstr Surg Glob Open*. 2023;11(9):e5245.

Fazeli S, et al. Cancer in pregnancy: breast cancer. *Abdom Radiol*. 2023;48(5):1645–1662.

Feng R, et al. A modified inverted nipple correction technique that preserves breastfeeding. *Aesthet Surg J*. 2019;39(6): NP165–NP175.

Frawley T, McGuinness D. Dysphoric milk ejection reflex (D-MER) and its implications for mental health nursing. *Int J Men. Health Nurs*. 2023;32(2):620–626.

Gada PB, Bakhshi G. Galactocele. In: *StatPearls*. Treasure Island, FL: StatPearls Publishing; 2024. https://www.ncbi.nlm.nih .gov/books/NBK578180/

Geddes DT, et al. 25 years of research in human lactation: from discovery to translation. *Nutrients*. 2021;13(9):3071.

Gnanavel H, et al. Inflammatory lesions. In: Dev B, Dennis Joseph L, eds. *Holistic Approach to Breast Disease*. Singapore: Springer Nature Singapore; 2023:187–210.

Grant A. *Ross & Wilson Pathophysiology E-Book*. St. Louis: Elsevier Health Sciences; 2023.

Haider R. Anatomy of the breast. *Int J Multidiscip Res*. 2023; 1(5):401–422.

Hannan F, et al. Hormonal regulation of mammary gland development and lactation. *Nat Rev Endocrinol*. 2023;19(1): 46–61.

Jaseem Hassan M, et al. Cytological diagnosis of crystallizing galactocele—report of an unusual case. *Breast Dis*. 2018; 37(3):159–161.

Jin X, et al. Causes of low milk supply: the roles of oestrogens, progesterone, and related external factors. *Adv Nutr*. 2024;15(1):100129.

Kantha SS. Montgomery glands in the areolar region: a clinical overview. *Int Med J*. 2023;*30*(3):128–131.

Kaya Ö, et al. The effect of interventions on flat and inverted nipple on breastfeeding: a systematic review. *J Ped Nursing*. 2024;74:e1–e13.

Kim TH, Wee SY. A new method for inverted nipple treatment with diamond-shaped dermal flaps and acellular dermal matrix: a preliminary study. *Aesthetic Plast Surg*. 2023;47(3):998–1006.

Kondracka A, et al. Occurrence, role, and challenges of microRNA in human breast milk: a scoping review. *Biomedicine*. 2023;11(2):248.

Lawrence RA, Lawrence RM. *Breastfeeding: A Guide for the Medical Professional*. St. Louis: Elsevier Health Sciences. 2021.

LeFort Y, et al. Academy of Breastfeeding Medicine position statement on ankyloglossia in breastfeeding dyads. *Breastfeed Med*. 2021;16(4), 278–281.

Liu H, et al. Dysphoric milk ejection reflex: report of two cases and postulated mechanisms and treatment. *Breastfeed Med*. 2023;18(5):388–394.

MAIN Trial Collaborative Group. Preparing for breast feeding: treatment of inverted and nonprotractile nipples in pregnancy. *Midwifery*. 1994;10:200–214.

Mariano L, et al. A pictorial exploration of mammary Paget disease: insights and perspectives. *Cancers*. 2023;15(21):5276.

Mesfin T, et al. Isolated breast hydatid cyst: a case report. *Clin Case Rep*. 2023;11(12).

Mohamad N, et al. Bloody nipple discharge post delivery: a case of "rusty pipe syndrome." *Korean J Fam Med*. 2021;42(4):339–341.

National Breast Cancer Foundation, Inc. Breast self-exam. 2024. https://www.nationalbreastcancer.org/breast-self-exam/

Neville MC, et al. Parental factors that impact the ecology of human mammary development, milk secretion, and milk composition—a report from "Breastmilk Ecology: Genesis of Infant Nutrition (BEGIN)" Working Group 1. *Am J Clin Nutr*. 2023;*117*:S11–S27.

Nguyen L, et al. Dysphoric milk ejection reflex: characteristics, risk factors, and its association with depression scores and breastfeeding self-efficacy. *Breastfeed Med*. 2024;19(6):467–475.

Ogata H, et al. Sonographic visualization of nipple blood flow can help differentiate Paget disease from benign eczematous nipple lesions. *PLoS One*. 2018;13(5):e0197156.

Otuneye AT, Audu LI. Breastfeeding: a basic strategy for health promotion (mini-review). *NJPNC*. 2023;3(1):12–15.

Polishwala S, et al. The assessment and comparison of the knowledge of breast self-examination and breast carcinoma among health care workers and the general population in an urban setting. *Cureus*. 2023;15(3):e36592.

Portnow LH, et al. Breast cancer screening in high-risk women during pregnancy and lactation. *JBI*. 2023;5(5):508–519.

Puerta-Alcalde P, et al. Breakthrough invasive fungal infection among patients with haematologic malignancies: a national, prospective, and multicentre study. *J Infect*. 2023;87(1):46–53.

Tekin-Guler T, et al. The association of pre-pregnancy obesity and breast milk fatty acids composition and the relationship of postpartum maternal diet, breast milk fatty acids and infant growth. *Breastfeed Med.* 2023;18(6):475–482.

Troupis T, Markopoulos C. Development, physiology and surgical anatomy of the breast. In: Markopoulos M, Karakatsanis A, eds. *Breast Cancer Management for Surgeons: An Examination Guide*. Cham, Switzerland: Springer International Publishing; 2023:3–18.

Ureño TL, et al. Dysphoric milk ejection reflex: a descriptive study. *Breastfeed Med.* 2019;14(9):666–673.

Uvnas-Moberg K, Kendall-Tackett K. The mystery of D-MER: what can hormonal research tell us about dysphoric milk-ejection reflex? *Clin Lact.* 2018;9(1):23–29.

Ventura AK, et al. Associations between variations in breast anatomy and early breastfeeding challenges. *J Hum Lact.* 2021;37(2):403–413.

CHAPTER 8

Nutrition in Pregnancy and Lactation

The quality of the food we consume has a major impact on our overall health. Pregnancy and lactation are often times of high motivation to improve eating habits for the baby and the parent's well-being. Body reserves, also known as *body fat*, created by the foods birth parents consume will provide the energy and nutrients babies need to grow and develop. An understanding of the nutrients needed in a healthy diet will help parents make the right food choices for their growing family. Caregivers with sound nutrition knowledge and effective counseling skills can confidently approach clients about their nutritional habits during pregnancy and lactation.

KEY TERMS

Allergen
Amino acids
Anemia
Arachidonic acid
Basal metabolic rate
Body mass index (BMI)
Caffeine
Calcium
Celiac disease
Complete protein complement
Complex carbohydrates
Dietary reference intake (DRI)
Fat-soluble vitamins
Fats
Genetically modified (engineered) food
Hemoglobin
Iron
Kilocalorie (kcal)
Metabolic syndrome
Minerals
Neural tube defects
Nutrients
Proteins
Retinoids
Simple carbohydrate
Vegan
Vegetarian
Vitamins
Water-soluble vitamins

Nutritional Knowledge

A combination of marketing practices and limited nutritional education results in many people reaching adulthood with meager skills to choose and prepare foods wisely. Formal nutrition education often ends in primary school, at a time when children have little control over their diets to put what they learn into practice. For many people, much of what they know about nutrition comes from media and social media, where many of the messages consist of product marketing rather than evidence-based knowledge. For example, an advertising campaign may tell us that a product has added **vitamins** but fails to explain that the added vitamins replace natural vitamins lost in processing or that added vitamins will not be as readily absorbed as those found in nature. Factors such as food content consisting of **genetically modified (engineered) foods** or irradiated foods may not be revealed (Karalis et al., 2020).

Concerns about the risks of genetically modified products to the environment and human health continue to be the subject of much debate. Because of these concerns, consumers want to know if the foods they purchase are genetically modified.

Health professionals and the internet are the most common sources of nutrition information during pregnancy (Lobo et al., 2020). However, many healthcare providers lack the knowledge to counsel parents on healthy nutrition for pregnancy and lactation (Bassin et al., 2020; Cuerda et al., 2021). Thus, many parents turn to the internet because of a lack of guidance and sound information from their healthcare providers (Daigle Millan et al., 2022; Snyder et al., 2020). Informed caregivers can guide clients of childbearing age toward sound nutritional principles and healthy choices.

Parents with dietary risk factors may need to be referred to a dietitian nutritionist for assessment. Referral is especially appropriate for a **body mass index (BMI)** of less than 19.8 (very underweight) or more than 26 (overweight), as well as for medical conditions such as diabetes, bariatric surgery, or metabolic disorders. Adolescent parents are at risk for poor nutrition inadequacies because they are still in a state of high growth, as well as their potentially unwise food choices. This can affect fetal growth and is associated with preterm birth (Yisahak et al., 2021).

Adolescent eating patterns and behaviors are influenced by many factors. The food habits of their parents and exposure to various flavors influence their behaviors throughout their lives (Scaglioni et al., 2018). Image-related social media messages may negatively affect their body image and food choices (Rounsefell et al., 2020). Referring expectant adolescents to a dietitian nutritionist can help ensure adequate nutrition.

Dietary Guidelines

Nutritional guidelines are issued by most countries' health ministries or departments. The World Health Organization (WHO) provides extensive nutritional education and information by region, including multiple online resources, such as an e-Library of Evidence for Nutrition Actions (WHO, 2019). **Table 8-1** presents recommendations for complementary feeding and child nutrition (United Nations Children's Fund [UNICEF], 2020a, 2020b). It presents key proven practices, services, and policy interventions for the prevention and treatment of stunting and other forms of undernutrition throughout the life cycle. Clinicians should be familiar with the dietary guidelines in their region.

In the United States, dietary guidelines are updated every 5 years by the U.S. Department of Agriculture (USDA) and Department of Health and

Table 8-1 United Nations Children's Fund Nutrition Guidance

Adolescence > Pregnancy	Birth	0–6 Months	6–23 Months
▪ Counseling on nutritious and safe diets, physical activity and rest, mental health, and monitoring of weight gain ▪ Supplementation with iron and folic acid or multiple micronutrients ▪ Deworming prophylaxis ▪ Calcium supplementation ▪ Care and support for nutritionally at-risk individuals	▪ Start nursing within 1 hour of delivery	▪ Exclusive nursing ▪ Vitamin A supplementation in first 8 weeks after delivery ▪ Multi-micronutrient supplementation ▪ Improved use of locally available foods, fortified foods	▪ Nutritionally adequate, age-appropriate, and safely prepared complementary foods ▪ Continued nursing until age 2 or longer ▪ Nutrition counseling and social and behavior change communication ▪ Responsive feeding and stimulation ▪ Diverse and nutritious complementary foods ▪ Vitamin and mineral supplements in settings where nutrient-poor diets prevail ▪ Fortified foods as needed ▪ Social protection programs and counseling services ▪ Safe water and clean household environments

Data from USDA. *Dietary Guidelines for Americans 2020–2025*. https://www.dietaryguidelines.gov/sites/default/files/2021-03/Dietary_Guidelines_for_Americans-2020-2025.pdf & UNICEF Nutrition Strategy 2020–2030. https://www.unicef.org/media/106511/file/%20Nutrition%20Strategy%202020-2030%20(Document)%20-%202021%20Edition..pdf

Human Services (USDHHS) and are available at https://www.dietaryguidelines.gov. Previous *Dietary Guidelines for Americans* provided guidance for pregnant individuals and nursing parents. Updated guidelines for 2020–2025 added dietary guidance for nursing infants and toddlers ages 0 to 24 months as well. The guidelines recommend nursing exclusively for 6 months and recommend when and how to introduce complementary foods and vitamin D supplements. They also recommend the introduction of allergen foods, including those containing peanuts, between 4 and 6 months to all infants. The newer guidelines also address the use of donor milk, including handling and storage. Further, they recommend nutrients and foods to meet the needs of parents and babies during pregnancy and lactation (USDA & USDHHS, 2020).

Basic Nutrients

A basic understanding of **nutrients** and their function in the body provides a foundation for educating parents about healthy nutrition. A nutrient is any nourishing substance in food that is released by digestion and then absorbed and used to promote body function. Macronutrients consist of protein, **fats**, and carbohydrates. Micronutrients consist of vitamins plus **minerals**, both macrominerals and microminerals.

Deficiencies in any of the micronutrients could decrease milk production and result in a nutritional deficiency in the infant (Lockyer et al., 2021). Micronutrient supplementation is recommended for positive birth outcomes in low- and middle-income regions where deficiencies are common or for individuals who would benefit from supplementation in addition to a well-balanced diet (Brown & Wright, 2020; Santander Ballestín et al., 2021; Tsakiridis et al., 2020).

Eating the required nutrients in proper quantities generally leads to a healthy nutritional status. Each nutrient has a specific function and relationship to the body. All nutrients must be present in the proper quantities to maintain health and a feeling of well-being. Recommendations for **dietary reference intake (DRI)** of key nutrients are increased during pregnancy and lactation (Aparicio et al., 2020).

Carbohydrates

Most foods contain carbohydrates, which the body breaks down into simple sugars. Carbohydrates are the main source of energy for all body functions and activities and help to regulate protein and fat metabolism. Sufficient carbohydrate intake avoids relying on protein as an energy source, allowing protein to perform other important body functions. The body converts excess carbohydrates into fat and stores it. Two major types of carbohydrates—simple and complex—are found in foods.

Simple Carbohydrates

Simple carbohydrates, or sugars, are digested easily and provide a quick burst of energy (also known as *glucose*) to the bloodstream. Simple carbohydrates include anything with sugar, which may be sugar, jams, honey, chocolate, and other sweets. Other simple carbohydrates can include foods made with refined white flour, such as crackers, cakes, cereals, and pastas. Because of the ease of body digestion, simple carbohydrates can cause a sudden rise in blood sugar level, which, after only a short time, drops rapidly and can create hunger cravings. When consumed alone, foods containing large amounts of simple carbohydrates may cause fatigue, dizziness, nervousness, or headache.

Complex Carbohydrates

Complex carbohydrates are longer sugar molecules that digest more slowly because of their complexity. Complex carbohydrates include starchy vegetables, legumes, and whole grains. These foods take longer to digest than simple carbohydrates and thus do not stimulate a craving for more food. Complex carbohydrates such as whole-grain foods and unprocessed vegetables and fruits contain important vitamins and minerals that are often missing in processed foods. Many complex carbohydrates provide needed fiber, which can control blood sugar levels, and promote gut health and bowel movements.

Proteins

Proteins are the major source of building material for all the body's internal organs, as well as for muscles, blood, skin, hair, and nails. The primary role of protein is to repair damaged tissues. Proteins are important to the production of hormones that, among numerous other functions, control sexual development and milk production during lactation. In moments of need, proteins are a source of heat and energy for the body. However, when the diet provides adequate energy from carbohydrates and fat sources, proteins can be used for important functions that other nutrients cannot perform.

Proteins are formed by combining the 22 building blocks called **amino acids**. The human body can synthesize 14 of these amino acids. The diet must supply the remaining ones in proportions that allow the body to synthesize proteins properly. Foods that contain all 22 essential amino acids are known as *complete protein foods*. Those that lack or have extremely low amounts of any of the essential amino acids are called *incomplete protein foods*.

Dietary sources of protein include meats, eggs, nuts, grains, legumes, and dairy products such as milk and cheese. Most meats and dairy products are complete protein foods with high biological value. In contrast, most vegetable or plant proteins, such as beans and grains, are incomplete protein foods with low biological value. Foods that are weak in an essential amino acid can be balanced with foods that have adequate amounts of that same amino acid. When combined with other incomplete protein foods that fill in the missing pieces (i.e., the other amino acids) an incomplete protein food becomes a **complete protein complement**. Examples of complement protein pairs include peanut butter and whole-grain bread, beans and rice, and hummus and pita bread. It may be a good idea to refer parents who follow a vegetarian or vegan diet to a dietitian nutritionist to confirm that adequate protein pairings are consumed during pregnancy.

DRI guidelines recommend 0.88 g per kg of weight per day of protein during pregnancy and 1.05 g per kg per day during lactation (USDA, 2019). In diets with sufficient protein, the additional needs during pregnancy and lactation are about 25 additional grams of protein daily. Excess protein intake from a high-protein diet could contribute to weight gain. Moreover, animal sources of protein contain saturated fat, which is linked to elevated low-density lipoprotein (LDL) cholesterol, a risk factor for heart disease. For parents with certain kidney disorders, high protein intake may affect kidney function (Narasaki et al., 2021). At times of stress—such as during surgery, hemorrhage, or prolonged illness—extra protein is needed to meet the body's increased requirements.

Fats

Fats, the most concentrated source of energy in the diet, act as carriers for the **fat-soluble vitamins** A, D, E, and K. Fats prolong the process of digestion by slowing the stomach's emptying. This creates a longer-lasting sensation of fullness after a meal. Fatty acids give fats their different flavors, textures, and melting points and are either saturated or unsaturated. A healthy diet should contain more unsaturated fats than saturated fats. Saturated fatty acids derive primarily from animal sources, such as meat, milk products, and eggs. Unsaturated fatty acids derive from vegetables, nuts, and seeds. Fish is a good source of omega fatty acids, although its benefit needs to be weighed against the potential for fish contamination (USDA & USDHHS, 2020).

Essential Fatty Acids

Two fatty acids—linoleic and alpha-linolenic—are known as *essential fatty acids* (EFAs). During digestion, these two EFAs are converted into nutrients that support neural and visual development in the fetus. A healthy diet contains a variety of types of oil in addition to animal sources of these EFAs. Large amounts of linoleic acid are found in most plant oils, which can include corn, sunflower, and walnut oils. This acid can be converted to **arachidonic acid** (AA) during digestion.

Arachidonic acid is directly available from beef, pork, poultry, and eggs. Vegetable oils such as canola and soybean oil contain large amounts of alpha-linolenic acid. This acid converts to docosahexaenoic acid (DHA) during digestion. DHA and eicosapentaenoic acid (EPA), another omega-3 fatty acid, are available in fatty fish such as mackerel, salmon, and sardines, as well as many fish oils. The USDA recommends a DHA/EPA intake of 250–400 mg per day during pregnancy and lactation. That can be met with 8 to 12 ounces of a variety of low-mercury seafood per week (USDA & USDHHS, 2020).

Vitamins

Vitamins are organic substances with special biochemical functions in the body. They convert fats and carbohydrates into energy and help to form bone and tissue. Adequate intake of essential vitamins before and during pregnancy is important for fetal development. A diet inadequate in vitamin content may require prescribed or over-the-counter supplements. See **Table 8-2** for recommended intake of vitamins during lactation.

Water-Soluble Vitamins

The body cannot store **water-soluble vitamins** so they need to be replenished frequently. These nutrients include vitamin C and the B vitamins B_1 (thiamin), B_2 (riboflavin), B_3 (niacin), B_5 (pantothenic acid), B_6 (pyridoxine), B_7 (biotin), B_9 (folic acid), and B_{12} (cyanocobalamin). Excess water-soluble vitamins are excreted through urine and are not stored in the body. Supplementation is unnecessary unless there is an established nutritional risk.

Table 8-2 Recommended Vitamins and Minerals During Lactation

Nutrient Name	RDA/DRI	Tolerable Upper Limit	Benefits	Good Sources
Biotin	Ages 14+: 35 µg	n/a	Helps convert food into energy and synthesize glucose. Helps make and break down some fatty acids. Needed for healthy bones and hair.	Whole grains, organ meats, egg yolks, soybeans, fish, almonds, mushrooms, sweet potato, spinach
Calcium	Ages 14–18: 1,300 mg Ages 19+: 1,000 mg	Ages 14–18: 3,000 mg Ages 19+: 2,500 mg	Builds and protects bones and teeth. Helps with muscle contractions and relaxation, blood clotting, and nerve impulse transmission. Good for strong bones and teeth, nerve function, muscle contraction, blood clotting.	Dairy and nondairy yogurt, cheese, dairy and nondairy milks, calcium-set tofu, sardines, salmon (with bones), beans and legumes, fortified juices, leafy green vegetables (broccoli, collards, kale)
Choline[a]	Ages 14+: 550 mg	Ages 14–18: 3.0 g Ages 19+: 3.5 g	Helps make and release the neurotransmitter acetyl-choline, which aids in many nerve and brain activities. Plays a role in metabolizing and transporting fats.	Milk, eggs, liver, peanuts, soy milk, tofu, quinoa, broccoli
Chromium	Ages 14–18: 44 µg Ages 19+: 45 µg	n/a	Enhances the activity of insulin, helps maintain normal blood glucose levels, and is needed to free energy from glucose. Used in the metabolism and storage of fats, proteins, and carbohydrates.	Meat, poultry, fish, some cereals, nuts, cheese, whole grains, bread, brown rice, broccoli, mushrooms, green beans, brewers' yeast, raw onions
Copper	Ages 14+: 1,300 µg	Ages 14–18: 8,000 µg Ages 19+: 10,000 µg	Plays an important role in iron metabolism. Helps make red blood cells.	Liver, shellfish, nuts, seeds, whole-grain products, beans, prunes, leafy greens (turnip greens, spinach, Swiss chard, kale, mustard greens), asparagus, summer squash
Fluoride	Ages 14+: 3 mg	Ages 14+: 10 mg	Encourages strong bone formation. Keeps dental cavities from starting or worsening.	Water that is fluoridated, toothpaste with fluoride, marine fish, teas, dried fruit, dried beans, cocoa powder, walnuts
Folic acid, folate	Ages 14+: 500 µg	Ages 14–18: 800 µg Ages 19+: 1,000 µg	Vital for new cell creation. Helps prevent brain and spine birth defects when taken early in pregnancy.	Fortified grains and cereals, asparagus, okra, spinach, carrots, turnip greens, broccoli, legumes (black-eyed peas, chickpeas), orange juice, tomato juice, yeast, liver, melon, apricots, pumpkin, beans, avocado

(continues)

Table 8-2 Recommended Vitamins and Minerals During Lactation *(continued)*

Nutrient Name	RDA/DRI	Tolerable Upper Limit	Benefits	Good Sources
Iodine[a]	Ages 14+: 290 µg	Ages 14–18: 900 µg Ages 19+: 1,100 µg	Part of thyroid hormone, which helps set body temperature and influences nerve and muscle function, reproduction, and growth.	Iodized salt, processed foods, seafood, cranberries, kelp, potatoes
Iron	Ages 14–18: 10 mg Ages 19+: 9 mg	Ages 14–18: 900 µg Ages 19+: 1,100 µg	Helps hemoglobin in red blood cells and myoglobin in muscle cells carry oxygen throughout the body. Needed for chemical reactions in the body and making amino acids, collagen, neurotransmitters, and hormones.	Red meat, poultry, eggs, fruits, green vegetables, fortified bread and grain products, oily fish, lentils, soybeans, tofu, tempeh, lima beans, grains (quinoa, fortified cereals, brown rice, oatmeal), nuts and seeds (pumpkin, squash, pine, pistachio, sunflower, cashews)
Magnesium	Ages 14–18: 360 mg Ages 19– 30: 310 mg Ages 31–50: 320 mg	Ages 14+: 350 mg	Works with calcium in muscle contraction, blood clotting, and regulation of blood pressure. Helps build bones and teeth.	Green vegetables (spinach, chard, broccoli), legumes, cashews, sunflower seeds, pumpkin seeds, almonds, black beans, halibut, whole-wheat bread, milk, nuts
Manganese	Ages 14+: 2.6 mg	Ages 14–18: 9 mg Ages 19+: 11 mg	Helps form bones. Helps metabolize amino acids, cholesterol, and carbohydrates.	Nuts, legumes, whole grains, tea, brown rice, bran, pecans, cooked spinach
Molybdenum	Ages 14+: 50 µg	Ages 14–18: 1,700 µg Ages 19+: 2,000 µg	Part of several enzymes, one of which helps ward off a form of severe neurological damage in infants that can lead to early death.	Legumes (beans, lentils, peas), nuts, grain products, milk
Phosphorus	Ages 14–18: 1,250 mg Ages 19+: 700 mg	Ages 14+: 4g	Helps build and protect bones and teeth. Part of DNA and RNA. Helps convert food into energy.	Milk and dairy products, meat, fish, poultry, eggs, liver, green peas, broccoli, potatoes, almonds
Potassium	Ages 14+: 5.1 g	n/a	Balances fluids in the body. Helps maintain a steady heartbeat and send nerve impulses. Needed for muscle contractions.	Meat, milk, fruits, vegetables, grains, legumes, winter squash, sweet potatoes, white beans
Selenium[a]	Ages 14+: 70 µg	Ages 14+: 400 µg	Acts as an antioxidant, neutralizing unstable molecules that can damage cells. Helps regulate thyroid hormone activity.	Organ meats, seafood, walnuts, Brazil nuts, spinach, white and shiitake mushrooms, grain products

Nutrient Name	RDA/DRI	Tolerable Upper Limit	Benefits	Good Sources
Sodium	Ages 14+: 1.5 g	Ages 14+: 2.3g	Balances fluids in the body. Helps send nerve impulses. Needed for muscle contractions.	Salt, soy sauce, processed foods, celery, beets
Sulfur	n/a	n/a	Helps form bridges that shape and stabilize some protein structures. Needed for healthy hair, skin, and nails.	Protein-rich foods (meats, fish, poultry), nuts, legumes, brussels sprouts, garlic, onions, asparagus, kale, wheat germ
Vitamin A[a]	Ages 14–18: 1,200 µg Ages 19+: 1,300 µg	Ages 14–18: 2,800 µg Ages 19+: 3,000 µg	Keeps tissues and skin healthy. Plays an important role in bone growth. Good for eyesight, growth, appetite, and taste.	Sweet potatoes, carrots, pumpkins, squash, spinach, mangoes, turnip greens, boiled carrots, raw kale, dandelion greens, dried apricots
Vitamin B_1 (thiamin)[a]	Ages 14+: 1.4 mg	n/a	Helps convert food into energy. Needed for healthy skin, hair, muscles, and brain. Good for nervous system, digestion, muscles, heart, alcohol-damaged nerve tissues.	Pork chops, ham, soy milk, watermelons, acorn squash, liver, yeast, egg yolk, cereal, red meat, nuts, wheat germ, black beans
Vitamin B_2 (riboflavin)[a]	Ages 14+: 1.6 mg	n/a	Helps convert food into energy. Needed for healthy skin, hair, blood, and brain. Good for the breakdown of protein, fat, and carbohydrates.	Milk, yogurt, cheese, whole and enriched grains and cereals, liver, yeast, green leafy vegetables, fish, mushrooms, almonds, quinoa
Vitamin B_3 (niacin)	Ages 14+: 2.0 mg	Ages 14–18: 30 mg Ages 19+: 35 mg	Helps convert food into energy. Essential for healthy skin, blood cells, brain, and nervous system.	Meat, poultry, fish, fortified and whole grains, mushrooms, potatoes, peanut butter, passion fruit, avocado
Vitamin B_5 (pantothenic acid)	Ages 14+: 7 mg	n/a	Helps convert food into energy. Helps make lipids (fats), neurotransmitters, steroid hormones, and hemoglobin.	Chicken, whole grains, broccoli, mushrooms, avocados, tomato products, sunflower seeds, corn, broccoli
Vitamin B_6[a]	Ages 14+: 2.0 mg	Ages 14–18: 80 mg Ages 19+: 100 mg	Helps convert tryptophan to niacin and serotonin, a neurotransmitter that plays key roles in sleep, appetite, and moods. Helps make red blood cells. Influences cognitive abilities and immune function.	Meat, fish, poultry, legumes, tofu and other soy products, potatoes, noncitrus fruits (bananas and watermelons), whole grains, dried beans

(continues)

Table 8-2 Recommended Vitamins and Minerals During Lactation *(continued)*

Nutrient Name	RDA/DRI	Tolerable Upper Limit	Benefits	Good Sources
Vitamin B_{12}[a]	Ages 14+: 2.8 μg	n/a	Assists in making new cells and breaking down some fatty acids and amino acids. Protects nerve cells and encourages their normal growth. Helps make red blood cells.	Meat, poultry, fish, milk, cheese, eggs, fortified cereals, fortified soy milk, shellfish, beans, mushrooms
Vitamin C[a]	Ages 14–18: 115 mg Ages 19+: 120 mg	Ages 14–18: 1,800 mg Ages 19+: 2,000 mg	Helps make collagen, a connective tissue that knits together wounds and supports blood vessel walls. Acts as an antioxidant, neutralizing unstable molecules that can damage cells.	Fruits and fruit juices (especially citrus), potatoes, broccoli, bell peppers, spinach, strawberries, tomatoes, brussels sprouts, berries, potatoes, green leafy vegetables, raw acerola, rosehips
Vitamin D[a]	Ages 14+: 15 μg	Ages 14+: 100 μg	Helps maintain normal blood levels of calcium and phosphorus, which strengthen bones. Helps form teeth and bones. Supplements can reduce the number of nonspinal fractures.	Fortified milk or margarine, fortified cereals, fatty fish, sunlight, cod liver oil, sardines, herring, salmon, tuna, mushrooms, tofu
Vitamin E	Ages 14+: 19 mg	Ages 14–18: 800 mg Ages 19+: 1,000 mg	Acts as an antioxidant, neutralizing unstable molecules that can damage cells. Protects vitamin A and certain lipids from damage.	Vegetable oils, salad dressings and margarines made with vegetable oils, wheat germ, leafy green vegetables, whole grains, nuts, soybeans, spouts, eggs
Vitamin K[a]	Ages 14–18: 75 μg Ages 19+: 95 μg	n/a	Activates proteins and calcium. Essential to blood clotting. May help prevent hip fractures.	Cabbage, liver, eggs, milk, romaine lettuce, collard greens, spinach, broccoli, sprouts, kale, brussels sprouts, scallions, prunes
Zinc	Ages 14–18: 13 mg Ages 19+: 12 mg	Ages 14–18: 34 mg Ages 19+: 40 mg	Helps form many enzymes and proteins and creates new cells. Frees vitamin A from storage in the liver. Needed for immune system, taste, smell, and wound healing.	Nuts, cashews, seeds, beans and legumes, eggs, red meat, poultry, oysters, fortified cereals, brown rice, whole grains, dark chocolate, sesame seeds, garlic, wheat germ

DRI = dietary reference intake; RDA = recommended daily allowance.
[a]Micronutrients in human milk that are influenced by parental intake and nutritional status.

A varied diet that meets energy needs generally provides enough water-soluble vitamins during lactation. Water-soluble vitamins can move easily from the blood to the milk. Thus, intake of most of these vitamins can affect the amounts in milk. When mammary tissue reaches a saturation level of water-soluble vitamins, levels in the milk reach a plateau for vitamin C, thiamin (B_1), and biotin.

Folate (vitamin B_9), which occurs naturally in leafy green vegetables and whole grains, contributes to cell growth and reproduction. It functions with vitamins B_{12} and C in the breakdown of proteins and the production of **hemoglobin**. Daily supplementation of folic acid is recommended during pregnancy to help prevent **neural tube defects** in the fetus (WHO, 2016). Folic acid is the synthetic form of folate used in dietary supplements. A large percentage of the population has a genetic mutation that prevents the conversion of synthetic folic acid into a usable form needed by the body. L-methylfolate is usually prescribed when there is a family history of neural tube defects or preterm births (Ferrazzi et al., 2020).

Fat-Soluble Vitamins

The fat-soluble vitamins A, D, E and K come primarily from animal and dairy products and are from some fruits and vegetables. They are important for vision, bone health, immunity and blood clotting. Fat-soluble vitamins are stored in the body's fatty tissues for long periods of time. Vitamin supplements that contain megadoses of these vitamins could lead to toxic levels.

Vitamin A. Vitamin A contributes to skeletal growth and promotes healthy mucous membranes and vision. **Retinoids**, the active form of vitamin A, derive from animal products such as dairy and liver. Other sources are foods rich in beta-carotene, such as green leafy vegetables, carrots, and cantaloupe. The body converts beta-carotene into vitamin A.

Vitamin A is a critical micronutrient, and deficiencies are particularly concerning for expectant parents and young children. Vitamin A deficiency during lactation reduces the amount of available vitamin A in the milk (Gannon, 2020). Inadequate stores of vitamin A can result in night blindness, anemia, and immunodeficiency (Imdad et al., 2022). In areas where vitamin A deficiency is a severe public health problem, daily supplementation is recommended to prevent night blindness (WHO, 2016).

Vitamin D. Vitamin D plays a role in immunity and control of cell growth. Primary food sources are milk and other dairy products fortified with vitamin D. The body manufactures vitamin D through sunlight exposure and converts it into a steroid that circulates in the blood. Thus, vitamin D deficiency is actually a deficiency of sunlight. Short walks in sunlight three times a week, starting before or during pregnancy, can help contribute to healthy vitamin D levels. Safe sunlight exposure and adequate dietary vitamin D intake are appropriate recommendations for most perinatal clients (Huang, 2023).

Low levels of vitamin D prenatally can result in a deficiency in the infant. Because the baby's body stores accumulate during gestation, if levels of vitamin D are low, the baby may be born with low levels. Individuals at the highest risk for deficiency are dark-skinned; avoid sunlight or spend little time outdoors; and wear clothes that cover most of their skin, as is the custom in many cultures. The Middle East and North Africa have some of the highest rates of vitamin D deficiency in the world (Chakhtoura et al., 2018).

Supplementation for vitamin D deficiency improves the nutritional status of both the nursing parent and baby. Researchers increasingly recommend higher doses of vitamin D for expectant and nursing parents (Chang & Lee, 2019; Gallo et al., 2020; Heo et al., 2022; Mansur et al., 2022). Higher dosing for parents is preferable to supplementing the baby alone. Otherwise, the parent's vitamin D levels would remain deficient, jeopardizing long-term health and placing the next baby at risk for deficiency. See **Chapter 9** for more information about vitamin D in nursing babies.

Vitamin E. Vitamin E acts as an antioxidant and protects vitamins A and C, red blood cells, and EFAs from destruction. Most vitamin E in the diet comes from vegetable oil (soybean, corn, cottonseed, and safflower) and products made with vegetable oil such as margarine and salad dressing. Other food sources include fruits and vegetables, grains, nuts (almonds and hazelnuts), sunflower seeds, and fortified cereals. Lactating parents may need to supplement their dietary intake of vitamin E to achieve the recommended daily intake of 19 mg (National Institutes of Health Office of Dietary Supplements, 2016). Studies on the effect of vitamin E supplementation vary in results.

Vitamin K. Vitamin K is essential for blood clotting. One form of vitamin K comes from green leafy vegetables, and another form comes from bacteria in the gut. Although vitamin K deficiency in adults is rare, infant stores at birth are low and can lead to a risk of vitamin K deficiency bleeding (also called *hemorrhagic disease of the newborn*). Supplementation during the final weeks of pregnancy may reduce the risk. Infants usually routinely receive an injection or oral dose of vitamin K at birth (Jullien, 2021).

Vitamin Supplements

Vitamin supplements should be complements to—not substitutes for—a healthy intake of foods rich in fiber, vitamins, and minerals. Prenatal vitamins target the needs of pregnancy and are not appropriate for lactation. Nursing parents may take multivitamin supplements that do exceed 20% of the recommended daily intake. Consumption of excess amounts of some vitamins, such as vitamin A, can be harmful. Vitamin supplements can be valuable in circumstances such as bariatric surgery, **anemia**, food intolerance, or allergies. Fact sheets on vitamin supplements are available in the U.S. at the National Institutes of Health Office of Dietary Supplements.

Minerals

Minerals contribute to overall mental and physical well-being. When present in adequate levels, they help physiological processes and strengthen skeletal structures. They also preserve the vigor of the heart, brain, muscles, and nerves. In addition, minerals play important roles in the production of hormones and help maintain the delicate water balance essential to mental and physical processes.

The diet must supply essential minerals. A varied and mixed diet of animal and vegetable origin that meets the recommended energy and protein needs will typically provide adequate minerals. A diet inadequate in mineral content may require prescribed or over-the-counter supplements. Refer to Table 8-2 for recommended intake of minerals during lactation. Three minerals—**calcium**, **iron**, and salt—are especially important during pregnancy and lactation.

Calcium

Calcium provides rigidity to bones and hardness to teeth. It aids in blood clotting and in controlling the action of the heart, muscles, and nerves. Consumption of adequate amounts of calcium maintains bones and provides for fetal bone development. Increased intestinal absorption during pregnancy provides the additional calcium needed at that time. Consumption of vitamin D along with calcium promotes optimal absorption and use of calcium.

Pregnancy and lactation are times of high calcium demand, particularly for individuals younger than 25, who are still experiencing increases in bone content. Daily supplementation of calcium is recommended in populations with low dietary calcium intake (WHO, 2016). Calcium mobilizes from the bones during lactation, with a recovery of bone mass after weaning (Capozzi et al., 2021; Lujano-Negrete et al., 2022). Lactation appears to increase bone mineral density, thereby helping to prevent osteoporosis (Briana et al., 2020). Calcium supplementation seems not to be useful for improving bone density during lactation (Tihtonen et al., 2022).

Calcium sources are listed in **Table 8-3**. In a diet that avoids all milk products, the protein, vitamins,

Table 8-3 Good Sources of Calcium

Food	Portion	Calcium (mg)
Yogurt, plain, nonfat or low fat	8 ounces	488
Yogurt, soy, plain	8 ounces	300
Yogurt, Greek, plain, low fat	8 ounces	261
Yogurt, Greek, plain, nonfat	8 ounces	250
Milk, low fat (1 %)	1 cup	305
Milk, fat-free (skim)	1 cup	298
Buttermilk, low fat	1 cup	284
Almond milk, unsweetened	1 cup	442
Rice milk, unsweetened	1 cup	283
Soy milk, unsweetened	1 cup	301
Cheese, cheddar	2 ounces	408
Collard greens, cooked	1 cup	268
Spinach, cooked	1 cup	245
Turnip greens, cooked	1 cup	197
Kale, cooked	1 cup	177
Mustard greens, cooked	1 cup	165
Beet greens, cooked	1 cup	164
Tofu, raw, regular, prepared with calcium sulfate	1/2 cup	434
Sardines, canned	3 ounces	325
Salmon, canned, solids with bone	3 ounces	181
Grapefruit juice, 100%, fortified	1 cup	350
Orange juice, 100%, fortified	1 cup	349

Data Source: U.S. Department of Agriculture, Agricultural Research Service. FoodData Central, 2019. fdc.nal.usda.gov and calories available in milk can be obtained from other calcium-rich foods. In a diet low in calcium-rich foods, calcium supplements may be needed to provide the recommended daily intake. Calcium carbonate is the safest supplement. Several brands of bone meal and dolomite contain high levels of lead or other toxic metals and should be avoided.

Iron

Dietary iron exists in two forms. Heme iron comes from meat, poultry, and fish and is easily absorbed. Nonheme iron comes from vegetables, iron-enriched cereals, and whole grains. Adding small amounts of heme iron or foods containing vitamin C to a meal can improve iron absorption from nonheme sources. Consumption of tea or coffee can reduce iron absorption from nonheme food sources. Cooking in a cast iron skillet helps increase overall iron in both heme and nonheme sources for those who are deficient.

Recommended dietary intake of iron varies among countries, as do practices regarding supplementation. Low levels of iron can reduce the oxygen-carrying capacity of the blood and cause constant fatigue, even after adequate rest. When iron stores are low, the body absorbs more available iron. Excess calcium, both in food and in supplements, can reduce iron absorption.

An individual who is anemic has poor tolerance to blood loss and is at greater risk in the event of surgery. Iron deficiency is mostly associated with low socioeconomic status, multiple gestations, and limited education. These individuals are also at risk of poor pregnancy outcome, independent of iron deficiency. Daily supplementation of iron is recommended during pregnancy to support the development of the placenta and fetus, as well as to prevent anemia (WHO, 2016).

A pregnancy that begins with sufficient iron stores and a varied diet does not require iron supplementation. During pregnancy and the early months of lactation, when menstruation is absent, the reduction in blood loss partially offsets additional needs. Many healthcare providers prescribe supplements routinely on the assumption that prepregnancy stores are low. A simple blood test can determine this need. Testing and treatment for anemia can begin before becoming pregnant.

Some individuals avoid iron supplements because of side effects such as heartburn, nausea, constipation, and diarrhea. Effective dietary counseling can help improve iron intake and absorption from foods. Supplements may be better tolerated when taken at bedtime and when consumed with water or juice and not with milk, tea, or coffee. Iron levels in the milk remain steady because iron is drawn from the body's stores and not the daily diet. Nevertheless, sufficient iron intake during lactation is important to rebuild long-term stores in the body.

Salt

Salt (sodium) helps control the body's fluid balance. Although salt usually causes the body to retain fluid in the bloodstream, pregnancy is one condition in which the body requires more salt so that it can function well. As a pregnancy progresses, the placenta requires increased blood flow to function efficiently. During a typical pregnancy, blood volume increases by more than 40% to meet this need. Most expectant parents can continue to consume the same amount of salt as is recommended for the general population.

Water

Water—the most abundant and important nutrient in the body—is involved in nearly every body process. Most foods contain water, which is absorbed by the body during digestion. Fruits and vegetables are especially good sources of water. The average adult female body contains about 50% water (approximately 30 quarts) and loses about 2 quarts daily through perspiration and excretion.

Adequate water consumption provides the fetus and nursing infant with sufficient fluids. Consumption of additional water-containing foods as part of the normal increase in food during these periods, combined with a natural sense of thirst, will usually provide the additional water needed. Having water nearby during feedings will remind parents to satisfy their thirst. Intake of approximately 6 to 8 cups of fluid per day during pregnancy and lactation will provide enough fluid to function and avoid constipation.

There is insufficient evidence to support increasing fluid intake during lactation beyond adequate levels. The notion that increasing fluid intake increases milk volume is a misconception. Failing to drink enough fluids will cause a decrease in urine output, not in milk production, except in cases of dehydration. Parents can monitor the adequacy of fluid intake by observing their urine. Except for the first morning void, the urine should be clear to light yellow. Just as for an infant, concentrated, dark yellow, or strong-smelling urine is the body's signal to increase fluid intake.

Nutritional Intake

Good nutritional status before conception and adequate nutrition during pregnancy and lactation contribute to the delivery of a healthy baby and long-term healthy outcomes for both the parent and child

(Marshall et al., 2022; Yisahak et al., 2021). Pregnancy and lactation are peak periods of interest in nutrition when expectant and nursing parents typically want to provide their babies with the best nourishment possible. They may also wish to give birth without a lasting change in body image. This can be a time when they begin to recognize the close relationship between what they eat and how they feel.

Most individuals do not meet dietary guidelines before conception or during pregnancy (Caut et al., 2020; Killeen et al., 2022). A high-fat diet during pregnancy and lactation affects the development of the infant's central nervous system (Gawlińska et al., 2021). A high-protein diet can significantly affect the infant's cerebral cortex and negatively affect behavioral performance (Silveira et al., 2022). Undernutrition as a child can result in short stature and a small pelvis, thereby increasing the risk of pregnancy complications (Stephenson et al., 2018). Throughout childhood, pesticides and heavy metals build up in the body. These contaminants can leach into the milk infants receive. Nutritional counseling can help increase the overall long-term health of the family, the community, and the whole population (Barker et al., 2018).

Preconception Nutrition

Preconception lifestyle changes toward a healthy, varied diet contribute to lower energy intake and BMI for many years (van Elten et al., 2019). Extremely low or high weight could decrease the ability to conceive. Preconception obesity is a significant predictor of many pregnancy complications and poor outcomes. Correction of grossly abnormal body weight can assist in conception and development of a healthy baby. Weight loss should be gradual—1 to 2 pounds per week—rather than the result of a crash diet.

Monitoring preconception iron levels ensures that treatment for anemia can begin early if levels are low. A folic acid supplement is frequently recommended before conception and during the first 3 months of pregnancy to reduce the risk of neural tube defects in the developing fetus. A later section discusses foods to avoid during pregnancy and lactation. An integrated approach to lifestyle changes can improve preconception health. This includes pregnancy prevention, planning, and preparation.

Nutrition During Pregnancy

Sound nutrition during pregnancy helps keep the body in prime condition for labor, delivery, and lactation and promotes optimal outcomes for the newborn. Increased amounts of most nutrients are needed during pregnancy. Folate, calcium, vitamin D, iron, and EFAs require special attention at this time. Individuals who are well nourished throughout their lives may not need to change their diet during pregnancy. An unhealthy diet can restrict fetal growth by reducing the number or size of fetal cells, including brain cells. Critically low nourishment during pregnancy can contribute to fetal death. For a person who has been poorly nourished before conception, pregnancy may provide an opportunity to improve diet to promote a healthy pregnancy outcome.

Prepregnancy weight should determine the target weight gain in pregnancy. Individuals older than 35 years of age may have a lower **basal metabolic rate** and therefore may not require as great an increase in energy intake while pregnant as younger individuals. Poor nutrition and including obesity during pregnancy may increase a baby's risk of developing obesity, hypertension, cardiovascular disease, and diabetes later in life (Mutamba et al., 2023). Collectively, this cluster of diseases is called **metabolic syndrome**. **Table 8-4** presents the target weight gain based on prepregnancy weight.

Expectant parents can begin working on healthy eating habits by learning the relationship of nutrition to the way they feel. Those who experience morning sickness and nausea can eat a cracker or a protein, such as turkey or cheese, before getting out of bed to settle their stomach. A high-protein breakfast and continued access to simple and healthy foods throughout the day will help avoid an empty stomach and the return of nausea. Opening a window or turning on a fan to remove food odors can also help avoid nausea. Regular exercise, drinking plenty of fluids, and consuming enough fiber in the form of fresh fruits and vegetables, whole grains, nuts, seeds, and bran can relieve constipation. Avoiding highly processed foods may also help.

Table 8-4 Target Weight Gain Based on Prepregnancy Weight

Status	BMI	Weight
Underweight	Less than 18.5	28–40 pounds
Normal weight	18.5–24.9	25–35 pounds
Overweight	25–29.9	15–25 pounds
Obese	30–39.9	Approximately 11–20 pounds

BMI = body mass index.

Data from Centers for Disease Control and Prevention. Weight Gain During Pregnancy: Pregnancy Weight Gain Recommendations. May 15, 2024. https://www.cdc.gov/maternal-infant-health/pregnancy-weight/index.html

Nutrition During Lactation

Lactation does not require special foods to maintain high-quality milk production. The normal healthy diet recommended for an average adult generally meets most lactation needs. An adolescent parent, one who is nursing two or more babies, or an expectant parent who is nursing another child may need to increase their food intake. These needs can be met by increasing serving sizes, adding more food at mealtimes, or eating extra foods between meals.

Lactation uses energy from body stores and the parent's diet. Nursing parents with a healthy diet and normal physical activity will lose an average of 1 to 2 pounds per month. Those whose intake exceeds their needs or who consume large amounts of sweet foods in place of nutritious foods will likely gain weight during lactation. Such practices can also prevent adequate consumption of the vitamins, minerals, and other nutrients the body needs. An overly restrictive diet may put a parent or baby at nutritional risk. In addition, arbitrary, rigid dietary restrictions during lactation may make nursing seem too difficult and increase the risk of early weaning.

Weight Loss While Nursing

Lactation appears to contribute naturally to postpartum weight loss, occurring gradually in the normal course of lactation. Parents who reduce caloric intake modestly can usually achieve gradual weight loss and continued appropriate infant growth. Substituting skim milk for whole milk, unsweetened yogurt for dessert foods, and low-calorie fluids for higher-calorie options will reduce caloric intake. Selecting lean meat, fewer eggs, and less or low-fat cheese will reduce fat intake and decrease calorie consumption. Parents can add more foods to their diet if they begin losing weight too rapidly or if they become easily fatigued.

Caloric intake during lactation should not go below 1800 **kilocalories (kcal)** per day. There is an association between intensity and duration of lactation and postpartum weight loss (Bazzazian et al., 2023; Foster, 2023). After lactation is established, parents with a higher body weight can safely reduce their intake by approximately 500 calories per day.

Parents are encouraged to follow sound nutritional diet plans rather than popular weight-loss diets. Combining diet reduction with exercise improves fitness while preserving muscle mass, whereas diet reduction alone reduces muscle mass (Carbone et al., 2019). Weight loss should not occur too quickly. Parents who consider restricting their diet while nursing are encouraged to discuss their plans with their healthcare provider. If they restrict food intake, they may need multivitamin and mineral supplements. Eating healthy may help them safely lose their pregnancy weight.

Low-Carbohydrate Diets

A healthy low-carbohydrate diet such as the Atkins and Paleo diets is compatible with lactation. Parents on these diets should consume fruits and vegetables and a limited amount of whole grains. To lose weight, they can reduce or eliminate high-carbohydrate foods such as sugar, flour, breads, cakes, pasta, junk foods, desserts, potatoes, and rice. Limiting carbohydrates decreases appetite, so parents need to ensure adequate caloric intake when following this type of diet regimen.

Ketogenic Diets

The ketogenic or "keto" diet originated in the 1920s to reduce epileptic seizures in children. The diet mimics carbohydrate starvation so that the body burns ketones for energy (McGaugh & Barthel, 2022). It calls for very high fat intake and minimal carbohydrates and fiber. Ketogenic diets are not recommended unless there is a medical indication. There have been several reports of nursing parents hospitalized with ketoacidosis from the restricted intake with this diet (Al Alawi et al., 2020). The South Beach Diet is a modified low-carbohydrate diet that is higher in protein and healthy fats than is a typical eating plan. Parents pursuing a diet that restricts carbohydrates need to consult their primary healthcare provider or a dietitian nutritionist when planning their diet.

Gluten-Free Diets

Many people believe they are gluten sensitive and eliminate gluten from their diets. Gluten is a protein found in many grains, including wheat, rye, barley, bulgur, farro, kamut, spelt, and triticale. Eliminating grains containing gluten can present dietary challenges because grains provide vitamins (including B vitamins), minerals, and fiber (National Digestive Disease Information Clearinghouse, 2020).

About 2% of the global population has **celiac disease**, an autoimmune disorder that damages the villi of the small intestine and interferes with the absorption of nutrients from food. People with celiac disease cannot tolerate gluten. Gas, bloating, diarrhea, constipation, headache, trouble concentrating, fatigue, and even weight loss and malnutrition (resulting from an inability to absorb vitamins and minerals) can occur. The disease is more common in females than males (Singh et al., 2018). The Academy of Nutrition and Dietetics (https://www.eatright.org) and other healthcare websites provide gluten-free food lists. Carefully checking food labels is important because many grains are used as fillers for packaged foods, sauces, and medicines.

Physical Exercise

Physical exercise contributes to emotional health, lowers stress, improves bone density, and manages weight. Increased physical activity can be achieved by using stairs instead of an elevator, parking farther from the building entrance when shopping, going for a walk with the baby, or participating in structured exercise programs. There is an association between increased physical activity during the first 4 months after birth and improved vitamin D status (Hall et al., 2018).

Exercising four to six times per week beginning 6 to 8 weeks postpartum is safe for most nursing parents. Moderate to high-intensity physical activity does not affect milk volume or its macronutrient content (Be'er et al., 2020). Although very strenuous exercise can increase lactic acid in the milk, there is no documented effect on the infant or on milk production or quality.

Obesity

Obesity is associated with a higher risk of nutritional deficiencies (Bima et al., 2021; Bjørklund et al., 2021; Chu et al., 2022; Mohapatra et al., 2020). Obesity before conception produces a greater risk of mixed feeding and shorter duration of exclusive nursing (Boudet-Berquier et al., 2018). Obesity in early pregnancy is associated with lower rates of exclusive nursing (Marshall et al., 2019; Nomura et al., 2019). Researchers recommend that weight control be encouraged both before and after pregnancy.

Lactation should be closely monitored in individuals with obesity. Parents with high body weight are at a greater risk of not initiating lactation compared with those with low or normal body weight (Fan & Molinaro, 2021; Nomura et al., 2020). The risk increases with the degree of obesity (Ramji et al., 2018). Overweight or obesity produces lower prolactin response to sucking and delays in stage II lactogenesis (Farah et al., 2021; Luzardo-Ocampo et al., 2023).

Eating Disorders

The changes that occur in the body during pregnancy and lactation can be distressing to someone with an eating disorder such as anorexia nervosa or bulimia nervosa. Anorexia is the deliberate restriction of calories to the point of starvation. A sign of this condition may be an individual who has extremely low weight and still complains about being "fat." People who are bulimic overfeed (binge) and then force themselves to vomit. They may use laxatives, diuretics, and extreme exercise to prevent weight gain (National Eating Disorders Association, 2018).

Parents with a history of disordered eating have a higher risk for birth complications and of giving birth to a preterm or low-weight infant (Mantel et al., 2020). They are also at risk for postpartum depression and anxiety about milk production and management of feedings (Kaß et al., 2021). The distress associated with body image may affect the transition to parenthood and lead to more serious health issues (Mancini, 2017; Urueña-Palacio et al., 2018). Clinical management and monitoring of the eating disorder and support from healthcare providers can help these parents, who have a higher risk of nursing problems, early weaning, and lower self-efficacy (Kapa et al., 2022; Kaß et al., 2021).

Parents with disordered eating may seem obsessed with the infant's feeding and elimination behavior and worry that their baby will grow up to be fat. They may refer to their eating habits in judgmental terms, such as "I was good today—I didn't eat breakfast," or "I was so bad last night—we ate fast food." It is appropriate to ask about dietary habits and any history of an eating disorder. The use of reflective listening, nonjudgmental language, and a gentle tone is important because harsh self-judgment and sensitivity to criticism are common. These parents need to be referred for specialized help. Maintaining a list of referral sources—mental health professionals and others with expertise in this area, local area support groups, licensed dietitians, and nutritionists—will ensure appropriate referrals.

Making Healthy Food Choices

Understanding the nutritional causes of hunger and fatigue can motivate parents to choose dietary practices that will enhance their health and well-being. Basing food selection and meal planning on nutritional guidelines will help improve their diets. An awareness of food labels, additives, and processing will help avoid unhealthy choices. Healthy eating is compatible with limited budgets and special diets such as vegetarianism (USDA & USDHHS, 2020). Education, marital status, and income are correlated with healthier dietary changes (Gete et al., 2022).

Food Selection

Many individuals become more conscious of the foods they eat during pregnancy and continue their nutritional awareness throughout lactation and beyond. A child's diet affects their food choices in later life. Healthy, diverse foods during pregnancy and lactation help infants learn to like many different food flavors (Spahn et al., 2019; Ventura et al., 2021). Food flavors pass to the developing infant through the amniotic fluid and, after birth, through the milk.

Fresh, unprocessed foods are typically the most nutritious and most desirable choices when selecting food for the family table. Food served directly after purchasing or picking is the most flavorful and nutritious. If perishable foods are not consumed immediately, proper storage will help to preserve their nutritional quality. Home gardening and local food growers offer an opportunity to save money and provide quality food in a family's diet. Many communities have community gardens, local farmers' markets, and low-income options to help families who are experiencing food insecurity. Some local food banks provide fresh produce to families in need. Many restaurants list nutritional and caloric data on their menus to help in selecting healthy foods when dining out.

Checking Food Labels

Economic uncertainty or practicality can lead parents to choose processed foods over fresh foods. Helping families understand nutrition labels will enable them to make the best food choices for their families. Nutritional information on food labels assists shoppers in healthy food selection, with ingredients listed in order of weight. When assessing the nutritional quality of a can of chicken stew, for example, chicken rather than water should be the main ingredient. Food labels identify additives such as sugar, salt, preservatives, flavoring, and coloring. They may also state whether a product is kosher, organic, or free from ingredients such as nuts or wheat.

Package labels offer information on the food's preparation and storage, as well as the percentage of the recommended daily allowances of nutrients the food provides. Nutritional claims on the label can be misleading, as in the case of a food that is marketed as low in fat but that is high in sugar and not a healthy food choice. Learning to check labels will help avoid additives such as corn syrup, sugar, and modified food starch, as well as large quantities of chemical preservatives, salt, and fat. **Figure 8-1** presents the U.S. Food and Drug Administration (FDA) food nutrition labels, which were updated in 2019 to provide clarity on serving size and calories.

Nutrition Facts	
8 servings per container	
Serving size	**2/3 cup (55g)**
Amount per serving	
Calories	**230**
	% Daily Value*
Total Fat 8g	**10%**
Saturated Fat 1g	**5%**
Trans Fat 0g	
Cholesterol 0mg	**0%**
Sodium 160mg	**7%**
Total Carbohydrate 37g	**13%**
Dietary Fiber 4g	**14%**
Total Sugars 12g	
Includes 10g Added Sugars	**20%**
Protein 3g	
Vitamin D 2mcg	10%
Calcium 260mg	20%
Iron 8mg	45%
Potassium 235mg	6%

*The % Daily Value (DV) tells you how much a nutrient in a serving of food contributes to a daily diet. 2,000 calories a day is used for general nutrition advice.

Figure 8-1 U.S. Food and Drug Administration food nutrition label.

Courtesy of the U.S. Food and Drug Administration.

Food Additives

The most nutritious foods will include limited highly refined or artificial ingredients. Chemical additives that color the food, enhance flavor, or preserve freshness can alter nutritional quality. Foods such as fresh fruits and vegetables may contain additives that are not obvious to the consumer. Vegetables may be treated with fungicides to retard mold growth. Foods such as peppers, cucumbers, and tomatoes are often waxed to preserve their freshness during long transport and storage times. Other foods, such as oranges, may be colored to enhance their visual appeal.

Although some changes to the food can improve quality, it is important to weigh the benefits of each ingredient against its possible harmful effects. It is nearly impossible to avoid purchasing treated foods. Washing or peeling such foods can avoid the consumption of undesirable ingredients. Washing with water and mild dish detergent can reduce pesticide residues in fruits and many vegetables. All produce should be washed well to remove harmful residues and bacteria. Additional information about toxins is presented in **Chapter 11**.

Vegetarian Diets

Most of the world's population consumes a **vegetarian** diet. A rice-and-beans combination has been a staple in China, India, Africa, and South America for centuries. Some families avoid meat because of cultural, philosophical, ecological, health-related, or economic factors. A balanced vegetarian diet may be more healthful than a meat-based diet. Vegetarians consume more volume and fiber with fewer calories and fats, thereby aiding digestion and decreasing the likelihood of accumulating excess weight.

A basic understanding of nutrition, careful meal planning, and selective food shopping are essential when following a vegetarian diet. A well-planned completely plant-based diet is suitable during pregnancy and lactation (Baroni et al., 2018). A poorly managed vegetarian diet can be deficient in protein and minerals. This imbalance may result in inadequate growth of the fetus and nursing infant and inadequate nourishment.

Extremely strict vegetarian regimens, such as a macrobiotic diet, raw foods diet, fruitarianism, or other restrictive eating pattern, may be harmful during pregnancy or lactation. These diets tend to be unbalanced, emphasizing one food group while neglecting others at the expense of needed proteins, vitamins, minerals, and calories. Nursing parents adhering to a vegetarian diet need guidance from a nutritionist or dietitian and need to inform both their primary healthcare provider and the baby's provider about their diet.

A vegetarian may be lacto-vegetarian (dairy but no eggs), ovo-vegetarian (eggs but no dairy), or lacto-ovo-vegetarian (both dairy and eggs). A **vegan** avoids all animal products, including eggs and dairy. The Mediterranean diet emphasizes plant-based foods but includes small amounts of fish and meat. A vegetarian diet that includes animal products such as milk and eggs can easily provide the nutrients needed for pregnancy, lactation, and healthy infant growth. Vegetarians and vegans produce milk of comparable nutritional value to nonvegetarians (Karcz & Królak-Olejnik, 2021). **Table 8-5** classifies several types of vegetarian diets based on the types of foods consumed.

Table 8-5 Classification of Vegetarian Diets

Type of Vegetarian Diet	Types of Foods Consumed
Vegan	Foods from plant sources (no animal products are consumed)
Lacto-vegetarian	Milk and milk products, such as cheese and ice cream, in addition to plant foods
Ovo-vegetarian	Plant foods and eggs
Lacto-ovo-vegetarian	Plant foods, dairy products, and eggs
Fruitarian	Fruits, nuts, olive oil, and honey

Balancing Foods in a Vegetarian Diet

The key to successful management of a vegetarian diet is to plan combinations of foods that provide the essential amino acids. An imbalance of amino acids prevents the body from synthesizing the proteins essential for building tissues. Combining bread or crackers with nut spreads or tofu (soybean curd) spreads creates healthy snack foods. If dairy products are not part of the diet, adding large quantities of green leafy vegetables, broccoli, almonds, molasses, tofu, and fortified soymilk can meet calcium needs. Iron requirements can be the most difficult to meet. Foods containing vitamin C—citrus fruit or juice and fresh vegetables eaten at the same meal with legumes and whole grains—help the body absorb the iron from these foods.

Supplements on a Vegetarian Diet

A vegan or vegetarian diet may require iodine supplementation during lactation to provide adequate amounts to the infant (Pawlak et al., 2023). in addition, because vitamin B_{12} is available primarily from animal sources, diets that exclude animal products such as milk, cheese, and eggs may be deficient in this vitamin. A small amount of vitamin B_{12} is present in fermented products and some seaweed. However, these foods may not be incorporated into the diet frequently enough to provide adequate amounts. Vitamin B_{12} supplementation during pregnancy and lactation is essential when a diet limits or excludes sources of the vitamin (Dror & Allen, 2018).

Low vitamin B_{12} intake leads to low levels in the milk. Signs of deficiency in an infant between 4 and 8 months of age include anemia, growth failure, neurologic delay, tremors, and excess skin pigmentation. Individuals who have had bariatric surgery are at higher risk for vitamin B_{12} deficiency. **Chapter 26** provides further discussion about bariatric surgery. Always refer to the primary healthcare provider or nutritionist for guidance to ensure optimal nutrition.

Avoiding Hunger and Fatigue

Expectant and nursing parents need at least three well-balanced meals and two snacks daily, consisting of a variety of foods and distributed throughout the day. Consuming enough protein and complex carbohydrates at breakfast avoids midmorning and midafternoon fatigue. Peanut butter on whole-grain toast, bread and cheese, yogurt and fruit, and whole-grain cereal and milk are simple breakfast meals that require little preparation. Consuming about one-third of the day's protein needs in the morning provides a feeling of well-being throughout the day.

Food should be consumed in response to hunger. Understanding the causes of hunger may help parents plan and control their food selection. An empty feeling in the stomach, talking about or seeing appealing foods, or a drop in blood sugar level can activate hunger. The body absorbs foods at varying rates, and food affects blood sugar in different ways. It is therefore possible to feel hungry even after consuming more calories than needed.

Refined sugar is absorbed directly and quickly, causing the blood sugar to rise and fall rapidly resulting in hunger soon afterward. Complex carbohydrates such as potatoes and grains into sugar enter the bloodstream more slowly than when sugar is consumed alone. The result is a slower rise and more gradual fall in blood sugar. Proteins and fats are digested even more slowly than carbohydrates. When these nutrients are consumed, blood sugar rises slowly and steadily, remains sustained for a longer period, and falls slowly.

Although many foods will result in a full stomach, fluctuating blood sugar levels will continue to cause feelings of hunger and lack of energy in the absence of adequate protein and fat. A breakfast of refined carbohydrate foods such as sweetened cereal, doughnuts, or sweet rolls causes blood sugar to rise rapidly and then plunge downward. Fatigue will follow 2 or 3 hours later, often leading to the consumption of more sugar, continuing the blood sugar swings.

Nonfood items may affect appetite as well. **Caffeine** and tobacco tend to suppress the appetite. Marijuana and alcohol stimulate appetite and promote indiscriminate snacking. When consumed in large amounts, empty calories from alcohol replace more nutritious foods and can result in nutritional deficiencies. Various over-the-counter and prescription medications can suppress or stimulate appetite depending on the drug.

Healthy Eating on a Budget

Families with limited finances to spend on food can employ cost-saving methods in purchasing, storing, and preparing foods for their families. Supermarket sales and coupons can help control grocery costs. Advanced meal planning and a carefully itemized shopping list help to avoid impulse purchases. Purchasing individual ingredients and preparing meals avoids the higher cost of convenience foods. Unit pricing labels can help identify better selections, with store-brand items generally being the same quality as popular brand names at substantially lower prices. The U.S. Center for Nutrition Policy and Promotion offers USDA food plans based on low-cost, moderate-cost, and liberal budgets (USDA, 2018).

Food in larger-sized packages is usually cheaper per serving and is practical when adequate storage is available and when the extra food in the house does not result in over-eating. An alternative may be to shop with a friend and divide large packages. Wholesale cooperatives are popular ways to save money on food purchases, especially for large families. Charitable organizations and community food banks are another option.

Meal Planning

Food costs can be reduced by basing meals on starchy foods such as pasta, rice, potatoes, or bread rather than building them around a higher-priced meat portion. Adding beans or vegetables to the main course stretches it to serve more people with less meat. Families who enjoy steak can purchase a beef chuck roast and slice it to half the thickness, making two steaks. When marinated and cooked with care, this option can be an appealing substitute for higher-priced cuts of beef. Canned fish is another alternative to more expensive fresh fish.

Food preparation methods and storage can help minimize waste and fuel costs—factors that are often overlooked when calculating food expenses. Stir-frying for a short time uses less fuel than boiling. Baking several items in the oven at the same time, such as a casserole, baked potatoes, and a dessert, minimizes fuel costs as well. Careful storage of fruits and vegetables reduces bruising and waste. Freezing leftovers in individual portions may help prevent waste.

Affordably of Healthy Foods

Globally, three billion people cannot afford a healthy diet, even if they spend most of their income on food (Ritchie & Rosado, 2021). The cost of a healthy diet is dependent on the affordability of lowest-cost foods that would meet dietary requirements. Food costs vary dramatically among countries. For example, consumer spending for food ranges from 1.5% in Norway, to 25% in Brail, to 55% in India, and to 92% in Madagascar. Food affordability for all countries is available at In Our World in Data (Ritchie et al., 2023). With the substantial variance in income and expenses among countries, healthy eating poses a challenge for low-income or "working poor" families.

A lack of grocery stores or supermarkets and a predominance of fast-food restaurants and convenience stores contribute to a poor diet. Food economists refer to urban and rural communities without easy access to fresh, healthy, and affordable food as *food deserts*. Food deserts can lead to higher levels of obesity and other diet-related diseases, such as diabetes and heart disease (WHO, 2020). Understanding such limitations within the communities in which your families live helps tailor your nutrition counseling.

Food Assistance Programs

Low-income families who are struggling with food insecurity may benefit from being linked to local not-for-profit agencies, school meal programs, community kitchens, or community nutrition programs. In the United States, the Supplemental Program for Women, Infants, and Children (WIC) provides supplemental foods and nutrition counseling to expectant and postpartum parents, nursing parents, and children from birth to age 6 when they meet basic requirements of low income or nutritional risk. Other U.S. food assistance programs include the food stamp program and Aid to Families with Dependent Children (AFDC). Canada's Prenatal Nutrition Program provides many of the same services as the U.S. WIC program. Other countries offer similar programs, usually through the ministry or department of health.

Foods to Limit or Avoid

Nursing babies can generally tolerate most foods the parent consumes. Traditional diets in many cultures include foods that parents may mistakenly believe will affect their baby. Acidic fruits, gas-forming vegetables and beans, milk, spices, and chocolate do not need to be avoided during lactation. A particular food that seems to cause a reaction in the baby can be omitted for a week and then reintroduced. A food consumed by the parent that seems to bother a newborn may have no effect a few months later or after the baby begins eating the food directly. A dietitian can help determine whether exclusion of a major food, such as wheat or cow's milk (the most common food **allergen** for humans), is warranted and ensure replacement of the nutrients in the excluded foods.

Alcohol

Alcohol enters the bloodstream and quickly migrates to the milk. Human milk metabolizes alcohol at about the same rate as the body metabolizes it—1½ to 2 hours per ounce of absolute alcohol. Occasional alcohol use timed around nursing does not seem to have any harmful effects on the infant (Hale & Krutsch, 2024). By comparison, moderate amounts of alcohol consumed regularly over time may slow brain growth in a nursing child. Consumption of large amounts of alcohol dramatically delays brain growth and limits parental effectiveness. Consuming excessive amounts of alcohol can cause life-threatening conditions in both the fetus and the nursing infant. Because alcohol is a carcinogen that can affect health, health officials assert that the safest option is to consume no alcohol (Anderson et al., 2023; WHO, 2023).

Caffeine

Caffeine passes to the infant through the milk. It is safe for nursing parents to drink coffee and other forms of caffeine in limited amounts just as it is during pregnancy. Up to 300 mg of caffeine per day is considered safe (Centers for Disease Control and Prevention, 2022). Caffeine passes to the infant through the milk. Very young infants cannot easily eliminate this toxin from the body. Infants who are particularly susceptible to caffeine's effects may experience fussiness or excessive wakefulness.

Allergens

Generally, most foods are acceptable during pregnancy and lactation unless they cause allergic reactions or are consumed in excessive amounts. Some evidence suggests that a fetus can be sensitized to allergens in utero, and an infant can be sensitized through nursing. A baby born to parents with a history of allergies has a greater possibility of developing the same allergies. A recent study suggests that nutrition during pregnancy and lactation can influence the risk of the infant developing allergies through epigenetic mechanisms (Di Costanzo et al., 2022). A more detailed discussion of substances found in milk and their effect on the infant can be found in **Chapter 11**.

Earlier guidelines suggested that avoidance of potentially allergenic foods during late pregnancy and lactation was associated with a lower incidence of allergy in children. However, the recommendation is now a healthy and diverse diet without eliminating or increasing allergenic foods during pregnancy and lactation (Sampath et al., 2021; USDA & USDHHS, 2020).

Foodborne Disease

Foodborne disease is an illness that results from eating contaminated food. Pesticides and heavy metals such as lead and mercury are stored in fatty tissue and later enter the milk. Individuals who are pregnant or considering pregnancy should avoid fish with the highest levels of mercury. These include orange roughy, shark, swordfish, king mackerel, marlin, bigeye tuna, and tilefish from the Gulf of Mexico (USDA & USDHHS, 2020). These fish could contain enough mercury to harm a fetus's nervous system. Young children and nursing parents should also avoid consuming those species of fish, which tend to live longer and have higher mercury concentrations in their tissues than other fish. Guidelines suggest it is permissible to eat as much as 12 ounces per week of shrimp, canned light tuna, salmon, pollock, and catfish. The FDA warns against eating more than 6 ounces of white albacore tuna, which contains more mercury than light tuna. Unpasteurized honey should be avoided because of the risk of botulism.

Food poisoning can be a serious illness when it occurs during pregnancy. The following practices will reduce the risk of contamination:

- When reheating food, make sure it is heated all the way through.
- Avoid raw eggs, and cook eggs until both the white and the yolk are solid.
- Store raw foods separate from cooked foods.
- Wash hands and utensils between preparing foods.
- Store food in a clean, dry, cool area away from flies, vermin, and household pets.
- Use pasteurized milk and discard it after its expiration date.
- Wash fruits and vegetables thoroughly rather than removing the skin, to preserve nutrients and fiber while eliminating toxins.
- Wear gloves when gardening or changing cat litter.
- Wash hands after using the toilet or changing diapers and before eating.

Summary

People are most receptive to improving their nutrition during pregnancy and lactation. Recognizing how nutrition affects overall health can motivate expectant and nursing parents to improve their eating habits for the baby's health and to feel good. Consuming sufficient nutrients and calories during pregnancy and lactation will provide the energy and nourishment babies need for healthy growth and development. Avoiding fad diets and maintaining a healthy weight will protect the health of both the parent and baby. Limiting the consumption of alcohol, caffeine, and potentially contaminated foods will preserve the safety of the milk. Awareness of food additives and processing will help parents select healthy foods and form sound nutrition practices. Integrating healthy nutrition gradually into parents' lifestyles increases the likelihood that these practices will continue to benefit family members for years to come.

What You Learned—At a Glance

Conversation Starters with Parents

- What vitamin and mineral supplements do you take?
- What does your typical diet include?
- How important is weight loss to you?
- What did you eat and drink in the past 24 hours?

Basic Nutrients

- Sugary foods can cause erratic blood sugar, fatigue, dizziness, nervousness, and headache.
- Complex carbohydrates take longer to digest and prevent cravings for more food.
- Protein is needed for the formation of hormones and milk production.
- Fats create a longer feeling of fullness.
- Folic or folate acid helps prevent prenatal anemia and neural tube defects.
- Low prenatal levels of vitamin D may result in low levels in the baby; supplementing the parent may improve the baby's vitamin D status.
- Newborns typically have low vitamin K levels and are supplemented at birth.
- Pregnancy and lactation are times of high calcium demand.
- Sufficient iron intake during lactation is important for rebuilding long-term stores.
- Nursing parents should drink to thirst.

Nutrition in Pregnancy and Lactation

- Pregnancy and lactation require increased nutritional intake to ensure good health.

- A normal, healthy diet will meet nutritional needs during lactation.
- Well-nourished nursing parents can safely lose about 1 pound (0.55 kg) per week.
- Parents with excess weight may experience delays in stage II lactogenesis (secretory activation).
- Disordered eating may cause concern about infant feeding, elimination, and weight.

Making Healthy Food Choices

- Pregnancy and lactation are times when families are receptive to nutrition education.
- A healthy diet includes three well-balanced meals a day with nutritious snacks as needed.
- Most foods are acceptable during pregnancy and lactation.
- Reading food labels will help avoid additives and processing that alter quality.
- Vegetarian diets that include milk and eggs provide necessary nutrients.
- Vegetarians may need vitamin B_{12} supplementation.
- Protein and complex carbohydrates at breakfast help prevent later fatigue.
- Expectant and nursing parents should avoid fish with high mercury levels.
- Limited alcohol consumption carefully timed around nursing is considered acceptable.
- Caffeine sensitivity may cause fussiness or excessive wakefulness in the infant.

References

Al Alawi AM, et al. Lactation ketoacidosis: a systematic review of case reports. *Medicina (Kaunas)*. 2020;56(6):299.

Anderson BO, et al. Health and cancer risks associated with low levels of alcohol consumption. *Lancet Public Health*. 2023;8(1): e6–e7.

Aparicio E, et al. Nutrient intake during pregnancy and postpartum: ECLIPSES study. *Nutrients*. 2020;12(5):1325.

Barker M, et al. Intervention strategies to improve nutrition and health behaviours before conception. *Lancet*. 2018;391(10132): 1853–1864.

Baroni L, et al. Vegan nutrition for mothers and children: practical tools for healthcare providers. *Nutrients*. 2018;11(1):5.

Bassin SR, et al. The state of nutrition in medical education in the United States. *Nutr Rev*. 2020;78(9):764–780.

Bazzazian S, et al. The relationship between social determinants of health and postpartum weight retention based on the World Health Organization model: path analysis. *BMC Public Health*. 2023;23(1):323.

Be'er M, et al. The effect of physical activity on human milk macronutrient content and its volume. *Breastfeed Med*. 2020;15(6): 357–361.

Bima A, et al. The interplay of vitamin D deficiency and cellular senescence in the pathogenesis of obesity-related comorbidities. *Nutrients*. 2021;13(11):4127.

Bjørklund G, et al. Iron deficiency in obesity and after bariatric surgery. *Biomolecules*. 2021;11(5):613.

Boudet-Berquier J, et al. Association between maternal prepregnancy obesity and breastfeeding duration: data from a nationwide prospective birth cohort. *Matern Child Nutr*. 2018;14(2): e12507.

Briana DD, et al. Inhibitors of osteoblastogenesis in early human milk and maternal serum: evidence for protective properties of mother's milk on bone. *J Matern Fetal Neonatal Med*. 2020;33(7):1095–1099.

Brown B, Wright C. Safety and efficacy of supplements in pregnancy. *Nutr Rev*. 2020;78(10):813–826.

Capozzi A, et al. Bone metabolism in pregnancy and lactation. *Minerva Obstet Gynecol*. 2021;73(6):697–703.

Carbone JW, et al. Recent advances in the characterization of skeletal muscle and whole-body protein responses to dietary protein and exercise during negative energy balance. *Adv Nutr*. 2019;10(1):70–79.

Caut C, et al. Dietary guideline adherence during preconception and pregnancy: a systematic review. *Matern Child Nutr*. 2020;16(2):e12916.

Centers for Disease Control and Prevention. Maternal diet. 2022. https://www.cdc.gov/breastfeeding/breastfeeding-special-circumstances/diet-and-micronutrients/maternal-diet.html

Chakhtoura M, et al. Vitamin D in the Middle East and North Africa. *Bone Rep*. 2018;8:135–146.

Chang SW, Lee HC. Vitamin D and health—the missing vitamin in humans. *Pediatr Neonatol*. 2019;60(3):237–244.

Chu BA, et al. Micronutrient deficiency as a confounder in ascertaining the role of obesity in severe COVID-19 infection. *Int J Environ Res Public Health*. 2022;19(3):1125.

Cuerda C, et al. Nutrition education in medical schools (NEMS) project: joining ESPEN and university point of view. *Clin Nutr*. 2021;40(5):2754–2761.

Daigle Millan K, et al. Information seeking behaviors, attitudes, and beliefs about pregnancy-related nutrition and supplementation: a qualitative study among US women. *Nutr Health*. 2022;28(4):563–569.

Di Costanzo M, et al. Nutrition during pregnancy and lactation: epigenetic effects on infants' immune system in food allergy. *Nutrients*. 2022;14(9):1766.

Dror DK, Allen LH. Overview of nutrients in human milk. *Adv Nutr*. 2018;9(Suppl 1):278S–294S.

Fan WQ, Molinaro A. Maternal obesity adversely affects early breastfeeding in a multicultural, multi-socioeconomic Melbourne community. *Aust N Z J Obstet Gynaecol*. 2021;61(1):78–85.

Farah E, et al. Impaired lactation: review of delayed lactogenesis and insufficient lactation. *J Midwifery Womens Health*. 2021; 66(5):631–640.

Ferrazzi E, et al. Folic acid versus 5-methyl tetrahydrofolate supplementation in pregnancy. *Eur J Obstet Gynecol Reprod Biol*. 2020;253:312–319.

Foster SF, et al. Breastfeeding, socioeconomic status, and long-term postpartum weight retention. *Int Breastfeed J.* 2023;18(1):1.

Gallo S, et al. Vitamin D supplementation during pregnancy: an evidence analysis center systematic review and meta-analysis. *J Acad Nutr Diet.* 2020;120(5):898–924.e4.

Gannon BM, et al. Vitamin A requirements in pregnancy and lactation. *Curr Dev Nutr.* 2020;4(10):nzaa142.

Gawlińska K, et al. Relationship of maternal high-fat diet during pregnancy and lactation to offspring health. *Nutr Rev.* 2021; 79(6):709–725.

Gete DG, et al. Changes in dietary patterns from preconception to during pregnancy and its association with socio-demographic and lifestyle factors. *Public Health Nutr.* 2022;25(9):2530–2540.

Hale T, Krutsch K. *Hale's Medications & Mothers' Milk 2025-2026: A Manual of Lactational Pharmacology 21st ed.* New York, NY: Springer Publishing Company; 2024.

Hall JT, et al. The relationship between physical activity and vitamin D status in postpartum lactating and formula-feeding women. *J Steroid Biochem Mol Biol.* 2018;177:261–265.

Heo JS, et al. Breastfeeding and vitamin D. *Clin Exp Pediatr.* 2022;65(9):418–429.

Huang YL, et al. Effects of climate, sun exposure, and dietary intake on vitamin D concentrations in pregnant women: a population-based study. *Nutrients.* 2023;15(5):1182.

Imdad A, et al. Vitamin A supplementation for preventing morbidity and mortality in children from six months to five years of age. *Cochrane Database Syst Rev.* 2022;3(3):CD008524.

Jullien S. Vitamin K prophylaxis in newborns. *BMC Pediatr.* 2021; 21(Suppl 1):350.

Kapa HM, et al. Body image dissatisfaction, breastfeeding experiences, and self-efficacy in postpartum women with and without eating disorder symptoms. *J Hum Lact.* 2022;38(4):633–643.

Karcz K, Królak-Olejnik B. Vegan or vegetarian diet and breast milk composition—a systematic review. *Crit Rev Food Sci Nutr.* 2021;61(7):1081–1098.

Karalis DT, et al. Genetically modified products, perspectives and challenges. *Cureus.* 2020;12(3):e7306.

Kaß A, et al. The impact of maternal eating disorders on breastfeeding practices: a systematic review. *Arch Womens Ment Health.* 2021;24(5):693–708.

Killeen SL, et al. Addressing the gaps in nutritional care before and during pregnancy. *Proc Nutr Soc.* 2022;81(1):87–98.

Lobo S, et al. Nutrition information in pregnancy: where do women seek advice and has this changed over time? *Nutr Diet.* 2020;77(3):382–391.

Lockyer F, et al. Breast milk micronutrients and infant neurodevelopmental outcomes: a systematic review. *Nutrients.* 2021; 13(11):3848.

Lujano-Negrete AY, et al. Bone metabolism and osteoporosis during pregnancy and lactation. *Arch Osteoporos.* 2022;17(1):36.

Luzardo-Ocampo I, et al. Obesity-derived alterations in the lactating mammary gland: focus on prolactin. *Mol Cell Endocrinol.* 2023;559:111810.

Mancini K. Body image, eating attitudes and breastfeeding intention: implications for mental health and maternal child nurses. *Issues Ment Health Nurs.* 2017;38(9):750–755.

Mansur JL, et al. Vitamin D: Before, during and after pregnancy: effect on neonates and children. *Nutrients.* 2022;14(9):1900.

Mantel Ä, et al. Association of maternal eating disorders with pregnancy and neonatal outcomes. *JAMA Psychiatry.* 2020;77(3): 285–293.

Marshall NE, et al. Impact of maternal obesity and breastfeeding intention on lactation intensity and duration. *Matern Child Nutr.* 2019;15:e12732.

Marshall NE, et al. The importance of nutrition in pregnancy and lactation: lifelong consequences. *Am J Obstet Gynecol.* 2022; 226(5):607–632.

McGaugh E, Barthel B. A review of ketogenic diet and lifestyle. *Mo Med.* 2022;119(1):84–88.

Mohapatra S, et al. Malnutrition in obesity before and after bariatric surgery. *Dis Mon.* 2020;66(2):100866.

Mutamba AK, et al. Therapeutic advances in overcoming intrauterine growth restriction induced metabolic syndrome. *Front Pediatr.* 2023;10:1040742.

Narasaki Y, et al. Dietary protein intake, kidney function, and survival in a nationally representative cohort. *Am J Clin Nutr.* 2021;114(1):303–313.

National Digestive Disease Information Clearinghouse, National Institute of Health. Definition & facts for celiac disease. October 2020. https://www.niddk.nih.gov/health-information/digestive-diseases/celiac-disease/definition-facts

National Eating Disorders Association. What are eating disorders? 2018. https://www.nationaleatingdisorders.org

National Institutes of Health Office of Dietary Supplements. Vitamin E fact sheet for health professionals. 2016. https://ods.od.nih.gov/factsheets/VitaminE-HealthProfessional/

Nomura K, et al. Prepregnancy obesity as a risk factor for exclusive breastfeeding initiation in Japanese women. *Nutrition.* 2019;62:93–99.

Nomura K, et al. Maternal body mass index and breastfeeding non-initiation and cessation: a quantitative review of the literature. *Nutrients.* 2020;12(9):2684.

Office of Dietary Supplements, National Institutes of Health. Vitamin and mineral supplement fact sheets. 2019. https://ods.od.nih.gov/factsheets /list-VitaminsMinerals/#m

Pawlak R, et al. Prevalence and predictors of low breast milk iodine concentration in women following vegan, vegetarian, and omnivore diets. *Breastfeed Med.* 2023;18(1):37–42.

Ramji N, et al. A comparison of breastfeeding rates by obesity class. *J Matern Fetal Neonatal Med.* 2018;31(22):3021–3026.

Ritchie H, et al. Food Prices. Published online at OurWorldinData.org. 2023. https://ourworldindata.org/food-prices

Ritchie H, Rosado P. Three billion people cannot afford a healthy diet. Published online at OurWorldinData.org. 2021. https://ourworldindata.org/diet-affordability

Rounsefell K, et al. Social media, body image and food choices in healthy young adults: a mixed methods systematic review. *Nutr Diet.* 2020;77(1):19–40.

Sampath V, et al. Food allergy across the globe. *J Allergy Clin Immunol.* 2021;148(6):1347–1364.

Santander Ballestín S, et al. Is supplementation with micronutrients still necessary during pregnancy? A review. *Nutrients.* 2021;13(9):3134.

Scaglioni S, et al. Factors influencing children's eating behaviours. *Nutrients.* 2018;10(6):706.

Silveira JS, et al. High-protein nutrition during pregnancy increases neuroinflammation and homocysteine levels and impairs behavior in male adolescent rats offspring. *Life Sci.* 2022; 310:121084.

Singh P, et al. Global prevalence of celiac disease: systematic review and meta-analysis. *Clin Gastroenterol Hepatol.* 2018;16(6): 823–836.

Snyder A, et al. A mixed-methods investigation of women's experiences seeking pregnancy-related online nutrition information. *BMC Pregnancy Childbirth.* 2020;20(1):377.

Spahn JM, et al. Influence of maternal diet on flavor transfer to amniotic fluid and breast milk and children's responses: a systematic review. *Am J Clin Nutr.* 2019;109:1003S–1026S.

Stephenson J, et al. Before the beginning: nutrition and lifestyle in the preconception period and its importance for future health. *Lancet*. 2018;391(10132):1830–1841.

Tihtonen K, et al. Calcium supplementation during pregnancy and maternal and offspring bone health: a systematic review and meta-analysis. *Ann N Y Acad Sci*. 2022;1509(1): 23–36.

Tsakiridis I, et al. Nutrition in pregnancy: a comparative review of major guidelines. *Obstet Gynecol Surv*. 2020;75(11): 692–702.

United Nations Children's Fund. Improving young children's diets during the complementary feeding period. UNICEF programming guidance. 2020a. https://www.unicef.org/media/93981/file/Complementary-Feeding-Guidance-2020.pdf

United Nations Children's Fund. Nutrition, for every child: UNICEF nutrition strategy 2020–2030. 2020b. https://www.unicef.org/media/106511/file/%20Nutrition%20Strategy%202020-2030%20(Document)%20-%202021%20Edition..pdf

Urueña-Palacio S, et al. Adult scurvy associated with psychiatric disorders and breast feeding. *BMJ Case Rep*. 2018;2018: bcr2017223686.

U.S. Department of Agriculture. The low-cost, moderate-cost and liberal food plans. Center for Nutrition Policy and Promotion. December 2018. https://www.cnpp.usda.gov/USDAFoodPlansCostofFood.htm

U.S. Department of Agriculture, National Agricultural Library. Lifecycle nutrition. Nutrition during lactation. June 18, 2019. https://www.choosemyplate.gov/moms-breastfeeding-nutritional-needs

U.S. Department of Agriculture, U.S. Department of Health Human Services. *Dietary Guidelines for Americans, 2020–2025*. 9th ed. December 2020. https://www.dietaryguidelines.gov/sites/default/files/2021-03/Dietary_Guidelines_for_Americans-2020-2025.pdf

van Elten TM, et al. Preconception lifestyle intervention reduces long term energy intake in women with obesity and infertility: a randomized controlled trial. *Int J Behav Nutr Phys Act*. 2019;16(1):3.

Ventura AK, et al. Maternal diet during pregnancy and lactation and child food preferences, dietary patterns, and weight outcomes: a review of recent research. *Curr Nutr Rep*. 2021;10(4):413–426.

World Health Organization. WHO recommendations on antenatal care for a positive pregnancy experience. 2016. https://www.who.int/publications/i/item/9789241549912

World Health Organization. Nutrition health topics. 2019. http://www.who.int/elena/en/

World Health Organization. Health and sustainable development. Nutrition insecurity and unhealthy diets. 2020. https://www.who.int/sustainable-development/cities/health-risks/nutrition-insecurity/en/

World Health Organization. No level of alcohol consumption is safe for our health. January 4, 2023. https://www.who.int/europe/news/item/04-01-2023-no-level-of-alcohol-consumption-is-safe-for-our-health

Yisahak SF, et al. Maternal diet patterns during early pregnancy in relation to neonatal outcomes. *Am J Clin Nutr*. 2021;114(1): 358–367.

CHAPTER 9

Health Factors in Lactation

Human milk is a species-specific first food that offers biologically natural nutrition and protects the infant's developing immune system. Human milk contains a host of **immunological** agents that protect infants against infections and allergens until their internal defenses develop more fully. This protection has a lifelong effect on the child's immune system. The individualized characteristics of the milk each baby receives provide the baby with nourishment that is ideally suited to their specific health needs and growth. Research continues to support the many short- and long-term health benefits of human milk and lactation for the newborn, older child, and nursing parent.

Although nonbinary, non-cisgender parents are able to nurse their children, research on human milk maternal health is based on the biologically female lactation model. Thus, some sections of this chapter may depart from the nongendered terminology used in the rest of this text.

KEY TERMS

Acrodermatitis enteropathica
Active immunity
Adiponectin
Antibacterial
Antibody response
Antigen
Antimicrobial
Antiviral
Bioavailability
Body mass index (BMI)
Calories
Carbohydrates
Casein
Centers for Disease Control and Prevention (CDC)
Cholecystokinin (CCK)
Colicky behavior
Colostrum
Cow's milk
Cytokines
Dehydration
Diarrhea
Enzyme
Epigenetics
Exogenous
Flora
Fluoride
Gene expression
Ghrelin
Glycan
Growth factors
Gut closure
Hemorrhagic disease
Humoral factors
Hypocalcemia
Immunoglobulin
Immunoglobulin A (IgA)
Immunological
Iron
Lactobacillus bifidus
Lactoferrin
Lactose intolerance
Leptin
Leukocytes
Lipase
Lipids
Long-chain polyunsaturated fatty acid
Lymphocytes
Lysozyme
Macrophages
Mature milk
Meconium
Microbiome
Mineral
Mucins
Myelin
Necrotizing enterocolitis (NEC)
Neutrophils
Nucleotides
Obestatin
Oligosaccharide
Otitis media
Passive immunity
Pathogen
Peptide
Phagocyte
Polysaccharides
Prebiotics
Probiotics
Prostaglandin
Protein
Resistin
Rickets
Rotavirus
Vaccine
Virus
Vitamin D
Vitamin K
Whey

Lactation and Maternal Health

Lactation is as much a women's health issue as it is an infant feeding issue. The biologically female body is designed to progress from pregnancy to birth and then lactation. Interrupting this normal cycle by not nursing interrupts the biological continuum. In their seminal work, the late anthropologist Ashley Montagu (1986) described gestation as an 18-month process, with a baby spending 9 months in utero and 9 months nursing. The first 12 weeks postpartum are described as the fourth trimester, a period of recovery and family adjustment (Verbiest et al., 2018).

Women's health has traditionally received little attention in the global healthcare arena. Part of the challenge in promoting lactation stems from this persistent failure in many healthcare systems. Healthcare professionals need to view lactation as an important part of women's health. The 2010 Affordable Care Act enacted in the United States considers lactation care as a preventive service, a welcome cultural signal recognizing lactation as a normal part of the female life cycle and not a temporary aberrance. Countries throughout the world have similar promotion efforts to protect and support nursing families.

Physical and Emotional Health

Lactation has a significant impact on a nursing parent's physical and emotional health. Endogenous oxytocin released during nursing contracts the uterus and helps stop postpartum bleeding. Prolactin and oxytocin each play a role in feelings of well-being, relaxation, and bonding with the infant. A positive nursing experience can contribute to self-confidence for parents, raising their self-esteem and empowering them. Numerous studies demonstrate the positive effects of lactation in minimizing postpartum depression (discussed in **Chapter 20**). Beginning nursing immediately after birth and continuing to nurse frequently will ensure the parent's biological continuum and enhance their emotional health.

Parents who nurse typically, although not always, experience delays in the return of fertility. Exclusive nursing is 98% effective in delaying pregnancy naturally without the use of artificial contraceptives for the first 4 to 6 months postpartum, as discussed in **Chapter 20**. Avoiding shorter birth intervals and a higher number of pregnancies over a life span protects against maternal and infant mortality (Calik-Ksepka et al., 2022; Molitoris et al., 2019; Starbird & Crawford, 2019).

Obesity is a growing global public health concern, with rates more than doubled since 1990. Currently, one in eight people across the globe live with obesity and the comorbidities associated with the condition (World Health organization [WHO], 2022a). Obesity during pregnancy is a major risk factor for developing gestational diabetes which increases the risk of developing lifelong issues with type 2 diabetes. Lactation lowers the risk of gestational diabetes developing into type 2 diabetes (Gunderson et al., 2018; Horta & de Lima, 2019).

Nursing lowers the risk for developing both premenopausal and postmenopausal breast cancer (Arriaga et al., 2019; Fan et al., 2023), ovarian cancer (Babic et al., 2020), and thyroid cancer (Jin et al., 2021). The protections are dose dependent. Lactation also provides protection against osteoporosis in later life (Duan et al., 2017). Continued research into the correlation between lactation and osteoporosis has provided reassurance to nursing parents that the bone loss experienced because of nursing regenerates after weaning (Ferreira et al., 2023; Winter, 2020).

Health Risks of Not Nursing

Birth parents who do not nurse are at greater risk for numerous health conditions. Low socioeconomic and ethnic group status increase multiple risk factors because they are correlated with higher rates of adverse health outcomes, including obesity, diabetes, and cardiovascular disease. The risks for hypertension (and stroke), hyperlipidemia (high cholesterol), and cardiovascular disease are higher among parents who do not nurse. **Table 9-1** outlines these and other health risks of not nursing. Maternal health organizations promote nursing because of the health protections it provides to nursing parents (American College of Obstetricians and Gynecologists [ACOG], 2018).

Lactation and Infant Health

There is global recognition of the impact of lactation on infant morbidity and mortality. Infants are born with immature immune systems. During uterine development, the fetus receives the parent's antibodies through the placenta. After birth, infants are designed to continue to receive the parent's immunities through their milk. Nursing—in particular, exclusive nursing for the first 6 months of a child's life—ranks among the most effective interventions for improving child survival and health (WHO, 2022b). The numerous infant health protections are a clear testament to the

Table 9-1 Health Risks of Not Nursing for Parents

Health Condition	Source
Arthritis, rheumatoid	Alotiby et al. (2021)
Breast cancer	Arriaga et al. (2019) Fan et al. (2023)
Cardiovascular disease and hyperlipidemia	Cho and Han (2018) Nguyen et al. (2017) Umer et al. (2019)
Diabetes, type 2	Horta and de Lima (2019) Gunderson et al. (2018)
Endometrial cancer	Jordan et al. (2017) Ma et al. (2018)
Hypertension	Chetwynd et al. (2017) Kirkegaard et al. (2018) Park and Choi (2018)
Nonalcoholic fatty liver disease	Ajmera et al. (2019)
Osteoporosis	Duan et al. (2017)
Ovarian cancer	Babic et al. (2020) Fan et al. (2023)
Postpartum blood loss	Karimi et al. (2019) Safari et al. (2018)
Postpartum depression	Alimi et al. (2022) Figueiredo et al. (2021)
Postpartum fertility (delayed ovulation and increased spacing between pregnancies)	Calik-Ksepka et al. (2022) Starbird and Crawford (2019)
Thyroid cancer	Jin et al. (2021)

significance of human milk in infant feeding. This protection is dose dependent, increasing with the period over which an infant nurses (Berlanga-Macías et al., 2020). The protections infants receive from infectious diseases and other negative health consequences continue into adulthood.

Secure Attachment

Nursing represents an important means for parents to form a secure personal connection with their new infant. The bonding that accompanies nursing enhances parents' sensitivity during early infancy. The early sensory stimulation from skin-to-skin contact that takes place during nursing helps develop the baby's perceptual and response mechanisms. Parents can respond intuitively to their baby's hunger cues without delays imposed by the need to prepare and heat bottles. The parent's immediate response to a baby's needs builds a sense of security and trust that contributes to healthy emotional and social development. A longer nursing duration is associated with parents' sensitive responsiveness, greater attachment security, and less attachment disorganization. Longer duration is also predictive of the parent's increased sensitivity toward the child up to 11 years old (Weaver et al., 2018).

Difficulty forming healthy interpersonal relationships and lack of parent–child bonding are some of the underlying causes of child neglect (WHO, 2022b). Nursing promotes the parent–child relationship and heathy attachment and may help to protect against child maltreatment, particularly neglect. For example, Kremer and Kremer (2018) found that adolescent parents who nursed for 9 months or more had reduced odds of neglectful and abusive behaviors compared with those who never nursed. The WHO 2022 report on violence against children estimates that across the globe, 1 billion children between the ages of 2 and 17 years experience neglect and abuse each year (WHO, 2022b). In the United States alone, 27.3% of victims of neglect and abuse are in the age range of birth through 2 years old. Infant victims younger than 1 year are 14.7% of all victims (U.S. Department of Health and Human Services, 2024). Supporting parents is one of the key interventions to help reduce the incidence of child neglect and abuse.

Intelligence and Neurological Development

The greatest growth of the human brain occurs during the second and third trimesters of pregnancy and the first 2 years of life. Nursing during the first year of life may promote growth in several cellular compartments in the cortex. Exclusive nursing duration leads to greater cortical thickness in regions of the brain involved in cognitive abilities (Grevet et al., 2023). The thickness of the cortex reflects the density and size of neurons. There is a positive association between nursing for more than 6 months and improved motor development outcomes at ages 10, 14, and 17 years, independent of sociodemographics (Grace et al., 2017). Cognitive ability, behavior, and executive function are modestly higher in children who were nursed (McGowan & Bland, 2023).

Nursing is positively associated with an infant's cognitive outcomes (Lovcevic, 2023; Pereyra-Elías et al., 2022). Infants bottle-fed human milk also exhibit better cognition than their formula-fed counterparts (Pang et al., 2020). Nursing reduces the odds of a low IQ score at age 5 years, with each month of nursing associated with modest but significant protection (Amiel Castro et al., 2021; Plunkett et al., 2021). Even short-term nursing results in a significant increase in IQ at 5 years of age (Lenehan et al., 2020). A meta-analysis suggests that nursing may supply fatty acid requirements for cognitive development, and longer duration is beneficial (Hartwig et al., 2019).

Craniofacial Development

The mechanics involved in nursing promote optimal development of the oral cavity. The longer children nurse, the less likely they are to have malocclusion (Abate et al., 2020; Thomaz et al., 2018). Being nursed exclusively for less than 6 months is associated with anterior open bite (Pereira Lopes et al., 2019). A child who is nursed also develops a proper swallowing pattern that extends into adulthood. Both outcomes may reduce the risk of obstructive sleep apnea in adulthood (Vinha & de Mello-Filho, 2017). The greatest increase in craniofacial development occurs in the first 4 years of life. Thus, the avoidance of bottles and artificial nipples during infancy can have far-reaching health consequences.

Table 9-2 Opportunities to Modulate Microbiota

Prenatally	Neonatally	Postnatally
▪ Placenta	▪ Mode of delivery ▪ Gestational age	▪ Fed human milk ▪ Geographic location ▪ Family members ▪ Host interactions ▪ Nursing parent's diet ▪ Weaning

Data from Milani C, et al. The first microbial colonizers of the human gut: composition, activities, and health implications of the infant gut microbiota. *Microbiol Mol Biol Rev.* 2017 Nov 8;81(4):pii:e00036-17.

Properties of Colostrum and Mature Milk

Human milk is a life-giving substance that provides much more than nutrition for the child. It is easily digested, efficiently used by the body, and fosters the infant's health and growth. The composition of human milk is ideally suited to human infants. Immune system protection and development, gut maturation, gut **microbiome** formation, and metabolic programming are key functions of human milk, in addition to providing energy. It is the only single food that meets all nutritional requirements to sustain human life.

The breast initially secretes protein-rich **colostrum**, which provides the infant with antibodies and other protection against disease. During the first few days after birth, colostrum mixes with increasing quantities of newly formed milk and eventually transitions to **mature milk**. Despite infant formula manufacturers' claims, no commercial parallel exists for this perfect infant nutrition. **Table 9-2** illustrates the microbiome development window from gestation to childhood.

Colostrum: The Early Milk

Colostrum, the first milk babies receive, is the residual mixture of materials present in the mammary glands and ducts. Colostrum production begins at approximately 120 days' gestation. It can be secreted prenatally and for several days after birth. Usually a sticky, rich-looking substance, colostrum comes in a range of colors and viscosity—from clear and thin to golden yellow, orange, and thick. New parents frequently need assurance that their newborn receives adequate nourishment and other important health benefits with their colostrum. This first milk is exactly what the newborn needs to make the transition to extrauterine life, both in amount and composition.

Colostrum Properties and Volume

Colostrum is rich in **protein**, which promotes the newborn's early rapid growth. It contains approximately 67 kcal per dL milk (18.76 kcal per oz). Compared with mature milk, it is richer in sodium, potassium, chloride, protein, fat-soluble vitamins, and **minerals**. Colostrum also contains less fat (2%) and lactose than mature milk. It has the appropriate level and balance of the essential fatty acids required by the newborn. The composition of the colostrum microbiome varies as a result of geography and ethnicity (Xie et al., 2022).

Total infant intake of colostrum in the first 24 hours ranges widely, with an average of 1.5 g (mL) per feeding (Santoro et al., 2010). Colostrum intake for a 7.5-pound baby in the first day of life differs dramatically, ranging from 10.2 to 108.8 mL (0.3–3.6 oz). The small amount of colostrum corresponds with the newborn's small stomach capacity, which is approximately 20 mL (Bergman, 2013). The removal of colostrum by the infant nursing stimulates further production of colostrum and milk.

Protective Qualities of Colostrum

Colostrum plays an important role in protecting the infant against bacteria and **viruses** and is considered a baby's first immunization. Living cells in colostrum engulf and digest disease organisms. Colostrum is composed of approximately 70% **leukocytes**, compared with less than 10% leukocytes in transitional and mature milk (Hanson, 2017). Leukocytes are white blood cells that mediate pain and defend the body against infectious disease and foreign materials. Colostrum aids in rapid **gut closure**, protecting the baby's intestinal wall against penetration by disease organisms and **antigens** (Bardanzellu et al., 2017). It provides protection against **pathogens** (disease agents), such as polio; Coxsackie B virus; several staphylococci; and *Escherichia coli,* the intestinal bacteria that can cause serious intestinal, urinary, and other infections in infants.

Colostrum provides the optimal beginning for the infant's gut microbiome. The gut microbiome is the bacterial ecosystem residing in the gastrointestinal (GI) tract and contains trillions of microorganisms—bacteria, yeast, and other fungi. The gut's microbiome has a lifelong impact on health and disease, including immune system development, infection prevention, nutrient acquisition, and possible brain and nervous system function. Imbalance of the microbiome is associated with obesity, as well as autoimmune and neurological diseases (McBurney et al., 2019). Gut bacteria are critical for gut metabolism regulation and for the immune system. Because the newborn gut is primarily sterile, it is crucial that the first microorganisms introduced be beneficial. The first few days of life prime the gut with either beneficial or unbeneficial bacteria (Ryan et al., 2019). Colostrum populates the immature newborn gut with beneficial microorganisms that have long-term health benefits.

Parents produce antibodies to all the diseases to which they have acquired relative immunity. Colostrum, in turn, contains many antibodies produced in response to a threat by a particular microbial invader, or antigen. The parent therefore passes many antibodies both to the fetus through the placenta and to the newborn through their colostrum and milk. The antibodies **immunoglobulin A (IgA)**, immunoglobulin G (IgG), and immunoglobulin M (IgM) are highly concentrated in colostrum and human milk. An **immunoglobulin** is a group of proteins that provide immunity. Of these immunoglobulins, IgA occurs in the highest concentrations in colostrum and human milk and is the most biologically active (Milani et al., 2017; Munblit et al., 2018). The high levels of IgA and other antibodies in colostrum protect the digestive tract against organisms that might otherwise invade it. Secretory IgA in human milk is essential for newborns. Babies only begin to produce secretory IgA around 4-6 weeks of age, and do not produce sufficient amounts to meet their needs until approximately 6 months of age.

Colostrum facilitates the establishment of bifidus **flora** (normal bacteria and other microbes) in the digestive tract. Bifidus flora promotes the growth of beneficial bacteria, primarily **Lactobacillus bifidus**, and facilitates the passage of **meconium**. Meconium is the newborn's thick, black, sticky first stools. Colostrum has a laxative effect that eliminates meconium from the infant's intestines. Bowel stimulation from meconium enables the infant's body to begin excreting waste products effectively. This elimination can be a critical factor in reducing the rate and severity of jaundice. Any water or artificial milk the baby receives will dilute colostrum's protective effects. Nursing newborns do not need water.

Transition to Mature Milk

Colostrum changes to transitional milk around day 6 of life and then to mature milk between 8 and 10 days postpartum. Detailed RNA microassays reveal that the milk change is driven by **gene expression** (Dastmalchi et al., 2022; Martin Carli et al., 2020). Thus, it is more precise to describe milk transition as being chemically stage dependent, not merely time dependent. The high ratio of sodium to potassium in colostrum lowers during transitional milk and is lowest in mature milk. This chemical transition provides the baby with **antimicrobial** protection and aids in the digestion of proteins.

Milk Appearance

Human milk has a naturally watery appearance that looks even more diluted when milk volume is high. As the baby's sucking stimulates oxytocin release and activates letdown, the milk flow washes fat that adheres to the walls of the milk ducts. This hindmilk is much higher in fat and therefore typically richer looking than the initial foremilk. Expressing milk at the end of a feeding, when fat content is higher, will produce a thicker and denser consistency.

Informing parents about color variations will help avoid unnecessary concern if they occur. Casein, a component of the proteins in milk, produces the typically bluish cast to human milk. A greenish color can result from additives in the parent's vitamins or **iron** supplements or from eating deep-green foods such as spinach and broccoli. Excessive amounts of vitamin A, either in foods or as a supplement, may color the milk yellow or orange. Black milk can result from the lactating parent ingesting the drug minocycline ("Minocycline," 2021). Milk that appears pink may be an indication of bleeding, either from the nipple or deeper within the breast. A discussion of bleeding in the breast appears in **Chapter 7**. Pink milk can also be associated with *Serratia marcescens*, a pathogenic bacterium (Moles et al., 2019).

Milk Volume

Milk volume is most heavily dependent on regular removal and the degree of drainage at each feeding or pumping session. Removal of milk at one feeding signals the amount of milk needed at the next feeding. Milk often seems most plentiful in the morning hours, especially immediately after waking. Expressing milk at that time and throughout the day will not decrease the amount of milk available to the baby. Volume is likely to increase with supplemental milk removal because removing milk signals more production. Minor variations may occur in the volume produced on each side, on different days, or in response to the infant's sucking pattern.

Babies have the ability to self-regulate feedings to meet their individual needs for optimal growth (Srivastava & Swati, 2023). They determine the amount they need from one feeding to the next through the amount of milk they remove. Reassure parents that milk intake can vary greatly from baby to baby. Milk intake for nursing babies typically does not match the large volumes (8 oz [240 mL]) that formula-fed babies consume. The average healthy nursing month-old baby will take approximately 2 to 4 oz per feeding (60–120 mL) or 24 to 32 oz (720–960 mL) of milk over 24 hours. During the second year of lactation, milk output is equivalent to about one 8-oz (240-mL) glass daily.

Milk volume is influenced to a lesser extent by the parent's nutrition and water intake. Babies whose parents nurse under challenging nutritional conditions have growth patterns similar to the baby of a well-nourished parent. It is important not to overemphasize the importance of diet during lactation, especially among first-time parents who may be unsure of their bodies' ability to nourish their newborn. A diet that includes all dietary reference intake (DRI) nutrients in sufficient amounts will avoid any significant decrease in milk volume or quality.

Sensory Qualities

Human milk provides richly changing experiences in taste and odor, bridging the transition from uterine nutrition to table foods. Variety in the infant's diet increases acceptance of foods later in life. The flavor of the milk is affected by the parent's diet, with sweetness being the most predominant basic taste. Interestingly, bitterness in the parent's diet correlates with bitterness in foremilk but not in hindmilk (Mastorakou et al., 2019). This may be because of the watery nature of foremilk or the fatty acid content in hindmilk that masks the bitterness. Studies have found that garlic's odor transmitted to the milk may increase infant sucking time and enhance the infant's food choices in the long term ("Garlic," 2023).

Nutritional Components in Human Milk

The milk of healthy, well-nourished parents contains almost all the necessary nutrients for an infant's growth and development. Milk composition changes throughout lactation and even during a given day or feeding. The milk continually adjusts to meet the needs of the growing child from the first few days of colostrum to beyond the child's second year. Early milk is high in immunoglobulins and protein. There is 4 to 5 times more fat and 1.5 times more protein present at the end of a feeding than at the beginning. Protein, lactose, iron, copper, **lactoferrin**, and secretory IgA remain stable during prolonged lactation. **Lysozyme** concentration increases, helping to fight infections, whereas zinc and calcium decline. Continuing a feeding until the baby ends it will ensure consumption of important nutrients. From 6 to 12 months of age, babies continue to receive three-fourths or more of their nutrient needs from human milk.

Scientists continue to make new discoveries about the many components of human milk. The next section describes the function **calories**, fat, fatty acids, **carbohydrates**, lactose, protein, vitamins, minerals, nitrogen, **enzymes**, growth factors, and hormones have in ensuring optimal nourishment of the infant.

Calories

The caloric content of human milk is ideally suited to the human infant. Colostrum contains approximately 18.76 kcal per oz. By 2 weeks, the average caloric content of mature human milk is 20 kcal per oz, increasing to 26 kcal per oz by 4 months. Differences in the caloric content result from variations in fat, and the caloric content changes throughout the day. Feedings must last long enough for the baby to receive sufficient calories from the fatty hindmilk. Babies typically consume nearly one-sixth of the available calories in the first 15 minutes of a feed. Over the day, with unrestricted nursing, a healthy infant takes in the calories needed.

Fat

Human milk fat provides as much as 50% of the infant's energy needs. It is the main source of fat-soluble vitamins and essential fatty acids needed for growth and development of the infant's central nervous system, brain, and immune system. Fat is an extremely variable constituent in human milk. The amount of available fat seems dependent on the parent's body fat stores (Bobiński & Bobińska, 2022; Bzikowska et al., 2018; Czank et al., 2017). Fat stores laid down during pregnancy are easier to mobilize for lactation than other fat stores. If the parent experiences severe food insecurity or is severely malnourished, their nutritional status does affect the composition of the milk, and milk fat levels may be lower (Bottin et al., 2022).

Fat content varies from lactating parent to parent and from feeding to feeding. Interestingly, the fat content of colostrum in parents 35 years or older is significantly higher than in younger parents (Argov-Argaman et al., 2017). This may be a result of increased fat synthesis and excretion in milk, lower water content, or a combination of both. There are significant day-to-day variations in both the macronutrients and caloric content of human milk (Kumar & Zumpf, 2021). Although we don't know exact percentages of fat and calories from feed to feed, the amount of fat a nursing infant receives is dependent on the length of time between feedings and the length of sucking time. Fat content in the milk decreases in the later months of lactation.

A baby who is not gaining sufficient weight may not be nursing long enough at feedings to receive sufficient fat. If a feeding on one side ends too early, the baby may fill up on foremilk from both sides and receive insufficient hindmilk. This could lead to behavior resembling colic, poor nourishment, or even growth faltering. Given the variance in fat content, allowing a baby to finish nursing on the first side and not restricting the length of the feeding helps the baby transfer the fat available in that feeding.

Fatty Acids

The **long-chain polyunsaturated fatty acids** in human milk aid in the development of the infant's immune response. Fatty acids in the human diet are crucial for neural development. To date, more than 200 types of fatty acids have been found in human milk, including both saturated and unsaturated fatty acids (*mono-* and *poly-* types), which are primarily medium- and long-chain in form. Like milk fat, the concentrations and types of fatty acids in the milk depend on the parent's stores and diet (Freitas et al., 2021; Giuffrida et al., 2022).

Two of the fatty acids in human milk are arachidonic acid (AA or ARA) from linoleic acid and docosahexaenoic acid (DHA) from linolenic acid. They are essential for infant growth, immune function, visual acuity, and brain development (Martin et al., 2016). Linoleic and linolenic acids have significance in the quality of **myelin** in nerve fibers. The development of myelin in infancy may be critical to preventing degradation later. Not nursing is associated with higher rates of multiple sclerosis, an autoimmune disease of the central nervous system that attacks the myelin sheath (Brenton et al., 2017; Holz et al., 2022).

Parents of preterm babies produce milk with higher fatty acid content than the milk of parents of term babies. Milk of parents delivering at term is comparable worldwide, despite regional dietary variations. There do not appear to be significant correlations between a parent's DHA and AA intake and their content in the milk, demonstrating the complexities of fatty acids in human milk. Essential fatty acids are available in fish (including salmon and sardines), fish oil, beef, eggs, nuts, flax seeds, and mushrooms. Parents do not need to buy expensive supplements containing acids produced from algae and fungi.

Carbohydrates

Lactose, also known as *milk sugar*, is the major sugar in mammalian milk and appears nowhere else in nature. Human milk also contains **glycans**, or **polysaccharides**. Polysaccharides are a class of carbohydrates (e.g., starch and cellulose) consisting of several monosaccharides joined by glycosidic bonds. Glycans are polysaccharides or **oligosaccharides**—that is, a type of complex carbohydrate. Oligosaccharides are the third-largest solid in human milk, after lactose and lipids, and the most diverse component (Bardanzellu et al., 2017).

Lactose

Human milk is 7% lactose, one of the highest levels among mammals. Lactose accounts for almost all the carbohydrates in the milk and provides 40 to 45% of the energy. Its concentration increases by about 10% over the first 6 months of lactation and is the least variable nutrient in milk. Nommsen et al.'s (1991) seminal study found that the lactose content of the milk of parents who produce high volumes of milk is higher than that of lower-producing parents. More recently, Ballard and Morrow (2013) validated these findings.

Lactose is specifically designed to promote newborn growth. It enhances calcium absorption, thereby helping to prevent **rickets**. It helps supply energy to the infant's brain and keeps the growth of harmful organisms in the intestine under control. It is also essential to the development of the central nervous system. Lactose is digested slowly, producing a steady release of glucose into the bloodstream. Sucrose is the sugar often used in milk substitute formulas such as soy. It is sweeter and splits rapidly, resulting in a high peak of glucose in the infant's bloodstream. The consequences of feeding a human infant a food without lactose, such as soy formula or milk-based lactose-free formula, are not clear.

Protein

The growth and development needs of all animal species determine their milk composition. Within the animal kingdom, human milk contains the least amount of protein, which results in the slow rate of growth. Colostrum contains approximately three times more protein than the amount of protein in mature milk. The protein content of human milk seems to remain relatively constant regardless of the parent's nutritional status or dietary practices. More than 1600 different proteins in human milk provide calories, immune and growth factors, hormones, and enzymes (Dekker et al., 2024).

The protein in human milk is digested easily and readily absorbed into the bloodstream. The distribution of specific proteins is ideally suited to infant growth, enabling the young child to use the proteins with extremely high efficiency. In one study, average protein concentration was significantly higher at 17 months postpartum than 11 months postpartum (Perrin et al., 2017).

Formula manufacturers have attempted to adjust their products to match the protein content of human milk as closely as possible. Infant formula, however, lacks certain proteins found in human milk, such as lactoferrin. The infant does not use lactoferrin completely and excretes some of these amino acids in the stool. The curd in **cow's milk** is tough and rubbery, whereas the curd of human milk is soft, small, and less compact, making it easier for the infant to digest.

Whey and Casein

Whey is the clear fluid in human milk, and **casein** is the curd portion. The ratio of these components changes from 90:10 in early milk to 60:40 in mature milk and to 50:50 in late lactation. By comparison, the ratio of whey to casein in cow's milk is 20:80. Ratios in infant formula vary depending on the manufacturer.

Lactoferrin

Lactoferrin, the iron-binding protein in whey, binds to receptors in the intestines, where it is internalized by the cell and binds to the nucleus. Lactoferrin then binds to DNA sites, where it regulates gene expression. It transports iron across the surface of the cell membrane to facilitate iron absorption. It inhibits the growth of iron-dependent bacteria (such as *E. coli*) in the GI tract, thus protecting the baby against GI infections.

Lactoferrin renders intestinal iron unavailable to pathogens in the baby's gut, thereby protecting the infant from such infections as those caused by *Salmonella* and *E. coli* bacteria and *Candida albicans* fungus. Protection from lactoferrin is impaired if the baby receives any other type of feeding. Giving iron supplements to newborns can saturate lactoferrin, thus allowing proliferation of *E. coli*.

Lysozyme

Lysozyme, another whey protein, is an important active enzyme present in human milk. It increases the levels of beneficial intestinal microflora and strengthens disease resistance in infants. Lysozyme provides an antimicrobial factor against Enterobacteriaceae and gram-positive bacteria.

Cytokines

Cytokines are proteins secreted by a variety of cells, especially those found in the immune system, including granulocyte colony-stimulating factor (G-CSF). The level is higher in colostrum and is thought to stimulate gut maturation, given that receptor cells are present in the infant intestine. Milk levels of osteopontin, a multifunctional cytokine, seem to be affected by the parent's dietary intake, **body mass index (BMI)**, and smoking (Aksan et al., 2021).

Taurine

Taurine, one of the eight essential amino acids in human milk, is a principal amino acid in many mammals. Taurine is important for vision and general development. It improves fat absorption in preterm infants. Infants have limited ability to synthesize taurine. Fetuses and infants depend on the taurine supplied via the placenta or the parent's milk. Excessive ingestion of β-alanine, a supplement to improve athletic performance, can inhibit taurine transfer via the parent's milk, whereas stress can enhance it (Tochitani, 2022).

Vitamins

Generally, all vitamins are available in sufficient quantities in human milk for infant growth. Some micronutrients are dependent in part on diet. These include vitamin B complex (thiamin, riboflavin, vitamin B_6, vitamin B_{12}, choline, but not folate), vitamin A, **vitamin D**, and **vitamin K** (Allen & Dror, 2018; Dror & Allen, 2018). Colostrum is particularly rich in vitamin E, and mature milk levels are high in this nutrient as well. Because a deficiency in vitamin E in infancy can result in anemia, nursing is considered to be a preventive measure against anemia in infancy. Excessive doses of vitamin B_6 (300–600 mg per day) have been reported to reduce milk production (Hale & Krutsch, 2024). Strict vegetarians and vegans may be deficient in vitamin B_{12}, which can result in megaloblastic anemia and neurological malfunction in the newborn (vegetarian diets are discussed in **Chapter 8**).

Multivitamin supplementation during pregnancy and lactation has been recommended for many years (Jouanne et al., 2021; Martin et al., 2016). The **Centers for Disease Control and Prevention** (CDC, 2022) cautions that routine continuation of prenatal vitamins during lactation may exceed the parent's iron and folic acid needs if they receive adequate nutrients through their diet. Healthcare providers should work with lactating parents to determine appropriate dietary supplements.

Vitamin D

Vitamin D is a steroid hormone produced in the body from a prosteroid that results from direct exposure of the skin to ultraviolet B (UVB) radiation in sunlight (Pludowski et al., 2018). Health recommendations regarding the cancer risk from sunshine have significantly reduced exposure. Insufficient sun exposure has led to a significant public health problem. Vitamin D deficiency in childhood can cause **hypocalcemia**, leading to rickets, which is characterized by abnormal bone growth, muscle pain, and weakness (Carpenter et al., 2017). Vitamin D deficiency is also linked to cancer, cardiovascular disease, diabetes, hypertension, autoimmune diseases, metabolic disorders, infectious diseases, and neurological conditions (Pludowski et al., 2018).

Vitamin D is present in both the water- and fat-soluble portions of human milk. Experts question whether the amount of vitamin D in human milk is sufficient to sustain the infant. The deficiency in the milk results from the lack of adequate sunlight exposure for the parent. Sun exposure varies by season, time of day, geographic latitude and altitude, air pollution, skin pigmentation, sunscreen use, rays passing through glass or plastic, and aging. Exclusive human milk feeding without adequate sun exposure or vitamin D supplementation places babies at risk for vitamin D deficiency. Modern lifestyles frequently do not provide sufficient vitamin D production through sun exposure.

Safe Exposure to Sunlight. Adults can safely acquire sun exposure for 30 minutes daily, depending on skin type and UV index (Alfredsson et al., 2020). The WHO recommends no sun exposure for babies younger than 1 year of age. The CDC and the AAP recommend avoiding sun exposure for older babies and children by keeping them out of direct sunlight and using sunscreen. More research is needed on healthy sun exposure for infants and young children because it would be helpful in maintaining adequate vitamin D status.

Supplementing the Parent and Infant. Most international guidelines recommend that exclusively or partially nursing infants be supplemented with 400 IU/day of vitamin D during their first year of life (Heo et al., 2022; Meek et al., 2022). Despite these recommendations, DelGuidice et al. (2018) found that fewer than half of the pediatricians they surveyed recommended vitamin D supplementation for their clients. Parents can supplement their diet to increase the level of vitamin D in their milk. Supplementing 6000 IU daily long term during lactation corrects vitamin D deficiency in both parents and babies, with no adverse effects (Dawodu et al., 2019; Kazemain et al., 2022). Clinicians who care only for infants are more likely to recommend supplementing the infant, whereas those who care for both infants and parents are more likely to recommend supplementing the parent (Aul et al., 2023).

Vitamin K

Vitamin K is present in small amounts in human milk. Fetal stores of vitamin K protect the infant in utero. The WHO and AAP recommend a prophylactic dose at birth for protection until the newborn receives sufficient milk and the child's intestine matures enough to manufacture its own (Meek et al., 2022; WHO, 2017). The prophylactic vitamin K newborns routinely receive promotes blood clotting and helps them avoid **hemorrhagic disease** of the newborn. Symptoms of hemorrhagic disease include convulsions, feeding intolerance and poor sucking, irritability, and pallor. This condition may also cause bulging or full fontanels, diminished or absent neonatal reflexes, and bruising (Majid et al., 2019). It is important to ensure that families understand the protective importance of vitamin K for newborns.

Vitamin K is administered by either intramuscular (IM) injection or oral dose. Oral dosing is less distressing to the newborn than an IM injection, making it an attractive option to some parents. Oral administration (initial dosing at birth, plus two or more follow-up doses) is used in several European countries (Löwensteyn et al., 2019). Although oral vitamin K is available in the United States, it is not widely used. The Canadian pediatric and family physicians' organizations state that IM vitamin K is more effective than oral dosing. These organizations recommend using oral vitamin K only for newborns whose parents decline IM vitamin K (Ng & Loewy, 2018). Most cases of hemorrhage involve nursing babies who receive no vitamin K prophylaxis (Sankar et al., 2016; Zurynski et al., 2019).

Minerals

The mineral balance in human milk meets the baby's needs perfectly and is not significantly affected by the parent's diet. Human milk has a low percentage of minerals, which minimizes the load placed on the baby's immature kidneys. The calcium in human milk is absorbed much more efficiently than the same nutrient in infant formula. The higher ratio of phosphorus to calcium in cow's milk can interfere with calcium absorption and potentially increase the risk of developing late neonatal hypocalcemia (Gonzalez Ballesteros et al., 2017). Under stressful situations, such as during hot weather or when an infant has diarrhea, the higher mineral content of an infant formula based on cow's milk is a significant contributor to **dehydration**.

The higher solute load of infant formulas may require additional water intake by the infant to expel the solutes. Parents often misinterpret the thirst induced by this type of food as hunger. Consequently, they feed more formula to their baby instead of the water the child needs. Babies who are nursed exclusively require no water supplements—not even in hot climates—because there is little waste to flush through the kidneys. Additional feedings will satisfy the infant's need for more fluids in hot weather. Part of the higher weight gains in artificially fed infants and subsequent excess weight in childhood and adulthood may result from greater sodium and water retention during infancy.

Iron

Iron is the most abundant metal in the human body. During the final 6 to 8 weeks of pregnancy, a healthy nonanemic expectant parent lays down iron stores to provide the baby with enough iron through their milk for the first few months postpartum. Blood from the umbilical cord also contributes iron that is stored in the infant's liver. Newborn iron stores remain sufficient until 4 to 6 months after birth or even later. Although iron is present in the milk in only small quantities, the level is sufficient to meet the iron requirements of the exclusively nursing full-term infant to approximately 6 months of age. A preterm infant may receive insufficient iron stores in utero and need iron supplementation.

Hemoglobin is the iron-containing portion of the red blood cell that carries oxygen to all parts of the body. The healthy infant's hemoglobin level is high at birth (18–20 g per dL) and then decreases rapidly as the child's body adjusts to extrauterine life. By 4 months of age, levels of hemoglobin typically range between 10.2 and 15 g per dL. Over this same period, the type of hemoglobin changes from a fetal to an adult form. Adult hemoglobin is more efficient in delivering oxygen to the tissues. Although the amount of hemoglobin decreases, the efficiency of each gram increases as this change takes place.

The iron in human milk is absorbed more efficiently than the iron in cow's milk, partly because of the high amount of vitamin C in human milk. Babies absorb 60% of the iron in human milk, compared with only 4% of the iron in infant formula. Routine supplementation of iron is of questionable value and may even be detrimental to a nursing infant. Lactoferrin, for example, loses its ability to inhibit the growth of bacteria when saturated with **exogenous** iron (Campos et al., 2013). When infants start receiving complementary foods while continuing to nurse, consuming iron-rich foods helps to maintain their iron status.

Fluoride

In communities with fluoridated drinking water, nursing babies receive **fluoride** through the milk. Nursing beyond 6 months protects them against developing fluorosis in their permanent teeth (Rojanaworarit et al., 2023). If the family's water supply contains less than 0.3 ppm of fluoride, infant fluoride supplementation is recommended after the age of 6 months. During the development of primary and secondary teeth, fluoride supplements ingested by the infant reduce cavities by 50% to 60%. Families are encouraged to learn their local community's water fluoridation levels, especially those with well water.

Trace Elements

Human milk contains a myriad of trace elements, including boron, chromium, cobalt, copper, iodine, zinc, manganese, selenium, silicon, sodium, aluminum, and titanium. Scientists continue to study the significance of these components. Concentrations of trace elements in the milk vary among populations' geography and lifestyle. They also vary between preterm and mature milk and diminish as lactation progresses (Klein et al., 2017). Some trace elements are associated with neurodevelopment in infants (Jia et al., 2022). Sodium may be associated with nursing self-efficacy (Noh & Lee, 2021). The increased **bioavailability** of zinc in the milk can be lifesaving in the inherited zinc-deficiency disorder known as **acrodermatitis enteropathica**.

Nitrogen

Nitrogen compounds in human milk are of key interest to researchers. **Nucleotides** in the form of non-protein nitrogen are an integral part of the immune system. These agents play key roles in many biological processes, including promoting optimal functioning and growth of the GI and immune systems. Nucleotides act as the host defense against bacteria, viruses, and parasites, as well as various malignancies. They are relatively absent in cow's milk and are added to infant formula (Albertos et al., 2023; De Almagro García et al., 2017; Hodgkinson et al., 2022). Other milk components under study include **prostaglandins**, bile salts, and epidermal growth factor (EGF).

Enzymes

More than 20 identified enzymes in human milk aid in the breakdown of macronutrients for easier absorption and provide additional bioactivity and protective effects to the milk (Carr et al., 2021). One enzyme, **lipase**, is essential for digesting fat and making it available to the infant as energy. Lipolytic activity is much higher in human milk than in bovine milk. Bile salt–stimulated lipase (BSSL) is the secondary lipase enzyme and comprises 1% of the total protein in human milk. BSSL is found only in the milk of higher primates. It is very important for the digestion of **lipids** by human babies. The fatty acids released by lipase and BSSL may also have an **antibacterial** effect. More research is needed into the full effects of enzyme activity as protective factors in infant gut and immune health (Carr et al., 2021).

Growth Factors

Growth factors enhance the infant's development and the maturation of the immune system, the central nervous system, and organs such as the skin. Digestive enzymes and many other important enzymes protect babies born with immature or defective enzyme systems. EGF is present in colostrum, preterm milk, and term milk. EFG promotes the growth and healing of gut mucosa. Vascular endothelial growth factor (VEGF) is present in human milk and has a role in angiogenesis (blood vessel growth and development). Concentrations are higher in preterm milk compared with milk for term babies (Szyller et al., 2024). In preterm babies, it may be significant in helping their guts mature more efficiently.

Lactase

Lactase in the milk converts lactose into simple sugars that the infant can assimilate easily. A deficiency in lactase can result in **lactose intolerance**, a condition that generally occurs because of diminishing activity of intestinal lactase after weaning. A person who is lactose intolerant is unable to digest milk sugar (lactose). The condition is more prevalent in adults and is rare in children younger than 3 years. As discussed earlier, lactose helps prevent the development of rickets and aids in calcium absorption and brain development.

Hormones

Increasingly sophisticated analytic methods have produced an explosion in the discovery and evolving understanding of the hormones in human milk. Over 300 **peptides** have been identified in human milk (Dekker et al., 2024). Peptide hormone levels change over time which may explain the large differences in rates of weight gain between nursing and artificially fed infants (Logan et al., 2019; Mazzocchi et al., 2019).

Cholecystokinin

Cholecystokinin (CCK) is a digestive hormone found in the digestive tract and brain. It is a peptide hormone of the GI system responsible for stimulating the digestion of fat and protein. CCK is triggered by the baby's sucking and may be responsible for the sleepiness parents and babies experience while nursing. Release of CCK was thought to create the feeling of satiety in babies. It is, however, not found in significant levels in human milk. It appears that **leptin**, discussed in the next section, registers satiety.

Thyroid

Human milk contains essential thyroid hormones that are absent in cow's milk and conventional infant formulas. These hormones may be responsible for preventing hypothyroidism, masking diagnosis, and providing protection until the baby weans. More protective factors are discussed in this section.

Leptin

Leptin is known as the "satiety hormone." It signals fullness and helps form neural circuits controlling food intake and fatness later in life. Leptin may play a role in helping newborns regulate their intake, as well as affecting long-term body weight and energy regulation. Artificially fed infants have much lower levels of leptin than nursing infants, with higher BMI in childhood. Thus, low leptin levels in infancy may potentially predict obesity in later life (Mazzocchi et al., 2019).

Ghrelin

Ghrelin, known as the "hunger hormone," is a peptide hormone that signals feelings of hunger. It is present in high levels in human milk (Zamanillo et al., 2019). Ghrelin is higher in foremilk than in hindmilk, whereas triglycerides and leptin are higher in the hindmilk. This difference may help nursing babies register feelings of fullness and regulate their intake (Larrosa Haro et al., 2019).

Adiponectin

Adipokine (cell-signaling proteins secreted by fat tissue) peptide hormones identified in human milk include **adiponectin** and leptin. Adiponectin regulates lipid and glucose metabolism and has anti-inflammatory effects (Choi et al., 2020; van Rossem et al., 2019). It is inversely related to fatness and insulin resistance in blood levels. Levels of adiponectin in human milk change over time. Studies have found both increases (Rio-Aige et al., 2023) and decreases (Brunner, 2014). Adiponectin in the milk may affect infant growth and development and possibly help preterm babies adapt metabolically (Gila-Diaz et al., 2019).

Other Peptides

Resistin is a protein peptide in human milk that is secreted by fat cells. It plays a role in fetal growth rate and aids in the baby's metabolic development (Kratzsch et al., 2018). Human milk contains **obestatin**, apelin, and nesfatin-1 (Filibeli et al., 2022; Suwaydi et al., 2021). Obestatin appears to regulate sleep, increase pancreas function, and reduce appetite. Apelin and nesfatin-1 could be important for growth, energy, and maturation of the newborn gut. These peptides are higher in mature milk than in colostrum and lower in the milk of parents with gestational diabetes.

Other peptides identified in human milk include copeptin, adropin, and irisin, associated with energy homeostasis and diabetes, as well as preptin, salusin, and hepcidin. These peptides may influence metabolic pathway regulation and postnatal organ growth. Additional peptides—Glucagon-like peptide-1 (GLP-1) and peptide YY (PYY)—may affect appetite and thus self-regulation of food intake (Larson Meyer et al., 2021). Research exploring the roles of these newly discovered components of human milk is published almost daily, especially in the studies of metabolic programming and obesity. Studies of specific components demonstrate that each parent's milk differs slightly because of individual genetic codes—further evidence that each infant receives milk uniquely made for them.

Immunological Protection

Human milk contains a wide variety of soluble, cellular, and **humoral factors** that affect maturation of the body's systems. These factors protect the infant against a host of diseases and confer lifelong immunities. As infants grow and their bodies begin to produce antibodies, they develop their own **active immunity**. Through this means, children are protected against bacterial infections, viral infections, protozoans, and allergies. The longer infants nurse, the greater the protection they receive. References for these protections are cited in **Table 9-3**.

Passive and Active Immunity

At birth, the infant is suddenly exposed to a variety of microorganisms to which the parent is already immune. This **passive immunity** transfers to the baby across the placenta before birth and in the colostrum and milk after birth. When a new microorganism enters the environment, the parent most likely produces corresponding antibodies to it. These antibodies pass

Table 9-3 Protection for the Child Against Infections

Infection	Evidence
Inside the gastrointestinal (GI) tract	
Gastroenterocolitis	Yang et al. (2019)
Diarrhea	Prentice et al. (2022); Sudarma et al. (2021)
Outside the GI tract	
Meningitis	Lyon and Doran (2022)
Otitis media	Al-Nawaiseh et al. (2022)
Respiratory syncytial virus (RSV)	Mineva et al. (2023); Tonon et al. (2024)
Rotavirus	Krawczyk et al. (2016)
Sepsis	Schreiner et al. (2023)
Respiratory infections (including sinus)	Hossain and Mihrshahi (2022)
Urinary tract infections	Frank et al. (2019)

to the baby through the milk. Protection from human milk extends beyond common childhood illnesses and illnesses of the parent to the infant's immediate environment. As the child grows, active immunity develops.

Antibody Response

Although some viruses pass into the milk, the presence of antibodies to counteract them offsets the potential harm to the baby. Antibodies in the milk are highly targeted against infectious agents in the environment, those to which the infant is likely to be exposed shortly after birth. When a parent contracts an infection, whether it be a cold, fever, or more serious illness, their body responds by producing antibodies in the milk that help protect the baby. The parent's body responds to and "remembers" for years specific infections it has encountered. Researchers believe this transmission may confer passive immunity on the infant (Myles & Datta, 2021; Singh et al., 2021). Additionally, parents receiving **vaccines** pass antibodies to the infant through their milk (Brady et al., 2018).

Another mechanism of disease transmission from parent to baby is through close contact, such as touching and through mouth and nose contact. When a nursing parent contracts an illness, it is likely that the baby was exposed through contact during the most contagious period. Therefore, the most effective treatment for the baby is to continue nursing while receiving any necessary medication. Parents can decrease the baby's exposure to the disease with careful handwashing before contact and, in extreme cases, by wearing a mask over their nose and mouth. A parent who develops a cold or fever can practice good hygiene and limit facial contact with the baby during the infectious period. Urge parents to rest and follow the treatment plan prescribed by their caregiver so that they can return to good health quickly. The breast itself also appears to produce antibodies to the organisms passed into it by the sucking infant. The mammary gland produces immunoglobulins locally and passes them to the infant in the milk, thereby protecting the child from the harmful effects of disease organisms.

Immunization Response

Human milk contains antibodies capable of enhancing infant **antibody response**. Nursing increases the probability of the infant's immune response after vaccination (Teni Nurlatifah et al., 2021). For example, the humoral response to measles is positively correlated with longer nursing duration (Ferreira et al., 2018).

Immunological Factors in Human Milk

Nursing confers both current and long-term immune-modulating effects on the child's developing cellular immune system (Garofoli et al., 2023; Le Doare et al., 2018). Ongoing research continues to uncover more details about the numerous factors in human milk that aid in protecting the infant from disease. **Mucins** protect against several viruses. Oligosaccharides serve as prebiotics to provide digestive protection. IgA provides GI protection. High levels of antibodies provide allergy protection. Key areas of current research in human milk focus on **epigenetics**, metabolic programming, and stem cell function.

Mucins

Mucins are high-molecular-weight glycoproteins. They are involved in many immune functions, including shielding the epithelium against pathogenic infection, regulating cellular signaling, and gene transcription. Mucin type 1 (MUC1) and type 4 (MUC4) are the primary mucins in human milk. MUC1 levels are significantly higher in colostrum than in mature milk. Mucins in the milk have a role in regulating inflammatory response and T-cell response. They protect against *Salmonella*, **rotavirus**, and human immunodeficiency virus (HIV) (Francese et al., 2023; Wu et al., 2023). They have also been linked to protection against **necrotizing enterocolitis (NEC)** (Wu et al., 2019) and *E. coli* (Wakinaka et al., 2013).

Oligosaccharides

Oligosaccharides are highly abundant in and unique to human milk. They represent the third-largest class of human milk components, after lactose and lipids. To date, up to 200 oligosaccharides have been identified in human milk (Sánchez et al., 2021). They comprise the once mysterious "bifidus factor" effect identified over 50 years ago that develops a healthy intestinal microbiota composition. *Lactobacillus* is present in high concentrations in both colostrum and mature milk (Bardanzellu et al., 2017). *Lactobacillus bifidus*, also called *Bifidobacterium*, represents the dominant microbiota of nursing infants and may protect newborn health.

Oligosaccharides are resistant to being digested and thus serve as prebiotics to populate the infant colon (Milani et al., 2017). Human milk oligosaccharides are antimicrobials that serve as decoys. They prevent pathogens from binding to receptor sites in the gut and lower the risk of viral, bacterial, and parasitic infections. Oligosaccharides provide protection throughout the baby's digestive system, passing into the stool and urine. This protects the baby against **diarrhea** and respiratory infections. Human milk oligosaccharides significantly lower the risk of NEC (Bering et al., 2018) and provide the baby with sialic acid, a potentially essential nutrient for brain and cognitive development (Bering et al., 2018; Liu et al., 2023).

Oligosaccharides vary among parents and over the course of lactation. Immunologically active factors may help prevent transmission of HIV from HIV-infected parents to their nursing babies, helping to explain the low transmission rates despite the babies' exposure. HIV-infected parents with high levels of oligosaccharides are less likely to transmit HIV via nursing (Doherty et al., 2018; Morozov et al., 2018).

The prebiotic and probiotic functions of human milk oligosaccharides have been studied extensively. **Prebiotics** are nondigestible food ingredients or supplements that selectively stimulate the favorable growth or activity of indigenous probiotic bacteria in the digestive system. Prebiotics for preterm infants are associated with significant decreases in sepsis and mortality rates, the length of hospital stays, and the time to full enteral feeding. No lower rates were demonstrated for NEC morbidity or feeding intolerance (Chi et al., 2019). A Cochrane review concluded that there is no reliable evidence that treating hyperbilirubinemia with prebiotics is effective (Armanian et al., 2019). **Probiotics** are supplements or foods containing viable microorganisms that cause alterations in the microflora of the host. These live microorganisms are thought to be beneficial to the health of the body. Lactic acid bacteria and bifidobacteria are the most common types of microbes used as probiotics. Certain yeasts and bacilli are also available for this purpose. There has been explosive research and marketing of prebiotics and probiotics in artificial baby milks and other foods, including preterm infant and toddler foods (Borewicz et al., 2019; Slattery et al., 2016).

Immunoglobulin A

The presence of IgA in colostrum and human milk protects the infant's GI tract against penetration by organisms and antigens. This immunoglobulin, probably the most important of the **antiviral** defense factors, is at its highest level immediately after birth. IgA binds to bacteria and prevents those pathogens from binding to receptor sites and invading the gut. Although it does not kill the bacteria, IgA surrounds them and prevents them from attacking or attaching to receptor sites, thereby preventing their invasion of the body. Levels of IgA remain relatively high for at least 6 or 7 months. IgA and sialic acid survive passage through the GI tract. They are found in much higher concentrations in the stools of nursing infants than in those of formula fed infants.

White Blood Cells

Colostrum and human milk contain living white blood cells (leukocytes) in the form of **phagocytes** (**neutrophils** and **macrophages**) and **lymphocytes**. Phagocytes are cells that engulf particles such as bacteria, other microorganisms, aged red blood cells, and foreign matter. Neutrophils are short-lived first responders that protect against foreign substances. Macrophages, the predominant phagocytes, release IgA and engulf and digest foreign cells and bacteria. The thymus, a small gland in the lymphatic system, is especially active in infancy and childhood. Its main function is to develop immature lymphocytes into immunocompetent T cells. The T cells recognize, target, and destroy specific foreign agents to help the immune system fight disease and infection, a process known as cell-mediated immunity. Human milk has a significant positive impact on thymic development (Huang et al., 2021).

Allergy Protection

Because there are almost no antibodies in the immature intestine of a newborn infant, the wall of the intestine is susceptible to invasion by foreign proteins. The IgA in human milk provides antiabsorptive protection to the lining of the infant's intestine. This effect shields the surface from the absorption of foreign protein and from bacterial invasion. Increased gut maturation prevents foreign proteins from entering the infant's system. Human milk nutrients such as zinc and long-chain polyunsaturated fatty acids aid in the development of the infant's immune response. Human milk is important for the development of the GI tract.

Allergens pass through the milk and may cause reactions such as spitting, vomiting, gas, diarrhea, **colicky behavior**, or skin rash. Human milk protects infants until the intestinal tract and immune system mature, regardless of allergic tendencies. An infant with galactosemia may have allergic symptoms in response to foods ingested by the parent and passed through the milk. These infants cannot process galactose (milk sugar) and cannot receive human milk. Although nursing does not eliminate all possible food allergies, formula feeding greatly increases their incidence and hastens their onset. Nursing confers the most protection against asthma development (Rosas-Salazar et al., 2022). **Chapter 10** discusses allergies and asthma, and **Chapter 27** discusses galactosemia.

Epigenetics

Colostrum and mature milk contain thousands of distinct bioactive molecules that protect against infection and inflammation. These components help the baby's immune system develop. They initiate metabolic functions (gene expression) that have lifelong health implications. Epigenetics studies factors that influence gene expression—the epigenome. The epigenome is the cellular layer that sits on top of the genome and is the mechanism that turns genes "on" or "off." Human milk microbiota contributes to the establishment of the infant's gut microbiome, which is implicated in brain development via epigenetic modifications (Gialeli et al., 2023). Nutrition received in the early postnatal period affects the endocrine system's response throughout life.

Stem Cells

Mammary stem cell research is an exciting arena that continues to grow. Human milk contains cells that display many of the properties typical of stem cells (Ninkina et al., 2019). Stem progenitor cells comprise up to 6% of human milk cells and migrate to the neonate's organs. Stem cells may play pivotal roles in a baby's immune development, growth and repair of intestinal tissue, and disease protection (Molès et al., 2018).

Human milk stem cells provide a growing alternative to embryonic stem cells for research. Stem cells isolated from human milk could potentially be "reprogrammed" to form many types of human tissues and provide a noninvasive source of stem cells for stem cell therapy (Pacheco et al., 2019; Tripathy et al., 2019). These cells in the milk decrease significantly as lactation progresses, with the greatest amount in days 3 to 5. This decrease may result from the increased quantity of milk, resulting in a relative decrease in the cells per unit of measured volume (Mane et al., 2022).

Anti-infective Protection

Human milk protects the infant, providing anti-infective agents and minimizing inflammation. The milk contains several anti-infective agents that maintain a very low bacterial level for many hours. Consequently, it destroys bacteria in the infant's GI tract before they affect the infant. Milk components also coat the GI tract, thereby preventing offending organisms and molecules from entering the infant's system. Human milk protects against infections both inside and outside the GI tract (Table 9-3), including childhood cancers (**Table 9-4**) and a variety of other conditions (**Table 9-5**). **Chapter 24** discusses the protection human milk provides to the preterm infant against NEC. Common conditions for which human milk provides protection are explored in more depth in the next section.

Otitis Media

Otitis media, or middle ear infection, is one of the most common infant infections. Human milk has a protective impact on the occurrence of otitis media in the first 3 years of life (Al-Nawaiseh et al., 2022; Prentice, 2022). The longer the baby nurses, the greater the protection the baby receives. Exclusive nursing for 6 months provides the greatest protection (van Ingen et al., 2021).

Diarrhea

Diarrhea is the second-leading cause of death in children under 5 years of age. The WHO (2019) estimates

Table 9-4 Protection for the Child Against Childhood Cancers

Type of Cancer	Evidence
Hodgkin's disease	Wang et al. (2013)
Leukemia and lymphoma	Ajrouche et al. (2015); Amitay and Keinan-Boker (2015); Arellano-Galindo et al. (2017); Gao et al. (2018); Güngör et al. (2019a); Küçükçongar et al. (2015); Ledesma-Martínez et al. (2019); Puumala et al. (2013); Rudant et al. (2015)
Soft tissue sarcomas, including rhabdomyosarcoma	Lupo et al. (2014)
Solid tumors (brain tumors, neuroblastoma, soft tissue sarcomas, germ cell tumors, renal tumor, bone tumor, retinoblastoma, hepatoblastoma)	Küçükçongar et al. (2015); Rios et al. (2016)

Table 9-5 Protection for the Child Against Chronic, Autoimmune, Neurological, Mental Health, and Other Conditions

Disease/Condition	Evidence
Allergies	Koukou et al. (2023); Rosas-Salazar et al. (2022); Wang et al. (2022); Zuurveld et al. (2020)
Arthritis (juvenile idiopathic and rheumatoid)	Alonso S, et al. (2023); Rocha et al. (2019)
Asthma	Kumar and Devgan (2021); Wilson et al. (2022)
Autism	Ghozy et al. (2020); Huang et al. (2021); Jenabi et al. (2023); Tseng et al. (2019)
Eczema/dermatitis	Mohammed Abouda and Berair (2023); Royal and Gray (2020)
High cholesterol and heart disease	Singhal (2019); Umer et al. (2019); Wong et al. (2018)
Hypertension	Lin et al. (2023); Umer et al. (2019)
Type 1 diabetes	Güngör et al. (2019b)
Type 2 diabetes	Bjerregaard et al. (2019)
Multiple sclerosis	Brenton et al. (2017); Holz et al. (2022)
Nonalcoholic fatty liver disease	Ayonrinde et al. (2017)
Obesity (childhood, adolescent, adult)	Pena-Leon et al. (2022); Qiao et al. (2020); Singhal (2019)
Pyloric stenosis	Kim et al. (2021)

that around 370,000 children under age 5 died in 2019 from this preventable and treatable disease. Human milk protects infants from digestive infections and decreases the severity of diarrhea (Nuzhat et al., 2019). Early initiation of nursing and avoidance of prelacteal feeds lower the prevalence of diarrhea. All babies, including those in the industrialized world, benefit from the protection human milk provides against diarrhea.

Obesity Protection

A person weighing more than what is considered healthy for their height is classified as overweight or obese, based on BMI. *Overweight* is defined as having a BMI greater than or equal to 25. Obesity describes a BMI over 30. Childhood and adult obesity are major health problems worldwide, causing staggering health and economic costs to society. Heart disease, stroke, type 2 diabetes, and certain types of cancer—leading causes of preventable death—are linked to obesity. A significant portion of the risk for adult metabolic conditions results from prenatal exposure. Thus, a parent's health during pregnancy may program the infant's risk for adverse long-term health outcomes, including cardiovascular disease or obesity (Geddes & Perrella, 2019; Schoppa et al., 2019).

Obesity Rates

Obesity is a global health crisis. Obesity nearly tripled worldwide between 1975 and 2016, with about 13% of the global adult population obese in 2016. In 2022, an estimated 37 million children under the age of 5 years were overweight or obese (WHO, 2024). Children and adolescents with obesity are at increased risk of becoming obese as adults. A 4-year-old child with obesity has a 20% chance of becoming obese as an adult, and a teenager with obesity has as much as an 80% chance of being obese as an adult (CDC, 2024).

Obesity Protection from Lactation

Lactation is associated with a lower risk of early obesity in children aged 2 to 6 years (Qiao et al., 2020; Rito et al., 2019). Protection against early childhood overweight and obesity through nursing is dose dependent, with longer exclusivity and duration conferring greater protection. Appetite peptides and hormones in human milk, such as ghrelin, leptin, and adiponectin, help the infant register satiety and self-regulate intake (Juan Castell et al., 2022).

Human milk helps the baby's immune system mature and protects against the onset of type 1 diabetes. The establishment of a healthy gut microbiome is also protective against diabetes development (Gurung et al., 2020; Zaky et al., 2021). The peptide hormones in human milk that promote appetite self-regulation help prevent excess weight gain during childhood and provide further protection against the development of type 2 diabetes (Horta & de Lima, 2019; Prentice, 2022).

Summary

Human milk is the biologically normal nutrition for the human infant. It is specific to the infant's age, and its composition changes throughout lactation to meet the child's changing needs. Researchers continue to uncover new functions of the many components in this rich and complex substance. Because of the health risks of not nursing, caregivers have a responsibility to promote human milk for all babies. The WHO, AAP, Canadian Paediatric Society, and other professional associations across the globe translate this responsibility into strong statements in support of nursing through the child's first year and beyond. You can encourage parents to regard nursing as the healthiest nutritional start possible for their children.

What You Learned—At a Glance

Conversation Starters with Parents

- What differences do you notice in your milk production throughout the day?
- How can you make sure your baby receives enough fat in your milk?
- How important is health protection for your baby in your feeding decision?
- How important is health protection for you in your feeding decision?

Health Protection for Parents

- Decreased risk of postpartum hemorrhage
- Protection from lactation hormones against stress
- Quicker return to prepregnancy weight and lower postpartum BMI
- Natural delay in ovulation
- Decreased risks of breast and ovarian cancer, osteoporosis, and type 2 diabetes
- Decreased risks of hypertension, stroke, hyperlipidemia, and cardiovascular disease

Colostrum

- Consists of residual materials in the breast mixed with newly formed milk
- Is richer in sodium, potassium, chloride, protein, fat-soluble vitamins, and minerals than mature milk
- Contains less fat and lactose than mature milk
- Has high concentrations of IgA, IgG, and IgM
- Engulfs and digests disease organisms and aids in rapid gut closure

Milk Volume and Composition

- Depends on regular removal
- Is most plentiful in the morning hours
- Meets ¾ of an infant's nutrient needs through the first 12 months
- Has at least 8 oz of daily output during the second year

- Changes in composition throughout lactation and during a day or feeding
- Is higher in immunoglobulins and protein during the first several weeks

Fat

- Varies from lactating parent to parent and feeding to feeding
- Is inversely proportional to the length of time between feedings
- Is related to the degree of breast fullness
- Decreases in later months of lactation
- May be up to four to five times higher at the end of a feeding
- Promotes optimal neural and visual development through hundreds of fatty acids

Lactose

- Enhances calcium absorption
- Supplies energy to the infant's brain
- Protects the infant's intestines from harmful organisms
- Is essential to development of the central nervous system
- Is the most constant of all milk constituents

Other Components in Milk

- Oligosaccharides prevent pathogens from binding to receptor sites in the gut.
- Protein level is relatively constant, regardless of the parent's diet.
- Curd is soft, small, less compact, and easy to digest.
- Lysozyme increases over the course of lactation and protects against Enterobacteriaceae and gram-positive bacteria.
- Vitamins are present in sufficient amounts if the parent has ample levels of vitamins D, K, and B.
- Healthy, nonanemic parents lay down sufficient iron stores for the first few months of nursing.
- Nucleotides promote the functioning and growth of the GI and immune systems.
- Peptides, including ghrelin, leptin, and obestatin, affect sensations of hunger and satiety, enabling infant self-regulation of appetite.
- Sucking triggers the release of digestive hormones, including CCK, promoting sleepiness in parents and babies.
- Stem cells are present in human milk.

Lifelong Protection to the Infant Against Disease

- Destroys bacteria in the GI tract
- Provides antiabsorptive protection for intestinal lining
- Protects against common cold, fever, and serious illness
- Protects against upper and lower respiratory infections, otitis media, diarrheal disease, urinary tract infections, sepsis, rotavirus, meningitis, leukemia, lymphoma, Hodgkin's disease, and neuroblastoma
- Lowers risk of breast cancer, chronic and autoimmune diseases, hypertension, high cholesterol, and heart disease
- Decreases risk of NEC and incidence of asthma
- Causes child to produce antibodies against organisms passed into the breast from sucking

Other Infant Protection

- Nursing increases IQ (dose dependent).
- Thyroid hormones prevent hypothyroidism and protect the hypothyroid baby until weaning.
- IgA protects the GI tract and is the most important of the antiviral defense factors.
- Lactase and lipase protect babies born with immature or defective enzyme systems.
- Lactase converts lactose into simple sugars that can be assimilated easily by the infant.
- Lysozyme breaks down bacteria in the bowel.
- Lactoferrin inhibits the growth of pathogenic bacteria, including *E. coli* (effects are reduced when saturated with exogenous iron).
- Bifidobacteria discourage the growth of pathogenic bacteria, including *E. coli*.
- Antibodies enhance the infant's antibody response.
- Mucins protect against bacterial infections.

References

Abate A, et al. Relationship between breastfeeding and malocclusion: a systematic review of the literature. *Nutrients*. 2020; 12(12):3688.

Ajmera VH, et al. Longer lactation duration is associated with decreased prevalence of non-alcoholic fatty liver disease in women. *J Hepatol*. 2019;70(1):126–132.

Ajrouche R, et al. Childhood acute lymphoblastic leukaemia and indicators of early immune stimulation: the Estelle study (SFCE). *Br J Cancer*. 2015;112(6):1017–1026.

Aksan A, et al. Osteopontin levels in human milk are related to maternal nutrition and infant health and growth. *Nutrients*. 2021;13(8):2670.

Albertos I, et al. Market research of infant formula milks in Spain. *Food Sci Nutr.* 2023;11(12):7957–7966.

Alfredsson L, et al. Insufficient sun exposure has become a real public health problem. *Int J Environ Res Public Health.* 2020; 17(14):5014.

Alimi R, et al. The association of breastfeeding with a reduced risk of postpartum depression: a systematic review and meta-analysis. *Breastfeed Med.* 2022;17(4):290–296.

Allen LH, Dror DK. Introduction to current knowledge on micronutrients in human milk: adequacy, analysis, and need for research. *Adv Nutr.* 2018;9(suppl 1):275S–277S.

Al-Nawaiseh FK, et al. Breastfeeding initiation and duration and acute otitis media among children less than two years of age in Jordan: results from a case-control study. *BMC Pediatr.* 2022; 22(1):370.

Alonso S, et al. Are patients with axial spondyloarthritis who were breastfed protected against the development of severe disease? *J Clin Med.* 2023;12(5):1863.

Alotiby A, et al. The relationship between breastfeeding and autoimmune diseases among children in Makkah City. *IJMRHS.* 2021; 10(8):107–113. https://www.ijmrhs.com/medical-research/the-relationship-between-breastfeeding-and-autoimmune-diseases-among-children-in-makkah-city-74378.html

American College of Obstetricians and Gynecologists. ACOG Committee Opinion No. 756 summary: optimizing support for breastfeeding as part of obstetric practice. *Obstet Gynecol.* 2018; 132(4):1086–1088.

Amiel Castro R, et al. Breastfeeding, prenatal depression and children's IQ and behaviour: a test of a moderation model. *BMC Pregnancy Childbirth.* 2021;21(1):62.

Amitay EL, Keinan-Boker L. Breastfeeding and childhood leukemia incidence: a meta-analysis and systematic review. *JAMA Pediatr.* 2015;169(6):e151025.

Argov-Argaman N, et al. Human milk fatty acids composition is affected by maternal age. *J Matern Fetal Neonatal Med.* 2017; 30(1):34–37.

Arellano-Galindo J, et al. Infectious agents in childhood leukemia. *Arch Med Res.* 2017 May;48(4):305–313.

Armanian AM, et al. Prebiotics for the prevention of hyperbilirubinaemia in neonates. *Cochrane Database Syst Rev.* 2019;8: CD012731.

Arriaga ME, et al. The preventable burden of breast cancers for premenopausal and postmenopausal women in Australia: a pooled cohort study. *Int J Cancer.* 2019;145(9):2383–2394.

Aul AJ, et al. Infant and maternal vitamin D supplementation: clinician perspectives and practices. *J Am Board Fam Med.* 2023; 36(1):95–104.

Ayonrinde OT, et al. Infant nutrition and maternal obesity influence the risk of non-alcoholic fatty liver disease in adolescents. *J Hepatol.* 2017;67(3):568–576.

Babic A, et al. Association between breastfeeding and ovarian cancer risk. *JAMA Oncol.* 2020;6(6):e200421.

Ballard O, Morrow AL. Human milk composition: nutrients and bioactive factors. *Pediatr Clin North Am.* 2013;60(1):49–74.

Bardanzellu F, et al. "Omics" in human colostrum and mature milk: looking to old data with new eyes. *Nutrients.* 2017;9(8).

Bergman NJ. Neonatal stomach volume and physiology suggest feeding at 1-h intervals. *Acta Paediatr.* 2013;102(8):773–777.

Bering SB. Human milk oligosaccharides to prevent gut dysfunction and necrotizing enterocolitis in preterm neonates. *Nutrients.* 2018;10(10).

Berlanga-Macías C, et al. Relationship between exclusive breastfeeding and cardiorespiratory fitness in children and adolescents: a meta-analysis. *Scand J Med Sci Sports.* 2020;30(5): 828–836.

Bjerregaard LG, et al. Breastfeeding duration in infancy and adult risks of type 2 diabetes in a high-income country. *Matern Child Nutr.* 2019;15(4):e12869.

Bobiński R, Bobińska J. Fatty acids of human milk—a review. *Int J Vitam Nutr* Res. 2022 Jul;92(3–4):280–291.

Borewicz K, et al. The effect of prebiotic fortified infant formulas on microbiota composition and dynamics in early life. *Sci Rep.* 2019;9(1):2434.

Bottin JH, et al. Food insecurity and maternal diet influence human milk composition between the infant's birth and 6 months after birth in Central-Africa. *Nutrients.* 2022;14(19):4015.

Brady RC, et al. Randomized trial comparing the safety and antibody responses to live attenuated versus inactivated influenza vaccine when administered to breastfeeding women. *Vaccine.* 2018;36(31):4663–4671.

Brenton JN, et al. Breastfeeding during infancy is associated with a lower future risk of pediatric multiple sclerosis. *Pediatr Neurol.* 2017;77:67–72.

Brunner S. Breast milk leptin and adiponectin in relation to infant body composition up to 2 years. *Pediatr Obes.* April 14, 2014;10(1):67–73.

Bzikowska A, et al. Correlation between human milk composition and maternal nutritional status. *Rocz Panstw Zakl Hig.* 2018;69(4):363–367.

Calik-Ksepka A, et al. Lactational amenorrhea: neuroendocrine pathways controlling fertility and bone turnover. *Int J Mol Sci.* 2022;23(3):1633.

Campos LF, et al. Effects of human milk fortifier with iron on the bacteriostatic properties of breast milk. J *Pediatr (Rio J).* 2013;89(4):394–399.

Carpenter TO, et al. Rickets. *Nat Rev Dis Primers.* 2017;3:17101.

Carr L, et al. Role of human milk bioactives on infants' gut and immune health. *Front. Immunol.* 2021;12:1–17.

Centers for Disease Control and Prevention. Breastfeeding maternal diet: should mothers take a multivitamin while breastfeeding? May 17, 2022. https://www.cdc.gov/breastfeeding/breastfeeding-special-circumstances/diet-and-micronutrients/maternal-diet.html

Centers for Disease Control and Prevention. Adult obesity facts. May 14, 2024. https://www.cdc.gov/obesity/adult-obesity-facts/index.html Chetwynd EM, et al. Cumulative lactation and onset of hypertension in African-American women. *Am J Epidemiol.* 2017;186(8):927–934.

Chi C, et al. Effects of prebiotics on sepsis, necrotizing enterocolitis, mortality, feeding intolerance, time to full enteral feeding, length of hospital stay, and stool frequency in preterm infants: a meta-analysis. *Eur J Clin Nutr.* 2019;73(5):657–670.

Cho S, Han E. Association of breastfeeding duration with dyslipidemia in women aged over 20 years: Korea National Health and Nutrition Examination Survey 2010–2014. *J Clin Lipidol.* 2018;12(2):437–446.

Choi HM, et al. Multifaceted physiological roles of adiponectin in inflammation and diseases. *Int J Mol Sci.* 2020;21(4):1219.

Czank C, et al. Chapter 4: Human milk composition: fat. In: Hale T, Hartmann P, eds. *Hale and Hartmann's Textbook of Human Lactation.* New York: Springer Publishing; 2017.

Dastmalchi F, et al. Assessment of human milk in the era of precision health. *Current Opinion in Clinical Nutrition and Metabolic Care.* 2022; 25(5): 292–297.

Dawodu A, et al. The effect of high-dose postpartum maternal vitamin D supplementation alone compared with maternal plus infant vitamin D supplementation in breastfeeding infants in a high-risk population. a randomized controlled trial. *Nutrients.* 2019;11(7):1632.

De Almagro García MC, et al. New ingredients in infant formula. Health and functional benefits. *Nutr Hosp.* 2017;34(suppl 4): 8–12.

Dekker PM, et al. Network analysis of the proteome and peptidome sheds light on human milk as a biological system. *Sci Rep* 2024;14:7569.

DelGiudice NJ, et al. Vitamin D prescribing practices in primary care pediatrics: underpinnings from the health belief model and use of web-based Delphi technique for instrument validity. *J Pediatr Health Care*. 2018;32(6):536–547.

Doherty AM, et al. Human milk oligosaccharides and associations with immune-mediated disease and infection in childhood: a systematic review. *Front Pediatr*. 2018;6:91.

Dror DK, Allen LH. Overview of nutrients in human milk. *Adv Nutr.* 2018;9(suppl 1):278S–294S.

Duan X, et al. A meta-analysis of breastfeeding and osteoporotic fracture risk in the females. *Osteoporos Int*. 2017;28(2):495–503.

Fan D, et al. Role of breastfeeding on maternal and childhood cancers: an umbrella review of meta-analyses. *J Glob Health.* 2023;13:04067.

Ferreira CSM, et al. Humoral immune response to measles and varicella vaccination in former very low birth weight preterm infants. *Brazilian J Infect Dis.* 2018;22(1):41–46.

Ferreira LB, et al. Lumbar spine bone mineral density in women breastfeeding for a period of 4 to 6 months: systematic review and meta-analysis. *Int Breastfeed J.* 2023;18(1):68.

Figueiredo B, et al. Exclusive breastfeeding moderates the association between prenatal and postpartum depression. *J Hum Lact.* 2021;37(4):784–794.

Filibeli BE, et al. The effect of breast milk nesfatin-1 and ghrelin levels on growth in infants with SGA. *Turk J Pediatr*. 2022;64(2):239–245.

Francese R, et al. Viruses and human milk: transmission or protection? *Adv Nutr.* 2023;14(6):1389–1415.

Frank NM, et al. The relationship between breastfeeding and reported respiratory and gastrointestinal infection rates in young children. *BMC Pediatr.* 2019;19:339.

Freitas RF, et al. Relationship between the diet quality index in nursing mothers and the fatty acid profile of mature breast milk. *Rev Paul Pediatr.* 2021;39:e2019089.

Gao Z, et al. Protective effect of breastfeeding against childhood leukemia in Zhejiang Province, P. R. China: a retrospective case-control study. *Libyan J Med*. 2018;13(1):1508273.

Garlic. LactMed [database online]. November 15, 2023. National Library of Medicine (US).

Garofoli F, et al. Anti-inflammatory and anti-allergic properties of colostrum from mothers of full-term and preterm babies: the importance of maternal lactation in the first days. *Nutrients.* 2023;15(19):4249.

Geddes D, Perrella S. Breastfeeding and human lactation. *Nutrients.* 2019;11(4).

Ghozy S, et al. Association of breastfeeding status with risk of autism spectrum disorder: a systematic review, dose-response analysis and meta-analysis. *Asian J Psychiatr.* 2020;48:101916.

Gialeli G, et al. Potential epigenetic effects of human milk on infants' neurodevelopment. *Nutrients.* 2023;15(16):3614.

Gila-Diaz A, et al. A review of bioactive factors in human breastmilk: a focus on prematurity. *Nutrients.* 2019;11(6).

Giuffrida F, et al. Human milk fatty acid composition and its association with maternal blood and adipose tissue fatty acid content in a cohort of women from Europe. *Eur J Nutr.* 2022;61(4): 2167–2182.

Gonzalez Ballesteros LF, et al. Unexpected widespread hypophosphatemia and bone disease associated with elemental formula use in infants and children. *Bone.* 2017;97:287–292.

Grace T, et al. Breastfeeding and motor development: a longitudinal cohort study. *Hum Mov Sci.* 2017;51:9–16.

Grevet LT, et al. The association between duration of breastfeeding and the trajectory of brain development from childhood to young adulthood: an 8-year longitudinal study. *Eur Child Adolesc Psychiatry.* 2023.

Gunderson EP, et al. Lactation duration and progression to diabetes in women across the childbearing years: the 30-year CARDIA study. *JAMA Intern Med.* 2018;178(3):328–337.

Güngör D, et al. Infant milk-feeding practices and childhood leukemia: a systematic review. *Am J Clin Nutr.* 2019a;109(suppl 7): 757S–771S.

Güngör D, et al. Infant milk-feeding practices and diabetes outcomes in offspring: a systematic review. *Am J Clin Nutr.* 2019b; 109(suppl 7):817S–837S.

Gurung M, et al. Role of gut microbiota in type 2 diabetes pathophysiology. *EBioMedicine.* 2020;51:102590.

Hale T, Krutsch K. *Hale's Medications & Mothers' Milk 2025–2026: A Manual of Lactational Pharmacology.* 21st ed. New York, NY: Springer Publishing Company; 2024.

Hanson L. Chapter 10: The role of breastfeeding in the defense of the infant. In: Hale T, Hartmann P, eds. *Hale and Hartmann's Textbook of Human Lactation*. New York: Springer Publishing; 2017.

Hartwig FP, et al. Effect modification of FADS2 polymorphisms on the association between breastfeeding and intelligence: results from a collaborative meta-analysis. *Int J Epidemiol*. 2019; 48(1):45–57.

Heo JS, et al. Breastfeeding and vitamin D. *Clin Exp Pediatr.* 2022;65(9):418–429.

Hodgkinson A, et al. Nucleotides: an updated review of their concentration in breast milk. *Nutr Res.* 2022;99:13–24.

Holz A, et al. Breastfeeding and risk of multiple sclerosis: a systematic review and meta-analysis of observational studies. *Neuroepidemiology.* 2022;56(6):391–401.

Horta BL, de Lima NP. Breastfeeding and type 2 diabetes: systematic review and meta-analysis. *Curr Diab Rep.* 2019;19(1):1.

Hossain S, Mihrshahi S. Exclusive breastfeeding and childhood morbidity: a narrative review. *Int J Environ Res Public Health.* 2022;19(22):14804.

Huang S, et al. Association of breastfeeding for the first six months of life and autism spectrum disorders: a national multi-center study in China. *Nutrients.*2021;23;14(1):45. Jenabi E, et al. Not breastfeeding and risk of autism spectrum disorders among children: a meta-analysis. *Clin Exp Pediatr.* 2023;66(1):28–31.

Jia K, et al. Breast-milk rubidium and other trace elements are associated with neurocognitive development in infants at age of 8 months. *J Nutr.* 2022;152(6):1507–1514.

Jin E, et al. Association between breastfeeding and breast, thyroid, and cervical cancer among Korean adult women based on the Korean Genome and Epidemiology Study: a cohort study. *Korean J Women Health Nurs.* 2021;27(4):368–378.

Jordan SJ, et al. Breastfeeding and endometrial cancer risk: an analysis from the epidemiology of endometrial cancer consortium. *Obstet Gynecol*. 2017;129(6):1059–1067.

Jouanne M, et al. Nutrient requirements during pregnancy and lactation. *Nutrients*. 2021;13(2):692.

Juan Castell MF, et al. A review of the relationship between the appetite-regulating hormone leptin present in human milk and infant growth. *Breastfeed Med*. 2022;17(2):98–111.

Karimi FZ, et al. The effect of mother-infant skin to skin contact on success and duration of first breastfeeding: a systematic review and meta-analysis. *Taiwan J Obstet Gynecol*. 2019; 58:1–9.

Kazemain E, et al. The Effect of maternal vitamin D supplementation on vitamin D status of exclusively breastfeeding mothers and their nursing infants: a systematic review and meta-analysis of randomized clinical trials. *Adv Nutr*. 2022;13(2):568–585.

Kim JH, et al. Breastmilk feeding during the first 4 to 6 months of age and childhood disease burden until 10 years of age. *Nutrients*. 2021;13(8):2825.

Kirkegaard H, et al. Breastfeeding and later maternal risk of hypertension and cardiovascular disease—the role of overall and abdominal obesity. *Prev Med*. 2018;114:140–148.

Klein LD, et al. Concentrations of trace elements in human milk: comparisons among women in Argentina, Namibia, Poland, and the United States. *PLoS One*. 2017;12(8):e0183367.

Koukou Z, et al. The effect of breastfeeding on food allergies in newborns and infants. *Children (Basel)*. 2023;10(6):1046.

Kratzsch J, et al. Adipokines in human breast milk. *Best Pract Res Clin Endocrinol Metab*. 2018;32(1):27–38.

Krawczyk A, et al. Effect of exclusive breastfeeding on rotavirus infection among children. *Indian J Pediatr*. 2016;83(3):220–225.

Kremer KP, Kremer TR. Breastfeeding is associated with decreased childhood maltreatment. *Breastfeed Med*. 2018;13(1):18–22.

Küçükçongar A, et al. Breastfeeding and childhood cancer: is breastfeeding preventative to childhood cancer? *Pediatr Hematol Oncol*. 2015;32(6):374–381.

Kumar P, Zumpf K. Challenges in providing adequate and reliable nutrition for extremely low birth weight infants *Clinical Nutrition ESPEN*. 2021;41,314–317.

Kumar PH, Devgan A. The association of breastfeeding with childhood asthma: a case-control study from India. *Cureus*. 2021; 13(11):e19810.

Larrosa Haro A, et al. Concentration of ghrelin and leptin in serum and human milk in nursing mothers according to the type of feeding. Version 2. *Nutr Hosp*. 2019 [revised 2019 Jan 1].

Larson-Meyer DE, et al. Appetite-Regulating hormones in human milk: a plausible biological factor for obesity risk reduction? *J Hum Lact*. 2021;37(3):603–614.

Le Doare K, et al. Mother's milk: a purposeful contribution to the development of the infant microbiota and immunity. *Front Immunol*. 2018;9:361.

Ledesma-Martínez E, et al. Casein and peptides derived from casein as antileukaemic agents. *J Oncol*. 2019;2019:8150967.

Lenehan SM, et al. The impact of short-term predominate breastfeeding on cognitive outcome at 5 years. *Acta Paediatr*. 2020; 109(5):982–988.

Lin D, et al. Breastfeeding is associated with reduced risks of central obesity and hypertension in young school-aged children: a large, population-based study. *Int Breastfeed J*. 2023; 18(1):52.

Liu F, et al. Sialic acid, the secret gift for the brain. *Crit Rev Food Sci Nutr*. 2023;63(29):9875–9894.

Logan CA, et al. Leptin in human milk and child body mass index: results of the Ulm birth cohort Studies. *Nutrients*. 2019;11(8).

Lovcevic I. Associations of breastfeeding duration and cognitive development from childhood to middle adolescence. *Acta Paediatr*. 2023;112(8):1696–1705.

Löwensteyn YN, et al. Increasing the dose of oral vitamin K prophylaxis and its effect on bleeding risk. *Eur J Pediatr*. 2019; 178(7):1033–1042.

Lupo PJ, et al. Allergies, atopy, immune-related factors and childhood rhabdomyosarcoma: a report from the Children's Oncology Group. *Int J Cancer*. 2014;134(2):431–436.

Lyon LM, Doran KS. Human milk oligosaccharides versus *Streptococcus*: how a human-made natural product protects us from pathogens. *mSphere*. 2022;7(1):e0004922.

Ma X, et al. Association between breastfeeding and risk of endometrial cancer: a meta-analysis of epidemiological studies. *Eur J Cancer Prev*. 2018;27(2):144–151.

Majid A, et al. Newborn vitamin K prophylaxis: a historical perspective to understand modern barriers to uptake. *Hosp Pediatr*. 2019;9(1):55–60.

Mane S, et al. Study of Stem Cells in Human Milk. *Cureus*. 2022;14(3):e23701.

Martin CR, et al. Review of infant feeding: key features of breast milk and infant formula. *Nutrients*. 2016;8(5):279.

Martin Carli JF, et al. Single cell RNA sequencing of human milk-derived cells reveals sub-populations of mammary epithelial cells with molecular signatures of progenitor and mature states: a novel, non-invasive framework for investigating human lactation physiology. *J Mammary Gland Biol Neoplasia*. 2020 Dec;25(4):367–387.

Mastorakou D, et al. Sensory characteristics of human milk: association between mothers' diet and milk for bitter taste. *J Dairy Sci*. 2019;102(2):1116–1130.

Mazzocchi A, et al. Hormones in breast milk and effect on infants' growth: a systematic review. *Nutrients*. 2019;11(8).

McBurney MI, et al. Establishing what constitutes a healthy human gut microbiome: state of the science, regulatory considerations, and future directions. *J Nutr*. 2019;149(11):1882–1895.

McGowan C, Bland R. The benefits of breastfeeding on child intelligence, behavior, and executive function: a review of recent evidence. *Breastfeed Med*. 2023;18(3):172–187.

Meek JY, et al. Policy statement: breastfeeding and the use of human milk. *Pediatrics*. 2022;150(1):e2022057988.

Milani C, et al. The first microbial colonizers of the human gut: composition, activities, and health implications of the infant gut microbiota. *Microbiol Mol Biol Rev*. 2017;81(4).

Mineva GM, et al. Impact of breastfeeding on the incidence and severity of respiratory syncytial virus (RSV)-associated acute lower respiratory infections in infants: a systematic review highlighting the global relevance of primary prevention. *BMJ Glob Health*. 2023;8(2):e009693.

Minocycline. LactMed [database online]. January 18, 2021. National Library of Medicine (US).

Mohammed Abouda MKM, Berair R. Association between breastfeeding and prevalence of allergies among children in the Academy Teaching Charity Hospital, Sudan. *Qatar Med J*. 2023; 2023(2):19.

Molès JP, et al. Breastmilk cell trafficking induces microchimerism-mediated immune system maturation in the infant. *Pediatr Allergy Immunol*. 2018;29(2):133–143.

Moles L, et al. Serratia marcescens colonization in preterm neonates during their neonatal intensive care unit stay. *Antimicrob Resist Infect Control*. 2019;8:135.

Molitoris J, et al. When and where birth spacing matters for child survival: an international comparison using the DHS. *Demography.* 2019;56(4):1349–1370.

Montagu A. *Touching: The Human Significance of the Skin*. New York: Harper & Row; 1986.

Morozov V, et al. Human milk oligosaccharides as promising antivirals. *Mol Nutr Food Res.* 2018;62(6):e1700679.

Munblit D, et al. Levels of growth factors and IgA in the colostrum of women from Burundi and Italy. *Nutrients.* 2018;10(9).

Myles IA, Datta SK. Frontline science: breast milk confers passive cellular immunity via CD8-dependent mechanisms. *J Leukoc Biol.* 2021;109(4):709–715.

Ng E, Loewy AD. Position statement: guidelines for vitamin K prophylaxis in newborns: a joint statement of the Canadian Paediatric Society and the College of Family Physicians of Canada. *Can Fam Physician.* 2018;64(10):736–739.

Nguyen B, et al. Breastfeeding and maternal cardiovascular risk factors and outcomes: a systematic review. *PLoS One.* 2017;12(11): e0187923.

Ninkina N, et al. Stem cells in human breast milk. *Hum Cell.* 2019; 32(3):223–230.

Noh S, Lee E. Relationship between selected trace elements in human milk and psychosocial characteristics in Korean early postpartum women. *Int J Environ Res Public Health.* 2021;18(1):350.

Nommsen LA, et al. Determinants of energy, protein, lipid, and lactose concentrations in human milk during the first 12 mo of lactation: the DARLING Study. *Am J Clin Nutr.* 1991;53(2): 457–465.

Nuzhat S, et al. Impact of Routine Counseling on Breastfeeding Status in Hospitalized Infants Below 6 Months: Observation from a Large Diarrheal Disease Hospital in Bangladesh. *Global Pediatric Health.* 2019;6.

Pacheco CMR, et al. In vitro differentiation capacity of human breastmilk stem cells: a systematic review. *World J Stem Cells.* 2019;11(11):1005–1019.

Pang WW, et al. Nutrients or nursing? Understanding how breast milk feeding affects child cognition. *Eur J Nutr.* 2020; 59(2):609–619.

Park S, Choi NK. Breastfeeding and maternal hypertension. *Am J Hypertens.* 2018;31(5):615–621.

Pena-Leon V, et al. Prolonged breastfeeding protects from obesity by hypothalamic action of hepatic FGF21. *Nat Metab.* 2022;4(7):901–917.

Pereira Lopes TS, et al. Association between duration of breastfeeding and malocclusion in primary dentition in Brazil. *J Dent Child (Chic).* 2019;86(1):17–23.

Pereyra-Elías R, et al. To what extent does confounding explain the association between breastfeeding duration and cognitive development up to age 14? Findings from the UK Millennium Cohort Study. *PLoS One.* 2022;17(5):e0267326.

Perrin MT, et al. A longitudinal study of human milk composition in the second year postpartum: implications for human milk banking. *Matern Child Nutr.* 2017;13(1).

Pludowski P, et al. Vitamin D supplementation guidelines. *J Steroid Biochem Mol Biol.* 2018;175:125–135.

Plunkett BA, et al. Association of breastfeeding and child IQ score at age 5 years. *Obstet Gynecol.* 2021;137(4):561–570.

Prentice AM. Breastfeeding in the modern world. *Ann Nutr Metab.* 2022;78(suppl 2):29–38.

Puumala SE, et al. Epidemiology of childhood acute myeloid leukemia. *Pediatr Blood Cancer.* 2013;60(5):728–733.

Qiao J, et al. A meta-analysis of the association between breastfeeding and early childhood obesity. *J Pediatr Nurs.* 2020;53:57–66.

Rio-Aige K, et al. Breast milk immune composition varies during the transition stage of lactation: characterization of immunotypes in the MAMI cohort. *Front Nutr.* 2023;10:1252815.

Rios P, et al. Risk of neuroblastoma, birth-related characteristics, congenital malformations and perinatal exposures: a pooled analysis of the ESCALE and ESTELLE French studies (SFCE). *Int J Cancer.* 2016;139(9):1936–1948.

Rito AI, et al. Association between characteristics at birth, breastfeeding and obesity in 22 countries: the WHO European childhood obesity surveillance initiative—COSI 2015/2017. *Obes Facts.* 2019;12(2):226–243.

Rocha FAC, et al. Long-term breastfeeding influences disease activity in a low-income juvenile idiopathic arthritis cohort. *Clin Rheumatol.* 2019;38(8):2227–2231.

Rojanaworarit C, et al. The protective effect of breastfeeding on dental fluorosis among children in rural fluoride-endemic areas. *Breastfeed Med.* 2023;18(7):540–548.

Rosas-Salazar C, et al. Exclusive breast-feeding, the early-life microbiome and immune response, and common childhood respiratory illnesses. *J Allergy Clin Immunol.* 2022;150(3):612–621.

Royal C, Gray C. Allergy prevention: an overview of current evidence. *Yale J Biol Med.* 2020;93(5):689–698.

Rudant J, et al. Childhood acute lymphoblastic leukemia and indicators of early immune stimulation: a Childhood Leukemia International Consortium study. *Am J Epidemiol.* 2015;181(8):549–562.

Ryan PM, et al. Paediatrician's perspective of infant gut microbiome research: current status and challenges. *Arch Dis Child.* 2019;104(7):701–705.

Safari K., et al. The effect of mother and newborn early skin-to-skin contact on initiation of breastfeeding, newborn temperature and duration of third stage of labor. *Int Breastfeed J.* 2018; 13:1–8.

Sánchez C, et al. Breast milk: a source of functional compounds with potential application in nutrition and therapy. *Nutrients.* 2021;13(3):1026.

Sankar MJ, et al. Vitamin K prophylaxis for prevention of vitamin K deficiency bleeding: a systematic review. *J Perinatol.* 2016;36(suppl 1):S29–S35.

Santoro W Jr, et al. Colostrum ingested during the first day of life by exclusively breastfed healthy newborn infants. *J Pediatr.* 2010;156(1):29–32.

Schoppa I, et al. Association of maternal prepregnancy weight with offspring adiposity throughout adulthood over 37 years of follow-up. *Obesity (Silver Spring).* 2019;27(1):137–144.

Schreiner C, et al. Microbiological screening of donor human milk. *Breastfeed Med.* 2023;18(12):901–907.

Singh KS, et al. Bio-therapeutics from human milk: prospects and perspectives. *J Appl Microbiol.* 2021;131(6):2669–2687.

Singhal A. The impact of human milk feeding on long-term risk of obesity and cardiovascular disease. *Breastfeed Med.* 2019; 14(S1):S9–S10.

Slattery J, et al. The significance of the enteric microbiome on the development of childhood disease: a review of prebiotic and probiotic therapies in disorders of childhood. *Clin Med Insights Pediatr.* 2016;10:91–107.

Srivastava A, Swati J. Appetite self-regulation in infancy—the role of direct breastfeeding. *World Nutrition.* March 2023;22–27.

Starbird E, Crawford K. Healthy timing and spacing of pregnancy: reducing mortality among women and their children. *Glob Health Sci Pract.* 2019;7(suppl 2):S211–S214.

Sudarma V, et al. Human milk oligosaccharides as a missing piece in combating nutritional issues during exclusive breastfeeding. *Pediatr Gastroenterol Hepatol Nutr.* 2021;24(6):501–509.

Suwaydi MA, et al. Human milk metabolic hormones: analytical methods and current understanding. *Int J Mol Sci*. 2021;22(16):8708.

Szyller H, et al. Bioactive components of human milk and their impact on child's health and development, literature review. *Nutrients*. 2024;16(10);1487–1505.

Teni Nurlatifah HR, et al. Determination factors associated with immune responses towards first dose Edmonston-Zagreb (EZ) measles vaccine in Indonesian infants. *Med Arch*. 2021;75(5):335–339.

Thomaz EBAF, et al. Breastfeeding versus bottle feeding on malocclusion in children: a meta-analysis study. *J Hum Lact*. 2018;34(4):768–788.

Tochitani S. Taurine: a maternally derived nutrient linking mother and offspring. *Metabolites*. 2022;12(3):228.

Tonon KM, et al. Human milk oligosaccharides and respiratory syncytial virus infection in infants. *Adv Nutr*. 2024;15(6):100218.

Tripathy S, et al. Potential of breastmilk in stem cell research. *Cell Tissue Bank*. 2019;20(4):467–488.

Tseng PT, et al. Maternal breastfeeding and autism spectrum disorder in children: a systematic review and meta-analysis. *Nutr Neurosci*. 2019;22(5):354–362.

Umer A, et al. Association between breastfeeding and childhood cardiovascular disease risk factors. *Matern Child Health J*. 2019;23(2):228–239.

U.S. Department of Health and Human Services, Administration for Children and Families, Administration on Children, Youth and Families, Children's Bureau. *Child Maltreatment 2022*. 2024. https://www.acf.hhs.gov/cb/data-research/child-maltreatment

van Ingen G, et al. Identifying distinct trajectories of acute otitis media in children: a prospective cohort study. *Clin Otolaryngol*. 2021;46(4):788–795.

van Rossem L, et al. Does breast milk adiponectin affect BMI and cardio-metabolic markers in childhood? *Br J Nutr*. 2019;121(8):905–913.

Verbiest S, et al. Elevating mothers' voices: recommendations for improved patient-centered postpartum. *J Behav Med*. 2018;41(5):577–590.

Vinha PP, de Mello-Filho FV. Evidence of a preventive effect of breastfeeding on obstructive sleep apnea in children and adults. *J Hum Lact*. 2017;33(2):448–453.

Wakinaka T, et al. Bifidobacterial α-galactosidase with unique carbohydrate-binding module specifically acts on blood group B antigen. *Glycobiology*. 2013;23(2):232–240.

Wang KL, et al. Breastfeeding and the risk of childhood Hodgkin lymphoma: a systematic review and meta-analysis. *Asian Pac J Cancer Prev*. 2013;14(8):4733–4737.

Wang S, et al. Association between breastmilk microbiota and food allergy in infants. *Front Cell Infect Microbiol*. 2022;11:770913.

Weaver JM, et al. Breastfeeding duration predicts greater maternal sensitivity over the next decade. *Dev Psychol*. 2018;54(2):220–227.

Wilson K, et al. The association between duration of breastfeeding and childhood asthma outcomes. *Ann Allergy Asthma Immunol*. 2022;129(2):205–211.

Winter EM, et al. Pregnancy and lactation, a challenge for the skeleton. *Endocr Connect*. 2020;9(6):R143–R157.

Wong PD, et al. The association of breastfeeding duration and early childhood cardiometabolic risk. *J Pediatr*. 2018;192:80.e1–85.e1.

World Health Organization. *WHO Recommendations on Newborn Health: Guidelines Approved by the WHO Guidelines Review Committee*. Geneva, Switzerland: World Health Organization; 2017.

World Health Organization. Diarrhoea. 2019. https://www.who.int/health-topics/diarrhoea#tab=tab_1

World Health Organization. Violence against children. 2022a. https://www.who.int/news-room/fact-sheets/detail/violence-against-children

World Health Organization. *WHO Recommendations on Maternal and Newborn Care for a Positive Postnatal Experience*. Geneva, Switzerland: World Health Organization; 2022b.

World Health Organization. Obesity and overweight. 2024. https://www.who.int/news-room/fact-sheets/detail/obesity-and-overweight

Wu J, et al. Exploring dynamic change and influencing factors of TGF-β1 and MUC1 in human breast milk, and their association with infantile diseases. *Transl Pediatr*. 2023;12(6):1139–1147.

Wu RY, et al. Human milk oligosaccharides increase mucin expression in experimental necrotizing enterocolitis. *Mol Nutr Food Res*. 2019;63(3):e1800658.

Xie W, et al. Contrasting diversity and composition of human colostrum microbiota in a maternal cohort with different ethnic origins but shared physical geography (island scale). *Front Microbiol*. 2022;13:934232.

Yang QH, et al. Clinical features of cow's milk protein allergy in infants presenting mainly with gastrointestinal symptoms: an analysis of 280 cases. *Zhongguo Dang Dai Er Ke Za Zhi*. 2019;21(3):271–276 [in Chinese].

Zaky A, et al. The role of the gut microbiome in diabetes and obesity-related kidney disease. Int J *Mol Sci*. 2021;22(17):9641.

Zamanillo R, et al. Breast milk supply of microRNA associated with leptin and adiponectin is affected by maternal overweight/obesity and influences infancy BMI. *Nutrients*. 2019;11(11).

Zurynski Y, et al. Vitamin K deficiency bleeding in Australian infants 1993–2017: an Australian Paediatric Surveillance Unit study. *Arch Dis Child*. 2019:13.

Zuurveld M, et al. Immunomodulation by human milk oligosaccharides: the potential role in prevention of allergic diseases. *Front Immunol*. 2020;11:801.

CHAPTER 10

Use of Infant Formula

Human milk is the optimal nutrition for babies, and nursing is the natural method of infant feeding for families. However, there are circumstances when babies cannot receive mammalian milk or need supplementation. There are also parents with health conditions that prevent providing their milk to their infants. The use of infant formula should be restricted to babies with a medical condition that precludes nursing or ingesting human milk. When used appropriately for medical reasons, infant formula is lifesaving and is a practical element of lactation care.

Health agencies worldwide recommend that babies who can nurse should receive human milk exclusively for the first 6 months. However, families are exposed to perpetual messaging about formula feeding. Many choose to feed their babies formula despite knowing that human milk is healthiest. Formula manufacturers lobby governments, promote their products through healthcare systems, and aggressively reach out to families. Parents who use formula receive little guidance and are challenged with selecting a formula brand, feeding it safely to their infant, and navigating costs and availability.

KEY TERMS

Colicky behavior
Cow's milk
Donor milk
Duarte's variant
Galactose
Galactosemia

Prevalence of Formula Feeding

The prevalence of formula feeding is largely attributable to the aggressive marketing of infant formula as safe, acceptable, and in keeping with the social norm (Mehmet, 2020; United Nations Children's Fund [UNICEF], 2024). Cultural conditioning and trust in the healthcare field foster a belief that healthcare providers would not recommend an alternative to human milk if it were not safe. Thus, most formula-feeding parents do not question what they feed their babies. The United States is one of the largest markets in the world for infant formula. The federally funded Women, Infants, and Children (WIC) program spent more than half a billion dollars on infant formula in fiscal year 2018 (Neuberger et al., 2022).

Legitimate Need for Infant Formula

Step 6 of the Ten Steps to Successful Breastfeeding states that newborns should not be given any food or fluids other than human milk unless it is medically indicated. This recommendation acknowledges that there are circumstances in which parents cannot nurse or feed their milk to their baby. Babies under 1 year of age should not consume **cow's milk**. Therefore, if parents are not a candidate for, or do not wish to use, **donor milk**, they will need to learn about the use of infant formula.

When formula supplementation is necessary, parents should receive it with written instructions tailored to their circumstances. Specific instructions might be, "Feed your baby 15 mL (½ oz) of formula after each time you nurse until your baby is seen in the clinic in 2 days." Parents also need to learn how to use a feeding method compatible with lactation, as described in **Chapter 22**. Instructions on the amount, frequency, and method for supplementing a baby enable parents to ensure their baby's health while protecting lactation. Without this guidance, parents could supplement too much or for too long and compromise their ability to establish or maintain full milk production.

Parent Circumstances That Preclude Nursing

Some parents are unable to establish full lactation. Insufficient milk production or delayed onset of full production may require formula supplementation. Some medical conditions and circumstances may prevent a parent from nursing (identified in **Figure 10-1**). These parents will benefit from sensitivity to their needs as they experience temporary or permanent weaning. **Chapter 26** discusses circumstances that affect a parent's ability to nurse. Circumstances that may require infant formula include the following:

- Sheehan's syndrome—Sheehan's syndrome (discussed in **Chapter 7**) prevents milk production.
- Physical condition—An acute condition such as eclampsia, sepsis, or shock can delay nursing until after sufficient healing. Lactation may not be emotionally or physically sustainable with a severe illness, such as unresolved congestive heart failure, insufficient renal function, or cancer.
- Cognitive condition—Postpartum depression or psychosis may render a parent functionally unable to care for the baby.

- Infection with the human immunodeficiency virus (HIV) in a developed country
- Taking antiretroviral medications in a developed country
- Untreated, active tuberculosis
- Infection with human T-cell lymphotropic virus type I or type II
- Using an illicit drug
- Taking prescribed cancer chemotherapy agents, such as antimetabolites that interfere with DNA replication and cell division
- Undergoing radiation therapies; however, some nuclear medicine therapies require only a temporary interruption in nursing

Figure 10-1 Medical conditions that prevent nursing.

Data from American Academy of Pediatrics. Breastfeeding and the Use of Human Milk, 2012.

- Herpes—An active herpes lesion where the baby may come in contact with it prevents nursing on the affected side until the lesion heals. The baby may continue to nurse on the other side. Milk can be expressed and discarded from the affected side.
- HIV—Most industrialized countries advise that HIV-positive parents should not nurse. The United States and United Kingdom say nursing is acceptable if viral load is undetectable (Clinicalinfo.HIV.gov, 2023; NHS Trust Imperial College Healthcare, 2021). Australia states that nursing is acceptable for 6 months if viral load is low and recommends stopping when solid foods begin (Better Health Channel, 2023).
- Medication—Medications such as cytotoxic, radioactive, or some antithyroid (other than propylthiouracil) drugs contraindicate nursing while the drug remains at a level that would harm the baby. This may necessitate temporary interruption of nursing with milk expression to maintain production. Sometimes total weaning may occur. A few long-term drug therapies, such as lithium or tamoxifen, rule out nursing because the substance or treatment would be dangerous to the infant (Hale & Krutsch, 2024).

Infant Circumstances That May Require Formula

Some nursing infants require a supplement, which, in order of preference, would be expressed milk, donor milk, or infant formula. In rare situations, nursing must be avoided altogether. **Chapter 27** discusses long-term infant conditions. Circumstances that may require formula include the following:

- Hypoglycemia or dehydration—Babies who experience hypoglycemia or dehydration need immediate calories. When possible, efforts should focus on expressing milk or increasing feedings to provide the needed nourishment. If the condition does not improve through increased nursing or expressed milk, the baby will need to be supplemented with either donor milk or formula until lactation is established.
- Jaundice—Phototherapy for jaundice makes babies sleepy. Therefore, milk expression may be necessary to protect milk production and supplement the baby. If there is not enough expressed milk, the baby will need to be supplemented with either donor milk or formula for the additional calories and fluids.

- Need for human milk fortifier—Babies with a low or extremely low birth weight or who are born preterm (less than 1000 g or 32 weeks' gestation) may require supplementation with human milk fortifier. **Chapter 24** discusses fortifiers, including fortifiers made from human milk.
- Phenylketonuria (PKU)—Babies with PKU need regular supplementation of a low-phenylalanine formula in addition to human milk (Pugliese et al., 2020).
- Maple syrup (sugar) urine disease (MSUD)—Infants with MSUD require lifelong monitoring and a protein-restricted diet to promote proper growth and development and prevent amino acid buildup.
- Galactosemia—Infants with **galactosemia** cannot metabolize lactose, which is the main carbohydrate in human milk. Therefore, they cannot consume human milk or any other mammalian milk (Badiu Tişa et al., 2022; Succoio et al., 2022). Galactosemia requires a special lactose-free formula, such as soy or amino acid formula. Galactosemia is an extremely rare condition (e.g., about 1 out of 60,000 births).
- Duarte's variant—Babies with **Duarte's variant**, a variation of galactosemia, can nurse (sometimes totally, sometimes partially) with careful monitoring of the baby's **galactose** levels (Carlock et al., 2019; Fridovich-Keil et al., 2021).

Composition of Infant Formula

Commercially prepared infant formula is an inert food product with slight differences depending on manufacturer. It is intended to meet the universal needs of infants. Regulation of infant formula production in the United States was enacted in 2014 by the U.S. Food and Drug Administration (FDA, 2014). Production is regulated internationally by the Codex Alimentarius of the United Nations Food and Agriculture Organization. This regulation was adopted as a worldwide standard in 1981 and has been revised regularly since then (Codex Alimentarius, 2023). Codex Alimentarius standards provide minimum and maximum concentrations of essential nutrients, including calories, protein, lipids, carbohydrates, vitamins, and minerals. The standards also indicate what food additives they recognize as safe.

Despite worldwide regulations, infant formulas remain deficient in many of the constituents essential for optimal infant growth and health. Unlike human milk, infant formulas do not mirror nature's adaptability to the baby's age and unique needs. Infant formulas provide no known protection against allergies and confer no immunity on the baby. Moreover, formula lacks human milk's sensory experience of various flavors despite efforts to improve the flavor (Chi et al., 2022).

Balance of Components

Infant formula manufacturers continually refine their products to simulate components in human milk. Advances have led to the addition of specialized protein, fatty acids, and complex carbohydrates (Ahern et al., 2019). The addition of polyunsaturated fatty acids (PUFAs) has produced significant improvement in lipid profile (Rivera-Pasquel et al., 2020). The addition of lactoferrin has not affected iron status (Björmsjö et al., 2020). Some researchers suggest that the addition of synthetic oligosaccharides has not demonstrated a benefit and that marketing it as "human milk oligosaccharides" is an inappropriate idealization of infant formula (Bührer et al., 2022). Other researchers suggest there is a subtle association with differences in stool microbiome and metabolome (Chichlowski et al., 2021). The successful separation of milk fat globule membrane (MFGM) from bovine milk has enabled it to be added to infant formulas. The addition of MFGM may lead to better cognitive development, reduction of infection risks, and modulation of the infant's gut microbiome (Hedrick et al., 2021; Lee et al., 2021; Mohamed et al., 2022; Zhao et al., 2022).

The imbalance of some components in infant formula carries health risks. Infant formula contains excessive protein, which is associated with childhood obesity and symptoms of metabolic syndrome in adults (Wazed & Farid, 2019). Vitamin D, which is toxic in high doses, appears in excessive amounts in many formulas. Some formulas are deficient in chloride. Some contain high levels of iodine, which could affect neonatal thyroid function. Arsenic, a semimetallic element found in soils, groundwater, surface water, and air, has been found in infant formula and infant foods (Igweze et al., 2020; Jallad, 2019). In its inorganic form, arsenic is a classified carcinogen (Chen & Costa, 2021; Palma-Lara et al., 2020).

Fatty Acids

No infant formula has replicated human milk's complex pattern of fatty acids, which are essential for brain development and visual acuity. Elevated free fatty acids in some formulas can contribute to intestinal injury in necrotizing enterocolitis (Sodhi et al., 2018). Formula manufacturers have added the long-chain polyunsaturated fatty acids (LCPUFAs) docosahexaenoic acid (DHA) and arachidonic acid (ARA or AA) from synthetic sources. Despite advertisements, these two synthetic sources are not equal to the over 200 fatty acids identified in human milk (Bobiński & Bobińska, 2022; Grunewald et al., 2019).

Although the infant food industry has advanced in recent years, there is no consensus on the effectiveness of adding bioactive ingredients to infant formulas (Almeida et al., 2021; Arija et al., 2022). Canadian regulations require manufacturers to minimize inflated health claims that these formulas' "enhancement" of brain and vision development makes them "closer than ever" to human milk (Canadian Food Inspection Agency, 2018).

Soy Formula

Soy formula, manufactured from soybeans, is marketed as an alternative to cow's milk formula. Because of the phytoestrogens in soy, children with congenital hypothyroidism who receive soy formula need adequate monitoring of thyroid function (Testa et al., 2018). Female infants fed soy formula exhibit estrogen-sensitive tissue and organ development consistent with responses to external estrogen exposure (Adgent et al., 2018). Female adults fed soy formula as infants have experienced higher rates of menstrual pain (Upson et al., 2019).

Soy milk contains approximately 80 times more manganese than human milk. High manganese intake is associated with adverse neurodevelopmental outcomes (Frisbie et al., 2019; Westmark, 2017). A 6-month-old infant ingesting soy-based formula consumes about 4 times the amount of aluminum consumed by an infant receiving human milk (Elaridi et al., 2020). Aluminum competes with calcium receptors, and excess amounts are associated with damage to the kidneys, liver, and bones.

The British Dietetic Association (2019) considers soy formula unsuitable as a first-line alternative for infants under 6 months of age. Health organizations in Canada recommend limiting soy formula use to infants with galactosemia or those who cannot consume dairy-based products for cultural or religious reasons (Government of Canada, 2015). The American Academy of Pediatrics (AAP) does not recommend soy formula for preterm infants weighing less than 1800 grams. Soy formula is also not recommended to prevent colicky symptoms or allergy or for infants with cow's milk protein-induced enterocolitis or enteropathy (AAP, 2018). Recent research recommends that soy formula not be used as a substitute for infant formulas or cow's milk in children younger than 24 months (Verduci et al., 2020).

Manufacturing Errors

Manufacturing errors and contamination of infant formula are devastating to families whose babies are harmed by them. The omission of vitamin B_1 (thiamine) from infant formula in Israel resulted in brain damage in 17 babies and at least two deaths in 2003 (Siegel-Itzkovich, 2003). The implications of omitted nutrients can have lifelong effects on health and overall well-being. In addition, there have been recalls of formula containing insect parts (FDA, 2010), metal particles (FDA, 2019; Hitti, 2006), inadequate iron (FDA, 2007), and rigid plastic (FDA, 2005). Faulty seals on bottles caused another recall (ABC News, 2022).

Contamination with bacteria has caused numerous formula recalls. A company in New Zealand exported 38 tons of potentially botulism-contaminated whey protein concentrate in 2012 (Backhouse, 2014). Multiple outbreaks of *Salmonella* infections due to infant formula occurred from 2017 through 2019 in France (Jones et al., 2019; Le Monde, 2023; Merieux Nutrisciences, 2019; Trompiz, 2019; Whitworth, 2019). There are several reported contamination cases with *Cronobacter sakazakii* (formerly called *Enterobacter sakazakii*). *C. sakazakii* is an opportunistic bacterium that survives and persists in dry and low-moisture environments, such as powdered infant formula. Infections caused by this pathogen are particularly fatal in infants born preterm and those younger than 2 months (Henry & Fouladkhah, 2019). Recalls occurred in 2022 after *C. sakazakii* and *Salmonella* infections occurred in five infants (two of whom died) (FDA, 2022). Possible *C. sakazakii* contamination caused two more recalls in 2023 (ABC News, 2023; NBC News, 2023).

Hazardous Practices

Some infant formula companies have deliberately used unsafe practices to decrease costs and increase profits. In 2008, more than 294,000 infants developed kidney stones when manufacturers in China added melamine (plastic) to food products. Over 50,000 infants were hospitalized, and 6 died (Chen, 2009). Furthermore, flour was used to mimic milk powder, causing malnutrition in at least 171 infants and 13 infant deaths in China (Chinaview, 2008). Iran recommends annually analyzing the country's food products, notably infant formula, for melamine contamination (Mirza Alizadeh et al., 2023).

Two large manufacturers exported infant foods with phthalates to several countries. Phthalates are a class of chemical compounds used to stabilize perfumes and solvents. They were added to the foods mimic emulsifiers (Tsai et al., 2016). A Swiss manufacturer mixed imported formula with out-of-date product, changing sell-by dates on packaging and relabeling formula for older babies as more expensive milk for younger children (*Daily Telegraph*, 2013). Animal feed containing dirt and flies was relabeled as baby formula and sold to Mexican food manufacturers (Gilot, 2004). Such questionable manufacturing tactics erode consumer confidence in food safety and increase public and private health costs.

Selecting an Infant Formula

Ideally, parents would make the choice of infant formula with their baby's caregiver, mindful of the health implications and allergy history of their entire family—siblings, parents, and other close blood relatives. However, parents typically receive little guidance when considering which formula to feed their baby. Brand choice often depends on which company left a case on their doorstep, which promotional discharge pack they received from their hospital, or which cents-off coupons are available. Parents may be influenced by their baby's caregiver being influenced by marketing of formula companies. Parents on a food assistance program may be limited to the manufacturer contracted by the organization. In addition to brand choice, parents have the option of using powdered, concentrated, ready-to-feed, or prescription formulas. Some may use soy or homemade formula.

- Powdered formula—This is the least expensive option with the longest shelf life. It is also the most easily contaminated, needs a safe water source, and is most at risk for incorrect preparation.
- Concentrated formula—This option is losing popularity, possibly because it is easily confused with ready-to-feed formula. Accidentally feeding concentrated formula without appropriate preparation poses serious health risks to an infant.
- Ready-to-feed formula—This is the most convenient and most expensive option. It is not dependent on a safe water source, making it suitable for travel.
- Soy formula—This is an option for infants who cannot consume cow's milk. Soy formula use varies globally, ranging from 2% to over 30% in various countries.
- Prescription specialized formula—This formula addresses health issues, such as low birth weight, food allergy or intolerance, and medical conditions, such as renal insufficiency. Contamination with aluminum is a concern (Redgrove et al., 2019).
- Homemade formula—Some families use homemade formula, both to save money and to know the components fed to their babies. Recipes abound online, including goat's milk and vegetarian recipes. Use of raw milk has increased in popularity, presenting bacterial and viral risks to the infant (Artursson et al., 2018; Willis et al., 2018). Because of health concerns, homemade formula is not recommended (Davis et al., 2020; McCarthy & Yale, 2023).

Precautions in Formula Use

Improper feeding and incorrect or inadequate use of infant formula account for approximately 1.5 million deaths annually worldwide (UNICEF, 2018). The potential for misuse of infant formula is especially worrisome in impoverished communities with substandard conditions and low education levels. When families cannot afford to purchase enough infant formula, parents may attempt to stretch the formula by diluting it. Families may lack access to refrigeration, clean water, or adequate waste facilities. Additionally, parents may not understand directions well enough to mix the formula correctly. It is important that parents receive instructions in a language they can understand and at an appropriate reading level.

Unsafe Water Supply

Water from a well or spring poses a risk of unsafe nitrate levels, placing babies at risk for methemoglobinemia. Methemoglobinemia is a blood disorder in which hemoglobin does not effectively release oxygen to body tissues. Expectant parents are urged to test their water before their baby arrives (Fossen Johnson, 2019). If they are unsure about the bacterial level in their water, they can boil it for 5 minutes. Boiling it any longer could increase the concentration of lead in the water, which is especially a concern in older homes where the water pipe joints may contain lead solder. Lead leaches out more easily in hot water, so individuals in older homes should obtain the water from the cold-water faucet, running it for at least 1 minute before collecting it and longer if the water has not been run for several hours.

Excessive fluoride from adding it to the community water supply could cause fluorosis, a condition in which teeth become mottled or discolored. Epidemiologic studies correlate elevated fluoride intake during early development with corresponding levels of neurotoxicity (Grandjean, 2019). One study found that formula-fed children in high-fluoride areas had lower IQ scores by 8.8 points on the Wechsler Primary and Preschool Scale of Intelligence–III, with significance remaining after accounting for prenatal exposure (Till et al., 2020). When there is concern about the safety of the water supply, families may need to use bottled water.

Unsafe Mixing

Inadequate guidance on formula use results in a high incidence of formula being mixed incorrectly (Altazan et al., 2019; Appleton et al., 2022; Kakoo Brioso et al., 2022). Each formula manufacturer has a particular set of instructions, and the size of the scoops for powdered formula is not uniform. Parents may not follow package directions or may fail to use the scoop that came with a particular brand of formula.

Because concentrated infant formula is a liquid, it is easy for parents to confuse it with ready-to-feed formula and feed their baby concentrated formula at ready-to-feed levels. Improving the readability of preparation instructions could improve accuracy (Gilmore et al., 2020). Furthermore, the higher cost may tempt parents to save unused portions rather than discard them after the specified period. They may overdilute expensive formula to last longer, resulting in poor nourishment and possible water intoxication.

Guidelines for Safe Practices

Families who use infant formula either as a supplement or as total nutrition need to know how to prepare and feed formula safely. Step 5 of the Ten Steps to Support Successful Breastfeeding addresses the safe preparation, handling, and storage of formula. Healthcare providers are responsible for ensuring that parents receive adequate instructions that are understandable by any individual caring for the infant. Safe practice formula-feeding guidelines are available from the World Health Organization (WHO, 2007). Guidelines for daycare settings, bottle feeding, and cup feeding are provided in multiple languages. Safety tips include the following:

- Monitor expiration dates.
- Follow instructions for mixing, storage, and how long the formula can remain at room temperature.
- Wash the can opener and the top and bottom of the can with hot, soapy water before opening the can.
- Use a clean bottle and utensils for every feeding.
- Discard formula mixed from concentrate after 48 hours.
- Discard formula mixed from powder after 24 hours.
- Discard formula removed from the refrigerator after 1 hour.
- Never save any unused portion of formula for a later feeding.

Infant Formula Industry Practices

Pharmaceutical companies own most formula manufacturers, and therefore they share common strategies. They frame their marketing in health messaging, lobby for favorable legislation, and use representatives to promote their products. Because human milk is their primary competitor, it is no surprise that formula manufacturers use strategies that compare their products to human milk. They acknowledge that human milk is "best" and promote their products by ostensibly promoting lactation. Companies use language appealing to parents and reach out to them in multiple ways. Their practices also focus on influencing decisions by healthcare facilities and professionals.

A study of Nestlé, the world's largest food company and one of the largest formula marketers, is illustrative of formula company marketing practices aimed at gaining respect and credibility, generating corporate goodwill, and increasing sales. Nestlé uses industry-funded research through academics, ghostwriters, their own research institutions, and front groups to produce information that is favorable to the infant formula industry. Front groups are organizations that purport to represent one agenda while serving the interests of another. The company establishes relationships with key opinion leaders, government agencies, health organizations, health professionals, and the media. They position themselves as corporate philanthropists, supporting events and community-level initiatives. Furthermore, they employ nutrition and health professionals to provide information to parents and health professionals free of charge (Tanrikulu et al., 2020).

Influencing Healthcare Decisions

Aggressive marketing by infant formula manufacturers targets the healthcare industry at all levels. Companies worldwide advertise their products in medical journals and use branding to promote them through healthcare workers and facilities. Pediatricians receive visits to their clinics, free formula samples, and sponsored meals and conferences (Werner et al., 2023). Hospitals receive free formula, equipment, architectural planning, and office supplies. Manufacturers know that parents who use a particular brand of formula in the hospital will be more likely to purchase that brand for continued use at home. Likewise, health workers are more likely to promote that product.

There are efforts to rein in the aggressive marketing by pharmaceutical companies. Legislation has made it more difficult to fund dinners, travel, medical fellowships, scholarships, educational grants, and other rewards. The Centers for Medicare and Medicaid Services Physician Payment Sunshine Act requires, as of 2014, that any manufacturer of medical supplies, medical equipment, or pharmaceuticals disclose to the U.S. Department of Health and Human Services (USDHHS) any payments, gifts, or "transfers of value" over $10 and the purpose of the payments (USDHHS, 2016).

Influencing Families

Marketing attempts to reach parents go far beyond the free formula given through hospitals. Mailing free samples of infant formula to families' homes is commonplace. Pervasive and invasive marketing tactics on social media and misleading messages are designed to keep parents as customers for as long as possible (WHO & UNICEF, 2022). Marketing campaigns use emotional appeals to build relationships with parents through social media, manufacturer websites, online retailers, blogs, mobile apps, and digital streaming services. Companies partner with online peer groups and social media influencers (Hastings et al., 2020; Horwood et al., 2022; Jones et al., 2022). Families in Mexico are highly exposed to formula marketing through healthcare professionals and on television and radio (Hernández-Cordero et al., 2022).

Violations of the International Code

The WHO's International Code of Marketing of Breastmilk Substitutes and advocacy organizations such as the Infant Feeding Action Coalition (INFACT), International Baby Food Action Network (IBFAN), and World Alliance for Breastfeeding Action attempt to hold formula companies accountable for their industry practices. The International Code aims to restrict the unethical marketing and promotion of infant formula. Formula company marketing strategies intentionally inhibit the enactment of the International Code worldwide.

Marketing violations that target families, health workers, and the public persist globally (Becker et al., 2022; Caicedo-Borrás et al., 2021; Hernández-Cordero, 2019; Rodríguez et al., 2023). Most noncompliance occurs with product labeling (Access to Nutrition Initiative, 2024). The formula industry continues to find new ways to violate the Code with digital marketing and newer types of human milk substitutes. Formula companies capitalized on fear related to COVID-19 by using health claims and misinformation about lactation. The pandemic and the boom in digital marketing provided a new entry point for donations and services to harness public sentiment (Ching et al., 2021).

Where the International Code led to country restrictions on the marketing of infant formula, the formula industry increased the promotion of baby food, toddler formula, and toddler food (Choi et al., 2020; Harris & Pomeranz, 2020). The promotion of toddler milk is confusing, with a wide range of categories, ages, and names. Labeling is similar to infant formula labels, increasing the potential for mistakenly feeding toddler formula to young infants.

The WHO and UNICEF (2022) reported on how the marketing of formula influences infant feeding decisions. They assert that formula manufacturers continue to do the following:

- Use marketing that is pervasive, personalized, and powerful
- Use manipulative marketing tactics that exploit parents' anxieties and aspirations
- Distort science and medicine to legitimize their claims and push their products
- Make false and incomplete scientific claims and position formula as close to, equivalent to, or superior to human milk
- Systematically target health professionals to build relationships and influence their practices and recommendations
- Undermine parents' confidence in nursing

Noncompliance with the Code involves more than the infant formula industry. Systemic failings occur at all levels of the implementation and monitoring process. When formula manufacturers interfere with the effective implementation of policies that protect, promote, and support lactation, they create personal and institutional conflicts of interest. The formula industry aggressively lobbies governments to influence and prevent lactation promotion. Formula advertising is prevalent in pediatric and obstetric offices, with posters and pamphlets promoting their products as optimal infant feeding. Hospitals globally continue to distribute infant formula discharge bags and samples. Many publications distributed by healthcare professionals continue to contain noncompliant advertisements (Hickman et al., 2021). Adoption of new World Health Assembly (WHA) resolutions are needed to address marketing gaps. **Chapter 1** provides more information on the Code.

UNICEF (2024) refutes numerous complaints about the Code by the formula industry. Formula manufacturers argue that the Code violates international trade agreements, intellectual property rights, and human rights. As a key stakeholder in infant feeding, they believe they have a role in developing and implementing policies. They claim that disallowing special pricing for parents increases the risk of unsafe feeding practices. They assert that resource-challenged health facilities need product donations. And they argue that the Code should not apply in emergencies.

Healthcare providers, facilities, governments, and international agencies can protect their independence, integrity, and credibility by rejecting the influence of formula manufacturers (Lhotska et al., 2020). Governmental regulatory processes must be transparent, open to public scrutiny, and free of conflicts of interest. In addition, companies, health workers, professional associations, and nongovernmental organizations (NGOs) can protect families from their influence by prohibiting the following (UNICEF, 2023):

- Free products or reduced-price foods to families through health workers or health facilities
- Donated equipment or services to health facilities
- Gifts or incentives to health workers
- Hosting events, contests, or campaigns using health facilities
- Gifts or coupons to caregivers and families
- Educating parents and other caregivers in health facilities
- Providing information for health workers other than that which is scientific and factual
- Sponsoring meetings of health professionals and scientific meetings

Consequences of Formula Use

The use of infant formula places an economic burden on families and has far-reaching effects on public resources and public health. Early exposure to infant formula in the first few days of life can increase the rates of cow's milk allergy (Oddy, 2017; Wazed & Farid, 2019). Allergic reactions may manifest themselves as **colicky behavior**; diarrhea; vomiting; malabsorption; skin irritation; ear infections; or respiratory reactions, including sneezing, congestion, coughing, and wheezing. Formula feeding increases the risk of asthma, respiratory disease, pneumonia, and gastroenteritis (Amazouz et al., 2021; Fang et al., 2021; Greer et al., 2019; Kim et al., 2023).

The risk of mortality due to diarrhea and other infections can increase in infants who are either partially nursed or not nursed at all (WHO, 2021). A lawsuit in the United States alleging that a formula manufacturer failed to warn consumers about the risk of necrotizing enterocolitis (NEC) associated with its product awarded $60 million to the parents of an infant who died from the disease (Pierson, 2024). Formula feeding also may negatively affect the normal development of the microbiota. There is increasing evidence that the intestinal microbiota plays a pivotal role in the maturation of the immune system and in the prevention of diseases throughout the life span (Ficara et al., 2020).

Family Finances

Families who formula feed their babies bear the expense of purchasing infant formula and feeding equipment, as well as potential medical costs when their baby lacks the health protection of human milk. Family finances often dictate the choice of formula, with name-brand formulas being more expensive than generic or store brands. Frequent changes in infant formula marketing, the continual so-called improvements in existing products, and rebranding result in frequent changes in prices and names.

The convenience of ready-to-feed packaging increases cost, as does the use of specialized formulas. Internet-savvy parents can easily compare the costs of formulas on manufacturer websites, discount websites, and the websites of retail giants. Parents in underdeveloped countries, or those without such resources, are more heavily burdened with the economic costs of formula feeding (WHO, 2017). **Figure 10-2** presents the percentage of young infants who are formula fed in UNICEF regions.

The baby food market generated a revenue of $71 billion worldwide in 2023 and it is projected to grow to $100 billion by 2028. China had the largest share of the market in 2023, with over 18.5 billion dollars in sales revenue. In 2022, U.S. revenue for milk formula was about $5.6 billion and revenue for prepared baby food was $2.4 billion (Statista, 2024).

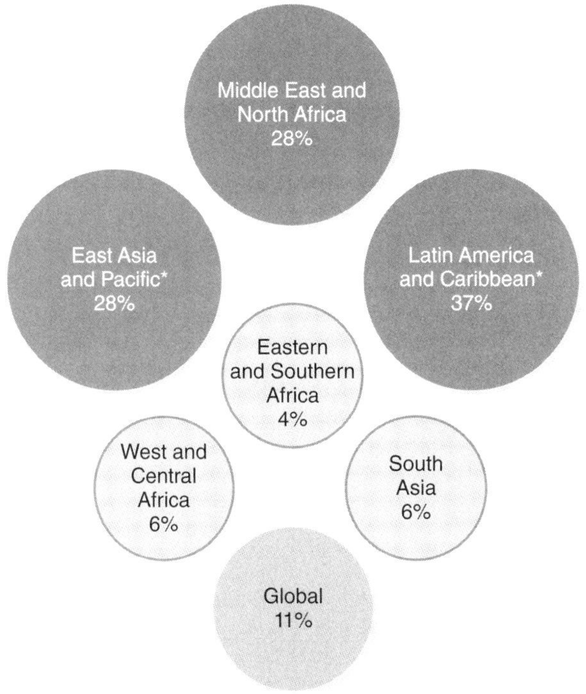

Figure 10-2 Percentage of Infants Aged 0 to 5 Months Fed Infant Formula, by UNICEF Region, 2018

Between 2008 and 2013, sales of (typically cow's) milk-based formula grew by 41% globally and by 72% in upper-middle-income countries such as Brazil, China, Peru, and Turkey. Analysis is based on a subset of 73 countries with available data between 2013 and 2018, covering 61% of the global population. Regional estimates are presented only where available data represent at least 50% of the region's population.

*To meet adequate population coverage, East Asia and the Pacific do not include China and Latin America, and the Caribbean does not include Brazil. Data are not available for Europe, Central Asia, and North America.

UNICEF global databases, 2019.

Impoverished families could spend as much as 100% of their cash income on these products if they were to follow the mixing instructions, especially in underdeveloped regions. All too often, to stretch their supply of formula, parents may dilute it or supplement their baby's diet with inappropriate foods, such as coffee, tea, sugared fruit drinks, and cow's milk.

Product Availability

The COVID pandemic presented a new crisis for families who rely on infant formula. When the pandemic struck in early 2020, restrictions on activity resulted in massive worker layoffs and the closing of factories. Ships were stuck at sea, warehouses overflowed, and trucks had no drivers. A global supply chain crisis affected the availability of infant formula. Adding to the crisis, a massive Abbott recall in February 2022 prompted the FDA to close the manufacturing facility in Sturgis, Michigan. By May, more than 40% of U.S. baby formula supplies were out of stock. Authorization of the Defense Production Act by the White House expedited the importation of infant formula to relieve domestic shortages (U.S. Mission Switzerland, 2022).

The Abbott plant did not reopen and resume production for another 2 months. The crisis hit Black and poor families disproportionately hard (Jung et al., 2023; Tomori & Palmquist, 2022). Parents faced uncertainty in safely feeding their babies. Some paid steep prices to scammers, not realizing they were purchasing from fraudulent sites until the formula they ordered never arrived. Some parents attempted to make their own formula (Kalaitzandonakes et al., 2023). Others diluted formula with extra water (Marino et al., 2023). There was a significant increase in lactation during the shortage (Imboden et al., 2022).

Community Resources

There are additional costs to the community beyond the expense of the infant formula itself. The production and packaging of the product consume valuable land and resources. The distribution process uses additional resources for fuel and contributes to environmental pollution. Even the disposal of waste products, such as infant formula cans, taxes the environment. Researchers estimate that nursing a baby for 6 months would save 95 to 153 kg of carbon dioxide per baby compared with formula feeding. For Great Britain alone, these reduced emissions would be equivalent to removing 50,000 to 77,500 cars from the road per year (Joffe et al., 2019). Furthermore, the ever-increasing need to improve infant formulas is a burden to research. It siphons off time and resources that might otherwise go toward mitigating unavoidable health concerns and facilitating lactation.

Healthcare Costs

Total global economic costs of not providing human milk to infants are calculated by analyzing deaths, increased morbidities, lost earnings, and cognitive losses. It is estimated that the increased morbidity, mortality, and lowered intelligence from not nursing could account for losses of about $341 billion annually, or 0.70% of world gross national income (Walters et al., 2019). In sub-Saharan Africa, a region with the highest under-5 mortality rates globally, the cost that nonexclusive and late lactation initiation attributed to child deaths was about $19.5 billion (Pretorius et al., 2021). Global economic losses from not providing human milk to infants result in $300 billion in avoidable annual costs (Jegier et al., 2024).

Lactation generates significant savings in healthcare costs (Camacho & Hussain, 2020; McLain et al., 2019; Santacruz-Salas et al., 2019; Unar-Munguía et al., 2019). It is estimated that the cost savings of a 10% increase in exclusive nursing in sub-Saharan Africa would be $27 billion in 2018 and $41 billion in 2030 (Pretorius et al., 2020). Globally, the disease protection that continues throughout lactation could prevent half of all deaths during the 12- to 23-month period (UNICEF, 2016).

Summary

Infant formula is an alternative for parents who cannot nurse and babies who cannot ingest human milk. Parents and caregivers require adequate education and resources to use formula safely. Excessive or inadequate levels of certain components can present serious health risks for infants. Errors and unsafe practices in manufacturing, aggressive marketing tactics, and the potential for preparation errors further increase infant risk. Promotion of infant formula use through the healthcare system compromises evidence-based, informed decisions on infant feeding. A family's reliance on infant formula creates financial burden and risks associated with product recalls and availability. Healthcare costs associated with formula use account for losses of billions of dollars of world gross national income.

What You Learned–At a Glance

Conversation Starters with Parents

- How familiar are you with the differences in infant formula brands?
- What health condition might prevent you from nursing your baby?
- What might require that your baby receive infant formula?
- What do you know about the risks of infant formula?

Parent's Legitimate Need for Formula

- Sheehan's syndrome
- Long-term contraindicated drug therapy
- Severe congestive heart failure
- Insufficient milk production
- Tuberculosis (until after treatment)
- HIV (when safe alternatives exist)
- Active herpes lesion
- Severe postpartum depression or psychosis that inhibits ability to care for baby
- Eclampsia or other severe illness or surgery preventing ability to care for baby
- Use of cytotoxic or radioactive drugs

Infant's Legitimate Need for Formula

- Hypoglycemia or dehydration if unimproved by increased nursing or expressed milk
- Jaundice if unimproved by increased nursing or expressed milk
- Prematurity
- Inborn errors of metabolism—galactosemia, maple syrup (sugar) urine disease, and PKU

Infant Health Risks from Formula

- Lower cognitive development
- Increased risk of childhood illnesses and death
- Contaminated water, mixing errors, and bacteria when left at room temperature too long
- Allergy from cow's milk

Concerns with Manufacturing and Use

- Slightly different among brands yet intended to meet the universal needs of infants
- Deficient or lacking in essential elements for optimal infant growth and health
- Excessive or deficient amounts of micronutrients or macronutrients
- Excessive amounts of vitamin D, which is toxic in high doses
- Lacking in most of the fatty acids present in human milk
- Contamination from processing
- Unsafe manufacturer practices
- Burden on family finances, community resources, and healthcare dollars

References

ABC News. Abbott launches new infant formula recall at another plant for faulty bottle cap seals. October 14, 2022. https://abcnews.go.com/Health/abbott-launches-infant-formula-recall-plant-faulty-bottle/story?id=91518369

ABC News. The maker of Enfamil recalls 145,000 cans of infant formula over bacteria risks. February 21, 2023. https://abcnews.go.com/US/wireStory/recalled-gerber-baby-formula-us-retailers-after-recall-99363937

Access to Nutrition Initiative. BMS marketing index 2024. March 2024. https://accesstonutrition.org/app/uploads/2024/03/BMS-Index-2024.pdf

Adgent MA, et al. A longitudinal study of estrogen-responsive tissues and hormone concentrations in infants fed soy formula. *J Clin Endocrinol Metab.* 2018;103(5):1899–1909.

Ahern GJ, et al. Advances in infant formula science. *Annu Rev Food Sci Technol.* 2019;10:75–102.

Almeida CC, et al. Bioactive compounds in infant formula and their effects on infant nutrition and health: a systematic literature review. *Int J Food Sci.* 2021;2021:8850080.

Altazan AD, et al. Unintentional error in formula preparation and its simulated impact on infant weight and adiposity. *Pediatr Obes.* 2019;14(12):e12564.

Amazouz H, et al. Infant feeding clusters are associated with respiratory health and allergy at school age in the PARIS birth cohort. *Allergy.* 2021;76(4):1223–1234.

American Academy of Pediatrics. Where we stand: soy formulas. August 7, 2018. https://www.healthychildren.org/English/ages-stages/baby/formula-feeding/Pages/Where-We-Stand-Soy-Formulas.aspx

Appleton J, et al. Informing infant nutrition: timing of infant formula advice, infant formula choice and preparation in the first 6 months of life. *J Nutr Educ Behav.* 2022;54(10):908–915.

Arija V, et al. Supplementation of infant formula and neurodevelopmental outcomes: a systematic review. *Curr Nutr Rep.* 2022; 11(2):283–300.

Artursson K, et al. Foodborne pathogens in unpasteurized milk in Sweden. *Int J Food Microbiol.* 2018;284:120–127.

Backhouse M. Botulism scare shook NZ's reputation—judge. *New Zealand Herald.* April 4, 2014. https://www.nzherald.co.nz/the-country/dairy-industry/news/article.cfm?c_id=168&objectid=11232363

Badiu Tişa I, et al. The importance of neonatal screening for galactosemia. *Nutrients.* 2022;15(1):10.

Becker GE, et al. Global evidence of persistent violations of the International Code of Marketing of Breast-milk Substitutes: a systematic scoping review. *Matern Child Nutr.* 2022;18(suppl 3): e13335.

Better Health Channel. HIV and women—having children. Reviewed September 28, 2023. https://www.betterhealth.vic.gov.au/health/conditionsandtreatments/hiv-and-women-having-children

Björmsjö M, et al. Reducing iron content in infant formula from 8 to 2 mg/l does not increase the risk of iron deficiency at 4 or 6 months of age: a randomized controlled trial. *Nutrients.* 2020;13(1):3.

Bobiński R, Bobińska J. Fatty acids of human milk—a review. *Int J Vitam Nutr Res.* 2022;92(3–4):280–291.

British Dietetic Association. Suitable milks for children with cow's milk allergy. Reviewed September 4, 2019. https://www.bda.uk.com/resource/children-with-cows -milk-allergy.html

Bührer C, et al. Infant formulas with synthetic oligosaccharides and respective marketing practices. *Mol Cell Pediatr.* 2022;9(1):14.

Caicedo-Borrás R, et al. Violations of the International Code of Marketing of Breastmilk Substitutes (WHO Code) in two Ecuadorian cities. *Nutrition.* 2021;87–88:111206.

Camacho EM, Hussain H. Cost-effectiveness evidence for strategies to promote or support breastfeeding: a systematic search and narrative literature review. *BMC Pregnancy Childbirth.* 2020; 20(1):757.

Canadian Food Inspection Agency. Labelling requirements for infant foods, infant formula, and human milk. Infant formula. August 16, 2018. https://inspection.gc.ca/food-label-requirements/labelling/industry/infant-foods-infant-formula-and-human-milk/eng/1393069958870/1393070130128?chap=3#s11c3

Carlock G, et al. Developmental outcomes in Duarte galactosemia. *Pediatrics.* 2019;143(1):e20182516.

Chen J. A worldwide food safety concern in 2008: melamine contaminated infant formula in China caused urinary tract stone in 290,000 children in China. *Chin Med J (Engl).* 2009;122(3): 243–244.

Chen QY, Costa M. Arsenic: a global environmental challenge. *Annu Rev Pharmacol Toxicol.* 2021;61:47–63.

Chi X, et al. E-nose, E-tongue combined with GC-IMS to analyze the influence of key additives during processing on the flavor of infant formula. *Foods.* 2022;11(22):3708.

Chichlowski M, et al. Effect of bovine milk fat globule membrane and lactoferrin in infant formula on gut microbiome and metabolome at 4 months of age. *Curr Dev Nutr.* 2021;5(5):nzab027.

Chinaview. China quality watchdog investigates baby milk powder scare. September 11, 2008. http://news.xinhuanet.com/english/2008-09/11/content_9920879.htm

Ching C, et al. Old tricks, new opportunities: how companies violate the International Code of Marketing of Breast-milk Substitutes and undermine maternal and child health during the COVID-19 pandemic. *Int J Environ Res Public Health.* 2021;18(5):2381.

Choi YY, et al. US toddler milk sales and associations with marketing practices. *Public Health Nutr.* 2020;23(6):1127–1135.

Clinicalinfo.HIV.gov. Recommendations for the use of antiretroviral drugs during pregnancy and interventions to reduce perinatal HIV transmission in the United States. Updated January 31, 2023. https://clinicalinfo.hiv.gov/en/guidelines/perinatal/infant-feeding-individuals-hiv-united-states

Codex Alimentarius. International food standards. Standard for infant formula and formulas for special medical purposes intended for infants. CXS 72-1981. United Nations Food and Agriculture Organization. 2023. https://www.fao.org/fao-who-codexalimentarius/sh-proxy/en/?lnk=1&url=https%253A%252F%252Fworkspace.fao.org%252Fsites%252Fcodex%252FStandards%252FCXS%2B72-1981%252FCXS_072e.pdf

Daily Telegraph (Sydney). Chinese "adulterated" Swiss baby formula (AAP News). March 29, 2013. http://www.dailytelegraph.com.au/chinese-adulterated-swiss-baby-formula/story-e6freuz9-1226608927320

Davis SA, et al. Homemade infant formula recipes may contain harmful ingredients: a quantitative content analysis of blogs. *Public Health Nutr.* 2020;23(8):1334–1339.

Elaridi J, et al. Determination of aluminum, chromium, and barium concentrations in infant formula marketed in Lebanon. *J Food Prot.* 2020;83(10):1738–1744.

Fang Y, et al. Associations between feeding patterns and infant health in China: a propensity score matching approach. *Nutrients.* 2021;13(12):4518.

Ficara M, et al. Changes of intestinal microbiota in early life. *J Matern Fetal Neonatal Med.* 2020;33(6):1036–1043.

Fossen Johnson S. Methemoglobinemia: infants at risk. *Curr Probl Pediatr Adolesc Health Care.* 2019;49(3):57–67.

Fridovich-Keil JL, et al. Acute and early developmental outcomes of children with Duarte galactosemia. *JIMD Rep.* 2021; 63(1):101–106.

Frisbie SH, et al. Manganese levels in infant formula and young child nutritional beverages in the United States and France: comparison to breast milk and regulations. *PLoS One.* 2019; 14(11):e0223636.

Gilmore LA, et al. Modifications to infant formula instructions improve the accuracy of formula dispensing. *Nutrients.* 2020; 12(4):1150.

Gilot L. Plant's baby formula called "filthy." *El Paso Times* (El Paso, TX). November 2, 2004:1.

Government of Canada. A joint statement of Health Canada, Canadian Paediatric Society, Dietitians of Canada, and Breastfeeding Committee for Canada. Nutrition for healthy term infants: recommendations from birth to six months. August 18, 2015. https://www.canada.ca/en/health-canada/services/canada-food-guide/resources/infant-feeding/nutrition-healthy-term-infants-recommendations-birth-six-months.html

Grandjean P. Developmental fluoride neurotoxicity: an updated review. *Environ Health.* 2019;18(1):110.

Greer FR, et al. Committee on Nutrition; Section on Allergy and Immunology. The effects of early nutritional interventions on the development of atopic disease in infants and children: the role of maternal dietary restriction, breastfeeding, hydrolyzed formulas, and timing of introduction of allergenic complementary foods. *Pediatrics.* 2019;143(4).

Grunewald M, et al. Variation and interdependencies of human milk macronutrients, fatty acids, adiponectin, insulin, and IGF-II in the European Prevent CD Cohort. *Nutrients.* 2019;11(9).

Hale T, Krutsch K. *Hale's Medications & Mothers' Milk 2025–2026: A Manual of Lactational Pharmacology*. 21st ed. New York, NY: Springer Publishing Company; 2024.

Harris JL, Pomeranz JL. Infant formula and toddler milk marketing: opportunities to address harmful practices and improve young children's diets. *Nutr Rev.* 2020;78(10):866–883.

Hastings G, et al. Selling second best: how infant formula marketing works. *Global Health.* 2020;16(1):77.

Hedrick J, et al. Infant formula with added bovine milk fat globule membrane and modified iron supports growth and normal iron status at one year of age: a randomized controlled trial. *Nutrients.* 2021;13(12):4541.

Henry M, Fouladkhah A. Outbreak history, biofilm formation, and preventive measures for control of *Cronobacter sakazakii* in infant formula and infant care settings. *Microorganisms.* 2019;7(3):77.

Hernández-Cordero S, et al. Exposure to marketing of breastmilk substitutes in Mexican women: sources and scope. *Int Breastfeed J.* 2022;17(1):16.

Hernández-Cordero S, et al. Violations of the International Code of Marketing of Breast-milk Substitutes in Mexico. *Matern Child Nutr.* 2019;15(1):e12682.

Hickman N, et al. Advertising of human milk substitutes in United Kingdom healthcare professional publications: an observational study. *J Hum Lact.* 2021;37(4):674–682.

Hitti M. Metal in infant formula prompts recall. February 22, 2006. https://www.webmd.com/parenting/baby/news/20060222/metal-in-infant-formula-prompts-recall

Horwood C, et al. An exploration of pregnant women and mothers' attitudes, perceptions and experiences of formula feeding and formula marketing, and the factors that influence decision-making about infant feeding in South Africa. *BMC Public Health.* 2022;22(1):393.

Igweze ZN, et al. Public health and paediatric risk assessment of aluminium, arsenic and mercury in infant formulas marketed in Nigeria. *Sultan Qaboos Univ Med J.* 2020;20(1):e63–e70.

Imboden A, et al. Impact of the infant formula shortage on breastfeeding rates. *J Pediatr Health Care.* 2022:S0891-5245(22) 00337-6.

Jallad KN. The hazards of a ubiquitary metalloid, arsenic, hiding in infant diets: detection, speciation, exposure, and risk assessment. *Biol Trace Elem Res.* 2019;190(1):11–23.

Jegier BJ, et al. The economic cost consequences of suboptimal infant and young child feeding practices: a scoping review. *Health Policy Plan.* 2024;39(9):916–945.

Joffe N, et al. Support for breastfeeding is an environmental imperative. *BMJ.* 2019;l5646. doi:10.1136/bmj.l5646

Jones A, et al. Digital marketing of breast-milk substitutes: a systematic scoping review. *Curr Nutr Rep.* 2022;11(3):416–430.

Jones G, et al. Outbreak of *Salmonella enterica* serotype Poona in infants linked to persistent *Salmonella* contamination in an infant formula manufacturing facility, France, August 2018 to February 2019. *Euro Surveill.* 2019;24(13):1900161.

Jung J, et al. The curious case of baby formula in the United States in 2022: cries for urgent action months after silence in the midst of alarm bells. *Food Ethics.* 2023;8(1):4.

Kakoo Brioso E, et al. Salt poisoning due to inadequate infant formula preparation: a rare cause of hypernatremia and massive cerebral hemorrhage in a newborn. *Cureus.* 2022;14(12): e33045.

Kalaitzandonakes M, et al. Coping with the 2022 infant formula shortage. *Prev Med Rep.* 2023;32:102123.

Kim JH, et al. Infant feeding pattern clusters are associated with childhood health outcomes. *Nutrients.* 2023;15(13):3065.

Le Monde. French company Lactalis charged over baby milk *Salmonella* scandal. February 16, 2023. https://www.lemonde.fr/en/france/article/2023/02/16/french-company-charged-over-baby-milk-salmonella-scandal_6016092_7.html

Lee H, et al. Milk fat globule membrane as a modulator of infant metabolism and gut microbiota: a formula supplement narrowing the metabolic differences between breastfed and formula-fed infants. *Mol Nutr Food Res.* 2021;65(3):e2000603.

Lhotska L, et al. Protecting breastfeeding from conflicts of interest. *J Hum Lact.* 2020;36(1):22–28.

Marino JA, et al. Impact of the COVID-19 pandemic on infant feeding practices in the United States: food insecurity, supply shortages and deleterious formula-feeding practices. *Matern Child Nutr.* 2023;19(3):e13498.

McCarthy JJ, Yale SC. Kwashiorkor in an 8-month-old infant due to homemade formula use. *WMJ.* 2023;122(1):67–69.

McLain AC, et al. Comparison of methods used to estimate the global burden of disease related to undernutrition and suboptimal breastfeeding. *Adv Nutr.* 2019 May 1;10(3):380–390.

Mehmet S. Governments failing to stop harmful marketing of breast-milk substitutes, warns report. June 2020. https://www.newfoodmagazine.com/news/111487/governments-failing-to-stop-harmful-marketing-of-breast-milk-substitutes-warns-report/

Merieux Nutrisciences. Market news. More babies infected with *Salmonella* in outbreak linked to rice milk formula. February 2019. https://www.merieuxnutrisciences.com/cn/sites/merieux_nutrisciences_cn/files/atoms/files/sinosilliker-market_news-201902.pdf

Mirza Alizadeh A, et al. Melamine in Iranian foodstuffs: a systematic review, meta-analysis, and health risk assessment of infant formula. *Ecotoxicol Environ Saf.* 2023;256:114854.

Mohamed HJJ, et al. Brain-immune-gut benefits with early life supplementation of milk fat globule membrane. *JGH Open.* 2022;6(7):454–461.

NBC News. Recalled Gerber baby formula was sent to U.S. retailers after recall began, wholesaler says. May 16, 2023. https://www.nbcnews.com/news/us-news/recalled-gerber-baby-formula-was-sent-us-retailers-recall-began-wholes-rcna84703

Neuberger et al. Infant formula shortage highlights WIC's critical role in feeding babies. Center on Budget and Policy Priorities. Updated June 22, 2022. https://www.cbpp.org/research/food-assistance/infant-formula-shortage-highlights-wics-critical-role-in-feeding-babies

NHS Trust Imperial College Healthcare. HIV and breastfeeding your baby. Reviewed November 2021. https://www.imperial.nhs.uk/-/media/website/patient-information-leaflets/maternity-services/postanatal-care/hiv-and-breastfeeding-your-baby.pdf

Oddy WH. Breastfeeding, childhood asthma, and allergic disease. *Ann Nutr Metab.* 2017;70(suppl 2):26–36.

Palma-Lara I, et al. Arsenic exposure: a public health problem leading to several cancers. *Regul Toxicol Pharmacol.* 2020;110:104539.

Pierson B. Reuters. Reckitt unit hit with $60 million verdict in Enfamil baby formula case in Illinois. March 15, 2024. https://www.reuters.com/legal/reckitt-unit-hit-with-60-million-verdict-enfamil-baby-formula-case-illinois-2024-03-14/

Pretorius CE, et al. Impact of breastfeeding on mortality in sub-Saharan Africa: a systematic review, meta-analysis, and cost-evaluation. *Eur J Pediatr.* 2020;179(8):1213–1225.

Pretorius CE, et al. Exclusive breastfeeding, child mortality, and economic cost in sub-Saharan Africa. *Pediatrics.* 2021;147(3):e2020030643.

Pugliese M, et al. Outcomes in pediatric studies of medium-chain acyl-coA dehydrogenase (MCAD) deficiency and phenylketonuria (PKU): a review. *Orphanet J Rare Dis.* 2020;15(1):12.

Redgrove J, et al. Prescription infant formulas are contaminated with aluminium. *Int J Environ Res Public Health.* 2019;16(5):899.

Rivera-Pasquel M, et al. Effect of milk-based infant formula fortified with PUFAs on lipid profile, growth and micronutrient status of young children: a randomized double-blind clinical trial. *Nutrients.* 2020;13(1):4.

Rodriguez R, et al. The idealization of infant formula: a longitudinal analysis of labels in Uruguay. *J Hum Lact.* 2023;39(3):519–528.

Santacruz-Salas E, et al. The economic influence of breastfeeding on the health cost of newborns. *J Hum Lact.* 2019;35(2):340–348.

Siegel-Itzkovich J. Police in Israel launch investigation into deaths of babies given formula milk. *BMJ.* 2003;327:1128.

Sodhi CP, et al. Fat composition in infant formula contributes to the severity of necrotising enterocolitis. *Br J Nutr.* 2018;120(6):665–680.

Statista Research Department. Revenue of the baby food market worldwide from 2018 to 2029. Oct 18, 2024. https://www.statista.com/statistics/249469/global-baby-food-market-size-2015/

Succoio M, et al. Galactosemia: biochemistry, molecular genetics, newborn screening, and treatment. *Biomolecules.* 2022;12(7):968.

Tanrikulu H, et al. Corporate political activity of the baby food industry: the example of Nestlé in the United States of America. *Int Breastfeed J.* 2020;15(1):22.

Testa I, et al. Soy-based infant formula: are phyto-oestrogens still in doubt? *Front Nutr.* 2018;5:110.

Till C, et al. Fluoride exposure from infant formula and child IQ in a Canadian birth cohort. *Environ Int.* 2020;134:105315.

Tomori C, Palmquist AEL. Racial capitalism and the US formula shortage: a policy analysis of the formula industry as a neocolonial system. *Front Sociol.* 2022;7:961200.

Trompiz G. Health news. Lactalis recalls baby milk from Spanish site linked to *Salmonella.* Reuters. January 25, 2019. https://www.reuters.com/article/business/lactalis-recalls-baby-milk-from-spanish-site-linked-to-salmonella-idUSKCN1PJ1YC/

Tsai HJ, et al. Intake of phthalate-tainted foods and microalbuminuria in children: the 2011 Taiwan food scandal. *Environ Int.* 2016;89–90:129–137.

Unar-Munguía M, et al. The burden of suboptimal breastfeeding in Mexico: maternal health outcomes and costs. *Matern Child Nutr.* 2019;15(1):e12661.

United Nations Children's Fund. From the first hour of life: making the case for improved infant and young child feeding everywhere. October 2016. https://data.unicef.org/resources/first-hour-life-new-report-breastfeeding -practices/

United Nations Children's Fund. Infant and young child feeding. July 2018. data.unicef.org/topic/nutrition/infant-and-young-child-feeding

United Nations Children's Fund. Protecting infant and young child nutrition from industry interference and conflicts of interest. 2023. https://www.globalbreastfeedingcollective.org/media/2126/file

United Nations Children's Fund. Countering industry arguments against code implementation: evidence and rights-based responses. 2024. https://www.globalbreastfeedingcollective.org/media/2581/file/Addressing-Industry-arguments-Code.pdf.pdf

Upson K, et al. Soy-based infant formula feeding and menstrual pain in a cohort of women aged 23-35 years. *Hum Reprod.* 2019;34(1):148–-154.

U.S. Department of Health and Human Services, Centers for Medicare & Medicaid Services. Open payments data. June 30, 2016. https://healthdata.gov/dataset /open-payments-data-0

U.S. Food and Drug Administration. Similac Advance with iron powdered infant formula. February 2, 2005. https://wayback.archive-it.org/7993/20170112170738/http://www.fda.gov/Safety/MedWatch/SafetyInformation/SafetyAlertsforHumanMedicalProducts/ucm150519.htm

U.S. Food and Drug Administration. Abbott Similac Special Care 24 Cal/fl. oz. Ready-to-feed premature infant formula with iron. May 29, 2007. https://wayback.archive-it.org/7993/20170112170435/http://www.fda.gov/Safety/MedWatch/SafetyInformation/SafetyAlertsforHumanMedicalProducts/ucm152999.htm

U.S. Food and Drug Administration. Similac powder infant formulas: recall. September 24, 2010. https://wayback.archive-it.org/7993/20170723102135/https://www.fda.gov/Food/RecallsOutbreaksEmergencies/SafetyAlertsAdvisories/ucm227339.htm

U.S. Food and Drug Administration. FDA sets standards for infant formula. February 6, 2014. https://www.fda.gov/consumers/consumer-updates/fda-takes-final-step-infant-formula-protections

U.S. Food and Drug Administration. Perrigo issues voluntary recall for parent's choice advantage infant formula milk-based powder with iron. June 21, 2019. https://www.fda.gov/safety/recalls-market-withdrawals-safety-alerts/perrigo-issues-voluntary-recall-parents-choice-advantage-infant-formula-milk-based-powder-iron

U.S. Food and Drug Administration. FDA investigation of *Cronobacter* infections: powdered infant formula (February 2022). 2022. https://www.fda.gov/food/outbreaks-foodborne-illness/fda-investigation-cronobacter-infections-powdered-infant-formula-february-2022

U.S. Mission Switzerland. Biden administration approves first operation fly formula mission. Press release, Washington DC. May 20, 2022. https://ch.usembassy.gov/biden-administration-approves-first-operation-fly-formula-mission/

Verduci E, et al. Use of soy-based formulas and cow's milk allergy: lights and shadows. *Front Pediatr.* 2020;8:591988.

Walters DD, et al. The cost of not breastfeeding: global results from a new tool. *Health Policy Plan.* 2019;34(6):407–417.

Wazed MA, Farid M. Hypoallergenic and low-protein ready-to-feed (RTF) infant formula by high pressure pasteurization: a novel product. *Foods.* 2019;8(9):408.

Werner KM, et al. Pediatricians' reports of interaction with infant formula companies. *Breastfeed Med.* 2023;18(3):219–225.

Westmark CJ. Soy-based therapeutic baby formulas: testable hypotheses regarding the pros and cons. *Front Nutr.* 2017;3:59.

Whitworth J. ANSES makes recommendations to ensure infant formula safety. Food Safety News. November 16, 2019. https://www.foodsafetynews.com/2019/11/anses-makes-recommendations-to-ensure-infant-formula-safety/

Willis C, et al. An assessment of the microbiological quality and safety of raw drinking milk on retail sale in England. *J Appl Microbiol.* 2018;124(2):535–546.

World Health Organization. Guidelines for the safe preparation, storage and handling of powdered infant formula. 2007. https://www.who.int/foodsafety/publications/powdered-infant-formula/en/

World Health Organization. *Guidance on Ending the Inappropriate Promotion of Foods for Infants and Young Children: Implementation Manual.* Geneva, Switzerland: World Health Organization; 2017. https://www.who.int/nutrition/publications/infantfeeding/manual-ending-inappropriate-promotion-food/en/

World Health Organization. Newsroom: infant and young child feeding. June 9, 2021. https://www.who.int/news-room/fact-sheets/detail/infant-and-young-child-feeding

World Health Organization and United Nations Children's Fund. How the marketing of formula milk influences our decisions on infant feeding. 2022. https://www.who.int/publications/i/item/9789240044609

Zhao J, et al. MFGM components promote gut *Bifidobacterium* growth in infant and in vitro. *Eur J Nutr.* 2022;61(1):277–288.

CHAPTER 11

Substances in Human Milk

Concern or confusion may arise when nursing parents consume medications or social toxicants or when they are exposed to environmental contaminants. When an exogenous substance is present in the milk, the most important consideration is the effect the substance will have on the infant. Tobacco, caffeine, alcohol, cannabis (marijuana), cocaine, and medications can travel through the milk to the baby. Environmental contaminants can be present in the milk, and some types transfer to the baby. The transfer of substances into the milk of nonbinary parents has not been well studied, and research is needed for this parent population. Discussion in this chapter focuses on maternal exposure based on historical studies.

KEY TERMS

Amphetamines
Bisphenol A (BPA)
Buprenorphine
Caffeine
Cannabis (marijuana)
Cocaine
Detoxify
Dichlorodiphenyldichloroethylene (DDE)
Dichlorodiphenyltrichloroethane (DDT)
Environmental contaminants
Half-life
Heroin
Naloxone
Naltrexone
Over-the-counter medication
Persistent organic pollutants (POPs)
Phencyclidine hydrochloride (PCP)
Phthalates
Polybrominated diphenyl ethers (PBDEs)
Social toxicant

Medications

Not long ago, experts believed that nursing parents should take no medications and that they would need to wean if a medication was necessary. As research in lactation and human milk has evolved, practitioners adopted a more moderate and practical approach toward medications during lactation. Very few medications require temporary or permanent weaning or other special considerations.

When reviewing the advisability of a substance, the primary considerations are the degree to which it is excreted into the milk and its possible effects on the infant. A maternal drug that is also used in pediatric care likely poses low risk to the infant. During pregnancy, the liver and kidneys **detoxify** and excrete substances for the fetus through the placenta. During lactation, however, the infant must metabolize the drug. Therefore, a medication such as pseudoephedrine that is considered safe during pregnancy may not be the best choice during lactation.

Nursing parents should consult the baby's health practitioner before taking any prescription drug, **over-the-counter medication**, herbs, vitamins, or supplements of any kind. Among the drugs for which information is available, few are contraindicated during lactation. Generally, a relative infant dose (RID) of less than 10% of the adult dose is considered safe (Hale & Krutsch, 2024). A drug that is safe for the fetus and the nursing infant may still affect the letdown reflex, milk production, or milk secretion. Parents need to remind the prescribing provider that they are nursing and confirm the drug's advisability. They can also consult with pharmacists for over-the-counter medications and other supplements.

Drug Entry into Milk

In many cases, substances are excreted into the milk in low concentrations and pose no danger to the infant. Additionally, the molecular weight or binding capacity of some substances does not allow them to enter the milk. When a substance passes into the milk, the infant's gastrointestinal (GI) tract often offers protection, either by not absorbing it or by altering it. The infant may experience some adverse effects, however, from substances in the milk that are not altered or eliminated by the GI system.

Figure 11-1 shows the factors that influence the complex process by which a substance passes from the bloodstream into the milk. **Figure 11-2** illustrates how medications transfer from the plasma through the capillary walls, past the alveolar epithelium, and into the milk. As illustrated in **Figure 11-3**, the gaps between alveolar cells are largest in the first few days postpartum, increasing the potential for drugs to enter the milk at that time. Fortunately, the volume of intake is small during the colostral phase. As the alveolar cells enlarge, they shut off many of the gaps and reduce the amount of drug entry.

- Size of the molecules in the substance (molecules over 800–1000 daltons have difficulty passing through alveolar cells).
- Solubility of the substance in water or fat (fat diffuses more easily into milk).
- Binding capacity of the substance with protein.
- pH of the substance.
- The milk/plasma ratio.
- Route of administration (oral, intramuscular, intravenous).
- Short- or long-acting version of the drug.
- Activity or inactivity of components of the substance.
- Rate of detoxification in the nursing parent's system.
- Whether the substance accumulates in the nursing parent's system.
- Duration of use.
- Time substance is ingested relative to a feeding.
- Number of days postpartum when substance is consumed.
- Age and size of the infant (preterm, full-term, older baby).
- Amount of milk the infant consumes (exclusively nursing or supplemented).
- Absorption of the substance in the infant's gut.
- Safety in giving the substance to the infant directly.

Figure 11-1 Potential for infant exposure to substances in human milk.

Infant Exposure

The potential effect of any substance on a nursing infant is of primary significance when medication is required during lactation. One consideration is whether the medication will pass into the milk and be absorbed in the baby's GI tract. Another is whether the infant can be exposed safely to the substance as it appears in the milk. Understanding the substance's characteristics can help resolve the dilemma faced by healthcare workers and parents when the need for a

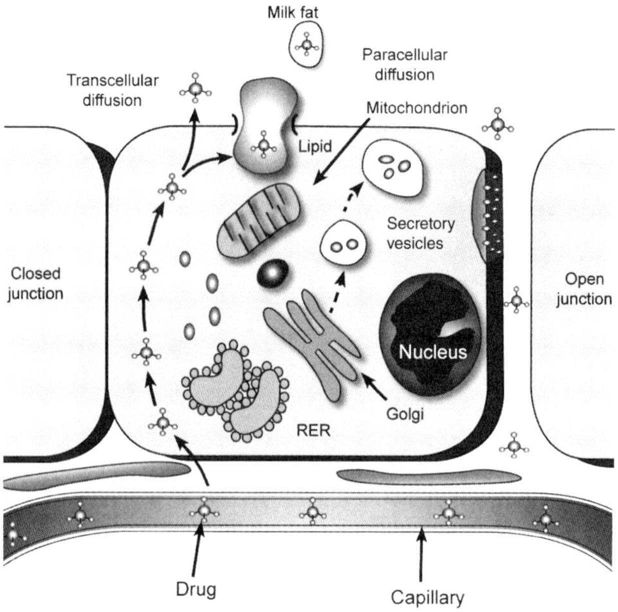

Figure 11-2 How drugs enter milk.

Printed with permission of Thomas Hale, Hale Publishing.

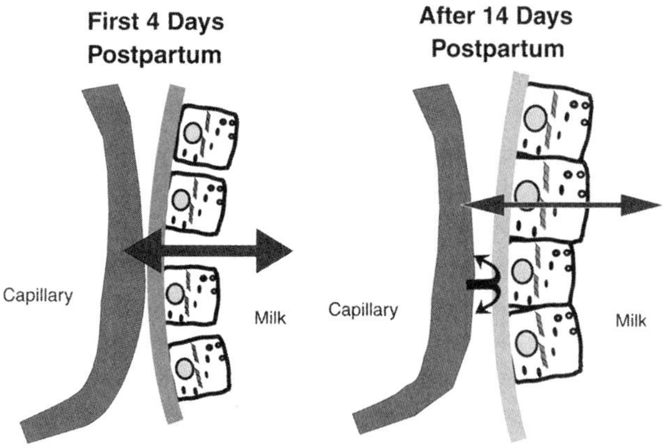

Figure 11-3 Alveolar cell gaps.

Printed with permission of Thomas Hale, Hale Publishing.

medication arises. Many factors influence the level of a substance found in the infant's bloodstream. Some factors relate to the infant, and others reflect characteristics of the drug itself.

How Soon After Birth

One safety consideration for the infant is how soon after birth a medication is consumed. The junctions between the alveolar cells in the mammary glands remain open for several days postpartum. Therefore, more of a medication can penetrate the milk at that time than in later weeks (Hale & Hartmann, 2017).

The amount of a substance that passes to the baby relates directly to the volume of milk that is consumed. Newborns consume small quantities of colostrum in the first few days. Thus, the amount of other substances ingested is small in comparison with later intake volumes. Likewise, infants who receive mixed feedings or solid food will receive a lesser amount of a substance through the milk than will an infant who nurses exclusively. The volume of milk consumed by a supplemented infant is lower, and less of the substance may be absorbed because of the supplemental food.

Gestational Age

The baby's age and size influence the effects of maternal medications. A preterm infant assimilates substances in the milk differently than a full-term infant or older infant. An older and larger baby may metabolize a substance more effectively, reducing its effect. A newborn's immature liver cannot efficiently detoxify a substance and excrete it in the urine or stool. Thus, in the early days postpartum, it may be difficult for a neonate to excrete even small amounts of a substance. A drug that depends on the liver for detoxification could pose a risk if not metabolized effectively.

Resistance to Detoxification

A substance that is particularly resistant to being destroyed in the infant's GI tract could accumulate to toxic levels and pose a danger to the infant. A maternal drug with poor oral bioavailability must be administered by injection so that the amount received in the milk is destroyed in the infant's GI tract. A drug that has reduced systemic absorption in the infant could theoretically cause GI symptoms such as diarrhea. Some substances compete for protein-binding sites and displace other toxic substances that are then free to migrate to other parts of the body (Hale & Hartmann, 2017). For example, sulfamethoxazole and trimethoprim are not recommended in babies with glucose-6-phosphate dehydrogenase (G6PD) deficiency or those who are jaundiced (Hale & Krutsch, 2024).

Over-the-Counter Medications

Questions often arise about consuming over-the-counter medications, such as pain relievers, cough medicines, cold remedies, suppositories, antacids, diarrhea remedies, and herbal preparations, during lactation. Many cold remedies contain antihistamines that dry up nasal secretions. Products containing pseudoephedrine can lower milk production by as much as 24% (Ceulemans et al., 2020; "Pseudoephedrine," 2020). Antihistamines may enter the milk and produce sedation in the baby. However, second-generation antihistamines have less sedating effects (Sanchez-Borges & Ansotegui, 2019).

Because these medications are more accessible than prescription drugs, there is a greater likelihood that parents will use them. Parents are encouraged to discuss the safety of over-the-counter medications. Healthcare providers need to know about present consumption of prescription drugs, over-the-counter medications, vitamins, herbs, and any other substances before they prescribe medications. This coordination will avoid possible interactions among the substances.

Minimizing the Effects of Medications

Some drugs present in the milk can either reduce or stimulate milk production or secretion. They may also cause reactions in the infant. Parents taking medications should watch for changes in milk production and any unusual changes in their baby's behavior, feeding, output, and sleeping patterns, such as fussiness, lethargy, rash, vomiting, or diarrhea. They can minimize the effects of drugs in the milk in many ways, as discussed in the following subsections.

Schedule Medications Around Nursing

Parents can schedule taking a drug around feedings to ensure the lowest amount of drug possible entering the milk. Considering the usual absorption rates and peak levels of most drugs, taking the medication toward the end of the dose cycle would be safest. As a general rule, it may be best to take the drug immediately after nursing or 3 to 4 hours before the next feeding. Depending on the drug, a brief pause in nursing may avoid the drug's peak level in the milk. Factors such as milk production, feeding frequency, and comfort will help determine whether to pump and discard the milk. One option may be to take a fat-soluble drug at bedtime, after which the baby usually does not feed as often.

Select the Least Offensive Drug

When possible, healthcare providers should prescribe a drug that produces the least amount in the milk and has the least potential for causing problems. **Table 11-1** provides an explanation of the lactation risk categories. **Table 11-2** rates drug safety on a scale of 1 to 5 for various families of drugs. Parents who must take a medication that has not been tested for safety during lactation can discuss options with the baby's healthcare provider. Medications with long plasma half-lives are more difficult for the baby to eliminate and could build up over time to higher concentrations in the baby's plasma. Enzyme action in the liver is usually required to metabolize a drug with a long half-life. This increases the possibility of its accumulation in a young baby.

For example, one older drug, lithium, is a drug of concern. It is rated L4 (the second-highest level of concern for lactation risk). In some instances, nursing has been allowed while taking lithium (Imaz et al.,

Table 11-1 Lactation Risk Categories

L1	Safest Drug: Controlled studies in nursing parents fail to show harm to infant or the product is not bioavailable to infant.
L2	Safe Drug: Studied in limited number of nursing parents, no increase in adverse effects to infant or evidence of risk to infant is remote.
L3	Moderately Safe: No controlled studies done on nursing parents. Drug should only be given if benefits justify potential risk to infant. New medications with no published data are included in this category.
L4	Possibly Hazardous: Known risk to infant or milk production, but benefits to nursing parent may still be acceptable.
L5	Contraindicated Studies: Documented evidence demonstrates risk to infant. Risk of drug outweighs benefits of nursing. The drug is contraindicated in nursing parents.

Source: Hale T, Krutsch K. *Hale's Medications & Mothers' Milk 2025-2026: A Manual of Lactational Pharmacology 21st ed.* New York, NY: Springer Publishing Company; 2024.

Table 11-2 Safety of Medications While Nursing

Pain Relievers:
Tylenol (*acetaminophen*) L1
Advil, Motrin (*ibuprofen*) L1
Limited aspirin (81–325 mg per day) L2

Antibiotic/Antifungal Meds:
Diflucan (*fluconazole*) L2
Monistat (*miconazole*) L2
Penicillins (*amoxicillin, ampicillin*) L1
Cephalosporins (*Keflex, Omnicef, Rocephin, Ceftin*) L1

Cough/Cold/Allergies:
Antihistamines:
Claritin®, Alavert (*loratadine*) L1
Allegra (*fexofenadine*) L2
Zyrtec (*cetirizine*) L2
Benadryl (*diphenhydramine*) L2

Decongestants:
Afrin Nasal Spray (*oxymetazoline*) L3—limit to 3 days
AVOID pseudoephedrine (may decrease milk production)

Steroid:
Medrol dose pack (*methylprednisolone*), oral prednisone
(<40 mg/day) L2
Kenalog shot (*triamcinolone*) L3
Rhinocort Nasal Spray (*budesonide*) L1
Other nasal sprays (*Flonase, Nasacort, Nasonex*) L3

Cough:
Sore throat spray (*Benzocaine*) L2
Cough drops (*limit menthol*)
Mucinex (*guaifenesin*) L2
Robitussin DM (*dextromethorphan*) L3
AVOID benzonatate (L4)

Birth Control:
Progestin only when establishing milk production
Mini Pill, Mirena (L3); after oral trials:
Depo-Provera, Implanon (L4)
Emergency contraception
Plan B (*levonorgestrel*) L2—withhold nursing for 8 hours

GI Meds:
Pepcid (*famotidine*) L1
Tagamet (*cimetidine*) L1
Colace (*docusate*) L2
Imodium (*loperamide*) L2
Limit Pepto-Bismol L3

Antidepressants:
Selective serotonin reuptake inhibitors—Zoloft (*sertraline*), Paxil (*paroxetine*), Lexapro
(*Escitalopram*), etc. L2
Bupropion (*Wellbutrin*) L3

Courtesy of InfantRisk Center/Texas Tech University Health Sciences Center.

2021). Because of prenatal lithium exposure, as well as other factors, it is difficult to tie adverse effects strictly to nursing. Recommendations on whether to continue lithium while nursing must be personalized to the individual parent and their infant. Personalized recommendations and close coordination with the parent's prescriber and the baby's healthcare provider, along with monitoring of the dyad's levels, are crucial in cases such as these (Imaz et al., 2021; Newmark et al., 2019).

Counseling About Medications

The role of lactation consultants regarding medications is to share information with parents and point out options. Parents often have questions about the safety of a particular medication while they are nursing. Unless you have prescribing privileges as a healthcare provider, your role is to educate parents to be active health consumers. They need to take responsibility for making decisions and taking specific action. You can help them pose questions and stimulate their thinking so that they will explore the facts and base their decisions on accurate and sound information.

A potential for conflict between specialties arises when lactation consultants have more education and information concerning lactation than do parents' healthcare providers. Lactation consultants have a responsibility to educate parents about practices that are supportive of nursing, including the use of medications. The International Board Certified Lactation Consultant (IBCLC) Scope of Practice includes the duty to provide evidence-based information regarding the potential impact on milk production and child safety of medications and other substances, as well as complementary and alternative therapies (International Board of Lactation Consultant Examiners [IBLCE], 2018). Furthermore, the IBCLC Code of Professional Conduct states that every IBCLC shall "supply sufficient and accurate information to enable clients to make informed decisions" (IBLCE, 2015, p. 2).

The internet provides a wealth of resources for researching medicines. Internet-savvy parents often will have researched their options before seeking advice. It is important that you present all drug information objectively and not in a manner that appears to recommend or provide advice about the safety of a particular medication. You can help clarify a situation, discuss options, and then encourage parents to consult their healthcare provider regarding questions or concerns. **Figure 11-4** presents some items you might discuss with parents.

After clarifying the situation, consider the following discussion points:

- Is there an alternative treatment course that would avoid any medication?
- Is there a safer medication or medical procedure?
- Do the benefits of the medication outweigh the possible risks to the baby?
- Does exposure to the medication pose less risk to the baby than the use of infant formula?
- Is the healthcare provider supportive of nursing?

Figure 11-4 Discussion points about medications.

Locating Drug Information

Information about the advisability of taking a drug during lactation needs to come from a reliable source. Become acquainted with each drug group and its potential risks and benefits. You can find the generic name of a drug's brand name with an internet search using "trade name generic" search terms. Reliable print resources include *Hale's Medications & Mothers' Milk* (Hale & Krutsch, 2024), *Nonprescription Drugs for the Breastfeeding Mother* (Nice, 2017), and *Drugs in Pregnancy and Lactation* (Briggs et al., 2021).

The market for mobile health applications has exploded. These apps include numerous offerings about medications and drug information. It is important that you consult bona fide resources for your clients' safety and that you dig deeper than the manufacturer's standard disclaimer. Popular apps include the U.S. National Library of Medicine's LactMed and the mobile app version of *Medications and Mothers' Milk* (Hale & Krutsch, 2024). Apps provide up-to-date information on new drugs as well as information about recalls or warnings.

The Infant Risk Center is a university-based call center and informational web resource for both healthcare professionals and consumers (Infant Risk Center, 2024). This key resource from Texas Tech University provides evidence-based information about new and existing drugs and their compatibility with nursing, as well as interactions among multiple medications in complex cases. Information about new drugs is posted as soon as studies or anecdotal observations become available. An online forum is free and accessible to the public. A nursing parent who is taking a medication that has not been studied or that has limited data can help further research by enrolling in the lactation research registry. The MommyMeds app is downloadable from the Apple store or Google Play for around-the-clock help, with a minimal cost to help fund the research and the service.

Newness of the data	There is much case reporting of drugs used during nursing that provides newer data, whereas most original data regarding drugs in human milk was published between 1920 and 1960.
Human versus animal data	Animal data may or may not apply to human lactation. The peer review process will assist in determining this relevance.
Completeness of screening	The reader should always look for whether the researcher mentions studying metabolites of the drug. If metabolites were not studied, justification is needed. Usually, researchers will justify that within their study. Consulting a pharmacologist will help you understand the significance and quality of a study about drugs.
Isolated cases	Much of the original data about a substance may be based on only 1 or 2 case reports, with insufficient controls. This occurs because ethics prevent experiments on humans. Clinicians must make decisions without complete data to guide them. If a nursing parent needs a medication and wants to continue nursing, physicians sometimes allow it, monitor it, and then write up the experience to share with colleagues. Such case reports have no control, but the medical community has at least a small amount of information instead of none. One cannot conclude universal safety from one case report. However, healthcare providers who support nursing even in difficult circumstances may be less reluctant to try a drug instead of stopping nursing. You can encourage nursing parents taking newer or little-used medications to register at the Infant Risk Center to benefit other parents and babies by providing milk samples for research. Nursing parents can register at www.infantrisk.com.
Sampling technique	Older studies may show random sampling of milk rather than samples based on drug peak and trough levels. Trough is the lowest blood or milk level achieved by the drug during its dosing period. Gentamicin, for instance, requires testing every 3 days or so to see what the highest and lowest levels of the drug are in the blood. This is done by testing an hour after a dose and an hour before the next dose is due. The timing of testing is different in different drugs. Some drugs have a narrow safety range, so it is important to keep the dose within that range. Although newer research is less problematic in this area, it is still important that you consider this when reading such research.
Personal correspondence	Although much personal correspondence is useful, the reader should be aware that the data may not be available for public inspection and could be biased. Often, personal correspondence is research in progress that lends support to the article.
Speculation	Speculation by the author of the original article may be interpreted as fact after several review articles have been written. This can be a problem, and readers should always beware of speculation.

Figure 11-5 Factors to consider in drug literature.

Sharing studies and research in an objective manner encourages parents to use the information to make informed decisions with their healthcare providers. When presenting information to parents, read the facts to them exactly as stated and cite the source for the information. Empower them to educate themselves about their condition and treatment. Responsive healthcare providers welcome a collaborative partnership with their clients and healthcare team members. Lactation consultants are a valued part of the healthcare team. Collaboration protects nursing while ensuring the infant's and parent's safety.

Critical Reading of Drug Studies

A legitimate evaluation of medical information must go beyond personal observation and withstand the test of scientific criticism. As part of this evaluation, the effectiveness of a drug or treatment should be compared with that of other treatments. A drug's safety should be determined after large numbers of observations over long periods. The burden of proof rests with the researcher—the one who is recommending a particular drug or treatment—especially if it involves a substance that is not well established in medical practice. Many review articles written in both lay and professional publications are helpful in providing background information on a drug's presence in human milk. When reading such articles, carefully consider each study's methods and conclusions. **Figure 11-5** identifies factors to consider when reading literature about drugs. Chapter 28 discusses research methods.

Social Toxicants

Social mood-changing toxicants—tobacco, coffee, tea, alcohol, **cannabis (marijuana)**, and other drugs—are consumed in varying degrees in most cultures. Parents need to understand how substances can negatively affect their milk quality or quantity or harm their babies through their milk. Some substances may be consumed in moderation, whereas others, such as recreational drugs, must be avoided during lactation (Meek, et al, 2022).

Nicotine and Tobacco

As many as 10% of birth parents who quit smoking during pregnancy resume smoking postpartum (Substance Abuse and Mental Health Services

Administration [SAMHSA], 2021). Smokers have over twice the probability of not initiating nursing as nonsmokers. There is a significant dose–response pattern, with the more cigarettes smoked per day resulting in a higher probability of formula feeding (Lechosa Muñiz et al., 2019). Smokers who initiate nursing have a higher probability of not continuing exclusive nursing (Tanda et al., 2018). They are also more likely to wean before 3 months than nonsmokers (Joseph et al., 2017). Despite higher initiation rates when parents quit smoking during pregnancy, early weaning is still a frequent outcome.

Smoking presents concerns about respiratory infections, chronic ear infections, sudden infant death syndrome (SIDS), low milk production, and poor weight gain. Parents may therefore believe they cannot nurse if they smoke. However, the American Academy of Pediatrics (AAP, 2019) and the Australian Breastfeeding Association (ABA, 2022) recommend nursing to protect babies from the harmful effects of smoking or vaping. The periods before and during pregnancy are opportunities for education about nursing and smoking and encouraging healthy practices. Motivation to overcome habits may be higher during pregnancy and even more so when planning to nurse. Nursing parents who smoke should be encouraged to quit or to smoke less.

Secondhand Smoke

All members of the baby's household need to be discouraged from smoking inside the home, especially anywhere around the baby. Prenatal exposure to secondhand smoke is associated with an increased risk of spontaneous abortion, stillbirth, low birth weight, preterm birth, congenital malformations, and neurobehavioral delays (Lee et al., 2019; Suzuki et al., 2019; Zheng et al., 2019). Children whose parents smoke in the home have a greater susceptibility to many respiratory ailments than children of nonsmokers. They are at increased risk of asthma (Brooks et al., 2021), acute respiratory infections (Singh et al., 2022), and otitis media (Lam et al., 2023; Wei et al., 2021; Yamada et al., 2019). Babies exposed to secondhand smoke are also at increased risk of SIDS (Brody et al., 2019; Brownstein et al., 2018; Tsai et al., 2018).

Nicotine in the Milk

Nicotine in the milk can cause fussiness, diarrhea, shock, vomiting, rapid heartbeat, and restlessness in an infant. Smoking 20 cigarettes daily can lead to relatively high levels of fat-soluble nicotine in the milk. This can harm the baby and cause vomiting and nausea. Even the milk of nonsmokers may be affected by environmental exposure to secondhand smoke. There is an increase in toxic metals in human milk as a result of environmental secondhand smoke exposure, which affects the bioactive substances needed for optimal growth and development of newborns and infants (Szukalska et al., 2021). Any of these factors could cause slow infant weight gain. For this reason, it is good practice to ask about smoking when a baby is not gaining weight adequately.

Smoking Cessation Programs

Providing a smoking cessation program in a pediatric setting offers a supportive, ongoing way to engage with parents for the health of their children. There are many interventions available to help with smoking cessation. Nursing parents may use nicotine replacement therapy (nicotine patch and chewing gum) and bupropion (an older antidepressant remarketed for smoking cessation) for nicotine withdrawal. Nicotine replacements are acceptable when nursing (Hale & Krutsch, 2024). Parents who use such replacements cannot smoke while using a nicotine patch or chewing gum. Doing so would further increase the baby's level of exposure to nicotine, in addition to making the parent very ill.

Continuing to Smoke

Parents are strongly encouraged to stop smoking and minimize secondhand smoke exposure (AAP, 2022; Suzuki et al., 2019). Many parents continue to smoke while they are nursing. Thus, their babies are exposed to secondhand smoke in the home. It is healthier for a baby exposed to secondhand smoke to receive protection from nursing. Nursing helps protect infants against illnesses and conditions resulting from exposure to secondhand smoke and nicotine in the milk, including asthma and respiratory infections, as discussed in **Chapter 9**.

Smoking parents who know it is unhealthy need education, support, and reassurance rather than condemnation or mixed messages. Encourage them to avoid smoking in the baby's presence. Even if they smoke only occasionally, they could affect the baby more by the smoke the baby inhales than by the amount of nicotine in the milk. Feedings can be timed to minimize the baby's exposure to the nicotine in the milk by smoking after a feeding rather than just before it.

Parents who smoke are advised to take a multivitamin because smoking depletes the body's vitamin stores.

Caffeine

Caffeine is present in coffee, tea, cola, energy drinks, and chocolate—substances often consumed in large quantities in Western culture. Moderate amounts of these foods are safe during lactation. The amount of caffeine present in human milk varies dramatically from one individual to another and according to the timing of ingestion ("Caffeine," 2019). Some people appear to have low absorption and efficient metabolism and excretion, so levels of caffeine in their milk remain low. Given these variations, each nursing dyad is unique in their response to caffeine. Acceptable levels of ingestion depend on the baby's reaction.

Effects on the Baby

Insufficient high-quality data are available to make good evidence-based recommendations on safe maternal caffeine consumption (McCreedy, 2018). Caffeine usually does not adversely affect the infant when consumed in low to moderate amounts (about 300 milligrams or less per day, which is about 2 to 3 cups of coffee). Very high caffeine intake, equivalent to about 10 or more cups of coffee daily, may cause infant wakefulness, hyperactivity, and colicky behavior.

Parents can watch for signs of caffeine sensitivity in their babies. If you learn of these behaviors, you can review caffeine use and suggest reduction in intake to determine whether it alleviates or resolves the symptoms. Newborn and preterm infants are particularly susceptible to caffeine's effects because their immature digestive systems take longer to eliminate caffeine from the body (Centers for Disease Control and Prevention [CDC], 2022). Even small amounts that pass into the milk can build up in the baby's body over time.

Caffeine Substitutes

Nursing parents may consume herbal teas as a substitute for caffeinated drinks. These substances can contain other active ingredients that have unpleasant effects. Cathartics in herbal teas, such as buckhorn bark and senna, can cause cramps and diarrhea in both infants and parents. Chamomile tea may sensitize the infant to ragweed pollen and cause an allergic reaction. Sage, parsley, and peppermint inhibit lactation and may therefore lower milk production. Some parents consume these herbs for weaning.

Alcohol

Alcohol reaches the same level in the milk as in the blood, with a high relative infant dose (RID) of 16% and a reduction of the amount of alcohol in the milk over time (Hale & Krutsch, 2024). The highest alcohol levels in milk occur 30 to 60 minutes after ingestion. One glass of alcohol per day is unlikely to cause problems in the nursing infant if nursing occurs after 2 to 2.5 hours per drink. It is generally considered safe to nurse when the parent feels normal again—that is, when the effects of the alcohol have worn off. By this time, levels in the bloodstream and the milk will be quite low (Hale & Krutsch, 2024). Eating food along with an alcoholic drink lowers alcohol absorption. A family history of alcoholism is a risk consideration in alcohol use by nursing parents.

Effects on the Baby

Moderate alcohol use is not associated with nursing duration, infant feeding, sleeping behavior at 8 weeks, or most infant developmental outcomes at 8 weeks or 12 months (Wilson et al., 2017). There are conflicting reports from prospective cohort studies that cognitive abilities are reduced based on the dose of alcohol consumed by the parent (Oei, 2020; Wilson et al., 2017). A reported dose-dependent reduction in cognitive abilities of 6- to 7-year-olds that was not sustained at 10 to 11 years of age. Drinking alcohol while nursing may result in a dose-dependent reduction in children's academic abilities, especially with frequent binge drinking (Gibson & Porter, 2020). Nursing should be avoided after moderate to high alcohol consumption. An interval of 2 hours after consuming more modest amounts of alcohol before resuming nursing is likely to be safe (Academy of Breastfeeding Medicine [ABM], 2023).

Excessive Alcohol Use

Excessive amounts of alcohol can lower prolactin levels (Pandey et al., 2022), block the release of oxytocin, and affect letdown ("Alcohol," 2023). Furthermore, excessive alcohol consumption can limit parental effectiveness and result in life-threatening conditions for the infant. A parent's impaired judgment and ability to care for the baby pose more serious risks than the baby's exposure to alcohol in the milk. A pattern of drinking is of greater concern than an occasional drink. Frequent alcohol intake of more than one or two drinks at a time or indications that alcohol is a problem may require a behavioral health referral. Local alcohol and substance treatment centers, drug counselors, and recovery groups such as Alcoholics

Anonymous are valuable resources. A parent's heavy alcohol use and depression can also be signs of intimate-partner aggression (Ward et al., 2021). Current local resources for these situations are crucial to provide families with options.

Drugs of Abuse

Healthcare providers care for an increasing number of infants experiencing the damaging effects of drug exposure. Prenatal illicit drug use is correlated to maternal age, with the highest incidence among the youngest people (SAMHSA, 2019). Prenatal illicit drug use and overuse of prescribed drugs are associated with intrauterine growth restriction, preterm birth, stillbirth, neonatal abstinence syndrome (NAS), and SIDS (Carlier et al., 2020; Prince et al., 2023). Children exposed prenatally to substances of abuse have increased rates of respiratory infections, asthma, and ear and sinus infections. These children are more irritable and have more attention difficulties and behavioral problems. They also incur a higher risk for childhood cancer (Auger et al., 2019).

Conducting research in this population is ethically challenging and difficult to perform. Thus, there is a lack of research on individual drugs of abuse in human milk. The AAP Committee on Drugs (2013) categorizes drugs of abuse as contraindicated during nursing. These drugs include cannabis, **amphetamines**, **cocaine**, **heroin** (and other opiates), and "designer drugs" with constantly changing chemical composition.

It is a common assumption that nursing parents are unlikely to abuse substances or develop a substance use disorder. However, surveys indicate that alcohol, cannabis, cocaine, and other illicit drugs are indeed used during lactation (SAMHSA, 2019). Understanding the risks that chronic use may pose to a nursing infant will help parents make informed decisions about the specific risks. The Academy of Breastfeeding Medicine (ABM) advises weighing the documented benefits of human milk against the risks associated with the substance that the infant may be exposed to during nursing (ABM, 2023).

Cannabis

Cannabis (marijuana) is the most commonly used illicit substance in the United States and many other countries internationally. The leaves and oils of the cannabis plant are smoked or added to food and eaten, primarily for the drug's pleasurable physical and psychotropic effects. Medicinal cannabis is increasingly used to treat chronic pain and nausea in Canada, parts of the United States, and Europe. Several countries and states in the United States have legalized the recreational use of cannabis. Thus, you may encounter parents more frequently than in the past who are using cannabis for medical reasons or recreationally.

Although it may be legal to consume cannabis, the safety of this activity in pregnancy and nursing and long-term consequences for the children need to be considered (Wang, 2017). The increased potency of Δ-9-tetrahydrocannabinol (Δ9-THC), the psychoactive component in cannabis, is a cause for concern for the developing infant (Bertrand et al., 2018; Grant et al., 2020). In light of data limitations, cannabis use in nursing parents should be discouraged. Healthcare professionals should encourage alternative treatment options for parents using marijuana for health conditions (ABM, 2023; Hale & Kutsch, 2024). A reduction in cannabis use to lower levels is associated with beneficial outcomes important to health (Mooney et al., 2018).

The risks and medical recommendations of cannabis consumption need to be individualized according to medical history, drug formulation, potency, duration, and route of ingestion. Parents should be educated on the potential adverse effects on fetal growth and development and encouraged to either stop or decrease its use. Healthcare providers have a critical role in educating families about cannabis use when nursing. This nonpunitive, collaborative approach aims to improve the health and quality of life for nursing families (Skelton et al., 2020).

Amphetamines

Amphetamines are stimulants that include popular street drugs such as ecstasy, harmony, love, and ice. There are scarce data on the use of nonprescribed stimulants among nursing parents. The AAP classifies nonprescribed amphetamines as contraindicated during lactation (ABM, 2023). Studies on the effects of such drugs conducted in laboratory animals, primarily rats, show that amphetamines enter milk (Franz et al., 2021). Hallucinations, hypothermia, extreme agitation, and seizures could occur from exposure to these drugs through the milk. If methamphetamine is used, the milk should be expressed and discarded for 48 to 100 hours (MotherToBaby, 2022).

Morbidity, characterized by cardiovascular disease, poor nutrition, and social stigma, has increased for methamphetamine users during pregnancy (Jarlenski et al., 2020). As with all illicit drugs, the key concern is that parents using these drugs may not be coherent enough to care for the baby appropriately.

A collaborative decision-making approach to supporting nursing is encouraged when working with these parents.

Medications to treat attention-deficit disorder and attention-deficit/hyperactivity disorder have amphetamine qualities. A parent may have been on these stimulants since childhood. Dexamphetamine readily enters human milk, although within a range that is generally accepted as being "safe" in the short term. Duloxetine and methylphenidate appear to have minimal levels in the milk and are considered likely to be compatible with nursing (ABM, 2023; Collin-Lévesque et al., 2018). Methylphenidate and bupropion are preferred during lactation over amphetamines (Ornoy, 2018). More research is needed to determine the long-term consequences of these agents for the developing child.

Cocaine

Cocaine is a powerful stimulant that acts on the central nervous system. It is easily absorbed and has a high milk–plasma ratio, making significant passage of cocaine into human milk probable (Hale & Krutsch, 2024). Although cocaine's "high" is brief, excreting the inactive metabolite from the body takes a long time. Traces can be present in exposed infants' urine for up to 60 hours. Secondhand inhalation of crack cocaine smoke may also cause a positive urine result in infants (D'Avila et al., 2016; Jones, 2015).

Effects of cocaine intoxication in the infant include irritability, jitteriness, tremors, increased heart and respiratory rates, and convulsions or seizures (National Institute on Drug Abuse [NIDA], 2016). The AAP classifies cocaine as contraindicated during lactation. Nursing parents who use cocaine intermittently should express and discard their milk for 24 to 48 hours after use.

Heroin

Heroin is a highly addictive drug that is converted to morphine after it enters the body. Although it is illegal in the United States, this drug is used for limited medical purposes in the United Kingdom and elsewhere. Heroin use has been on the rise because of increased opiate addiction in the general population. Individuals cut off from their supply of opiate pain medications may turn to street heroin because it is cheaper than buying opiate prescription drugs illegally (Cicero & Ellis, 2017).

The AAP categorizes heroin as contraindicated during lactation. Heroin may pass to the infant through the milk. It can cause increased sleepiness, respiratory depression (Ito, 2018), and poor appetite in the infant, resulting in an undernourished baby. An uncoordinated and ineffective sucking reflex, tremors, restlessness, and vomiting may result from heroin ingestion.

Opiates

There is a global increase in the use and abuse of prescription and nonprescription opiates (Morrow, 2018). The use and abuse of prescription opiates during pregnancy is a public health problem that disproportionately affects rural, non-White, and public insurance–dependent populations (MacMillan, 2019). Opiate pain medications include oxycodone, hydrocodone, tramadol, fentanyl, and hydromorphone.

Increased opiate abuse has resulted in a corresponding increase in NAS, with related annual hospital costs amounting to $1.5 billion (American College of Obstetricians and Gynecologists, 2017. Severe infant withdrawal occurs most often because of maternal opiate use. Infants exposed to opiates in utero are likely to exhibit symptoms such as irritability (which increases in severity), hypertonia, tremors, feeding intolerance, emesis, watery stools, seizures, and respiratory distress (Khan, 2020). These babies are at risk for low birth weight, respiratory problems, and longer inpatient stays.

Health practitioners who know in advance about prenatal use of opiates or other drugs can anticipate neonatal withdrawal and plan appropriate care. If the history is unknown, symptoms in the newborn may take a while to diagnose. Feeding difficulty is one of the first symptoms in an affected baby. Nursing reduces the severity of NAS for drug-exposed babies and is considered a key nonpharmacologic intervention to improve care (Clemans-Cope et al., 2020; Holmes et al., 2017). Infants who receive their parent's milk experience less severe opioid withdrawal symptoms, have shorter hospital stays, and are less likely to be treated with medication for withdrawal (Bogen & Whalen, 2019).

Opiate Maintenance Therapy. Many individuals in recovery from opiate dependency are placed on maintenance doses of opiate-agonist drugs—primarily methadone and **buprenorphine**. These drugs pass into the milk; however, babies exposed to maintenance drug dosing experience lower rates of NAS and require shorter treatment than exposed babies who are not nursed. Infants exposed to these drugs should be monitored for increased sleepiness and breathing difficulty (MotherToBaby, 2021, 2023a). Methadone is a micro-opioid receptor agonist commonly used to treat opiate dependency and addiction. It is considered acceptable during lactation (AAP, 2013; ABM, 2023). Levels of methadone in nursing infants are dependent on maternal dosage.

Buprenorphine is a partial micro-opioid receptor agonist and a kappa-opioid receptor antagonist drug sometimes used instead of methadone for opiate dependency. Prenatal buprenorphine treatment results in a clinically significant less severe NAS than with methadone (Kushnir et al., 2023). A third agonist used to treat opiate dependency, **naltrexone**, is a nonselective opioid receptor antagonist. The relative infant dose of naltrexone received by an exclusively nursed infant is about 0.86% of the maternal dosage. Naltrexone is considered compatible with nursing ("Naltrexone," 2018). Naltrexone should not be confused with a similarly named drug, **naloxone**, which is used in emergency care to counteract drug overdoses.

Parents describe inner conflict between wanting to nurse and concerns about the social stigma surrounding opiate maintenance therapy (McGlothen et al., 2018). Parents on opioid maintenance tend to discontinue nursing sooner than nondependent parents. This may be a result of misinformation from health practitioners and minimal support for nursing (Clark, 2019). Key concerns with early weaning are infant exposure to medications or other substances and concerns about milk production (Yonke et al., 2020).

Hallucinogens

There are many hallucinogens and dissociative drugs available. The pharmacology and popularity of various compounds waxes and wanes. These drugs change a user's perceptions of time, motion, colors, sounds, and self. Street names include acid, angel dust, vitamin K, and psilocybin (the psychoactive substance in magic mushrooms, also known as caps, shrooms, and buttons). The ability to think and communicate rationally is impaired, sometimes resulting in bizarre or dangerous behavior (NIDA, 2020). Hallucinogens are associated with flashbacks and psychotic behaviors long after use.

Although little understood, psilocybin is used in parts of the world to treat anxiety, depression, and psychosis. A study at Monash University in Australia used brain scans of healthy adults under the influence of psilocybin to understand the drug's effect on brain connectivity (Stoliker, et al., 2024. Psilocybin studies being undertaken at Johns Hopkins University do not focus on nursing parents (Nayak et al., 2023). There is no current research on the use of magic mushrooms during pregnancy and lactation (MotherToBaby, 2023b).

Phencyclidine hydrochloride (PCP), or angel dust, is stored in fat tissue and excreted very slowly from the body. The AAP categorizes PCP as contraindicated during lactation unless there is a negative urine toxicology at birth or the parent has abstained for 90 days and is in a substance abuse treatment program ("Phencyclidine," 2021).

Counseling Implications

Regardless of the pharmacologic effects or safety of illicit drugs for infants, the overriding concern is the inhibition of parents' ability to care for their baby. Given the risks, both known and unknown, parents should be educated about the dangers of using such drugs, both prenatally and while nursing. Although you can educate parents and warn them about harmful practices, you cannot take responsibility for their actions. If they disregard your advice, you can remind them of the potential danger to the baby and urge them to tell their baby's healthcare provider about the substance they are using.

If there is a reported history of a substance use disorder, or if it is suspected, a urine and/or blood culture is done. In most areas, it is mandatory to refer a parent who tests positive for illegal drugs to a social services worker or child protective services. If child endangerment, abuse, or neglect is suspected, most governments mandate reporting to a child protective services agency. Familiarize yourself with resources and the reporting requirements where you live, as well as your institution's policies, concerning this difficult area of parental–child health care.

Environmental Contaminants

Unlike social toxicants, we have little control over exposure to contaminants in the environment. Many chemicals strongly resist breakdown into more benign components, often leading to environmental pollution. In the body, these chemicals primarily deposit in fat, accumulate, and pass into the milk. Human milk is naturally rich in fat and therefore contains traces of many **environmental contaminants**. The analysis of human milk is not as invasive as blood tests, making human milk a popular medium for environmental contamination testing (Brajenović et al., 2018).

Environmental contaminant exposure may influence the development of infant gut microbial function

(Iszatt et al., 2019). Diet, especially the consumption of fish, is a major factor in levels of certain pollutants in human milk. Most studies reaffirm the superiority of human milk, and nursing is generally not discouraged because of exposure to environmental contaminants. Exclusive nursing for 6 months protects infants from trace elements present in water and foods (Linares et al., 2024). A global WHO survey of contaminants emphasizes that exposure in utero is greater than exposure through human milk. The WHO asserts that the proven health advantages of nursing far outweigh any potential adverse effects (van den Berg et al., 2017).

Polybrominated Diphenyl Ethers

Flame-retardant chemicals—specifically, **polybrominated diphenyl ethers (PBDES)**—are an ongoing environmental concern. Some of these chemicals—which are used in many computer plastics, foam cushions, textiles, and other products—accumulate in animals and people. Levels of PBDEs in North America are substantially higher than those in many regions of Europe, Asia, Oceania, and Africa (Tang & Zhai, 2017).

In animal studies, PBDEs are shown to affect thyroid, liver, and brain development. Concentrations in human milk are inversely associated with mental and psychomotor development in children aged 1 to 2 years. PBDEs are also associated with child behavioral problems (Kim et al., 2018). Researchers estimate that human milk contributes 95.2% of children's accumulation of PBDEs at 6 months and 92.2% at 1 year of age (Shin et al., 2018). Pollutant sources, body mass index, and metabolism may all affect accumulative load (Caspersen et al., 2016).

Persistent Organic Pollutants (POPs)

Persistent organic pollutants (POPs) are organochlorine pesticides that include a class of chemicals known as *polychlorinated biphenyls* (PCBs). Although widely banned, these substances are still used worldwide. PCBs can impede a child's mental development and immune system. Increased POP blood levels were found in pregnant people who had low parity and low body mass index. The negative effects of these pesticides on infant neurodevelopmental outcomes appear mostly because of prenatal exposure. There is some association with nursing (Kao et al., 2019). These chemicals accumulate in fat tissue and have a great affinity for high lipids, which human milk contains in abundance.

Infants who nurse exclusively have higher levels of PCBs than those who receive mixed feedings. Longer nursing duration in 3-year-old children is associated with increased POP concentrations (Caspersen et al., 2016). Increasing age of nursing parents, fish consumption, and heavy alcohol consumption are significant factors as well. Highly sensitive test assaying can determine the different types of PCBs in the milk by region, including proximity to an industry or a contaminated body of water. It can also account for the type of milk (colostrum, foremilk, and hindmilk) and the number of past pregnancies (Šimić et al., 2020).

Because of the relatively short period of time infants nurse, the risk of potentially higher consumption is outweighed by the health benefits of nursing. The amount of exposure from human milk is less than the tolerable daily intake (Pajewska-Szmyt et al., 2019). Nursing appears to be protective against environmental contaminants.

DDT and DDE

The potential for harm caused by **dichlorodiphenyl trichloroethane (DDT)** has been a concern for years. Restrictions on this pesticide's use since 1950 have resulted in a decline in the levels of **dichlorodiphenyldichloroethylene (DDE)**, the main breakdown product of DDT, in human milk. Despite this trend, many low-income countries still use these chemicals in farming (Mansouri et al., 2017).

There is a significant association between reduced neurodevelopmental performance in children and DDT in human milk (Al-Saleh et al., 2019; Kao et al., 2019). However, the benefits of nursing outweigh the potential risks of low levels of pollutants in human milk (Hassan et al., 2022). More research is needed to identify the main exposure sources and explore ways to decrease exposure.

Bisphenol A (BPA)

Bisphenol A (BPA) is a chemical used in the lining of food and beverage packaging to protect food from contamination and extend shelf life. It has been used in the manufacture of baby bottles and the lining of metal containers of infant formula. Levels of this chemical entering liquid formula from cans are likely far higher than those that leach from baby bottles. BPA migration in baby bottles remains a health concern for babies (Dehdashti et al., 2023). Most adults in the United States have detectable levels of BPA in their urine. BPA can be detected at higher levels in human milk, with ensuing developmental concerns (Fahrenkopf & Wagner, 2020).

BPA binds to estrogen receptors and, in animal studies, has been shown to damage reproductive, neurologic, and immune systems during critical stages of development, including mammary gland development. It is also linked to breast cancer and the early onset of puberty (Atlas & Dimitrova, 2019; Jung et al., 2019). Perinatal exposure to BPA appears to be associated with anxiety and depression (Wiersielis et al., 2020).

BPA's interaction with estrogen receptors plays a role in the development of metabolic disorders, including polycystic ovary syndrome (PCOS) (Urbanetz et al., 2023). BPA exposure may predispose subsequent generations to the risk of developing BPA-related disease, including PCOS (Pivonello et al., 2020). **Chapter 26** provides more information on PCOS, a condition that is related to low milk production.

The U.S. Food and Drug Administration (FDA) banned BPA materials in baby bottles and sippy cups in 2012 and from infant formula packaging in 2013 (FDA, 2023). Canada and the European Union phased out the use of BPA in some products in 2018 and re-evaluated the risk in 2023 (Food Standards Australia New Zealand, 2023). These actions were based on discontinuation of its use by manufacturers rather than the safety of BPA.

Phthalates

Phthalates are chemicals used in the manufacture of products to increase the softness and flexibility of the plastic. Phthalates are considered semivolatile organic compounds. They can be found in most products, such as cosmetics, toothbrushes, soaps, toys, and gloves used for food handling, and in food that is in contact with plastics used in production, packaging, or delivery (Wang & Qian, 2021). These plasticizers are chemically unbounded and evaporate slowly but permanently from the products (CDC, 2017).

Phthalates are endocrine disruptors, and ingestion is linked to reproductive tract defects, primarily in males. Phthalates have been identified in human milk with the highest amounts in the first month of nursing, and decreasing levels thereafter (Hung et al., 2021). Levels are less than those found in previous studies, perhaps because of restrictions put in place in Japan, Australia, the United States, and China, among other countries.

Exposure to Environmental Contaminants

Environmental contaminants and resulting health implications vary globally depending on local pollution sources, diet, and occupation. The number of studies worldwide has grown exponentially. The WHO global study summarizes these studies and calls for measures to reduce human exposure (van der Berg et al., 2017). Where countries ban or regulate these chemicals, trends show a decline in pollutants such as organochlorine pesticides, PCBs, and dioxins in human milk (Thomas et al., 2019).

Healthcare providers who suspect that a contaminant in the milk may be the cause of illness in a child should ask about occupational exposure. Large numbers of parents continue to nurse after returning to work. Some of these parents have jobs that expose them to chemical pollutants, such as lead, mercury, cadmium, pesticides, plastics, or solvents. Testing the milk is usually not necessary unless the healthcare providers suspects illness in the parent or baby that may be due to chemical exposure.

Reducing Exposure to Environmental Contaminants

Parents can take precautions to reduce their exposure to environmental contaminants and the potential for chemical pollutants to enter their milk:

- Avoid occupations that involve potential exposure, or consult an occupational medicine expert to evaluate an occupation's safety.
- Avoid mothproofed garments and hobbies that involve the use of oil-based paints, paint or varnish removers, glues, and other solvent-based chemicals.
- Limit the use of domestic sprays such as pesticides and household cleaners.
- Limit the consumption of freshwater fish to reduce exposure to chemical wastes in lakes and streams.
- Because contaminants concentrate in fatty tissue, avoid fatty meats and remove excess fat when possible.
- Avoid eating organ meats (e.g., liver, gizzards, hearts, brains, intestines), where contaminants are stored in greater concentrations.
- Thoroughly wash or peel fresh fruits and vegetables to remove chemicals.
- Choose certified organic produce when practical and economically feasible.

Guidelines for safe fish consumption during pregnancy and lactation suggest 8 to 12 oz

- Give well-documented facts in an objective manner.
- Explain options concerning potential impurities.
- Explain that water and infant formula may sometimes be contaminated with impurities.
- Urge parents to seek caregiver advice and to share concerns openly.
- Urge parents to remind the caregiver that they are nursing.
- Cite references for facts that you share.
- Discuss drug substitutes in a neutral manner, citing reliable sources.
- Suggest ways to minimize the effects of drugs.
- Urge parents to avoid unnecessary exposure to contaminants.

Figure 11-6 Issues to address about impurities.

- Refrain from giving personal opinions.
- Do not interpret drug information unless you have prescriptive privileges.
- Do not offer advice about a drug's safety; read straight from the literature.
- Do not indicate that you disagree with advice from the healthcare provider or other medical resources unless you are medically qualified.
- Do not suggest refusing a drug when it is needed.
- Do not encourage parents to act against the healthcare provider's advice.

Figure 11-7 Precautions in discussing impurities.

(approximately 230–340 mg) of a variety of fish each week and 8 oz in young children, from choices that are lower in mercury (FDA, 2021). Fish low in mercury include salmon, shrimp, pollock, tuna (light canned), tilapia, catfish, and cod. Tilefish from the Gulf of Mexico, shark, swordfish, and king mackerel should be avoided because they are the highest in mercury. When eating fresh fish from streams, rivers, and lakes, it would be helpful to check with local authorities on those water bodies for current consumption safety advisories. Carp, catfish, trout, and perch are more likely to have fish advisories resulting from mercury or other contaminants. Toxicity and regulatory information related to pesticides is available online at www.pesticideinfo.org and www.pan-international.org.

Counseling Parents About Impurities

A primary concern about research on impurities in human milk is that parents may perceive their milk as "bad" for their babies and decide not to nurse. Sensationalistic media reports may cause parents to think that they should have their milk tested and wean. There is a compelling need for ethical considerations as researchers conduct studies and interpret, communicate, and act on findings (Thurston et al., 2019). Your guidance to parents trying to assimilate and contextualize media information about environmental pollution and contaminants may help prevent untimely weaning. You can also inform them that most contaminant exposure occurs during gestation (van den Berg et al., 2017).

The guidelines in **Figures 11-6** and **11-7** will assist you when you are counseling parents concerning the potential for impurities in their milk. These guidelines apply to any of the substances that may compromise the safety or quality of the milk and are especially important when discussing medications with parents.

Summary

Most substances in parents' blood appear to some degree in their milk. The relevant considerations are whether a substance will be absorbed in the baby's GI tract and whether the infant's exposure to the substance as it appears in the milk is safe. Factors that influence the level of a substance in the infant's bloodstream include how soon after birth the medication is consumed, how the medication is metabolized, and the baby's age and weight.

Drugs in the milk may increase or decrease milk production and secretion. They may also cause changes in the baby's behavior, feeding, and sleeping patterns—such as fussiness, lethargy, rash, vomiting, or diarrhea. The effects of drugs in the milk can be minimized by selecting the least offensive drug, adjusting the timing for taking the drug, and avoiding medications with a long plasma half-life. When counseling parents, present drug information objectively from well-documented sources.

Environmental contaminants in human milk reflect exposure and accumulation in the general population. Environmental toxins deposit primarily in fat and excrete through the milk. Parents can take precautions to reduce their exposure to contaminants and the potential for chemical pollutants in their milk. Diet, especially fish consumption, is a factor in milk levels of certain pollutants. All recreational drugs are contraindicated during lactation.

What You Learned—At a Glance

Conversation Starters with Parents

- What questions do you have about taking medications while you are nursing?
- How much do you smoke or consume alcohol each day?
- What recreational drugs do you consume?
- How much exposure do you have to environmental and foodborne contaminants?

Considerations Regarding Drug Entry into Milk

- Will it pass into the milk and be absorbed in the baby's GI tract?
- Can the baby be safely exposed to the substance as it appears in the milk?
- How soon after birth will the medication be taken?
- What is the baby's gestational age?

Minimizing Effects of a Drug

- A relative infant dose of less than 10% of the adult dose is generally considered safe.
- Take immediately after nursing or 3 to 4 hours before the next feeding.
- Avoid nursing when the drug is at its peak level in the milk.
- Avoid drugs with a long half-life.
- Select the least offensive drug.

Deciding to Take a Drug

- Are there treatment alternatives that do not involve medication?
- Is there a safer medication?
- Do the benefits of a medication outweigh possible risks to the baby?
- Do the risks of a medication to the baby outweigh the risks of formula?

Social Toxicants and Nursing

- Nicotine and tobacco use should be avoided or timed to minimize the baby's exposure through the milk.
- It takes newborn and preterm infants a long time to eliminate caffeine.
- Generally, one to two alcoholic drinks will not pose a problem; nursing may occur when the effects have worn off.
- Recreational drugs are contraindicated in nursing.

Environmental Contaminants and Nursing

- Contaminants primarily deposit in fat and leach into the milk.
- PCBs affect mental development.
- DDE reduces protection against asthma, eczema, and hay fever.
- PBDEs may affect learning, memory, behavior, thyroid hormones, and bodily functions.

Reducing Exposure

- Avoid occupations, hobbies, and fabrics that involve possible exposure.
- Avoid eating organ meats, shark, swordfish, king mackerel, and tilefish.
- Limit consumption of canned albacore tuna and other fish.
- Wash or peel fresh fruits and vegetables.

References

Academy of Breastfeeding Medicine, et al. Clinical Protocol #21: breastfeeding in the setting of substance use and substance use disorder (revised 2023). *Breastfeed Med.* 2023;18(10):715–733.

Alcohol. LactMed [database online]. September 15, 2023. National Library of Medicine (US).

Al-Saleh I, et al. Selenium status in lactating mothers-infants and its potential protective role against the neurotoxicity of methylmercury, lead, manganese, and DDT. *Environ Res.* 2019;176:108562.

American Academy of Pediatrics. Updated AAP guidance recommends longer breastfeeding due to benefits. 2022. https://publications.aap.org/aapnews/news/20528/Updated-AAP-guidance-recommends-longer?autologincheck=redirected

American Academy of Pediatrics. E-cigarette use during pregnancy and breastfeeding FAQ. 2019. https://www.healthychildren.org/English/ages-stages/prenatal/Pages/E-Cigarette-Use-During-Pregnancy-Breastfeeding.aspx

American Academy of Pediatrics (AAP), Committee on Drugs. Clinical Report: The transfer of drugs and therapeutics into human breast milk: an update on selected topics. *Pediatrics.* 2013;132(3):e796–e809.

American College of Obstetrics and Gynecologists. Opioid use and opioid use disorder in pregnancy. 2017. https://www.acog.org/clinical/clinical-guidance/committee-opinion/articles/2017/08/opioid-use-and-opioid-use-disorder-in-pregnancy

Atlas E, Dimitrova V. Bisphenol S and bisphenol A disrupt morphogenesis of MCF-12A human mammary epithelial cells. *Sci Rep.* 2019;9(1):16005.

Auger N, et al. Maternal use of illicit drugs, tobacco or alcohol and the risk of childhood cancer before 6 years of age. *Drug Alcohol Depend.* 2019;200:133–138.

Australian Breastfeeding Association. Breastfeeding and smoking or vaping. Updated 2022. https://www.breastfeeding.asn.au/resources/breastfeeding-and-smoking-or-vaping

Bertrand KA, et al. Marijuana use by breastfeeding mothers and cannabinoid concentrations in breast milk. *Pediatrics.* 2018; 142(3).

Bogen DL, Whalen BL. Breastmilk feeding for mothers and infants with opioid exposure: what is best? *Semin Fetal Neonatal Med.* 2019;24(2):95–104.

Brajenović N, et al. Levels of polychlorinated biphenyls in human milk samples in European countries. *Arh Hig Rada Toksikol.* 2018;69(2):135–153.

Briggs G, et al. *Drugs in Pregnancy and Lactation: A Reference Guide to Fetal & Neonatal Risk.* 11th ed. Baltimore, MD: Lippincott Williams & Wilkins; 2021.

Brody DJ, et al. Secondhand smoke exposure among nonsmoking youth: United States, 2013–2016. *NCHS Data Brief.* 2019; (348):1–8.

Brooks CC, et al. NAT1 genetic variation increases asthma risk in children with secondhand smoke exposure. *J Asthma.* 2021; 58(3):284–292.

Brownstein CA, et al. Chapter 31. The genetics of sudden infant death syndrome. In: Duncan JR, Byard RW, eds. *SIDS Sudden Infant and Early Childhood Death: The Past, the Present and the Future.* Adelaide, AU: University of Adelaide Press; May 2018.

Caffeine. LactMed [database online]. June 30, 2019. National Library of Medicine (US).

Carlier J, et al. Testing unconventional matrices to monitor for prenatal exposure to heroin, cocaine, amphetamines, synthetic cathinones, and synthetic opioids. *Ther Drug Monit.* 2020;42(2):205–221.

Caspersen IH, et al. Determinants of plasma PCB, brominated flame retardants, and organochlorine pesticides in pregnant women and 3 year old children in the Norwegian Mother and Child Cohort Study. *Environ Res.* 2016;146:136–144.

Centers for Disease Control and Prevention. National biomonitoring program. Factsheet: phthalates. April 7, 2017. http://www.cdc.gov/biomonitoring/phthalates_factsheet .html

Centers for Disease Control and Prevention. Maternal diet. Last reviewed May 17, 2022. https://www.cdc.gov/breastfeeding/breastfeeding-special-circumstances/diet-and-micronutrients/maternal-diet.html

Ceulemans M, et al. Prevalence and characteristics of pregnancy- and lactation-related calls to the National Poison Centre in Belgium: a retrospective analysis of calls from 2012 to 2017. *J Eval Clin Pract.* 2020;26(3):911–917.

Cicero TJ, Ellis MS. The prescription opioid epidemic: a review of qualitative studies on the progression from initial use to abuse. *Dialogues Clin Neurosci.* 2017;19(3):259–269.

Clark, RRS. Breastfeeding in women in opioid maintenance therapy: a review of policy and practice. *J Midwifery Womens Health.* 2019;64(5):545–558.

Clemans-Cope L, et al. Neonatal abstinence syndrome management in California birth hospitals: results of a statewide survey. *J Perinatol.* 2020;40(3):463–472.

Collin-Lévesque L, et al. Infant exposure to methylphenidate and duloxetine during lactation. *Breastfeed Med.* 2018; 13(3):221–225.

D'Avila FB, et al. Cocaine and crack cocaine abuse by pregnant or lactating mothers and analysis of its biomarkers in meconium and breast milk by LC-MS—a review. *Clin Biochem.* 2016;49(13–14):1096–1103.

Dehdashti B, et al. Health risk assessment of exposure to bisphenol A in polymeric baby bottles. *Environ Health Insights.* 2023;17:11786302231151531.

Fahrenkopf A, Wagner CK. Bisphenol A (BPA) induces progesterone receptor expression in an estrogen receptor α-dependent manner in perinatal brain. *Neurotoxicol Teratol.* 2020;78: 106864.

Food Standards Australia New Zealand. Bisphenol A (BPA). December 2023. https://www.foodstandards.gov.au/consumer/chemicals/bpa

Franz T, et al. Findings of illicit drugs in hair of children at different ages. *Int J Legal Med.* 2021;135(2):465–471.

Gibson L, Porter M. Drinking or smoking while breastfeeding and later academic outcomes in children. *Nutrients.* 2020;12(3):829.

Grant KS, et al. Update on the developmental consequences of cannabis use during pregnancy and lactation. *Birth Defects Res.* 2020;112(15):1126–1138.

Hale T, Krutsch K. *Hale's Medications & Mothers' Milk 2025–2026: A Manual of Lactational Pharmacology.* 21st ed. New York, NY: Springer Publishing Company; 2024.

Hassan HF, et al. Persistent organic pollutants in human milk: exposure levels and determinants among lactating mothers in Lebanon. J Food Prot. 2022;85(3):384–389.

Holmes AP, et al. Breastfeeding considerations for mothers of infants with neonatal abstinence syndrome. *Pharmacotherapy.* 2017;37(7):861–869.

Hung SC, et al. Phthalate exposure pattern in breast milk within a six-month postpartum time in Southern Taiwan. *Int J Environ Res Public Health.* 2021;18(11):5726.

Imaz ML, et al. Case report: clinical and pharmacokinetic profile of lithium monotherapy in exclusive breastfeeding. a follow-up case series. *Front Pharmacol.* 2021;12:647414.

Infant Risk Center. Texas Tech University Health Sciences Center. 2024. http://www.infantrisk.com

International Board of Lactation Consultant Examiners. Code of professional conduct for IBCLCs. Updated September 2015. https://iblce.org/wp-content/uploads/2017/05/code-of-professional-conduct.pdf

International Board of Lactation Consultant Examiners. Scope of practice for International Board Certified Lactation Consultant® (IBCLC®) certificants. Dissemination and effective date. December 12, 2018. https://ibclc-commission.org/wp-content/uploads/2023/05/2018_Scope_of_Practice.pdf

Iszatt N, et al. Environmental toxicants in breast milk of Norwegian mothers and gut bacteria composition and metabolites in their infants at 1 month. *Microbiome.* 2019;7(1):34.

Ito S. Opioids in breast milk: pharmacokinetic principles and clinical Implications. *J Clin Pharmacol.* 2018;58(suppl 10): S151–S163.

Jarlenski M, et al. Substance use disorders and risk of severe maternal morbidity in the United States. *Drug Alcohol Depend.* 2020;216:108236.

Jones W. Cocaine use and the breastfeeding mother. *Pract Midwife.* 2015;18(1):19–22.

Joseph HM, et al. The influence of smoking on breast feeding among women who quit smoking during pregnancy. *Nicotine Tob Res.* 2017;19(5):652–655.

Jung N, et al. Early steps of mammary stem cell transformation by exogenous signals; effects of bisphenol endocrine disrupting chemicals and bone morphogenetic proteins. *Cancers (Basel).* 2019;11(9).

Kao CC, et al. Residue levels of organochlorine pesticides in breast milk and its associations with cord blood thyroid hormones and the offspring's neurodevelopment. *Int J Environ Res Public Health.* 2019;16(8):1438.

Khan L. Neonatal abstinence syndrome. *Pediatr Ann.* 2020; 49(1):e3–e7.

Kim S, et al. Association between maternal exposure to major phthalates, heavy metals, and persistent organic pollutants, and the neurodevelopmental performances of their children at 1 to 2 years of age—CHECK cohort study. *Sci Total Environ.* 2018;624:377–384.

Kushnir A, et al. neonatal abstinence syndrome in infants with prenatal exposure to methadone versus buprenorphine. *Children (Basel).* 2023;10(6):1030.

Lam TK, et al. Association of e-cigarette exposure with pediatric otitis media recurrence. *Ann Otol Rhinol Laryngol.* 2023;132(9): 1018–1025.

Lechosa Muñiz C, et al. Impact of maternal smoking on the onset of breastfeeding versus formula feeding: a cross-sectional study. *Int J Environ Res Public Health.* 2019;16(24):4888.

Lee M, et al. Exposure to prenatal secondhand smoke and early neurodevelopment: Mothers and Children's Environmental Health (MOCEH) study. *Environ Health.* 2019;18(1):22.

Linares AM, et al. Concentrations of lead and arsenic in mother's milk and children's blood in Peruvian breastfeeding dyads. *J Hum Lact.* 2024;40(1):69–79.

MacMillan KDL. Neonatal abstinence syndrome: review of epidemiology, care models, and current understanding of outcomes. *Clin Perinatol.* 2019;46(4):817–832.

Mansouri A, et al. The environmental issues of DDT pollution and bioremediation: a multidisciplinary review. *Appl Biochem Biotechnol.* 2017;181(1):309–339.

McCreedy A, et al. Effects of maternal caffeine consumption on the breastfed child: a systematic review. *Swiss Med Wkly.* 2018;148:w14665.

McGlothen KS, et al. "I'm doing the best that I can for her": infant-feeding decisions of mothers receiving medication-assisted treatment for an opioid use disorder. *J Hum Lact.* 2018;34(3):535–542.

Meek J, et al. AAP Policy Statement: breastfeeding and the use of human milk. *Pediatrics.* 2022;150(1):e2022057988.

Mooney LJ, et al. Reduction in cannabis use and functional status in physical health, mental health, and cognition. *J Neuroimmune Pharmacol.* 2018;13(4):479–487.

Morrow P. The American opioid death epidemic—lessons for New Zealand? *NZ Medical Journal.* 2018;131(1469):59–62.

MotherToBaby. Buprenorphine. October 1, 2021. https://mothertobaby.org/fact-sheets/buprenorphine/

MotherToBaby. Methamphetamines. September, 1, 2022. https://mothertobaby.org/fact-sheets/methamphetamine/

MotherToBaby. Methadone. July 1, 2023a. https://mothertobaby.org/fact-sheets/methadone/

MotherToBaby. Psilocybin mushrooms ("magic mushrooms"). May 1, 2023b. https://mothertobaby.org/fact-sheets/magic-mushrooms/

Naltrexone. LactMed [database online]. October 31, 2018. National Library of Medicine (US).

National Institute on Drug Abuse. Cocaine. What are the effects of maternal cocaine use? May 2016. https://drugabuse.gov/publications/research-reports/cocaine/what-are-effects-maternal-cocaine-use

National Institute on Drug Abuse. Hallucinogens. February 8, 2020. https://www.drugabuse .gov/drugs-abuse/hallucinogens

Nayak, SM, et al. Naturalistic psilocybin use is associated with persisting improvements in mental health and wellbeing: results from a prospective, longitudinal survey. *Front Psychiatry.* 2023;14:1199642.

Newmark RL, et al. Risk-benefit assessment of infant exposure to lithium through breast milk: a systematic review of the literature. *Int Rev Psychiatry.* 2019;31(3):295–304.

Nice F. *Nonprescription Drugs for the Breastfeeding Mother.* 2nd ed. Derwood, MD: Nice Breastfeeding, LLC; 2017.

Oei JL. Alcohol use in pregnancy and its impact on the mother and child. *Addiction.* 2020;115(11):2148–2163.

Ornoy A. Pharmacological treatment of attention deficit hyperactivity disorder during pregnancy and lactation. *Pharm Res.* 2018;35(3):46.

Pajewska-Szmyt M, et al. QuEChERS extraction coupled to GC-MS for a fast determination of polychlorinated biphenyls in breast milk from Polish women. *Environ Sci Pollut Res Int.* 2019;26(30):30988–30999.

Pandey S, et al. Sex-specific factors associated with lifetime suicide attempt among patients with alcohol use disorders. *BJPsych Open.* 2022;8(4):e135.

Phencyclidine. LactMed [database online]. July 19, 2021. National Library of Medicine (US).

Pivonello C, et al. Bisphenol A: an emerging threat to female fertility. *Reprod Biol Endocrinol.* 2020;18(1):22.

Prince MK, et al. Substance use in pregnancy. In: *StatPearls.* Treasure Island, FL: StatPearls Publishing; July 2023. http://www.ncbi.nlm.nih.gov/books/NBK542330/

Pseudoephedrine. LactMed [database online]. April 20, 2020. National Library of Medicine (US).

Sánchez-Borges M, Ansotegui IJ. Second generation antihistamines: an update. *Curr Opin Allergy Clin Immunol.* 2019;19(4):358–364.

Shin MY, et al. Prenatal contribution of 2, 2′, 4, 4′-tetrabromodiphenyl ether (BDE-47) to total body burden in young children. *Sci Total Environ.* 2018;616–617:510–516.

Šimić I, et al. Optimization of gas chromatography-electron ionization-tandem mass spectrometry for determining toxic non-ortho polychlorinated biphenyls in breast milk. *Biomed Environ Sci.* 2020;33(1):58–61.

Singh PK, et al. Does secondhand smoke exposure increase the risk of acute respiratory infections among children aged 0–59 months in households that use clean cooking fuel? A cross-sectional study based on 601 509 households in India. *Indoor Air.* 2022;32(1):e12980.

Skelton KR, et al. Management of cannabis use in breastfeeding women: the untapped potential of International Board Certified Lactation Consultants. *Breastfeed Med.* 2020;15(2):1–4.

Stoliker D, et al. Neural mechanisms of psychedelic visual imagery. *Molecular Psychiatry.* 2024;11:1–8.

Substance Abuse and Mental Health Services Administration. 2018 National Survey on Drug Use and Health: annual national report. August 20, 2019. http://www.samhsa.gov/data/release/2018-national-survey-drug-use -and-health-nsduh-releases

Substance Abuse and Mental Health Services Administration. Highlights for the 2021 National Survey on Drug Use and Health. 2021. https://www.samhsa.gov/data/sites/default/files/2022-12/2021NSDUHFFRHighlights092722.pdf

Suzuki D, et al. Secondhand smoke exposure during pregnancy and mothers' subsequent breastfeeding outcomes: a systematic review and meta-analysis. *Sci Rep.* 2019;9(1):8535.

Szukalska M, et al. Toxic metals in human milk in relation to tobacco smoke exposure. *Environ Res.* 2021;7:111090.

Tanda R, et al. Factors that modify the association of maternal postpartum smoking and exclusive breastfeeding rates. *Breastfeed Med.* 2018;13(9):614–621.

Tang J, Zhai JX. Distribution of polybrominated diphenyl ethers in breast milk, cord blood and placentas: a systematic review. *Environ Sci Pollut Res Int.* 2017;24(27):21548–21573.

Thomas A, et al. Application of ensemble methods to analyse the decline of organochlorine pesticides in relation to the interactions between age, gender and time. *PLoS One.* 2019;14(11):e0223956.

Thurston AM, et al. Results communication in breast milk biomonitoring studies: a scoping review and stakeholder consultation. *Health Hum Rights.* 2019;21(1):63–79.

Tsai J, et al. Exposure to secondhand smoke among nonsmokers—United States, 1988–2014. *MMWR Morb Mortal Wkly Rep.* 2018;67(48):1342–1346.

Urbanetz LAML, et al. Does bisphenol A (BPA) participate in the pathogenesis of polycystic ovary syndrome (PCOS)? *Clinics (Sao Paulo).* 2023;78:100310.

U.S. Food and Drug Administration. Advice about eating fish for women who are or might become pregnant, breast feeding mothers, and young children. Revised October 2021. https://www.fda.gov/food/consumers/advice-about-eating-fish

U.S. Food and Drug Administration. Bisphenol A (BPA): use in food contact application. April 20, 2023. http://www.fda.gov/newsevents/publichealthfocus/ucm064437.htm

van den Berg M, et al. WHO/UNEP global surveys of PCDDs, PCDFs, PCBs and DDTs in human milk and benefit-risk evaluation of breastfeeding. *Arch Toxicol.* 2017;91(1):83–96.

Wang GS. Pediatric concerns due to expanded cannabis use: unintended consequences of legalization. *J Med Toxicol.* 2017;13(1):99–105.

Wang Y, Qian H. Phthalates and their impacts on human health. *Healthcare (Basel).* 2021;18;9(5):603.

Ward N, Correia H, McBride N. Maternal psycho-social risk factors associated with maternal alcohol consumption and fetal alcohol spectrum disorder: a systematic review. *Arch Gynecol Obstet.* 2021;304(6):1399–1407.

Wei CF, et al. Associations between infant developmental delays and secondhand smoke exposure modified by maternal prepregnancy overweight and obesity status. *Nicotine Tob Res.* 2021;23(9):1475–1483.

Wiersielis KR, et al. Perinatal exposure to bisphenol A at the intersection of stress, anxiety, and depression. *Neurotoxicol Teratol.* 2020;79:106884.

Wilson J, et al. Alcohol consumption by breastfeeding mothers: frequency, correlates and infant outcomes. *Drug Alcohol Rev.* 2017;36(5):667–676.

Yamada M, et al. Association between lifestyle, parental smoke, socioeconomic status, and academic performance in Japanese elementary school children: the Super Diet Education Project. *Environ Health Prev Med.* 2019;24(1):22.

Yonke N, et al. Breastfeeding motivators and barriers in women receiving medications for opioid use disorder. *Breastfeed Med.* 2020;15(1):17–23.

Zheng Z, et al. Congenital malformations are associated with secondhand smoke among nonsmoking women: a meta-analysis. *Birth.* 2019;46(2):222–233.

PART 3

Prenatal Through Postpartum

CHAPTER 12

Prenatal Considerations

The decision for new parents on how they will feed their baby is often made before the baby is born. The prenatal period is an excellent opportunity to provide accurate information and dispel myths about nursing and human and artificial milk. A key message to convey is that providing human milk to infants is the biological way to nourish human infants. Although nursing is the natural continuation of fetal life, it is a learned behavior for both parents and infants. Because of this, parents can benefit from early education about infant feeding. Healthcare professionals have a moral and ethical obligation to provide evidence-based, informed consent to expectant families. To make a fully informed decision, parents need to understand the importance of providing human milk as well as the consequences of *not* doing so. Educating parents before birth will help them make informed feeding decisions. They will benefit from prenatal infant feeding education, tips on preparing to nurse, and assistance with selecting caregivers who are supportive of and knowledgeable about lactation.

KEY TERMS

Hospital privileges

Self-efficacy

Standing orders

Infant Feeding Choice

Factors involved in infant feeding decisions are complex and involve influences from a variety of sources. To understand these dynamics and provide appropriate guidance, the decision needs to be seen in relation to life circumstances and immediate sociocultural context. Social support has a significant effect on infant feeding choice, especially among low-income populations (Bich et al., 2019; Schmied et al., 2019). Prenatal and postpartum healthcare providers have an important role in assisting new parents to make informed decisions about feeding their newborn infants.

The decision to nurse usually occurs before the baby's birth, often before pregnancy (McKinley et al., 2019). In a Spanish study of 5671 women, over 97% decided to nurse their infant before giving birth. Within that subgroup, 81.1% were exclusively providing their own milk to their infant at discharge (Ballesta-Castillejos et al., 2020). The intent to nurse may even be formed as early as adolescence (Reyes et al., 2019). Prenatal intentions regarding infant feeding are often aligned with actual infant feeding practice (Ballesta- Castillejos et al., 2020). This highlights the importance of early education and support. When they give birth, some parents are still undecided about whether they will nurse and, if so, for how long. Thus, the early weeks postpartum are pivotal in shaping infant feeding plans. Acknowledging this dilemma will help in guiding parents who have committed to an infant feeding decision prior to delivery and those at risk for not continuing.

Nursing as an infant feeding choice has evolved over the centuries. Two hundred years ago, wealthy families were more likely to employ wet nurses, and in some cultures, only the lower classes nursed their babies. More recently, that paradigm has reversed in developed nations, where educated, upper-middle-class parents are more likely to nurse, and lower-income and marginalized parents disproportionately formula feed. The pediatric profession began in part from a desire to give artificial milk to infants who were not nursed. Families visited the new professional, a pediatrician, at periodic intervals in their babies' growth and acquired the appropriate recipe, or "formula," to sustain their children (Hess, 1923; Wolf, 2003). Despite the introduction of commercial proprietary infant formulas in the 1920s, most parents continued to nurse or use home recipes because they were easy to prepare and affordable. Commercial formulas became more popular in the 1950s through manufacturing and marketing.

The lactation profession arose several decades later as part of a movement that sought to reverse the trend toward formula feeding and return infant feeding to its biological imperative. Researchers began to debunk the myths surrounding many unsubstantiated practices that had carried over from formula feeding to nursing. Lactation practitioners continue to correct misconceptions among members of the health profession and the public regarding lactation care. As the paradigm continues to shift, previously accepted practices and thinking about infant feeding will change as well.

Making the Decision to Nurse

Table 12-1 describes factors that influence a parent's decision to nurse their baby. Many of these factors pertain to social norms and influence from family and friends rather than medical or scientific reasons (Ballesta-Castillejos, et al., 2020; Cato et al., 2020; Ragusa et al., 2020; Schroeder et al., 2019). The decision to nurse for working parents can be linked to workplace practices. If parental leave is short, parents may wonder if it's worth the effort to start nursing their baby. The employer may not support pumping at the workplace. Countries with government-supported parental leave allow parents to make infant feeding choices without the burden of going back to work.

Parents report that the decision to nurse was made because it was healthier for the baby, and the choice to bottle feed was made to avoid being tied down by the baby (Cato et al., 2020). Convenience plays a large role in the decision to nurse. Some parents believe that nursing their baby will be more flexible and provide bonding time. Others believe that bottle feeding allows them to share the infant feeding responsibility with their partners (Cato et al., 2020). A loss of freedom can deter some parents from nursing. They might feel that they can never leave their baby or can only leave them for short periods of time. Having the other parent feed the baby by bottle is thought to provide more bonding time for the non-nursing parent. Health professionals should be sensitive to these conflicting emotions and assist their clients in the transition to their new role as parents. On the other hand, some parents find that they can go anywhere with their infant because they can nurse anytime without a schedule or various feeding supplies (Rodriguez-Vazquez et al., 2020).

Toledo and Cianelli (2019) note the important role self-objectification plays in the decision to nurse. Self-objectification stems from the intense cultural

Table 12-1 Factors Influencing the Infant Feeding Decision

Supports Nursing and Human Milk	Supports Artificial Infant Milk
Previous successful nursing experience	Previous unsuccessful nursing experience
Longer and paid parental leave	Short, unpaid parental leave
Supportive partner	Unsupportive partner
Positive stories and support from family and friends	Negative stories from family and friends
Healthcare provider's recommendation and promotion of lactation	Healthcare provider's lack of knowledge and promotion of artificial infant milk
Professional support with feeding challenges	Lack of support when experiencing infant challenges
Prenatal education specific to lactation	Lack of prenatal education on infant feeding
Cultural acceptance of nursing in public	Cultural criticism of nursing in public
High education level of nursing parent	Low education level of nursing parent
Vaginal delivery, low birth intervention	Cesarean delivery, high birth intervention
Birth setting: trained and supportive staff, Baby-Friendly Hospital Initiative (BFHI) designation, supportive protocols	Birth setting: untrained or unsupportive staff, non-BFHI designation, unsupportive protocols

Source: Woods Barr et al. (2021a); Cato et al. (2020); Jefferson et al. (2021); Ragusa et al. (2020).

sexualization and emphasis placed on physical appearance. These internalized beliefs can prioritize breast appearance over nursing benefits and thus negatively influence the initiation and duration of nursing, as well as nursing in public. Parents receive conflicting messages in societies where the female body is sexualized. They are told that human milk is healthiest for infants. At the same time, they are told to cover up because nursing in public is indecent (Cato et al., 2020). More work needs to be done to support parents who nurse their babies in any public or private setting. Influence may also come from the historical experience of parents within their specific culture. In a study of African American parents, their decision to nurse was influenced by the generations of parents before them in their families and communities (Woods Barr et al., 2021b). Previous generations' infant feeding experiences are often passed through oral tradition. Historically, African American parents have low rates of nursing their infants. According to recent data from the U.S. Centers for Control and Disease Prevention (CDC), 66% of African Americans initiated nursing compared with 82% of non-Hispanic Whites (CDC, 2020).

The disparity in initiation rates is connected to historical events that prevented parents from having the autonomy to nurse their infants. Slave women were often separated from their own children and forced to nurse their masters' babies. Newly freed slaves commonly left their children behind as they settled into new jobs during the Great Migration to northern states in the early 20th century. Low economic opportunities forced parents to return to work soon after the birth of their infant, without the option to express their milk (Devane-Johnson et al., 2022).

Historically, Indigenous cultures of North America supported human milk for infants. Families and communities ensured that infants were kept close to their parents, provided nourishing food to those who were lactating, and passed on wisdom about the use of herbs for breast issues. However, the impact of colonization resulted in the loss of traditional knowledge about nursing, the destruction of many family units, and the increased use of infant formula. Thus, nursing rates of Indigenous families have consistently decreased since the 1960s (Schroeder et al., 2019). Respecting this intergenerational history is imperative to delivering nonjudgmental support so that parents can change the narrative around infant feeding practices in their communities.

Disparities and inequities persist that affect the decision to nurse. Rates of nursing are lower among parents who are less educated, are under 20 years old, are unmarried, have incomes below the poverty level, and are living in countryside areas (Segura-Pérez et al., 2021). Rates of initiating and continuing to nurse are low among non-White parents. Because ethnic and racial disparities are often found with social and economic inequities, interventions to support nursing should be targeted to communities with fewer lactation and postpartum resources. Infant feeding recommendations by lactation experts *from* the community can also influence the decision to nurse. There has been a call to increase the diversity among lactation professionals to include those from different ethnicities and racial groups who speak the same language as the families they serve (Rhodes et al., 2021).

Healthcare professionals can influence their clients' decision to nurse as well. By acknowledging the cultural and social context of this decision, healthcare professionals can support the decision by providing education to the client, their partner, and extended family if appropriate. Presenting positive images of nursing dyads can normalize their feeding choice. Reserving the recommendation of formula for medical indications highlights the expectation that nursing is the "normal" way to feed an infant.

Parents Who Nurse

Parents who are most likely to nurse are in their mid-30s, college educated, married, and in the middle-income level. In the United States, White parents have higher rates of nursing, whereas, in the United Kingdom, parents of Black, Asian, and mixed or other ethnic groups are more likely to nurse. This is attributed to denser communities where parents of the same ethnic groups support each other (Simpson et al., 2022). Support programs can target specific groups of parents to increase the number of nursing dyads.

The infant feeding decisions of parents who choose to nurse tend to be evidence based and centered on infant health (Cato et al., 2020). A belief in the importance of providing human milk is the underlying motivator in the decision to nurse. Nursing also facilitates bonding between the nursing parent and baby that is unique to this kind of feeding experience.

A positive attitude toward nursing prior to pregnancy has the greatest influence on initiation. A continued positive attitude and confident commitment enable parents to withstand a lack of support and lactation/nursing challenges. *Self-efficacy* is the term used to describe a person's belief in their ability to accomplish a certain task. The higher a person's self-efficacy is, the higher their success in achieving their goals. A parent's self-efficacy in their ability to provide nourishment to their baby from their own milk will lead to a satisfying lactation experience.

Combination Feeding. Many parents combine nursing and formula feeding methods. Combination feeding is influenced by family and cultural beliefs and practices that may not support exclusive nursing (Hackman et al., 2022; Horwood et al., 2022; Matriano et al., 2022). Although Hispanic people initiate nursing, they are less likely to exclusively nurse. *Las dos cosas* ("both things") is a common feeding practice among newly immigrant, low-income Hispanic women in the United States who believe that *las dos cosas* is a healthy option (Linares et al., 2019). Prenatal education about the sufficiency of human milk, presented in a culturally humble and sensitive manner, is needed. Correcting misinformation from family and friends, as well as consistent messaging from healthcare professionals, may help families make healthy infant feeding choices.

Mixed messages from healthcare providers may imply that both are equivalent health options and lead parents to believe that supplementing with formula is just as healthy as exclusive nursing. Families might think that they are choosing between two equal milks (Horwood et al., 2022). False and misleading messages imply that infant formula is equal to human milk in terms of nutrition. Infant formula companies market to healthcare providers in hopes that they will influence their clients' infant feeding decisions to include their product (World Health Organization [WHO] and United Nations Children's Fund [UNICEF], 2022).

Healthcare providers also have a duty to present infant feeding education that includes the benefits of human milk, risks of formula, and management of lactation issues common among all parents. Assumptions cannot be made about which parents nurse their babies and which parents use formula.

Parents Who Formula Feed

Infant feeding decisions of parents who formula feed tend to be based more on perceptions, lifestyle, and the opinions of others than on evidence-based information (Bookhart et al., 2022; Roberts et al., 2023). In one study, the most common reasons parents fed their infants formula while still in the hospital were medical indications, parental preferences, lactation management-related issues, and social influences (Bookhart et al., 2021). Early formula supplementation is also associated with smoking (Tanda et al., 2018; Taşhan et al., 2017). Education on infant feeding is imperative before the hospital stay. Healthcare professionals also play a large role in whether families receive formula in the first few days postpartum. Lactation support given for early feeding issues such as pain and perceived low milk production can prevent the unnecessary use of infant formula.

Parents who gave formula to their older children or had a previous negative nursing experience are more likely to choose formula again. These parents often report frustration and low self-efficacy with nursing (Bookhart et al., 2021). Nursing in public is also a deterrent for many parents. In the United Kingdom, discreet nursing in public is supported. This contradiction gives formula companies an opportunity to market their product by taking advantage of parents' insecurities and conflicted feelings around nursing (Roberts et al., 2023). **Chapter 3** discusses health inequities and other factors related to low nursing rates.

Mental Health Issues

A history of mental health disorders can be a barrier to nursing. Historically, mental health disorders during pregnancy and the postpartum period escaped being assessed or treated. Perinatal anxiety disorders and depression affect 17% and 7% to 20% of parents, respectively. Up to one in three parents experiences childbirth trauma, which leads to depression and posttraumatic stress disorder (Pezley et al., 2022).

You can normalize mental health issues by asking all your clients about their mental health history and emotional state. Stay up to date on new mental health medications and their compatibility with nursing. Provide referrals for mental health therapists and online resources. Encourage clients to have adequate sleep, proper nutrition, and help with household obligations. Support their mental and emotional needs as you would for their physical needs. **Chapter 20** discusses postpartum mood disorders.

Influence of Others

Significant people in parents' lives can exert a substantial influence over the decision to nurse. Perceived social support from personal relationships, employers, and government affect a family's infant feeding decisions (Ballesta-Castillejos, 2020; Roberts et al., 2023). Opinions of family members play an important role in nursing decisions after the infant's birth. It is important to recognize these influences and include family members in prenatal education about infant feeding practices. Likewise, the attitude and knowledge level of healthcare practitioners influence the choice (Meek, 2019; Seyyedi et al., 2021).

Family

The family serves as the primary agent for passing along basic cultural beliefs, values, and customs to society's newest members. Thus, family is often in the best position to influence decisions. Because we generally have frequent contact with family members, they are instrumental in establishing our values, attitudes, and behavior. Positive perceptions of family members, such as nursing being the more natural and healthier choice, encourage parents to choose to nurse (Chang et al., 2021; Matriano et al., 2022). Family members who prefer formula might think that formula feeding is easier and will help the infant sleep better (Horwood et al., 2022).

Grandmothers often take on the role of "wise educator," and give advice in support of nursing. First-time parents, especially, might look to their own mothers for advice (Woods Barr et al., 2021a). Even the paternal grandmother can influence nursing decisions and duration (Wallenborn et al., 2019).

There can be conflict if the grandmother had a negative nursing experience or if their advice contradicts evidence-based information the parents learned. Because parenting recommendations have changed over the years, parents might feel that the grandmother's ways are "old-fashioned." Lack of grandmother support for nursing negatively affects the continuance of human milk provision for extremely low-weight infants after neonatal intensive care unit (NICU) stay (Patel et al., 2019).

Many grandmothers want to receive more knowledge about lactation and human milk (Chang et al., 2021). Optimal nursing practices are higher in families where grandmothers have the correct knowledge of nursing. You can enhance grandmothers' knowledge and support of nursing by including them in conversations about nursing practices if they are present and if you have the parents' permission.

Partner

Support from partners (**Figure 12-1**) plays a pivotal role in the infant feeding decision. A partner's attitudes are often a strong influence on the decision to nurse, as well as on its continuation when working through challenges (Roberts et al., 2023). Understanding the attributes of partner support can help determine how to approach the nursing decision. Partners want to be involved in caring for their infant, and they often consider feeding as an important interaction.

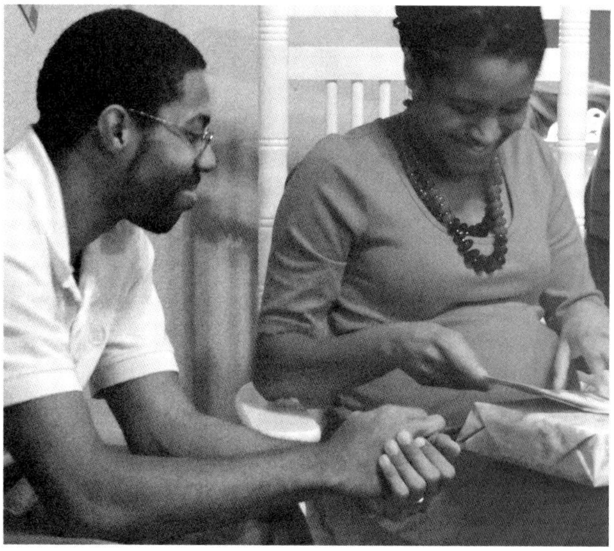

Figure 12-1 Expectant couple.

Printed with permission of Anna Swisher.

Efforts are needed to involve partners in decision-making about nursing because nursing duration tends to be longer when the partner prefers exclusive nursing. Conversely, if there are nursing obstacles, an uneducated partner will be more likely to think formula is easier. This can lead to early cessation of nursing (Chang et al., 2021). Acknowledgment of the partner's involvement in the infant feeding choice needs to be included in lactation promotion campaigns. Offering classes and support groups that accommodate the partners' work schedules can encourage their engagement in infant feeding decisions and increase infant bonding (Bich et al., 2019). In Vietnam, a club for fathers provides a space for peer education and social support (Bich et al., 2019; Wang et al., 2018).

Friends

Second to family, friends are an important influence on our decisions. We are more likely to seek information from friends who share our values or outlook. It is important to recognize these sources of influence on parents and consider what will be most helpful to them. Separation of generations, frequent relocation, little experience caring for children, and lack of nursing as the cultural norm can compromise new parents' confidence in their ability to nurse or their understanding of how the process works.

Exposure to nursing within their friend group increases the likelihood of a new parent nursing (Roberts et al., 2023). In the absence of nursing role models, young parents may "try" to nurse with an expectation of difficulties and even failure. When artificial feeding is widespread among family and friends, a problem with any aspect of nursing may lead to early weaning. You can help parents recognize the important contribution they make to society in their roles as nurturers of the next generation.

Online Support Groups and Social Media Influencers

New parents often turn to social media and online support groups for advice and support from other parents, either in addition to or in lieu of seeking advice from their healthcare providers. Participation in online support groups provides incentives to continue nursing. Parents value providing social and emotional support as much as receiving it from the groups. A shared experience in an online community seems to create strong connections and meet the needs of the participants (Morse & Brown, 2022). The use of social media for lactation support during the COVID-19 pandemic allowed connection to other parents at a time when in-person support groups were not available.

Online support groups can be convenient and provide access to help when healthcare professionals are not available. These groups promote emotional well-being and increase self-efficacy. Although parents trust online resources, they are aware of the lack of regulation and need to be discerning about advice. However, joining an online support group can help parents feel included in a group within a specific social context. This can be especially important for underrepresented groups of parents, such as single parents and LGBTQ+ parents.

It is important to recognize that in online support groups parents receive information from other parents. This can lead to the dissemination of inaccurate information, especially when the groups' advice is more trusted than advice coming from healthcare professionals. In addition, these groups exist because there is an overall lack of lactation support. Healthcare professionals might consider using a social media platform to provide education to the public. By doing so, their expertise will have a wider reach and affect more parents by encouraging long-term nursing.

Healthcare Providers

Caregivers exert a tremendous influence on a family's infant feeding choice. Provider encouragement to nurse has a major effect on initiation and duration (American College of Obstetricians and Gynecologists, 2016). Some healthcare professionals fail to recognize the value of nursing despite the vast body of evidence supporting its importance. The approach taken during pregnancy can move expectant parents in the direction of nursing—or away from it. Asking if they plan to nurse or asking how they plan to feed their baby implies equality between human milk and substitutes. Instead, asking, "What questions do you have about nursing?" conveys the health importance of nursing and opens the door to learning more about it.

Quality improvement learning collaborations have demonstrated the ability to transform hospital system delivery of care. In the United States, hospitals participating in the Best Fed Beginnings learning collaborative obtained a three-fold increase in Maternity Practices in Infant Nutrition and Care (mPINC) scores compared with other hospitals (Grossniklaus et al., 2017). The mPINC score, as discussed in **Chapter 1**, measures hospital practices that support nursing families.

Hospital personnel are ideally positioned to promote nursing at the time of admission and correct any misconceptions that may prevent parents from nursing their babies. Parents who indicate they do not plan to nurse or who seem ambivalent about nursing provide opportunities for hospital staff to discuss concerns or misconceptions. For example, they can discuss pumping and storing milk with parents who plan to return to work. Helping with the nursing decision conveys a caregiver's belief in the importance and normalcy of lactation.

Society

Society influences the decision to nurse, with cultural norms having a strong influence on feeding choice (Cohen et al., 2018; Simpson et al., 2019). Therefore, approaching the general population is an essential factor in promoting lactation. Many social barriers in developed nations fail to recognize nursing as the natural way to nourish babies or openly discourage nursing. The portrayal of bottle feeding as the model in Western culture influences professionals and laypersons alike. Drawing attention to public nursing and the sexualization of breasts can affect the infant feeding decision (Hauck et al.,

2021). Mixed images of the breasts as sexual—as opposed to a means of nurturing babies—can create internal conflicts for parents. Although the maxim "breast is best" is freely spoken, many of society's infant feeding messages imply equality between human milk and artificial baby milk. When parents receive such mixed signals, they may become even more confused and question whether nursing will fit into their lifestyle.

Employers

Employer policies and practices influence their employees' decisions regarding their families. Greater employer support for nursing employees is needed. Creating a business environment supportive of lactating employees is a key aspect of legislation protecting the nursing rights of employees. **Chapter 25** offers a detailed discussion of ways that lactation consultants can help working parents continue nursing.

Realistic Expectations

It is important to neither minimize nor dismiss concerns as parents work through their infant feeding decisions. Acquainting them with the realities of nursing will help them develop realistic expectations. Formula feeders often choose bottle feeding because they perceive nursing as disagreeable in some respect. Anticipatory guidance will help find ways to decrease discomfort and minimize any inconveniences. Learning how to fit nursing into their lifestyle will be the first of many accommodations parents will make as they blend their new child into their family. **Figure 12-2** presents information that will help parents in their decision to nurse. **Figure 12-3** describes common misconceptions about nursing that you can help dispel.

- The nursing parent has a free hand to attend to other needs or activities such as reading, snacking, and helping other children.
- Nursing is possible almost anywhere.
- Travel and other activities are more convenient when the baby accompanies the nursing parent. Traveling "with" the baby, instead of "away from" the baby can be very empowering and liberating for nursing parents.
- Parents can nurse modestly in front of others.
- Nursing requires no special equipment and avoids the expense of infant formula.
- The stools and spit-up of nursed babies have a less offensive odor than those of formula-fed babies; they also do not stain clothing.
- Engorgement, nipple pain, and other challenges can be avoided or minimized with sound lactation management and help from experts.
- Frequent feedings required by a nursed baby require a nursing parent to be available to her young baby for nourishment. Frequency diminishes as the baby grows.

Figure 12-2 Information to help with the infant feeding decision.

Preparation for Nursing

Babies throughout history have been nurtured primarily with human milk without the aid of detailed scientific knowledge or special devices. The decades from 1930 to 1980 saw an increase in the popularity of formula feeding and a decline in nursing in the United States and many other industrialized countries. Fewer family members know enough about nursing to offer today's parents the practical nursing information and support they need. Consequently, many expectant parents benefit from learning how to prepare for and manage nursing.

Lactation rates increased after 1980, and many of those parents now have grandchildren. They are influential in solidifying the world's cultural return to nursing as the norm for babies. Parents who were nursed are more likely to nurse their own infants (Grassley et al., 2012) or support their partners in nursing. The educational process and parents' active participation in planning for a nursed baby are effective means of preparing psychologically for nursing. Parental **self-efficacy** will increase through these activities and help overcome minor discomfort and obstacles associated with nursing a baby.

Learning About Nursing

Learning the reasons to nurse, as well as the risks of not nursing, enables parents to make informed decisions about how they will feed their babies. The earlier they receive information, the greater the likelihood they will nurse for a substantial period. Attentiveness and retention of information may be greater in the later months of pregnancy as the delivery date nears. Although natural, nursing an infant is a learned behavior for both the parent and the infant. Like any new skill, education provides the best foundation for success. Expectant parents can develop a sound base for nursing practices by seeking information online, taking a prenatal infant feeding class, and reading books or articles. In addition, meetings of a community breastfeeding support group enhance confidence, increase nursing knowledge, and provide

- *A nursed baby will be too dependent on the nursing parent.* Nursed babies actually seem to display more independence because their needs are met (Chapter 14).
- *Nursing is too time-consuming.* There is actually less work involved in nursing than in bottle feeding if the nursing parent is doing the bottle feeding. Nursing frees the nursing parent to spend valuable time with the baby and other family members (Chapter 20).
- *My sister didn't have enough milk, so maybe I won't either.* A well-nourished parent produces the amount of milk the baby needs. The nursing experience of female relatives has little bearing on the parent's ability to nurse, barring genetic hormonal conditions. Between 1930 and 1980, parents received little effective advice or support to nurse, which led to many failing to nurse during those decades (Chapter 1).
- *Maybe my milk won't agree with my baby.* Each parent's milk is ideally suited to their baby. Nursed babies rarely experience negative reactions to their parent's milk. Conversely, many babies are unable to tolerate cow's milk (Chapter 10).
- *My breasts are too small to nurse my baby.* Breast size is determined primarily by fatty tissue, not functional breast tissue. Breast size usually has little bearing on the ability to produce sufficient milk (Chapter 7).
- *I am too high-strung to nurse.* Nursing can be calming to a high-strung parent because of the hormones (prolactin, oxytocin, and cholecystokinin) activated by nursing. The added skin contact with the baby can have a calming effect as well (Chapter 7).
- *If I nurse, my diet will be too restricted.* Nursing babies generally can tolerate the same foods the nursing parent tolerates. The only foods a parent may need to restrict are those that seem to produce signs of intolerance in the baby (Chapter 8)
- *If I have a cesarean birth, I won't be able to nurse.* The type of birth a has no effect on the ability to nurse, although pain and separation may cause initial obstacles. Nursing parents who deliver by cesarean birth are able to nurse (Chapter 13).
- *Nursing will drain my energy too much.* All parents find caring for a newborn tiring, regardless of which feeding method is used. Nursing encourages a parent to relax during feeding times and helps them get even more rest than a parent who bottle feeds. A nursing parent can recoup their energy by resting while the baby sleeps.
- *Nursing parents lose their figures and get sagging breasts.* Breast sagging results from pregnancy and loss of muscle tone from aging, not from having nursed (Chapter 7). Additionally, the caloric demands of nursing can help parents control their weight (Chapter 8).
- *Infant formula is just as healthy as human milk.* There are substantial differences between formula and human milk. Human milk is a live substance that provides immunity from disease to the child and has antibacterial properties (Chapter 9). By comparison, formula is inert and susceptible to contaminants (Chapter 9).
- *Nursing is essentially an alternative to infant formula.* Nursing is much more than the milk the baby receives. It is a dynamic process, a bonding relationship between a nursing parent and baby (Chapter 4).
- *I'll have to wean when I return to work anyway.* Nursing parents who are separated from their babies have many options, whether for a return to work, school, or other activity. They can express milk for the caregiver to feed to the baby or provide formula for the baby during the separation. Unrestricted nursing when the parent and baby are together will help maintain milk production (Chapter 25).

Figure 12-3 Misconceptions about nursing.

opportunities to share common interests with others in the community.

Attending childbirth classes and practicing relaxation techniques can enhance expectant parents' awareness of their bodies and help them learn ways to overcome tension and discomfort. The information and skills obtained during pregnancy will be especially useful during the trial-and-error period of establishing a comfortable nursing routine. Associating with families of young babies and occasionally caring for babies can familiarize expectant parents with baby care and nursing. In this way, they will develop proficiency in handling babies, build parenting confidence, and be prepared to overcome worries they encounter when the baby arrives.

Giving expectant parents information will help them blend nursing into their lives, and assist them in avoiding or minimizing problems. Helping them identify aspects that will be useful personally leads to the development of useful strategies to apply postpartum. Such education can increase lactation rates and help healthcare providers form effective relationships with parents. **Figure 12-4** identifies questions that are helpful in gathering the information necessary to assess a need for lactation education and support. Open-ended questions such as these encourage expectant parents to respond with information that is more descriptive.

Infant Feeding Classes

A large part of teaching about infant feeding occurs through group instruction. Classes enable you to reach large numbers of families at various stages. Education can be given during the prenatal period, through in-hospital nursing support, and through postpartum support. Prenatal lactation education meets Step 3 of the Ten Steps to Successful Breastfeeding.

Attendance in prenatal education classes is declining among young adults, who often seek education from online sources. However, these parents do not want passive learning experiences and they

- How do you feel about the prospect of nursing?
- What practical knowledge do you have about nursing?
- What prior experience or exposure do you have to nursing?
- How many friends or relatives have nursed?
- What nursing resources have you used (websites, mobile apps, online or in-person classes, support groups, or books)?
- Have you attended an infant feeding class?
- What have healthcare providers discussed with you about nursing?
- Have you selected a physician for the baby's care (pediatrician or family practice)?
- What have you done to prepare for nursing?
- Have you checked for inverted nipples?
- What have you learned about breast care?
- What currently owned clothing will allow the baby easy access to nurse?
- What arrangements have you made for help at home?
- Have you arranged for rooming-in if delivering in a hospital?
- Are you interested in attending group discussions with other parents?
- Will you be returning to work or school, and if so, how soon after birth?
- What are your specific questions or concerns?

Figure 12-4 Questions to ask prenatally about lactation and nursing.

value social learning environments with hands-on and direct involvement. Many hospitals and educational organizations offer online courses to reach these parents. Interactive gaming apps, such as Kahoot!, provide the interactive digital experiences this generation expects. It can be especially important to create ice-breakers in an online class to engage people and build a sense of community among participants.

The purpose of a class will determine its content. Ideally, childbirth classes will include discussions about lactation and infant formula to help them make an informed infant feeding decision. A discussion of expectations followed by getting off to a good start with nursing is then helpful. A postpartum class or support group after the baby arrives provides continued support and information to parents.

Teaching an Infant Feeding Class

Much of what you teach during the prenatal period will focus on attitude and expectations. Expectant parents may remember little of the particulars of establishing lactation and nursing their baby. However, they will recall the impressions they gain regarding the health benefits and long-term ease of nursing, as well as the risks of not nursing. These perceptions will reinforce their decision about how they will feed their baby.

The most important rule in teaching a class is to "keep it simple." There are no hard-and-fast rules in nursing. All that is required is that the baby gains weight appropriately and the parent is comfortable in the process. Encourage parents to trust their instincts and respond to their baby's cues. Help them focus on the positive aspects of nursing and regard it as a learning and growth process for both them and their baby. Such education may help couples recognize that any challenges they encounter with nursing are usually resolvable.

Capitalize on teachable moments, and tailor your teaching methods to adult learners. During a prenatal class, expectant parents may focus on the imminent delivery of their baby and have difficulty projecting beyond that point. To engage them in the educational process, include activities that will involve them actively to enhance their learning. Use a variety of activities that appeal to different learning styles—visual, auditory, and kinesthetic (tactile). Be sure to limit the length of a class. Classes that go longer than an hour are too long for busy parents-to-be, given that most parents continue to work or attend school until the baby's birth. **Chapter 4** discusses adult learning principles.

Because much of what parents learn prenatally may not be retained after the birth, reinforcing learning with resources on specific issues helps overcome the tendency to forget. Visual learning from other nursing parents and short video clips can also promote retention. Ideas from creative lactation consultants and support groups abound. You can pass around infant formula samples to taste compared with condensed milk. (Human milk is the sweetest of all mammalian milks.) A tablespoon of water in a disposable diaper helps prospective parents sense the weight of an ample void. Concocting a human milk stool look-alike from mustard and sesame seeds is a humorous teaching tool as well.

Because both parents are instrumental in a decision to nurse the baby, be sure to encourage both to participate in classes. Partners' physical and mental health benefits from parenting involvement and prenatal education facilitate this involvement (Bourget et al., 2017). A prenatal class can help some undecided couples choose nursing. You can dispel any misconceptions the couples have and address information they will need for making their decision. Discuss the risks of not nursing and the convenience, economics, and ease of travel with a nursing infant.

Often, couples express a concern that the partner will feel left out when the baby nurses. Help partners learn ways they can be involved with their nursed baby (**Chapter 20**).

Prenatal Lactation Education

Many hospitals offer prenatal infant feeding classes. If such a class does not exist, you might initiate one or refer families to community, and online classes. Working in cooperation with area childbirth education classes will ensure that information about lactation is included and is consistent with what you teach. Information delivered in such a forum can reach expectant parents who may not otherwise receive it. In addition, you might work with healthcare providers in obstetric and family practice and health clinics to increase correct and consistent information about nursing during prenatal visits.

In a prenatal class, you can also discuss how parents can prepare for nursing. Present the health benefits of nursing and human milk while also discussing the risks of formula. Explain the importance of eating when hungry and drinking when thirsty without strict dietary regimens. Encourage resting with the baby to facilitate recovery after the birth. Identify infant feeding behaviors, pointing out that babies communicate through distinct cues before, during, and after feedings. Help parents identify how these cues will enable them to understand and best meet their babies' needs. **Chapter 14** provides a more detailed discussion of infant hunger cues.

Use visual examples to demonstrate nursing positions commonly used for feeding babies and give couples dolls to practice their own positioning. Show them through interactive media and pictures how to recognize when their baby has good positioning and latch. Explain how an effective latch is the key to milk transfer and avoiding nipple soreness. Be sure your visuals represent families from all backgrounds. Present the health benefits of nursing and human milk while also discussing the risks of formula.

Help couples understand supply and demand in relation to milk production and how to determine when their baby is receiving enough milk. Encourage them to be alert to signs of good intake, such as audible swallows, satiety, and ample wet diapers and stools. Provide reputable smartphone feeding log apps, or print feeding logs for use during the first 2 weeks of nursing to identify the appropriate number of feedings, voids, and stools.

The first 2 weeks after childbirth are a time of learning for both parents and baby. You might suggest the analogy of the first time the couple danced together, awkwardly testing where to place their hands and feet. Help them recognize that a nursing parent and baby are new dance partners learning how to fit together in the same way. Remind them that although nursing is natural, it is also a learned behavior. Open, honest discussions will help couples achieve a smooth transition to initiating nursing.

Figure 12-5 presents a sample outline for a prenatal infant feeding class. Remember to include information parents will need from birth to the first 2 weeks. A prenatal class is not the time to discuss introducing solids, returning to work issues, or weaning. Instead, provide appropriate classes for parents of older babies, support groups, or written material to be used

1. Welcome—10 minutes
   a. List couples' questions to address in class (list on board)
   b. List couples' reasons for nursing (list on board)
2. Lactation as a biological norm—10 minutes
   a. How infant feeding evolved
   b. Benefits of nursing for baby and parent
   c. Consequences of formula use
3. Milk production—20 minutes
   a. Colostrum: normal amounts and importance to baby
   b. Milk "coming-in" (avoiding engorgement, establishing robust production)
   c. Supply and demand (growth spurts, poop and pee/pass around diapers)
4. Positioning and latch—20 minutes
   a. Latch: skin-to-skin and nursing after birth (video)
   b. Positions: reclined (laid-back), cradle hold, cross-cradle hold, side-sitting (football or clutch) hold, side-lying position (practice with dolls)
   c. Knowing what is NOT normal

BREAK—10 minutes

5. Factors that affect milk production—10 minutes
   a. Delayed onset of milk production: C-section, hypertension, edema, gestational diabetes, retained placenta, theca lutein cyst
   b. Parent's hormonal issues: infertility, PCOS, hypothyroidism, androgen disorders
   c. Baby issues: prematurity, oral anomalies, difficult births, interventions
6. Potential early challenges—5 minutes
   a. Engorgement: Reverse pressure softening
   b. Hypoglycemia: Supplementing with colostrum
7. Returning to work or school—10 minutes
   a. Employer/school support
   b. Expressing and storing milk
8. Caregiver selection—5 minutes
9. Community resources and wrap-up (resource sheet)—5 minutes

Figure 12-5 Sample outline for a prenatal infant feeding class.

later. It might be useful to think of the material in a prenatal class as covering pregnancy, birth, the golden hour (first hour of life), first 4 days postpartum (onset of lactogenesis II), and days 5 to 14 postpartum.

Postpartum Infant Feeding Education

New parents benefit from a postpartum class where they can receive support and information after they have begun feeding their babies. Discuss what parents can expect in the next several months. Help them anticipate typical infant behavior, growth spurts, crying, and teething. Discuss nursing in public, and returning to work or school, complementary foods, and weaning. Expectant parents can be encouraged to attend postpartum classes or support groups as well, where they can talk with nursing families and observe dyads in the different stages of nursing. Because so many parents search for answers to their questions online, it is important to remind parents of reputable resources.

Allow some time for group problem-solving and prevention of problems such as engorgement, ductule narrowing, and mastitis. Review the importance of exclusive nursing and the question of supplementing with infant formula. Make sure parents understand that early supplementation with formula is a key predictor of early weaning. Finally, make sure they know where they can get help with questions or concerns. **Figure 12-6** provides a sample outline for a postpartum infant feeding class.

1. Welcome—10 minutes
   a. Icebreaker (cards or online game with smartphones)
   b. Current questions or concerns (list on board and check off as addressed)
2. New family adjustments—10 minutes
   a. Self-care
   b. Incorporating new baby into daily life
3. Feeding frequency and duration—20minutes
   a. Exclusive nursing, baby-led feeding
   b. Normal frequency, cluster feeding, growth spurts
   c. Duration of feedings
   d. Supply and demand (growth spurts, poop and pee/pass around diapers)
4. Positioning and latch—20 minutes
   a. Latch: Knowing what is NOT normal
   b. Positions: reclined (laid-back), cradle hold, cross-cradle hold, side-sitting (football or clutch) hold, side-lying position (practice with dolls)

BREAK—10 minutes

5. What to expect over the first year—10 minutes
   a. Developmental milestones
   b. Starting complementary foods
6. Returning to work or school—15 minutes
   a. Legal rights
   b. Employer/school support
   c. Breast pump demos
   d. Pumping routines
   e. Home feeding routine
7. Ongoing support—5 minutes
   a. Working with baby's caregiver
   b. Community and online support
   c. Professional help
8. Community resources and wrap-up (resource sheet)—5 minutes

Figure 12-6 Sample outline for a postpartum infant feeding class.

Prenatal Breast Care

The breast undergoes many changes during pregnancy. Hormones act on the breast tissue to prepare it for lactation. The skin stretches and becomes more pliable to accommodate internal breast tissue development. Increasing pigmentation protects the nipple and areola, which may become enlarged. This pigmentation is due to increased melanin, which may strengthen the skin. The Montgomery glands lubricate the nipple and areola to protect the keratin from drying out and flaking off.

Prenatal contact is an opportunity to assess breast anatomy and provide recommendations as needed to prepare for nursing. Near the beginning of the third trimester, the pinch test (described in Chapter 22) can determine whether the nipples will need any assistance with latch. A nipple that protrudes when stimulated makes it easiest for the baby to get a good mouthful of breast tissue. A nipple that remains flat or inverts may require assistance to improve latch. The last trimester is the best time to manipulate flat or inverted nipples. The skin has gained elasticity and stretches more easily at that time than earlier in pregnancy.

Nipple Correction

The pliability or elasticity of the breast tissue plays a role in whether a flat or inverted nipple needs intervention. If breast tissue is soft, the baby may nurse on an inverted nipple without difficulty. If breast tissue is taut and firm, the baby may have difficulty drawing in enough breast tissue to elicit a sucking response. Any history of preterm birth, miscarriage, or false labor should be addressed with the client's prenatal caregiver regarding the advisability of nipple preparation, breast foreplay, or intercourse. Such stimulation could theoretically trigger oxytocin release, cause the uterus to contract, and induce labor.

Inverted and flat nipples are caused by shortened lactiferous ducts in fibrous bands. Commercial products such as breast shells and nipple everters exist to exert gentle negative pressure, slowly breaking up the fibrous bands and releasing the nipple tissue. However, these have limited success in fully everting the nipple. The infant's sucking may increase skin elasticity sufficiently. Surgery for correcting inverted nipples has also become common. Historically, the surgery damaged the milk ducts in the areolar complex, affecting milk release. Newer surgical techniques preserve lactation function by not severing milk ducts (Byun et al., 2022). **Chapter 22** discusses devices in detail, including benefits and cautions.

Colostrum During Pregnancy

Colostrum production begins during pregnancy. Leaking may occur, sometimes in copious amounts. Prenatal leakage of colostrum is not a predictor of the amount of milk production. If breasts become uncomfortably full with colostrum, gentle expression to the point of comfort will help. Colostrum that leaks during pregnancy can be frozen for later use. If there is no desire to collect colostrum that leaks prenatally, it can be rubbed into the areola. If colostrum causes the bra to stick to the nipple, moistening the bra with warm water before attempting to remove it will prevent skin irritation. Disposable or cotton nursing pads will absorb the colostrum and protect nipple skin.

Expectant parents whose babies are at risk for supplementation at birth can begin to express their colostrum during late pregnancy (after 37 weeks' gestation), freeze it, and take it to the hospital with them. These include individuals with gestational, type 1, or type 2 diabetes and those who plan to have a scheduled cesarean delivery. A baby who is born large for gestational age (LGA) or who is separated from the biological parent because of a cesarean birth is at high risk for being supplemented with formula in the hospital. If the client is interested in collecting and storing their colostrum while pregnant, refer them to their prenatal provider to discuss any risks to the pregnancy caused by increased nipple stimulation.

Expectant parents can avoid formula risks by arranging with their healthcare provider for colostrum to be used in the event of a need for supplementation. They can express colostrum prenatally and bring it to the hospital or obtain milk from a donor milk bank. Some may bring donated milk from peers or family members. Hospitals can accommodate these parents' wishes by having them sign a consent form releasing the hospital from any liability for the use of the milk. Hospitals are increasingly providing donor human milk for medical supplementation of an otherwise healthy newborn.

Parents who are lactating at the time of pregnancy may continue to tandem nurse their newborn and older baby. During the last trimester, their milk will change to colostrum. Some toddlers wean when the taste of the milk changes and the quantity decreases. Others continue to nurse throughout the pregnancy without incident. **Chapter 15** discusses tandem nursing in more depth.

Practices to Avoid

Caution expectant parents against rubbing their nipples with a towel to toughen them—an old recommendation that could damage breast tissue and does not need to be practiced. They should avoid wearing a tight bra or other clothing that binds their breasts. Such localized pressure on breast tissue can cause discomfort and result in inflammation. In addition, discourage the use of drying agents, plastic liners in breast pads, unnecessary lubricants, and lubricants that do not allow the skin to breathe or that must be washed off (being careful to read labels for ingredients).

Practical Planning Suggestions

An expectant parent can prepare for nursing in the early days by planning a quiet place for feedings, initial sleeping arrangements for the baby, and clothing that will accommodate nursing. You can encourage them to arrange household help for the early weeks at home. These plans and preparations, as well as learning about nursing, can be instrumental in building confidence about feeding choice. At the same time, you can reassure expectant parents that nursing will become second nature after a few weeks and that they will be able to easily nurse anytime, anywhere.

Nursing Area

Planning a quiet, convenient space for feedings will help parents relax undisturbed. Having several pillows available for support will help them find a comfortable position. A chair with armrests will assist in supporting the baby during feedings. A footstool will elevate their knees to provide additional support. A small table within arm's reach will provide a place for a beverage, snack, reading materials, laptop or tablet, cell phone, remote control, and other items they may need. A cozy nursing corner can help parents feel confident and prepared for feeding their newborn at home. However, if parents want the flexibility to nurse in different areas of the house, they can create a "mobile nursing nook" by keeping items they will need in a basket to take with them anywhere they choose to nurse.

Clothing Suggestions

Although many representations of nursing show the upper chest area uncovered, nursing can be discreet, with little of the body visible. Shirts and blouses will cover the upper torso and allow the baby easy access for latching. The baby covers the lower chest and abdomen so that very little skin is visible. The wardrobes of most expectant parents already include many items suitable for nursing, and few clothing purchases are necessary. Layered outfits, tank tops, blouses, pullovers, sweaters, and dresses with front or side openings are ideal. Blouses that button in the front can be unbuttoned from the bottom for good coverage. Dark-patterned materials readily hide spots caused by milk leakage. Natural fiber materials are the most comfortable because synthetic materials tend to hold moisture and do not allow the skin to breathe. For nighttime feedings, front-opening gowns, pajamas, or special nursing nightgowns with layered bodices provide easy access.

Special nursing apparel is widely available but these clothes tend to be very expensive. Nursing fashions typically have openings such as flaps or zippers to make nursing easy and discreet in public. Altering clothing parents already have is a more cost-effective approach. Good values for clothes are available through online resale groups, stores, and garage sales. During feedings, any exposed area of the breast can be covered with an open sweater, jacket, blanket, or diaper. Nursing covers are unnecessary and can make it difficult to see the baby's face. Ironically, nursing tents and blankets draw attention and announce, "Look at us; we're nursing!"

Nursing Bra

New bras may be needed during pregnancy, especially if there is significant breast growth. The last trimester is generally the earliest time for selecting a nursing bra. New bras may be delayed until after delivery, when full milk production occurs. The ideal bra provides support yet does not bind. A practical approach is to purchase one bra and wear it for a while to determine whether it is a good fit before purchasing more.

Bra cups should be made from cotton or a cotton–polyester blend. A bra with simple cup fasteners allows easy access to the breast. Practicing unfastening and fastening the cup several times will help determine whether it will be easy to manage with one hand. Velcro fasteners, although convenient, are sometimes noisy and may attract attention when nursing in public. Sports bras may provide enough support while accommodating changes in breast size during the early days of lactation. Bras with underwires and elastic around the cups should be avoided because they might press on milk ducts and prevent sufficient drainage. For the same reason, the bra seams need to be well past the front of the breast, toward the underarm.

Help at Home

New parents typically receive offers of help during the first several weeks after delivery. Clarifying the roles of potential helpers before accepting help can avoid misunderstandings or hurt feelings. The goal of accepting offers of help is for the parents to relax, rest, and care for their new baby. It is important that helpers understand that the parents will be caring for and bonding with their baby. Helpers can assist with household tasks, errands, and grocery shopping.

Some parents arrange for the services of a doula—a Greek term referring to an experienced woman who helps other women during childbirth and in the early postpartum period. Birth doulas may extend their services to assisting new families at home. Postpartum doulas typically provide services in the home rather than attending the birth. They provide the care that the extended family would historically provide but that today's scattered families may not be able to give. Having doula support at birth or at home during the postpartum period can have a positive effect on the duration of nursing (Acquaye & Spatz, 2021).

Sleeping Arrangements

Parents will need to consider sleeping arrangements for their baby, especially during the early weeks after delivery. The sleep surface should be firm, with no soft objects or loose bedding such as pillows or blankets. Bumper pads should not be used because of the potential risk of suffocation, strangulation, or entrapment.

The American Academy of Pediatrics (AAP) recommends that parents and babies sleep in proximity to each other in the early weeks, but on separate sleep surfaces (Moon et al., 2022). Keeping the baby near where the parents sleep helps them respond to their baby's needs and facilitates nighttime feedings. It also limits disruptions and makes it more likely that they all quickly return to sleep. A bassinet or crib can be placed in the parents' room in the early weeks. Some parents opt for a commercial side-sleeper crib that hooks safely to the parents' bed.

Some families prefer to sleep with their infants in the same bed. Although the AAP recommends that babies not sleep in the parents' bed, cosleeping is the norm in most of the world. The Academy of Breastfeeding Medicine (Blair et al., 2020) published guidelines for safe bed sharing for nursing families. It is important to provide the risks and benefits of different sleep arrangements so that parents can make an informed decision that is best for their situation. See **Chapter 14** for further discussion of cosleeping and other sleep issues.

Selecting a Healthcare Provider

Expectant parents will need to select caregivers for their pregnancy and birth and for their baby. Establishing a relationship with a healthcare provider before pregnancy can help determine whether that same caregiver will meet the needs for both prenatal care and birth. Selection of a caregiver for the baby should include consideration of whether the caregiver will support plans to nurse and provide appropriate advice. In countries that provide insurance coverage, the insurance company may dictate the choice of caregiver. Low-income families are constrained by the number of providers who accept Medicaid or sliding-scale fees for service for those without insurance. Families in countries with single-payer or government-provided health care may not have these constraints.

Selecting a Prenatal and Baby Provider

Pregnancy, birth, and the postpartum period are intimate times in a person's life. It is important for parents to choose a provider with whom they feel confident and who can support them through these life changes. If they doesn't already have an established relationship with a provider, they might request a "meet-and-greet" visit. This visit can be approached as an "interview" where the parents ask the provider questions about their background, experience, and philosophy on topics that matter most to them. Meet-and-greet visits are common, although they might not be offered by busy practices. **Table 12-2** suggests considerations to explore during such a visit with a baby provider.

Table 12-2 Considerations for Selecting Healthcare Providers

Child's Care Provider	Hospital or Birth Center Where Baby Will Be Born
▪ How soon after birth the first office visit will occur ▪ Number of times the caregiver expects to see the baby for health maintenance ▪ Privileges at the hospital where the baby will be born, and, if none, how the caregiver refers clients to another caregiver ▪ After-hours coverage, billing and payment policies, and same-day appointments ▪ Parent involvement in nonmedical decisions, such as those related to feeding schedule, sleep patterns, supplemental foods, and weaning ▪ Postdischarge treatment of newborn jaundice ▪ Viewpoint on circumcision ▪ Policy on vitamin, iron, and fluoride supplements ▪ Policy on initial vaccinations (such as immunization against hepatitis B) ▪ Percentage of nursing babies in the practice and the average duration of nursing ▪ Willingness to support the parents' desired nursing practices ▪ Management of nursing problems ▪ The person who answers nursing questions ▪ Whether there are IBCLCs on staff or parents are referred to an IBCLC ▪ Criteria for starting solid foods ▪ Guidelines for weaning, including support for child-led weaning ▪ Relationship with and referrals to breastfeeding support groups in the community	▪ Whether the facility is Baby-Friendly ▪ Policy regarding delay of routine newborn procedures until after the first nursing session (e.g., weight, length, vitamin K prophylaxis, hepatitis B immunization, antibiotic ointment in the baby's eyes, bath) ▪ Policy regarding how soon the baby can nurse after delivery ▪ Encouragement of rooming-in ▪ Nursing policy ▪ Policy on water and formula supplementation ▪ Whether there are IBCLCs on staff and available ▪ Relationship with and referrals to breastfeeding support groups in the community

Parents might select a provider based on their insurance/fee, setting for the birth (hospital, birth center, or home), location, and the availability of provider after hours. Consumer reviews of providers are available online. Prenatal providers could be obstetricians, midwives, or family practice healthcare providers. Providers for infants could be pediatricians, nurse practitioners, or family practice healthcare providers. Lactation education varies among medical and nursing programs. The type of provider chosen will depend on the philosophy of care, medical history, insurance/cost, and location.

Providers are required to have **hospital privileges** to care for the patients in the facility. If a particular hospital is preferred by a parent, having hospital privileges might determine their choice of providers. Hospitalists (hospital-only healthcare providers) are increasingly used in hospitals instead of community healthcare providers. Knowing if their community practice provider makes hospital rounds will help expectant parents as they plan for their child's arrival and care.

Expectant parents might choose a provider or hospital based on their support of nursing and providing human milk to infants. They can ask the providers about their **standing orders** related to lactation and how comfortable they are supporting and managing nursing issues. **Figure 12-7** contains a checklist for determining whether a healthcare professional is supportive of nursing; the full text of this checklist appears in the article by Newman (2009). If this is not their area of expertise, parents might ask what continuing education they have received and whether they refer clients to a lactation consultant. They can ask if the hospital is Baby-Friendly with protocols that support and promote lactation. **Chapter 30** has more information about BFHI. Lactation consultants can work with the community's prenatal and baby providers by providing services support either in their offices or as a referral for their clients. Collaborating with other providers will benefit both practices, as well as the families you serve.

- Provides formula samples or formula company literature.
- Considers nursing and bottle feeding as essentially equal.
- Recommends a brand of formula.
- Says it is not necessary to feed the baby immediately after the birth because you are (will be) tired and the baby is often not interested anyway.
- Discredits nipple confusion and recommends giving bottles early to make sure that the baby accepts a bottle nipple.
- Recommends not nursing when you or your baby is sick.
- Is surprised to learn that your 6-month-old child is still nursing.
- Believes that human milk has no nutritional value after the baby is 6 months or older.
- Advises that you never allow your baby to fall asleep while nursing.
- Advises you that you not stay in the hospital to nurse your sick child because it is important that you rest at home.
- Fails to help if you have trouble with nursing.

Figure 12-7 Actions that indicate a health professional is not supportive of nursing.

Communicating with Caregivers

Parents and caregivers must be able to develop a mutually respectful, adult working relationship. Parents need to communicate their wishes to the baby's caregiver and be prepared to share any concerns that arise. Caregivers can record the birth and nursing plan in the baby's chart and reflect any changes that occur. Often, the caregiver will be flexible when parental concerns are presented with confidence and self-assurance. Make sure families understand that it is never too late to raise a concern. If second thoughts arise after a visit, encourage contacting the provider's office. While in the hospital, if parents have questions that cannot wait until the scheduled rounds, they can ask the nursing staff to contact the caregiver. If staff members are busy, they may not get to this task as quickly as parents would like. In such circumstances, parents may want to contact the provider's office directly rather than wait.

Often, a concern may arise from a misunderstanding or misinterpretation of what a provider said. You can help formulate questions and clarify the caregiver's response. Parents who believe they must supplement feedings with formula can clarify exactly what was said. Did the caregiver say, for example, "You must supplement with formula" or "You need to supplement"? Encourage parents to share tactfully any confusion they have about the care plan. Parents might also need more education to fully understand the provider's recommendations. Empower parents to ask questions to gain clarity while still communicating their commitment to nursing their baby.

Conflicting Advice

Parents who are knowledgeable about nursing are keenly attuned to advice from their caregiver that seems questionable. You can offer suggestions for times when advice seems detrimental to nursing (e.g., early complementary foods, emphasis on sleep training, or restricting feedings). Providing evidence-based information with research and resources to share with the caregiver will help when discussing concerns. If the provider is part of a medical team or group, it may be possible to work with a supportive member of the team who has more knowledge of lactation.

Encourage parents to work with and inform their caregiver about their day-to-day nursing. Nursing decisions are, for the most part, not medical in nature. Responsible, informed parents will make responsible, informed decisions regarding the care of their baby. If a healthcare provider's advice about nursing conflicts with what a parent has learned from other informed sources, the parent's responsibility is to choose what is best for the baby. You can communicate to the parents that caregivers and parents alike want the same outcome: a healthy, thriving child.

Working Through Conflicts

When conflicts arise with a caregiver, you can provide support while respecting the primary healthcare relationship. Prepare parents before a visit by reminding them of typical nursing patterns at their baby's present stage of development. Encourage them to write down specific questions prior to office visits. Urge parents to ask for the reason behind the advice and question whether alternative treatment is possible. Help them work out solutions and adapt advice to their nursing. If the caregiver recommends formula supplements because of low weight gain, for example, they can ask whether verifying intake during a feeding or supplementing with expressed milk will meet this goal. The parent might use a nursing supplementer so that the baby receives any needed supplement while nursing. If this is not agreeable, you can suggest that they give the supplements after nursing.

In the case of low weight gain, the caregiver may agree to a short trial period with increased nursing frequency to increase the baby's caloric intake. This could be followed by a weight check to determine whether supplements are needed. Another alternative might be a full feeding assessment with prefeed/postfeed intake measurements to verify the baby's ability to transfer milk and to protect milk production if the baby is not transferring effectively.

When parents overcome nursing challenges, encourage them to share their success with the caregiver so that both can learn from the experience. The caregiver will then be better able to help families with similar problems in the future. You can also send your chart notes to the provider (with the parents' consent) to share your care plan and follow up. This strengthens the collaborative relationship between the provider and lactation consultant and provides better continuity of care for the parent.

Recommending Caregivers

Parents who are always at odds with their caregiver might consider changing to a new provider. Caregiver choices for families on public medical assistance or without insurance coverage may be very limited. Families with adequate health insurance may have more options available to them if they wish to change caregivers.

If parents ask you to recommend a provider, suggesting the names of several local providers will avoid the impression of recommending a particular individual. This helps ensure that nursing families in your community work with a variety of caregivers, thus increasing the caregivers' practical experience with lactation care. It also maintains your professionalism and objectivity in making recommendations and preserving collaborative, respectful relationships with medical providers in your community.

When providing provider referrals, you can share information without expressing personal preferences. You can suggest pertinent questions to ask and use what you know about caregivers to help prepare parents for their hospital experiences and pediatric checkups. For example, you can share what a caregiver usually tells parents at the first checkup and suggest that they have any questions or concerns ready. Most medical practices have websites describing their services, including patient forms and online appointment-setting capabilities. An informed and prepared parent is more likely to be satisfied with the visit's outcome, better understand and follow recommendations, and be less apt to contact the caregiver for clarification. It also empowers parents, allowing them to be proactive in their family's health care.

Summary

Healthcare providers are instrumental in helping parents make and be satisfied with their infant feeding decisions. Families are entitled to facts that enable them to make informed choices. Teaching parents prenatally will help them acquire this information at a time when they are considering a method of infant feeding. Provide practical suggestions regarding breast care, preparations at home, and selecting a caregiver who is knowledgeable about and supportive of nursing.

Classes on nursing will give prospective parents relevant information at key times. Early prenatal education on nursing will help in the decision-making process. A later class on practical lactation management helps parents prepare for the baby's arrival. Postpartum education and networking can reinforce effective practices and address questions parents may have as they establish nursing. These early interventions lay a strong foundation of support as parents anticipate their baby's birth and the beginning of nursing.

What You Learned—At a Glance

Conversation Starters with Parents

- What is most important in your infant feeding choice?
- How supportive are your partner and other family members of your feeding choice?
- How will nursing fit into your life?
- What have you done to prepare for nursing your baby?
- How confident do you feel with your healthcare provider's knowledge about nursing?

Infant Feeding Choice

- Social support has a significant effect on infant feeding choice.
- Most families make their infant feeding decision before the baby is born.
- Parents may question their decision not to nurse if the consequences appear to be detrimental.
- The intention to nurse and self-efficacy are predictors of successful nursing outcomes.
- Parents who formula feed or supplement nursing with formula report feelings of guilt, stigma, and defensiveness for their feeding choice.
- Opinions of family members and healthcare providers are important in nursing decisions.

Lactation Education

- Encouraging partner involvement recognizes their pivotal role in the nursing decision and outcome.
- Parents need to know the health risks of not nursing, as well as the health, emotional, and financial protections of nursing.
- Parents need to know the realities of breast fullness, nipple tenderness, and being available to the baby for feedings.
- Dispelling misconceptions will increase confidence in the decision to nurse.
- Discussing individual goals and giving practical information will help families blend nursing into their lives.
- Classes should keep messages simple, actively involve parents in learning, and reinforce knowledge retention with visual aids and multiple learning modalities.
- Combining infant feeding classes with a breastfeeding support group allows for individual problem-solving and prevention of common problems.

Prenatal Preparation

- Performing the pinch test will determine whether nipples may need assistance with latch.
- Colostrum expressed prenatally can be saved for use after the baby's birth.
- Colostrum should not be expressed prenatally if there is a history of preterm birth, miscarriage, or false labor until approved by the healthcare provider.
- Avoiding drying agents and tight bras will help preserve breast and nipple health.
- Plan a quiet place for feedings, initial sleeping arrangements, clothing to accommodate feedings, and help at home.

Selecting Caregivers

- Caregiver attitude and lactation knowledge greatly influence parents' decisions and confidence.
- Prenatal support and postpartum contact increase the likelihood of continuing nursing.
- Confidence in and a good working relationship with caregivers are important to parents.
- To ensure compatibility, parents can ask about healthcare providers' nursing knowledge, hospital affiliation, and accessibility.
- Families need an open, collaborative, mutually respectful relationship with their caregivers.
- Referring families to at least three potential caregivers avoids the appearance of making a recommendation.

References

Acquaye SN, Spatz DL. An integrative review: the role of the doula in breastfeeding initiation and duration. *J Perinat Educ.* 2021;30(1):29–47.

American College of Obstetricians and Gynecologists' Committee on Obstetric Practice, Breastfeeding Expert Work Group. Committee Opinion No. 658 summary: optimizing support for breastfeeding as part of obstetric practice. *Obstet Gynecol.* 2016;127(2):420–421.

Ballesta-Castillejos, et al. Factors that influence mothers' prenatal decision to breastfeed in Spain. *Int Breastfeed J.* 2020;5(1):1–9.

Bich TH, et al. Community-based father education intervention on breastfeeding practice—results of a quasi-experimental study. *Matern Child Nutr.* 2019;15(S1):e12705.

Blair PS, et al. Academy of Breastfeeding Medicine. Bedsharing and Breastfeeding: The Academy of Breastfeeding Medicine Protocol #6, Revision 2019. *Breastfeed Med.* 2020;15(1):5–16. Erratum in: Breastfeed Med. 2021 Aug;16(8):662.

Bookhart LH, et al. A nation-wide study on the common reasons for infant formula supplementation among healthy, term, breastfed infants in US hospitals. *Matern Child Nutr.* 2022;8(2): e13294.

Bourget M, et al. An educational intervention to support the development of a sense of mastery of the anticipated paternal role in expectant fathers: a clinical project. *J Perinat Educ.* 2017; 26(1):23–36.

Byun IH, et al. Double triangle suture technique for inverted nipple correction while preserving the lactiferous ducts. *J Cutan Aesthet Surg.* 2022;15(4):371–374.

Cato K, et al. Breastfeeding as a balancing act—pregnant Swedish women's voices on breastfeeding. *Int Breastfeed J.* 2020; 5;15(1):16.

Centers for Disease Control and Prevention. Breastfeeding and special circumstances. 2020. https://www.cdc.gov/breastfeeding/breastfeeding-specialcircumstances/index.html

Chang YS, et al. Relatively speaking? Partners' and family members' views and experiences of supporting breastfeeding: a systematic review of qualitative evidence. *Philos Trans R Soc Lond B Biol Sci.* 2021;376(1827):20200033.

Cohen SS, et al. Factors associated with breastfeeding initiation and continuation: a meta-analysis. *J Pediatr.* 2018;203:190. e21–196.e21.

Devane-Johnson S, et al. Historical research: the history of African American breastfeeding in the United States. *J Hum Lact.* 2022;38(4):723–731.

Grassley JS, et al. A grandmothers' tea: evaluation of a breastfeeding support intervention. *J Perinat Educ.* 2012;21(2):80–89.

Grossniklaus DA, et al. Participation in a quality improvement collaborative and change in maternity care practices. *J Perinat Educ.* 2017;26(3):136–143.

Hackman N, et al. Paternal education and its impact on breastfeeding initiation and duration: an understudied and often overlooked factor in US breastfeeding practices. *Breastfeed Med.* 2022;17(5):429–436.

Hauck YL, et al. Women's experiences with breastfeeding in public: an integrative review. *Women Birth.* 2021;34(3):e217–e227.

Hess J. *Infant Feeding: A Handbook for the Practitioner.* Chicago, IL: American Medical Association; 1923.

Horwood C, et al. An exploration of pregnant women and mothers' attitudes, perceptions and experiences of formula feeding and formula marketing, and the factors that influence decision-making about infant feeding in South Africa. *BMC Public Health.* 2022;25;22(1):393.

Jefferson UT, et al. Infant feeding exposure and personal experiences of African American mothers. *Breastfeed Med.* 2021; 16(2):124–130.

Linares AM, et al. Las dos cosas versus exclusive breastfeeding: a culturally and linguistically exploratory intervention study in Hispanic mothers living in Kentucky. *J Pediatr Health Care.* 2019;33(6):e46–e56.

Matriano MG, et al. Factors that influence women's decision on infant feeding: an integrative review. *Women Birth.* 2022;35(5): 430–439.

McKinley EM, et al. The prenatal rating of efficacy in preparation to breastfeed scale: a new measurement instrument for prenatal breastfeeding self-efficacy. *J Hum Lact.* 2019;35(1):21–31.

Meek JY. Educational objectives and skills for the physician with respect to breastfeeding, revised 2018. *Breastfeed Med.* 2019;14(1):5–13.

Moon RY, et al. Sleep-related infant deaths: updated 2022 recommendations for reducing infant deaths in the sleep environment. *Pediatrics.* 2022;150(1):e2022057990.

Morse H, Brown A. The benefits, challenges and impacts of accessing social media group support for breastfeeding: A systematic review. *Matern Child Nutr.* 2022;18(4):e13399.

Newman J. How to know a healthcare practitioner is not supportive of breastfeeding, revised. 2009. ibconline.ca/information-sheets/how-to-know-a-healthcare-practitioner-is-not-supportive-of-breastfeeding/

Patel AL, et al. Mediators of racial and ethnic disparity in mother's own milk feeding in very low birth weight infants. *Pediatr Res.* 2019;85(5):662–670.

Pezley L, et al. Efficacy of behavioral interventions to improve maternal mental health and breastfeeding outcomes: a systematic review. *Int Breastfeed J.* 2022; 5;17(1):67.

Ragusa R, et al. Breastfeeding in hospitals: factors influencing maternal choice in Italy. *Int J Environ Res Public Health.* 2020; 20;17(10):3575.

Reyes C, et al. Investigating the effectiveness of school-based breastfeeding education on breastfeeding knowledge, attitudes and intentions of adolescent females. *Midwifery.* 2019;70: 64–70.

Rhodes EC, et al. Promoting equity in breastfeeding through peer counseling: the US Breastfeeding Heritage and Pride program. *International Journal for Equity in Health.* 2021;20(1): 1–12.

Roberts D, et al. Exploring the reasons why mothers do not breastfeed, to inform and enable better support. *Front Glob Womens Health.* 2023;12;4:1148719.

Rodriguez-Vazquez R, et al. Intergenerational transmissible meanings in breastfeeding in Spain: a phenomenological study. *J Pediatr Nurs.* 2020;51:e108–e114.

Schmied V, et al. Place of sanctuary: an appreciative inquiry approach to discovering how communities support breastfeeding and parenting. *Int Breastfeed J.* 2019;14:25.

Schroeder D, et al. Rediscovering empowerment with breastfeeding in an urban First Nation's population. *BMC Pregnancy Childbirth.* 2019;19;19(1):509.

Segura-Pérez, S, et al. Impact of breastfeeding interventions among United States minority women on breastfeeding outcomes: a systematic review. *Int J Equity Health*. 2021;20:72.

Seyyedi N, et al. Effectiveness of a smartphone-based educational intervention to improve breastfeeding. *Int Breastfeed J*. 2021;16(1):70.

Simpson DA, et al. Twenty-five-year trends in breastfeeding initiation: the effects of sociodemographic changes in Great Britain, 1985–2010. *PLoS One*. 2019;14(1):e0210838.

Simpson, DA, et al. Trends and inequalities in breastfeeding continuation from 1 to 6 weeks: findings from six population-based British cohorts, 1985–2010. *Eur J Clin Nutr*. 2022;76: 671–679.

Tanda R, et al. Factors that modify the association of maternal postpartum smoking and exclusive breastfeeding rates. *Breastfeed Med*. 2018;13(9):614–621.

Taşhan T, et al. Maternal smoking and newborn sex, birth weight and breastfeeding: a population-based study. *J Matern Fetal Neonatal Med*. 2017;30(21):2545–2550.

Toledo C, Cianelli R. Self-objectification in the context of breastfeeding: a concept analysis. *Public Health Nurs*. 2019;36(2): 207–214.

Wallenborn JT, et al. Importance of familial opinions on breastfeeding practices: differences between father, mother, and mother-in-law. *Breastfeed Med*. 2019;14(8):560–567.

Wang S, et al. When fathers are perceived to share in the maternal decision to breastfeed: outcomes from the Infant Feeding Practices Study II. *Matern Child Health J*. 2018;22(11): 1676–1684.

Woods Barr AL, et al. "...[T]his is what we are missing": the value of communicating infant feeding information across three generations of African American women. *J Hum Lact*. 2021a;37(2):279–288.

Woods Barr AL, et al. EveryGenerationMatters: intergenerational perceptions of infant feeding information and communication among African American women. *Breastfeed Med*. 2021b;16(2):131–139.

Wolf J. Low breastfeeding rates and public health in the US. *Am J Pub Health*. 2003;93(12):2001–2010.

World Health Organization, United Nations Children's Fund. More than half of parents and pregnant women exposed to formula milk marketing. 2022. https://www.who.int/news/item/22-02-2022-more-than-half-of-parents-and-pregnant-women-exposed-to-aggressive-formula-milk-marketing-who-unicef

CHAPTER 13

Hospital Practices That Support Lactation

Throughout much of the world, childbirth occurs within a midwifery model of family-centered care, with babies born in birth centers or at home. Recognizing nursing as a continuation of the normal birth process, these cultures respect a person's ability to give birth and minimize labor "management." In contrast, births in most industrialized nations occur in hospitals, which vary in practices that support or hinder the establishment of lactation. Hospital practices directly influence nursing for parents who give birth there. An environment that is supportive and encourages exclusive nursing builds self-confidence in parents' ability to nourish their newborn infants.

The **Ten Steps to Successful Breastfeeding** provide a foundation for evidence-based maternity practices to support nursing for all individuals globally. Topics in this chapter highlight each of the Ten Steps. Supportive routines reflect a belief in lactation as the biologic and cultural norm and facilitate sound lactation care. Policies are evidence-based and support best nursing practices to achieve positive outcomes for families. Because there is little research into hospital practices that support nursing for nonbinary parents, the focus of this chapter is maternally based. Research on and policies to support nonbinary families is needed to fill the knowledge gaps and provide appropriate and inclusive care for all families.

KEY TERMS

Analgesia
Assisted vaginal delivery (or operative vaginal delivery) (AVD or OVD)
Baby-Friendly Hospital Initiative (BFHI)
Bonding
Clutch hold
Combined spinal–epidural (CSE)
Doula
Edema
Epidural analgesia
Epidural anesthesia
Episiotomy
Football hold
Forceps
Hunger cues
Hydration
Induction
Kangaroo care
Nipple shield
Patient-controlled epidural anesthesia (PCEA)
Placenta accreta
Placenta previa
Rooming-in
Side-sitting hold
Spinal anesthesia
Supplementary feeding
Ten Steps to Successful Breastfeeding
Vacuum extraction
Vernix

Setting the Stage for Nursing Prior to Birth

Step 3 of Ten Steps to Successful Breastfeeding: Discuss the importance and management of breastfeeding with pregnant women and their families.

A birth environment supportive of nursing begins with educating expectant parents about lactation and empowering them at a time when they are most vulnerable. Informed parents thrive in a climate of acceptance, cared for by supportive lactation practices. Healthcare providers are typically viewed as authority figures, and their opinions are valued because of their extensive training and experience. Thus, caregiver attitudes about nursing greatly influence parents' attitudes and, indirectly, the quality of their nursing experiences. Informing expectant parents about lactation promotes healthy feeding practices.

Supportive Birth Environment

Almost all babies in industrialized countries today are born in hospitals. In the United States, 98.3% of parents give birth in hospitals, 1.1% give birth at home, and 0.5% give birth in freestanding birth centers (Martin et al., 2019). Similarly, in England, Wales, and Canada, 98% of births occur in hospital or birth center settings (Office of National Statistics, 2019; Statistics Canada, 2020). The Netherlands has the highest rate of home births of industrialized countries with one in eight babies born at home (van Mulligen, 2019). The number of U.S. birthing centers doubled from 170 in 2004 to 344 in 2018 (American Association of Birth Centers, 2020; MacDorman & Declercq, 2019).

Healthcare provider fear of distance to emergency care, barriers resulting from midwives and healthcare providers working across different care models, rising cesarean rates, and healthcare systems affect birthing practices (Caughey & Cheyney, 2019). These factors make choosing natural birth challenging for families in many industrialized nations, especially for those who are underserved or marginalized.

Many of the world's poorest parents living in low-income countries give birth at home. Home birth rates are 28% in low- to middle-income countries (Hernández-Vásquez et al., 2021). There is a need to seek methods to improve birth outcomes and decrease maternal mortality on a global basis (WHO, 2021).

Supportive Policies

Step 1 of Ten Steps to Successful Breastfeeding: Comply fully with the International Code of Marketing of Breast-milk Substitutes *and relevant World Health Assembly resolutions; have a written infant feeding policy that is routinely communicated to staff and parents; and establish ongoing monitoring and data-management systems.*

Part of prenatal decision making for families is the selection of a birth facility that supports and promotes sound lactation practices. That means having lactation policies in all areas of the facility that care for nursing parents and babies. A supportive facility would also comply with the *International Code of Marketing of Breast-milk Substitutes*. The WHO established the Code in 1981 to regulate the marketing of human milk substitutes. One of the most important recommendations in the Code is that human milk substitutes should only be used when medically indicated and that they be purchased through the normal channels used to purchase all other medical supplies. This is to ensure that formula companies cannot market directly to hospitals and undermine practices that promote early nursing. Healthcare providers should practice within the guidelines of the Code and World Health Assembly (WHA) resolutions (WHO, 1981b; WHO & UNICEF, 2018). These are discussed in **Chapter 1**.

Parents need to receive consistent, accurate, and positive messages from all hospital staff and volunteers. Developing lactation policies in all patient care settings based on current scientific knowledge can help eliminate barriers to establishing early lactation and nursing. These policies need to be communicated routinely to all healthcare staff who encounter nursing families. This includes maternity staff, other healthcare providers, ancillary staff, patient care technicians, and administrative staff of all units that care for nursing families. It also includes the neonatal intensive care unit (NICU), labor and delivery, pediatrics, and with surprising frequency, the emergency department and medical–surgical units.

The collection of data regarding the feeding status of newborns is essential for a healthcare facility. Evidence-based practice and quality improvement initiatives depend on collecting and evaluating practice data. Therefore, facilities should monitor practices and collect data (through electronic or paper charting) related to infant feeding and care, especially for small and preterm infants. Recommended indicators for data collection include growth parameters, type of feeding, feeding measurement, skin-to-skin care, and other related information (WHO & UNICEF, 2018).

Knowledgeable Staff

Step 2 of Ten Steps to Successful Breastfeeding: Ensure that staff have sufficient knowledge, competence and skills to support breastfeeding.

It is important that healthcare staff know why and how to implement lactation policies. Understanding the rationale and scientific basis behind these policies may increase their acceptance by the medical and nursing staff. In addition, learning basic lactation care reinforces the normative nature of lactation and improves productivity and the ability to focus on complex cases. Basic instruction should include positioning and latch, evaluating the quality of a feeding, and knowing when and how to supplement infants. It should also include teaching and initiating milk expression when the baby is unable to nurse, for example, when a baby is in a special care nursery (SCN) or NICU. Having knowledgeable staff helps ensure that parents receive appropriate and consistent help when a lactation consultant is not available. **Chapter 28** discusses staff education.

Supportive Labor and Delivery Practices

The labor and delivery experience can affect both early initiation and continuation of nursing. Intrusive labor and delivery practices create obstacles to initiating lactation. Policies that routinely separate birth parents and infants interfere with nursing and are not in the best interests of families. Institutional support and trained healthcare providers are essential in providing supportive labor and delivery practices.

Nurses in obstetrics typically support the normal physiologic process of birth. Unfortunately, however, there are time constraints on a labor unit in a hospital. Understaffing and increased workloads can result in less time to help a birth parent labor without medications and medical interventions. The WHO's goal of initiating nursing within 1 hour after birth is not being met. Globally, only half of all infants are nursing within 1 hour after birth, with no country exceeding the 80% mark (Shrimpton, 2017).

Provide Labor Support

Having a support person such as a labor nurse, a midwife, or a **doula** increases the rates of nursing initiation and exclusive nursing (WHO, 2018b). Ideally, hospitals will encourage the presence of an experienced labor support person throughout the entire labor and delivery. Having a companion of choice increases birth satisfaction and does not negatively affect neonatal outcomes. Care by certified nurse midwives (CNMs) results in lower rates of epidurals, **inductions**, perineal lacerations, episiotomies, and cesarean deliveries (Declercq et al., 2020). Midwifery care also results in significantly higher rates of vaginal birth, including vaginal birth after previous cesarean delivery (Carlson et al., 2019).

A doula provides emotional, physical, and informational support to new and expectant parents before, during, and after birth. They are experienced in the use of comfort measures to decrease the pain of labor without the use of medications or anesthesia. Doula support results in fewer interventions and can increase Apgar scores (Alexandria et al., 2023). It can reduce the cesarean rate, labor length, Pitocin use, pain medication use, the need for **forceps**, and requests for **epidural anesthesia** (Sobczak et al., 2023). Babies are more alert and responsive after an unmedicated birth, which is a much more likely outcome with doula support. Alert and responsive babies usually latch and nurse robustly within 1 to 2 hours after birth.

Limit Birth Interventions

Families should be given cultural and emotional support to birth with as few interventions as possible. The use of medications, anesthesia, and other interventions during labor and birth can negatively affect early nursing and influence feeding duration. Normal and optimal postpartum lactation management can be difficult after labor and delivery interventions. Any policy that routinely and unnecessarily separates a nursing dyad interferes with lactation and contradicts good medical care. Complications resulting from routine interventions tend to normalize the abnormal and lead to high volumes of sleepy, lethargic babies who have difficulty latching and sucking. They may also render parents less responsive to their baby. The Policy Statement from the American Academy of Pediatrics (AAP; Meek et al., 2022) recommends avoidance of routine procedures until completion of the first feeding.

Nonessential Routine Interventions

Events surrounding birth have a direct impact on early nursing. Labor and birth, although normal biologic processes, are not treated as such in many hospitals. The medicalization of childbirth in many countries has led to a culture of normalizing unnecessary interventions during low-risk, uncomplicated births. Hospitals increasingly rely on technology as a strategy to reduce litigation, lower staffing levels, and decrease costs. As a consequence, there has been an unprecedented rise in the scheduling of births, including elective inductions and elective cesarean sections (Lothian, 2019).

Elective Cesarean Section

Some parents want the convenience of a scheduled cesarean section. The increased incidence of elective cesarean deliveries in some countries is troubling, especially in terms of the ethics of surgically removing a baby based on maternal request rather than medical necessity. Cesarean deliveries increase the risk of neonatal death and maternal death. In low- to middle-income countries, maternal death rate is 7.6 per 1000 cesareans, and the perinatal death rate is 84.7 per 1000 cesareans (Sobhy et al., 2019). The risks for maternal complications and death are almost five times greater than with vaginal birth, including hemorrhage, sepsis, blood clots, and embolisms.

Parents who deliver via cesarean section exhibit less sensitivity to their baby's cry than those who deliver vaginally (Kasser et al., 2019). Cesareans require longer hospital stays and involve risks of bladder and bowel injuries and serious complications for future pregnancies (American College of Obstetricians and Gynecologists [ACOG], 2019). Cesarean delivery increases risks in future pregnancies for **placenta previa** (the placenta lies low in the uterus and covers all or part of the cervix), **placenta accreta** (the placenta grows too deeply into the uterine wall), and uterine rupture (De Mucio et al., 2019; Narava et al., 2020).

China recently changed its one-child policy to two children and made a concerted effort to lower its cesarean rates. From 2007 to 2016, the cesarean rate in China fell from 46% to 32% at county-level hospitals and from 68% to 44% at provincial-level hospitals. Low-risk parents increasingly chose vaginal birth, with new encouragement from healthcare providers and nurse midwives (Wang & Hesketh, 2017). However, with the 2016 two-child policy, cesarean rates plateaued and increased in rural areas versus cities. This may be partly explained by increased birth rates for older parents and parents with a history of cesarean delivery, as well as increased rural health services (Li et al., 2020). Other potential reasons for the higher cesarean rate in rural areas include sociological issues, such as superstitious culture, and lack of anesthesiologists to administer **epidural analgesia**, as noted by a low rate of labor epidural analgesia in rural China (Zhao et al., 2021). Globally, one in five births is cesarean, a rate that puts birthing parents and infants at risk if a cesarean is performed when there is not a medical indication (WHO, 2021).

Labor Induction

In an ironic twist, the fear of pain and loss of control during birth has resulted in a true loss of control for countless expectant parents. Elective induction frequently leads to hours of failure-to-progress labor and an unplanned cesarean surgery (Neal et al., 2019). The cesarean rate for parents with obesity who have labor inductions is almost 50% (Paidas Teefey et al., 2020). Parents who are older are also at increased risk for induction resulting in a cesarean birth, with a risk that is three to five times higher across 5-year age spans in first-time birth parents compared to parents with previous births (Bergholt et al., 2020). Limiting unnecessary technology surrounding their baby's birth helps parents get nursing off to a good start. This approach requires parents to educate themselves and advocate for their needs.

Some parents choose the convenience of labor induction. Pitocin, the brand name for synthetic oxytocin, is a hormone administered via an intravenous (IV) line to induce or stimulate labor. This exogenous oxytocin has different effects than the endogenous oxytocin a birthing person's body produces during labor. Exogenous oxytocin has an antidiuretic effect and can cause **edema** in extremities, such as the breast and nipple tissue. The result can be "meaty" and "flat" nipples that make latch difficult until the edema is relieved. It can take as long as 2 weeks for this edema to resolve. **Chapter 22** discusses softening the areolae to assist with latch. The potential for edema increases further when combined with additional IV fluids in conjunction with epidurals and exogenous oxytocin. **Figure 13-1** illustrates severe edema in a birth parent's ankles and feet. Breast edema from the use of synthetic oxytocin may also cause a delay in lactogenesis II (Lian et al., 2022).

Concern has been expressed about the effect of flooding the body with exogenous oxytocin as a new parent is acquiring the maternal/parental role. Studies yield conflicting results on the effect of exogenous oxytocin on lactation initiation and duration. In one review, 50% of studies reported an association between exogenous oxytocin and less optimal lactation

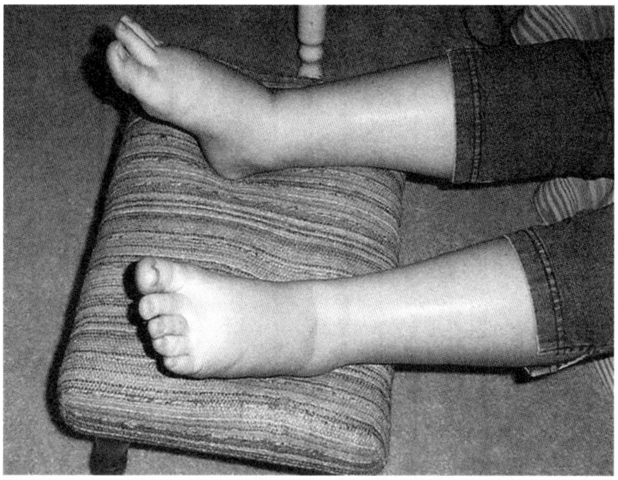

Figure 13-1 Edema resulting from excessive fluids.
Printed with permission of Anna Swisher

outcomes, 23% revealed no association, and 26% had mixed results. These variances demonstrate the complexity and confounders with exogenous oxytocin augmentation versus natural labor and endogenous oxytocin release (Erickson & Emeis, 2017).

Low concentrations of endogenous plasma concentration are associated with birth anxiety and prolonged labor (Walter et al., 2021). Researchers found a relationship between exogenous oxytocin use and inhibition of the infant feeding in the first hour after birth. At discharge, 97.3% of babies whose birth parent did not receive exogenous oxytocin were exclusively nursing compared with 87.1% of the babies whose birth parent received exogenous oxytocin. At 3 months, the rates were 72.5% compared with 65.9%, respectively. Maternal obesity was also predictive of impaired lactation at 3 months postpartum, suggesting that obesity may confound the effects of exogenous oxytocin (Gomes et al., 2018).

The Epigenetic Impact of Childbirth Collaborative (EPIIC) studies how intrapartum events affect the epigenetic remodeling processes and subsequent health of the birth parent and offspring. These events include the use of exogenous oxytocin, antibiotics, and cesarean section. The researchers posit that normal labor and birth provide eustress (a healthy, positive form of stress) on the baby. This process has an epigenomic effect on the genes that program immune responses, weight regulation, and tumor suppression. Reduced or elevated levels of cortisol, adrenalin, and oxytocin during labor may influence abnormal gene expression. Thus, labor and birth conditions may affect epigenetic remodeling, influencing the child's future development and risk of morbidities (Qiu et al., 2023; Zuccarello et al., 2022).

Pain Relief in Labor

The use of support persons, walking, showers, bathing, birthing balls, and other comfort measures can help with pain control to avoid the unnecessary use of drugs. However, many expectant parents desire a medicated birth with assurances of minimal pain. Medications received during labor can create feeding difficulties or delay the onset of full milk production. Studies on epidural anesthesia and feeding outcomes are conflicting. One review found 12 studies with negative lactation outcomes associated with epidurals, 10 studies reported no effect, and 1 study associated epidurals with positive lactation (French et al., 2016). There are limitations in studies examining causal relationships, and many of the variables are not well defined. *Hale & Hartmann's Textbook of Human Lactation* (Hale & Hartman, 2017) provides a comprehensive primer on analgesic and anesthetic medications, including how they work and their effects on the parent and infant.

Systemic Analgesia. Analgesics relieve pain without a total loss of feeling, muscle movement, and consciousness. These drugs are used to lessen pain and usually do not stop it completely. Systemic analgesics are not usually given immediately before delivery to avoid slowing the baby's reflexes and breathing at birth (American Society of Anesthesiologists [ASA], 2020). Pain relief medications diminish early sucking. Consequently, parents who receive such medications during labor are more likely to leave the hospital without having established lactation.

Epidural Analgesia and Anesthesia. Epidural analgesia causes some loss of feeling in the body from the uterus down. The amount of numbing is dependent on the drug and the amount given. Epidural anesthesia is used for cesareans and provides complete loss of physical sensation. A needle passed through the epidermal space within the spinal canal delivers anesthetic drugs, such as morphine, fentanyl, or sufentanil. A catheter is inserted for additional infusion (ASA, 2020). The option of **patient-controlled epidural anesthesia (PCEA)** allows the patient to control the amount of medicine and is associated with lower dosages and reduced hypotension. Perceived as fast and effective, epidurals are commonly used in both vaginal and cesarean section births. Complication rates related directly to anesthesia are estimated at about 3% (Maronge & Bogod, 2018).

Epidurals lead to increased use of exogenous oxytocin and increased risk of **assisted or operative vaginal delivery** using forceps or a vacuum device.

A Cochrane Review found a correlation of an increased risk of cesarean section for fetal distress, although the overall rate of cesareans did not increase. Parents who received epidurals during labor had increased incidents of fever, possibly because of an inflammatory response (Anim-Somuah et al., 2018).

Epidurals can also affect a parent's nursing ability, either directly through the medication (Hale & Hartmann, 2017) or through the chain of events triggered by anesthesia use. Several large studies have documented that epidural analgesia use in labor affects nursing at exclusivity and duration (Newnham et al., 2021; Oommen et al., 2021; Orbach-Zinger et al., 2019).

Spinal Anesthesia. Parents who deliver surgically typically receive **spinal anesthesia**. A needle injects an anesthetic, such as bupivacaine, and a narcotic, such as fentanyl, into the cerebrospinal fluid (CSF). Spinal anesthesia is a stronger block than epidural anesthesia, is more evenly distributed, is easier to administer, and has a quicker onset of action. However, it carries the risk of lowering blood pressure, which can distress the baby. It also has a higher incidence of nausea and vomiting and a shorter duration of anesthesia. Complications can affect the parent's ability to breathe, cough, and swallow. Other risks include loss of arm movement, severe bradycardia, and cardiac arrest (ASA, 2020). The most common complication is a "spinal headache," estimated at 1% of procedures and associated with accidental dural puncture (Janvier & Russell, 2022).

Combined Spinal-Epidural Anesthesia. A **combined spinal-epidural (CSE)** places a needle into the epidural space, followed by another small-gauge needle into the spinal space, with a catheter placed into the epidural space for additional drug administration. CSE causes very rapid numbing and requires smaller amounts of the drugs. It enables walking during labor and may create the sensation to push if it is given late in labor. This procedure is sometimes called a "walking epidural" (ASA, 2020).

Nitrous Oxide. Nitrous oxide gas provides pain relief during labor and delivery. Popularly known as "laughing gas," nitrous oxide slows the body's reaction time, lowers anxiety, and dulls pain sensitivity. Positive nursing outcomes are associated with the use of nitrous oxide for labor pain relief. One study found that over 83% of the parents surveyed reported positive pain relief. Higher lactation rates were reported at 1 week, 1 month, and 3 months after birth (Zanardo et al., 2018).

Interventions During Delivery

Medical intervention during delivery can increase the risk of lactation difficulties. Episiotomies are performed to increase the size of the vaginal opening. The use of forceps or vacuum extraction assists in removing the baby from the birth canal when labor is not progressing or when the parent's or baby's health are at risk from prolonged labor. Interventions after delivery include suctioning and separating the dyad before they have an opportunity to nurse.

Episiotomy. An **episiotomy** is a surgical incision through the perineum to enlarge the vaginal opening and avoid tearing of the surrounding skin. This procedure increases the risk of a fourth-degree laceration—namely, a tear through the rectal mucosa. Parents who have had an episiotomy often find it difficult to get comfortable, particularly when they sit upright. Pain when sitting makes it difficult to relax enough to position the baby comfortably for feeding. Medications such as hydrocodone and ibuprofen can safely relieve the discomfort. The baby's low milk intake in the first few days prevents exposure to large quantities of these medicines if the parent needs to take them (Hale & Krutsch, 2024).

Mechanical Devices. Complications with delivery can result in the use of forceps or **vacuum extraction** to help remove the baby from the birth canal. Forceps grasp the baby inside the birth canal and help guide them out. Vacuum extraction applies suction and traction to the baby's head to help pull the baby out. Both of these procedures increase the risk of bruising, injury, sensitivity to the infant's head, and discomfort when nursing. Bruising increases the risk of jaundice, which can cause sleepiness and a lack of interest in feeding (Centers for Disease Control and Prevention, 2019). Clinicians have also noted increased chomping and inability to suck in babies who have been subjected to forceps and vacuum extractions.

Suctioning. In a vaginal birth, fluids in the baby's nose and mouth are normally squeezed out by labor and birth. Babies born by cesarean will typically need to have their nose and mouth suctioned to remove these fluids. Suctioning may also be necessary after a quick delivery. It is best not to attempt to nurse immediately after deep suctioning. This practice can cause some babies to appear to associate nursing with the discomfort that preceded their first feeding experience and to react negatively when feedings are initiated (Widström et al., 2019).

Removing the Baby to a Radiant Warmer. Babies are often placed in radiant warmers after delivery because of an inability to self-regulate their temperatures. Warmers are usually unnecessary, however, when the nursing dyad remains together. Babies who are held skin to skin warm faster, stay warm longer, and exhibit greater sucking competence. Skin-to-skin care, or **kangaroo care**, allows for adequate temperature maintenance without increased fluid loss. It reduces the risk of hypothermia as compared with conventional incubator care for infants weighing 1800 g or more. When placed against the parent's skin, the infant breathes warm, humidified air rather than dry hospital air, as with artificial warmers. Covering the dyad with blankets while they remain skin to skin will help prevent neonatal hypothermia and initiate early nursing. The infant's armpit or forehead temperature can be monitored while one of the parents holds the newborn.

Delayed First Nursing. The longer feeding is delayed, the greater the likelihood that the baby will receive formula in the first few days of life. Standard routines that delay feeding for more than an hour after birth include weighing, measuring, bathing, warming, dressing, and wrapping the baby. Standard treatments include administration of antibiotic eye drops, vitamin K shot, and hepatitis B shot (the first vaccination). Babies who are born by cesarean are frequently separated from their birth parent and given formula as a first feeding. Babies born large for gestational age (LGA) are also vulnerable to formula use. These babies are frequently subjected to multiple prefeed blood glucose heel sticks even when asymptomatic for hypoglycemia because of their size, especially if the birth parent has gestational diabetes (Academy of Breastfeeding Medicine [ABM], 2021). The labor and delivery staff can preserve and protect nursing by avoiding unnecessary separation, which can hinder subsequent lactation. Many procedures can be delayed until after the first nursing.

Promote Bonding Immediately After Birth

Ideally, parents will spend the initial moments after delivery holding and **bonding** with their baby. After leaving the comfortable, secure confines of the womb, the newborn enters an unfamiliar and perhaps unsettling environment. When placed in the comfort of their parent's arms, newborns respond to the warmth of their parent's body and familiar smell by nuzzling against their skin. If the parent is the first person to hold the infant, their normal body bacteria will colonize the baby's body. Furthermore, an infant is attuned to their parent's smell, and the odor of the milk may reduce pain response (Baudesson de Chanville et al., 2017; Zhang et al., 2018).

Bonding is strongest in the first 1 or 2 hours of life. Soon after birth, staff will need to observe and assess the baby's overall health. These assessments can be done quietly without disruption while the parent holds the baby. Many countries require treatment of newborn infants' eyes with an antibiotic to safeguard against the effects of sexually transmitted disease. Postponing antibiotic treatment of the baby's eyes allows eye contact and enhances bonding between the parents and the baby. Staff can delay this procedure to allow the parents and baby at least 1 hour of uninterrupted time together.

The Bonding Process

The term *bonding* was popularized in the classic book *Maternal–Infant Bonding* (Klaus & Kennell, 1982) and later in *Bonding: Building the Foundations of Secure Attachment and Independence* (Klaus et al., 2000). Bonding describes the close physical contact between the parent and the baby soon after birth. The most favorable time to initiate bonding is in the first minutes after birth, when the baby is alert and the parents are eager to touch their new child. This period is described as the "golden hour," "magical hour," or "sacred hour," highlighting the impact of bonding, attachment, and nursing during the first hour of life. Routine birth practices that delay this contact, strict feeding schedules, and separation from the baby all limit opportunities for early bonding. This separation also delays acquisition of the parental role (discussed in **Chapter 20**).

The process of bonding begins with the first parent–infant contact in the hours following birth and continues as parents and infants interact to form a unique and lasting relationship. This intimacy develops through exchanging messages and feelings with all five senses—sight, touch, smell, taste, and sound. Parents often express attachment through touching, fondling, talking to, and kissing their babies while holding them face to face. Babies reciprocate through recognizing and responding to the parents' overtures. They may smile, follow their parents' image with their eyes, and display signs of contentment and acceptance. Skin and eye contact, the parent speaking and the baby responding, and other interchanges help to build a loving relationship. This time spent together soon after birth encourages affectionate contact between parent and child throughout the child's formative years.

Positive Results of Bonding

Bonding enables babies to begin nursing immediately after birth. It may be that the infant locates the nipple through a pheromone-like effect. The vomeronasal organ (VNO) located in the bottom of the nasal cavity detects pheromones. These chemical cues may trigger newborn arousal, motivation, and attraction. They may provide assistance in latching and boost the neural circuitry for learning (Coombes et al., 2018). Fatty acids in amniotic fluid may provide the sensory cue that guides newborns in their first feeding. Whether it is pheromones that mimic amniotic scent, fatty acids, or a combination, studies report that newborns are attracted to their source of nourishment (Hanser et al., 2017). This reaffirms the importance of beginning nursing immediately after birth before bathing the baby and removing any olfactory cues.

Extended parent–infant contact during the first days of life is associated with long-term behavioral and developmental advantages. There is a dose–response relationship between early skin-to-skin contact and exclusive nursing (Giang et al., 2022). Immediate nursing after birth may reduce the risk of cognitive impairment (Krol & Grossmann, 2018). A study found that children with specific language impairments were significantly less likely to have nursed directly after birth compared with neurotypical children (Diepeveen et al., 2017).

Over time, nursing parents exhibit more positive moods, lower stress, and more effective emotional responsiveness. This in turn is likely to influence maternal behaviors positively. A recent longitudinal study of birth parents' habitual use of a smartphone while nursing did not reveal any negative emotions or problems bonding at 9 months postpartum (Inoue & Hashimoto, 2021).

Non-Birth Parent Bonding

Non-birth parents who touch, fondle, and talk to their newborn babies form close emotional ties. The needs of non-birth parents (typically the father) are often neglected during the childbearing experience. Yet, 2 out of 10 men may experience postpartum depression, which can affect bonding and long-term family functioning. Thus, it is beneficial for caregivers to include the non-birth parent when facilitating bonding.

A qualitative study found that attending the birth fostered perceptions of increased bonding with the partner and newborn and increased family togetherness (Lwanga et al., 2017). Holding their newborn skin to skin in the NICU reduced partner's stress significantly, with lowered cortisol stress levels and lowered blood pressure (Varela et al., 2018). Skin-to-skin care helps partners feel more included and just as important as the birth parent, encouraging a more equal parenting role (Olsson et al., 2017).

Bonding encompasses the affectionate attachment of both parents to their newborn infant. Bonding by the birth parent earlier in pregnancy or the postpartum period is positively associated with quality dual parent-to-infant bonding moving forward. A desired pregnancy and good social support are also associated with bonding quality in most studies (Tichelman et al., 2019). A study of non-birth parents involved in prenatal support programs reports greater attachment to their infants right from birth. They demonstrated more affection, caregiving, and play with their babies. Their babies displayed higher motor, language, and personal and social development at 9 months of age than the nonintervention group (Rempel et al., 2017).

Secure attachment as a couple promotes positive parenting. A non-birthing parent, although fascinated with their baby, can experience some jealousy about the more intimate relationship between the birth parent and the nursing baby. Bonding and the building of love for the baby help partners adjust to the new family relationships. Fostering and supporting these caregiving behaviors can help families acquire confidence (Fonseca et al., 2018). **Chapter 20** discusses changes in the family with a baby's birth.

Help with Initiating Nursing

Step 4 of Ten Steps to Successful Breastfeeding: Facilitate immediate and uninterrupted skin-to-skin contact and support mothers to initiate breastfeeding as soon as possible after birth.

Initiating nursing as early as possible confers many health advantages. Digestion of colostrum clears meconium from the baby's gut and provides immunologic protection. Delaying the first bath until after the first nursing allows the **vernix** to soak into the baby's skin, lubricating and protecting it. This prevents temperature loss and facilitates nursing by preserving amniotic scent. Initiating nursing immediately after birth also increases duration. One Baby-Friendly hospital reported a 97.4% initiation rate, with 60.1% nursing within the first hour. Six-month exclusive nursing rates were 38.9% (Yılmaz et al., 2017).

The increased oxytocin secretion from sucking contracts the uterus more quickly and controls bleeding immediately after delivery, reducing the need for exogenous oxytocin. Caution parents that exogenous oxytocin may be given routinely postpartum to prevent hemorrhaging without their knowledge. Supportive practices during labor can facilitate early nursing. Maintaining **hydration** preserves the parent's energy, which in turn may have a subtle impact on the birth experience and early feedings. Allowing birthing parents to labor in any position they choose rather than requiring that they labor while lying down employs gravity and assists second-stage labor. Creating an environment that facilitates second-stage labor and delivery enhances the initiation of nursing.

Skin-to-Skin Care

Immediate skin-to-skin contact at birth enhances bonding, birth parent sensitivity, the infant's self-regulation, and nursing (Widström et al., 2019). A newborn's rooting and sucking reflexes are particularly strong in the first few hours following an unmedicated delivery. Unmedicated babies who remain undisturbed on the parent's abdomen will crawl to the breast, search out the nipple, latch, and suck. This typically can be accomplished within about 1 hour of birth. When held quietly skin to skin, newborns will typically work through nine distinct behaviors, including head bobbing, bringing their hands to their mouth, making sucking motions, and nuzzling and licking the breast (Brimdyr et al., 2018; Widström et al., 2019). **Chapter 15** discusses these behaviors and the postbirth approach to care.

Early skin-to-skin contact establishes earlier effective sucking and feeding behaviors (Widström et al., 2019). It increases exclusive nursing and nursing duration. Early skin-to-skin care also stabilizes blood glucose levels, increases attachment behavior and affectionate touch, and enhances infant recognition of the parent's milk odor. It reduces infant crying, provides better maintenance of infant temperature, and improves cardiorespiratory stability in late preterm infants. Skin-to-skin contact and nursing provide **analgesia** for painful neonatal procedures (Aydin & İnal, 2019; Dar et al., 2019). Skin-to-skin care of preterm infants is associated with positive parent–child reciprocity and enhanced cognitive development and organized sleep from 6 months to 10 years of age (Bigelow & Power, 2020). There is an increase in maternal–infant mutuality 1 year after birth when the dyad has skin-to-skin contact immediately after delivery (Widström et al., 2019).

Removing the baby during this sensitive time to be bathed, suctioned, and weighed and to receive medical procedures interferes with the instinctual bonding process. Birth attendants can help the natural postpartum process by drying and placing the baby skin to skin near the chest immediately after birth, covering the dyad together with a warm blanket. If the baby does not spontaneously begin to lick and explore feeding within the first hour, gently stroking the baby's mouth with the nipple can help initiate the rooting reflex. This is an optimal time to teach parents about **hunger cues** (discussed in **Chapter 14**) and encourage parents to respond to them. A caregiver can be made available if the baby seems ready to nurse and needs help. Moving the dyad to a postpartum room allows them to remain together during transport with continued contact. The goal is not necessarily to accomplish a feeding but rather to provide the opportunity and foster self-confidence. Babies should not be rushed or forced to nurse.

Nursing After a Cesarean Delivery

Cesarean delivery does not preclude early nursing. Practical protocols and policies have been developed for hospitals to provide skin-to-skin care after a cesarean (Crenshaw et al., 2019; Stevens et al., 2019). These proven quality improvements can be used by facilities to support providing baby-friendly, family-centered care after an operative birth. Parents who deliver surgically can nurse as soon as they are awake and able to respond to their baby. If they have any post-operative delays, the partner or other family member can provide skin-to-skin contact until the dyad can be reunited.

A positive experience with initiating nursing can help to normalize the postpartum experience for parents who may feel a sense of failure or disappointment that they did not give birth vaginally. Holding the baby skin to skin and encouraging closeness can lower anxiety and help them connect with their new baby. Skin-to-skin contact in the operating room after a cesarean has resulted in higher satisfaction with birth experiences and lower cortisol stress levels. No negative effects on newborn stability were observed (Crenshaw et al., 2019).

Parents who deliver by cesarean may have limited mobility, frustration at needing help, fatigue, pain, and impaired infant feeding abilities. Cesarean delivery also increases the risk of supplemental feedings in the hospital, which are associated with early weaning. In addition, these parents have been through major trauma and may be hearing only how "lucky" they are to have a "healthy baby." Posttraumatic stress disorder can occur after difficult births, and healthcare providers need to address this with their patients (Benton et al., 2019; Dekel et al., 2019).

Surgical delivery can make it difficult to nurse comfortably. Assisting with positioning will help them find what works best for them and their baby. Lying side to side facing the baby helps avoid incision pain in the first few hours. It also accommodates nursing when the parent's head must remain down because of spinal anesthesia. Pillows behind their back and under their knees will support their abdomen. If reclining on their back, they can place their baby on top with the baby's legs angled away from the incision site. In a sitting position, a pillow placed over the surgical incision will cushion it from the pressure of the baby's body. Pillows under the parent's knees will provide further support when sitting in bed. Another sitting position that many nursing parents find comfortable is with the baby tucked along the parent's side under their arm (**side-sitting hold**, also known as a **clutch hold** or **football hold**). Pillows placed under the baby will bring the baby level with the breast.

Supportive Postpartum Environment

Parents have vocalized dissatisfaction with postpartum care worldwide and even with different care models (Crowther et al., 2019). First-time nursing parents are novices, as are their babies. Although nursing is instinctive by nature, it is also a learned skill and often requires new knowledge and practice. Parents need time and patience to adjust to each other's idiosyncrasies as they learn to work together as a team.

A relaxed and supportive climate encourages parents to seek help and laugh at any missteps as they and their baby learn together. Although a parent may feel awkward and clumsy at times, in an accepting atmosphere, their awkwardness will not deter them from persevering. Demonstrating a willingness to listen to parents' concerns reinforces the importance of nursing and helps you provide anticipatory guidance.

Eliminate Negative and Unnecessary Practices

Negative and unnecessary postpartum practices can compromise nursing in both the short and long term. Routines that inhibit interaction, practices that imply possible failure, and ineffective problem-solving often stem from tradition and misinformation. Lactation advice and support from healthcare providers may derive from personal experience (Wright & Hurst, 2018) or misconceptions rather than being rooted in evidence-based information. Support from a healthcare professional significantly increases the probability of nursing initiation. Healthcare provider education leads to innovations in evidence-based practice and supports and helps to eliminate negative practices (Wallenborn et al., 2018).

Limit Interruptions

Despite global support for early and frequent nursing after delivery, new parents are not always provided with a hospital environment that allows them to spend adequate time on early nursing. Hospital routines and procedures often create continual interruptions that interfere with the time parents need for sleeping and learning how to care for their baby. Parents experience numerous interruptions on their first day postpartum in the hospital. One study determined that new parents spend only 20% of their time on lactation-related actions during the postpartum stay (Mitsui & Saito, 2019). The postpartum hospital stay needs to be protected from routine and/or unnecessary interruptions by healthcare providers and other hospital staff that interfere with parents learning how to care for and feed their baby.

The typical patient care routine in most birth facilities includes daily visits by the parent's and baby's providers to check on the dyad's progress. Nurses will visit periodically throughout the day and night to check the baby; monitor the parent's temperature and blood pressure; examine any incision sites and IV lines; check the fundus, perineum, and breasts; provide medications and snacks; help with toileting or bathing, and change bed linens.

Dietary personnel will bring meals. Housekeeping personnel will clean and empty trash. A photographer may stop by to take pictures. Additional interruptions may occur from maintenance, media services, volunteer services, and clergy—not to mention friends and relatives who visit. These interruptions are doubled if the room is shared with another patient.

The simple use of a privacy sign may reduce unnecessary interruptions. Such a sign is especially useful to ensure privacy for individuals who are nursing or pumping their milk. Encouraging parents to request that visitors wait until the family goes home will help them get the rest they need and allows more time for teaching parents about infant care and lactation.

Place No Restrictions on Feedings

Step 8 of Ten Steps to Successful Breastfeeding: Support mothers to recognize and respond to their infants' cues for feeding.

Baby-Friendly hospitals and other facilities that promote lactation place no rules or restrictions on feedings and keep dyads together (ABM, 2018). Free access and early feeding during hospitalization are key indicators for exclusively nursing infants for the first 3 months of life (Zhang et al., 2020). Expectant parents can be encouraged to inquire about the hospital's infant feeding policy before delivery and to negotiate changes if needed. They can also ask about policies to keep parents and babies together for unrestricted feeding. **Rooming-in** is discussed later in this chapter.

Parents need to know how their baby signals a readiness to nurse, and the importance of responding to their signals. Feeding babies on a rigid schedule or ignoring natural hunger cues fails to help parents learn how to respond to hunger cues. The baby may become agitated and frantic by the time a feeding is initiated. There is an increase in the incidence of jaundice and hypoglycemia in infants when feedings are limited (ABM, 2017b, 2021). Clinicians refer to this effect as *lack-of-breastfeeding jaundice*, indicating that the jaundice is a result of lactation mismanagement. Parents who are governed by a rigid schedule may not be nursing often enough to stimulate milk production or satisfy the baby. Some hospitals schedule feedings every 2 to 3 hours and require blood glucose testing after a certain number of hours if the baby has not fed. Many babies are sleepy the first few days postpartum and *do* need to be awakened to feed.

Give No Unnecessary Supplements

Step 6 of Ten Steps to Successful Breastfeeding: Do not provide breastfed newborns any food or fluids other than breast milk, unless medically indicated.

Unnecessary supplementation of nursing babies is all too common in many birth facilities. Nursing infants should receive no foods or liquids other than human milk for approximately the first 6 months of life (AAP, 2022). The only time they should receive any type of supplement is for a specific medical need, such as hypoglycemia, weight loss of 10% or more, signs of dehydration, prematurity, or lethargy. When a supplement is needed, the first choice should be the parent's expressed colostrum or milk (ABM, 2017a). **Chapter 22** discusses teaching hand expression.

Newborns who nurse frequently from birth, at least every 2 to 3 hours, usually 8 to 12 times in 24 hours, or in response to hunger cues never need water and seldom need supplemental formula. Routine use of glucose water or formula for nursing babies should be discouraged. In addition, formula use can negatively affect the establishment of milk production and increase the child's risk of developing long-term negative health outcomes, as discussed in **Chapter 10**.

Infants who receive supplements for nonmedical reasons are at increased risk for early nursing cessation (AAP, 2022). Non–medically indicated supplementation sends the message to parents that their milk alone is not sufficient to nourish their baby. This undermines their confidence in their ability to exclusively nurse their baby. Even in a Baby-Friendly hospital, 15% of nursing infants were supplemented during their hospital stay. Reasons for supplementation included obesity, first birth, late preterm infant, low birth weight, and the use of exogenous oxytocin to stimulate labor. Uninterrupted skin-to-skin care at birth for 65 plus minutes reportedly reduced the risk for supplementation (Kalmakoff et al., 2018). Parents can reduce the risk of unnecessary supplementation by keeping their baby with them or instructing the nursery to bring their baby to them for feedings and to give no supplements unless medically indicated.

Give No Artificial Teats to Infants

Step 9 of Ten Steps to Successful Breastfeeding: Counsel mothers on the use and risks of feeding bottles, teats and pacifiers.

Babies suck differently on artificial nipples than on the parent's nipple. Consequently, the use of bottles and pacifiers appears to cause confusion for some babies. Although not all babies are confused when given an artificial nipple, they may tend to prefer the smaller, longer, rigid latex or silicone nipple that fits into their mouth like their fingers. This can negatively affect their latch when attempting to nurse.

Bottle feeding is the most common supplementation method (Penny et al., 2018, 2019). However, when more nourishment is needed, the baby can receive it by a method other than a bottle and artificial nipple. Researchers endorse cup rather than bottle feeding as a temporary substitute for nursing in healthy, term newborns (Feldman-Winter et al., 2020). Masseter activity is highest in nursing newborns and lowest in bottle-fed babies. Cup-feeding masseter activity ranks between the nursing and bottle-feeding groups. Cup feeding is associated with higher nursing rates after discharge and can be done safely. **Chapter 22** discusses alternative feeding methods.

Bottle feeding of preterm infants is a complex issue. Direct nursing of preterm infants in the hospital is significantly associated with nursing for 6 or more months, as well as with the duration of exclusive nursing (Pinchevski-Kadir et al., 2017). Higher weight gain has been found in infants who are fed human milk via bottle rather than by directly nursing (Azad et al., 2018; Holmes, 2018). Some healthcare providers believe that bottle feeding is a helpful transition to direct nursing (Penny et al., 2018). Manufacturers continue to develop artificial teats that they claim mimic sucking during nursing (Perrella et al., 2019).

A Cochrane review reported low to moderate evidence that avoiding bottle use in preterm infants during the establishment of nursing increases the rates of full nursing, along with any nursing, at discharge. Higher continued nursing rates were reported at 3 and 6 months after discharge as well (Penny et al., 2018). A multidisciplinary approach is needed for compromised or preterm babies.

Extended use of pacifiers can affect the child's craniofacial development. However, pacifier use for preterm infants helps with transitioning from gavage feeds to oral feeds. Occupational therapists, speech-language therapists, lactation consultants, and other clinicians may also use bottles as therapeutic transitional tools. **Chapter 24** discusses preterm and high-risk infants. Caution about artificial teats also applies to the use of pacifiers (discussed in **Chapter 16**) and **nipple shields** (discussed in **Chapter 22**).

Promote Practices That Support Nursing

Lactation-friendly protocols and practices encourage the dyad to be together as much as possible and create an environment that is conducive to nursing. A supportive culture reinforces the belief in parents' ability to nurse and provides sound principles of lactation care. As part of these practices, parents and babies remain together from the moment of birth, followed by rooming-in for the remainder of the hospital stay. Parents learn how to recognize when their baby is hungry and respond with frequent feedings. They learn about lactation management, how to care for their breasts, and continued nursing after they return home.

Keep Parents and Babies Together

Step 7 of Ten Steps to Successful Breastfeeding: Enable mothers and their infants to remain together and to practise rooming-in 24 hours a day.

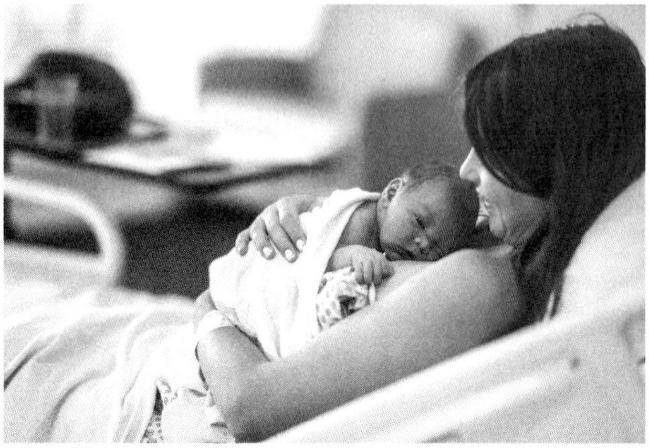

Figure 13-2 Baby rooming-in with birth parent.

Many birthing facilities embrace the concept of 24-hour rooming-in, recognizing that healthy newborns do not need to be cared for in a nursery. Family-centered birthing practices keep parents and babies together as much as possible, with babies staying in the parent's room, as depicted in **Figure 13-2**. Healthcare providers and hospital staff perform required procedures at the bedside to encourage parents to ask questions and discuss concerns. Baby-Friendly Guidelines for Facilities specify that healthy term infants should room-in day and night with the exception of up to 1 hour per 24-hour period unless there are compelling reasons related to medical needs, safety, or informed decision by the parent requesting separation (Baby-Friendly USA, 2021).

Parents with an uncomplicated delivery often remain with their baby with no interruption. If the baby was born by cesarean delivery, having a support person present will facilitate early rooming-in. Some hospitals offer partial rooming-in, taking the baby to the nursery when the parent is sleeping or showering. Flexible rooming-in permits parents to keep the baby in their room and take the baby to the nursery as the need arises. Expectant parents can inquire about rooming-in policies in the hospital where they plan to give birth.

Many facilities accommodate the parent's partner sleeping in the room, thus maximizing the opportunity for both parents to interact with their infant. This increases their self-confidence in handling their baby as they both learn to diaper, clean, burp, and hold their baby. Being able to see, hear, and respond to their baby is reassuring for parents. Parents who know their babies' abilities are better able to notice and respond to them. Rooming-in incorporates the baby into the family unit immediately after birth and promotes bonding and parent responsiveness.

Parents who care for their babies throughout the day and night in the hospital are more likely to have babies who are better nursers. Rooming-in enables parents to recognize and respond to their babies' hunger cues. This increases feeding frequency, promotes early milk production, and increases infant weight gain. The baby experiences less crying and movement, thereby conserving energy. These babies have less disorganized cries, startle less frequently, and feed more often than babies who are cared for in central nurseries.

Keeping parents and babies together during the postpartum stay also promotes learning and enhances the parents' self-efficacy. In this supportive environment, parents learn hunger cues and nursing techniques in a setting where they can have their questions answered and their techniques evaluated. Additionally, human milk provides antibodies to the microbes in the vicinity. If a baby remains in a nursery with its set of pathogens, the parent's milk will not reflect this.

Teach Parents Hunger Cues

Parents need to learn how to read and respond to the messages their babies send to communicate their needs for nourishment and comfort. There is a clear relationship between this type of responsive behavior and the establishment of sound lactation practices. The ideal feeding pattern allows babies to nurse in response to hunger cues. In addition to meeting the baby's needs and encouraging bonding, this enables nursing to get off to a good start and ensures the early establishment of milk production through frequent milk removal. Feeding in response to hunger cues helps to avoid milk stasis and problems such as engorgement or issues along the mastitis spectrum. Lack of knowledge about hunger cues can cause parents to misinterpret infant behavior and supplement unnecessarily.

Parents can begin to recognize their babies' hunger cues at delivery while they hold their baby skin to skin. Pointing out the baby's mouthing movements and other cues will help parents recognize them. Calling attention to hunger cues throughout the postpartum stay will reinforce their learning. Watching the baby for early hunger cues will help parents know when and how often to feed their baby. Newborns typically become hungry every 1½ to 3 hours, and sometimes sooner. They may feed every 1 to 1½ hours three or four times in a row and then sleep for 4 or 5 hours.

Make sure parents understand that cue-based feeding does not mean responding to their baby's cries. Most babies demonstrate hunger cues such as mouthing and hand-to-mouth activity before starting to cry. Babies who have been crying will have difficulty nursing because they are unable to organize themselves to focus on feeding. Crying compromises and disorganizes their suck and reduces their sucking strength. Recognizing that a baby's cry is a means of communication that is not always associated with hunger will help parents understand that their baby's cry is signaling a need. Urge parents to watch for early hunger cues before their baby progresses to crying. **Chapter 14** describes an infant's progressive hunger cues.

Teach Parents How to Nurse

Step 5 of the Ten Steps to Successful Breastfeeding: Support mothers to initiate and maintain breastfeeding and manage common difficulties.

The postpartum hospital stay is a pivotal learning time for new parents. Every nursing parent should receive basic instruction in early lactation management and newborn behavior. A knowledgeable caregiver, optimally, will be present to assist with the first feeding, observe technique, and answer questions. Some parents may require no help beyond that. Others will need more help learning how to manage feedings. The time taken by hospital staff to ensure early nursing initiation will help establish sound lactation practices. This investment in anticipatory guidance helps avoid time spent problem-solving for later difficulties that might have been avoided.

Lack of time prevents some hospital staff from providing adequate assistance to new parents. This is a valid concern with managed care, staffing shortages, and minimal staff–patient coverage ratios. The needs of nursing parents for emotional and practical support go largely unmet because of time constraints imposed on healthcare providers. This deficit underscores the importance of postpartum follow-up and support.

When infants have difficulty in their initial feeding attempts, parents will need assistance, perhaps at every feeding. Newborns typically sleep most of the time, and it is common for a baby to show little interest in nursing in the first few attempts. It is also common for a baby to nurse regularly and eagerly on the first day postpartum and then appear sleepy or fussy on the second day. Encourage parents to approach this time as an opportunity to practice their nursing skills and become acquainted with their baby.

A quiet and comfortable environment with minimal interruptions will help parents learn new skills and establish confidence with nursing before leaving the hospital. Nursing parents who are separated from their infants need special assistance with establishing milk production. They need to learn hand expression and effective milk removal, including pumping with a hospital-quality pump at least eight times in a 24-hour period (ABM, 2018). Make sure they know where to obtain a breast pump and that they understand human milk storage requirements, especially NICU protocols. **Chapter 22** provides information on pumping.

Teach Breast Care

Teaching birth parents breast care related to lactation will help them minimize the discomfort of nipple soreness and keep their breast tissue healthy. Healthy skin contains sufficient moisture to keep it soft and pliable. Nipples require no treatment unless they are tender or sore. In fact, a healthy nipple needs no special attention other than observing practices that will preserve the health of the skin. Primary among these practices is positioning the baby to facilitate a good latch. Expressing a drop or two of colostrum or milk and gently rubbing it into the nipple and areola after feeding will help with any initial tenderness. Information on nipple pain is provided in **Chapter 17.**

Provide Effective Discharge Planning

> *Step 10 of Ten Steps to Successful Breastfeeding: Coordinate discharge so that parents and their infants have timely access to ongoing support and care.*

A short hospital stay leaves little time to assess lactation knowledge, teach basic techniques, and evaluate feedings. Discharge planning will help parents plan realistically to meet both the baby's and their own needs when they return home. Some parents will have help from relatives or friends or through a postpartum doula service. Some parents will access community support groups, clinics, or services from their local public health department. Many parents, however, must manage on their own. Internet sites, online education, in-hospital learning TV channels, DVDs, and simple visual handouts are resources that support new parents.

The postpartum hospital stay is a time when parents are eager to listen and learn—teachable moments. Prior to hospital discharge, the postpartum staff must ensure that the parents understand how to nurse and how to assess if the baby is nursing well and thriving. Many parents begin nursing with no prior knowledge of lactation or normal infant development. Some may not decide to nurse until after the baby arrives. It is important not to assume a new parent will automatically know what to do, even if they have previously learned about lactation. Once parents are caring for their baby, a review of nursing techniques will help them relate to the information more readily than they did before the baby arrived.

Observing a nursing session on the day of discharge will provide a final opportunity to evaluate parents' understanding of nursing technique before they take their baby home. Parents need to know how to tell when their baby is receiving sufficient nourishment. Worry about not having enough milk is the primary reason for supplementing with formula and for early weaning. Teaching parents the signs that their baby is transferring milk, including being well hydrated and gaining weight within normal limits, will help increase their confidence in nursing. **Chapter 17** describes the signs of adequate milk production and milk transfer.

Parents need to leave the hospital with contact information for available resources, including local lactation consultants, support groups, their insurance plan's pump provision, and breast pump rental, if necessary. If concerns about potential feeding issues remain at discharge, the baby's caregiver needs to be informed, and the parents need to leave with a feeding plan that addresses the concerns. Parents will also need to schedule an appointment for their baby to be checked for weight and bilirubin level within 2 days of discharge. Many hospitals document the scheduling of this appointment by parents before discharge.

Refer Parents to Resources for Support

All parents benefit from receiving information about community resources and support. The volume of information they receive in the hospital can be overwhelming. Knowing how to access support in the community when concerns or questions arise will facilitate continued nursing. The first weeks with a new baby are challenging for many parents. A parent who is unfamiliar with newborn behavior may not know what to expect. Learning about normal feeding and behavior patterns and lactation milestones will help parents know what to anticipate and help prevent problems.

Many parents find the one-on-one peer support provided by breastfeeding support groups (discussed in **Chapter 2**) to be especially helpful. Peer counseling is positively associated with both initiation of nursing and duration of up to 12 months (McCoy et al., 2018). If there are no community support groups, the hospital might consider creating one. Peer online groups, social media, and internet "lactation cafés" are also popular avenues for seeking ongoing lactation support. An up-to-date list of recommended sites will be useful for new parents. Families who qualify will benefit from guidelines and contact information for public health assistance. Learning about community-based lactation support in your area will enable you to refer families who need their help.

The need for sensitivity and individualized care is a high priority in lactation support (Blixt et al., 2019). Parents benefit from individualized follow-up after discharge. Nursing duration increases with early contact and telephone follow-up from knowledgeable caregivers. Lactation support and education provided by both professionals and peers are associated with increased nursing duration and exclusivity (Gavine et al., 2022). Some hospitals provide contact for nursing parents after discharge when questions or concerns arise. The Affordable Care Act in the United States requires most insurance companies to provide lactation support as a preventive care measure. In many other countries, health ministries provide home health visits for a certain period after birth.

Postpartum Care Plans

A postpartum care plan helps staff efficiently utilize their time with nursing parents and provides a guide for evidence-informed decision-making related to lactation. A care plan can ensure that each hospital shift has assigned responsibilities to support early nursing. Coordination of care and instruction helps ensure that families receive the information they need. Care plans should cover all areas in which nursing parents and babies receive care, from labor and delivery through postpartum care. The ABM provides evidence-based model protocols for peripartum lactation management for the healthy parent and term infant and for a model hospital lactation policy (ABM, 2018).

The AAP recommends that someone knowledgeable about lactation observe a feeding at least once every 8 hours during the hospital stay. In hospitals where lactation consultants visit all nursing parents, at least one observation daily is recommended. In some hospitals, lactation consultants visit only first-time parents; in other hospitals, they visit only those who are referred for assistance. Lactation consultants can teach staff what to anticipate when observing nursing, how to help with technique, and what to teach prior to discharge. Teaching should include hand expression, alternate feeding methods, how to know when nursing is going well (as in **Figure 13-3**), and warning signs that indicate a problem (as in **Figure 13-4**).

Lactation Consultant Name and Phone: ______________________________

NURSING IS GOING WELL IF:

- Your baby is nursing at least 8 times in 24 hours.
- Your baby has at least 5–6 good wet diapers every 24 hours by the 4th day of age.
- Your baby has at least 3 tablespoon-size stools every 24 hours by the 4th day of age.
- Your baby gulps or swallows at feedings.
- Your breasts feel softer after a feeding.
- Your nipples are not painful.
- Nursing is an enjoyable experience.

If you go home from the hospital in 72 hours or less, your baby should be seen by their healthcare provider 2 or 3 days after discharge and again at 10 days to 2 weeks of age. It is your responsibility to schedule these visits, and to notify them and/or your board certified lactation consultant if at any time you feel nursing is not going right for either you or your baby.

WARNING SIGNS!

CALL YOUR BABY'S DOCTOR OR LACTATION CONSULTANT IF:

- Your baby is having fewer than 5–6 good wet diapers a day by the 4th day of age.
- Your baby is having fewer than 3 or 4 stools ("scoopable poops" of at least 1 tablespoon) by the 4th day of age, or is still having black tarry stools on day 5.
- Your baby is nursing fewer than 8 times a day.
- You have milk but you do not hear your baby gulping or swallowing frequently during nursing.
- Your nipples are painful throughout the feeding.
- Your baby seems to be nursing "all the time," or consistently falls asleep within a minute or two.
- You do not feel that milk production has started by the 5th day.

Baby's birthdate and time______________________________

Your baby will be 4 days old on ______________________________

Baby's birth weight ______________________________

Baby's discharge weight______________________________

Figure 13-3 Determining whether nursing is going well.

Issues that have a negative impact on lactation are set in **bold**.
In general, the more checkmarks the dyad has, the greater the risk for lactation problems or failure.
If an issue that is set in bold or multiple issues are checked, it is suggested that the dyad receive a lactation referral within 1–3 days of discharge.

Risk factors for nursing parent:

- ☐ no breast changes during pregnancy
- ☐ thyroid or pituitary problems
- ☐ **breast abnormalities, e.g., hypoplastic breasts, wide angle, tubular, marked asymmetry**
- ☐ prior lactation failure(s)
- ☐ flat or inverted nipples
- ☐ diabetes: Type 1, Type 2, or gestational diabetes
- ☐ poorly controlled diabetes
- ☐ hypertension, essential or pregnancy induced
- ☐ eclampsia, preeclampsia
- ☐ antenatal administration of betamethasone
- ☐ **PCOS/other infertility problems**
- ☐ **obesity (BMI > 29)**
- ☐ adolescent
- ☐ advanced age
- ☐ first time parent
- ☐ psycho/social stress/problems, e.g., depression, lack of support for nursing
- ☐ smoking
- ☐ **breast surgery or trauma, including radiation**
- ☐ plans to nurse and formula feed
- ☐ plans to return to work early

Risk factors for parent while in the hospital:

- ☐ stressful labor or delivery
- ☐ unscheduled cesarean section
- ☐ separated from infant(s)
- ☐ **delivery of multiples**
- ☐ **persistent nipple pain**
- ☐ edema of nipple/areolar complex
- ☐ **Sheehan's syndrome**
- ☐ anemia
- ☐ **no transitional milk by 72 hours**
- ☐ **breast pump dependent at the time of discharge**

Risk factors with infant's birth:

- ☐ male infant
- ☐ stressful delivery
- ☐ born after a long running epidural
- ☐ **one of a multiple**
- ☐ **oral anatomical abnormality, e.g., tongue tie, cleft, macroglossia**
- ☐ **neurological problem, e.g., Down syndrome, hypotonia, hypertonia**
- ☐ **preterm (<34 weeks gestation)**
- ☐ late preterm:
  - ☐ **born at 34 weeks gestation**
  - ☐ **born at 35 weeks gestation**
  - ☐ **born at 36 weeks gestation**
  - ☐ **born at 37 weeks gestation**
- ☐ post-term (41 weeks or more gestation)
- ☐ small for gestational age (SGA)
- ☐ large for gestational age (LGA)
- ☐ intrauterine growth restriction (IUGR)

Risk factors for infant while in the hospital:

- ☐ less than 2 hours of skin-to-skin contact with nursing parent immediately after delivery
- ☐ separated from nursing parent for a procedure
- ☐ medical problem, e.g., jaundice, hypoglycemia, hypothermia, respiratory problem
- ☐ inadequate caloric intake
- ☐ pacifier use
- ☐ **requires a special feeding plan**
- ☐ **using a feeding device at the time of discharge. e.g., nipple shield, nursing supplementer**
- ☐ **weight loss of more than 7% on the 3rd day of life**
- ☐ **inability to latch and transfer milk at the time of discharge**
- ☐ **receiving supplementation**
- ☐ supplemented with a bottle nipple more than 3 times
- ☐ **transferring less than 9 ml per feeding at 60 hours of life**
- ☐ **effective nursing not established at time of discharge**
- ☐ discharged from hospital in less than 48 hours

Figure 13-4 Red flags and risk factors for nursing.

A key sign that a baby is feeding effectively is long drawing sucking, which indicates milk transfer (swallowing will not necessarily be audible). Signs in the parent include uterine cramping, thirst, and sleepiness—all of which indicate that the milk is letting down. These indicators should all be present by 2 or 3 days postpartum. Hospitals usually have protocols for the length of time they will allow a baby to go without feeding before supplementing or testing blood glucose. The ABM has a protocol on the use of **supplementary feedings** in the healthy, full-term, human milk–fed neonate (ABM, 2017).

Care Plan for a 48-Hour Hospital Stay

A 48-hour stay leaves minimal time for teaching nursing before discharge. It does, however, allow numerous

Table 13-1 Lactation Care Plan for a 48-Hour Hospital Stay

Labor and Delivery	■ Keep room quiet, dim the lights, and reduce stimulation. ■ Delay visitors for at least 1 hour. ■ Place baby skin to skin with parent. ■ Point out baby's hunger cues. ■ Help with latch as needed if baby is ready to feed.
Hours 1–8	■ Keep baby and parent together for remainder of hospital stay. ■ Baby should nurse at least one time during this period. ■ Observe and document a feeding; point out nutritive and nonnutritive sucking. ■ Show parent how to record feedings and output in a nursing diary/log or phone app. ■ Teach positioning, latch, and hunger cues. ■ If baby has not fed by 8 hours, express milk and feed it to baby.
Hours 9–16	■ Baby should nurse two or more times during this period, ■ Observe and document a feeding, ■ Teach normal healthy diet, eat to hunger, and drink to thirst, ■ If baby is not nursing, continue to express milk and feed it to baby.
Hours 17–24	■ Baby should nurse two or more times during this period. ■ Observe and document a feeding; have parent identify nutritive and nonnutritive sucking. ■ Parent should be able to demonstrate effective positioning and latch. ■ If baby is not nursing well, continue to express milk and feed it to baby; refer the dyad for a lactation consultant consultation.
Hours 25–32	■ Baby should nurse two or more times during this period. ■ Observe and document a feeding. ■ Teach appropriate numbers of feedings, wet diapers, and stools, and how to know when nursing is going well (Figure 13-3). ■ Review the nursing diary/log with parent. ■ Teach warning signs that indicate a problem, as well as how to prevent nipple soreness and engorgement and when to contact a lactation consultant (Figure 13-3).
Hours 33–40	■ Observe and document a feeding. ■ Parent should be able to position and latch baby without help. ■ Teach cluster feedings, avoidance of artificial nipples, and risks of formula. ■ Discuss support person's role, safe sleeping, and what to expect during the first few nights home.
Hours 41–48	■ Parent should be able to identify nutritive sucking and swallowing. ■ Review sequence of hunger cues and how crying disorganizes the baby's suck. ■ Baby should be latching and feeding well. ■ Parents should appear comfortable holding, burping, dressing, and diapering baby.
Discharge	■ Ensure that baby is latching and feeding well before discharge. ■ Review signs of adequate milk production and transfer. ■ Give contact information for resources and any necessary feeding plan. ■ Notify baby's caregiver of any potential problems based on risk factors. ■ Ask parent to confirm when baby will be checked for weight and bilirubin levels.

opportunities for hospital staff to observe and help with nursing. Teaching can be divided into several short segments to avoid overwhelming parents at any one time. Parents will have 2 days to practice nursing with the support of knowledgeable staff, who can help them work through any difficulties prior to discharge. **Table 13-1** presents a sample care plan for a 48-hour hospital stay.

Care Plan for a 24-Hour Hospital Stay

Some hospitals discharge their postpartum parents after a 24-hour stay. The AAP identified milestones for discharging families less than 48 hours after delivery (Sullivan & Cruz-Rivera, 2020). These milestones state that the infant must complete at least two

Table 13-2 Lactation Care Plan for a 24-Hour Hospital Stay

Labor and Delivery	■ Keep room quiet, dim the lights, and reduce stimulation. ■ Delay visitors for at least 1 hour. ■ Place baby skin to skin with parent. ■ Point out hunger cues as the baby exhibits them. ■ Help with latch as needed if baby is ready to feed.
Hours 1–8	■ Keep baby and parent together for remainder of hospital stay. ■ Observe and document a feeding; point out nutritive and nonnutritive sucking. ■ Baby should nurse at least one time during this period. ■ Show parent how to record feedings and output in a nursing diary/log. ■ Teach positioning, latch, and hunger cues. ■ If baby has not fed by 8 hours, express milk and feed expressed milk to baby. ■ Teach appropriate numbers of feedings, wet diapers, and stools and how to know when nursing is going well (Figure 13-3). ■ Review nursing diary/log with parents.
Hours 9–16	■ Baby should nurse two or more times during this period. ■ Observe and document a feeding. ■ Teach normal healthy diet, eat to hunger, and drink to thirst. ■ If baby is not nursing, continue to express milk and feed expressed milk to baby.
Hours 17–24	■ Baby should nurse two or more times during this period. ■ Observe and document a feeding; have parent identify nutritive and nonnutritive sucking. ■ Parent should be able to position and latch their baby without help. ■ Teach warning signs that indicate a problem, as well as how to prevent nipple soreness and engorgement and when to contact a lactation consultant. ■ Review sequence of hunger cues and how crying disorganizes baby's suck. ■ If baby is not latching by mid-shift, delay discharge until at least two effective feedings; refer parent to lactation consultant for a feeding plan.
Discharge	■ Baby should be latching and feeding well before discharge. ■ Review signs of adequate milk production and transfer. ■ Give contact information for resources and any necessary feeding plan. ■ Notify baby's caregiver of any potential problems based on risk factors. ■ Ask parent to confirm when baby will be checked for weight and bilirubin levels. ■ Confirm if baby will return the next day to check weight and bilirubin levels.

successful feedings and be able to coordinate sucking, swallowing, and breathing while feeding. Parents must receive training and demonstrate competency in feeding the infant. Prior to discharge, trained staff should assess nursing dyads for position, latch, and adequacy of swallowing. Because the brevity of 24-hour hospital stays requires abridged teaching, parents should be encouraged to visit a caregiver at 48 hours to compensate for the early discharge. **Table 13-2** presents a sample care plan for a 24-hour hospital stay.

Summary

The course of a family's lactation journey takes root in their experiences during and immediately after their baby's birth. This chapter has explored elements covered by all Ten Steps to Successful Breastfeeding within the context of the parent's hospital experience. You can support families during their early postpartum days by being alert to the potential for any complications, providing appropriate anticipatory guidance, and ensuring they have information on community support to help when challenges arise. Make sure parents understand the importance of sound lactation practices. Encourage them to regard this time as a period of learning and adjustment and not to feel discouraged by any obstacles they encounter. Supporting the new family through this transitional time will help them transition smoothly to home.

What You Learned—At a Glance

Conversation Starters with Parents

- How soon did you nurse after your baby was born?
- How much time do you spend holding your baby skin to skin?
- What birth or postpartum interventions did you experience?
- How often does your baby nurse?
- How do you know when your baby is hungry?

Labor and Delivery Practices

- A relaxing and supportive environment will increase parents' comfort and self-confidence.
- Parent–infant bonding and infant rooting and sucking reflexes are strongest in the first 1 or 2 hours after birth.
- Immediate, continuous skin-to-skin care maintains newborn temperature and increases bonding.
- Delaying treatment of the infant's eyes and vitamin K injection up to 1 hour allows for bonding.
- Parents benefit from noninterfering help with positioning and latch.
- Parents who had a cesarean delivery may need help finding a comfortable feeding position.

Effect of Birth Medications and Interventions

- Labor medications diminish early sucking, lower blood pressure, and increase intrapartum fever.
- Forceps and vacuum extraction increase the risk of bruising and pain in the infant.
- Exogenous oxytocin and other IV medications may cause breast/nipple edema, and delay onset of full milk production.
- Delaying the first nursing increases the risk of non–medically indicated supplementation.

Postpartum Environment

- Extended parent–infant contact promotes exclusive nursing.
- A relaxed, supportive learning climate encourages parents to seek help when needed.
- Supplements should not be given routinely or without medical reason.
- Artificial nipples should be given to infants only when requested by the parents.
- Nipple shield use requires guidance of staff instructed in appropriate use and follow-up.
- Rooming-in and unrestricted feedings help get lactation off to the best start.
- Teaching hunger cues helps parents learn and respond to them.
- Care plans based on length of hospital stay will ensure parents receive the lactation support they need prior to discharge.

References

Academy of Breastfeeding Medicine. ABM clinical protocol #3: supplementary feedings in the healthy term breastfed neonate, revised 2017. *Breastfeed Med.* 2017a;12:188–198.

Academy of Breastfeeding Medicine. Clinical protocol #22: guidelines for management of jaundice in the breastfeeding infant 35 weeks or more of gestation—revised 2017. *Breastfeed Med.* 2017b;12(5):250–257.

Academy of Breastfeeding Medicine. Clinical protocol #7: model maternity policy supportive of breastfeeding. *Breastfeed Med.* 2018;13(9):559–574.

Academy of Breastfeeding Medicine. ABM clinical protocol #1: guidelines for blood glucose monitoring and treatment of hypoglycemia in term and late preterm neonates, revised 2021. 2021. *Breastfeed Med.* 2021;15(5):1–13.

Alexandria S, et al. The effect of doulas on maternal and birth outcomes: a scoping review. *Cureus.* 2023;15(5).

American Academy of Pediatrics. Newborn and infant breastfeeding. May 31, 2022. https://www.aap.org/en/patient-care/newborn-and-infant-nutrition/newborn-and-infant-breastfeeding/

American Academy of Pediatrics, Section on Breastfeeding. Breastfeeding and the use of human milk. *Pediatrics.* 2022;150(1): e2022057988.

American Association of Birth Centers. Birth centers are growing. 2020. https://www.birthcenters.org/page/bcgrowth

American College of Obstetricians and Gynecologists. Cesarean delivery on maternal request. ACOG Committee Opinion No. 761. *Obstet Gynecol.* 2019;133:e73–e77.

American Society of Anesthesiologists. Lifeline to modern medicine. Types of pain relief in labor and delivery. 2020. http://www.lifelinetomodernmedicine.com/Anesthesia-Topics/Types-of-Pain-Relief-in-Labor-and-Delivery.aspx

Anim-Somuah M, et al. Epidural versus non-epidural or no analgesia for pain management in labour. *Cochrane Database Syst Rev.* 2018 May;5(5):CD000331.

Aydin D, İnal S. Effects of breastfeeding and heel warming on pain levels during heel stick in neonates. *Int J Nurs Pract.* 2019; 25(3):e12734.

Azad MB, et al. CHILD Study Investigators. Infant feeding and weight gain: separating breast milk from breastfeeding and formula from food. *Pediatrics.* 2018;142(4):e20181092.

Baby-Friendly USA, Inc. *Guidelines and Evaluation Criteria for Facilities Seeking Baby-Friendly Designation.* 6th ed. Albany, NY: Baby-Friendly USA; 2021. https://www.babyfriendlyusa.org/wp-content/uploads/2021/07/Baby-Friendly-GEC-Final.pdf

Baudesson de Chanville A, et al. Analgesic effect of maternal human milk odor on premature neonates: a randomized controlled trial. *J Hum Lact.* 2017;33(2):300–308.

Benton M, et al. Women's psychosocial outcomes following an emergency caesarean section: a systematic literature review. *BMC Pregnancy Childbirth.* 2019;19(1):535.

Bergholt T, et al. Maternal age and risk of cesarean section in women with induced labor at term-A Nordic register-based study. *Acta Obstet Gynecol Scand.* 2020;99(2):283–289.

Bigelow AE, Power M. Mother-infant skin-to-skin contact: short- and long-term effects for mothers and their children born full-term. *Front Psychol.* 2020;11:1921.

Blixt I, et al. Women's advice to healthcare professionals regarding breastfeeding: "offer sensitive individualized breastfeeding support"—an interview study. *Int Breastfeeding J.* 2019;14(1):1–12.

Brimdyr K, et al. An implementation algorithm to improve skin-to-skin practice in the first hour after birth. *Matern Child Nutr.* 2018;14(2):e12571.

Carlson NS, et al. Influence of midwifery presence in United States centers on labor care and outcomes of low-risk parous women: a Consortium on Safe Labor study. *Birth.* 2019;46(3):487–499.

Caughey AB, Cheyney M. Home and birth center birth in the United States: time for greater collaboration across models of care. *Obstet Gynecol.* 2019;133(5):1033–1050.

Centers for Disease Control and Prevention. Jaundice & kernicterus. Facts about Jaundice and kernicterus. November 26, 2019. http://www.cdc.gov/ncbddd/jaundice /facts.html

Coombes HA, et al. Female chemical signaling underlying reproduction in mammals. *J Chem Ecol.* 2018;44(9):851–873.

Crenshaw JT, et al. Effects of skin-to-skin care during cesareans: a quasiexperimental feasibility/pilot study. *Breastfeed Med.* 2019;14(10):731–743.

Crowther S, et al. Policy, evidence and practice for post-birth care plans: a scoping review. *BMC Pregnancy Childbirth.* 2019; 19(1):1–16.

Dar JY, et al. Analgesic effect of direct breastfeeding during BCG vaccination in healthy neonates. *J Ayub Med Coll Abbottabad.* 2019;31(3):379–382.

De Mucio B, et al. A systematic review and meta-analysis of cesarean delivery and other uterine surgery as risk factors for placenta accreta. *Int J Gynaecol Obstet.* 2019;147(3):281–291.

Declercq ER, et al. Intrapartum care and experiences of women with midwives versus obstetricians in the Listening to Mothers in California Survey. *J Midwifery Womens Health.* 2020;65(1): 45–55.

Dekel S, et al. Delivery mode is associated with maternal mental health following childbirth. *Arch Women's Ment Health.* 2019;22(6):817–824.

Diepeveen FB, et al. Specific language impairment is associated with maternal and family factors. *Child Care Health Dev.* 2017;43(3): 401–405.

Erickson EN, Emeis CL. Breastfeeding outcomes after oxytocin use during childbirth: an integrative review. *J Midwifery Women's Health.* 2017;62(4):397–417.

Feldman-Winter L, et al. Evidence-based updates on the first week of exclusive breastfeeding among infants ≥ 35 weeks. *Pediatrics.* 2020;145(4):e20183696.

Fonseca A, et al. Mothers' and fathers' attachment and caregiving representations during transition to parenthood: an actor-partner approach. *J Reprod Infant Psychol.* 2018;36(3):246–260.

French CA, et al. Labor epidural analgesia and breastfeeding: a systematic review. *J Hum Lact.* 2016;32(3):507–520.

Gavine A, et al. Remote provision of breastfeeding support and education: systematic review and meta-analysis. *Matern Child Nutr.* 2022;18(2):e13296.

Giang, HTN, et al. Prevalence of early skin-to-skin contact and its impact on exclusive breastfeeding during the maternity hospitalization. *BMC Pediatr.* 2022;22(1):395.

Gomes M, et al. Intrapartum synthetic oxytocin and breastfeeding: a retrospective cohort study. *J Obstet Gynaecol.* 2018; 38(6):745–749.

Hale T, Hartmann P. *Hale & Hartmann's Textbook of Human Lactation.* New York: Springer; 2017.

Hale T, Krutsch K. *Hale's Medications & Mothers' Milk 2025–2026: A Manual of Lactational Pharmacology.* 21st ed. New York, NY: Springer Publishing Company; 2024.

Hanser HI, et al. Odorant-odorant metabolic interaction, a novel actor in olfactory perception and behavioral responsiveness. *Sci Rep.* 2017;7(1):10219.

Hernández-Vásquez A, et al. Prevalence of home birth among 880,345 women in 67 low-and middle-income countries: a meta-analysis of demographic and health surveys. *SSM-Population Health.* 2021;16:100955.

Holmes AV. Is breast still best from a bottle? *Pediatrics.* 2018;142(4): e20182297.

Inoue C, et al. Mothers' habitual smartphone use, infants during breastfeeding, and mother–infant bonding: a longitudinal study. *Nursing & Health Sciences.* 2021;23(2):506–515.

Janvier AS, Russell R. Postpartum headache—diagnosis and treatment. *BJA Educ.* 2022;22(5):176–181.

Kalmakoff S, et al. Predictors of supplementation for breastfed babies in a Baby-Friendly hospital. *Women Birth.* 2018; 31(3): 202–209.

Kasser S, et al. Birth experience in newborn infants is associated with changes in nociceptive sensitivity. *Science Report.* 2019;9(1):1–8.

Klaus M, et al. *Bonding: Building the Foundations of Secure Attachment and Independence.* New York: Perseus; 2000.

Klaus M, Kennell J. *Maternal-Infant Bonding.* 2nd ed. St. Louis, MO: CV Mosby; 1982.

Krol KM, Grossmann T. Psychological effects of breastfeeding on children and mothers. Psychologische effekte des stillens auf kinder und mütter. *Bundesgesundheitsblatt Gesundheitsforschung Gesundheitsschutz.* 2018;61(8):977–985.

Li H, et al. Trends in cesarean delivery rates in China, 2008–2018. *JAMA.* 2020;323(1):89–91.

Lian W, et al. Determinants of delayed onset of lactogenesis II among women who delivered via cesarean section at a tertiary hospital in China: a prospective cohort study. *Int Breastfeeding J.* 2022;17(1):81.

Lothian JA. Healthy birth practice #4: avoid interventions unless they are medically necessary. *J Perinat Educ.* 2019;28(2):94–103.

Lwanga H, et al. An exploratory study of men's companionship, perceptions and experiences during pregnancy and delivery in Uganda. *BMC Pregnancy Childbirth.* 2017;17(1):196.

MacDorman MF, Declercq E. Trends and state variations in out-of-hospital births in the United States, 2004–2017. *Birth.* 2019;46(2):279–288.

Maronge L, Bogod D. Complications in obstetric anaesthesia. *Anaesthesia.* 2018;73(suppl 1):61–66.

Martin JA, et al. Births: final data for 2018. *Natl Vital Stat Rep.* 2019;68(13):1–47.

McCoy MB, et al. Associations between peer counseling and breastfeeding initiation and duration: an analysis of Minnesota Participants in the Special Supplemental Nutrition Program for Women, Infants, and Children (WIC). *Matern Child Health J.* 2018;22(1):71–81.

Meek JY, et al. Policy statement: breastfeeding and the use of human milk. *Pediatrics*, 2022;150(1):e2022057988.

Mitsui Y, Saito I. Mothers' breastfeeding-related durations and nursing management during the early postpartum period in a mixed hospital ward with an obstetrics department: a prospective observational study. *Kobe J Med Sci.* 2019;64(5):e160–e169.

Narava S, et al. Outcome of multiple cesarean sections in a tertiary maternity hospital in the United Arab Emirates: a retrospective analysis. *Eur J Obstet Gynecol Reprod Biol.* 2020;247:143–148.

Neal JL, et al. Midwifery presence in United States medical centers and labor care and birth outcomes among low-risk nulliparous women: a Consortium on Safe Labor study. *Birth.* 2019;46(3):475–486.

Newnham EC, et al. Comparison of labour and birth outcomes between nulliparous women who used epidural analgesia in labour and those who did not: a prospective cohort study. *Women Birth.* 2021;34(5):e435–441.

Office of National Statistics. Birth characteristics in England and Wales: 2018. December 6, 2019. https://www .ons.gov.uk/people populationandcommunity/birthsdeathsandmarriages/livebirths /bulletins/birthcharacteristicsin englandandwales/2018

Olsson E, et al. Skin-to-skin contact facilitates more equal parenthood—a qualitative study from fathers' perspective. *J Pediatr Nurs.* 2017;34:e2–e9.

Oommen H, et al. The association between intrapartum opioid fentanyl and early breastfeeding: a prospective observational study. *Acta Obstetricia Et Gynecologica Scandinavica.* 2021; 100(12):2294–2302.

Orbach-Zinger S, et al. The effect of labor epidural analgesia on breastfeeding outcomes: a prospective observational cohort study in a mixed-parity cohort. *Anesth Analg.* 2019;129(3): 784–791.

Paidas Teefey C, et al. Risk factors associated with cesarean delivery after induction of labor in women with Class III obesity. *Obstet Gynecol.* 2020; 135(3):542–549.

Penny F, et al. Cup feeding as a supplemental, alternative feeding method for preterm breastfed infants: an integrative review. *Matern Child Health J.* 2018;22(11):1568–1579.

Penny F, et al. International Board Certified Lactation Consultants' practices regarding supplemental feeding methods for breastfed infants. *J Hum Lact.* 2019;35(4):683–694.

Perrella SL, et al. Effect of vacuum-release teat versus standard teat use on feeding milestones and breastfeeding outcomes in very preterm infants: a randomized controlled trial. *PLoS One.* 2019;14(3):e0214091.

Pinchevski-Kadir S, et al. Direct feeding at the breast is associated with breast milk feeding duration among preterm infants. *Nutrients.* 2017;9(11):1202.

Qiu C, et al. Association of labor epidural analgesia, oxytocin exposure and the risk of autism spectrum disorders in children. *JAMA Netw Open.* 2023;6(7):e2324630.

Rempel LA, et al. Influence of father-infant relationship on infant development: a father-involvement intervention in Vietnam. *Dev Psychol.* 2017;53(10):1844–1858.

Shrimpton R. Early initiation of breastfeeding. World Health Organization. 2017. https://www.who.int/tools/elena/commentary /early-breastfeeding

Sobczak A, et al. The effect of doulas on maternal and birth outcomes: a scoping review. *Cureus.* 2023;15(5):e39451.

Sobhy S, et al. Maternal and perinatal mortality and complications associated with caesarean section in low-income and middle-income countries: a systematic review and meta-analysis. *Lancet.* 2019;393(10184):1973–1982.

Statistics Canada. Live births and fetal deaths (stillbirths), by place of birth (hospital and non-hospital), Canada, provinces and territories. February 10, 2020. https://www150 .statcan.gc.ca /t1/tbl1/en/tv.action?pid=1310042901

Stevens J, et al. Skin-to-skin contact and what women want in the first hours after a caesarean section. *Midwifery.* 2019;74:140–146.

Sullivan CK, Cruz-Rivera SD. Hospital discharge of the healthy term and late preterm infant. In: Campbell DE, ed. *Neonatology for Primary Care.* Itasca, IL: American Academy of Pediatrics; 2020:341–364.

Tichelman E, et al. Correlates of prenatal and postnatal mother-to-infant bonding quality: a systematic review. *PLoS One.* 2019;14(9):e0222998.

van Mulligen A. What to expect in the Netherlands. Expatica.com. November 14, 2019. https://www.expatica.com/nl/health care /womens-health/what-to-expect-in-the-nether lands-101827/

Varela N, et al. Cortisol and blood pressure levels decreased in fathers during the first hour of skin-to-skin contact with their premature babies. *Acta Paediatr.* 2018;107(4):628–632.

Wallenborn JT, et al. The impact of the professional qualifications of the prenatal care provider on breastfeeding duration. *Breastfeed Med.* 2018;13(2):106–111.

Walter M, et al. The role of oxytocin and the effect of stress during childbirth: neurobiological basics and implications for mother and child. *Front Endocrinol.* 2021;12:742236.

Wang E, Hesketh T. Large reductions in cesarean delivery rates in China: a qualitative study on delivery decision-making in the era of the two-child policy. *BMC Pregnancy Childbirth.* 2017;17(1):405.

Widström AM, et al. Skin-to-skin contact the first hour after birth, underlying implications and clinical practice. *Acta Paediatr.* 2019; 108(7):1192–1204.

World Health Organization. The International Code of Marketing of Breast-milk Substitutes. 1981. https://www.who.int/publications /i/item/9241541601

World Health Organization. Ten Steps to Successful Breastfeeding. 2018a. https://www.who.int/teams/nutrition-and-food -safety/food-and-nutrition-actions-in-health-systems/ten -steps-to-successful-breastfeeding

World Health Organization. *WHO Recommendations: Intrapartum Care for a Positive Childbirth Experience.* Geneva, Switzerland: World Health Organization; 2018b.

World Health Organization. Caesarean section rates continue to rise, amid growing inequalities in access. 2021. https://www

.who.int/news/item/16-06-2021-caesarean-section-rates-continue-to-rise-amid-growing-inequalities-in-access

World Health Organization, United Nations Children's Fund. *Protecting, Promoting and Supporting Breastfeeding in Facilities Providing Maternity and Newborn Services: The Revised Baby-Friendly Hospital Initiative*. Geneva, Switzerland: World Health Organization; 2017. https://www.unicef.org/media/95191/file/Baby-friendly-hospital-initiative-implementation-guidance-2018.pdf

Wright AI, Hurst NM. Personal infant feeding experiences of postpartum nurses affect how they provide breastfeeding support. *J Obstet Gynecol Neonatal Nurs*. 2018;47(3):342–351.

Wu JL, et al. The mothers' breastfeeding behaviour within six weeks postpartum: new scale development and psychometric validation study. *BMC Pregnancy Childbirth*. 2023;23(1):1–13.

Yılmaz E, et al. Early initiation and exclusive breastfeeding: factors influencing the attitudes of mothers who gave birth in a baby-friendly hospital. *Turk J Obstet Gynecol*. 2017;14(1):1–9.

Zanardo V, et al. Nitrous oxide labor analgesia and pain relief memory in breastfeeding women. *J Matern Fetal Neonatal Med*. 2018;31(24):3243–3248.

Zhang S, et al. The analgesic effects of maternal milk odor on newborns: a meta-analysis. *Breastfeed Med*. 2018;13(5):327–334.

Zhang Y, et al. Effects of baby-friendly practices on breastfeeding duration in China: a case-control study. *Int Breastfeeding J*. 2020;15(1):92.

Zhao P, et al. Why is the labor epidural rate low and cesarean delivery rate high? A survey of Chinese perinatal care providers. *PLoS One*. 2021;16(5):e0251345.

Zuccarello D, et al. Epigenetics of pregnancy: looking beyond the DNA code. *J Assist Reprod Genet*. 2022;39(4):801–816.

CHAPTER 14

Infant Assessment and Development

A newborn's abilities and behaviors are closely linked to feeding. Therefore, an understanding of healthy newborn development, characteristics, and reflexes is important when assessing nursing. You can help parents learn to watch, identify, and interpret their babies' hunger cues and other behaviors. Patterns of behavior, growth, sleeping, crying, and digestion vary from one baby to another. Certain infant conditions may require a change in your approach to assisting a family. A complete medical history and thorough assessment of nursing parents and infants will help you identify situations that could negatively affect lactation.

KEY TERMS

Acrocyanosis
Alveolar ridge
Ankyloglossia
Apgar
Approach behavior
Asymmetry
Average baby
Avoidance behavior
Bauer crawling reflex
Bifurcated or bifid
Bovine immunoglobulin G (IgG)
Buccal frenula
Buccal pads
Candidiasis
Caput succedaneum
Cephalhematoma (also spelled *cephalohematoma*)
Clavicle
Cleft lip
Cleft palate
Constipation
Cosleeping
Cow's milk protein allergy
Cradle cap
Dancer hand position
Diaper rash
Diarrhea
Down syndrome
Epiglottis
Epstein pearls
Erythema toxicum
Flatulence
Flexion
Fontanel
Food sensitivity
Frenotomy
Frenuloplasty
Gastroenteritis
Gastroesophageal reflux (GER)
Gastroesophageal reflux disease (GERD)
Hirschsprung's disease
Hunger cues
Hydration
Hypertonic
Hypotonic
Infant acne
Infant states
Intravenous
Labial frenum
Lactase
Lactase deficiency (lactase nonpersistence)
Lactose overload
Lingual frenulum
Macroglossia
Macular
Micrognathia
Milia
Molding
Mottling
Natal tooth
Neonatal adaptation syndrome (NAS)
Neonatal tooth
New Ballard Scale (NBS)
Palate
Periosteum
Peristalsis
Philtrum
Placid baby
Projectile vomiting
Prone
Pyloric stenosis
Rapid eye movement (REM)
Reflexes
Rooting reflex
Submucosal cleft
Sucking
Sudden infant death syndrome (SIDS)
Sudden unexplained infant death (SUID)
Supine
Swaddling
Thrush
Turgor
Voiding
Yeast infection

Assessment of the Newborn

A newborn's first assessment will be documented with an **Apgar** score, which ranges from 0 to 10 (**Table 14-1**). The Apgar score is performed at 1 minute of life and again at 5 and 10 minutes. Heart rate, respiratory effort, muscle tone, reflex irritability, and color each receive a score of 0, 1, or 2. The Apgar score provides a quick status of the newborn and the response to resuscitation if needed (American Academy of Pediatrics [AAP], 2015). Scores can be influenced by drugs, trauma, congenital anomalies, infections, hypoxia, hypovolemia, and preterm birth. Apgar scores are an intrinsic part of the newborn's postpartum status and have less relevance after hospital discharge. However, low 5-minute scores, with other markers, may identify infants at risk for developing seizures (Persson et al., 2018). The Apgar score also provides a snapshot of a baby who had a challenging transition at birth and is at increased risk for feeding difficulties.

Generally, an initial contact with a nursing infant will include a full infant assessment. This especially applies when there are concerns such as poor weight gain, food intolerance, irritability, lethargy, or sucking difficulties. The baby should be completely undressed for the assessment and lying on a flat, firm surface. Evaluate posture, skin, head, oral structure, **clavicle**, **reflexes**, color, elimination, and **hunger cues**. Be alert for any areas on the baby's body that may cause pain or discomfort.

The **New Ballard Scale (NBS)** is helpful in assessing the normal newborn. This gestational assessment tool evaluates the tone of the infant's total body, wrist, biceps muscle, knee joint, shoulder girdle, and pelvic girdle. Girdle refers to the bones that encircle the shoulder and pelvis. A detailed description and free online illustration of the scale are available at www.ballardscore.com. Chapter 24 addresses preterm and other high-risk infants. Chapter 27 discusses a variety of long-term infant medical conditions. Another useful assessment tool, the Queensland Clinical Guidelines Newborn Baby Assessment (Queensland Health, 2021), provides an excellent overview of routine newborn assessment. Detailed descriptions and charts are available free from http://www.health.qld.gov.au/qcg.

Table 14-1 Apgar Score

Evaluate each of these five factors of the baby's condition with a score of 0, 1, or 2, with 2 being the best score.

1. Activity and muscle tone
2. Pulse (heart rate)
3. Grimace response (medically known as *reflex irritability*)
4. Appearance (skin coloration)
5. Respiration (breathing rate and effort)

Posture

Babies favor the fetal position, and healthy, full-term newborns generally hold their arms and legs in moderate **flexion**, often tucked under the body. Their fists are closed and usually held near the face. When awake, babies resist having their extremities extended and may cry at attempts to do so. As they mature, they spend less time in the fetal position and more time comfortably in semi-extension.

Observing a baby's body tone will provide clues about potential problems. When held in the prone (abdominal) position, healthy infants lie on their abdomen, draped over the examiner's hand, and alternate between trying to bring their head up and putting it down again. A baby whose body tone appears too loose (**hypotonic**) or too rigid (**hypertonic**) may have difficulty feeding effectively.

A baby whose birth parent has taken antidepressants in the selective serotonin reuptake inhibitor (SSRI) class may exhibit **neonatal adaptation syndrome (NAS)**. NAS may occur from exposure to substances in utero. It is characterized by one or more of the following signs and symptoms: jitteriness, irritability, lethargy, hypotonia, hypertonia, hyperreflexia, apnea, respiratory distress, vomiting, poor feeding, or hypoglycemia (Grossman & Berkwitt, 2019). Note that these babies can exhibit either hypotonia or hypertonia.

Hypotonia

A hypotonic infant has very low body tone. In the **prone** position, a hypotonic baby lies over the examiner's hand with their head hanging down, unable to bring it up. Their extremities are in extension, and there is minimal resistance to passive movement. The baby appears floppy, sluggish, and flaccid. Compare the hypotonic infant in **Figure 14-1** with the infant in **Figure 14-2** demonstrating normal tone. A hypotonic baby may have difficulty staying latched because of a weak suck. These babies may find it difficult to maintain intraoral negative pressure, even when sucking on the examiner's finger. They may nurse with their shoulders elevated to just beneath their ears to support their neck and chin (Academy of Breastfeeding Medicine [ABM], 2016).

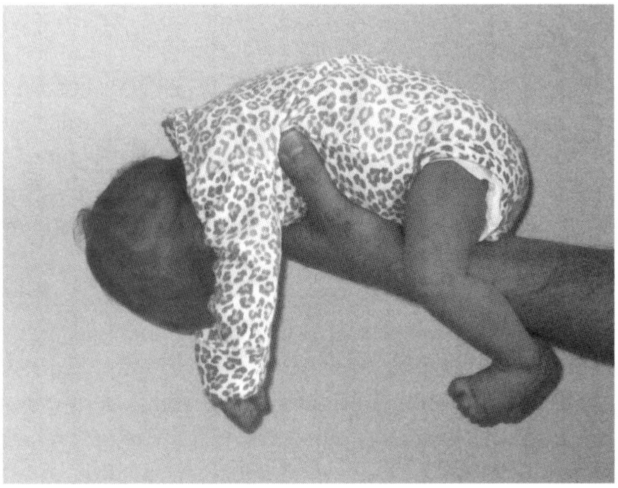

Figure 14-1 Hypotonic baby.

Printed with permission of Anna Swisher.

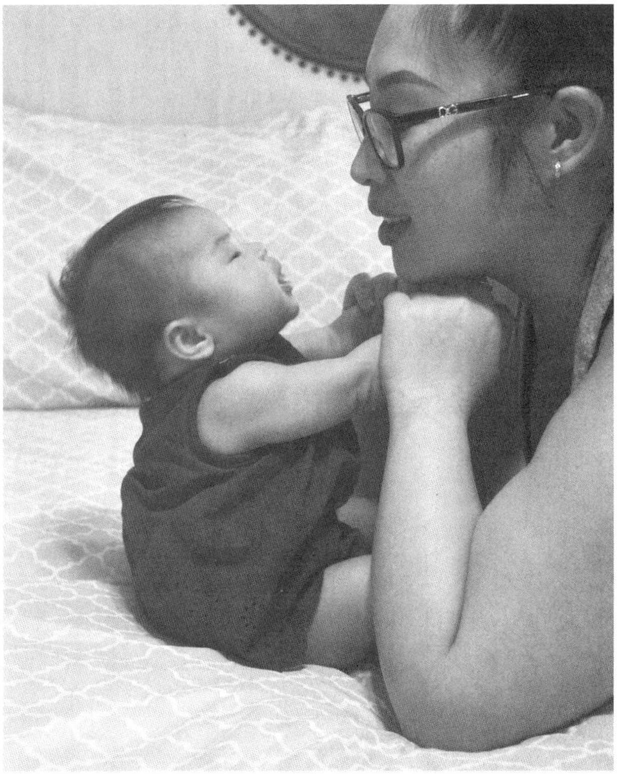

Figure 14-2 Baby with good muscle tone.

Printed with permission of Lyly Tran.

Hypotonia is a marker for certain syndromes and neurological disorders. Ineffective sucking and hypotonia are often symptoms of an underlying problem, not the problem itself. It may be associated with preterm birth, **Down syndrome**, autism spectrum disorder (ASD), Prader–Willi phenotype of fragile X syndrome, or botulism infection (Ersen et al., 2023; Kamity, 2019).

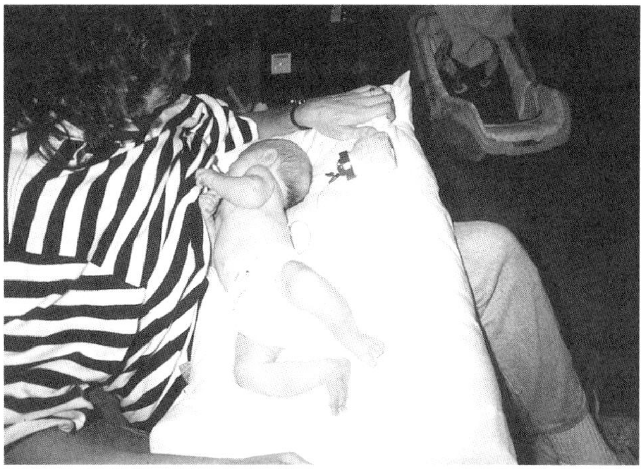

Figure 14-3 Hypertonic baby who arches away from the parent.

Printed with permission of Linda Kutner.

Hypertonia

Hypertonia is associated with neurological damage or disorders such as cerebral palsy (Straathof et al., 2022), neonatal infection, and prenatal drug exposure to cocaine and methamphetamines (Conradt et al., 2019; Evans et al., 2017). A hypertonic infant has a rigid body tone. When held in the prone position, a hypertonic baby will be virtually straight, lifting both the head and buttocks and maintaining them on a horizontal plane. The baby is often in hyperextension and arching away (**Figure 14-3**).

Many hypertonic babies cannot tolerate being held and prefer to interact from a safe distance. They may be difficult to comfort, pull away from contact, and do not snuggle into the parent's chest or neck. Instead, the baby leans back and away from the parent. They are often alert and squirmy, and they will hold their heads erect from a prone (face-down) position or on the shoulder. Hypertonic babies often arch the back when pressure is placed on the head or neck—for example, when positioning for feeding.

Skin

A healthy newborn's skin is warm and dry, with a pink or ruddy appearance depending on skin tone. The ruddiness is a result of an increased concentration of red blood cells in the blood vessels, coupled with minimal subcutaneous fat deposits. Small moles and birthmarks are common. Large congenital moles, although rare, can develop into skin cancer and should be referred for medical assessment.

Birthmarks may be simple, such as small red dots or "stork bites," which usually fade away within a year or so. The baby may have pigmented birthmarks or a cluster of pigment cells, with colors ranging from tan to brown, gray to black, and even blue. Mongolian spots are large blue to gray pigmented birthmarks usually found on the lower back and buttocks of newborns. They occur most often in dark-skinned infants and usually fade away within a few years.

Vascular birthmarks, which are due to abnormal blood vessel development, include port wine stains and hemangiomas. They may be associated with syndromes and glaucoma. Disfiguring or debilitating conditions may be treated with laser or steroid therapies (Smith et al., 2017). A hemangioma near or on the infant's lips or nose could interfere with nursing (see **Color Plate 14**). Alternative feeding methods may be needed until treatment is obtained.

Lanugo

In newborns, *lanugo* describes the fine, downy hair covering the body. It usually appears in utero at about 5 months' gestation. It typically is shed at 7 to 8 months' gestation. Lanugo is most abundant in preterm babies who are born at 5 to 6 months' gestation (Verhave et al., 2023).

Hydration

Hydration can be assessed by evaluating the **turgor** (elasticity) of the baby's skin. Turgor is the normal strength and tension of the skin, caused by outward pressure of the cells and the fluid that surrounds them. The baby's chest, abdomen, or thigh is a good area on which to test skin turgor. When gently grasped between a finger and thumb, the skin should spring back to its original shape when the tissue is released. It should not leave an indentation, fold, or wrinkled appearance. Loose skin that slowly returns to a position level with the tissue next to it is a sign of dehydration (Zakerihamidi et al., 2023). The baby's skin may be dry, flaky, or peeling, especially by the end of the first or second week after birth. This appearance is normal and not a sign of dehydration.

Color

There are wide natural variations in a newborn's skin tone. A significant increase in bilirubin level creates a yellowing in the skin color from jaundice, also called *hyperbilirubinemia* (see **Color Plate 15**). You can assess for jaundice in natural light by pressing the baby's skin with your index finger and noting the color when you lift your finger.

Visual observation of jaundice is an effective method of identifying infants who will need referral and laboratory measurement of bilirubin levels. Jaundice usually presents in the face first and then progresses from the infant's head to the trunk (chest) and extremities (Kamphuis et al., 2021). This is called *cephalocaudal* (head-to-toe) progression. Jaundice of the distal extremities (far from the center of the body), such as the palms and soles of the feet, or dark jaundice of the trunk or head is associated with higher bilirubin levels. These visual observations indicate the need for further investigation and possible treatment (Darmstadt et al., 2021). Visual assessment of jaundice is much less reliable in newborns with darker skin tones (Dionis et al., 2021). Progression of color occurs only when the bilirubin level is rising. When it begins to fall, the skin color fades gradually in all affected areas at the same time (Kamath-Rayne et al., 2021). If you observe jaundice in an infant, refer the parents to the baby's primary healthcare provider immediately so that the infant's bilirubin levels can be measured with a blood test. **Chapter 23** provides an in-depth discussion of jaundice and its implications.

Acrocyanosis describes a bluish tinge to the newborn's hands and feet (see **Color Plate 16**). It may be present after birth because of poor peripheral circulation (Stanford School of Medicine, 2018). The bluish color typically disappears after a few days. Parents often need reassurance that this condition is normal and does not indicate that their baby is cold.

Erythema Toxicum

Erythema toxicum is a pink to red **macular** area with a yellow or white center (**Color Plate 17**). It is the most common skin eruption in newborns, occurring in as many as 70% of infants. It is common on the newborn's trunk or limbs and is temporary. It may be present at birth but usually appears during the second or third day after birth and then disappears within about 1 week. Erythema toxicum has no apparent significance and requires no treatment (Narendran, 2020).

Infant Acne

Infant acne resembles adolescent acne. It appears on the face, primarily on the nose, forehead, and cheeks (**Color Plate 18**). The appearance changes depending on whether the baby is hot, cool, crying, or quiet. In most cases, infant acne starts at about 2 weeks of age and disappears at 8 to 10 weeks. It is believed to be the result of sebaceous gland stimulation by maternal or infant hormones (Samycia et al., 2016). If newborn acne does not resolve on its own, the baby's healthcare provider can explore for underlying causes.

Mottling

Mottling (cutis marmorata) is a white and reddish skin coloration on the baby's trunk and extremities (**Color Plate 19**). This condition is a vascular response to cold and usually clears when the skin is warmed. Some babies' skin may mottle easily for several weeks, months, or even into early childhood. No treatment is needed (Narendran, 2020).

Milia

Milia are very small "whiteheads" that are keratin deposits within the dermis (**Color Plate 20**). As many as half of all newborns exhibit milia. They usually occur on the forehead, cheeks, nose, and chin and may also occur on the trunk and in the diaper area (Narendran, 2020). Milia usually resolve without intervention by the end of the first month.

Diaper Rash

Diaper rash appears as a small, reddened, pimplelike rash in the diaper area. Frequent diaper changes, careful washing, air drying (leaving the diaper off for a while), and over-the-counter ointments or creams aid in healing. A diaper rash that does not clear up with appropriate treatment may indicate a **yeast infection**. Yeast infection rashes tend to be raised, larger red patches and appear more like welts than small red dots. Any diaper rash that does not clear quickly should be checked by a healthcare provider to rule out a bacterial or yeast infection (Fölster-Holst, 2018).

Cradle Cap

Cradle cap (seborrheic dermatitis) is a thick, scaly dandruff mostly found on the infant's scalp (**Color Plate 21**) and sometimes on the face, ears, neck, and even in the diaper area. It usually occurs within the first 6 weeks of life. Cradle cap is unattractive and can be distressing to parents. It may be caused by overactive sebaceous glands, although a yeast infection should also be ruled out (Chadha & Jahnke, 2019). Cradle cap is usually self-limiting and goes away as the baby matures. The healthcare provider may prescribe an antifungal shampoo if regular cleansing does not help. The baby should be evaluated for immunodeficiency in the event of unresolved scaling accompanied by diarrhea and low weight gain or faltering growth.

Head

The newborn's head is large, accounting for approximately one-fourth of their total body size. The skull bones are soft and pliable. The skull, or cranial, bones remain unfused at birth to accommodate the infant's descent through the birth canal during second-stage labor. After birth, the head may appear asymmetric because of the overlap of cranial bones, referred to as **molding**. Severe molding may cause temporary difficulty with latch. You can help parents with positioning the baby during nursing to avoid pressure on the baby's head. Laid-back (reclined) or side-lying positions may be most comfortable for the infant.

Caput Succedaneum

Caput succedaneum is a collection of fluid between the newborn's skin and cranial bone (**Figure 14-4**). It usually forms during labor on the presenting area of the head in the cervical opening. The longer the head is engaged during labor, the greater the swelling can

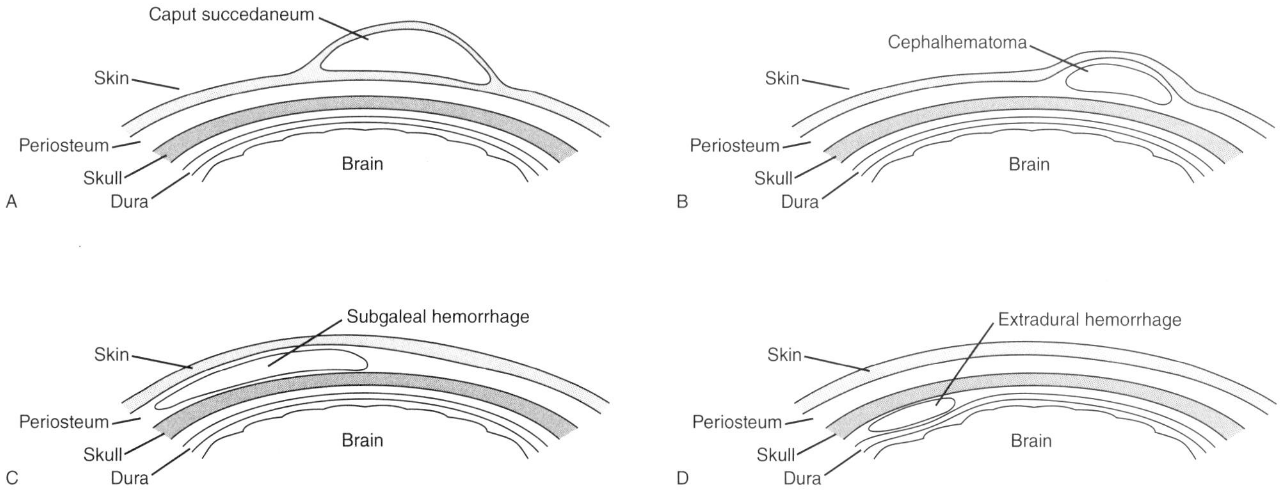

Figure 14-4 Common hematomas of the newborn scalp.

Printed with permission of Anna Swisher.

be. There may be red or bruised discoloration, and the baby may be sensitive to pressure on the affected area. Swelling begins to subside soon after birth. This condition occurs in 20% to 40% of vacuum extractions (Volpe, 2018). Severe caputs and cephalhematomas (discussed next) are associated with feeding difficulties (Genna, 2017).

Cephalhematoma

A **cephalhematoma** is a pool of blood between the bones of the head and the **periosteum**, the covering of the bone (**Color Plate 22**). The resultant swelling may begin to form during labor and slowly become larger in the first few days after birth. It may take up to 6 weeks to resolve completely. A cephalhematoma is usually a result of trauma, often from an extended second stage of labor, forceps, or vacuum extraction. Because the area may be sensitive to touch, a nursing position that avoids contact with the baby's head will work best. Be aware that bruising increases the risk of feeding difficulties and jaundice as the blood is reabsorbed into the infant's blood vessels.

Fontanel

The **fontanel** is a space between the bones of an infant's skull that is covered by tough membranes. The posterior fontanel closes at about 2 months. The anterior fontanel remains soft until the baby reaches about 18 months. Increased brain pressure may cause a fontanel to become tense or to bulge. The fontanel of a dehydrated infant may be soft and sunken, especially when the infant is held in the **supine** position.

Facial Asymmetry

Facial **asymmetry** may occur in utero when the infant's face is wedged against their body or the uterus, or from injury to the nerves because of birth trauma. The asymmetry usually resolves over several days following birth, depending on the severity. You may encounter infants with facial asymmetry when crying (known as *asymmetric crying facies*). These babies' faces appear symmetrical at rest, but the lower lip droops on one side when crying. Crying facies may be due to birth injury; muscle deformity; or neurological issues, including syndromes (Arya et al., 2017). Asymmetry may also be a marker for genetic disorders.

Some babies with facial asymmetry respond well to chiropractic care (International Chiropractic Pediatric Association, 2018) or to physical or occupational therapy (Michalska et al., 2019). If the baby's tongue is not centered in the mouth as a result of asymmetry, the nipple can be positioned over the center of the tongue rather than the center of the mouth. These babies may respond well to feeding in the clutch or football hold position.

Eyes

The majority of babies' eyes are grayish blue at birth. Final eye color typically develops at 6 to 12 months of age. Some babies will have broken capillaries in the sclera resulting from the birth. These usually resolve within the first 10 days postpartum. Jaundice can cause a yellow staining in the sclera (the white portion) of the eye. There is no clear consensus as to the bilirubin level at which scleral jaundice first appears. It is typically evident by the time the bilirubin levels reach 3 mg/dL (Abel & Hrishikesh, 2023). Some infants may have swollen eyelids, which typically recede by a few days after birth.

Neck

The neck surrounds the infant's esophagus and trachea. The **epiglottis**, the cartilage that overhangs the trachea, closes during swallowing to prevent food from entering the trachea (**Figure 14-5**). An infant's neck is short. Because a newborn's neck is too weak to consistently provide head support, the head must always be supported. Supporting the baby's neck and shoulders at feedings helps prevent pushing on their head, which can be counterproductive. The parent can run their arm along the infant's back, neck, and head as they bring the infant in for nursing. This avoids pressure on the head while still supporting the head's weight during a feeding.

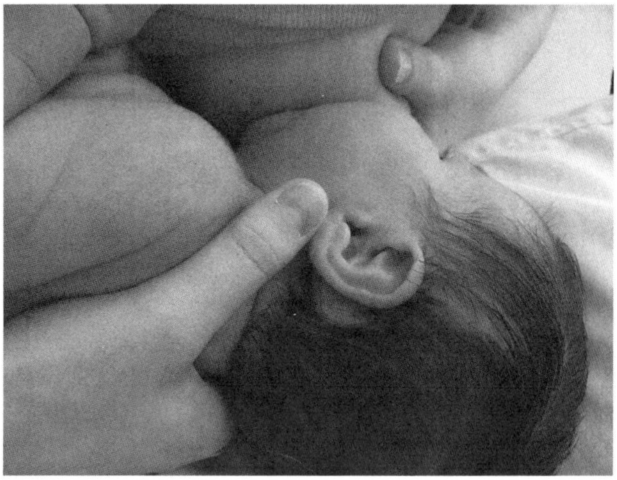

Figure 14-5 Swallowing anatomy.

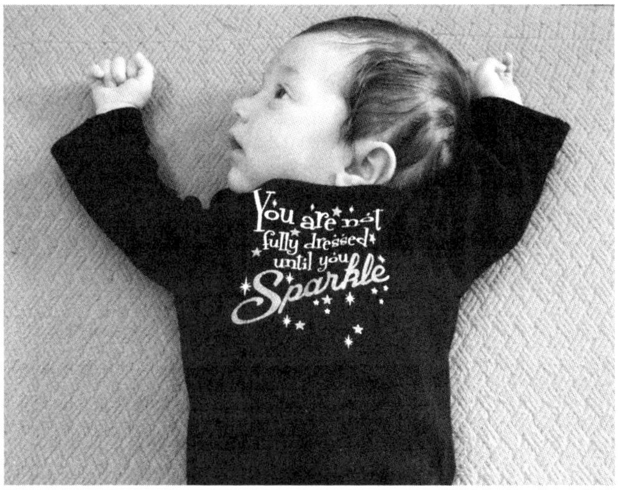

Figure 14-6 Baby with torticollis.

Printed with permission of Anna Swisher.

Torticollis. A baby whose head is continually turned to the side, usually to the right, may have torticollis—literally, "twisted neck" (**Figure 14-6**). Torticollis in infants is caused by a shortening of the muscle that extends from the base of the ear down to the clavicle. The cause may be the baby's position or lack of space in the womb, birth trauma, or low amniotic fluid. Rarely, torticollis can be a marker for serious problems, so it warrants assessment by the primary care practitioner. Congenital torticollis can be associated with neurodevelopmental conditions (Kim et al., 2022).

A baby with torticollis may be comfortable nursing only when their head is turned to the side. Feeding in a side-sitting position (also called *football* or *clutch hold*) can provide control over the infant's neck position. Some infants with torticollis may feed well in the cradle hold for one side and not the other. In such a case, they can shift to the other side without changing the angle of the neck. Nursing lying down provides postural support. Other nursing positions can be added as range of motion improves through physical therapy or chiropractic care.

Jaw

The jaw (mandible) provides stability for movements of the tongue, lips, and cheeks. It is the part of the head that moves for feeding. All babies are born with degrees of receding jaws. As the baby grows, the jaw usually comes forward. Achieving a deep latch can be challenging when the jaw is severely recessed or very small (**micrognathia**). A severely receding or small jaw is a marker for a variety of genetic conditions, including Pierre Robin sequence (Zhen et al., 2021). Consult **Chapter 27** for further discussion of infant conditions.

The impact of bottle feeding on oral-facial development and later dental development is unclear. Some studies indicate that bottle feeding interferes negatively with oral-facial development (Sánchez-Molins et al., 2010) and later dental development (Boronat-Catalá et al., 2017; Wilkins, 2020). Other research questions these findings, stating that the impact of bottle feeding on dental occlusions cannot be substantiated (Parker & Chia, 2020).

Oral Structure

Visual inspection of the mouth is an important element of an infant assessment. Check for gum lines that are smooth and a **palate** that is intact and gently arched. The tongue should be able to extend over the lower **alveolar ridge** (gum line) and up to the middle of the baby's mouth when it is open wide. There should be sufficient fat inside the cheeks (buccal pads) to facilitate sucking and milk transfer.

Lips

When assessing a baby's lips, inspect them for friction blisters, which are typically seen on the midline of the top lip. Known as *sucking blisters*, they can be signs that the baby is not generating enough negative pressure to maintain latch. The baby compensates by using the lip muscles (orbicularis oris) to compress the breast. If you observe sucking blisters in a newborn, ask if the baby was born with the blister or whether it developed after birth. Babies can be born with lip blisters from sucking on their hands in utero. If it occurred after birth, check the baby's latch to determine if assistance is needed.

Lip tone is an important consideration in nursing. A baby's lips close around the breast and form a seal to create negative pressure. Tight, pursed lips are a marker for impaired intraoral pressure in the baby. They may also be an indication of a labial (upper) lip tie, although the impact of the lip tie on nursing remains controversial (Carnino et al., 2023). Soft, flaccid lips with a poor seal and little resistance can be a sign of low muscle tone. This deviation occurs in babies with neurological conditions (Yozawitz et al., 2018) or genetic conditions such as Down syndrome (Gur et al., 2023). It may also occur in babies affected by drugs and medications in utero (Desaunay et al., 2022) or birth trauma, such as facial nerve injury (Sardesai, 2019). Be aware that the **philtrum**—the midline space between the upper lip and the nose—has a slight dip. A flat philtrum can be a marker for neurological issues, especially fetal alcohol syndrome.

A **cleft lip** is the most noticeable defect involving the lips. A cleft (opening or split) may be unilateral (one side) or bilateral (both sides). A cleft lip may be combined with a cleft in the hard or soft palate, or there may be normal palatal development. A baby may also have a **cleft palate** with no lip defect—often called a *hidden cleft*, which can interfere with nursing. **Chapter 27** discusses clefts in more depth.

Tongue

While nursing, the baby's tongue draws the breast into the mouth to form a groove or trough. Sucking draws a bolus of milk through the trough toward the back of the mouth, where it is swallowed. Evaluate the size and shape of the baby's tongue for any anomalies that could affect troughing or movement, especially when there is pain when nursing.

Assess whether the tongue is short or humped, unusually thick or thin, or long or abnormally large. **Macroglossia** (large tongue) is a marker for genetic disorders, including Down syndrome and Beckwith–Wiedemann syndrome. It is also associated with the low muscle tone found in children with neurological damage (Núñez-Martínez et al., 2016).

Alveolar Ridge (Gumline)

The baby's alveolar ridge should be smooth and uniform. Occasionally, a baby has a bumpy gumline, from which it appears teeth are about to erupt. These bumps may be white or yellowish gingival cysts (**Epstein pearls**), a benign condition. Epstein pearls may also occur on the palate. These cysts resolve a few weeks or months after birth, and no treatment is required (Diaz de Ortiz & Mendez, 2020).

Approximately 1 in 2000 babies are born with an erupted **natal tooth**. Another 1 in 3500 infants will have a **neonatal tooth** erupt within the first month of life (Kalra et al., 2019). Most natal and neonatal teeth are primary teeth. They are occasionally extra, or supernumerary, teeth. Natal and neonatal teeth can cause feeding difficulties, traumatic injuries, and even aspiration risk as a result of excessive tooth mobility (Kérourédan et al., 2018). Because of the risk of aspiration, it is important that a dental care provider evaluate a baby with a natal or neonatal tooth. Occasionally, treatment may include extraction of the tooth (Holden et al., 2022). Positional changes or use of a nipple shield may be helpful when nursing. If nursing is too painful, the parent can pump to protect milk production while the baby is evaluated and treatment is planned.

Lingual Frenulum

The **lingual frenulum** is the string of skin, a midline fold in a layer of fascia, under the tongue. It tethers the tongue to the floor of the mouth and controls the tongue's motion (Mills et al., 2019). Frenula can vary in position, thickness, and length. A tongue that cannot extend over the alveolar ridge may be due to **ankyloglossia**—a tight frenulum, also referred to as *tongue-tie* (**Color Plate 23**).

Ankyloglossia, a midline defect, may restrict movement of the tongue. Anterior restriction (tethering to the tip of the tongue) may cause a classic heart-shaped appearance when crying. Mid-tongue and posterior restriction may be subtler. Posterior restriction may affect tongue mobility and range of motion (Ghaheri et al., 2017). It is also possible to have a sublingual tongue-tie, referred to as *hidden*. The Bristol Tongue Attachment Tool (BTAT) can assist with identifying this condition (Ingram et al., 2019).

Ankyloglossia occurs in about 4% to 11% of infants and seems to be more common in males (O'Shea et al., 2017). There may be a familial link (Lenormand et al., 2018), so ask if there is any family history of tongue-tie. Genetic factors are also associated with tethered oral tissues, including the methylenetetrahydrofolate reductase *(MTHFR)* gene variation (U.S. Department of Health and Human Services [USDHHS], 2017).

Feeding difficulties are associated with this condition, including ongoing nipple pain (Cordray et al., 2023). A tight frenulum can make it difficult for the baby to stay latched and may result in poor milk transfer and low weight gain (Campanha et al., 2019; Cordray et al., 2023). Be alert to the possibility of a tight frenulum as the cause of chronic nipple pain, cracked and bleeding nipples with a "positional stripe" bruising or scabbing, slow weight gain, long feedings, low milk production, or issues along the mastitis spectrum.

Ankyloglossia occurs in stages and varies in severity, including its effects on both the form and function of the child's mouth. Types 1 and 2 can be resolved by clipping or by laser cautery. Clipping the frenulum (**frenotomy** or frenectomy) releases the lingual frenulum and usually improves tongue movement. A frenotomy is the incisional release of the frenulum. A frenectomy, or frenulotomy, is the removal of the frenulum tissue. Clipping is an in-office procedure in which a small cut is made at the anterior portion of the frenulum (**Figure 14-7**). This enables the baby's tongue to extend adequately to produce a good latch and milk transfer. Laser techniques have increased in popularity for tongue-tie release (Komori et al., 2017).

More severe cases (types 3 and 4) may require **frenuloplasty** (also called *frenoplasty*), a more invasive procedure that involves deeper cutting and stitches (Shekher et al., 2021).

A seminal study by Ballard et al. (2002) brought attention to the effect of ankyloglossia on nursing. Infant latch has been shown to improve significantly after treatment for posterior ankyloglossia, with positive nursing outcomes (Ghaheri et al., 2017). However, there is significant professional disagreement as to whether tethered oral tissues warrant release (Carnino et al., 2023; Nakhash et al., 2019). Like many areas in lactation, best practice depends on careful assessment of each nursing dyad. Although subjective, improvements in nursing are reported in most infants who have frenotomies, with high parental satisfaction and few reported complications (Cordray et al., 2023; Muldoon et al., 2017).

A list of healthcare providers in your community who are knowledgeable about evaluating and treating tethered oral tissues is a useful resource for parents. Some practitioners recommend bodywork for infants before and/or after the procedure. Bodywork includes craniosacral therapy, chiropractic care, massage, and/or occupational therapy (Ankyloglossia Bodyworkers, 2019). Further research is needed before a consensus can be reached (Batista Borges Pereira, 2022).

Encourage parents to share the results of their child's evaluation and treatment with their primary care provider. Such sharing helps raise awareness and support in the medical community for treating ankyloglossia and other oral anomalies. Resources for healthcare providers include a position statement and protocol on neonatal ankyloglossia in nursing dyads developed by the ABM (LeFort et al., 2021).

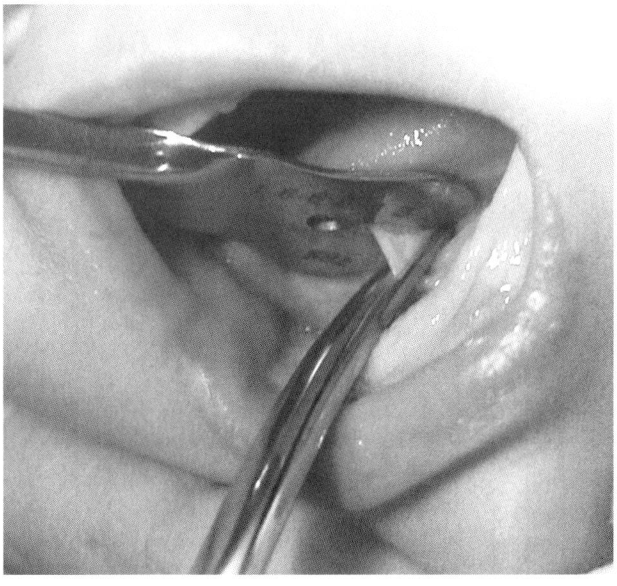

Figure 14-7 Frenotomy procedure.

Printed with permission of Catherine Watson Genna, BS, IBCLC.

Labial (Maxillary) Frenum

The **labial frenum**, also called the *maxillary*, *upper*, or *superior frenum*, is the fold of skin that anchors the upper lip to the top gum (see **Color Plate 24**). A large, thick labial frenum may eventually form a gap between the two top front teeth, although it does not usually interfere with latch. If the frenum is especially short or tight, it may be difficult for the baby to flange the upper lip. Restricted labial movement can result in lip curling, reduced mobility, or a poor seal for feeding. It can also cause nipple compression, discomfort while nursing, and compromised milk transfer.

Clipping and treatment of a tight labial frenum are usually done for aesthetic reasons. If there are no apparent dental or nursing difficulties, treatment is not always necessary (Benoiton et al., 2016). Clinicians report good results from clipping when the constriction interferes with latch (Ghaheri et al., 2017). Laser treatment is increasingly the method of choice for labial frenum release because it prevents bleeding and offers faster healing (Dioguardi et al., 2023).

Buccal Pads

Buccal pads inside the cheeks (also called *fat pads* or *sucking pads*) add to the thickness of the cheek wall (see **Figure 14-8**). They help decrease the space within the infant's mouth, thereby increasing negative pressure and facilitating milk transfer. Buccal pads may not be present in an infant who is malnourished or born preterm. When working with a thin or preterm baby with feeding difficulties, you can place

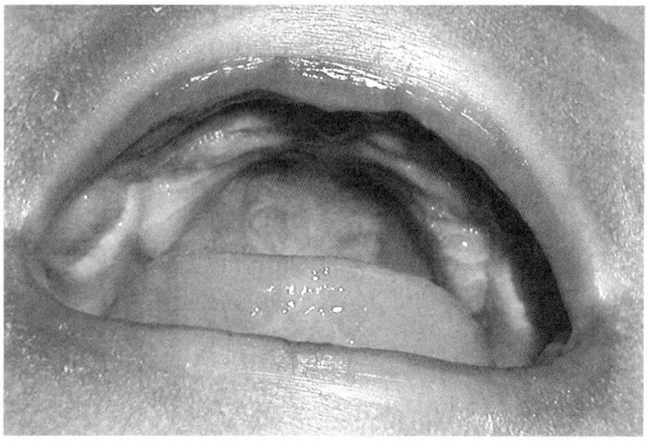

Figure 14-8 Buccal pads.

Printed with permission of Catherine Watson Genna, BS, IBCLC.

your gloved finger inside the mouth and your thumb on the outside of the cheek to feel the thickness of the fat pads. When the pads are extremely thin, your fingers will almost touch.

Buccal frenula are folds of mucous membranes connecting the buccal mucosa to the alveolar mucosa. Some practitioners believe that buccal frenula affect nursing. There has been limited research on buccal ties and their association with nursing difficulties (Baxter et al., 2018). The Academy of Breastfeeding Medicine asserts there is no evidence for surgically treating buccal frenula (LeFort et al., 2021).

To facilitate nursing for infants who lack well-developed buccal pads, positioning the infant while holding a finger against the baby's cheeks will compensate for the lack of fat. This is referred to as the **Dancer hand position**, as shown in Figure 15-6 in Chapter 15. As the baby grows, the cheek muscles become stronger and provide more stability and the size of the fat pads diminishes.

Palates

The roof of the mouth contains a hard palate and soft palate. The hard palate is in the front of the mouth. The soft palate lies behind hard palate, in line with the end of the upper alveolar ridge. The condition and shape of the palates can become a factor in establishing nursing. Note whether the hard palate has a smooth slope or is highly vaulted, grooved, or bubble-shaped. Some high palates may result from the tongue being unable to reach the roof of the mouth to spread the palate during uterine development. If the palate is high, explore under the tongue for a tight frenulum. Sometimes, a palate is grooved, high, or channeled because of extended intubation with preterm or ill babies. However, high palates typically occur naturally.

A high, arched, or bubble palate can sometimes cause the nipple to "catch" in the groove and therefore not elongate for nursing. This type of palate makes it more difficult for the tongue to compress the breast tissue adequately to feed effectively. It can result in nipple pain, long feedings, and an unsatisfied infant who nurses frequently.

When the tissue in the roof of the mouth does not close fully in the womb, the baby is born with a cleft palate. In most cases, a cleft is also present in the lip. When an infant has a cleft lip, the condition is immediately obvious to everyone. A cleft palate may not be as obvious. A cleft can involve the hard palate and/or the soft palate. Occasionally, a cleft of the soft palate escapes initial diagnosis. A cleft of the soft palate may cause the baby to choke and gag while nursing. Milk can escape from the baby's nose when letdown occurs, and stridor or wheezing may be heard. Changing positioning is often helpful in identifying this kind of cleft palate.

Some infants may have **submucosal clefts**, in which skin covers a cleft of the hard or soft palate. In this condition, a notched V shape may be observed on the hard palate. These babies often have a **bifurcated** uvula (**bifid** uvula, or split in two parts) (**Figure 14-9**). Submucosal clefts and bifid uvulas are markers for a variety of genetic disorders, with differing rates of severity (FACES: The National Craniofacial Association, 2016; Hanny et al., 2016). Babies with submucosal clefts may not feed effectively, resulting in low weight gain. Be alert for nasal regurgitation, which may indicate a submucosal cleft or a weak soft palate seal (Eshete et al., 2016). Submucosal clefts frequently escape diagnosis until speech impediments occur and are generally diagnosed later than cleft palates (Smit et al., 2021). Other markers are eustachian tube dysfunction, hearing loss, and swallowing difficulties (Fairmont et al., 2024). Chapter 27 provides more information on nursing an infant who has a cleft of the lip, palate, or both.

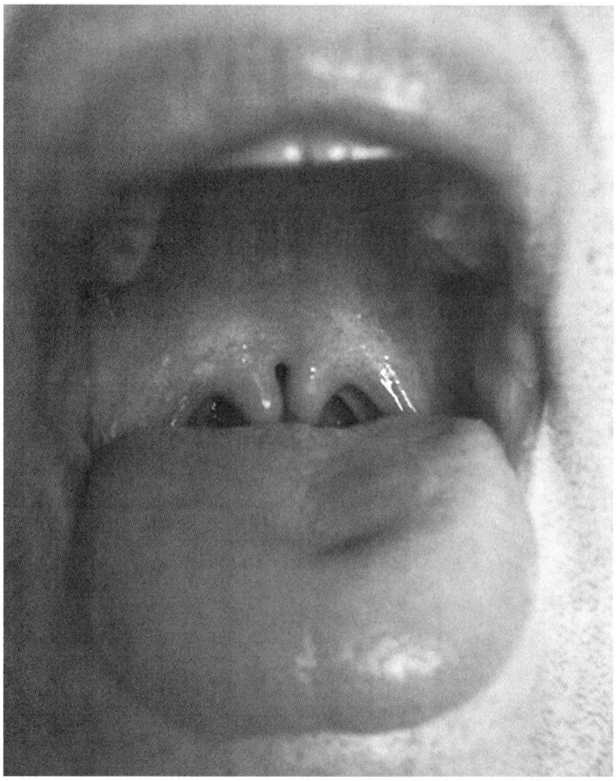

Figure 14-9 Bifurcated uvula.

Thrush

Thrush is a yeast infection often characterized by white patches that cannot be removed without causing bleeding (**Color Plate 25**). This kind of infection may occur between the baby's gums and lips, on the inside of the cheeks, and on the tongue. It is thick and patchy as opposed to the thin, uniform white coating usually found on an infant's tongue. Thrush, which is most frequently caused by the organism *Candida albicans*, is also known as **candidiasis** (Taylor et al., 2023). The infection may appear on the nipples as well as in the baby's mouth, making it imperative that both the parent and baby are treated at the same time. Refer to **Chapter 17** for more information on yeast as a cause of nipple pain.

Clavicle

An injured clavicle (collarbone) is a common birth trauma that is typically identified during the baby's initial examination. In some cases, it may escape detection until later. In response to the injury, the baby may restrict the use of the affected arm and resist nursing in a position that places pressure on the fractured area. For example, a baby with a fractured left clavicle may be uncomfortable feeding on the right side in the cradle hold. Imaging will confirm the fracture. Treatment typically consists of immobilizing the arm by pinning it in a shirt or blanket. Clavicle fractures usually heal quickly within 2 months and without special care. After healing, there may be a callus on the clavicle, which will disappear as the baby grows.

Chest

Observe the infant breathing while bare-chested. Labored breathing—evidenced by marked retractions or observable indentations in the chest—may be a symptom of respiratory or cardiac problems. If you work with a baby who exhibits this type of breathing, the baby needs to be promptly assessed by a healthcare provider.

Nipple appearance on the baby's chest is a sign of maturation. The more preterm the baby is, the flatter the nipple bud will be. Supernumerary nipples (accessory nipples along the milk line) may be present either bilaterally or unilaterally and can be mistaken for moles. The infant breast may be swollen and even leak "witch's milk," a fluid caused by transplacental transfer of maternal hormones, as discussed in **Chapter 7** (Shah et al., 2021). This term, found in multiple languages, stems from ancient beliefs in witches (Forbes, 1950). The fluid usually disappears within the first 3 weeks after birth and occurs in both males and females.

Reflexes

Newborn reflexes are present until the central nervous system has matured. They serve as a form of communication that tells us much about what babies need and how they are developing (Scannell & Puka-Beals, 2019). It is important to carefully assess the infant's reflexes because the presence or absence of a reflex can be an indication of neurological impairment.

The Moro (or startle) reflex results when the infant is exposed to a loud noise, causing the infant's legs to draw up and arms to fling out. The grasp reflex is initiated by touching the palm of the baby's hand. Arching resembles the positioning of a hypertonic infant (Figure 14-3). If pressure exerted on the back of the head pushes the baby's face into the breast during a feeding, the baby may arch backward. Pressure on the soles of the baby's feet will elicit spontaneous crawling efforts and extension of the baby's head, referred to as **Bauer crawling reflex**. When positioning for a feeding, be careful not to press the baby's feet against the back or side of the couch or chair, pressure that could cause the baby to arch away.

Rooting

A full-term healthy newborn has many reflexes that aid nursing (**Table 14-2**). The **rooting reflex** is at the forefront of these reflexes. Lightly stroking the baby's cheek will cause their head to turn in the direction of the stimulus. The mouth will open, and the tongue will come forward, as illustrated in **Figure 14-10**. Gently touching the baby's upper lip causes their mouth to open. Brushing the nipple against the baby's cheek will initiate the rooting reflex and stimulate the baby to turn toward and search for the nipple. Gently brushing the baby's nose or philtrum can encourage a deeper, asymmetrical latch with the baby's head tilting back slightly.

Sucking

An object placed sufficiently far into the baby's mouth, near the juncture between the hard and soft palate, will elicit sucking. Babies demonstrate two types of **sucking**. A high-flow nutritive suck—characterized by a long, deep suck–swallow–breathe pattern—elicits about one suck per second. A low-flow nonnutritive suck elicits about two sucks per second.

Table 14-2 Gestational Development of Newborn Reflexes

Baby's Age	Nutritive Sucking
9 weeks	Mouth and lower face movement
12 weeks	Swallow
18–24 weeks	Nonnutritive suck
32–34 weeks	Nutritive suck and swallow
Baby's Age	**Associated Reflexes and Responses**
26–27 weeks	Gag accompanied by tongue protrusion, head and jaw extension, contraction of the pharynx
28 weeks	Phasic bite in response to gum stimulation, with rhythmic opening and closing of the jaw
28 weeks	Transverse tongue response when the surface is touched, with movement of the tongue toward the stimulation
32 weeks	Rooting (searching) progressively toward a stimulation
40 weeks	Tongue protrusion when the anterior tongue is touched (inhibited as the infant grows)

Printed with permission of the International Lactation Consultant Association.

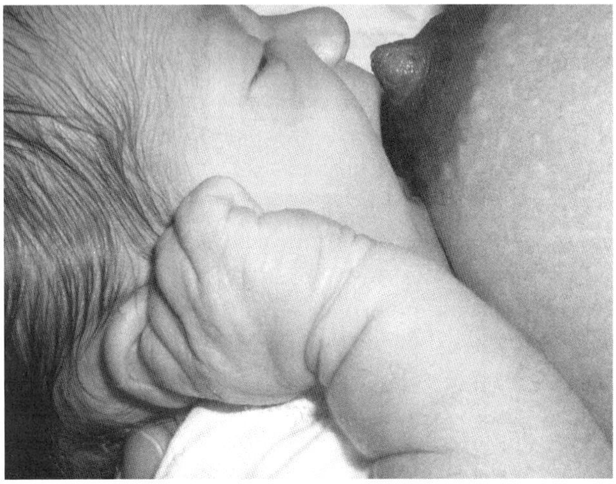

Figure 14-10 Rooting for the nipple is a feeding readiness signal from the baby.

Printed with permission of Catherine Watson Genna.

It is characterized by a light suck, almost a flutter, with short jaw excursions and little or no audible swallowing (Batista et al., 2019). **Chapter 16** provides a detailed discussion of sucking.

Digestion

Babies exhibit their own unique growth and activity patterns. The manner in which they digest food and expel waste are equally individualized. Encourage parents to become familiar with their baby's digestive patterns and needs. The baby's disposition, eating and sleeping patterns, and body temperature influence their digestion. A change in pattern can alert parents to a problem or illness before it becomes serious. Encourage them to consider the baby's overall pattern before contacting the caregiver. This will help them determine whether the current issue represents one small change in their baby's habits or a more significant change. The parents should also observe skin color; changes in breathing; and other signs of illness, such as glassy eyes or abdominal cramping. Four functions that occur during digestion—burping, spitting or vomiting, **voiding**, and stooling—are discussed in the following sections.

Burping

Babies may become uncomfortable from taking in air during feeding or when crying. Burping will release the air from the baby's stomach. Nursing babies usually do not take in as much air as bottle-fed babies. However, babies who suck vigorously may gulp air when they nurse. When parents respond to hunger cues before the baby becomes ravenous, crying and swallowing air will be prevented or minimized.

Positioning the baby at a 45-degree angle after feeding (with a baby sling, infant seat, or swing) will help bring up air before laying them down to sleep. Gently rocking, patting, or rubbing the baby's back will help air bubbles coalesce and rise to the top of the baby's stomach to be expelled. The parent can hold the baby against their shoulder and massage or pat the middle of the baby's back with firm pressure from the bottom up. Another technique is to lay the baby on their stomach across the parent's lap, turn their head to one side so that the nose is free, and gently rub their back from the bottom up. If a baby consistently spits up after nursing, more time for burping may be needed. A baby who has been crying will need to be burped before attempting a feeding. A vigorous feeder will need to nurse before becoming upset to reduce the amount of air intake.

Spitting Up

The passage between a baby's stomach and mouth is extremely short. The muscle valve at the upper end of the stomach (the cardiac sphincter, or lower esophageal sphincter) is not as efficient as it will be later in life. Thus, spitting up is quite common in the early months. Although spitting up is messy and inconvenient, unless there are concerns with growth or development, there usually is no reason for worry. The parent can try burping the baby more often, both before and during a feeding. More frequent feeding may also help to reduce spitting up.

Frequent spitting up could be a sign of overfeeding or overactive milk production. Limiting the baby to one side per feeding may help reduce overproduction. Spitting up can occur if the baby is upset and gulps air with the milk when feeding intervals are too far apart. Responding to hunger cues will help avoid this. Mucus in the baby's stomach can also cause spitting up, especially directly after birth and when the baby has an upper respiratory infection. Cow's milk protein intolerance and nicotine can cause spitting up. Thus, lifestyle and diet adjustments may be advisable, including avoiding smoking or reducing the number of cigarettes smoked. The force with which the baby expels milk will determine whether they are spitting up or have a problem with vomiting.

Projectile Vomiting

A violent expulsion of milk is considered **projectile vomiting** and requires a healthcare provider's attention. Even nursing babies can experience **gastroenteritis** (inflammation of the stomach and intestines) or stomach flu that could cause vomiting. Babies become dehydrated much faster than older children or adults. Thus, if a baby vomits more than twice in a 4-hour period, parents need to contact their healthcare provider immediately.

A baby several weeks old who suddenly begins vomiting or in whom vomiting becomes progressively worse may have **pyloric stenosis**. With pyloric stenosis, the outflow valve of the baby's stomach does not open satisfactorily to permit the contents of the stomach to pass. The condition, which can lead to dehydration and weight loss, is treated with surgery. Babies with pyloric stenosis may seem to be hungry all the time. Your role in supporting the family is to help protect milk production until the baby can nurse again.

Pyloric stenosis occurs more frequently in firstborns, Caucasians, males, preterm infants, and multiples (Kapoor et al., 2019). Formula-fed and nonexclusively human milk–fed (mixed feeding) infants have higher rates of pyloric stenosis (Li et al., 2018). Infant exposure to macrolides (a class of antibiotics that includes erythromycin, azithromycin, clarithromycin, and roxithromycin) prenatally and possibly postnatally through human milk has been associated with pyloric stenosis (El-Gohary et al., 2018). A more recent review and meta-analysis found a significant correlation only with direct postnatal exposure to macrolides (Almaramhy & Al-Zalabani, 2019).

It is important to take a complete history of both the parent and the baby, including the use of any medications. Projectile vomiting is associated with the use of the steroid prostaglandin for cyanotic congenital heart disease (Tandırcıoğlu et al., 2023). A sudden onset of vomiting can indicate an obstruction of the intestines or a strangulated hernia. Both conditions require immediate medical evaluation and may result in surgery (Tatekawa, 2018). **Chapter 25** provides more information on a baby who is ill or hospitalized.

Gastroesophageal Reflux

Some infants spit up only occasionally, whereas others seem to spit up all the time. Spitting up multiple times in 1 day can be a sign of **gastroesophageal reflux (GER)**. GER is a backflow of the contents of the stomach into the esophagus. It often occurs when the lower esophageal sphincter fails to close or is soft so that it does not stay securely closed. Acidic gastric juices may produce burning pain in the esophagus. Reflux is a common physiological occurrence in infancy and is also known colloquially as *posseting*. It is age related, with reduced frequency as the baby grows. GER resolves in most infants by 12 months of age (Leung & Hon, 2019).

GER is distinct from **gastroesophageal reflux disease (GERD)**, which is a medical diagnosis. GERD is defined as GER that is associated with persistent symptoms or complications. Symptoms include pain, wheezing, apnea, stridor, recurring bronchiolitis, oxygen desaturation, aspiration pneumonia, swallowing dysfunction, frequent vomiting, choking and gagging, lower energy intake, excessive weight loss, disorganized and dysfunctional sucking or swallowing, delayed readiness for solid foods, food refusal, and delayed development (Friedman et al., 2021). Always be diligent in referring parents to their baby's healthcare provider immediately if symptoms do not improve with coping strategies.

Identifying Gastroesophageal Reflux. Infants with reflux may spit up several times after feeding. Some may spit up even during feeding. Silent reflux may also occur, a condition in which the stomach contents fail to come all the way back up. In such a case, the infant does not spit up but may experience burning and discomfort. Infants who nurse experience a more rapid resolution of GER compared with those who do not (Mairuhu et al., 2021). Food allergies can contribute to GERD, excessive crying (discussed later in this chapter), or **constipation** in infancy. Infants with these conditions often respond to the parent's dairy elimination diet or a non–bovine-based formula if they are supplemented (Rajani et al., 2020).

Weaning to formula, as is often suggested by care providers, is counterproductive. GER is associated with, and sometimes induced by, **cow's milk allergy** or protein sensitivity (Salvatore et al., 2021). The protein that the baby is reacting to may come either from the parent's diet or from formula. The use of antireflux medications is associated with the development of food allergies, leading researchers to urge caution in prescribing these medications for infants (Noh at al., 2023).

Effects on the Infant. Constant regurgitation of milk into the esophagus can cause severe irritation or pain for the infant. Some infants with GER learn to limit their intake after associating a full stomach with the pain that accompanies reflux. Regurgitating human milk is not as irritating as regurgitating formula. Infants digest human milk more quickly than infant formula and absorb more milk in the same amount of time. It is not appropriate to switch a human milk–fed infant to formula as a treatment for GER. Formula-fed and mixed-feeding infants have higher rates of GER (Mairuhu et al., 2021).

Frequent spitting up and limited intake can lead to poor weight gain. If an infant with reflux has been self-limiting intake because of discomfort, milk production may decrease because the baby removes only small amounts of milk at each feeding. Therefore, an infant with no or slow weight gain coupled with limited milk production may experience an exacerbation of symptoms when milk intake increases. Some infants with reflux may display signs of discomfort that resemble hunger signs and so may be overfed, with excessive weight gain of 2 or more ounces per day. It is important to pay attention to signs of reflux in any infant whose weight gain is outside the normal range in either direction.

Coping Strategies for GER. Infants who experience GER need to be fed in an upright position with the head above the belly so that gravity can help the milk stay down. Holding the baby upright after feeding will also help keep the milk down. These babies benefit from smaller, more frequent feedings to limit the amount of milk the infant takes in at a feeding. Similarly, the baby could nurse from only one side at a feeding, provided there is adequate milk production. Limiting the amount of milk at a feeding also ensures that the infant consumes the fatty hindmilk and is able to digest and retain more calories.

Some parents find it helpful to put the infant to sleep on an incline and using a pacifier after feedings. Like many interventions, these approaches have mixed results (Bellaïche et al., 2017; Chabra & Peeples, 2020). Positions that avoid pressure on the abdomen but keep the trunk supported and extended are preferred when the child has GER. The use of a car seat for positioning should be avoided because that can place a lot of pressure on the infant's abdomen, contributing to more discomfort and reflux. Therefore, car-seat use should be limited to travel. Burping positions can be limited to ones that avoid pressure on the baby's stomach. Some parents find relief from infant massage and chiropractic care.

Some healthcare providers may recommend adding cereal to the parent's milk to produce a thicker fluid that will stay down better. A commercial thickener made with rice, cornstarch, carob bean gum, soybeans, or xanthan gum produces the same result. It is difficult to thicken human milk with rice cereal because the enzymes in human milk begin digesting starches almost immediately. Elevated levels of arsenic in rice cereal are also a concern (Rosen et al., 2018). Attempting to compensate for the slowness of feeding with thickened milk by using bottle nipples with larger holes defeats the purpose of thickening. Furthermore, the fact that the milk is not spit up does not mean that the reflux and pain have been treated effectively. Feeding expressed milk with thickening may lead to early weaning. The use of thickeners has been associated with necrotizing enterocolitis (Abdulezer et al., 2022). For infants who are formula fed, commercially thickened formulas are increasingly preferred by nutritionists versus adding thickeners to standard formulas (Salvatore et al., 2021).

The stress of having an infant with reflux can cause parents to feel that their baby cries and fusses all the time. In some cases, the baby may be upset only at feeding time, which can feel like personal rejection. Parents need validation that reflux is stressful and that caring for their child is draining. Acknowledge the parents' grief that their baby is not the pleasant, cooing, cuddly baby they had envisioned. Reassuring them that it is not a reflection of their parenting can help them enjoy the moments when their baby is content. Support from other parents, friends, and relatives helps alleviate the sense of isolation parents may feel. Symptoms related to reflux usually decrease in the second half of the first year of life and subside by the child's first birthday.

Medications. Medications for severe reflux may be prescribed to decrease acid in the infant's stomach or increase milk flow from the stomach into the intestines. A systematic review of randomized controlled trials did not find that these medications significantly decreased infant crying and irritability (Gieruszczak-Białek et al., 2015). The efficacy of these medications continues to be questioned (Wicaksono et al., 2023). Most healthcare providers will usually try medications before resorting to more invasive tests such as barium swallow studies, endoscopy, pH probe, or other imaging exams. These tests are indicated when the baby has poor weight gain or does not respond to medications.

Overprescribing of antireflux medications is a concern, and many babies prescribed these drugs do not meet the diagnostic criteria for GERD (Rosen et al., 2018). Long-term toxicity risks of reflux medications (specifically, proton pump inhibitors) include gastrointestinal and respiratory tract infection, vitamin B_{12} deficiency, hypomagnesemia, bone fractures, and rebound hyperacidity (De Bruyne & Ito, 2018). Researchers caution against the overuse of medications without confirmed esophageal reflux (Lopez & Lemberg, 2019; Vandenplas & Kindt, 2022).

Elimination

Elimination patterns are significant indicators of an infant's intake. There is wide variability in stooling and voiding among infants in the early days after birth, especially when there are differences in feeding patterns. Keeping a diary of feedings, voids, and stools for the first week or two postpartum helps parents assess patterns in their new baby's behavior. When concerns arise about intake, a diary provides a helpful record for medical care providers. It also builds parents' confidence that exclusive nursing provides sufficient nourishment for their baby.

Voiding

Healthy newborns have small, frequent voids that range from pale yellow to clear. Full-term babies typically void when they are awake. In the first week of life, the baby should have an increasing number of voids daily. Many hospitals correlate the number of voids and stools with the number of days old the baby is, up to day 4 or 5. By 4 or 5 days of age, the baby should be voiding at least six times in 24 hours.

Pink (copper or "brick-dust") stains that appear with urination are urate crystals, whose presence indicates excess uric acid (**Color Plate 26**). Urate crystals generally are not significant in the first 1 to 3 days of life. Assessment of the baby's hydration status is necessary if the stains appear after this.

Stooling

The color, consistency, and volume of a nursing baby's stools differ greatly from those of a formula-fed baby. A nursing newborn's first stools are a black, tarry meconium, usually passed within the first 24 to 36 hours (**Color Plate 27**). Transitional stools are greenish black to greenish brown as the meconium gives way to brown and then to a golden or mustard yellow color when the baby is approximately 48 to 72 hours old (**Color Plate 28**). Texture can range from watery to seedy yellow to a toothpaste consistency. There is no strong odor to the stools of an exclusively nursing infant. This is all very different from the stools of a formula-fed infant. Their stool color is yellow-brown, tan-brown, and green-brown with a consistency similar to peanut butter. The stool is also more odorous.

Infants in the first month of life will typically have a minimum of three or more soft, yellow, runny stools each day. An infant who has fewer than three stools in a 24-hour period may not be getting enough to eat and will need to be weighed, examined, and monitored for adequate intake. Encourage parents to become familiar with their baby's stooling patterns. Every baby's digestive system, and thus the pattern for expelling waste, is individual to that baby. In one study, nursing infants stooled less than once every 24 hours without any negative effect (Moretti et al., 2019). The underlying causes for infrequent stooling in some nursing infants are unclear. In general, stooling frequency is higher in nursing infants than formula-fed infants (Moretti et al., 2019).

By around 4 to 6 weeks of age, the baby will begin going longer between stools. Frequency of elimination in older nursing infants can range from several stools per day to stooling only once every few days. Both patterns are acceptable. Stooling may decrease to once a day in the second month of life, a pattern that could continue until complementary foods are started. Stool characteristics of healthy nursing infants are described in **Table 14-3**, along with variations and their possible causes.

Table 14-3 Stool Patterns of a Nursing Baby

Characteristics	Normal Stool	Variations	Possible Causes
Color	First stool (meconium) is black, brown, or green in the first 3 days. Later, color ranges from brown or green to mustard yellow.	Unexplained color changes: black, brown, or red spots.	Parent or infant diet. Cracked nipples (possible bleeding—there is no harm to the baby). Bleeding from baby's rectum. If no known cause, consult the healthcare provider.
Consistency	Ranges from a toothpaste-like texture to a liquid with curds.	Very watery.	Foods in diet other than human milk, antibiotics, or illness.
		Hard pellets.	Foods in diet other than human milk, insufficient fluids, or baby tense or ill.
		Mucous.	Newborn mucus, cold, congestion, or allergy to parent's or baby's diet.
		Fibrous.	Bananas and cereal present in the baby's diet.
Odor	Very little, not unpleasant.	Unpleasant.	New foods in addition to human milk, antibiotics, or illness.
Frequency	Ranges from 1 with every feeding to 4 or more per day under 1 month of age; average of 3 per day. Decrease in frequency after the first month of life.	Sudden change in frequency. Watch carefully and assess for other symptoms.	Foods, maturity, or illness.
Volume	Varies with frequency. More frequent stools mean less volume per diaper.	Any sudden change. Watch carefully and be alert to other symptoms.	Foods, maturity, or illness.
Ease of expulsion	Easy and semicontrolled with some straining by the baby.	Flows out continually.	Foods other than human milk, illness, or antibiotics.
		Very difficult, with extreme straining.	Foods other than human milk or insufficient fluids.

Infrequent Stooling. An infant who does not stool adequately in the first month of life needs a complete feeding assessment. Infrequent stooling in the first month may result from insufficient milk intake. A baby who is voiding but does not stool or gain weight may not be feeding frequently enough or may be feeding ineffectively. Infrequent stooling is sometimes the first indication of low milk production. Stooling frequency usually corrects itself with additional feeding or longer feedings to ensure that the infant receives more hindmilk. This intervention works when there is adequate milk production and the baby transfers milk well.

Infrequent stooling could be caused by **Hirschsprung's disease**, a condition in which a part of the infant's intestines lacks proper innervation for the stool to pass easily. Hirschsprung's disease occurs in about 2 out of 10,000 births. It is more common in males and African American and Asian/Pacific Islander infants (Anderson et al., 2018). Symptoms in infants include difficult bowel movements; poor feeding; poor weight gain; and a large, bloated abdomen from the impacted stool and gas.

Cow's milk allergy can both mimic and influence Hirschsprung's disease (Arakoni et al., 2023). Early diagnosis can prevent serious complications, including enterocolitis and colonic rupture (Ostertag-Hill et al., 2024). Nursing infants may escape detection until the parents add solid foods to their diet and their stools become more bulky. Although this is a rare condition, any exclusively nursing infant who is gaining adequate amounts of weight but not stooling frequently needs careful evaluation and monitoring.

Constipation. Constipation is rare in nursing infants and is unrelated to stooling frequency. Lack of a daily stool and straining at stooling are normal aspects of toileting and not signs of constipation. Constipation in infants is identified by stool consistency, with stools that are molded and firm like pellets or marbles. Iron supplements taken by the nursing parent have been reported anecdotally to contribute to an infant's constipation. However, there are no research studies to support this belief. Discontinuing these supplements for a few days may return the child's digestive system to normal.

Constipation sometimes occurs when solid foods are added to the baby's diet. If the baby is receiving large amounts of cereal, it can be stopped or decreased for several days until normal stooling is reestablished and then reintroduced in smaller amounts less frequently. Adding more fruits and vegetables and, when the baby is old enough, yogurt, oatmeal, or prunes may help. Parents should not treat their infant with suppositories without consulting the baby's healthcare provider.

Diarrhea. The typically loose stools of a nursing baby may be mistakenly interpreted as diarrhea by parents who were supplementing with formula and then return to exclusive nursing. The same is possible if they are familiar with the stools of previous children who were formula-fed. Likewise, grandparents or other caregivers who are unfamiliar with nursing may worry that a normal human milk stool is diarrhea.

With **diarrhea**, the stool is much looser than normal and may be greenish and foul-smelling. Diarrhea may indicate the beginning of an illness or a reaction to antibiotics taken by either the parent or the baby. If diarrhea is suspected, it is important that nursing continue and that the parent contact the baby's caregiver immediately to avoid the baby becoming dehydrated. Diarrhea removes valuable intestinal bacteria that aid in the digestion of food. Such bacterial colonization can be restored with human milk feedings. Human milk provides all the electrolytes a baby needs so supplemental electrolytes are not necessary.

Infant Communication

A full-term, nonmedicated baby is biologically equipped to nurse. Respecting the baby's innate ability to nurse capitalizes on their neurobehaviors and is empowering to parents. Infants communicate their needs and their willingness to interact through their behavior. You can help parents understand, interpret, and respect their infants' communication so that they respond accordingly. Recognizing and responding to these communication cues is important to developing a bond between parents and their infant. New parents with anxiety or fear of attachment have higher rates of depression than those with feelings of security and attachment (Kinser et al., 2018). There is also a correlation between postpartum depression and early nursing cessation (Islam et al., 2021).

The concept of mutually responsive orientation, in which parental responsiveness elicits responses from infants, is associated with the development of self-regulation and self-representation (Kim & Kochanska, 2019). For example, social smiling emerges out of attentive engagement with an interactive parent. Smiling and other developmental milestones are addressed in **Chapter 18**. Postpartum depression is discussed in **Chapter 20**.

Approach and Avoidance Behaviors

Infants exhibit behavior that indicates a willingness to be approached. **Approach behavior** is integrated, stable, balanced, exploratory, and self-regulated. The signals illustrated in **Figure 14-11** are characteristic of a more mature infant. Conversely, infants display **avoidance behavior** that indicates a desire to withdraw, as depicted in **Figure 14-12**. Recognizing these behaviors will help parents know how to respond to their baby. **Tables 14-4** and **14-5** describe infant approach and avoidance behaviors.

Hunger Cues and Stages of Alertness

Many infant approach behaviors signal an interest in being fed, though they can also indicate a need

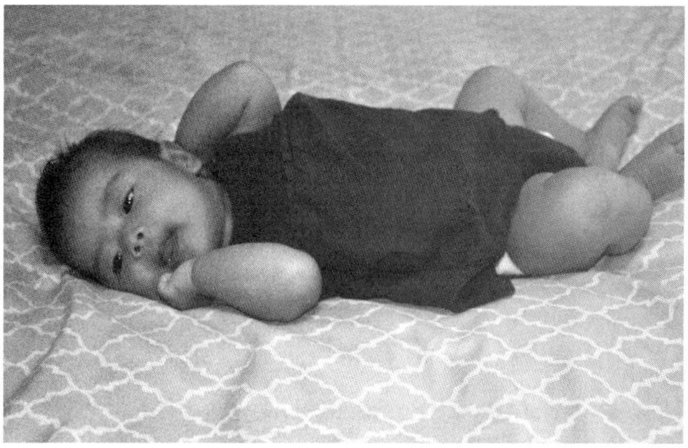

Figure 14-11 An infant exhibiting approach behavior.
Printed with permission of Lyly Tran.

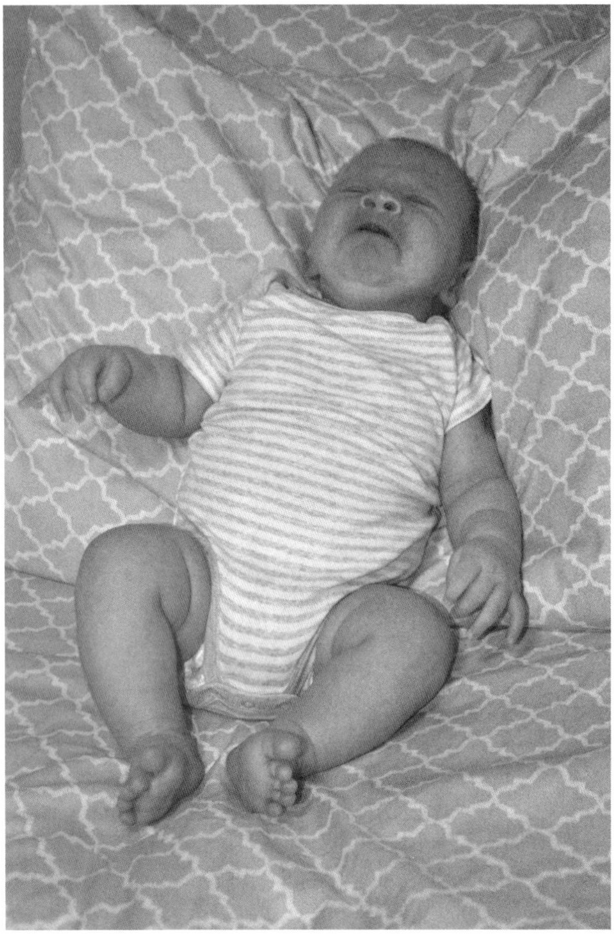

Figure 14-12 An infant exhibiting avoidance behavior.

to be comforted. Because approach behaviors can have various motives, learning hunger cues will help parents know when their baby is ready to nurse. If parents wait until their baby cries to initiate feeding, the baby will already be exhibiting the final sign of hunger. Pointing out hunger cues during a feeding assessment will help parents recognize the cues. An interest in feeding depends on the baby's level of alertness, as described in the **infant states** in **Table 14-6**.

Knowing When to Initiate a Feeding

Hunger cues may be evident when the baby is in a light sleep, drowsy state, or quietly alert. The baby will begin to wriggle, and tightly closed eyes may exhibit **rapid eye movement (REM)**. Cues progress to passing one or both hands over the head, bringing a hand to the mouth (**Figure 14-13**), and making sucking motions. The baby will begin to root if the cheek or mouth is touched. Soon, more vigorous sucking begins. The baby will then settle back into a less active state.

A baby may exhibit hunger cues several times in the span of 20 to 30 minutes. If these signals remain unheeded, they could become frustrated and cry. Conversely, the baby might become exhausted and fall back asleep without having received any

Table 14-4 Infant Approach Behaviors

Behavior	Description
Tongue extension	Infant's tongue extends toward a stimulus or repeatedly extends and relaxes.
Hand on face	Infant's hand or hands are placed onto the face or over the ears and remain there briefly.
Sounds	Infant's vocalizations are undifferentiated and may sound like a whimper.
Hand clasp	Infant grasps own hands or clutches hands to the body. Infant's hands may be closed and touch each other.
Foot clasp	Infant positions feet against each other, sole to sole. Infant's legs may fold in a crossed position with the feet grasping the legs or resting on them.
Finger fold	Infant interweaves one or more fingers of each hand.
Tuck	Infant curls or turns trunk or shoulders, pulls up legs, and tucks arms into torso. Infant uses the examiner's hands or body to attain tuck flexion.
Body movement	Infant adjusts body, extremities, or head into a more flexed position. Infant may turn to the side or attempt to attain a tonic neck response.
Hand to mouth	Infant attempts to bring hands or fingers to the mouth and may or may not achieve it.
Grasping	Infant's hands make grasping movements toward own face or body, in midair, toward the examiner's hands or body, or toward the side of the bassinet or crib.

Behavior	Description
Leg and foot brace	Infant extends legs and/or feet toward an object to self-stabilize. Infant may push against the examiner's body or hands, the examination surface, or the sides of the bassinet. Once touching, infant may flex legs or may restart the bracing.
Mouthing	Infant makes mouthing movements with their lips or jaws.
Suck search	Infant extends their lips forward or opens their mouth in a searching fashion, usually moving their head at the same time.
Sucking	Infant sucks on their own hands or fingers, clothing, the examiner's fingers, a pacifier, or other object they obtained or that the examiner inserts into their mouth.
Hand-holding	Infant's hands actively holds on to the examiner's hand or finger. The infant or the examiner may have positioned them there.
"Ooh" face	Infant rounds their mouth and purses their lips or extends them in an "ooh" configuration. Their eyes may be open or closed.
Locking visually	Infant visually locks onto the examiner's face or something in the environment and maintain the gaze for observable periods. The sound component of an environmental stimulus may contribute to their looking.

Printed with permission of Sarah Coulter Danner.

Table 14-5 Infant Avoidance Behaviors

Behavior	Description
Spit up	Infant spits up, with more than a passive drool. The amount of vomit may be minimal.
Gag	Infant appears to momentarily choke, gulp, or gag with unsynchronized swallowing and respiration patterns. This is often accompanied by mild mouth opening.
Hiccough	Infant hiccoughs.
Bowel movement grunting or straining	Infant's face and body display straining and infant emits the grunting sounds often associated with bowel movements.
Grimace, lip retraction	Infant's lips retract noticeably and the face is distorted in a retracting direction.
Truncal arching	Infant arches the trunk (torso) away from the bed or the parent's body.
Finger splay	Infant's hands open strongly with the fingers extended and separated.
Airplane	Infant's arms are fully extended out to the side at approximately shoulder level or the upper and lower arm are at an angle to each other and extended out at the shoulder.
Salute	Infant's arms are fully extended into midair, either singly or simultaneously.
Sitting on air	Infant's legs are extended into midair, either singly or simultaneously. This may occur when the infant is lying flat in a supine position or upright.
Sneezing, yawning, sighing, or coughing	Infant sneezes, yawns, sighs, or coughs.
Averting	Infant actively averts gaze and may momentarily close eyes.
Frowning	Infant knits or furrows brows or darkens the eyes by contracting muscles (squinting).
Startle	Infant's limbs jerk once, occasionally followed briefly by a slight amount of jitteriness and possibly crying.

Printed with permission of Sarah Coulter Danner.

Table 14-6 The Six Infant States

Infant State	Description
Deep sleep	Baby lies very still, with an occasional twitch or sucking movement, and cannot easily be aroused. Characterized by limp extremities, a placid face, quiet breathing, and no rapid eye movement (REM).
Light or active sleep	Baby awakens easily and is likely to remain awake if disturbed. Characterized by resistance in the extremities when moved, mouthing or sucking motions, body movement, and facial grimaces. Most of the baby's sleep is spent in this state, with less regular breathing and REM (eyes flutter beneath the eyelids). Although the baby may stir, they can return to sleep if left undisturbed.
Drowsy	Baby is aroused easily and may drift back to sleep. Eyes may open and close intermittently, and they may murmur, whisper, yawn, and stretch.
Quiet alert	Baby looks around, interacts with others, and is extremely responsive. Their body is still and watchful, eyes are bright, and breathing is even and regular. This is an excellent time to initiate nursing.
Active alert	Baby moves extremities and plays. They are more attentive, being wide-eyed, with rapid and irregular breathing. They may become fussy and more sensitive to the discomfort of a wet diaper or excessive stimulation.
Crying	Baby is agitated and needs comforting.

Adapted from Brazelton TB, Cramer, BB. *The Earliest Relationship*. Boston, MA: De Capo; 1990.

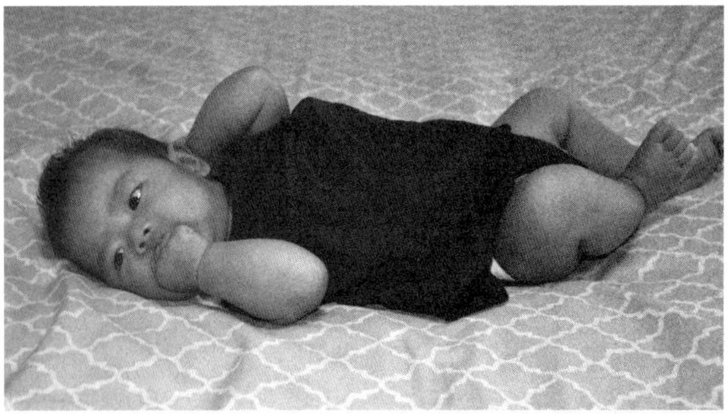

Figure 14-13 An infant exhibiting hunger cues.

Printed with permission of Lyly Tran.

nourishment. A missed feeding opportunity can have consequences for the next feeding. This pattern is common in infants who are born preterm, health compromised, or fed on a schedule despite hunger cues.

Crying can disorganize a newborn's motor functions and it can take several minutes for the infant to settle enough to nurse. Some infants may be unable to nurse until they have slept again for a while. If parents need to wake the baby for a feeding, they can do so when the baby is drowsy or in a light sleep. Most babies move from deep sleep to light sleep in approximately 20- to 30-minute cycles.

Infant Behavior Patterns

The first few weeks of a baby's life are a series of adjustments for everyone. For parents, it is a time when love, patience, and understanding for their infant are most important. Because newborns rely on their parents to meet their needs, a parent may spend nearly all their time and energy during the first month caring for their baby. While enjoying the closeness and warmth of their growing relationship, they may also feel physically drained and emotionally frustrated by the infant's helplessness.

An infant's temperament is innate, and their disposition and pattern of sleeping and eating can affect the nourishment they receive. Inexperienced parents sometimes become concerned about their babies' dispositions. It helps them to learn that babies experience a variety of behavior patterns, ranging from easygoing and undemanding to active and fussy. Understanding the various behavior patterns, dispositions, and sleeping and eating patterns will help you offer appropriate suggestions. It may take some time for parents to discover all the variations and subtle nuances in their baby's behavior.

The Average Baby

An **average baby** who is exclusively nursed typically nurses between 8 and 12 times in 24 hours. They sometimes cluster their feedings so that feedings blend together with few distinctions between starting and stopping. They usually sleep from 12 to 20 hours per day, possibly with one or two longer periods of sleep balanced by one or two fussy periods. Fussy periods typically occur in the early evening. The baby is usually responsive when handled and is generally quiet, alert, and listening while awake. Some babies learn self-soothing by sucking on a fist or displaying some other type of comfort measure.

The Easy Baby

Some babies have a nursing pattern typical of an average baby, consisting of approximately 8 to 12 feedings in 24 hours. However, they have longer sleep periods and are less demanding, with relatively little or no fussiness. Parents, who often refer to their easy baby, may need to make a conscious effort to give tactile stimulation and attention to foster the baby's emotional growth and physical development. These parents need to devote time to their baby even in the absence of bids for attention.

The Placid Baby

Some babies demonstrate a lack of engagement and cue for feeds as few as four to six times in 24 hours. Parents of a **placid baby** will need to be alert to possible undernourishment. The baby sleeps as much as 18 to 20 hours per day and is usually quietly alert and tranquil when awake. Despite making few demands for attention, the infrequent feedings do not indicate a lack of hunger. The baby may wake, feel hungry, and need to nurse but does not cry or demonstrate specific hunger cues. Rather, they soon return to sleep and later wake again and repeat the same pattern. Infants who do not feed frequently and sleep more than 12 to 16 hours per day should be evaluated for any underlying health issues.

Lack of attention and stimuli for a placid baby can lead to poor emotional development. The parent may not meet the infant's needs for nourishment and social interaction because the baby does not give overt cues. With such vital physical and emotional needs going unfulfilled, the baby may become withdrawn and lethargic. Parents often describe a placid baby as being "such a good baby" who does not cry and who sleeps through the night. You can discreetly ask the parents of a "good" baby about feeding and elimination patterns. These babies may be slow weight gainers and can be undernourished.

The parents of a placid baby must meet their baby's needs without receiving the necessary cues. Parents can use a monitor or place a noise device on the crib, such as a safe rattle, bell, or squeaky toy, to alert them to movement. A placid baby will benefit from being carried in a sling or baby carrier and being kept close to a parent or other family member, even without bids for attention. Parents can take advantage of natural waking by picking up their baby to nurse. They should avoid soothing techniques such as pacifiers, cradles, or swings. Babies who pacify themselves through thumb sucking can be encouraged to satisfy their sucking needs through nursing instead.

The Active and Fussy Baby

Active, fussy babies may nurse more frequently than the average baby, perhaps because of a greater need for comfort. Such a baby may seem insatiable and impatient for the milk to let down. They will sleep fewer hours than average. When awake, they will be active and frequently unable to self-soothe. In addition, there may be several periods of inconsolable crying during the day. The baby may overreact to freedom and stimulation and will need gentle, slow, and soothing movements as a calming measure. They may respond to **swaddling**, being kept warm, frequent holding, and being held close to the caregiver's body.

An active, fussy baby may respond well to nursing, dozing, and playing at the breast for generous periods. The greater need to be comforted, combined with increased milk intake, may result in frequent spitting up from being overly full. Nursing on only one side at a feeding may allow leisurely sucking after milk is removed to reduce the amount of milk to a level the baby can handle. Air swallowed because of overeagerness at feedings may require frequent burping. The baby may do well when carried in a sling and held upright after nursing (**Figure 14-14**). When using a baby sling, parents are cautioned to make sure the baby's face is visible and is not pressed so tightly against the wearer that it obstructs their breathing.

Infant Growth

Caloric intake will determine an infant's growth. In assessing growth, note the baby's weight gain since the last weight check, as well as the rate of weight gain since the baby's lowest weight (rather than birth weight). Record their growth in length and head circumference. Monitor signs of adequate intake in

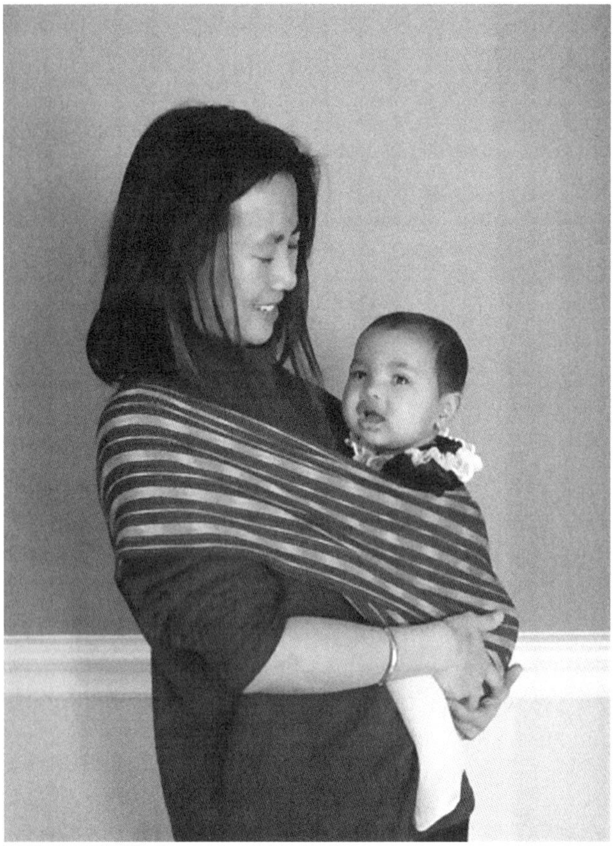

Figure 14-14 Parents can wear their baby in a sling for comforting.

Printed with permission of Anna Swisher.

relation to weight gain, including alertness, skin turgor, moist mucous membranes, and adequate output. Use growth charts that reflect nursing children as opposed to those based on infants raised on infant formula.

Caloric Intake

The calories in human milk depend on its fat content, given that half of the energy content of milk comes from the fat. Fat content varies between lactating parents, the time of day, and fullness. Most parents report that one side makes more milk than the other. Calorie content depends on the infant nursing long enough to receive the rich, fatty hindmilk. Healthy, full-term infants self-regulate their food intake, provided no arbitrary scheduling or time limits are imposed on feedings. Over the course of the day, the baby will take in the amount of milk needed for growth. Giving babies water can affect their caloric intake because the volume makes them feel full. Sterile water has no calories, and sugar (dextrose) water (D_5W) has only a limited amount of energy—6 kcal per 29.57 mL (1 oz). Calorie content of the milk is an issue for preterm babies or babies with illness, low weight gain, faltering growth, or disorders. High risk infants are discussed in **Chapter 24**.

Nursing infants typically have a leaner body mass than artificially fed infants because they utilize human milk efficiently. Their energy intake is lower throughout their first year as compared with formula-fed infants (Huang et al., 2018). Energy needs per day decrease as the baby gets older. Artificially fed infants have higher sleeping metabolic rates, higher rectal temperatures, and higher heart rates than nursing infants. This may account for the differences in energy intake and expenditure rates. The link between formula feeding and obesity is explored in **Chapters 9** and **10**.

Weight Gain

Growth patterns vary from one baby to the next. Newborns initially may lose as much as 7% to 10% of birth weight because of a loss of fluids and the passage of meconium. Excessive **intravenous** fluids received during labor can cause a fluid shift to the infant that artificially increases initial birth weight (Kellams et al., 2017). Infants who experience fluid shifts typically void large amounts of urine in the first 24 hours of life and can lose more weight than a baby born without intravenous interventions. Exposure to medications during labor can depress the baby's central nervous system and lead to fewer feedings in the first days of life—another factor that will affect weight gain in the early days.

A weight loss of more than 7% to 10% of birth weight indicates a need for evaluation and possible assistance with nursing. A weight loss of 10% or more requires thorough infant and feeding assessments (Flaherman et al., 2017). By day 3, a full-term infant who nurses without restrictions usually does not continue to lose weight. The baby's weight should stabilize by the end of the first week, and birth weight should be regained by 10 to 21 days after birth. Infants who have not regained to their birth weight by this time require evaluation before a supplementation is considered (Sarmiento-Aguilar et al., 2022). **Table 14-7** presents monthly weight ranges and weekly weight gain ranges for infants through the first year based on the World Health Organization (WHO) growth charts (**Figure 14-15**).

Nursing infants gain weight at a slightly higher trajectory in the first 3 months of life as compared with infants who are fed formula. After 3 months, formula-fed infants exhibit a higher weight gain than nursing infants (Azad et al., 2018; Centers for Disease Control and Prevention [CDC], 2023).

Table 14-7 Typical Infant Weight Gain

Range of Weekly Infant Weight Gain				
Girls (Grams)	**Boys (Grams)**	**Month**	**Girls (Ounces)**	**Boys (Ounces)**
175–325	225–350	1	6.2–11.5	7.9–12.3
200–300	225–350	2	7.1–10.6	7.9–12.3
150–225	175–225	3	5.3–6.2	6.2–7.9
100–200	150–200	4	3.5–7.1	5.3–7.1
100–150	100–150	5	3.5–5.3	3.5–5.3
75–125	75–125	6	2.6–4.4	2.6–4.4
75–125	75–125	7	2.6–4.4	2.6–4.4
50–100	75–100	8	1.8–3.5	2.6–3.5
50–100	50–75	9	1.8–3.5	1.8–2.6
50–75	50–100	10	1.8–2.6	1.8–3.5
50–100	50–75	11	1.8–3.5	1.8–2.6
50–75	50–75	12	1.8–2.6	1.8–2.6
Infant Weight Range				
Girls (Grams)	**Boys (Grams)**	**Month**	**Girls (Ounces)**	**Boys (Ounces)**
2.3–4.4	2.3–4.6	Birth	5.1–9.11	5.1–10.1
3.0–5.7	3.2–6.0	1	6.9–12.9	7.1–13.3
3.8–6.9	4.1–7.4	2	8.6–15.3	9.0–16.4
4.4–7.8	4.8–8.3	3	9.11–17.3	10.9–18.4
4.8–8.6	5.4–9.1	4	10.9–19	11.14–20.1
5.2–9.2	5.8–9.7	5	11.8–20.4	12.12–21.6
5.5–9.7	6.1–10.2	6	12.1–21.6	13.8–22.8
5.8–10.2	6.4–10.7	7	12.12–22.8	14.1–23.9
6.0–10.6	6.7–11.1	8	13.3–23.6	14.12–24.8
6.2–11.0	6.9–11.4	9	13.11–24.4	15.3–25.1
6.4–11.3	7.1–11.8	10	14.1–24.14	15.11–26.0
6.6–11.7	7.3–12.1	11	14.9–25.12	16.1–26.11
6.8–12.0	7.5–12.4	12	15.0–26.8	16.5–27.3

Data from 2006 World Health Organization Growth Charts.

Formula-fed infants consume a higher volume and more energy-dense milk in early life, leading to faster growth (Appleton et al., 2018; Huang et al., 2018). There do not appear to be significant height differences between adults who were nursed or formula fed (Bell et al., 2017).

Obesity

Assessing infant growth is of key interest in view of the obesity epidemic among youth. The role of nutrition early in life is increasingly recognized as contributing to growth and metabolic changes in later life. A recent

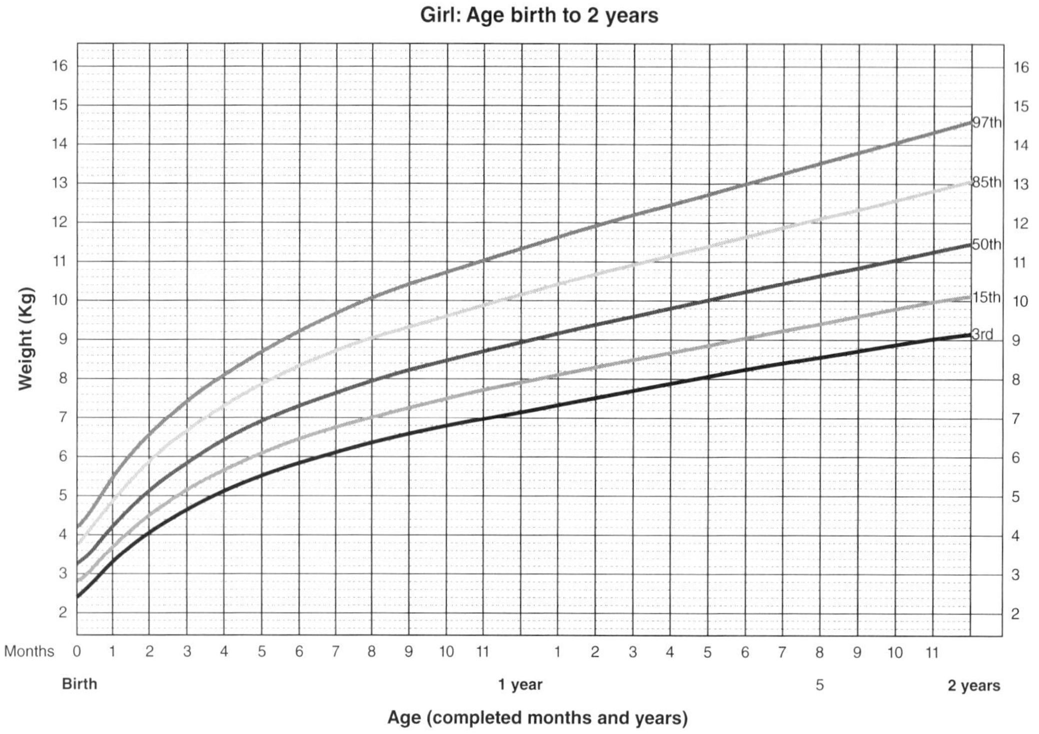

A

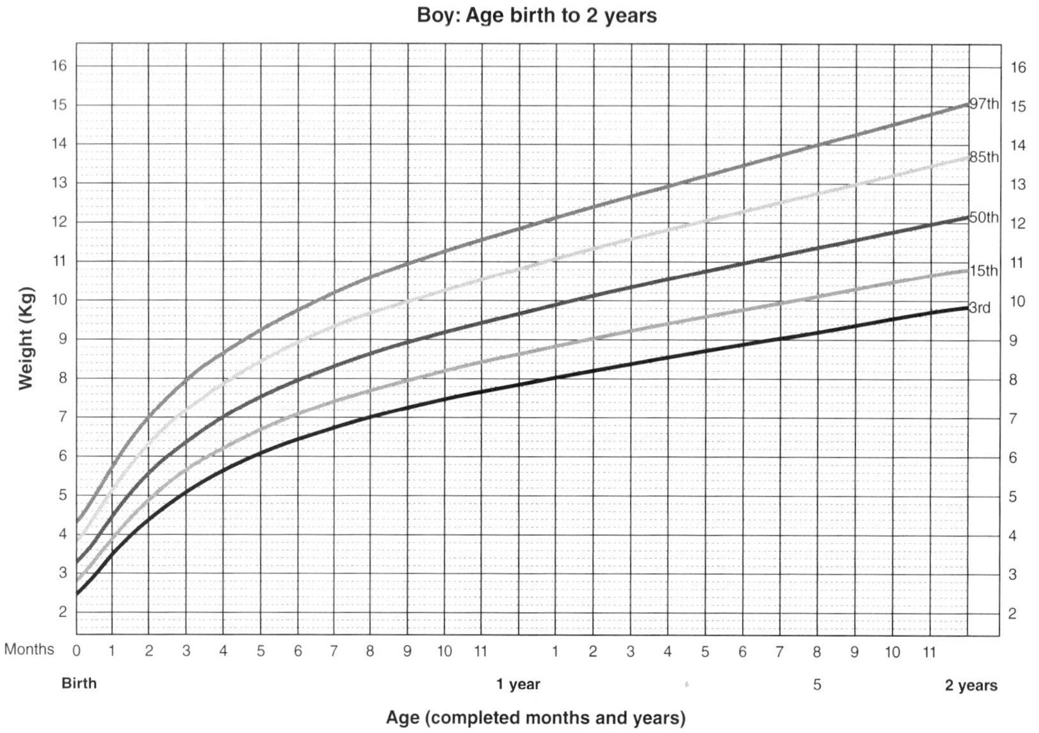

B

Figure 14-15 World Health Organization (WHO) weight charts. **(A)** Weight-for-age, girls. **(B)** Weight-for-age, boys.

systematic review of the association between nursing and obesity concluded that nursing reduces the odds of obesity later in life (Horta et al., 2023). Formula feeding appears to be a predictor of obesity in both infancy and adulthood. **Chapters 9** and **10** discuss formula feeding, the gut microbiome, and the role of metabolic programming for lifelong health.

Growth Charts

Infant growth charts produced by formula companies depict growth of primarily formula-fed infants and are not reliable for charting growth in nursing babies. They are based on 1977 growth charts from the U.S. National Center for Health Statistics (NCHS). CDC charts released in 2000 exhibited notable differences between the typical growth pattern of nursing infants and the expected growth curve. WHO growth charts released in 2006 are based on the growth of exclusively or predominantly nursed children (WHO, 2006). The CDC recommends the use of the WHO growth charts for all infants until the age of 2 years.

Sleeping Patterns

All babies require a lot of sleep, and the amount varies from baby to baby. Some babies sleep as few as 8 hours in a 24-hour period, whereas others sleep as many as 20 hours per day. Understanding typical sleep patterns will help parents adapt to their child's unique needs. There are no clear data on the impact of infant feeding method and sleep duration. One study concluded that exclusively nursed infants had overall longer nighttime and total amount of sleep in 24 hours as compared to formula-fed infants (Abdul Jafar et al., 2021). Likewise, feeding method is not associated with parental sleep or fatigue (Ataŝ & Özerdoğan, 2021). Variations may be developmental, environmental, or nutritional in nature. For example, overtiredness or overstimulation can cause fretfulness before and during sleep. Sounds, lights, the temperature of the room and bedding, and low humidity (which causes difficulty in breathing) can affect (and sometimes interfere with) sleep.

Babies who sleep separated from their nursing parent may wake at night to seek nourishment and physical contact. The absence of the parent's body warmth and skin contact can make it more difficult for the baby to fall asleep and sleep undisturbed. A baby may also have trouble sleeping if the parent consumes too much caffeine. Caffeine passes through the milk and accumulates in the infant because of their inability to metabolize it efficiently (Hale & Krutsch, 2024). Developmental factors that affect sleep are discussed in **Chapter 18**.

Encouraging the Baby to Sleep

When parents voice concerns about their babies' sleep habits, you can help them determine how realistic their expectations are. A smartphone app or written record can track several days of the baby's sleep patterns, including even 5-minute naps. Gaining a better understanding of normal newborn behavior can help parents relax and not allow uninterrupted sleep to be such an important goal. Sleeping when the baby sleeps will help recoup lost sleep, especially in the early postpartum period. During the night, the parent's partner can bring the baby to bed for nursing, allowing the parent to stay in bed. If the baby sleeps for longer periods during the day than at night, parents can try waking them more frequently during the day to discourage longer sleep periods. This enables the baby to nurse more often and helps the baby's rhythm come into harmony with the rest of the family.

Establishing a bedtime ritual can be enjoyable for both parents and baby. A routine helps the baby associate the ritual with going to sleep at an established time every night. Quiet, soothing activities directly before bedtime—such as a bath, story, rocking, and nursing—can prepare the baby for sleep. In colder climates, parents can warm the baby's sleeping area with a heating pad or hot water bottle and remove it right before laying the baby down. Flannel sheets can help keep the infant from waking because of the initial coolness of cotton sheets. It is important to note that parents should be cautious not to overheat their baby.

Issues with Sleep and Nursing

A well-nourished baby can usually sleep for long periods at night. Nursing frequently during the day will accomplish this goal. Nursing directly before bedtime ensures a full stomach and helps soothe the baby. A parent who returns to work or school can retire early in the evening and take their baby to bed with them. Nursing while lying in the middle of the bed makes it easy to move the baby to the crib when they are in a deeper sleep. Some parents keep the baby in their bed until morning or until after the next feeding. When the baby wakes in the middle of the night to nurse, avoiding stimulation will facilitate a return to sleep. A nightlight near the baby's bed eliminates the need to turn on a bright light. A soiled diaper can be changed before nursing on the second side so that the baby can nurse back to sleep undisturbed.

Cosleeping

Worldwide, most infants sleep with their parents. The cultural expectation in many industrialized countries is that babies sleep through the night separate from their parents. This practice does not support human babies' biological need to be close to their parents for a feeling of safety, including during sleeping (Yoshida & Funato, 2021).

Many parents opt for a family bed shared by the parents and baby. **Cosleeping**, also called bed sharing, helps babies fall asleep more easily, and babies wake readily when moved (**Figure 14-16**). Cosleeping is helpful with a baby who wakes frequently during the night. In the absence of hazardous factors, there are significant differences in bedsharing between nursing and non-nursing dyads (McKenna & Gettler, 2016).

Cosleeping infants become aroused more often and in greater synchrony with their parents than do separate sleepers. This relationship suggests that safe cosleeping may reduce the risk of **sudden infant death syndrome (SIDS)**. More frequent arousals promote nighttime nursing. Thus, parents who cosleep with their babies nurse more frequently than parents whose babies sleep in a separate room (Blair et al., 2020). Bed sharing is associated with a longer duration of nursing as well (Baddock et al., 2019; Kural & Gökçay, 2022).

The AAP recognizes the need for closeness to facilitate nursing and recommends that nursing parents and babies sleep in proximity to each other. However, the AAP Task Force on SIDS advises against parent–infant bed sharing and supports the generic use of pacifiers (AAP, 2016; Moon et al., 2022). The ABM issued revised guidelines for safe cosleeping (**Figure 14-17**).

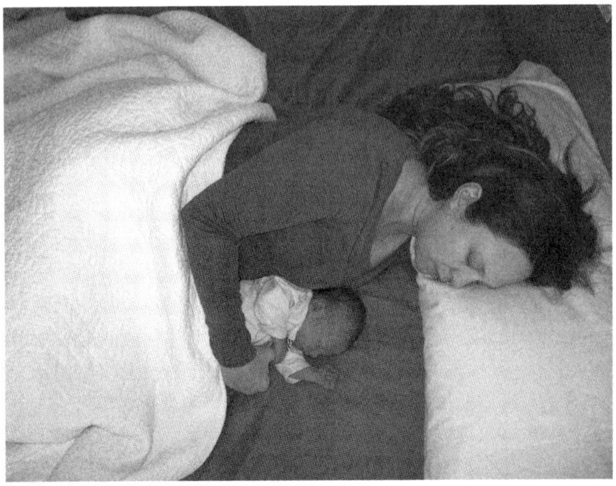

Figure 14-16 Parent cosleeping with baby.

Printed with permission of Anna Swisher.

Exclusively nursing parents get more nighttime sleep than those who feed formula during the first month after birth. A recent meta-analysis indicated that nighttime sleep in nursing parents was significantly higher than in non-nursing parents and that cosleeping increased the overall sleeping hours of parents (Srimoragot et al., 2022). As an alternative to sharing their bed with their child, some parents use a crib, or cosleeper, that attaches to their bed. For more information on this topic, **Chapter 20** discusses responsive parenting.

Prevalence of Cosleeping

Cosleeping was the cultural norm in most of the world until the 20th century, and in many places, it still is. Sweeping cultural changes in the global north brought mechanistic, scientific, and behavioristic models of child development that defined "normal" behavior

Precautions for cribs and adult beds:

- Use a firm mattress to avoid suffocation.
- Have no gaps between the mattress and the frame.
- Keep bedding tight around the mattress.
- Avoid strings or ties on baby's and parents' night-clothes.
- Avoid soft items such as comforters, pillows, stuffed animals, lambskins, and bean bags.
- Do not sleep with infant in a waterbed.
- Keep baby's face uncovered.
- Put the baby on their back to sleep.
- Do not overheat the room or overdress baby.
- Do not place a crib near window cords or sashes.

Additional precautions for co-sleeping:

- Parents pull back and fasten long hair to prevent the hair from tangling up with the baby.
- Refrain from the use of alcohol or other drugs, including over the counter or prescription medications.
- Have no head or food board railings with spaces wider than allowed in safety approved cribs.
- Place crib away from walls and furniture to prevent the infant's head or body from being wedged.
- Keep infant away from secondhand smoke; parents who smoke should not sleep with their infants.
- The baby should never be left alone on an adult bed.
- Adopt the "C" sleeping position, with the infant's head across from the parent's chest and the parent's arms and legs curled around the infant.
- Avoid bed sharing if parent is morbidly obese; consider the use of a side car or in-bed device to be placed adjacent to the parent's bed.
- When bedsharing cannot be done safely, discuss the importance of room sharing.
- Encourage partner and other support persons' involvement in infants sleep activities.

Figure 14-17 Creating a safe infant sleep environment.

Data Source: Blair PS, et al. Bedsharing and breastfeeding: The Academy of Breastfeeding Medicine Protocol #6, Revision 2019. *Breastfeed Med.* 2020;15(1):5-16. Mother-Baby Behavioral Sleep Laboratory. Safe Cosleeping Guidelines. University of Notre Dame. 2023. https://cosleeping.nd.edu/safe-co-sleeping-guidelines/

based on bottle-feeding babies. Despite recommendations by public health authorities, cosleeping continues to be common in Western culture (Cole et al., 2020; D'Souza et al., 2023). This mirrors non-Western cultures, where an infant and parent remain together continually, both day and night (Mileva-Seitz et al., 2017).

Reasons parents give for cosleeping include nursing, comforting, better sleep, monitoring, bonding, environmental, crying, tradition, disagree with danger, and parental instinct (Barry & McKenna, 2022). The warmth and familiar smell of the parent comforts the infant when sleeping in the parents' bed. The infant can nuzzle and nurse ad lib, and the parent does not have to leave the bed to nurse a hungry infant. Thus, the nursing parent can get the sleep they need while meeting their infant's needs.

Concerns About Cosleeping

Some parents worry that it is emotionally unhealthy to share their bed with their infant or that the habit may be difficult to break once formed. Some authorities fear a parent could inadvertently roll over onto the infant while they are asleep. Authorities in many countries do not universally advise against bed sharing in the absence of high-risk conditions (Blair et al., 2020). Some cultures have high rates of bed sharing and low rates of SIDS, whereas others have high rates of bed sharing and high rates of SIDS (AAP, 2016). While it is a cultural norm in the United States for infants to sleep separated from their parents, it is not the biological norm.

With appropriate education and support, parents who cosleep with their infant can evaluate their sleep environment and make it as safe as possible for their baby. Both parents should feel comfortable with the decision to cosleep with their baby and be committed to following appropriate safety precautions. Although no one sleep environment is guaranteed to be risk-free, there are ways of reducing risks in both cribs and adult beds. Admonishing parents who cosleep fails to respect their responsiveness to their babies. A more reasonable approach is to recognize the need to increase infant safety by following safe co-sleeping guidelines while protecting nursing (Blair et al., 2020; Mother-Baby Behavioral Sleep Laboratory [MBBSL], 2025).

Sudden Infant Death Syndrome

Sudden infant death syndrome (SIDS) is the sudden death of an infant younger than 1 year of age that remains unexplained after an autopsy, examination of the death scene, and review of the clinical history. An expanded version, **sudden unexplained infant death (SUID)** encompasses both SIDS and other sudden explainable infant mortality cases. The three most frequently reported causes of death in infants younger than one year are SIDS, unknown cause, and accidental suffocation/strangulation in bed. In 2020, 41% of unexplained deaths were attributed to SIDS (CDC, 2023). For example, in 2020, there were about 1380 deaths due to SIDS, 1046 due to unknown causes, and about 900 deaths due to accidental suffocation and strangulation in bed (Shapiro-Mendoza et al., 2023). Research suggests that brainstem abnormalities and genetic variations may contribute to SIDS (Kinney & Haynes, 2019; Vincent et al., 2023).

SIDS occurs in all socioeconomic, racial, and ethnic groups. Most SIDS deaths occur when a baby is between 2 and 4 months of age. Ninety percent of all SIDS deaths occur before the child reaches 6 months of age. Most babies who die of SIDS appear to be healthy prior to death. There are significant racial/ethnicity differences in SIDS rates. It is important to note that in global north countries the incidences of SIDS is higher in poor and marginalized populations (Bartick et al., 2019).

Protection Against SIDS

Nursing for at least 2 months is associated with reducing the risk of SIDS by 50%. Greater protection is conferred with increased nursing duration (Thompson et al., 2017). A baby who is not nursed may be at greater risk because of the lack of immunological protection and differences in breathing and arousal patterns (Thompson et al., 2017). Nursing infants arouse more easily from active sleep at 2 to 3 months of age. Given that this age coincides with the peak incidence of SIDS, this behavior may represent a protective mechanism of nursing.

The position in which the baby is placed for sleep is a major factor in the risk of SIDS. Placing them in a supine position (on their back) rather than in a prone position (on their stomach) substantially reduces the incidence of SIDS. Nursing parents who cosleep predominantly put their infants on their backs to facilitate feedings. Multiple countries throughout the world, including (but not limited to) Australia, Canada, Denmark, Ireland, New Zealand, the United Kingdom, and the United States, have implemented safe sleep policies, although they differ in their specific recommendations (Deering et al., 2018). SIDS rates have declined by more than 50% in the United States since 1994, when the "Back to Sleep" public information campaign began.

The campaign was later rebranded as "Safe to Sleep" to focus on both SIDS and other sleep-related infant deaths (National Institutes of Health [NIH], 2024).

Parental smoking is a significant risk factor for SIDS. An estimated one-third of SIDS deaths are associated with the nursing parent smoking during pregnancy (Cerda et al., 2017). Another risk factor is the baby's inhalation of passive smoke. Parents who smoke around their baby need to learn the dangers to their baby. One study found that tobacco-using families practice less safe sleeping behaviors. They put their infants on their backs to sleep less often (75% vs. 88%), bed shared more (62% vs. 44%), and used soft bedding more (50% vs. 32%) than families without tobacco use (Hussain et al., 2018).

Small-at-birth infants who sleep in a separate room are at increased risk for SIDS compared with similar infants who sleep in the same room with their parents. Keeping the baby in the parents' room (room sharing) may reduce the risk of SIDS by as much as 50% (Moon et al., 2022). Sleeping on sofas increases the risk of SIDS and comprises almost 13% of infant sleep-related deaths (MacFarlane et al., 2022). Soft bedding, blankets, pads, pillows, and stuffed toys are also risk factors. Bed sharing should be avoided if parents consume alcohol, smoke, or take drugs or if the infant is born preterm (Blair et al., 2020; Moon et al., 2022).

The AAP Task Force on SIDS states that using a pacifier to go to sleep may be protective against SIDS and recommends that all babies be put to sleep with pacifiers (Moon et al., 2022). This recommendation, however, is based on studying babies who typically used pacifiers and were more at risk for SIDS if they did not use one. Babies who nurse themselves to sleep do not fit that profile.

Crying

Crying is an infant's first language, a powerful communication tool used by babies to interact with their environment. In a cause-and-effect relationship, babies learn that crying elicits parental response to meet their needs. This enhances attachment to the parents, develops trust more readily, and reduces crying. In response to their baby's cry, the parent's heart beats louder, their blood pressure increases, and the temperature increases in their breasts. The sound of a crying infant is disturbing and aggravating (**Figure 14-18**). It is biologically designed to ensure that the newborn receives the attention they need (Etherton et al., 2016). The decibel level of a baby's cry is higher than street noise and can be 20 decibels louder than normal speech. **Table 14-8** describes several combinations of temperament that can affect a baby's disposition. **Chapter 15** discusses the baby who is fussy during feeding.

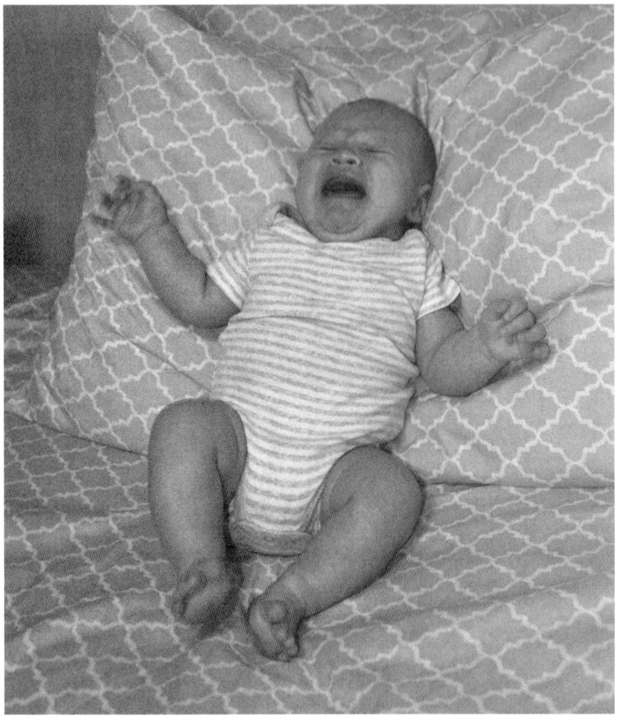

Figure 14-18 A crying infant needs to be settled before attempting a feeding.

The crying pattern of a preterm infant is different from that of a full-term infant (Orlandi et al., 2016; Shinya et al., 2017). Preterm infants have a different rhythm, pause, and inhalation–exhalation pattern. Their cry is a full octave higher than that of a full-term infant, signaling a greater urgency. Preterm infants have been found to fuss and cry more frequently when they reach term-adjusted age (Shinya et al., 2017).

Parental Reactions to Crying

New parents envision a baby who smiles, coos, and snuggles, not one who is fussy and cries. Worry about the infant's crying in the first 3 months accounted for 20% of pediatric visits in one study (Barr et al., 2015). Often, parents are dissatisfied with healthcare providers who fail to take their concerns seriously (van der Veek & van Rosmalen, 2023). Therefore, they may worry that their baby's crying reflects poor parenting.

Table 14-8 Influences on Baby's Disposition

Baby's Disposition	Parent's Disposition	Probable Outcome
Easy	Responsive	The baby is predictable and cuddly and the parent is in tune with the baby's rhythms. The parent feels good about their parenting based on the positive interactions with the baby.
Easy	Restrained	The baby is not too demanding. The parent may not develop comfort skills, believing they are unnecessary. The baby may, in time, exhibit more fussy behavior.
High needs with good attachment-promoting behaviors	Responsive	The parent cannot ignore the needs of their baby and responds to them. The baby exhibits occasional satisfied responses. The parent will continue to explore alternative responses for one that draws a reaction. The parent's responsiveness leads to the baby developing attachment-promoting skills, resulting in mutual sensitivity.
High needs with poor attachment-promoting skills	Responsive	The baby may show little or no effort to respond to or be comforted by the parent's efforts. The parent's nurturing responses are fine-tuned by their baby's reactions. The baby's lack of responsiveness may jeopardize the parent–baby relationship. The parent may need assistance from a professional who is trained in interaction counseling or therapy.
High needs	Restrained	The parent–baby relationship is at risk. Often, the parent has been advised to let the baby cry it out. Continued lack of response to the baby's needs will lead them to intensify the high-need behaviors or give up. The baby shuts down communication efforts, withdraws, and is prone to attach to objects rather than persons.

Data from Sears W, Sears M. *The Fussy Baby Book: Parenting Your High-Need Child from Birth to Age Five*. New York: Little Brown & Company; 1996.

Help parents recognize that babies fuss and cry because they need something and that this is normal. Encourage them to focus on the positive attributes of this behavior rather than considering their baby to be difficult or spoiled. A fussy baby is alert, responsive to the environment, and a good communicator.

Parents are vulnerable to people reacting negatively to their crying baby. When others stare at the parents of a crying baby or make rude or personal comments, the parents may feel out of control or judged. Often, the problem lies in their expectations of what parenting will be like. Parents are often advised not to pick up their crying infant and are encouraged to let the child "cry it out." See **Chapter 20** for a discussion of "baby training" and its negative impacts on nursing. Babies repeatedly left to cry alone learn that their needs will not be met. Failing to understand or respond to infants' messages can compromise their care, as well as parental effectiveness, thereby undermining the relationship between parents and their baby.

Parents who are restrained in their response to crying stop nursing sooner and have infants who cry more overall. They may perceive infant fussiness as dissatisfaction with nursing and conclude that supplementing with formula or cereal will provide a solution. Short nursing duration or formula use from birth is significantly associated with low nurturance levels and high anxiety levels. Longer nursing duration is associated with parents being more responsive to their infant's cues (Little et al., 2018). Educating parents that crying is a baby's method of communicating with the world will help reassure them that nursing is not the cause and that their baby is doing what is normal for their age.

The Effect of Crying on the Infant

Crying increases the newborn's heart rate and blood pressure, which in turn increases intracranial pressure. Poorly oxygenated blood flows back into circulation rather than into the lungs. Large fluctuations in blood flow increase cerebral blood volume and decrease cerebral oxygenation, increasing the risk of respiratory difficulty. Crying for a preterm infant requires great effort, which can cause distress and lower blood oxygenation.

Metabolically, crying leads to increased glucose expenditure. In the immediate postpartum period this could result in hypoglycemia. Crying also increases gastric distention and may result in a discontented baby because of gas pain. In addition, crying raises infants' stress hormones. Continually elevated stress hormone levels are believed to contribute to infant illness (Hernandez-Reif & Gungordu, 2022). Babies who have been crying have difficulty organizing their behavior to nurse.

Identifying the Cause of Crying

A baby's cry often indicates some form of physical discomfort. As parents become accustomed to their baby, they will learn to distinguish whether the cry indicates hunger, pain, or a reaction to the environment. Too often, a parent immediately assumes that hunger is the cause and may blame the quantity or the quality of milk for their baby's fussy disposition. If the baby nursed recently and does not appear to be hungry, parents can investigate other causes of the crying.

Crying from Hunger

In the early weeks after birth, it is common for a baby to require frequent feedings and to sleep sporadically for short periods. Parents will learn to recognize a hunger cry as they tune in to their baby's pattern of sleeping and waking. They can consider how recent and long the previous feeding was, the baby's hunger cues and general disposition, and whether the baby soothes easily or with difficulty.

A newborn may cry from hunger approximately 1½ to 2 hours or more after feeding. A hunger cry may be more prevalent in the evening hours when milk production seems lowest and the environment feels harried. Because of this, it is common for babies to cluster feedings in the early evening. When a baby cries from hunger, parents may have failed to respond to earlier cues before the baby resorted to crying. Nursing in response to early hunger cues, also known as *nursing on demand*, tends to produce more contented babies. These babies will cry less frequently than those on a strict feeding schedule that disregards their cries. You can teach parents to recognize and respond to hunger cues rather than waiting until the baby cries.

Crying from Discomfort

Wet or soiled diapers by themselves may not be sufficient to cause crying. However, when the diaper cools, the temperature drop can cause discomfort, leading to increased crying. Babies may also cry from excessive heat. First-time parents tend to overdress a new baby even on the hottest summer day, fearing they may become chilled. In warm weather and cold weather alike, healthy, full-term babies can be dressed in the same type of clothing that an adult wears.

Babies may cry when they are undressed and lose the warm, secure feeling of clothing and blankets. A baby who is especially sensitive to this effect may benefit from swaddling. The texture of the cloth that touches the child's body is important as well. For example, plastic or rubber is more irritating than soft toweling or blanketing. Other skin irritations, such as heat rash or **diaper rash**, can be a cause of a baby's cries.

A baby's crying may be from gasiness or overfullness. A baby who is constantly fussy during feedings may need to bring up a bubble of air. Parents can help the baby pass gas in the intestines by using the techniques described later in this chapter. Additionally, some babies take in more milk than they can handle. Such overfeeding causes pressure, which in turn can produce discomfort. Nursing long enough for the baby to drain one side before offering the other one will help avoid ingesting excessive amounts of milk at a feeding.

If parents have ruled out hunger and discomfort, their baby may settle after a few minutes. Focusing on the cues their baby gives in response to their parenting approach will help them know how to proceed. If their baby is responding positively to a technique, it can be encouraged. If their baby exhibits withdrawal or avoidance behaviors, they will want to try a new approach.

Crying from External Stimuli

When parents have tended to the physical needs of their baby and the crying continues, something external may be the cause. Babies may startle and cry in reaction to sudden movement, touch, smell, light, noise, or excessive handling. This often accounts for the initial fussiness babies demonstrate when transitioning from hospital to home. Constant soft, soothing noise can be an effective comfort measure. The steady movement of being rocked is comforting, as is the motion of a car ride. Re-creating the sounds and feeling of the womb comforts a newborn.

Swaddling. Some babies respond well to swaddling, which reduces their movements and therefore the amount of stimulation they receive. Confining the arms and legs prevents the infant from startling and provides a feeling of warmth, security, and constant touch stimulation. Although swaddling may increase the time a baby sleeps and decrease the time spent crying, it does not necessarily do so at the expense of time spent quietly awake.

Swaddling should be done with the baby's legs together in normal flexion to prevent hip dysplasia (Vaidya et al., 2021). Parents should be wary of some commercial swaddlers and wearable blankets because injuries and deaths have been reported with these. Decreasing infants' natural ability to arouse may lead to an increase in sudden unexplained infant deaths (Dixley & Ball, 2022). SIDS researchers recommend that parents discontinue swaddling as soon as an infant's earliest attempts to roll over are observed (Moon et al., 2022).

Some babies dislike being swaddled and will cry or squirm when they are wrapped or held too tightly. The baby may push away when held too closely and may prefer a position that allows body movement. Nursing in a side-lying position while lightly supporting the baby from behind with a hand or a pillow will allow the baby more freedom of movement. The parent can also nurse while leaning above the reclining infant.

Baby Sling. Figure 14-14 shows a comforting technique of "wearing" the baby in a sling. This practice provides the infant with the secure feeling of swaddling, with the added benefit of closeness to the person who wears the sling. Infant deaths have occurred in slings, either from compression of the baby into a forward-flexed position or from suffocation. Thus, it is important to teach parents to use the sling safely, ensuring that they keep the baby upright and the baby's head clear of the material (Moon et al., 2022).

Excessive Crying

Excessive infant crying is often referred to as *colic* or *colic-like* behavior. The term *colic* derives from the Greek word *kolikos*, an adjective derived from *kolon*, meaning "large colon." In defining colic, duration is more significant than frequency. Colic has classically been defined by the "rule of threes," characterized by inconsolable crying for which no physical cause can be found that lasts more than 3 hours per day, occurs at least 3 days per week, and continues for at least 3 weeks. The baby experiences spasmodic contractions of the smooth muscle, causing pain and discomfort.

More recently, diagnostic criteria have been further refined using the Rome classification of functional GI disorders. The duration of 3 weeks has been reduced to a 7-day duration (Zeevenhooven et al., 2018). Symptoms can last up to 12 to 16 weeks of age. The prevalence is about 20% during the first 6 weeks of life, declining to about 11% of infants at 8 to 9 weeks and fewer than 1% at 12 to 14 weeks of age (Wolke et al., 2017). Rather than attempting to cure infants with excessive crying, the challenge may be to help parents reduce their stress during the challenging months and minimize the impact on the family.

PURPLE Crying

Excessive crying is also referred to as the *period* aspect of PURPLE crying, as described in **Table 14-9**. The term—now often used to replace the term *colic*—may help parents understand what they can expect from their baby related to excessive crying. It describes the period in the first few months of a baby's life when they cry excessively. Using the term *period* can help parents understand that their baby's crying has a beginning and an end. Therefore, they can recognize that what their baby is experiencing is short-lived and normal and that they are not doing anything wrong (Power & Sharif, 2021).

The pattern of periods of PURPLE crying is quite different from the one or two fussy periods a day experienced by most infants. Infants who cry excessively

Table 14-9 PURPLE Crying

Description	Infant's Behavior
Peak of crying	Crying may increase until age 2 months and lessen at 3 to 5 months.
Unexpected	Crying can come and go, and the parent may not know why.
Resists soothing	Crying may not stop no matter what the parent tries.
Pain-like face	The baby may appear to be in pain, even when they are not.
Long lasting	Crying can last as much as 5 hours a day, sometimes more.
Evening	Crying may occur more in the late afternoon or evening.

exhibit unexplained fussiness, fretfulness, and irritability. They appear to suffer from severe discomfort, with cries that are piercing, explosive attacks. Excessive **flatulence** (gas) and apparent abdominal pain may cause their legs to draw up sharply into the abdomen or their body to stiffen and twist. The baby may awaken easily and frequently and appear intense, energetic, excitable, and easily startled—with clenched fists and a facial grimace. Continuous crying can cause the baby to swallow air and further aggravate the discomfort.

The exact cause of excessive infant crying has not been determined medically. There are likely multiple biopsychosocial factors involved (Mai et al., 2018). It may result from an immature digestive and intestinal system or allergies. Possible causes are explored in the following sections.

Parental Influences

Psychosocial factors have been suggested as causes of excessive infant crying. It is found in higher proportions in families with less education, smoking, domestic violence, impaired bonding, hostility, and postpartum depression (Firooz et al., 2021). There appear to be higher rates of excessive crying in infants of parents who experienced depression and anxiety during pregnancy and after childbirth. A partner's depression leading to decreased interaction with the parent and the infant is associated with excessive crying. Decreased nursing self-efficacy is also a factor, potentially due to incorrect feeding technique.

Immature Gastrointestinal and Neurological Systems

Compared with other mammals, a human baby is born in an extremely immature state—essentially neurologically incomplete. Excessive crying may be a symptom of neurological distress, such as a headache or migraine (Gelfand, 2016). These infants may have more permeable intestinal linings (Daelemans et al., 2018). **Peristalsis** (wavelike rhythmic contractions of smooth muscle) may be irregular, faint, forceful, or spasmodic. A lack of muscle tone can cause food to move up out of the stomach, as well as down into the intestines. The colon in normal infants takes several hours to empty. For infants with excessive crying, the colon can empty very quickly and contract violently.

Drugs

A parent's prenatal use of heroin, marijuana, barbiturates, or cocaine can result in excessive crying in the infant (Mai et al., 2018), or NAS. Infants born with NAS often exhibit signs of nervous system instabilities. Symptoms may not appear until a week or more after birth. They can include excitability, trembling, restlessness, ravenous appetite, jitteriness, hyperactivity, shrill scream, feeding problems, and either hypertonia or hypotonia. **Chapter 11** provides more information on the effects of drugs on the newborn.

Nicotine

There is a correlation between infant fussiness and parental use of nicotine. Tobacco metabolites can be transmitted through the placenta during pregnancy, as well as after birth through the milk and secondhand smoke. This increases motilin hormone levels in the infant's gut, which can lead to increased motility and abdominal pain (Firooz et al., 2021). Infants of parents who smoke are more excitable, with lower muscle tone than other infants (Froggatt et al., 2020). Therefore, they require more careful handling, show more signs of stress, and have more difficulty with self-regulation. Supporting nursing is an important intervention for these dyads.

Food Sensitivity

An infant who reacts to something in the milk is typically calm at the start of a feeding and then begins to pull off, stiffens their body, cries, and then relatches. This pattern may repeat several times during a feeding. Symptoms of **food sensitivity** can be continuous or may start after the feeding. It is rare for symptoms to show up before 3 weeks. **Figure 14-19** presents signs of food sensitivity.

- Stuffy or drippy nose without any other sign of having a cold
- Frequently pulling off during a feeding
- Arching and crying while feeding
- Itchy nose
- Red, scaly, oily rash on the forehead or eyebrows, in the hair, or behind the ears
- Eczema
- Red rectal ring
- Fretful sleeping or persistent sleeplessness
- Frequent spitting up or vomiting
- Diarrhea or green stools, perhaps with blood in them
- Wheezing
- Coliclike symptoms and behaviors

Figure 14-19 Signs of food sensitivity in an infant.

Cow and Soy Milk Intolerances

Cow's milk protein is a common cause of intolerance in infants. Almost all mammal milks contain **bovine immunoglobulin G (IgG)**. One research study found that nursing parents of babies who cry excessively have high levels of bovine IgG in their milk (Clyne & Kulczycki, 1991). The high bovine IgG levels may contribute to an increase in GI upset in infants. Levels in human milk range from 0.1 to 8.5 mg per mL compared with 0.6 to 128 mg per mL in cow's milk formulas. There is no bovine IgG in soy or amino acid formulas.

Intolerance to cow's milk protein in the parent's milk contributing to excessive crying and irritability in infants continues to be reported (Al-Beltagi et al., 2022). Because of the length of time it may take for bovine IgG to clear from the milk, a 2- to 4-week dairy-free trial may be necessary to identify if cow's milk protein is contributing to the infant's symptoms (Al-Beltagi et al., 2022; Gordon et al., 2018).

A nursing parent who suspects an intolerance to cow's milk might try eliminating dairy foods from their diet for 2weeks. If cow's milk is the cause of the infant's excessive crying, they may see some improvement in 48 hours. Full resolution of the symptoms could take 2 to 4 weeks. The parent can then reintroduce dairy slowly into their diet. They can start with hard cheeses or yogurt the first week, add soft cheeses in the second week, add butter and ice cream in the third week, and add cow's milk in small quantities in the fourth week. If the baby becomes fussy or other symptoms return, the parent can once again reduce their intake of dairy products.

A completely dairy-free diet eliminates all dairy products, including whey, casein, and sodium caseinate. Parents who use a dairy elimination diet need to read food labels because casein is used as a binder in many processed foods. Be cautious in recommending an elimination diet so that the parent does not perceive that their milk is harmful to the infant because this can lead to early weaning (McWilliam et al., 2023). Recent systematic reviews have found little significant clinical efficacy for dietary modifications (Gordon et al., 2018; Perry et al., 2019).

Lactose Overload

Lactose, the sugar in human milk, is crucial for brain development. The amount of lactose in the milk is independent of the parent's diet. Approximately 20% of lactose passes undigested into the large intestine, where it promotes the proliferation of healthy bacteria (Mikkelsen, 2014). The enzyme **lactase** breaks down lactose. Damage to the gut lining resulting from the infant receiving cow's milk protein may compromise lactase production (Heine et al., 2017). Alternatively, the increase in the amount of lactose may be too rapid for the lactase to break down the lactose, resulting in **lactose overload** symptoms. An infant with lactose overload may produce green, frothy, loose, and frequent stools. Poor weight gain, a bloated abdomen, and excessive of gas are also symptoms and are very similar to the symptoms of food intolerance.

Causes of Lactose Overload. Ending a feeding from one side before letdown has occurred results in the baby ingesting a larger ratio of foremilk on the first side and then filling up on foremilk again on the second side. Although the amount of lactose is the same in both foremilk and hindmilk, fat concentrations are low in foremilk and high in hindmilk. An infant who consumes an excessive amount of foremilk receives a higher percentage of lactose in comparison with the percentage of fat. The excess lactose then ferments in the baby's gut, which can lead to gassiness and fussiness. Fat intake varies between feedings, and the emptier the breast, the higher the fat content. Thus, allowing the baby to remain on each side long enough to drain it will ensure adequate fat intake. Some babies may need to nurse repeatedly on the same side before they switch to the other side. **Chapter 9** discusses milk composition.

Overabundant milk production can cause the baby to take in more lactose than their gut can digest. When the extra lactose reaches the lower bowel, normal gut bacteria release gas and causes pain. A parent with overabundant milk production might try nursing on one side for several feedings before switching. This should be recommended only after a full feeding assessment that includes before- and after-feeding (ac/pc) weights measured on a digital scale. This intervention may be combined with pumping residual milk. For example, a baby might present with markers for overabundant milk production, but when ac/pc weights are done, the baby will have had an intake of only 2 or 3 ounces. In this case, the fussy behavior may be unrelated to nursing.

Lactose Intolerance. Lactose overload should not be confused with lactose intolerance. You may encounter a parent who says their baby is "lactose intolerant." This is a misconception propagated by superficial media and formula companies selling "lactose-free" products. Lactose intolerance occurs when a person does not produce enough lactase—the enzyme required to digest lactose—and therefore cannot digest lactose. Thus, lactose intolerance is a result of insufficient lactase, not a condition in and of itself. As people age, their bodies begin to produce less lactase. Up to 70% of the world's population has **lactase deficiency**, or **lactase nonpersistence**. This is indicative of the body's maturation as a child matures and weans from human milk. It is rare for children to have primary lactase deficiency before 3 years of age, even in populations with genetic propensities for it, such as Asians, South Americans, and Africans (Heine et al., 2017). This is also reflective of the biologically normal ages for weaning.

Treatment of Excessive Crying

Treatments for excessive crying range from folk remedies to prescription medication. Successful calming techniques for fussiness include holding, nursing, walking, and rocking. Carrying the infant taps into neurophysiological responses and is especially effective (Zeevenhooven et al., 2018). Excessive crying correlates with a shorter duration of exclusive nursing. Giving anticipatory guidance about infant feeding, crying, and recommended nursing duration will help ensure that parents continue nursing as long as desired.

Physical Therapy

Many parents seek help from chiropractic care, massage therapy, or craniosacral therapy for excessive crying (Perry et al., 2019). Referral to occupational or physical therapy may help reduce parental distress by addressing the baby's symptoms. Chiropractic care involves gentle pressure to relieve nerve compression that impairs the affected system. Most parents find an improvement in symptoms. Massage has relaxing effects on both the baby and the parent, enhances parent–infant interaction and infant sleep, and lowers levels of stress hormones. Massage of preterm babies in the neonatal intensive care unit is linked to greater weight gain, earlier discharge, and increased developmental scores (Campbell & Jacobs, 2021; Pados & McGlothen-Bell, 2019). **Figure 14-20** describes one effective technique for infant massage. Sometimes, the baby will cry throughout the massage but be calm by the end. Other infants may respond immediately. Many resources for infant massage abound online, through community classes, and in print media. Resources from the International Association of Infant Massage (IAIM, 2019) can be helpful for parents.

- Hold the naked baby on the parent's lap, supine, with the baby's head resting on the parent's knees.
- Gently massage the baby's stomach, shoulders, head, hands, and feet.
- Turn the baby over and massage the back.
- Hold and soothe the baby against the parent's shoulder until the crying ceases.

Figure 14-20 Technique for infant massage.

Home Remedies

Some parents use homeopathic preparations for excessive crying. Many cultures promote home remedies such as chamomile, catnip, fennel, dill, and anise. A recent review found some evidence that fennel preparations may be effective, with no reported adverse effects (Çetinkaya, 2021). However, results from various studies are not conclusive (Perry et al., 2019). Parents should discuss their options with their baby's caregiver before they use any over-the-counter, herbal, or folk remedy. Such treatments may even be dangerous. The use of Japanese star anise has resulted in infant poisoning (Obando Pacheco et al., 2016).

Medication

Prescription medication is available for relieving excessive crying. Dicyclomine, an anticholinergic agent used to treat the symptoms of irritable bowel syndrome, relieves muscle spasms in the GI tract. Some caregivers prescribe simethicone (Mylicon) drops or cimetropium bromide. The use of medication such as simethicone reportedly has little to no effect on crying duration (Ellwood et al., 2020; Hjern et al., 2020). Supplementing the infant with probiotics, *Lactobacillus reuteri* in particular, may help to reduce crying (dos Reis Buzzo Zermiani et al., 2021; Perry et al., 2019).

Comfort Techniques

Table 14-10 identifies interventions parents can try while they seek the cause of excessive crying. **Figure 14-21**, depicts one technique, with the parent placing the baby across their lap. If all measures used to comfort the baby fail, the parents should consult their baby's caregiver to rule out a medical condition. The potential harm associated with diagnosis and treatment may surpass any harm from the excessive crying. Families will benefit from reassurance, social support, and the tincture of time (Zeevenhooven et al., 2018).

Table 14-10 Measures for Comforting a Crying Baby

Holding techniques	"Wear" the baby around the house in a cloth baby sling, making sure the nose is not blocked. Walk and dance in a soothing manner. Hold the baby upright against the parent's shoulder near the neck. Place the baby on their stomach across the parent's lap or knees. Carry the baby against the parent's hip. Lay the baby face down on the parent's chest. Lay the baby face down on the inside of the parent's forearm with the baby's head held in the crook of the parent's arm. The pressure on the stomach feels good, and the parent's free hand can pat and rub the baby's back. Pick up the baby as soon as they start to fuss to decrease the length of fussiness and prevent it from escalating.
Sounds and motion	Provide a steady noise from a vacuum, clothes dryer, music, humming, or a recording of the parent's heartbeat. Speak closely and softly in whispers. Position baby to gaze at the parent's face. Provide an unexpected distraction to startle the baby to cease crying. Take the baby for a car ride to provide soothing, rhythmic motion. Bounce, swing, rock, and walk in slow, rhythmical movements.
Security and warmth	Place the baby in a warm bath. Check for any rashes that could indicate a reaction to the fiber or detergent in clothing or blankets. Swaddle the baby to provide closeness and security, or unswaddle them if the blanket seems too constricting. Check the diaper for dampness and keep the baby warm with sweaters or blankets. Place a warmed hot water bottle against the baby's stomach area to help them release tension and pass gas. Fold the baby's legs up to their stomach in a bicycle motion to help eliminate gas.

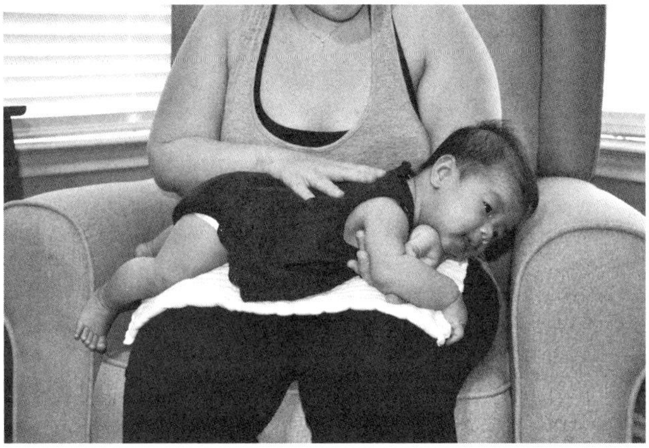

Figure 14-21 Placing the baby on their stomach across the parent's lap can help relieve excessive crying.

Printed with permission of Lyly Tran.

Supporting the Parents

When a baby cries excessively, parents' stress and concern naturally increase. They will need support, frequent contact, reassurance, and resources to assist them in caring for their child. Many online parenting resources are available. Breastfeeding support groups and online meetings can provide a support network to help families get through this intense and difficult beginning to their baby's life.

Physical exhaustion is common from constantly trying to comfort a crying baby. Parents who experience excessive crying may feel frustration and guilt for resenting their child. The baby may sense the parent's emotional state and be comforted immediately when another person picks them up. This can further add to a parent's feelings of guilt and inadequacy. They may feel that their baby is rejecting them and that they are the cause of the baby's crying. During this time, parents need a great deal of emotional support.

Caring for an infant with unexplained, persistent crying is one of the most stressful and common concerns for new parents. Interaction between parents and their infant is compromised, and tension can further aggravate the baby's condition. Parents need an avenue for venting anger and frustration. Encourage them to seek help if they feel they cannot cope with their baby's crying. They will benefit from the support of someone who is receptive, caring, and reassuring.

Home-based healthcare intervention and support, when available, help reduce parenting stress and improve interactions between parents and their infants.

Parents may need to take a break and spend some time away from the baby to keep their perspective. These time outs are critical to keeping their baby safe. Persistent crying places babies at risk for shaken baby syndrome (Zeevenhooven et al., 2018). Shaking can cause brain damage, blindness, and death (Laurent-Vannier, 2022). Time outs and support are especially critical in preventing shaking the baby in frustration. No baby was ever hurt by being put safely in a crib while the parent took a much-needed break. Parents need to recognize the causes and dangers of shaken baby syndrome and know never to shake or handle the baby roughly.

Summary

Infant assessment is a significant part of caring for nursing families. Recognizing deviations from normal in the infant's body, posture, skin, head, and reflexes provides important information about the child's condition. Assessment of the infant's oral structure and elimination patterns will help determine whether changes are needed in feeding management. Learning about normal baby behavior and how to recognize and interpret infant signals helps parents stay tuned in to their baby's needs. As parents learn about their infant's behavior, growth, sleeping, crying, and digestion patterns, they become proficient in interpreting their babies' behaviors and more confident in their parenting abilities.

What You Learned—At a Glance

Conversation Starters with Parents

- How do you know when your baby is hungry?
- How do your nipples feel when your baby sucks?
- How can you tell that your baby is receiving milk during a feeding?
- How is your baby's pattern of burping ... wet and dirty diapers ... weight ... sleep?
- How comfortable does your baby seem between and after feedings?

Elements of Newborn Assessment

- Body tone can indicate possible congenital anomalies or the need for assistance with positioning for feedings.
- Skin turgor indicates hydration status.
- Severe caput succedaneum or cephalhematoma can lead to feeding difficulties or jaundice.
- Facial asymmetry or torticollis can lead to potential latch and sucking difficulty.
- Low-fat buccal pads indicate a possible need to assist with latch.
- Short tongue, tight frenulum or frenum, or other inability to extend the tongue over the alveolar ridge can interfere with latch and cause nipple damage.
- High palate or palatal defects, such as a cleft of the soft palate, a submucosal cleft, or a bifurcated (bifid) uvula, could interfere with latch or sucking.
- Fractured clavicle or sensitivity from forceps or vacuum can cause feeding discomfort or impairment.
- Nutritive and nonnutritive sucking indicate whether the baby is receiving milk.

Digestion

- Burping decreases gas pain and reduces spitting up.
- The amount, frequency, and force of spit-up indicates whether a change in lactation management is needed.
- Spitting up multiple times in a day can be a sign of GER.
- GERD is associated with esophagitis, low weight gain, faltering growth, and respiratory disorders.
- Monitoring voids and stools ensures adequate nourishment.
- Recognizing normal stool consistency helps parents rule out constipation or diarrhea.

Infant Communication and Behavior

- Infants communicate through approach and avoidance behaviors.
- Hunger cues are most evident in a light sleep, drowsy, or quiet and alert state.
- If hunger cues are unheeded, the baby may cry or fall back asleep.
- The infant's behavior pattern, which ranges from easygoing to active and fussy, may affect nursing.
- Knowing how to stimulate a sleepy or undemanding baby and comfort a fussy baby will help parents ensure the baby's adequate nourishment.

Infant Growth

- Healthy, full-term infants self-regulate food intake.
- Passage of meconium and urine may result in up to 7% to 10% of newborn birth weight.
- Weight loss over 10% requires careful assessment of feeding and possible intervention.
- Heavy maternal load of IV fluids is associated with faster and greater infant weight loss.
- Weight should stabilize by the end of the first week, with birth weight regained by 10 to 21 days.
- WHO growth charts provide normal weight patterns in nursing babies.

Sleep

- The AAP recommends that nursing parents and babies sleep in proximity to each other.
- Guidelines are available for parents to create a safe environment for cosleeping.
- Nursing reduces the risk of SIDS by approximately 50%.
- Sleeping in a prone position and parental smoking are risk factors for SIDS.

Crying

- Infants cry to elicit parental response to meet their needs.
- A newborn may cry from hunger approximately 1½ to 2 hours or more after a feeding.
- Some babies settle when swaddled or carried in a sling.
- A baby who cries excessively has severe abdominal discomfort, piercing cries, and explosive attacks.
- Infants born preterm and small for gestational age are at risk for excessive crying.
- Prenatal drug use and parental intake of nicotine can cause excessive crying.
- Cow's milk protein accounts for up to 30% of excessive crying in nursing infants.
- Babies are usually not bothered by foods in the nursing parent's diet.
- Consuming an unbalanced amount of foremilk and hindmilk can cause excessive crying.
- Infant massage may help relieve excessive crying.
- Herbal preparations for excessive crying should be used with caution because of the possible toxicity of some substances.

References

Abdul Jafar NK, et al. Association between breastfeeding and sleep patterns in infants and preschool children. *Am J Clin Nutr*. 2021;114(6):1986–1996.

Abdulezer A, et al. Xanthan- and rice cereal-based thickeners in infants: a multidisciplinary single-center experience. *J Pediatr Gastroenterol Nutr.* 2022;3(2):e190.

Abel J, Hrishikesh S. Jaundice. In: *StatPearls*. Treasure Island, FL: StatPearls Publishing; August 8, 2023. https://www.ncbi.nlm.nih.gov/books/NBK544252/

Academy of Breastfeeding Medicine. Clinical protocol #16: breastfeeding the hypotonic infant. Revision. August 2016. https://www.bfmed.org/protocols

Al-Beltagi M, et al. Cow's milk-induced gastrointestinal disorders: from infancy to adulthood. *World J Clin Pediatr*. 2022;11(6):437–454.

Almaramhy HH, Al-Zalabani AH. The association of prenatal and postnatal macrolide exposure with subsequent development of infantile hypertrophic pyloric stenosis: a systematic review and meta-analysis. *Ital J Pediatr.* 2019;45(1):20.

American Academy of Pediatrics. Policy statement. The Apgar score. American Academy of Pediatrics Committee on Fetus and Newborn, American College of Obstetricians and Gynecologists Committee on Obstetric Practice. *Pediatrics*. 2015;136(4):819–822.

American Academy of Pediatrics, Task Force on Sudden Infant Death Syndrome. SIDS and other sleep-related infant deaths: updated 2016 recommendations for a safe infant sleeping environment. *Pediatrics*. 2016;138(5):e20162938.

Anderson JE, et al. Epidemiology of Hirschsprung disease in California from 1995 to 2013. *Pediatr Surg Int*. 2018;34(12):1299–1303.

Ankyloglossia Bodyworkers. Benefits of bodywork. 2019. https://www.ankyloglossiabodyworkers.com/benefits-of-bodywork.html

Appleton J, et al. Infant formula feeding practices associated with rapid weight gain: a systematic review. *Matern Child Nutr.* 2018;14(3):e12602.

Arakoni R, et al. Very early onset perinatal constipation: can it be cow's milk protein allergy? *World J Gastroenterol*. 2023;29(33):4920–4926.

Arya S, et al. Facial asymmetry in a crying newborn: a comparison of two cases and review of literature. *Case Rep Pediatr.* 2017;2017:6368239.

Ataş AN, Özerdoğan N. Perceived sleep quality and fatigue in a population of new mothers: a cross-sectional study comparing relationships with breastfeeding and bottle feeding. *Breastfeed Med*. 2022;17(2):155–162.

Azad MB, et al. CHILD Study Investigators. Infant feeding and weight gain: separating breast milk from breastfeeding and formula from food. *Pediatrics*. 2018;142(4).

Baddock SA, et al. The influence of bed-sharing on infant physiology, breastfeeding and behaviour: a systematic review. *Sleep Med Rev.* 2019;43:106–117.

Ballard JL, et al. Ankyloglossia: assessment, incidence, and effect of frenuloplasty on the breastfeeding dyad. *Pediatrics*. 2002;110(5):e63.

Barr R, et al. Education about crying in normal infants is associated with a reduction in pediatric emergency room visits for crying complaints. *J Dev Behav Pediatr*. 2015;36(4):252–257.

Barry ES, McKenna JJ. Reasons mothers bedshare: a review of its effects on infant behavior and development. *Infant Behav Dev*. 2022;66:101684.

Bartick M, Tomori C. Sudden infant death and social justice: A syndemics approach. *Matern Child Nutr.* 2019;15(1):e12652

Batista CLC, et al. Nutritive and non-nutritive sucking patterns associated with pacifier use and bottle-feeding in full-term infants. *Early Hum Dev*. 2019;132:18–23.

Batista Borges Pereira M. Tongue-and lip-tie beyond breastfeeding difficulties. *JFOCG*. 2022;2(2):64–72.

Baxter R, et al. *Tongue-Tied: How a Tiny String Under the Tongue Impacts Nursing, Speech, Feeding, and More*. Pelham, AL: Alabama Tongue-Tie Center; 2018.

Bell KA, et al. Associations of infant feeding with trajectories of body composition and growth. *Am J Clin Nutr*. 2017;106(2):491–498.

Bellaïche M, et al. Gastroesophageal reflux and sleep position of infants. A survey conducted in France by 493 pediatricians. *Arch Pediatr.* 2017;24(1):17–23 [in French].

Benoiton L, et al. Management of posterior ankyloglossia and upper lip ties in a tertiary otolaryngology outpatient clinic. *Int J Pediatr Otorhinolaryngol*. 2016;88:13–16.

Blair PS, et al. Bedsharing and breastfeeding: the Academy of Breastfeeding Medicine Protocol #6, Revision 2019. *Breastfeed Med*. 2020;15(1):5–16.

Boronat-Catalá M, et al. Association between duration of breastfeeding and malocclusions in primary and mixed dentition: a systematic review and meta-analysis. *Sci Rep*. 2017;7(1):5048.

Campanha SMA, et al. Association between ankyloglossia and breastfeeding. *Codas*. 2019;31(1):e20170264.

Campbell M, Jacobs L. The effect of parent-administered infant massage on the developmental outcomes of premature infants. *SAJOT*. 2021;51(1).

Carnino JM, et al. The effect of frenectomy for tongue-tie, lip-tie, or cheek-tie on breastfeeding outcomes: a systematic review of articles over time and suggestions for management. *Int J Pediatr Otorhinolaryngol*. 2023;171:111638.

Centers for Disease Control and Prevention. Data and statistics—SIDS and SUID. March 8, 2023. https://www.cdc.gov/sids/data.htm

Cerda J, et al. Infant morbidity and mortality attributable to prenatal smoking in Chile. *Rev Panam Salud Publica*. 2017;41:e106.

Çetinkaya B. Complementary and alternative therapies for infantile colic: a systematic review of the literature. *Altern Ther Health Med*. 2021;27(2):42–47.

Chabra S, Peeples ES. Assessment and management of gastroesophageal reflux in the newborn. *Pediatric Annals*. 2020;49(2):e77–e81.

Chadha A, Jahnke M. Common neonatal rashes. *Pediatr Ann*. 2019;48(1):e16–e22.

Clyne P, Kulczycki A. Human breast milk contains bovine IgG: relationship to infant colic? *Pediatrics*. 1991;87:439–444.

Cole R, et al. Infant care practices and parent uptake of safe sleep messages: a cross-sectional survey in Queensland, Australia. *BMC Pediatr*. 2020;20(1):27.

Conradt E, et al. Prenatal opioid exposure: neurodevelopmental consequences and future research priorities. *Pediatrics*. 2019;144(3):e20190128.

Cordray H, et al. Severity and prevalence of ankyloglossia-associated breastfeeding symptoms: a systematic review and meta-analysis. *Acta Paediatr*. 2023; 112(3):347–357.

Daelemans S, et al. Recent advances in understanding and managing infantile colic. *F1000Res*. 2018;7:F1000 Faculty Rev-1426.

Darmstadt GL, et al. Validation of visual estimation of neonatal jaundice in low-income and middle-income countries: a multicentre observational cohort study. *BMJ Open*. 2021;11(12):e048145–e048145.

De Bruyne P, Ito S. Toxicity of long-term use of proton pump inhibitors in children. *Arch Dis Child*. 2018;103(1):78–82.

Deering JJ, et al. A comparison of infant sleep safety guidelines in nine industrialized countries. *J Community Health*. 2018;44(1):81–87.

Desaunay P, et al. Neonatal hypotonia following in utero exposure to antidepressant drugs. *J Pediatr*. 2022;245:222–226.e2.

Diaz de Ortiz LE, Mendez MD. Epstein pearls. PubMed. 2020. https://www.ncbi.nlm.nih.gov/books/NBK493177/

Dioguardi M, et al. Labial frenectomy using laser: a scoping review. *Int J Dent*. 2023:7321735.

Dionis I, et al. Reliability of visual assessment of neonatal jaundice among neonates of Black descent: a cross-sectional study from Tanzania. *BMC Pediatrics*. 2021;21(1).

Dixley A, Ball HL. The effect of swaddling on infant sleep and arousal: a systematic review and narrative synthesis. *Front Pediatr*. 2022;10:1000180.

dos Reis Buzzo Zermiani AP, et al. Evidence of *Lactobacillus reuteri* to reduce colic in breastfed babies: systematic review and meta-analysis. *CAM*. 2021;63:102781.

D'Souza L, et al. Understanding motivations and satisfaction with sleep location among co-sleeping (including bed-sharing) parents. *Fam Relat*. 2023;73(2):661–682.

El-Gohary Y, et al. Pyloric stenosis: an enigma more than a century after the first successful treatment. *Pediatr Surg Int*. 2018;34(1):21–27.

Ellwood J, et al. Comparison of common interventions for the treatment of infantile colic: a systematic review of reviews and guidelines. *BMJ Open*. 2020;10(2):e035405.

Ersen A, et al. Approach to the differential diagnosis of hypotonia in infancy. In: Diniz G, ed. *Clues for Differential Diagnosis of Neuromuscular Disorders*. New York: Springer; 2023:275–284.

Eshete M, et al. Congenital palatal fistula associated with submucous cleft palate. *Plast Reconstr Surg Glob Open*. 2016;4(2):e613.

Etherton H, et al. Discussion of extinction-based behavioral sleep interventions for young children and reasons why parents may find them difficult. *J Clin Sleep Med*. 2016;12(11):1535–1543.

Evans SH, et al. Hypertonia. *Curr Probl Pediatr Adolesc Health Care*. 2017;47(7):161–166.

FACES: The National Craniofacial Association. What is velo-cardio-facial syndrome? February 18, 2016. https://www.faces-cranio.org

Fairmont I, et al. The presence of a submucous cleft palate in patients with isolated cleft lip and middle ear dysfunction. *Am J Otolaryngol*. 2024;45(4):104281.

Firooz M, et al. Parental factors affecting the incidence of infantile colic: a systematic review. *J Pediatrics Review*. 2021;9(2):105–114.

Flaherman VJ, et al. Newborn weight loss during birth hospitalization and breastfeeding outcomes through age 1 month. *J Hum Lact*. 2017;33(1):225–230.

Fölster-Holst R. Differential diagnoses of diaper dermatitis. *Pediatr Dermatol*. 2018;35(suppl 1):s10–s18.

Forbes TR. Witch's milk and witches' marks. *Yale J Biol Med*. 1950;22(3):219–225.

Friedman C, et al. Understanding gastroesophageal reflux disease in children. *JAAPA*. 2021;34(2):12–18.

Froggatt S, et al. Infant neurobehavioural consequences of prenatal cigarette exposure: a systematic review and meta-analysis. *Acta Paediatr*. 2020;109(6):1112–1124.

Gelfand AA. Infant colic. *Semin Pediatr Neurol*. 2016;23(1):79–82.

Genna CW. *Supporting Sucking Skills in Breastfeeding Infants*. 3rd ed. Burlington, MA: Jones and Bartlett Learning; 2017.

Ghaheri BA, et al. Breastfeeding improvement following tongue-tie and lip-tie release: a prospective cohort study. *Laryngoscope*. 2017;127(5):1217–1223.

Gieruszczak-Białek D, et al. No effect of proton pump inhibitors on crying and irritability in infants: systematic review of randomized controlled trials. *J Pediatr*. 2015;166(3):767–770.e3.

Gordon M, et al. Dietary modifications for infantile colic. *Cochrane Database Syst Rev*. 2018;10:CD011029.

Grossman M, Berkwitt A. Neonatal abstinence syndrome. *Semin Perinat*. 2019;43(3):173–186.

Gur S, et al. Radiological and genetic evaluation in hypotonic Infants. *J Coll Physicians Surg Pak*. 2023;33(9):1028–1034.

Hale T, Krutsch K. *Hale's Medications & Mothers' Milk 2025–2026: A Manual of Lactational Pharmacology*. 21st ed. New York, NY: Springer Publishing Company; 2024.

Hanny KH, et al. Late detection of cleft palate. *Eur J Pediat*. 2016;175:71–80.

Heine RG, et al. Lactose intolerance and gastrointestinal cow's milk allergy in infants and children—common misconceptions revisited. *World Allergy Organ J*. 2017;10(1):41.

Hernandez-Reif M, Gungordu N. Infant sleep behaviors relate to their later cognitive and language abilities and morning cortisol stress hormone levels. *Infant Behav Dev*. 2022;67:101700.

Hjern A, et al. A systematic review of prevention and treatment of infantile colic. *Acta Paediatr*. 2020;109(9):1733–1744.

Holden E, et al. Natal and neonatal teeth: a review and management recommendations. *J Neonatal Nurs*. 2022;28:240–243.

Horta BL, et al. Systematic review and meta-analysis of breastfeeding and later overweight or obesity expands on previous study for World Health Organization. *Acta Paediatr*. 2023;112(1):34–41.

Huang J, et al. Early feeding of larger volumes of formula milk is associated with greater body weight or overweight in later infancy. *Nutr J*. 2018;17(1):12.

Hussain S, et al. You can have your breastmilk and safe sleep too: a preliminary analysis of infant safe sleep data in a Midwestern home visiting program. *Inj Epidemiol*. 2018;5(suppl 1):14.5.

Ingram J, et al. The development and evaluation of a picture tongue assessment tool for tongue-tie in breastfed babies (TABBY). *Int Breastfeed J*. 2019;14:31.

International Association of Infant Massage. 2019. Home page. https://www.iaim.net

International Chiropractic Pediatric Association. Advancing the family wellness lifestyle. 2018. https://www.icpa4kids.org

Islam MJ, et al. Early exclusive breastfeeding cessation and postpartum depression: assessing the mediating and moderating role of maternal stress and social support. *PLoS One*. 2021;16(5):e0251419.

Kalra N, et al. Neonatal molar in a child with Langerhan cell histiocytosis. *J Indian Soc Pedod Prev Dent*. 2019;37(1):107–109.

Kamath-Rayne BD, et al. Neonatal hyperbilirubinemia. In: Garder SL, et al., eds. *Merenstein & Gardner's Handbook of Neonatal Intensive Care: An Interprofessional Approach*. 9th ed. St. Louis: Elsevier; 2021:662–691.

Kamity R. Hypotonia in the newborn. In: Martin GI, Rosenfeld W, eds. *Common Problems in the Newborn Nursery*. Cham: Springer; 2019:171–182.

Kamphuis ASJ, et al. Cephalocaudal progression of neonatal jaundice assessed by transcutaneous bilirubin measurements. *Early Hum Dev*. 2021;160:105418.

Kapoor R, et al. Prevalence and descriptive epidemiology of infantile hypertrophic pyloric stenosis in the United States: a multistate, population-based retrospective study, 1999–2010. *Birth Defects Res*. 2019;111(3):159–169.

Kellams A, et al. ABM clinical protocol #3: supplementary feedings in the healthy term breastfed neonate, revised 2017. *Breastfeed Med*. 2017;12(4):188–198.

Kérourédan O, et al. Diagnosis and management of natal and neonatal teeth: case report of three newborns. *J Dent Child (Chic)*. 2018;85(2):79–82.

Kim OH, et al. Neurodevelopmental outcomes and comorbidities of children with congenital muscular torticollis: evaluation using the National Health Screening Program for Infants and Children database. *Clin Exp Pediatr*. 2022;65(6):312–319.

Kim S, Kochanska G. Evidence for childhood origins of conscientiousness: testing a developmental path from toddler age to adolescence. *Dev Psychol*. 2019;55(1):196–206.

Kinney HC, Haynes RL. The serotonin brainstem hypothesis for the sudden infant death syndrome. *J Neuropathol Exp Neurol*. 2019;78(9):765–779.

Kinser PA, et al. Depressive symptom prevalence and predictors in the first half of pregnancy. *J Women's Health (Larchmt)*. 2018;27(3):369–376.

Komori S, et al. Clinical study of laser treatment for frenectomy of pediatric patients. *Int J Clin Pediatr Dent*. 2017;10(3):272–277.

Kural B, Gökçay G. Association between infant sleep location and breastfeeding. *Breastfeed Med*. 2022;17(4).

Laurent-Vannier A. Shaken Baby Syndrome (SBS) or Pediatric Abusive Head Trauma from Shaking: Guidelines for Interventions During the Perinatal Period from the French National College Of Midwives. *J Midwifery Womens Health*. 2022;67:S93-S98

LeFort Y, et al. Academy of Breastfeeding Medicine position statement on ankyloglossia in breastfeeding dyads. *Breastfeed Med*. 2021;16(4):278–281.

Lenormand A, et al. Familial autosomal dominant severe ankyloglossia with tooth abnormalities. *Am J Med Genet A*. 2018;176(7):1614–1617.

Leung AK, Hon KL. Gastroesophageal reflux in children: an updated review. *Drugs Context*. 2019;8:212591.

Li J, et al. Epidemiological and clinical characteristics of 304 patients with infantile hypertrophic pyloric stenosis in Anhui Province of East China, 2012–2015. *J Matern Fetal Neonatal Med*. 2018;31(20):2742–2747.

Little EE, et al. Mother infant physical contact predicts responsive feeding among U.S. breastfeeding mothers. *Nutrients*. 2018;10(9).

Lopez RN, Lemberg DA. Gastro-oesophageal reflux disease in infancy: a review based on international guidelines. *Med J Austr*. 2019;212(1):40–44.

MacFarlane ME, et al. Infant sleep hazards and the risk of sudden unexpected death in infancy. *J Pediatr*. 2022;245:56–64.

Mai T, et al. Infantile colic: new insights into an old problem. *Gastroenterol Clin North Am*. 2018;47(4):829–844.

Mairuhu MA, et al. Exclusive breastfeeding lowers incidence of gastroesophageal reflux in infants: a 12-month cohort study. *IJRP*. 2021;82(1):58–62.

McKenna JJ, Gettler LT. There is no such thing as infant sleep, there is no such thing as breastfeeding, there is only breastsleeping. *Acta Paediatr.* 2016;105(1):17–21.

McWilliam V, et al., World Allergy Organization (WAO) Diagnosis and Rationale for Action against Cow's Milk Allergy (DRACMA) guidelines update - X - Breastfeeding a baby with cow's milk allergy. *World Allergy Organ J.* 2023;16(11):1-14.

Michalska A, et al. Asymmetric crying facies: its meaning in the differential diagnosis of congenital developmental abnormalities. *Medical Studies.* 2019;35(4):312–318.

Mikkelsen A. Children's hypersensitivity to cow's milk. Public health aspects and impact on families. Public Health Epidemiology Unit, Institute of Medicine Sahlgrenska Academy at University of Gothenburg. 2014. https://gupea.ub.gu.se/handle/2077/34816

Mileva-Seitz VR, et al. Parent-child bed-sharing: the good, the bad, and the burden of evidence. *Sleep Med Rev.* 2017;32:4–27.

Mills N, et al. What is a tongue tie? Defining the anatomy of the in-situ lingual frenulum. *Clin Anat.* January 30, 2019;32(6):749–761.

Moon RY, et al. Sleep-related infant deaths: updated 2022 recommendations for reducing infant deaths in the sleep environment. *Pediatrics.* 2022;150(1):e2022057990.

Moretti E, et al. The bowel movement characteristics of exclusively breastfed and exclusively formula fed infants differ during the first three months of life. *Acta Paediatr.* 2019;108(5):877–881.

Mother-Baby Behavioral Sleep Laboratory. Safe cosleeping guidelines. University of Notre Dame. 2025. https://cosleeping.nd.edu/safe-co-sleeping-guidelines/

Muldoon K, et al. Effect of frenotomy on breastfeeding variables in infants with ankyloglossia (tongue-tie): a prospective before and after cohort study. *BMC Pregnancy Childbirth.* 2017;17(1):373.

Nakhash R, et al. Upper lip tie and breastfeeding: a systematic review. *Breastfeed Med.* 2019;14(2):83–87.

Narendran V. The skin of the neonate. In: Martin RJ, Fanaroff AA, Walsh MC, eds. *Fanaroff & Martin's Neonatal-Perinatal Medicine: Diseases of the Fetus and Infant.* 11th ed. St. Louis: Elsevier; 2020:1898–1933.

National Institutes of Health. Campaign history. Safe to Sleep. https://safetosleep.nichd.nih.gov. 2024. https://safetosleep.nichd.nih.gov/campaign/history#:~:text=Led%20by%20the%20Eunice%20Kennedy

Noh Y, et al., Prenatal and infant exposure to acid-suppressive medications and risk of allergic diseases in children. *JAMA Pediatr,* 2023;177(3):267–277.

Núñez-Martínez PM, et al. Congenital macroglossia: clinical features and therapeutic strategies in pediatric patients. *Bol Med Hosp Infant Mex.* 2016;73(3):212–216.

Obando Pacheco P, et al. Liver failure secondary to poisoning by a homemade product made of star and green anise in a 4-month-old infant. *Rev Esp Enferm Dig.* 2016;108(12):819–821.

Orlandi S, et al. Application of pattern recognition techniques to the classification of full-term and preterm infant cry. *J Voice.* 2016;30(6):656–663.

O'Shea JE, et al. Frenotomy for tongue-tie in newborn infants. *Cochrane Database Syst Rev.* 2017;3:CD011065.

Ostertag-Hill CA, et al. Late diagnosis of Hirschsprung disease: clinical presentation and long-term functional outcomes. *J Pediatr Surg.* 2024;59(2):220–224.

Pados BF, McGlothen-Bell K. Benefits of infant massage for infants and parents in the NICU. *Nurs Women's Health.* 2019;23(3):265–271.

Parker K, Chia M. Breastfeeding: does it affect the occlusion? *Prim Dent J.* 2020;9(1):32–36.

Perry R, et al. An overview of systematic reviews of complementary and alternative therapies for infantile colic. *Syst Rev.* 2019;8(1):271.

Persson M, et al. Five and 10 minute Apgar scores and risks of cerebral palsy and epilepsy: population based cohort study in Sweden. *BMJ.* 2018;360:k207.

Power E, Sharif F. Period of purple crying program for the prevention of abusive head trauma/shaken baby syndrome. *Ir Med J.* 2021;114(7):415.

Queensland Health. Queensland clinical guidelines. Newborn baby assessment (routine). Guideline No. MN21.4-V6-R26. 2021. http://www.health.qld.gov.au/qcg

Rajani PS, et al. Presentation and management of food allergy in breastfed infants and risks of maternal elimination diets. *J Allergy Clin.* 2020;8(1):52–67.

Rosen R, et al. Pediatric gastroesophageal reflux clinical practice guidelines: joint recommendations of the North American Society for Pediatric Gastroenterology, Hepatology, and Nutrition and the European Society for Pediatric Gastroenterology, Hepatology, and Nutrition. *J Pediatr Gastroenterol Nutr.* 2018;66(3):516–554.

Salvatore S, et al. Cow's milk allergy or gastroesophageal reflux disease—can we solve the dilemma in infants? *Nutrients.* 2021;13(2):297.

Samycia M et al. Infantile acne. *CMAJ.* 2016;188(17–18):e540.

Sánchez-Molins M, et al. Comparative study of the craniofacial growth depending on the type of lactation received. *Eur J Paediatr Dent.* 2010;11(2):87–92.

Sardesai, S. Newborn birth injuries. In: Martin G, Rosenfeld W, eds. *Common Problems in the Newborn Nursery.* Cham: Springer, 2019. https://link.springer.com/book/10.1007/978-3-319-95672-5

Sarmiento-Aguilar A, et al. Percentage of birth weight loss as a reference for the well-being of the exclusively breastfed newborn. *Bole Méd Hospital Infant.* 2022;79(6):341–349.

Scannell M, Puka-Beals E. A guide to newborn assessment. *Nursing Made Incredibly Easy!* 2019;17(4):26–33.

Shah A, et al. Neonatal milk production (witch's milk). In: Knoop KJ, Stack LB, Storrow AB, Thursman R, eds. *The Atlas of Emergency Medicine.* 5th ed. New York: McGraw Hill; 2021. https://accessemergencymedicine.mhmedical.com/content.aspx?bookid=2969&sectionid=250460136

Shapiro-Mendoza CK, et al. Sudden unexpected infant deaths: 2015–2020. *Pediatrics.* 2023;151(4):e2022058820.

Shekher R, et al. How to treat a tongue-tie: an evidence-based algorithm of care. *Plast Reconstr Surg Glob Open.* 2021;9(1):e3336.

Shinya Y, et al. Fundamental frequency variation of neonatal spontaneous crying predicts language acquisition in preterm and term infants. *Front Psychol.* 2017;8:2195.

Smit JA, et al. Incidence of symptomatic submucous cleft palate in the Netherlands: a retrospective cohort study over a period of 22 years. *Cleft Palate Craniofac J.* 2021;58(9):1121–1127.

Smith CJF, et al. Infantile hemangiomas: an updated review on risk factors, pathogenesis, and treatment. *Birth Defects Res.* 2017;109(11):809–815.

Srimoragot M, et al. Infant feeding type and maternal sleep during the postpartum period: a systematic review and meta-analysis. *J Sleep Res.* 2022;32(2):e13625.

Stanford School of Medicine, Newborn Nursery at LPCH. Acrocyanosis. 2018. med.stanford.edu/newborns/professional-education/photo-gallery/general.html#acrocyanosis

Straathof EJM, et al. Development of muscle tone impairments in high-risk infants: associations with cerebral palsy and cystic periventricular leukomalacia. *Eur J Neurol*. 2022;37:12–18.

Tandırcıoğlu UA, et al. Effect of prostaglandin-E1 treatment on pyloric wall thickness in newborns with ductal-dependent critical congenital heart diseases. *Pediatr Surg Int*. 2023;39(1):144.

Tatekawa Y. Food protein-induced eosinophilic enteritis with intestinal stricture in a neonate: a case report and review of the literature. *J Surg Case Rep*. 2018;2018(7):rjy170.

Taylor M, et al. Oral candidiasis. In: *StatPearls*. Treasure Island, FL: StatPearls Publishing; 2023.

Thompson JMD, et al. Duration of breastfeeding and risk of SIDS: an individual participant data meta-analysis. *Pediatrics*. 2017;140(5).

U.S. Department of Health and Human Services, National Institutes of Health, National Center for Advancing Translational Sciences. *MTHFR* gene variant. September 22, 2017. https://rarediseases.info.nih.gov/diseases/10953/mthfr-gene-mutation

Vaidya S, et al. Developmental dysplasia of hip and post-natal positioning: role of swaddling and baby-wearing. *Indian J Orthop*. 2021;55(6):1410–1416.

van der Veek SMC, van Rosmalen L. Maternal satisfaction with professional health care for excessive infant crying: does it meet maternal needs? *Early Child Development and Care*. 2023;193(4):602–615.

Vandenplas Y, Kindt S. Gastroesophageal reflux. In: Guandalini S, Dhawan A, eds. *Textbook of Pediatric Gastroenterology, Hepatology and Nutrition*. Cham: Springer; 2022:125–155. https://link.springer.com/book/10.1007/978-3-030-80068-0

Verhave BL, et al. Embryology, lanugo. In: *StatPearls*. Treasure Island, FL: StatPearls Publishing; 2023. https://www.ncbi.nlm.nih.gov/books/NBK526092

Vincent A, et al. Sudden infant death syndrome: risk factors and newer risk reduction strategies. *Cureus*. 2023;15(6):e40572.

Volpe J. *Neurology of the Newborn*. 6th ed. Philadelphia, PA: Elsevier; 2018.

Wicaksono Y, et al. Pediatric gastroesophageal reflux disease (GERD): a literature review. *APGHN*. 2023;2(2):46–60.

Wilkins, MB. Common preventable defects of childhood. *NZMJ*. 2020;133(1520):157–161.

Wolke D, et al. Systematic review and meta-analysis: fussing and crying durations and prevalence of colic in infants. *J Pediatr*. 2017;185:55–61.e4.

World Health Organization. *WHO Multicentre Growth Reference Study Group: WHO child growth standards*. 2006. https://www.who.int/childgrowth/standards/en

Yoshida S, Funato H. Physical contact in parent-infant relationship and its effect on fostering a feeling of safety. *iScience*. 2021;24(7):102721.

Yozawitz E, et al. Neonatal hypotonia. *NeoReviews*. 2018;19(8):e445–e455.

Zakerihamidi MF, et al. Prevalence, risk factors, and prognosis of neonatal hypernatremia dehydration among full-term newborns: a systematic review. *JPNIM*. 2023;12(2):e120207.

Zeevenhooven J et al., Infant colic: mechanisms and management. *Nat Rev Gastroenterol Hepatol*. 2018;15(8):479–496.

Zhen L, et al. Fetal micrognathia in the first trimester: an ominous finding even after a normal array. *Eur J Obstetr Gynecol Reprod Bio*. 2021;263:176–180.

CHAPTER 15

Getting Nursing Started

With support, most parents and babies are able to nurse. Nursing is a combination of instinct and learned skill for the dyad. Parents have the innate desire to snuggle and cuddle with their newborns. They often instinctively hold their babies in positions that are similar to nursing, even at nonfeeding times. Some babies have difficulty in their initial attempts at nursing. Others begin feeding with little or no help. Both parents and babies will master nursing with time, patience, and gentle guidance as they learn to coordinate their natural behaviors with each other. You can support each family based on their distinct goals and needs.

KEY TERMS

Assisted reproductive technology (ART)
Asymmetrical latch
Biological nurturing
Calming techniques
C-hold
Clutch hold
Cradle hold
Cross-cradle hold
Dancer hand position
Dominant hand hold
Flange
Football hold
Fussy baby
Laid-back nursing
Latch
Modified side-sitting hold
Primitive neonatal reflexes (PNRs)
Rooting reflex
Searching response
Side-lying position
Side-sitting hold
Tandem nursing

Getting Ready to Nurse

New parents typically anticipate their first feeding with anticipation and excitement. Some may feel anxious or unprepared. Ideally, a parent and baby remain together and begin nursing shortly after the baby is born. The earlier feedings begin, the earlier the baby will receive colostrum, which promotes stooling. This early sucking also triggers milk production. Parents and babies should not be subjected to unnecessary separation that interferes with this process. Delays in initiating nursing can contribute to engorgement, low milk production, and shorter nursing duration (Froh et al., 2021; Wu et al., 2019).

Establishing a Nursing Routine

Parents may feel awkward with their newborn and with early feedings. Reassure them that this feeling of awkwardness is normal. It takes time to learn the nuances of holding and positioning the baby for feeding. These first sessions are ideal times for parents and babies to learn about each other and how they best work together. Nursing an infant usually becomes second nature very quickly.

A few simple preparations can help parents develop self-confidence and increase their comfort with nursing. Gathering a basket of items to have nearby during a feeding can be helpful. These items may include pillows to help with comfortable positioning, something to drink, a cloth for burping a cell phone, a tablet or laptop, remote control, reading material, breast pads, diapers, and baby wipes. Similar items can be kept in a diaper bag for feeding on the go. Silencing the phone will contribute to an undisturbed feeding. However, some parents find a feeding to be a quiet time to catch up with friends after the baby has settled in to nurse. Suggestions for relaxing and creating an optimal climate for feedings appear in **Table 15-1**.

Encouraging Baby-Led Feedings

Full-term, healthy newborns have the innate ability to tell their parents when they need to nurse and when they are finished. Imposing limits on feeding frequency and length can lead to frustration for everyone. Such restrictions create an unnecessary burden at a time when parents are becoming acquainted with their newborn. Babies, just like adults, are not always hungry at the same times every day as other babies. Allowing them to self-regulate their feedings will meet their individual needs for optimal growth.

Time restrictions on feedings can lead to engorgement for the parent and underfeeding for the baby. Moreover, not following babies' hunger cues overrides a baby's natural ability to self-regulate their feedings. This can lead to negative reactions and behaviors, including refusal to nurse. Interfering with the balance

Table 15-1 Creating a Relaxing and Effective Climate for Nursing

Issue	Suggestions
Relaxation techniques	■ Spend a few minutes before going to sleep and at other times to analyze your relaxation techniques (e.g., movements, positions, and room darkness). ■ Remove distractions (e.g., find a quiet spot and silence the phone). ■ Get comfortable (e.g., empty your bladder; find a cozy chair or bed; get pillows for support; remove eyeglasses, shoes, or tight clothing; adjust room temperature). ■ Listen to relaxing music. ■ Take a deep breath and let it out slowly. Repeat this several times. ■ Breathe steadily and rhythmically, noting the faint movement of your body. Breathe slowly to relax further. ■ Take a warm shower or bath prior to a feeding. ■ Close your eyes and move them back and forth or up and down. Then rest your eyes and feel the release of tension. Relax your eyes by envisioning a ship sailing away from you and disappearing over the horizon. ■ Allow your mind to drift into a sleepy state by thinking pleasant thoughts (e.g., enjoyable moments, pleasures, or dreams). ■ Think about your baby, milk flowing, or water rushing. ■ Think about, write down, or talk with someone about your fears, stresses, tensions, and what you think causes them. Then let your mind drift or think of pleasant thoughts and feel the release of tension. ■ Meditate on a passage of a text from a favorite author.
Creating an optimal climate	■ Nurse in a quiet spot away from distractions. ■ Avoid embarrassing or stressful situations when feeding. ■ Drink a favorite beverage before and during feeding. ■ Set up a routine for beginning feedings.
Self-care	■ Nap or rest when the baby rests. ■ Simplify daily chores and establish priorities around the baby. ■ Get help with household tasks, child care, and other responsibilities. ■ Take a break from the daily routine with an evening out, shopping, a walk, or lunch with a friend.
Feeding-related techniques	■ Use warm compresses before feeding. ■ Rub expressed milk onto the nipple to gently stimulate it. ■ Hold the baby skin to skin. ■ Lean back in a comfortable, reclined position to nurse, with baby prone on chest. ■ Use breast compression while baby is nursing. ■ Lie down to nurse. ■ Nurse baby in bed at night.

of foremilk and hindmilk intake can also lead to colic-like symptoms from lactose overload (Iacovou et al., 2021). Lactose overload in the small intestine causes fermentation and, consequently, increased gas and gut motility in the gastrointestinal tract. This can lead to a very uncomfortable, **fussy baby**. **Chapter 14** discusses lactose overload and excessive crying.

Encourage parents to watch their babies for hunger cues—not the clock. Babies cannot tell time. They simply know that they are unhappy when they are hungry and content when they are full. Scheduling feedings when the baby is not ready to nurse can produce frustration and cause the baby to be wary of the process. Hunger cues help parents know when their baby is ready for a feeding, as described in **Chapter 14**. A healthy, full-term baby exhibits a progression of signs that indicate a desire to feed. Help parents learn how to recognize their baby's feeding readiness. When they learn how to recognize hunger signs, they can trust their baby to lead the way.

Babies are equally able to indicate when a feeding is finished on one side. Encourage parents to begin a feeding on the side that received the least stimulation at the previous feeding and to continue nursing on that side until the baby releases the nipple. If the baby unlatches after only a short time, they can try burping or addressing any other discomfort the baby may have and then resume nursing on the same side. If feeding on one side seems especially lengthy, the parent can switch the feeding to the other side if sucking has become nonnutritive. Infants may not nurse from both sides at every feeding. In the early days of nursing, however, stimulating both sides equally will ensure optimal milk production.

Exceptions to Baby-Led Feedings

There are some instances when parents may need to monitor the time between feedings rather than relying on their baby to determine frequency. Babies born after long medicated labors can exhibit sleepiness and feeding challenges, as discussed in **Chapter 13**. In addition, many birthing parents have medically complex pregnancies. Preexisting issues with diabetes, hypertension, and obesity are associated with more difficult births and nursing difficulties (Feldman-Winter et al., 2020; Mallan et al., 2018). Other occurrences presenting feeding challenges include preterm or late preterm birth; birth trauma; and neurological or congenital issues such as Down syndrome, Turner syndrome, or cerebral palsy (Feldman-Winter et al., 2020; Hookway et al., 2021).

Babies with these conditions are sleepy, difficult to rouse, and ineffective at milk transfer. They frequently develop jaundice, which increases their sleepiness even further. These babies need a lot of stimulation and encouragement to nurse. They need frequent feedings and often require supplementation. Parents need to "watch the clock" temporarily and be vigilant that their baby receives sufficient calories for growth. Very early preterm babies often have significant health problems, such as cardiac or respiratory issues, that require continual monitoring and care by the parents. **Chapter 24** discusses these feeding issues.

Late preterm babies, born at 34 to 36 weeks' gestation, need to be monitored carefully as well. They do not always demonstrate strong hunger cues and need help with nursing skills (Carpay et al., 2021; Muelbert et al., 2019). The parents of a late preterm infant will benefit from targeted healthcare professional support for their nursing (Vizzari et al., 2023). Parents can focus on three goals: Feed the baby, protect milk production, and transition the baby to full nursing. Usually, as the due date approaches, the baby suddenly seems to "wake up" and begins to nurse robustly.

Beginning the Feeding

Newborns can be trusted to find their source of nourishment when they enter the world. If placed on the parent's abdomen at birth, babies' innate reflexes enable them to search for the nipple and **latch**. As feedings progress, parents can find a comfortable position that supports the baby's weight and enables the baby to maintain an effective, sustained latch. In most cases, the baby will suck effectively when placed in a comfortable position and when helpers are not overly intrusive. Holding the baby skin to skin in the early days will facilitate feedings and calm a fussy baby who is struggling to latch.

Newborn Reflexes

Babies are neurologically primed to nurse. They have an innate ability after birth to root, find, and latch onto the nipple when given time and the opportunity to do so (Bergman, 2017; Widström et al., 2019; Yin et al., 2021). Newborns use a series of innate neurosensory cues to search for and independently find the teat, grasp it, and suck (Smillie, 2023). Newborn behaviors include the stepping response to scoot up the parent's body to the breast, bobbing the head, rooting to find the nipple, grasping to achieve latch, and commencing sucking, as classically documented by Righard and Alade in 1990. As feedings begin in the postpartum period, birth attendants should provide "hands-off" support to allow infants an opportunity to self-attach (Yin et al., 2021).

Rooting Reflex

When the baby's head is turned away from the nipple, stimulating the **rooting reflex** entices the baby to turn back toward the nipple. Touching the baby's cheek with the nipple causes their head to turn toward the stimulus, with their mouth opened wide and their tongue extended. Caution parents to avoid stimulating any other part of the baby's face. The baby will instinctively root toward the new source of the stimulation and may become confused and frustrated. Licking movements precede rooting when the infant is in an alert state.

Attempting to start a feeding when the baby is not ready to nurse can disturb the rooting–tongue reflex process. When crying, the baby's tongue moves up toward the palate. If pushed to latch (even with gentle pressure), a crying infant may remember the sensation and defensively place their tongue up toward the palate at subsequent feedings. This reaction may also occur if a parent attempts a feeding when the baby is not demonstrating signs of hunger. The action may cause the infant to pull their head back or lead to feeding aversion (Smillie, 2023).

Other Primitive Neonatal Reflexes

Although much research has focused on rooting, sucking, and swallowing, other individual newborn reflexes play important roles in robust nursing behavior as well. **Primitive neonatal reflexes (PNRs)** can either stimulate or impair nursing. They include 20 feeding behaviors and positions classified into four types (endogenous, motor, rhythmic, and antigravity) and two functional clusters (finding/latching and milk transfer). For example, rather than the newborn preferring to lie on a side with pressure along the back, researchers postulate that the newborn is an abdominal feeder and, like some other animals, displays antigravity reflexes that aid latch.

The reflexes most significantly involved in the immediate postpartum period are described in **Figure 15-1**. They are beautifully detailed in a video, *Breast Crawl*, available free online in several languages (United Nations Children's Fund, 2019). Playing a brief video clip can help familiarize parents with these innate abilities before the baby is born in preparation for providing immediate skin-to-skin care.

Healthcare providers need to respect the newborn's early hours and not attempt to intervene unless medically indicated. Providing uninterrupted time to allow these reflexes to be expressed can be challenging in hospitals with time constraints and medicated deliveries that blunt newborn instinctive behaviors. Every healthy parent and vigorous baby should be given the time and support for remaining together skin to skin to begin nursing.

Positioning at Feedings

Effective positioning will provide the optimal circumstances for the baby to nurse. The parent's position and the baby's body position are both important elements in feeding. The parent needs to be comfortable and relaxed, with support for the baby's weight. The baby needs the opportunity to find the nipple independently, open their mouth wide (**Figure 15-2**), latch onto a large mouthful of breast tissue, and remain latched. **Chapter 16** discusses latch in detail.

- Rooting
- Sucking
- Swallowing
- Hand to mouth
- Mouth gaping/opening
- Tongue licking
- Arm and leg cycling
- Head lifting
- Head bobbing
- Stepping/crawling

Figure 15-1 Significant infant reflexes in the immediate postpartum period.

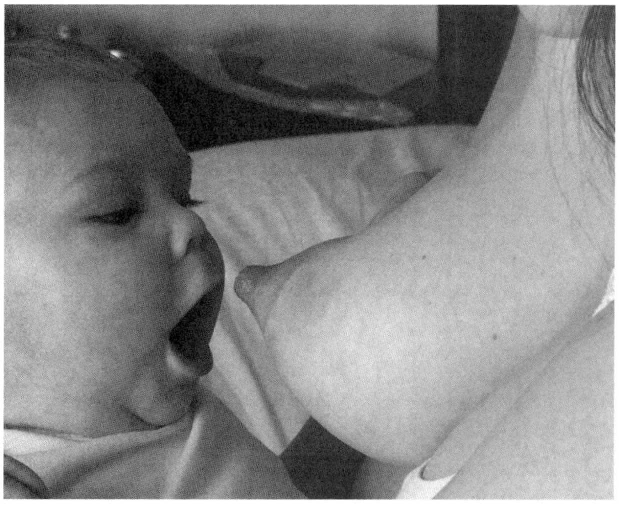

Figure 15-2 Baby opening mouth wide to latch.

Printed with permission of Nelia Box.

The Parent's Position

Regardless of how a parent holds their baby for feeding, they need to be comfortable with support for their baby's weight. Pillows will help support the parent's arms, as illustrated in **Figure 15-3**. The parent should be relaxed, with shoulders resting comfortably and their back supported. Reclining enables the baby to rest prone on the parent's torso, helping to trigger a **searching response**. A pillow placed under the parent's back may increase comfort and relieve back strain. When sitting, the parent's feet should be supported on the floor or on a footstool. Positioning the knees higher than the hips places the baby close to the parent's chest and helps prevent back strain from leaning over the baby to nurse.

Typical postpartum discomforts need to be addressed in early feedings to increase the parent's comfort, particularly in the perineal and incision areas. If the parent is in pain, you may note facial grimacing or hunched shoulders. Parents may also become uncomfortable remaining in the same position for a long time. Positioning should place the least stress on any sore areas. Following a cesarean section, the abdominal incision can be protected with a pillow or folded blanket. Alternatively, the parent can position the baby at their side in the **side-sitting hold** (also called the **football hold** or **clutch hold**), with pillows to raise the baby to a level near the breast and protect the abdomen.

The Baby's Position

Postural stability is important for a baby to initiate feeding behaviors. The baby needs to be well supported and held closely. When latching, the baby may respond best when placed vertically in the middle of the parent's chest, with their head below or at the same height as the nipples. As the baby reaches for the nipple to latch, the parent can continue to support their body.

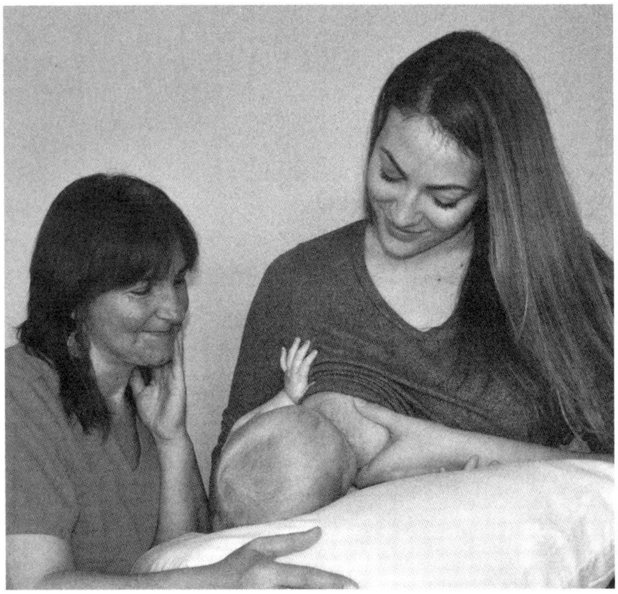

Figure 15-3 Using pillows to help with positioning and comfort.

Printed with permission of Anna Swisher.

The baby's body should be flexed, with their ears, shoulders, and hips in alignment. The tops of their cheeks should be in line with the nipple, with the chin pressed deeply into the breast. If the breast tissue obstructs breathing, gently lifting the baby's hips and legs will angle their head slightly away from the breast to ease breathing. Parents with soft breast tissue can depress the tissue slightly away from the baby's nose with their thumb. Effective sucking within the first hour of life is associated with positioning infants so that their chin can instinctively nudge the underside of the breast as they approach to latch the nipple and suck (Kellams, 2024).

The baby's mouth should be positioned slightly below the nipple (as in Figure 15-2) so that the baby reaches up to it. Lining up the baby's nose with the nipple is a helpful visual reference. In this position the lower lip covers more of the areola than the upper lip, known as an **asymmetrical latch**. Some babies latch better with the nipple angled up toward the hard palate. This helps trigger the baby's suck reflex and encourages the baby to take in more of the areola below the nipple (Scott & Kirkland, 2023; Tiruye et al., 2018). The baby's tongue will extend over the lower gum (alveolar ridge), often out to the lower lip. However, many babies will latch in the middle (like a bull's-eye target). The key consideration is how the latch feels to the parent. If they are comfortable, it works!

Incorrect positioning at feedings is the major cause of nipple soreness. When the baby's positioning avoids pulling on the nipple, the potential for pain is lessened. That is not to say that parents will not react with surprise at the sensation of the first latch, as evidenced in **Figure 15-4**. It is common for parents to describe a certain amount of discomfort when they first begin nursing. This sensation typically subsides in time and should not escalate to prolonged pain. Note that the helper's hand in this figure is placed on the baby's head. It is important not to push the baby's head toward the breast and could cause the baby's chin to be flexed toward their chest, making opening wide and swallowing more difficult.

Supporting the Breast

Supporting the breast may help facilitate feedings in the early days to help the baby maintain latch. This is especially the case when the weight of a heavy breast pulls the nipple away from the baby's mouth. The parent can provide support by cupping the breast with their fingers to form the letter *C*. Referred to as the **C-hold**, the thumb is on top with the fingers curved below the breast well behind the areola, as in **Figure 15-5**. A rolled blanket or towel can be placed underneath a large breast to provide adequate support and free a hand. After the nursing dyad has mastered positioning and latch, it may no longer be necessary to provide this support.

Depending on the baby's positioning, the angle of the C-hold may need to change to prevent compressing the tissue vertically to the baby's mouth. The hold should parallel the angle of the baby's mouth so that the shape of the tissue is parallel to the shape of the baby's mouth. Using the analogy of holding the breast as one would hold a sandwich—that is, parallel to the mouth and not vertical—will help parents visualize this. Pictures, drawings, a breast model, handouts, or other visual aids can augment verbal instructions for better understanding. Kinesthetic learners may be receptive to you gently putting your hand around their hand to demonstrate the technique.

A slight variation of the C-hold works well with preterm infants and other babies who have weak muscle development and find it difficult to hold their jaw steady while they suck. This position, known as the **Dancer hand position**, begins in the C-hold. The parent brings their hand forward to support the breast with the first three fingers. The baby's chin is supported by resting on the parent's hand between the thumb and index finger, as illustrated in **Figure 15-6**. The parent then bends their index finger slightly so that it gently holds the baby's cheek on one side while their thumb holds the other cheek. This hold helps decrease the available space in the baby's mouth and increases negative pressure. Used with steady, equal

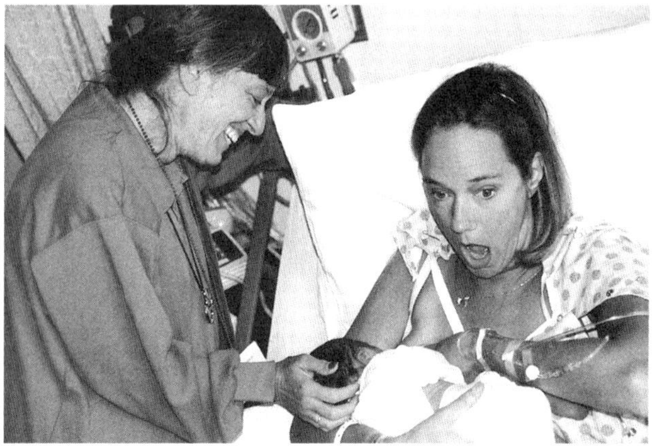

Figure 15-4 The surprise of a baby's first latch.
Printed with permission of Tammy Arbeter.

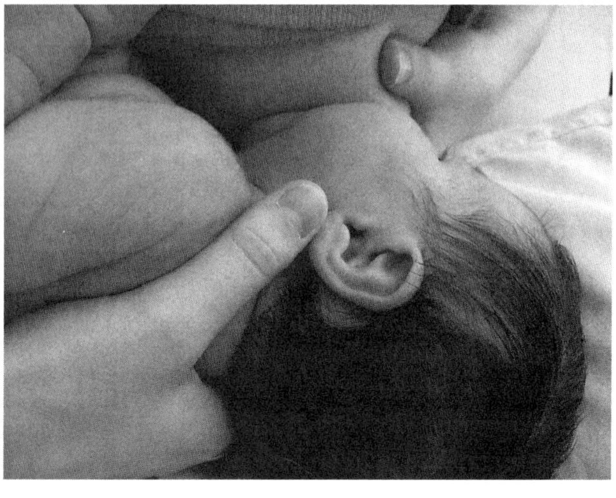

Figure 15-5 Using the C-hold to support the breast for nursing.
Printed with permission of Anna Swisher.

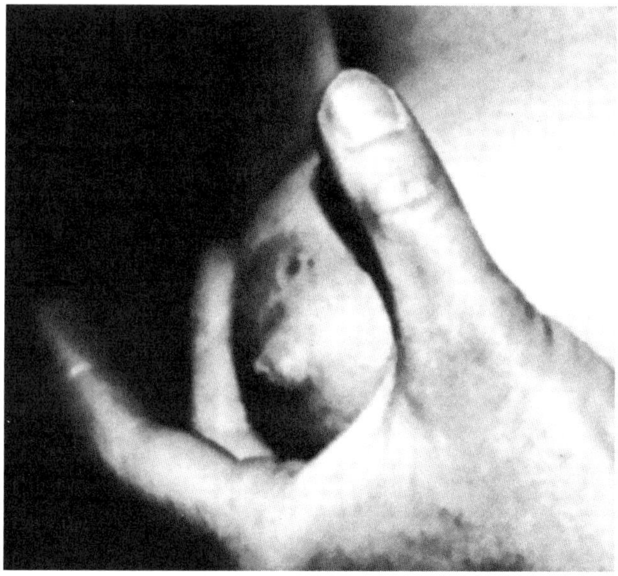

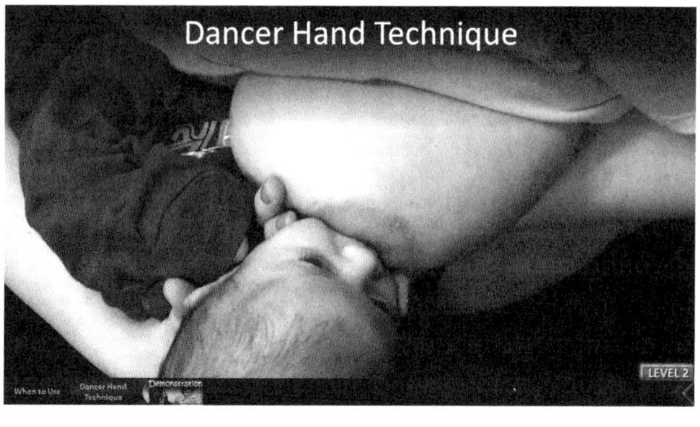

Figure 15-6 Dancer hand position supports the baby's mouth and gently compresses their cheeks.
Printed with permission of Sarah Coulter Danner.

pressure it does not interfere with the infant's rooting response. As the baby's muscle tone begins to improve, the parent can place their thumb back on top of the breast, leaving the index finger to support the baby's chin.

Parents have been depicted in art throughout the centuries positioning their fingers like open scissors to hold the nipple. This was later discouraged because of a concern that placing a finger near each side of the areola would block the lactiferous sinuses, affect milk flow, and possibly cause plugged ducts. In the mid-2000s, it was discovered that lactiferous sinuses do not even exist and that the ducts beneath the nipple are shallow and branch into a network. **Chapter 7** discusses breast anatomy. If a parent intuitively places their fingers in this way, offer alternative placement suggestions *only* if the technique interferes with latch.

Nursing Positions

Parents nurse their infants in a variety of positions. Considering the innate and instinctive behavior of the nursing dyad, this flexibility helps new parents as they become acquainted with their baby. It is important to affirm a parent's positioning for feeding and offer alternatives only when something is not working. Avoid making negative comments or touching the parent or baby during the initial positioning. Such intervention could undermine the parent's confidence or increase their anxiety.

Some parents become frustrated that there is no one "right" answer to their questions or that they are told different things by different caregivers. In the early days following birth, the baby's abilities and responsiveness can vary greatly from feeding to feeding. Parenting and learning to nurse are ongoing processes that continually unfold. Encourage parents to recognize that they have the capacity to discover what works for them and their baby at each stage of their baby's growth. It is natural to feel pressure to "fix" a feeding. Respecting each dyad as unique will neutralize your expectations. What works best for one dyad may be very different from what works for another.

If a nipple sore develops, the parent will need to find a position that minimizes irritation. Figure 17-3 in **Chapter 17** depicts the analogy of the breast as a clock as the parent experiments with different positions. When offering advice, always remember to account for variations in breast anatomy, as well as comfort and self-efficacy levels. If a particular analogy does not resonate with a parent, change it to something that works.

Learning about typical infant patterns for each developmental stage will help parents adapt their routines and find nursing positions that work as their baby grows and matures. The most common positions are **laid-back nursing** or the laid-back position, the **cradle hold**; side-sitting hold; **cross-cradle hold**; and **side-lying position**. Parents find other creative variations as well. If a less traditional position leads to an effective latch, there is no reason to intervene.

Laid-Back Position

Laid-back nursing, also referred to as **biological nurturing**, capitalizes on the innate intuition and instinct of parents and babies. There are significantly more PNRs as stimulants in semireclined postures than when parents are upright or side-lying (Colson, 2019). Thus, when a parent is semireclined with the infant prone on their chest, instinctive nurturing behaviors and PNRs are triggered, thereby stimulating nursing. It is for this reason that parents are encouraged to use this position for feedings in the early postpartum period. In the laid-back position illustrated in **Figure 15-7**, the parent lies semireclined on their back, with the baby lying in a stomach-to-stomach position on top. In addition to facilitating newborn reflexes, this positioning may be useful when overabundant milk production causes excessive amounts of milk to gush into the baby's mouth.

Healthcare professionals are encouraged to incorporate a biological nurturing approach within a framework of care that provides parents with a range of skills to enable them to adapt their nursing to a variety of situations (Milinco et al., 2020). If a baby who is held in a laid-back position fails to settle into robust nursing, some assistance will be needed.

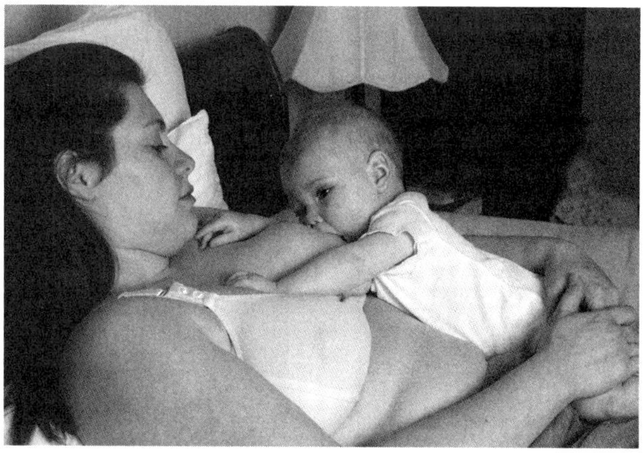

Figure 15-7 Prone (laid-back or posture) position.

Printed with permission of Nelia Box.

Sometimes a baby's latch can be adjusted by gently shifting the baby's body or using a different hold. The ideal approach is the intuitive response that works best for the parent. Babies can nurse in a variety of positions, and there is no one right way to hold a baby. Over time, the baby will self-latch and nurse in a variety of positions, especially in later months. Older nurslings often find creative positions that new parents cannot envision!

Cradle Hold

The cradle hold is a commonly used position in which the parent sits with the baby's body across their abdomen. With the baby on the right side, they place the infant's head in the crook of the right arm and support their body with their right hand, as illustrated in **Figure 15-8**, and vice versa for the left side. Sometimes called the *Madonna and Child* hold because of the many depictions of mothers and babies in art, this position is very intuitive.

When using the cradle hold, the parent has limited control over the movement of the baby's head. It works well for older babies with good head control. However, it is not ideal in the early newborn period when the baby's weak neck can flex forward and interfere with swallowing. It may also not be optimal if the dyad has any problems with latch. Parents cannot easily assist or guide the baby to a better latch. Even so, the cradle hold is the position used instinctively by many parents, and you should not interfere with it unless it is clearly ineffective. If an infant is struggling with latching when held in the cradle hold, parents can consider another position that provides better control during the feeding.

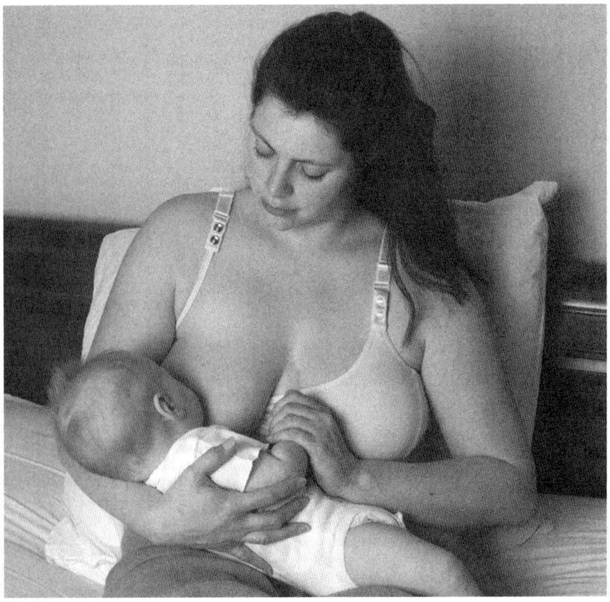

Figure 15-8 Cradle-hold nursing position.

Printed with permission of Nelia Box.

Side-Sitting Hold

In the side-sitting (also called *football* or *clutch*) hold, the parent places the baby under their arm much in the same way that one would clutch a purse under the arm or like an American football player holds the ball while running. The baby lies along their side with their feet toward the parent's back. Holding the baby's neck with their hand, the parent supports the child's body with their forearm and raises their head to nipple level, as illustrated in **Figure 15-9**. Pillows can help support the baby and the parent's arm. Many parents find that their baby will nurse best in the side-sitting position if the baby's body is angled with the torso and feet lower than the head.

The side-sitting position is especially effective for nursing a preterm baby, who fits snugly under the parent's arm. It is also useful for full-term infants who have difficulty latching. The parent can hold the baby's entire body on their arm and respond to the baby's body movements better. This hold is helpful in tricking a baby into nursing after resisting the traditional sitting position. It helps for babies with a short tongue or ankyloglossia, for nursing multiple children (e.g., twins, triplets), and for parents with a cesarean incision. It works well for parents with very large breasts, along with a firm pillow or folded blanket for support. It also allows the parent's opposite hand to support the breast if needed.

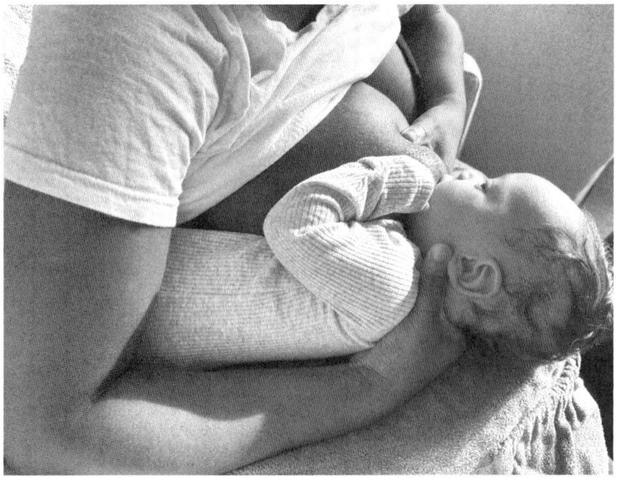

Figure 15-9 Side-sitting (football or clutch) nursing hold.

Used with permission from Kristina Chamberlain.

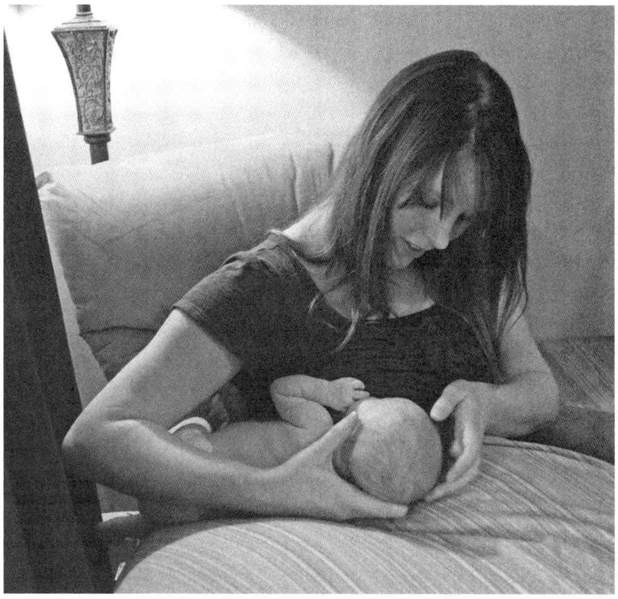

Figure 15-10 Modified side-sitting hold.

Printed with permission of Anna Swisher.

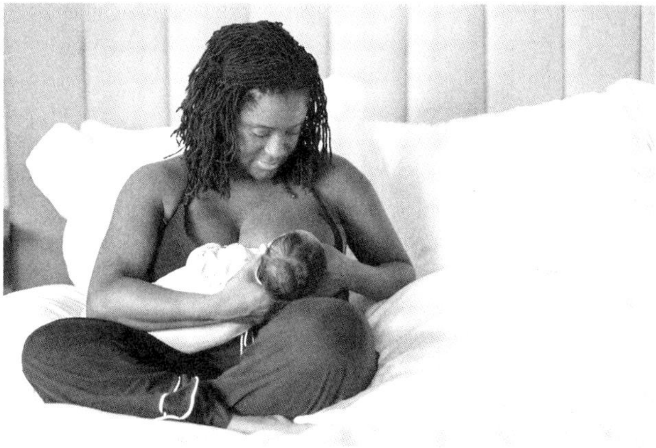

Figure 15-11 Cross-cradle dominant hand hold nursing hold.

Printed with permission of Jenny Jimenez.

Some parents have difficulty ensuring good positioning with their baby's body in a side-sitting hold. A **modified side-sitting hold** places the baby on the parent's side with the top of the baby's head toward the middle of the parent's chest and the feet facing away. As illustrated in **Figure 15-10**, the modification allows the parent to observe more of the baby's body.

Cross-Cradle Position

The cross-cradle hold (also called **dominant hand hold**) combines the side-sitting hold and the cradle hold, with the baby's head resting in the parent's hand. When latching using the right arm, the parent supports the baby's neck and shoulders with the right hand and supports the child's body with their forearm. The parent then moves their arm along with the baby across their body to the opposite side, as illustrated in **Figure 15-11**. They can support the breast with their free hand if needed. This position can be reversed using the left arm for feeding on the right breast.

Holding the baby with the dominant hand in the cross-cradle position can be especially helpful in early feedings or when a baby is not latching well. This position enables the parent to help a preterm, small, or otherwise disorganized baby latch and stay latched well enough to initiate sucking. Feedings are easier to manage, which increases the parent's self-confidence. Some parents begin a feeding in a cross-cradle position and then bring the other arm around to hold the baby in a cradle position after the baby has a firm latch and is sucking more robustly.

Side-Lying Position

Lying down to nurse helps parents obtain needed rest and allows the baby to self-latch. In this position, the parent lies on their side, with their knees slightly bent. Pillows placed under their head, between their legs, and behind their back will help them achieve a comfortable position. The lower arm can be placed under their head, using the top arm to support the baby's head and back. Alternatively, the lower arm can lie under the baby's head or along the back of the child's body to provide support.

The parent can first latch the baby and then raise or lower the breast by rolling their body. A pillow, rolled towel, or blanket placed behind the baby's back will help keep them lying on their side for an effective latch. To nurse on the top breast, the parent can roll toward the baby so that the nipple is level with the baby's mouth. Another method for changing sides is for the parent to hug the baby against their chest and roll on their back to the opposite side, as illustrated in **Figure 15-12**.

Other Creative Positions

Parents devise numerous creative positions to nurse their babies when conventional positions do not work. Two variations are illustrated here. The position in **Figure 15-13** places the baby on the bed with the parent leaning over the baby on their hands and knees. This position is useful when a parent has a sore spot on the nipple and for babies who are in traction

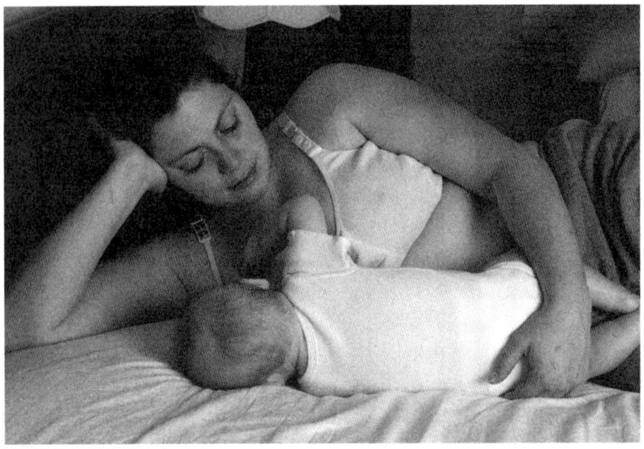

Figure 15-12 Lying-down nursing position.
Printed with permission of Nelia Box.

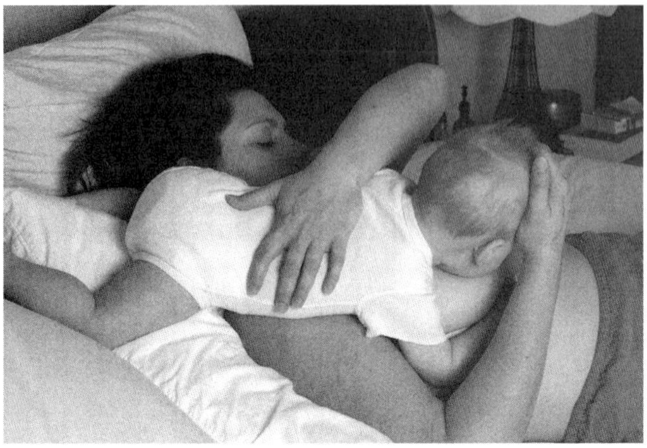

Figure 15-14 Baby lying over the parent's shoulder.
Printed with permission of Nelia Box.

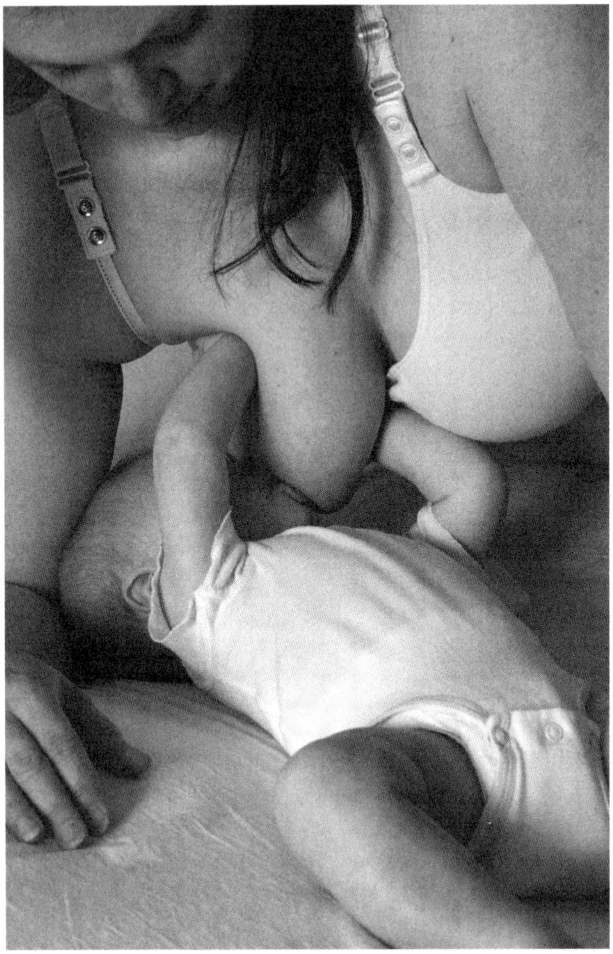

Figure 15-13 Leaning over the baby to nurse.
Printed with permission of Nelia Box.

or who have undergone surgery. It allows positioning the nipple in the baby's mouth by rotating the baby's body. The position in **Figure 15-14** places the parent on their back with the baby lying on their stomach and their feet over the parent's shoulder. This position can relieve ductal narrowing, inflammation, and other mastitis-related symptoms. Such variations demonstrate that there is no one correct position for nursing. If the baby can maintain a firm latch and the parent is comfortable, they can continue to be creative in their approaches.

Assisting with Feedings

In the early days of nursing, it is common for a baby to seem unresponsive to the parent's attempts to nurse. Sleepiness in newborns is common, perhaps from labor medications or simply because of the immaturity of the baby's system. Parents can try several techniques to rouse a sleepy baby and stimulate more interest in feeding. At times, a baby may cry and seem to resist feeding. The longer the parent tries, the more the baby cries and fights, and the more frustrated the parent can become.

Quietly watching the dyad nurse will help identify whether assistance is needed. A baby who nurses robustly and effectively will usually gently release the nipple at the end of a feeding. Sometimes a parent may need to break suction to interrupt a feeding. Do not be in a hurry to assist or say anything until you have determined a need for help.

Observing Nursing

As you observe a feeding, note the parent's posture and whether they appear comfortable. Note how the baby is held and whether the parent would benefit from holding their breast to assist with latch. Note the position of the baby's body, the position of the mouth on the nipple, the placement of the tongue, and the position of the baby's head and hands.

The baby should appear comfortable, with their body in alignment. The baby's lips should **flange** out, and the cheeks should be smooth and rounded, without any dimpling or hollowing. If the baby is deeply latched, depending on the size of the breast, lip placement may not be observable. There is no reason to disrupt the feeding by pulling the baby back to view the lips. It could create a shallow latch or cause the baby to unlatch completely.

The baby should settle into long, deep sucks in a rhythmic suck–swallow–breathe pattern. With copious amounts of milk, swallowing may be evident. Babies suck about once per second when a large volume of milk is flowing and about twice per second when there is little milk flow. A faster sucking pattern may reflect the time between milk ejections or signal the end of the feeding on that side. If the baby exhibits a faster sucking pattern throughout an entire feeding, the latch may need to be adjusted, or there may be little milk available. If clicking occurs when the baby sucks, repositioning may help the baby maintain a better latch. Observing the dyad at a feeding can help you assess whether any intervention is needed.

Sleepy Baby

A sleepy infant who is medically stable may go up to 24 hours without feeding. Being alert to the baby's hunger cues will help parents determine the most receptive times for feeding. If a sleepy baby displays no hunger cues, the parent may need to gently rouse the baby to nurse every 2 to 3 hours to establish and protect milk production. The parent can use the rousing techniques described in **Figure 15-15**. These techniques are helpful both before and during a feeding as necessary.

You can help parents explore possible causes for their baby's sleepiness, as described in **Figure 15-16**. The baby may be sleepy or medicated from the delivery or from postpartum pain medication. Newborns who sleep for long periods during the day will typically nurse more at night. Waking these babies to nurse periodically during the day will help encourage longer sleep periods at night. Parents will need to be patient because it may take several weeks to reverse the baby's rhythm. If sleepiness continues for several feedings, the parent will need to express milk to maintain production and prevent engorgement until the infant is ready to actively feed.

A sleepy newborn benefits from 24-hour rooming-in and being held skin to skin. Rooming-in enables parents to distinguish between deep sleep and light sleep and to observe and respond to their baby's hunger cues. Initiating a feeding when the baby demonstrates hunger cues is more effective than trying to feed a baby who is in a deep sleep. Parents can attempt to nurse every half hour to an hour when the infant demonstrates signs of a light sleep state. Cuddling the baby skin to skin on the parent's chest often increases the baby's interest in nursing. Dimming the lights may encourage the baby's eyes to open. If the baby does not waken enough to nurse, the parent can try again in another half hour to an hour.

It is important to monitor a sleepy baby's output and watch for symptoms of dehydration or hypoglycemia. The baby may need supplemental

- Talk to the baby and try to make eye contact.
- Loosen or remove blankets.
- Hold the baby upright in a sitting or standing position.
- Partially or fully undress the baby.
- Change the baby's diaper.
- Stimulate the baby through increased skin contact, such as massage or gently rubbing the baby's hands and feet.
- Stimulate the baby's rooting reflex.
- Stimulate the baby's sense of smell by bringing them close to the breast so they can detect the scent of the parent's skin.
- Stimulate the baby's sense of taste by expressing milk onto the nipple or into the baby's mouth.
- Wipe the baby's forehead and cheeks with a cool, moist cloth.
- Manipulate the baby's arms and legs by playing pat-a-cake, doing baby exercises, and so on.
- Give the baby a bath or, better yet, take a bath with the baby to provide increased skin-to-skin contact.
- If the baby latches but does not maintain a rhythmic suck-swallow-pause pattern, try stroking under the baby's chin from front to back. Also, compress the breast, as with manual expression.
- Express colostrum onto a finger and elicit sucking with the finger.

Figure 15-15 Infant rousing techniques.

- Medications given during labor.
- A traumatic birth resulting from a long labor or long second-stage labor.
- The baby is preterm.
- It is the baby's usual sleepy period.
- The first feeding was delayed.
- Hunger cues were overlooked.
- The baby has sensory overload from bright lights, loud noises, or painful procedures.
- Response to interventions, particularly circumcision.
- The baby is jaundiced.
- A schedule was imposed on feedings.
- Birth was by cesarean delivery.
- The baby is experiencing hypothermia.

Figure 15-16 Possible causes of infant sleepiness.

feedings until nursing is well established. When small amounts of colostrum are available, hand expression is usually most effective and easier for removing milk (Becker et al., 2016; Morton, 2024; Steurer & Smith, 2018). Feeding colostrum to a sleepy baby may rouse them to latch. If the parent's expressed milk or donor milk is not available, supplementation with infant formula may be necessary. The ABM provides a protocol for the appropriate supplementation of healthy, full-term nursed infants (ABM, 2017).

Fussy Baby

Some babies seem to be fussy and irritable, and easily stimulated and excited during the first month of life. They may cry frequently and require continuous attention during their waking hours. Swaddling a fussy baby to restrict startling and movement can provide a sense of security and calm. If a baby is fussy at feedings, encourage parents to hold them calmly, in skin-to-skin contact on their chest. If latching attempts cause resistance or crying, limit the attempts to no more than a few minutes at a time and try again 10 or 15 minutes later when the baby has calmed. **Figure 15-17** presents possible causes of fussiness.

A crying baby may have difficulty coordinating breathing and swallowing and may choke or swallow air. If crying is because the baby is overly hungry, the baby may choke and gag because of overeagerness to nurse. Carefully observing and responding to the newborn's behavior will ensure that feedings begin before the baby becomes upset or overly hungry. A crying, fussy baby cannot latch well and needs soothing before feeding. Parents with a fussy baby will benefit from suggestions for **calming techniques** as presented in **Figure 15-18**. They can use these techniques before and during a feeding, as well as at other times during the day. It is important that the parent express milk to maintain production. The expressed milk can be fed to the baby until nursing is well established.

When a baby is fussy, parents may become tense and frustrated by the behavior. If the baby responds to parental tension by crying even more, changing the parents'

- Caregivers have handled the baby too much.
- The baby is in pain or has experienced pain.
- Medication given during labor or postpartum passed to the baby.
- The baby has discomfort from forceps, vacuum extraction, internal monitor lead, or cephalhematoma.
- The baby has oral aversion because of deep suctioning or other invasive procedures.
- The baby is irritable.
- The baby received an artificial nipple or pacifier, leading to nipple preference.
- Lack of confidence causes the parent to hold the baby tentatively.
- The baby needs to be swaddled to provide boundaries or to be soothed by being cuddled skin-to-skin.
- The baby has shut down from too much intervention, such as someone attempting to push the child on the nipple.
- The dyad was separated, resulting in missed hunger cues and missed imprinting.
- Rarely, fussiness in a baby can be a sign of serious problems, such as neurologic disorders.
- The baby is withdrawing from nicotine or other drugs passed in utero.

Figure 15-17 Possible causes of infant fussiness.

- Limit invasive procedures to minimize crying.
- Hold the baby skin to skin.
- Cuddle without pushing the baby to nurse.
- Work with the baby for short periods.
- Be sensitive to and respect the baby's cues.
- Use slow, calm, deliberate movements in caring for the baby.
- Cuddle, hold, and walk with the baby.
- Talk or sing to the baby in a soft voice.
- Swaddle the baby.
- Nurse in a dark, quiet room.
- Relax in a rocking chair.
- Burp the baby often (unless burping seems upsetting). Burp before switching to the other side at a feeding.
- Carry the baby in a position that puts gentle and firm pressure on their abdomen—for example, on the parent's hip or shoulder.
- Play music, create a monotonous noise by running a vacuum cleaner or dishwasher, or play a recording of such sounds.
- Change the baby's diaper when it becomes damp or soiled.
- Sleep or nap together so the baby is comforted by the parent's body warmth and heartbeat.
- Massage the baby for 10 to 15 minutes (the baby may fuss during the massage and then become quiet afterward).
- Use a sling to carry the baby close to the parent's body.
- Use a baby swing for times when individual attention is not possible.
- If the baby was born at full term and has good temperature control, remove their clothes to provide air exposure for limited amounts of time.
- Lay the baby on their stomach on the parent's lap while they bounce their knees or move them back and forth.
- Take a bath together.
- Get help from others—partner, grandparents, or other support person. The baby may calm when held by someone who is calm.
- Provide monotonous movement with a stroller or car ride.
- Remove allergens from the parent's diet.

Figure 15-18 Infant calming techniques.

response can help break the cycle. The parent can leave the room for several minutes and use relaxation and breathing techniques to calm down. It may be helpful to emphasize to parents the importance of caring for themselves during any periods of stress. Enlisting the help of a family member or friend to care for the baby may help the parent feel less overwhelmed. Nursing while lying down and enlisting the help of others to care for the baby will allow the parent to nap or take a break. Talking about possible feelings of anger, frustration, or inadequacy may help relieve their tension. A walk outdoors or a soothing bath may help, although in some cases, leaving the baby for any length of time may actually increase parental anxiety. Accessible meals and snacks that are easily prepared will promote a nutritious diet. **Chapter 14** discusses crying and the care of a fussy baby.

Ending a Feeding

A baby who nurses robustly and effectively will usually gently release the nipple spontaneously at the end of a feeding. The baby can then be latched to the other side and continue to nurse on both sides, one after the other, for as long as they want. There is always milk available, except in cases of certain medical conditions, as discussed in **Chapter 21**. Unless the parent feels pain or discomfort, there are problems with milk transfer, or the infant has a medical problem such as reflux, babies can continue to nurse for as long as nutritive sucking and swallowing are observed.

If the parent needs to interrupt a feeding before this point (e.g., to achieve a better latch), teach them how to break the suction. One technique is to insert a finger gently into the corner of the baby's mouth between the gums. **Figure 15-19** illustrates this technique. Another technique is to press a finger against the areola near the corner of the baby's mouth to release suction pressure, allowing the nipple to slip out easily.

If the baby begins to chew or tug on the nipple toward the end of a feeding or to the extent that it causes discomfort, the parent may need to end the feeding. Often when touching the baby's lips to break suction, a baby may instinctively begin to suck faster—a reflexive response to having the lip touched while latched. The parent can gently continue efforts to unlatch the baby. Keeping the infant latched when feedings are painful can lead to nipple damage (Douglas, 2022).

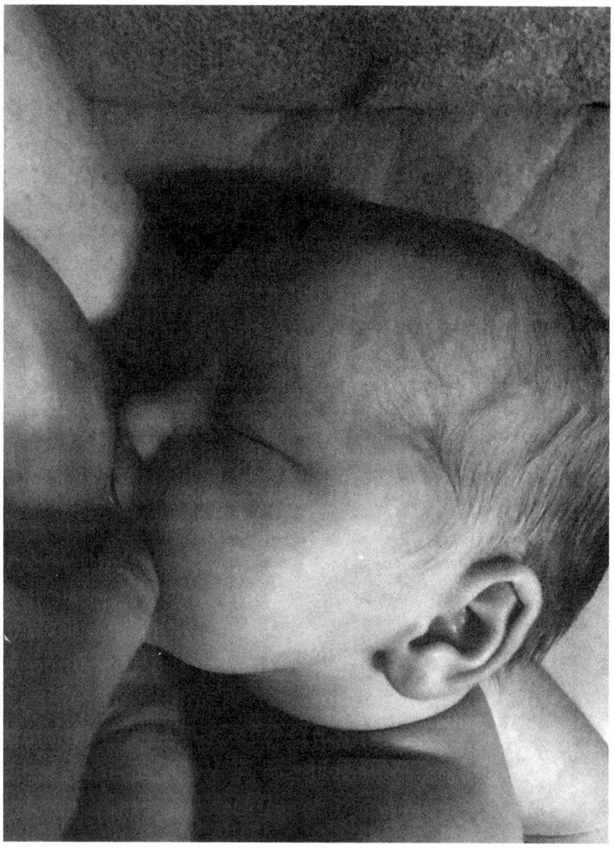

Figure 15-19 A finger placed in the corner of the baby's mouth helps break suction to gently remove the nipple.

Printed with permission of Lindsay Doyal.

Nursing Multiples

The immunological properties of human milk are especially important to multiples, who experience increased pregnancy, birth, and postnatal complications (Bartick et al., 2017b). Preterm or very preterm birth is more common in twin pregnancies. Most twin deliveries occur between 32 and 33 weeks' gestation. The prevalence of delivery prior to 32 weeks reported in the United States is 5% to 10% (Cobo et al., 2020). Multiples are at substantially greater risk than singletons for low birth weight and neurological impairments. Fetal, neonatal, and infant morbidity is greater for multiples as well (Ward & Caughey, 2021).

Twin pregnancies place parents at a fourfold increased risk for severe complications before and after delivery, including acute morbidity (Madar et al., 2019). Parents of multiples have often used fertility treatments to help them conceive. Fertility treatments—also known as **assisted reproductive technology (ART)**—increase the likelihood of multiple births. ART has doubled over the past decade, with over 2.26% of all infants born in the United States every year conceived using ART (Centers for Disease Control and Prevention [CDC], 2024).

Parents of twins and higher-order multiples (triplets or more) can attain the same nursing outcomes as parents of singletons. Although there may be more demands on their time and they face some special challenges, nursing can bring a calming element to an otherwise hectic life. It reduces the expense of buying double or triple the amount of infant formula and the increased medical expenses associated with more frequent illnesses from not having human milk (Bartick et al., 2017a, 2017b; Walters et al., 2019).

Parents expecting more than one baby may be told they should not nurse, that they will not have enough milk to support the babies, or that the babies will need to be fed on a schedule to monitor weight gain (Cassidy et al., 2024). You can reassure prospective parents that they can make enough milk for multiple babies. Records from 1900 reveal that wet nurses in France were able to furnish 2230 g (78 oz) of milk per day. One woman yielded as much as 2840 g (100 oz) in 1 day (Budin, 1907)! The few possible exceptions to ample milk production include hormonal problems, breast surgery or injury, and insufficient glandular development. Some parents who conceive through reproductive technology have difficulty with milk production. **Chapter 26** discusses insufficient milk production.

Parents of multiples are less likely to initiate nursing than parents of singletons, and they nurse for a shorter duration (Ayton & Hansen, 2023; Whitford et al., 2017). Nevertheless, they increasingly want to nurse their babies. Families using ART to achieve pregnancy tend to be highly educated and have higher incomes (Sunderam, 2020)—the key demographic of families who nurse in industrialized countries. Nursing preterm and even full-term multiple-birth infants is complex and demanding for these families. Higher-order multiples are frequently induced or delivered by cesarean as early as 36 weeks' gestation. These families will encounter more feeding problems resulting from the infants' preterm birth than from having two babies to feed. Parents who carry their twins to 39 weeks have fewer feeding issues.

Assisting with Nursing Multiples

Families with multiples require ongoing help from healthcare providers who are committed to the provision of human milk for these children. The most influential factor for nursing twins exclusively is a high level of nursing self-efficacy, which increases the parents' confidence. Additional factors include family and healthcare provider support, as well as peer counseling throughout their nursing journey (Anjarwati et al., 2019).

The International Council of Multiple Birth Organizations (ICMBO, 2022), an advocacy coalition, has outlined a declaration of rights and statement of needs for twins and higher-order multiples. The ICMBO advocates for education regarding the nutritional, psychological, and financial benefits of nursing for preterm and full-term infants. It cites the need for encouragement and coaching in nursing techniques, as well as simultaneous bottle feeding of comultiples, adequate resources, support systems, and family work leave for parents of multiples.

Nursing Routines for Multiples

While in the hospital, having the babies together for feedings enables parents to learn the practical aspects of nursing multiples. A helper can keep one baby positioned while the parent latches the second baby onto the other side. If there are more than two babies, the third baby can be fed with an alternative method while two are nursing. Rotating babies at each feeding will give all of them equal time nursing. If one baby must remain in a special care nursery, the parent can nurse the other baby and express milk for the one in special care. Pillows can help with positioning. There are several commercially available pillows for use with twins that parents may find useful.

Some parents consider co-bedding or cosleeping helpful for night nursing of multiples. Evidence on the safety of this practice is mixed. A 2023 integrative review of co-bedding infant twins found potential benefits and no evidence of harm for the infants. However, the researchers found that the quality of evidence was low and insufficient to provide recommendations for practice (Mann et al., 2023). The American Academy of Pediatrics, in its updated 2022 safe sleep guidelines, cautions that the potential benefits of co-bedding twins are outweighed by the risks and recommends against co-bedding of twins or higher-order multiples (Moon et al., 2022).

Nursing multiples born preterm usually requires close attention until the babies reach their "full-term" date and are robust feeders. With creative planning and flexibility, a routine will develop that works best for the family. Nursing encourages parents to regard each baby's needs individually. It promotes more time in close physical contact, enabling maximum skin contact with each baby. Nursing the babies separately at least once a day and spending other time alone with each baby will foster a unique connection with each baby and help parents get to know their babies' individual personalities.

Household priorities will need to accommodate the demands of more than one baby. Time-saving techniques will be essential in establishing a daily routine.

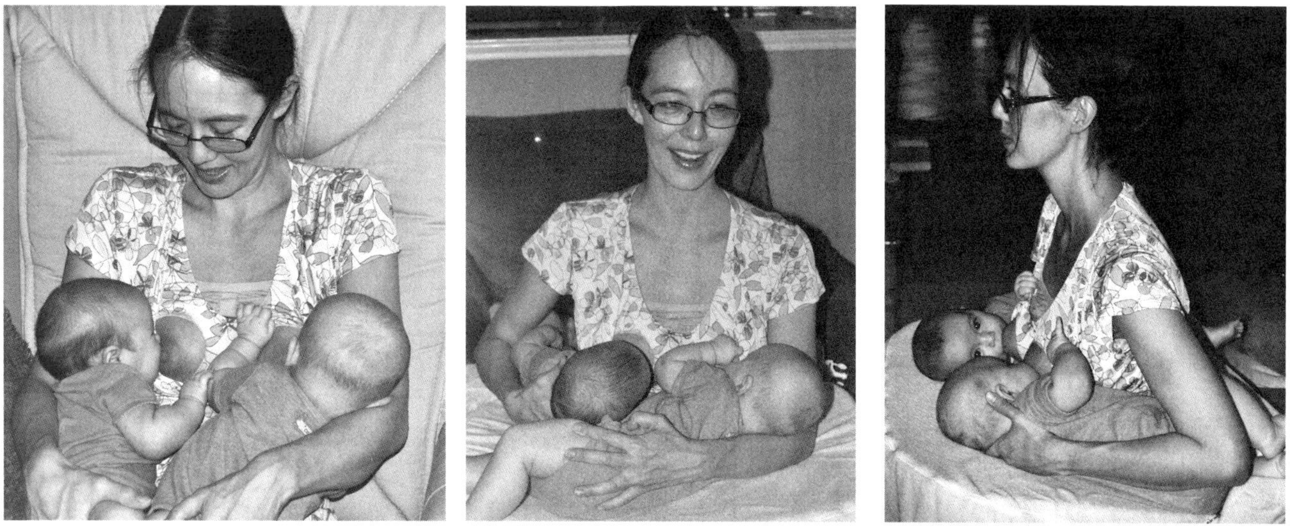

Figure 15-20 Positions for nursing multiples simultaneously.
Printed with permission of Anna Swisher.

Higher-income families may hire others to help with child care or use shopping and cleaning services to assist them with tasks of daily living. Families who do not have these options may enlist family members, friends, or volunteers to help them for a few hours during the day. Seasoned parents of older multiples are ideal resources for new parents. You can help by linking families to peer support groups for parents of multiples or online resources for parents of multiples.

Simultaneous Feedings

Some parents find that nursing their babies at the same time is overwhelming and prefer to nurse them separately, especially when in public (Cassidy et al., 2024). Others prefer to nurse their twins simultaneously to avoid the hunger cries of the other baby waiting to be fed. **Figure 15-20** illustrates positions for nursing two babies simultaneously. Some parents limit each baby to one side only and reserve the same side for the same baby for all feedings. If one baby has a stronger suck, one side will experience increased milk production, leading to breast asymmetry. This can be avoided by nursing each baby on one side per day and switching to the other side the next day.

On some occasions, one baby may want to nurse at a time when the other baby is not hungry. Parents may feed the hungry baby separately or wait until the second baby is ready to nurse and feed them simultaneously. At an appropriate time, you can discuss each baby's individual needs, the effect of stress hormones from crying, and the importance of responding to babies' early cues. It is the parents' decision on how they will approach feedings. Healthcare providers should not add to feeding challenges by criticizing how parents manage caring for their babies. Each family needs to be supported in finding a routine that works best for them.

Feeding Challenges with Multiples

Mastitis may be more common among parents of multiples because of both fatigue and abundant milk production. A missed feeding by one or more babies can result in engorgement more quickly than in the case of nursing a singleton. Given this possibility, these parents will need to be accessible to their babies for feedings or be able to express milk easily. When separated, expressing milk will avoid engorgement and the possibility of mastitis-related issues. A manual pump or portable electric pump is helpful in case of travel, appointments, and other separations. Learning hand expression will ensure milk removal in the absence of a breast pump.

Multiples develop and grow at varying rates, just as other siblings do. Although growth spurts may occur simultaneously, it is more likely that these events will come at slightly different times for each baby. They may be ready for solid foods and weaning at different times as well. Some parents of multiples nurse exclusively for several months, whereas others elect to supplement every day. Parents of multiples may feel pressured by well-meaning friends and family to begin supplemental foods early or to wean at an earlier age (Mikami et al., 2018; Wang et al., 2023).

Supplemental feedings are common with higher-order multiples, mostly for time management or to allow some self-care time for the nursing parent. In a classic case study a parent of five babies provided milk for approximately half of their intake and supplemented with donor milk (Szucs et al., 2009a, 2009b). At 5 to 6 months postpartum, the parent was nursing each baby once and one baby twice daily while continuing to pump six or seven times per day. At 16 months, the parent continued to lactate, making 700 mL milk per day and nursing two of the five babies once a day.

When multiples are born preterm, the family may be able to obtain insurance coverage for donor milk through commercial or state-run insurance coverage. The amount of coverage varies significantly from country to country. For example, in the United States, most Medicaid insurance does not cover the cost of donor milk, even when medically necessary (Bai & Kuscin, 2021; Rose et al., 2022). Some families seek donor milk from online sources and informal milk-sharing groups. They will benefit from information about milk safety and heat treatment so that they may home-pasteurize donated milk.

Nursing higher-order multiples requires even more creativity than nursing twins. The help of another person at feedings will most likely be needed regularly in the early days. It is time-consuming to nurse each baby separately. The parent can nurse two infants simultaneously while someone else feeds the other baby or babies with an alternative feeding method. Another option is to nurse the first two babies simultaneously and then nurse the other(s) afterward. Parents will eventually become adept at managing feedings on their own. Optimally, all babies will receive the same amount of nursing time, and both sides will receive equal stimulation. Keeping a log of each baby's voiding, stooling, and feeds will help monitor each child's growth.

Although exclusive nursing is the optimal choice for infants, nursing does not have to be an "all or nothing" proposition for parents of multiples. Infants are able to establish a unique connection with their parents through nursing which is a rewarding and comforting element in the lives of babies whose individual personalities are emerging. The nurturing obtained through nursing and feeling the close special attention of the parent is reassuring to each individual baby.

Supporting Parents of Multiples

Parents' reactions to having multiples can range from delight to dismay. The quality of their support system is a major factor in their coping abilities. Both parents' emotions—and especially the birth parent's feelings—are likely to fluctuate, depending on how each day goes. The nursing parent may feel more stressed by the constant demands on their time and energy. The partner may feel shunted aside, wondering what happened to their identity as a couple.

Establishing an emotional connection with each baby may be challenging with multiples. It can be especially complicated when one baby remains hospitalized longer than the other(s). In such cases, the parents may form an attachment with one baby and find it difficult to establish the same attachment with the other(s) when they come home. As each baby is discharged home, the parent can make arrangements that will allow them to spend more time getting to know the new arrival.

Most parents know they are carrying multiples before they deliver, especially when the pregnancy results from ART. Anticipatory guidance and information are especially important to these families. Success stories from parents who have nursed triplets and quadruplets are empowering and can help reassure expectant parents about their abilities. Online resources, including websites, support forums, and virtual groups, can provide emotional and practical support. Helping parents of higher-order multiples access support systems of volunteers will assist their long-term adjustments after the babies arrive. **Table 15-2** provides suggestions for counseling parents of multiples.

Lactation support will be important in helping parents accommodate nursing to the busy routine of parenting multiples. Not-for-profit organizations that offer support and advice about caring for multiples are around the world. The ICMBO at https://icombo.org/ has links to many international support groups and may be helpful for finding support for families in your region. Support for parenting multiples can occur simultaneously with support from a lactation consultant or breastfeeding support group, preferably one that includes other parents who are nursing multiples.

Tandem Nursing

The term **tandem nursing** describes the nursing of two or more children of different ages, as illustrated in **Figure 15-21**. A nursing parent who begins another pregnancy may be reluctant to give up the special relationship they enjoy with their nursing child. Additionally, their child may resist attempts at weaning. Most parents who nurse throughout pregnancy and

Table 15-2 Counseling Parents of Multiples

Concern	Suggestions
Lack of time for all tasks	Plan feeding schedule. Carefully evaluate priorities. Use time-saving methods for household chores. Prepare simple, nutritious meals. Enlist help from others.
Emotionally connecting with babies	Nurse separately at least one time every day. Spend additional time alone with each baby every day.
Emotionally connecting with a baby who has a delayed homecoming	Regard babies as individuals and meet their separate needs. Obtain help with babies who are already settled in and spend more time with the new arrival.
Nursing two babies simultaneously	Put babies on alternate sides at each feeding. Let each baby nurse on one side for the entire day and alternate sides daily.
Spending too much time nursing babies separately	When one baby is hungry, nurse both.
Nursing three or more babies	Nurse two at a time and get help from another person to feed the other baby. Alternate babies so that a different one is fed with alternate means at each feeding. Nurse two babies simultaneously and the other baby on both sides afterward.
Greater susceptibility to mastitis	Avoid long periods away from the babies. Express milk when feedings are missed.

then tandem nurse do so to meet their child's emotional needs and allow the older child to self-wean (O'Rourke & Spatz, 2019). Tandem nursing may also occur when a child who had previously weaned indicates a renewed interest in nursing after witnessing the new baby nursing. Nursing can provide a good lesson in sharing and help adjust to having a new sibling.

Health Concerns with Nursing During Pregnancy

Parents may be advised to wean their nursing child when they become pregnant. There may be concern that oxytocin released during nursing will stimulate uterine contractions. However, there is evidence that high levels of progesterone block the uterus from sensitivity to the effects of oxytocin until the end of the pregnancy (Choi, 2017; Conde-Agudelo et al., 2018). Concern is also expressed that tandem nursing may cause undernourishment in the developing baby. However, a 2021 study found that tandem nursing did not adversely affect the health of the newborn, and that tandem-fed children gained weight sufficiently (Sinkiewicz-Darol et al., 2021).

Another concern expressed with continuing to nurse during pregnancy is whether short spacing between children allows the parent's body to recover to a healthy nutritional status. It is prudent to encourage clients to consult their healthcare provider if there are any concerns with their nutritional status. Increased rates of preterm births, lower birth weights, maternal anemia, and certain vitamin depletions have been

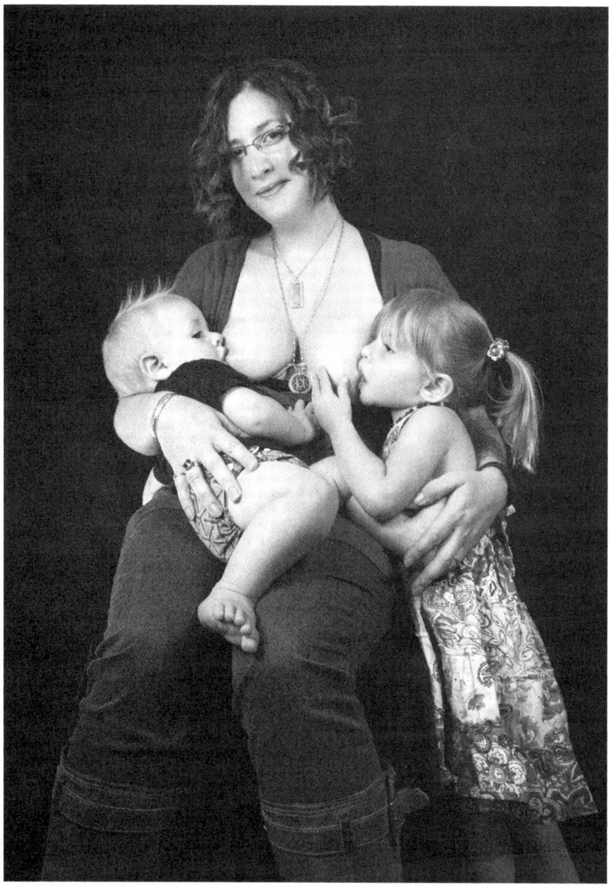

Figure 15-21 Tandem nursing.

Courtesy of Mandi Chase Wolfe.

noted in parents with short birth spacing (Ahrens et al., 2019; Hutcheon et al., 2019; Zhang et al., 2018). The American College of Obstetricians and Gynecologists (ACOG) states that the optimal interval between delivery and a subsequent pregnancy is 18 months to 5 years. The greatest risk of preterm birth and low birth weight occurs with intervals under 6 months (ACOG, 2019). Because of the potential impact on nutritional needs during pregnancy, encourage pregnant parents who continue to nurse to consume enough nutrients to meet their nutritional needs and those of the fetus and the nursing child.

A parent who has experienced a preterm birth or who is at risk for preterm labor is not a good candidate for tandem nursing (Molitoris, 2019). The oxytocin released during nursing could theoretically trigger premature labor. Thus, it may be prudent to wean to avoid the possibility of miscarriage. Encourage parents to discuss specific circumstances with their healthcare provider for guidance, and be available to help with weaning if needed.

Effects During Pregnancy

Nipple tenderness is common in early pregnancy and may cause discomfort when nursing the older child. Parents may also feel nauseated when the older child nurses. These discomforts can discourage some parents from nursing when they are pregnant. In addition, the older child may wean because of the changed composition and taste of the milk caused by pregnancy hormones.

Parents who tandem nurse may experience a decrease in milk yield about the fourth or fifth month of pregnancy. If the sibling is younger than 1 year old when the parent conceives, frequent weight checks will help monitor the child for adequate intake. The reduced yield can cause some children to lose interest in nursing and self-wean (Stalimerou et al., 2023). Supplementation may be necessary if milk production decreases to the point that it does not meet the child's needs.

Nursing Siblings

Parents may worry about having sufficient milk to sustain both an older child and a new infant at the same time. This is rarely an issue because the increased sucking will continue to increase milk production. The more important factors are the emotional needs of the older child and the parent's comfort. A parent who believes that their older child will benefit from the emotional nurturing may choose to continue nursing. For a parent who is uncomfortable with tandem nursing, it may be better to wean the older child rather than feel resentment when the toddler nurses. It is important that parents do what works for the unique needs of their family.

Toddlers who continue to nurse can position themselves easily, making simultaneous feedings with an older child and a newborn manageable. In addition, the child may be old enough to understand the need to wait to nurse and the concept of taking turns, which can facilitate separate feedings. Each child will indicate a preference to nurse at a particular time of day. Nursing them separately at their preferred time can give them close individual attention.

Because the older child is receiving additional nutrients from other foods, the parent needs to nurse the younger baby first, when milk production and release are greatest. The older child can then nurse on the less full side, thereby obtaining less milk. The parent needs to let the baby finish a feeding first to obtain adequate hindmilk. Another option is to reserve a particular side for each child and alternate sides daily to equalize production. The toddler's more efficient nursing will increase milk production, perhaps so much that the younger baby receives too strong a flow of milk and chokes when attempting to nurse. In this event, the parent can allow the older child to nurse briefly before beginning to nurse the younger child.

A parent who chooses to wean the older child will want to do so gradually, as in any other weaning situation. If the older child wants to nurse when the baby nurses, the parent can nurse the baby when the older child is not present or when they are happily occupied with other things. Substituting other special activities and snacks in place of nursing can help the older child move easily toward weaning. The nursing parent's partner or other family member can take over evening rituals, such as baths and bedtime stories, to avoid the child wanting nurse at that time. Encourage parents to substitute ample amounts of hugs, cuddles, and touching to help the older child feel included.

Summary

The early days with a new baby are important in forming a strong foundation for nursing. Learning to recognize newborn instincts, reflexes, and responses will guide parents in meeting their baby's needs. Establishing a routine for feedings may facilitate the process. Recognizing hunger cues will enable parents trust their baby to initiate and end feedings. Understanding the principles of positioning and latch encourages parents to trust their instincts when feeding their babies.

New parents benefit from professional guidance as they begin their lactation journey. Make it a goal to observe every dyad at an early nursing session and offer any necessary assistance. Be available to assist with babies who have difficulty latching. Provide support for babies who are sleepy or fussy, and offer suggestions for rousing or calming the baby. Support parents of multiples and those who tandem nurse an infant and older child. The time spent assisting parents in establishing nursing will influence the course of their long-term experience.

What You Learned–At a Glance

Conversation Starters with Parents

- How do you know when to feed your baby?
- How much help do you need with feedings?
- How do you position your baby at feedings?
- What determines when feedings end?

Beginning a Feeding

- Healthy, alert term infants will self-regulate feedings with no restrictions.
- Sleepy and late preterm infants need to be monitored and stimulated for feedings.
- Innate feeding reflexes include rooting, sucking, swallowing, hand to mouth, mouth gaping, tongue licking, arm and leg cycling, head lifting and bobbing, and stepping and crawling.
- Parents need to be relaxed, with back and arm support as needed for comfort.
- Breast support may help some parents with latch in the early days.

Positioning

- The baby should be well supported and held closely in flexion.
- The baby's ears, shoulders, and hips should be in alignment.
- The baby's chin should press deeply into the breast, with their mouth slightly below the center of the nipple (nipple to nose).
- A reclined (laid-back) position triggers neonatal reflexes to search, latch, and nurse.
- The cradle hold is effective for babies with good head control.
- The side-sitting (football or clutch) hold is effective with a preterm baby or a baby with latch difficulty.
- The cross-cradle hold is helpful with a baby who has latch difficulty.
- The side-lying position helps parents rest.

Managing Feedings

- Observe an entire feeding to reveal adjustments that may be needed.
- Allow the baby to pace feedings.
- Impose no rules on feedings, and limit unnecessary interventions.
- Teach parents to respond to hunger cues and to watch their baby for signs to end a feeding.
- Help parents find a comfortable position for effective latch and milk transfer.
- Teach parents how to stimulate a sleepy baby or comfort a fussy baby for feeding.
- Help parents of multiples with simultaneous feedings.

Tandem Nursing

- Parents can produce enough milk to feed both an infant and older child.
- The new baby should be nursed first, when milk production and release are greatest, and allowed to end the feeding to receive the hindmilk.
- Parents at risk for preterm labor should discuss nursing their older baby with their healthcare provider for guidance.

References

Ahrens KA, et al. Short interpregnancy intervals and adverse perinatal outcomes in high-resource settings: an updated systematic review. *Paediatr Perinat Epidemiol.* 2019;33(1):O25–O47.

American College of Obstetricians and Gynecologists, Committee on Committee on Gynecologic Practice, American Society for Reproductive Medicine. Committee Opinion No. 762: prepregnancy counseling. *Obstet Gynecol.* 2019;133(1):e78–e89. https://www.acog.org/-/media/project/acog/acogorg/clinical/files/committee-opinion/articles/2019/01/prepregnancy-counseling.pdf

Anjarwati N, et al. Exclusive breastfeeding for twin babies and its influencing factors: a study in East Java, Indonesia. *Compr Child Adolesc Nurs.* 2019;42(suppl1):261–266.

Ayton J, Hansen E. Breastfeeding multiples. In: Abduljabbar H, ed. *Multiple Pregnancies—New Insights.* IntechOpen; February 15, 2023.

Bai Y, Kuscin J. The current state of donor human milk use and practice. *J Midwifery Womens Health*. 2021;66(4):478–485.
Bartick MC, et al. Disparities in breastfeeding: impact on maternal and child health outcomes and costs. *J Pediatr.* 2017a;181:49–55.e6.
Bartick MC, et al. Suboptimal breastfeeding in the United States: maternal and pediatric health outcomes and costs. *Matern Child Nutr.* 2017b;13(1).
Becker GE, et al. Methods of milk expression for lactating women. *Cochrane Database Syst Rev.* 2016;9:CD006170.
Bergman N. Breastfeeding and perinatal neuroscience. In Genna CW. *Supporting Sucking Skills in Breastfeeding Infants*. 3rd ed. Burlington, MA: Jones & Bartlett Learning; 2017:49–63.
Budin P. *The Nursling: The Feeding and Hygiene of Premature and Full-Term Infants*. Paris; 1907. Lecture 3. Malony WJ, trans. London, UK: Caxton. https://www.neonatology.org/classics/nursling/nursling.3.html
Canada. Nutrition for healthy term infants: recommendations from six to 24 months. 2024. https://www.canada.ca/en/health-canada/services/canada-food-guide/resources/nutrition-healthy-term-infants/nutrition-healthy-term-infants-recommendations-birth-six-months/6-24-months.html
Carpay NC, et al. Barriers and facilitators to breastfeeding in moderate and late preterm infants: a systematic review. *Breastfeed Med*. 2021;16(5):370–384.
Cassidy H, et al. A qualitative investigation of experiences of breastfeeding twins and multiples. *Midwifery*. 2024:135:104048.
Centers for Disease Control and Prevention (CDC). ART Surveillance. December 10, 2024. https://www.cdc.gov/art/php/surveillance/index.html
Centers for Disease Control and Prevention. Fortified cow's milk and milk alternatives. October 10, 2024. https://www.cdc.gov/infant-toddler-nutrition/foods-and-drinks/cows-milk-and-milk-alternatives.html
Choi SJ. Use of progesterone supplement therapy for prevention of preterm birth: review of literatures. *Obstet Gynecol Sci*. 2017;60(5):405–420.
Cobo T, et al. Risk factors for spontaneous preterm delivery. *Int Jour Gynecol Obstet*. 2020;150(1):17–23.
Colson S. *Biological Nurturing: Instinctual Breastfeeding.* 2nd revised and updated ed. Amarillo, TX: Praeclarus Press; 2019.
Conde-Agudelo A, et al. Vaginal progesterone is as effective as cervical cerclage to prevent preterm birth in women with a singleton gestation, previous spontaneous preterm birth, and a short cervix: updated indirect comparison meta-analysis. *Am J Obstet Gynecol.* 2018;219(1):10–25.
Dewey KG, Cohen RJ. Does birth spacing affect maternal or child nutritional status? A systematic literature review. *Matern Child Nutr*. July 2007;3(3):151–173.
Douglas P. Re-thinking lactation related nipple pain and damage. *Women's Health*. 2022:18:17455057221087865.
Feldman-Winter L, et al. Evidence-based updates on the first week of exclusive breastfeeding among infants ≥35 weeks. *Pediatrics*. 2020;145(4):e20183696.
Froh EB et al. The critical window of opportunity: lactation initiation following cesarean birth. *Breastfeed Med.* 2021;16(3):258–263.
Healthychildren.org. Cow's milk alternatives: parent FAQs. Updated June 2, 2022. https://www.healthychildren.org/English/healthy-living/nutrition/Pages/milk-allergy-foods-and-ingredients-to-avoid.aspx
Hookway L, et al. The challenges of medically complex breastfed children and their families: a systematic review. *Matern Child Nutr*. 2021;17(4).
Hutcheon JA, et al. Short interpregnancy intervals and adverse maternal outcomes in high-resource settings: an updated systematic review. *Paediatr Perinat Epidemiol*. 2019;33(1):O48–O59.
Iacovou M, et al. Dietary changes among breastfeeding mothers. *J Hum Lact*. 2021;37(3):566–576.
International Council on Multiple Birth Organizations. Declaration of rights and statement of needs of twins and higher order multiples. 2022. https://icombo.org/wp-content/uploads/2024/01/Declaration-of-Rights-2022.pdf
Kellams A. Initiation of breastfeeding. UpToDate. 2024. https://www.uptodate.com/contents/initiation-of-breastfeeding/print.
López-Fernández G, et al. Breastfeeding during pregnancy: a systematic review. *Women Birth*. 2017;30(6):e292–e300.
Madar H, et al. Severe acute maternal morbidity in twin compared with singleton pregnancies. *Obstet Gynecol*. 2019;133(6):1141–1150.
Mallan KM, et al. Comparing barriers to breastfeeding success in the first month for non-overweight and overweight women. *BMC Pregnancy Childbirth*. 2018;18(1):461.
Mann P, et al. Integrative review of cobedding of infant twins. *JOGNN*. 2023;52(2):128–138.
Mikami FCF, et al. Breastfeeding twins: factors related to weaning. *J Hum Lact*. 2018;34(4):749–759.
Milinco M, et al. Effectiveness of biological nurturing on early breastfeeding problems: a randomized controlled trial. *Int Breastfeed J*. 2020;15(21).
Molitoris J. Breast-feeding during pregnancy and the risk of miscarriage. *Perspect Sex Reprod Health*. 2019;51(3):153–163.
Moon RY, et al. Sleep-related infant deaths: updated 2022 recommendations for reducing infant deaths in the sleep environment. *Pediatrics*. 2022;150(1).
Morton J. ABC for professionals: part 1. Firstdroplets.com. 2024. https://firstdroplets.com/professionals/
Muelbert M, et al. Nutritional policies for late preterm and early term infants—can we do better? *Semin Fetal Neonatal Med*. 2019;24(1):43–47.
Oommen H, et al. The association between intrapartum opioid fentanyl and early breastfeeding: a prospective observational study. *Acta Obstetricia Et Gynecologica Scandinavica*. 2021;100(12):2294–2302.
O'Rourke MP, Spatz DL. Women's experiences with tandem breastfeeding. *MCN Am J Matern Child Nurs*. 2019;44(4):220–227.
Righard L, Alade M. Effect of delivery room routines on success of first breastfeed. *Lancet*. 1990;336:1105–1107.
Rose AT, et al. US state policies for Medicaid coverage of donor human milk. *J Perinatol*. 2022:42:829–834.
Scott, A., Kirkland, T. Rethinking breastfeeding management. *Nurse Pract*. 2023;48(3):11–19.
Sinkiewicz-Darol E, et al. Tandem breastfeeding: a descriptive analysis of the nutritional value of milk when feeding a younger and older child. *Nutrients*. 2021;13(1):277.
Smillie C. How infants learn to feed: a neurobehavioral model. In: Genna CW, ed. *Supporting Sucking Skills in Breastfeeding Infants*. 4th ed. Burlington, MA: Jones & Bartlett Learning; 2023:89–106.
Stalimerou V, et al. Breastfeeding during pregnancy: a systematic review of the literature. *Maedica (Bucur)*. 2023;18(3):463–469.
Steurer LM, Smith JR. Manual Expression of Breast Milk: A Strategy to Aid in Breastfeeding Success. *J Perinat Neonatal Nurs*. 2018;32(2):102-103
Sunderam S. Assisted reproductive technology surveillance—United States, 2017. *MMWR Surveillance Summaries*. 2020;69(9):1–20.
Szucs KA, et al. Quintuplets and a mother's determination to provide human milk: it takes a village to raise a baby—how about five? *J Hum Lact*. 2009a;25(1):79–84.

Szucs KA, et al. The quintuplets receiving human milk: an update. *J Hum Lact*. 2009b;25(3):269.

Tiruye G, et al. Breastfeeding technique and associated factors among breastfeeding mothers in Harar city, Eastern Ethiopia. *Int Breastfeed J*. 2018;13:5.

United Nations Children's Fund. Breast Crawl. Initiation of breastfeeding by breast crawl. 2019. https://www.breastcrawl.org

Vizzari G, et al. Feeding difficulties in late preterm infants and their impact on maternal mental health and the mother-infant relationship: a literature review. *Nutrients*. 2023;15(9):2180.

Walters DD, et al. The cost of not breastfeeding: global results from a new tool. *Health Policy Plan*. 2019;34(6):407–417.

Wang S, et al. Analysis on the current situation of twin breastfeeding and its influencing factors. *Medicine*. 2023;102(38):e35161–e35161.

Ward C, Caughey AB. Late preterm births: neonatal mortality and morbidity in twins vs. singletons. *J Mater-Fetal Neonatal Med*. 2021;35(25):7962–7967.

Whitford HM, et al. Breastfeeding education and support for women with twins or higher order multiples. *Cochrane Database Syst Rev*. 2017;2:CD012003.

Widström AM, et al. Skin-to-skin contact the first hour after birth, underlying implications and clinical practice. *Acta Paediatr*. 2019;108(7):1192–1204.

Wu X, et al. Modifiable individual factors associated with breastfeeding: a cohort study in China. *Int J Environ Res Public Health*. 2019;16(5).

Yin C, et al. Effect of baby-led self-attachment breastfeeding technique in the postpartum period on breastfeeding rates: a randomized study. *Breastfeeding Med*. 2021;16(9):734–740.

Zhang L, et al. Effect of interpregnancy interval on adverse perinatal outcomes in southern China: a retrospective cohort study, 2000–2015. *Paediatr Perinat Epidem*. 2018;32(2):131–140.

CHAPTER 16

Infant Latch and Sucking

An awareness of the mechanics of infant sucking will help healthcare providers understand the transfer of milk to the baby during nursing. The parent and the baby play influential roles in milk transfer. A functioning letdown and effective positioning, latch, and sucking by the infant are key to milk transfer. The mechanics of nursing are substantially different from those of bottle feeding. With nursing, the way a baby sucks, the baby's sucking needs, and the feeding pattern all affect milk transfer. Although some infants have difficulty sucking, most difficulties can be resolved with adjustments to latch and positioning. This chapter explores infant sucking related to the baby's latch and milk transfer.

KEY TERMS

Bolus
Carpal tunnel syndrome
Chiropractic care
Craniosacral
Dysfunctional suck
Flange
Hard palate
Intubation
Latch
Masseter muscle
Milk-ejection reflex (MER)
Milk transfer
Nasopharynx
Neuromotor dysfunction
Nonnutritive sucking (NNS)
Nutritive sucking (NS)
Oral structure
Orbicularis oris muscle
Small for gestational age (SGA)
Soft palate
Sucking pattern
Trough

Baby Latching

A deep **latch** enables babies to draw a large amount of tissue into their mouth to suck and remove milk. Latching describes the moment of contact of the baby's mouth on the breast for nursing. The baby needs to latch well behind the nipple and take in as much of the areola and surrounding tissue as possible. This enables the baby to generate a strong enough vacuum to suck, elicit letdown, and obtain milk. Removal of milk, in turn, relieves fullness and maintains milk production. Failing to take in enough tissue could cause the baby to have difficulty extracting milk and result in failure to gain adequate weight. The baby might attempt to compensate by increasing suction and compressing their lips to hold the nipple securely, possibly resulting in nipple pain. A change in positioning can improve the latch.

When latched well, the baby will demonstrate long, drawing, nutritive, high-flow sucks. After copious milk production begins, audible swallows will occur. In the first 24 to 48 hours after birth, the baby's swallows often sound like small puffs of air after 3 to 4 nutritive sucks. There is usually minimal discomfort associated with latch, although transient soreness with the initial latch is common during the first few days postpartum. It is important to validate and explore any reports of discomfort and not to minimize or discount them. If pain occurs, the baby's latch or position needs to be adjusted. **Figures 16-1** and **16-2** illustrate the differences between a baby who has a good latch and one who needs to be repositioned, respectively.

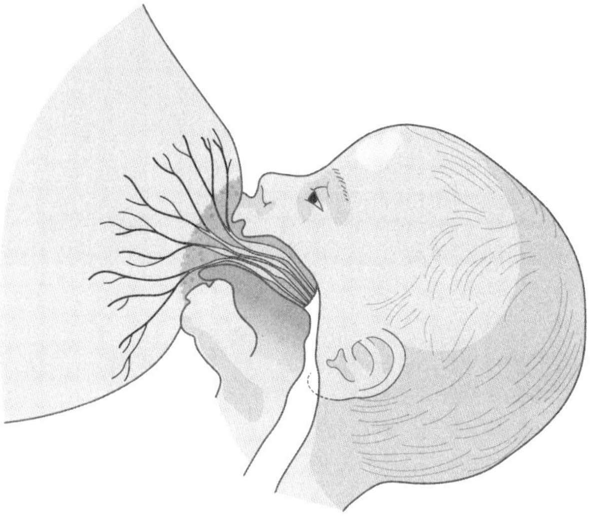

Figure 16-1 A baby positioned well for feeding.

Reproduced from King FS. *Helping Mothers to Breastfeed*, Revised Edition, p. 14. Nairobi, Kenya: AMREF. Reprinted with permission.

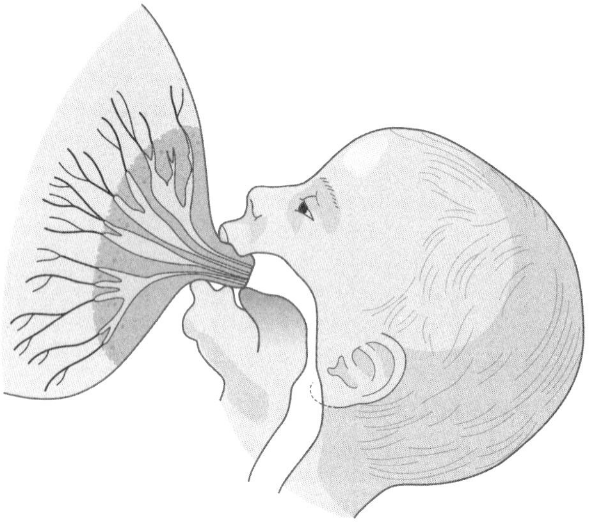

Figure 16-2 A baby poorly positioned for feeding.

Reproduced from King FS. *Helping mothers to breastfeed*, revised edition, p. 14. Nairobi, Kenya: AMREF. Reprinted with permission.

Principles of an Effective Latch

A solid latch begins with holding the baby closely with their head and body in alignment and their head facing the parent's body. Many babies self-latch easily, especially when parents recline and lay the baby prone on their chest. Reclining to feed is called by various terms, including *prone*, *Aussie*, *laid-back*, *baby-led*, and *Biological Nurturing* (Colson, 2019). Effective positioning helps the baby draw in adequate tissue surrounding the nipple and areola. In the position for optimal sucking, the nipple is slightly above the center of the baby's open mouth. For babies who struggle with latch, suggesting to parents that they position their baby "nipple to nose" may help them achieve optimal alignment. With the baby's nose and the nipple aligned, the parent can brush the upper lip with the nipple, causing the baby to aim up and not down, as illustrated in **Figure 16-3**.

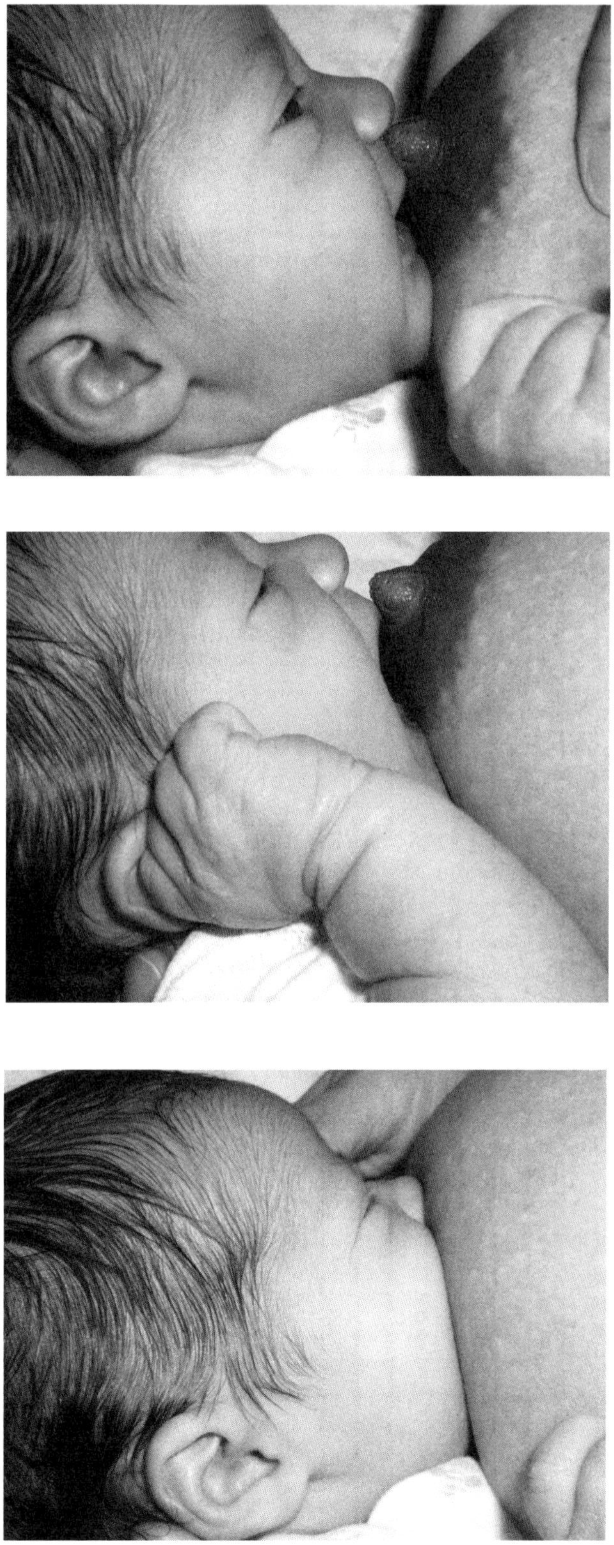

Figure 16-3 Positioning the baby nipple to nose.

Printed with permission of Catherine Watson Genna, BS, IBCLC.

With an effective latch, the baby's lips **flange** (curve) out and open wide to take in a large mouthful of tissue. The bottom lip covers more of the areola, and the top lip covers somewhat less of the areola in what is called an *asymmetrical latch*. An asymmetrical, or slightly off-center, latch can aid in achieving a deep latch. The nipple, areola, and surrounding tissue completely fill the baby's oral cavity. The baby's tongue will be under the breast and will extend outward far enough to cover the alveolar ridge (bottom gumline). The tongue forms a **trough** through which the milk will flow and draws the nipple into the center of the mouth or tongue. The baby's jaws will be well behind the nipple and compress the areola rhythmically, establishing a pattern of repeated bursts of suck–swallow–breathe. These wide jaw excursions characterize **nutritive sucking (NS)** in a nursing baby, whereas they may appear to be dysfunctional when sucking on a bottle.

The Baby's Latch in the First Few Days

It is common for babies to need help with latch in the early days of nursing, especially if labor and birth involved interventions and medications (refer to Chapter 13). If the baby misses the initial latch attempt, the parent can wait a few seconds and allow proximity to the nipple to possibly trigger the baby's search response. Stroking the upper lip or philtrum with the nipple may help a baby who seems disorganized. If the rooting reflex appears weak, expressing milk onto the baby's lips may help the baby locate the nipple.

If these attempts fail to achieve latch, the parent can stop, relax, reposition the baby, and repeat the rooting stimulus. Establishing a routine will help the baby develop a pattern for latching. Encourage parents to think of the early days as a learning period and not to become discouraged if difficulties occur. If the baby continues to be disorganized or becomes frantic, the parent can try to stimulate sucking with a finger after hand expressing colostrum on it. This action may calm the infant and encourage rooting. Once the baby is sucking on the finger, the baby can be moved to the nipple to continue sucking. Often, this helps achieve a good latch and sustained sucking.

Infant Sucking

The terms "sucking" and "suckling" are often used interchangeably, and individual disciplines assign different meanings to them. Descriptions within the lactation profession vary as well. One source defines sucking as the act of feeding, and sucking as the oral-motor activity that transfers milk (Genna, 2022). This text uses the term "sucking" throughout.

Sucking provides both physical and emotional pleasure and is a primary means of comfort for a baby. It can also provide positive feelings for the parent. The baby's sucking releases oxytocin, which signals a **milk-ejection reflex (MER)** in the parent, also referred to as *letdown*. Continued oxytocin release promotes affectionate and protective feelings in the parent towards their baby (Floricica et al. 2021). Oxytocin also helps the uterus return to its prepregnancy state.

Sucking promotes digestion by stimulating saliva and promoting gut motility, which helps the infant pass stool and gas. Sucking has a calming effect on infants, although sucking needs vary from one baby to another. Many babies are born with lip "sucking blisters" and red marks or blisters on the hands or wrists from sucking in utero. Babies use their thumbs, fingers, and hands to soothe and calm themselves. The need for sucking is usually greater in the first 3 months after birth than at any other time. You can encourage parents to be sensitive to this important aspect of their babies' health. Satisfying a baby's sucking needs enhances the baby's physical growth and well-being.

Sucking and Swallowing

Sucking and feeding develop in a predictable and organized way after birth. Sucking and swallowing are coordinated in a rhythmic and repeated suck–swallow–breathe pattern. Babies regulate their breathing by pausing between bursts of sucking. In functional suck–swallow–breathe sequencing, swallowing does not occur simultaneously with breathing. Swallowing while breathing would result in aspiration—that is, taking foreign matter into the lungs. A pattern of increased sucks per minute is associated with fewer swallows. Therefore, a higher sucking frequency correlates with more breaths and higher oxygen saturation.

Respiratory rate during sucking is related to both the duration of the suck burst and the rate of sucking. The infant's respiration rate is lower during active sucking bursts and is more marked with longer sucking bursts. Sucking develops on a continuum, with preterm infants having fewer sucks per burst and longer pauses than full-term infants and older children. Nursing patterns are often characterized by a consistent rhythm and maintaining steady oxygen levels, whereas bottle feeding disrupts this pattern.

Bottle-fed infants may therefore demonstrate irregular patterns of suck–swallow–breathe, risking more episodes of apnea (Cresi et al., 2024).

A baby's **sucking pattern** will indicate the degree of milk transfer. Studies illustrate that effective and efficient sucking and swallowing are reliant on the suck–swallow–breathe pattern. The suck–swallow–breathe pattern can range from 1:1:1 up to 12:1:4. These ratios vary because of alternating milk flow rates during milk ejection. Infants can adapt to the changing rates when nursing (Geddes et al., 2021). Shorter sucking bursts and sucking times usually result in more feeding difficulties than patterns of longer, more frequent sucks. Sucking pressure is an important part of sucking efficiency in newborns and can be used to measure adequate milk intake. (McGrath et al., 2020). The greater the pressure, the greater the amount of milk that is transferred.

Sucking Rate

A nursing baby sucks with both nutritive sucking (NS) and **nonnutritive sucking (NNS)**. NS releases more milk with varying milk flow rates, whereas NNS has limited milk flow. High rates of milk flow result in slower sucking rates of about 1 suck per second, described as NS. The rate of NNS is faster than NS, averaging 2 sucks per second. Examples of NNS include babies sucking on their hands and fingers, a parent's finger, a pacifier, or at the end of a feeding when milk volume is low. Drugs administered during labor can affect NS in the newborn. The impact of labor medications is discussed in **Chapter 14**.

The volume of milk and the flow rate can affect sucking rates. When colostrum is present in low volumes, the number of sucks per swallow will be greater. As milk production increases, the sucking rate gradually slows. Babies suck rapidly at the beginning of a feeding to promote milk flow. After letdown occurs and the infant swallows, the sucking pace slows. The sucking pattern will continue to alternate between NS and NNS throughout the feeding. Babies suck rapidly to stimulate milk flow and then slow the sucking rate to collect and swallow milk. When babies nurse on the second side, the same pattern resumes; however, the duration of active sucking and milk intake is usually less (Genna, 2022).

Full-term neonates younger than 24 hours old exhibit less rhythmic sucking than older term infants. During the first 2 or 3 days, a neonate sucks with several short, rapid bursts per swallow, indicating that the volume of colostrum is relatively small. A regular feeding rhythm becomes established around day 3 or 4. This indicates the arrival of transitional milk with increased volume. At around 4 to 5 days, a full-term infant may or may not swallow with every suck after the parent's letdown. As they age, infants become more efficient at nursing and extend their sucking bursts with fewer pauses.

Assessing Infant Suck

Functional sucking in an infant is a complex process. Infant sucking is explored in-depth in *Supporting Sucking Skills in Infants* (Genna, 2022). Genna references a behavioral sequence that describes the pattern of getting a baby to nurse:

- Hand-to-mouth movements
- Tongue movements
- Mouth opening
- Focusing on the nipple
- Crawling to the nipple
- Massaging to evert the nipple
- Licking and latching

Preterm Infant Sucking Ability

A preterm infant's ability to suck on a nipple will determine their readiness to nurse. Two tools are commonly used for evaluating the progression of oral feeding (Azuma et al., 2020). The Neonatal Oral-Motor Assessment Scale (NOMAS) focuses on observation of oral-motor sucking patterns and can detect early risks for neurodevelopmental delays. The Infant-Driven Feeding Scale assesses an infant's readiness for nipple feeding as well as their feeding abilities. This tool includes the infant's interests in oral feeding and their neurobehavioral state, which is important in NS.

It is important to encourage NNS in preterm infants with the use of a pacifier if nursing is not possible (Shandley et al., 2021). Initiating NNS for an infant born preterm helps establish the suck–swallow–breathe pattern. NNS can be performed between 28 and 33 weeks with a pacifier. The associated pattern of short, rapid bursts will slow down as NS becomes more established between 32 and 34 weeks' adjusted age and the suck pressure matures (Kamity et al., 2021).

Lactation is influenced by the neonatal intensive care unit (NICU) environment, such as diseases, maternal-infant separation, and challenges in managing expressed milk. Because of these obstacles, the frequency of nursing, milk volume, and milk output for preterm infants are lower compared with full-term infants (Lin et al., 2020). NNS or nursing after milk has been removed will lead to more successful nursing sessions (Fucile et al., 2021). Preterm infants who begin NNS at the breast can achieve earlier and more effective nursing outcomes. This increases oral feeding success (Azuma et al., 2020). There is no evidence to support postponing preterm infants from nursing until they can successfully feed on a bottle. In fact, high flow rates from artificial nipples force the preterm infant to continuously swallow, thus limiting their chance to breathe.

Preterm infants can coordinate the suck–swallow–breathe pattern while nursing as early as when bottle feeding. The relationship between the central nervous system, respiratory system, and neuromuscular system should be considered for oral feeding success. If one of a preterm infant's systems is dysfunctional, oral feedings will be compromised, causing a prolonged hospital stay because of feeding difficulties (Azuma et al., 2020). **Chapter 24** explores NICU feeding issues and ability-sensitive protocols that help establish nursing in this population.

Sucking Physiology

Assessment of an infant's suck includes the oral, pharyngeal, and esophageal phases of feeding. The movement and activation of the tongue during nursing can be observed with the use of ultrasound. Ultrasound imaging allows visualization of the tongue in an upward position while nursing, with the mid-tongue resting at the **hard palate**. The **soft palate** connects the oral cavity to the pharynx at the junction of the hard palate and soft palate.

The oral cavity seal is essential to create a vacuum or suction when the infant is latched. Intraoral vacuum with a lack of tongue movement allows **milk transfer**. Simultaneously, the alveolar glands contract and dilate the milk ducts, and milk fills the intraoral space between the hard palate and the surface of the tongue.

Ultrasound studies of sucking physiology reveal less nipple pain and increased milk transfer when the following are present (Douglas, 2022):

- Reduced distance between the nipple tip and junction of the hard and soft palates when the mandible is up and when depressed
- Expansion of the nipple and surrounding tissue
- Increase in the intraoral dimensions
- Decreased movement of the nipple when the tongue moves up and down

Sucking Mechanics During Nursing

Sucking action in nursing involves the baby's entire mouth—lips, gums, tongue, cheeks, jaw, and hard and soft palates. The infant grasps the nipple, areola, and surrounding tissue with the anterior part of the tongue, and the lips form a seal. The soft palate and the muscles of the tongue create a tight seal at the back of the mouth. The baby actively sucks to receive milk, with the jaw having a primary role. Jaw movements involve muscles under the chin (submental), around the mouth (orbicularis oris), and those along the neck that flex and rotate the head (sternocleidomastoid). The inspiratory muscles (diaphragm and external intercostal muscles) are believed to help generate intraoral vacuum during nursing. **Figure 16-4** illustrates the sagittal (vertical) view of the muscles and nerves used in sucking and swallowing. **Figure 16-5** illustrates the lateral view of the muscles and nerves.

During nursing, the baby's tongue draws in the nipple, areola, and surrounding tissue to conform to the shape of the baby's mouth, as illustrated in **Figure 16-6**. When the baby draws in sufficient tissue,

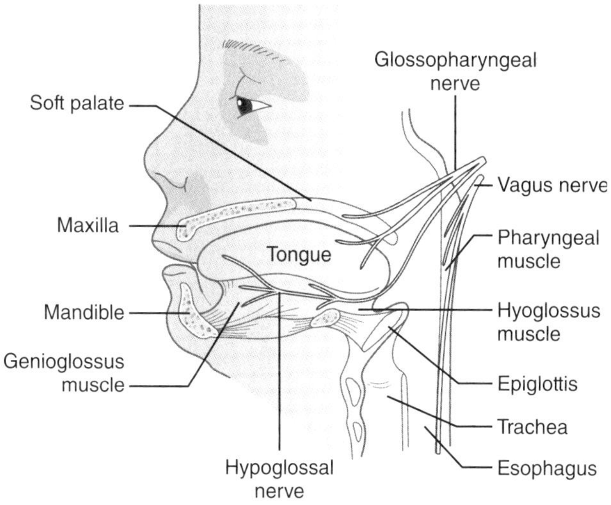

Figure 16-4 Muscles and nerves used in sucking and swallowing—sagittal view.

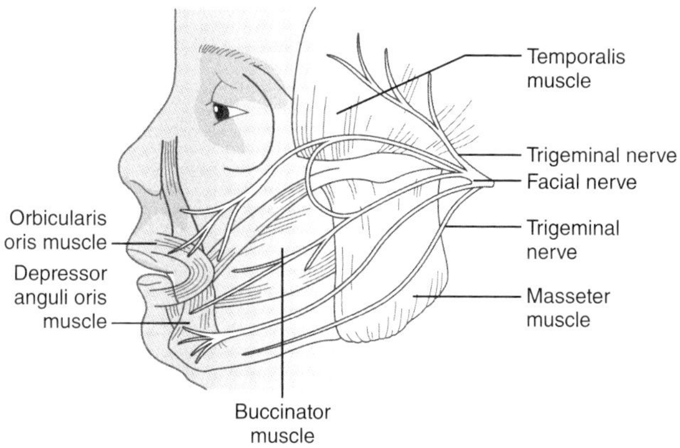

Figure 16-5 Muscles and nerves used in sucking and swallowing—lateral view.

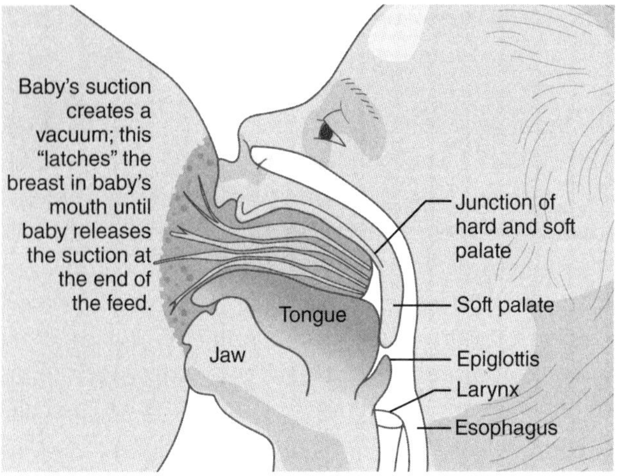

Figure 16-6 Sucking action in nursing.

Printed with permission of Rebecca Glover, IBCLC.

the tongue is free from frictional movement against the skin. No significant in-and-out movement should occur. If the baby appears to slide back and forth on the nipple during feeding, the parent may experience discomfort.

When the baby sucks, the areola and nipple press upward against the upper gum and the hard palate. The nipple does not appear to completely reach the juncture of the hard and soft palates. When the tongue drops in a downward motion, it creates a strong vacuum, which releases milk. This is created by the negative pressure of the baby's mouth (Geddes et al., 2021). The negative pressure created by the baby's suck transfers milk with much greater flow when the tongue is down than when the tongue is up. This negative pressure, along with the alternate compression and release of the gums, moves the milk through the ducts and out the nipple. When the baby's jaw drops, the increased negative pressure moves the milk into the baby's mouth.

Sucking and Milk Ejection

Milk ejection is essential to the regulation of milk production. The MER is a neuroendocrine response originating from the posterior pituitary gland, releasing oxytocin into the bloodstream. Babies with strong sucking patterns stimulate the release of prolactin, which creates more prolactin receptors. Concurrently, oxytocin is released by contracting the myoepithelial cells, leading to milk ejection. As the myoepithelial cells contract, milk flows through the ducts into the nipple, ready to be removed. The MER occurs bilaterally within 60–90 seconds after beginning nursing or pumping. It can last from 45 seconds to 3.5 minutes and can occur multiple times in a feeding or pumping session (Geddes et al., 2021).

Sucking and Milk Transfer

Milk transfer occurs when the baby's sucking delivers a **bolus** of food to the **nasopharynx** (part of the throat behind the nose) and is swallowed. The nipple, areola, and surrounding tissue form a teat within the baby's mouth. The baby's tongue cups along the sides of the teat to form a trough. Milk reaching the back of the baby's mouth stimulates swallowing. Negative pressure maintains latch and may help milk move down the ducts. Thus, the amount of tissue the baby takes in plays a role in how easily milk is extracted.

The baby alternately compresses the nipple and swallows when the back of the mouth fills with milk. Sucking typically occurs in a continuous cycle of suck–swallow–breathe. The baby's tongue continually covers the alveolar ridge throughout the sucking cycle. The end of the nipple is drawn back to within a few centimeters of the soft palate, and the lower jaw and tongue rise to compress the tissue. Milk enters the nipple because of positive pressure in the alveoli created by the MER and suction caused by the jaw lowering. Although some milk is released during compression, more is released when compression ends and the baby's jaw opens.

Evaluating milk transfer is a key element of a feeding assessment. Many babies transfer milk remarkably well while some may require assistance. One way to evaluate milk transfer is by assessing the rhythm of a baby's suck–swallow–breathe pattern. A consistent and rhythmic suck–swallow–breathe pattern indicates milk transfer. A more objective evaluation method is to conduct test weights, which determine the volume of milk transferred after nursing (Geddes et al., 2021). For example, measuring the baby's prefeed and postfeed weights on a sensitive calibrated digital scale can precisely identify the volume of milk transferred. This is helpful with a preterm infant or an infant with rapid and high weight loss or low weight gain. The use of test weights to determine milk transfer is helpful in assessing a particular nursing session but does not predict milk transfer for future nursing sessions. **Figure 16-7** presents signs of effective milk transfer.

Use of Artificial Teats

The sucking motion used for extracting milk from a bottle is very different from nursing, as illustrated in **Figure 16-8**. In bottle feeding, babies draw the nipple into the mouth and must alter the mouth to accommodate the shape of the bottle nipple. The long, firm

- The baby moves from short, rapid sucks to slow, deep sucks early in the feeding.
- Letdown is felt or observed.
- No dimpling or puckering of the baby's cheeks is noted.
- Breast tissue does not slide in and out of the baby's mouth when the baby sucks or pauses.
- No smacking or clicking sounds are evident with sucking.
- Swallowing is apparent every 1 to 2 sucks.
- The baby maintains a latch throughout the feeding.
- The breast softens as the feeding progresses, noted after lactogenesis II (secretory activation).
- The baby spontaneously unlatches and is satiated.
- The nipple does not appear blanched, compressed, or misshapen when the baby unlatches.
- There is no nipple pain during or after feeding.
- The baby is content between most feedings.
- The baby's voiding, stooling, and weight gain are appropriate for age.

Figure 16-7 Signs of effective milk transfer.

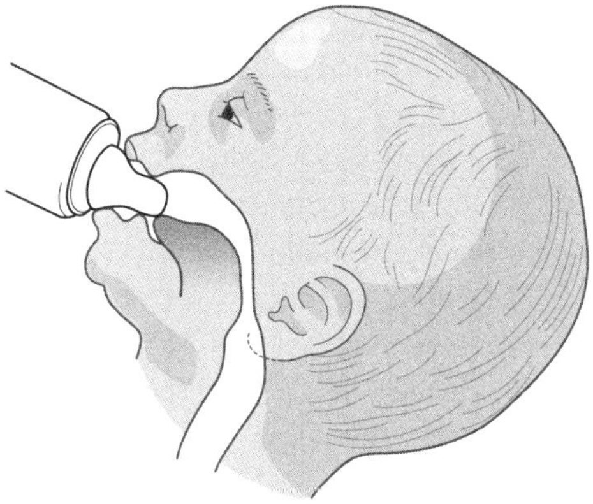

Figure 16-8 Bottle-feeding sucking action.

object stimulates the baby's palate and initiates a suck almost immediately. The baby must compress the nipple for milk to flow freely from the bottle. Any kind of sucking stimulus on the bottle nipple will cause fluid to flow into the baby's mouth, thus preventing NNS. The baby will have to hump the tongue at the front of the nipple to control milk flow. It is important to observe a baby who is bottle feeding as part of an overall feeding assessment. Parents should be educated on how to pace feedings when they use a bottle. Paced feeding is described more in **Chapter 22**.

Bottle feeding results in stronger sucking bursts partly because of fast flow from the nipple. Faster flowing nipples lead to larger volumes and fewer sucks, which affects the swallow and breathing pattern. Longer pauses allow swallowing and breathing to occur. Unlike nursing, bottle-feeding infants are less able to self-regulate their feedings. Infants feeding via bottle are typically fed the same volume each time throughout the day regardless of the time in between feeds (Kotowski et al., 2020).

Alternating Nursing and Bottle Feeding

Because of the very different ways in which babies nurse and suck on a bottle, alternating between the two may potentially create challenges for some babies. This is especially true in the early weeks when the baby is mastering feeding technique. Nursing babies must suck actively to receive milk. While bottle feeding, they rely on the compression of the nipple to remove milk (Kotowski et al., 2020). Milk flows immediately and faster from a bottle nipple. This immediate gratification with bottle feeding may cause the baby to develop a preference for bottles over nursing. Bottle feeding is associated with reduced lactation rates when combined with nursing (Wu et al., 2019). Infants are increasingly being fed via bottle without parents understanding its effects on exclusive nursing. Globally, 59% of infants by 5 months of age are fed with human milk or formula via bottle feeding (Kotowski et al., 2020).

Pacifier and Artificial Nipple Use

Parents will want to watch their baby for feeding cues. They also need to protect their milk production by not allowing pacifier use to replace the sucking needed to stimulate the nipple and maintain production. Use of pacifiers has been thought to have a negative impact on nursing duration and early weaning. However, a meta-analysis of studies conducted via randomized control trials found that early pacifier use is not associated with nursing ability. It concluded that recommendations should include discussing the consequences of pacifier use with parents while recognizing it is the parent's decision (Tolppola et al., 2022). This reflects recommendations by the Baby-Friendly Hospital Initiative and the AAP regarding appropriate pacifier use.

There is a benefit to pacifier use for preterm infants and with transitions from gavage feeds to oral feeds. That said, the use of bottles and artificial nipples during infancy can have far-reaching health consequences. Extended periods of pacifier use create a reliance on it and can have potential dental health concerns (Rocha et al., 2020). Because of the continued development of the craniofacial structures into childhood, extended use of pacifiers poses more harm than good.

Orofacial Muscles

There are differences in infant oral muscle movements between nursing and bottle feeding. Use of the buccinator (cheek) and **orbicularis oris muscles** (around the mouth) is more predominant with bottle feeding compared to nursing. A vacuum builds up in a standard bottle as the baby withdraws milk. As the feeding continues, negative pressure increases, opposing the suction exerted by the infant until the nipple seal is broken. This can lead to difficulty in generating suction or decreased suction strength for the baby. A weakened suck, in turn, reduces the strength of the **masseter muscle** (a muscle in the face and jaw) and increases the strength of the orbicularis oris muscles. With bottle feeding, facial muscles subsequently develop in a pattern that is exactly the opposite of what nature intended. In contrast, nursing requires the baby to use all the muscles of the mouth and jaw, thereby involving all the perioral musculature and leading to its proper development.

Swallowing. The act of swallowing involves the coordination of several oral and neck muscles. An adult swallowing pattern mirrors that of a nursing baby. The tongue does not exert pressure on any teeth and rests against the hard palate until the next swallow. In bottle feeding, babies place their tongue at the back of the throat to prevent too much liquid from being swallowed. To limit the flow, the baby's tongue may exhibit a thrusting motion against the bottle nipple. Because of the different patterns of oral muscle use, bottle feeding has the potential to alter the natural development of swallowing. Tongue thrusting can continue into adulthood, causing an adult to push against the teeth and create spaces. Nursing babies who are given bottles may use this same thrusting motion when attempting to nurse.

Malocclusion. The increase in the prevalence of dental problems in toddlers is attributed to the prolonged use of bottles. Tongue thrusting may be the greatest contributor to the development of malocclusion (improper alignment of the upper and lower teeth). The use of pacifiers and other artificial nipples can lead to malocclusion due to overactivity of the buccinator muscle. This leads to impaired growth of the maxillary arch because of repetitive malformation (Felipe de Deus et al., 2020). Extended use of bottles beyond 6 months when paired with pacifier use creates negative health outcomes for infants. The higher sucking action with bottle feeding can alter the natural U shape of the dental arch and form a V shape. Over time, this could lead to an increased risk of obstructive sleep apnea in adulthood. Protecting the oral cavity early in life can avoid health conditions in later life (Amer et al., 2022).

Problems with Latch

It can sometimes take several feedings before a nursing dyad achieves an effective latch. Approaching early feedings calmly and with a sense of humor decreases potential frustration for both parents and babies. If difficulties arise, encourage parents to keep feeding attempts short. Depending on the baby's tolerance, they can attempt to establish a good latch for about 10 minutes. If the baby cries, pushes away, or demonstrates other withdrawal or avoidance behaviors such as hiccoughing, coughing, gagging, or sneezing, it can be more productive to stop the current attempt, calm the baby, and try again later.

The parent may also try feeding on the other side or holding the baby in a different position (**Chapter 15** discusses positioning). If the baby rejects nursing after several attempts, suggest stopping all efforts for that feeding. The parent can snuggle skin to skin with the baby on their chest and watch for the return of approach behaviors, such as tongue extension, mouthing movements, or rooting. If the baby fails to latch at that point, the parent can continue holding the baby skin to skin near the nipple and watch for hunger cues. If latching difficulty persists, milk expression will help establish milk production and ensure the infant is fed. The information in **Table 16-1** will help you explore the possible causes of latch difficulty so that you can determine the appropriate measures for a particular dyad.

Identifying a Shallow Latch

An effective latch can be determined through various assessments and observations. The baby needs to latch onto ample tissue surrounding the nipple to settle into a sucking rhythm and nurse until satiated. With a shallow latch, the baby may be unable to stay latched for more than several sucks. They may develop a pattern of the nipple sliding in and out of the mouth throughout sucking. Dimpling or puckering of the baby's cheeks when sucking is another sign of a shallow latch. Clicking or smacking noises during sucking can also indicate a need to improve the latch, although some babies who are latched well also make these noises. A shallow latch can result in the nipple

Table 16-1 Helping a Baby Who Has Difficulty Latching

Cause	Suggestions for Management
The baby must twist their neck to nurse.	Hold the baby close, directly facing and slightly lower than the nipple.
The baby's mouth does not open wide enough.	Tease the baby with the nipple by gently touching the upper lip until the mouth opens wide before latching.
The baby has used an artificial nipple and has a sucking preference. The tongue may thrust or hump when trying to latch and suck.	Give no artificial nipples, and allow the baby to suck only when nursing. If supplementation is necessary, use a small spoon, cup, or a nursing supplementer.
The nipples are flat because of engorgement.	Express milk to help the nipple protrude and soften the areola. Try reverse pressure softening.
The nipples are inverted to the point that the baby cannot latch.	Draw out an inverted nipple with mild suction before feeding using an everter or pump.

appearing flattened, creased, or blanched after the baby unlatches. It is the primary cause of nipple pain, so it is important to assess the baby's latch anytime a parent reports pain during or after feedings.

Observing little or no swallowing during a feeding indicates low milk transfer and possibly a poor latch. Latch should be assessed if the baby is fussy during or after feeding, behavior that could indicate low milk transfer. Inadequate voiding or stooling is another sign of poor milk transfer that requires latch assessment. Little or no change in fullness from the beginning to the end of a feeding is another sign of poor milk transfer. This outcome would be apparent after secretory activation (lactogenesis II), when there is copious milk.

Feeding Adjustments to Improve Latch

When a baby continues to have difficulty latching, alternative ways to manage feedings are needed. The parent can recline back and place the baby on their chest, just as the baby would be placed immediately after birth. If rooting occurs, they can help guide the baby to nurse, making sure not to exert pressure. Laid-back nursing is discussed in **Chapter 15**. Parents may have more success getting their baby latched using a position where the dominant hand is in control. A right-handed parent could use the side-sitting (also football or clutch) hold on the right side of their body or the cross-cradle hold. The positions would be reversed for a left-handed parent. Such positions will give the parent control over head movement and help bring the baby in for feeding as soon as the baby's mouth is opened wide enough.

If the baby attempts to latch without a wide-open mouth, parents can encourage a wider opening. Babies often imitate facial expressions. When the baby is awake and content, parents can tickle the baby's upper lip with a finger, talking to the baby, saying slowly, "o . . p . . e . . n . . w . . i . . d . . e" while opening their mouth wide so that the baby will mirror the action. When the baby responds, they can gently put a finger into the baby's mouth, pad side up, to suck on as a reward. Dipping the finger into expressed colostrum or milk serves as an added incentive.

One way to help a baby improve latch is to make the nipple easier to grasp. The nipple may be flat or inverted or might be poorly defined because of fullness. Parents can void overfullness by not restricting feeding frequency or duration. If the nipple is inverted, it should be noted that nipple inversion does not necessarily interfere with nursing. Babies latch onto the tissue surrounding the nipple, not just the nipple. **Chapter 22** describes techniques and tools that help to define the nipple better for improving latch. A flexible approach will limit suggestions to only what a particular parent can tolerate at one time. This flexibility may require providing more alternatives in some cases than in others.

Assisting a Baby Who Cannot Stay Latched

Some babies initially may achieve a good latch and then form a pattern of popping on and off during feeding. The baby may latch and begin to nurse but releases the nipple after a short time and cries or chokes. This might happen several times during a feeding. **Table 16-2** presents the possible causes of this behavior and measures to address each cause. Difficulty maintaining a latch sometimes happens before full milk production is established, although it could occur after as well. A strong letdown can result in overactive milk production and overwhelm the baby with large amounts of milk.

Some situations can cause a baby to have trouble latching and generating enough sucking pressure to

Table 16-2 Helping a Baby Who Cannot Stay Latched

Cause	Suggestions for Management
The baby must reach or twist the neck to maintain latch.	Hold the baby close, directly facing and slightly lower than the nipple, with the nose and chin touching the breast and the ear, shoulder, and hip in alignment.
The baby is unable to breathe when attempting to nurse.	Avoid flexing the baby's head forward in such a way that the nose is occluded. Ensure that the baby's head is slightly extended so that the chin and nose are just touching the breast. Pull the baby's bottom in more, and the head will angle out.
The parent or baby is moving, or there is insufficient support to maintain latch.	Use a side-sitting position with the head cradled in the parent's hand for greater head control. Use pillows or rolled blankets for support so that a fatigued arm will not let the baby slip. Check for a deep latch; unlatch to encourage a wide-open mouth and try again.
Milk flow is too forceful.	Avoid overfullness resulting from limited feedings. Express milk before feeding to lessen the force of the flow. Nurse on only one side per feeding with no time limits; express milk from the other side for comfort. For an overabundance of milk, nurse on the same side two or three times before changing to the other side.

maintain latch. For example, a parent with very large breasts whose baby is born late preterm or **small for gestational age (SGA)** may experience this difficulty. The parent can help the baby stay latched by gently compressing the tissue and holding it horizontally in line with the baby's mouth, as an adult would eat a sandwich. This technique can help the baby take in a substantial amount of tissue by flattening it so that it fits parallel to the baby's mouth. This type of assistance is usually needed only in the early days after birth or until the preterm or late-preterm baby reaches the original due date.

Figure 16-9 illustrates a parent using a sandwich hold, cupping the tissue in the C-hold with the thumb on the outer part of the areola. The thumb and index finger flatten the tissue so that the baby can take in a mouthful. Parents are usually advised to place their fingers behind the areola. However, if the areola is large, this placement might be too far back to provide

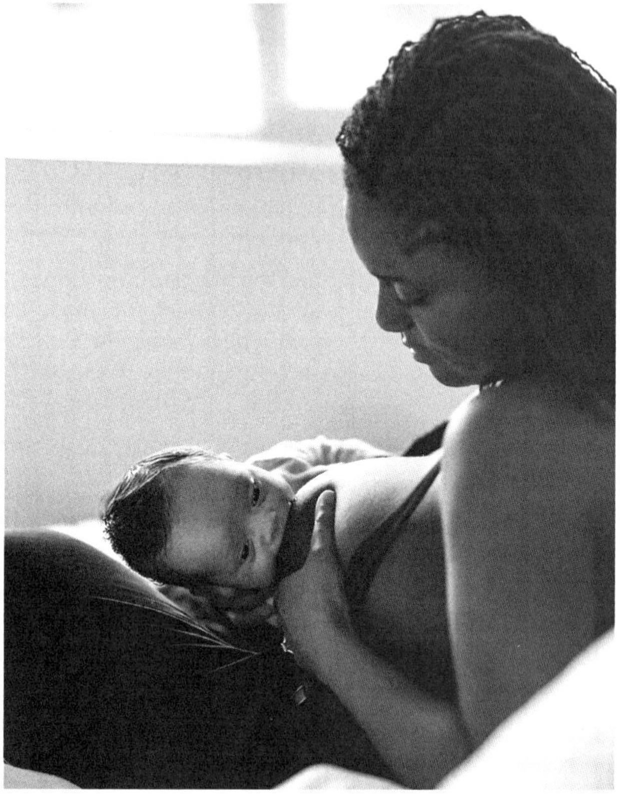

Figure 16-9 Assisting the baby with the sandwich hold.

Printed with permission of Jenny Jimenez.

the necessary compression and result in the baby sliding down on the nipple. This is an example of the uniqueness of each dyad. Flexibility and creativity are two of a parent's most important tools!

Consequences of a Poor Latch

As mentioned earlier, a shallow latch is the primary cause of nipple pain. In turn, the pain—or anticipation of pain—when the baby latches can inhibit letdown and prevent sufficient milk transfer. A poorly latched baby cannot remove milk adequately, placing the parent at risk for engorgement, ductal narrowing, and mastitis. Milk production will diminish, and lactation failure is likely to result in the absence of any intervention. Frequent milk expression is important when a baby is not latching and nursing effectively.

Consequences of a shallow latch can occur for the baby as well. Because of the parent's decreased letdown, the baby may receive primarily foremilk, possibly resulting in increased hunger, fussiness, and the potential for high lactose intake and excessive crying. The baby's urine and stool output may be low, and jaundice may occur. A baby who cannot obtain enough high-fat hindmilk may fail to gain adequate weight or may even experience weight loss. If human milk is not available, formula supplements may be necessary to preserve the baby's health. Supplementation can lead to the end of nursing unless the care plan includes suggestions on ways to simultaneously increase milk production. Adjusting the baby's latch early on can help prevent the potential need for supplementation and the risk of early weaning.

Physical Issues That Can Affect Latch

In some cases, difficulty with latch may result from physical conditions in either the parent or the baby. Size or shape of a parent's breast or nipple can make it difficult for the baby to latch. An acute or chronic physical condition such as low back pain; **carpal tunnel syndrome**; or pain related to delivery, particularly perineal or cesarean incision pain, can affect latch. Physical issues related to the baby that can affect latch include a cleft lip or palate, neurological or orthopedic problems, Down syndrome, a fractured clavicle, torticollis, ankyloglossia (tight frenulum), or a high palate. These factors need to be explored as possible causes for a baby's difficulty with latch.

Some babies engage in rapid side-to-side head movements, making it difficult to achieve and maintain a productive latch. This movement is one of the primitive neonatal reflexes, as discussed in **Chapter 15**. Parents can avoid feeding positions that place them on their side to restrict the baby's head movement. They can lean back and lay the baby prone on their chest, which allows the baby's head to bob up and down purposefully.

Problems with Sucking

Most feeding difficulties result from poor latch or from positioning that interferes with the baby's ability to suck and transfer milk. In many cases, patience, practice, and repositioning of the baby to facilitate latch will alleviate sucking difficulties. Babies who experience early sucking problems are at risk for early weaning. Parents will need specific strategies and postdischarge support to help develop sound practices. If a problem with a baby's suck does not respond to simple adjustments in positioning and latch, a full assessment is needed.

Most latch or sucking difficulties resolve with the passage of time when the baby receives sufficient calories. A baby may have a weak or ineffective suck because of insufficient nourishment. Often, a baby's sucking can improve simply by consuming more calories. **Intubation** and other respiratory therapies are other factors to consider when evaluating an infant's suck, especially with preterm infants. Preterm or ill newborns may have a longer process in establishing adequate sucking. Infants with neonatal abstinence syndrome, discussed in **Chapter 11**, will have sucking patterns similar to those of preterm infants regardless of their gestational age.

Absence of Nutritive Sucking

A baby may appear to achieve a good latch and then suck ineffectively or not at all. First, determine whether the baby is simply sleepy and not hungry. Sucking can be affected if a baby is being supplemented or is exerting energy with NNS on a pacifier. Therefore, explore whether the baby is receiving any artificial feedings and, if so, the frequency and amount of any supplement per day. If the baby spends sucking time on a pacifier, learn when and for how long.

A key part of your assessment is learning why the baby is being supplemented or why the parents are using a pacifier. Many times, these factors can be corrected simply by eliminating the problematic practices or reminding parents of the risks of constant pacifier use hiding hunger cues. Clarification of the parents' motives and education about early bottle and pacifier use can help a baby return to exclusive nursing, if that is the parents' goal.

Disorganized Sucking

Some babies have initial difficulty in mastering sucking. Babies may exhibit an uncoordinated suck in the first few days of life because of sucking habits in utero, birth interventions, or early artificial nipple feedings. Disorganized sucking can result from a delay in the first nursing session at birth, late-preterm birth, prematurity, medications, or illness. **Neuromotor dysfunction** and variations in oral anatomy can affect sucking ability as well. Disorganized sucking does not imply a **dysfunctional suck**. Often, uncoordinated or disorganized sucking resolves soon after birth with sucking practice and protected caloric intake.

Causes of Sucking Problems

Table 16-3 identifies causes of sucking problems and suggests measures to rectify them. Careful assessment is an integral part of determining the appropriate course of action. Many nursing problems relate to an ineffective latch rather than dysfunctional sucking.

Table 16-3 Causes of Sucking Problems

Cause	Suggestions for Management
Medication received during labor	Encourage expectant couples to learn about the effects of labor medications, including epidurals and cesarean births.
Forceps delivery or vacuum extraction	Monitor positioning of the baby to avoid pressure on the head.
Postbirth interventions such as deep laryngeal suctioning or circumcision	Avoid nursing immediately after deep suctioning or other oral insult. Avoid circumcision until after at least three good feedings, preferably after 24 hours of life.
Prolonged crying, especially due to interventions	Comfort the baby before nursing. Feed on cue rather than waiting for the baby to cry. Keep the dyad together skin to skin to calm the baby.
Fractured clavicle or cephalohematoma	Position the baby in a manner that prevents pressure on the affected area.
Tight, taut tissue with flat or inverted nipples	Massage breast before feeding. Use a hold that controls the baby's head movement and ensures a deep latch. Use an eversion technique to form the nipple (**Chapter 22**). A nipple shield may be needed (**Chapter 22**).
Incorrect positioning	Make sure parent and baby are comfortably positioned for a deep latch.
Lack of confidence in handling baby and nursing	Help parents recognize that they will become more comfortable with practice and time. Demonstrate how to handle the baby and initiate feeding. Avoid putting the baby in position for them unless the parent is incapacitated.
High-arched or bubble palate	Use the side-sitting hold. Remove the baby 30–60 seconds after latching and then latch again. The second latch helps draw tissue farther back into the baby's mouth.
Short or tight frenulum/ frenum	Contact the pediatrician, dentist, oral surgeon, or ear–nose–throat specialist for evaluation and possible release.
Cleft lip	Mold baby's lip around the tissue or cover the cleft with a finger to form suction. Massage before and during the feeding to promote milk flow.
Cleft palate	Use a semi-upright position. Hold the nipple in the baby's mouth during feedings. Place an obturator feeding plate over the cleft. Interrupt feeding as necessary to allow the baby to burp or breathe. Supplement nursing. A referral to a cleft palate team will be needed.
Hypoglycemia	Feed expressed colostrum or milk, or formula if they are not available. Nurse at regular intervals, waking the baby if necessary.
Hypotonia or hypertonia	Provide postural support or allow the baby to find a comfortable position. Decrease external stimulation and use rousing techniques, starting with gentle infant massage. Nurse frequently (every 1.5–2 hours) for short times. Establish a routine for latching, especially if the rooting reflex is not well developed. Express milk and supplement the baby until the condition improves. These babies respond well to being fed through nursing supplementers.
Tongue sucking or tongue thrust	A baby who consistently sucks their tongue may have been doing so in utero for months. Teach the baby to suck progressively on the parent's small finger, middle finger, and then thumb to gradually increase size. Finger feed until the baby can latch.
Bottle use caused a preferance for an artificial nipple	Discontinue bottle use and supplement with a cup, spoon, syringe, or medicine dropper.
Stuffy nose due to a cold or allergies	Use an upright position. Place saline drops or expressed milk in the baby's nostrils to clear stuffiness. Avoid a bulb syringe which may irritate delicate mucous membranes and cause swelling.
Maternal medication in the milk affects the baby	Change to a medication that will have less effect on the baby. Nurse when the drug in the milk is lowest. If possible, delay the medication until the baby is older. If reactions are serious, pump and discard the milk to maintain lactation until nursing is safe.

Management of Sucking Problems

Management of sucking problems involves peeling away the layers of the symptoms to find the root cause. For example, poor weight gain is a symptom of an underlying sucking problem, not the problem itself. Determining the root cause of poor weight gain can more quickly resolve the cause of the baby's sucking problem. Feeding the baby formula, in contrast, simply treats the symptom of low weight and fails to address the underlying cause of the sucking problem. Considering conditions for both parent and baby, such as anatomy, oral restrictions, or low milk production, can help in determining the cause of a sucking difficulty.

Sensitivity to the family's emotional states and lifestyle will help relieve the stress parents feel when they experience a feeding problem with their baby. Collaborate with the parents on a feeding plan, and avoid overwhelming them with too many things to do. Consider any long-term consequences of the feeding plan, such as possible stress from a bottle causing nipple preference or the comfort of using a nipple shield. Ask parents what will work for them and enlist their input in discussing options. A practical, participatory plan that is workable, given the family's unique needs, will encourage parents to comply with the plan.

When there is a true need for assistance, start with a technique that places the baby in control of the feeding whenever possible. Progress to the next level only when you determine that the less invasive technique failed. Any intervention in the hospital for a healthy term infant can result in poor or ineffective feeding behaviors. Some babies develop an oral aversion because of unpleasant experiences. Given these possibilities, be sensitive to how you examine the baby, including the way you touch the baby's mouth and **oral structure**. Refer to Chapter 22 for further details on the techniques described in the remainder of this section.

Noninterventive Techniques

The first and least invasive approach to resolving a sucking difficulty is to determine the probable cause and then consider whether the situation is one that will improve with time. If the way the baby is being held is the cause, help parents find more effective positioning. Then wait for the "golden moment," the time when the baby is hungry and rooting with a wide-open mouth. Dripping expressed colostrum or

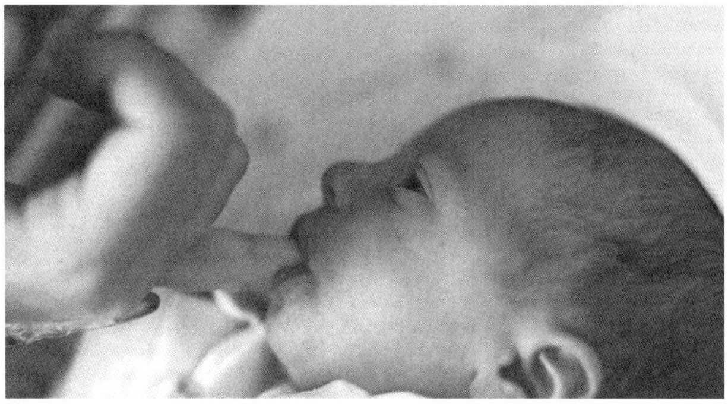

Figure 16-10 Index finger inserted pad side up into the baby's mouth.

glucose water onto the nipple can entice the baby to latch and suck. The sweeter the solution, the more vigorously the baby may suck. Caution parents not to use honey because contaminants in honey can cause botulism in infants.

Minimal-Level Intervention

If enticing the baby has been unsuccessful, an index finger placed pad side up on the baby's tongue may initiate rhythmic sucking, as illustrated in **Figure 16-10**. This also works as a pacifying technique when the baby is fussy and unable to settle into feeding. A supplemental feeding device may be useful for a baby who latches and maintains a seal but does not suck adequately. It provides calories for the baby and stimulates sucking at the same time. If the baby cannot latch and maintain a seal, a nursing supplementer will not be helpful.

Low-Level Intervention

Inserting an index finger into the baby's mouth to evaluate oral structure and suck constitutes a low-level intervention. In addition, assessing the baby's oral structure visually may identify a bubble palate, short tongue, or tight lingual frenulum. Observation can also indicate whether the baby's tongue elevates to the roof of the mouth. Sometimes a tight frenulum is more subtle and requires more than observing its appearance. Placing the little finger in the corner of the baby's mouth between the gums should elicit reflexive bites. The tongue should also lateralize (move side to side). A tongue that dips or cannot move laterally may be tethered. If sweeping the little finger under the tongue from side to side encounters resistance, the baby may have an oral restriction of the lingual frenulum (Lefort et al., 2021).

Moderate-Level Intervention

If less intrusive measures are unsuccessful, an index finger placed in the baby's mouth with the pad side up can help organize the infant's sucking. This technique involves the caregiver placing light pressure on the midline of the baby's tongue and then pulling the finger out slowly to encourage the baby to suck it back in. Provide verbal reinforcement when the baby sucks correctly. With this higher level of intervention, the caregiver exerts more control through manipulation of the finger in the baby's mouth. Its use is appropriate only after other measures have failed to elicit effective sucking.

Parents can use finger feeding to provide nourishment until the baby is nursing effectively. Some babies respond well to finger feeding with a supplemental nursing system. The feel of the parent's finger may resemble the sensory stimulation of nursing more closely than a silicone or latex nipple. **Chapter 22** discusses finger feeding. A nipple shield may be a successful bridge to direct nursing if the nipples are flat or inverted, as well as when the baby is preterm. Nipple shields can also be used for engorgement, nipple trauma, or when the baby has a recessed chin (Almeida dos Santos et al., 2023).

High-Level Intervention

The highest degree of intervention involves stimulating specific parts of the baby's tongue, mouth, and lips to train the infant to suck. A specialized clinician such as an occupational therapist or speech therapist with training in this area may use digital manipulation to improve a dysfunctional suck. The therapist places an index finger in the baby's mouth, pad side up, and stimulates certain portions of the oral anatomy to train the baby to suck. There are different types of stimulation, including the therapist's finger "walking" back on the tongue. Various tools and textures are also used. If there is a need for this type of intervention, other neurological problems, such as cerebral palsy, may be present, with the suck being the first area in which the problem presents. This is beyond the scope of practice for most lactation care providers unless they have been trained in the technique.

In a hospital setting, speech-language therapists and occupational therapists may be available to work with rehabilitating inpatients. A hospital with a NICU or pediatric intensive care unit (PICU) should have therapists trained to work with infants who can assess sucking and swallowing problems. Some parents find that their babies' feeding ability improves with **chiropractic care**, massage therapy, or **craniosacral** therapy (**Figure 16-11**). Developing a list of reliable allied health professionals will enable you to refer parents appropriately.

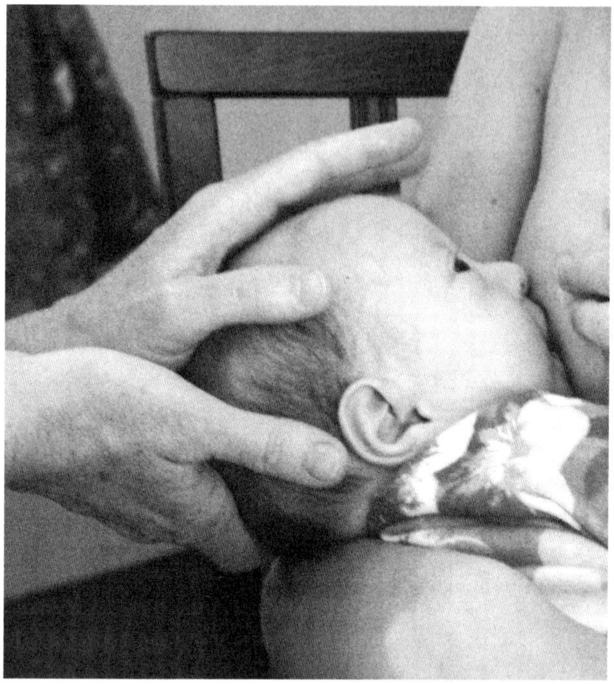

Figure 16-11 Infant receiving craniosacral therapy.

Printed with permission of Anna Swisher.

Close coordination of care and communication between the therapist, the lactation consultant, and the baby's primary healthcare provider helps to ensure that the family obtains appropriate help and protects lactation. If the baby is diagnosed with neurological or other physical problems, community groups are a good source of support and education. Referral to an organization that assists families of neurologically impaired children may be helpful as well.

Summary

The baby's latch and sucking ability and the parent's MER all interact to establish effective milk transfer. The use of bottles and pacifiers can interfere with this symbiotic relationship. Although some babies need assistance with latching and effective sucking, the majority need no help. Many initial sucking difficulties resolve with the passage of time and increased caloric intake. When intervention is needed to improve the baby's suck, caregivers should begin with the least invasive method and increase involvement only when those methods are unsuccessful. Partnering with therapists trained in suck and swallow disorders can help parents resolve significant feeding problems.

What You Learned—At a Glance

Conversation Starters with Parents

- How can you tell that your baby is removing milk?
- How often does your baby suck on an artificial nipple?
- How do your nipples feel when your baby latches?
- How do you know when your baby needs a better latch?
- What problems have you noticed with your baby's sucking?

Signs of an Effective Latch

- Parent and baby are comfortable.
- Nipple is slightly above the center of the mouth.
- Mouth is open wide.
- Chin is pressed into the breast.
- Lips are flanged outward.
- Lower lip covers a large part of the areola.
- Tongue is between the nipple and alveolar ridge.
- Tongue forms a trough for the milk.
- Baby maintains latch throughout the feeding.

Sucking

- Sucking stimulates saliva, gastrointestinal secretions, hormones, motility, milk production, and maternal yearning.
- Sucking is calming and helps the baby pass gas and stool.
- Sucking stimulates multiple milk ejections and facilitates milk transfer.
- NS averages 1 suck per second with wide jaw excursions.
- NNS averages 2 sucks per second.
- Several short, rapid sucking bursts per swallow may indicate low milk volume or ineffective sucking.
- Sucking rhythm is suck–swallow–breathe, with periodic pauses.
- Suction (negative pressure) combined with wavelike tongue movement (positive pressure) removes milk and initiates swallowing.
- Jaw movements and oral muscles help generate intraoral vacuum.
- The tongue draws the nipple and areola into the mouth and forms a trough for the milk.

Use of Bottles

- The baby's mouth must accommodate the shape of the bottle nipple.
- Milk flows freely unless the baby's tongue thrusts forward to block the flow.
- Early introduction of a bottle can compromise lactation.
- Extended bottle use may alter the development of the masseter muscle and dental arch and cause malocclusion and sleep apnea in adulthood.

Signs That Help Is Needed with Latch

- Dimpling or puckering of the baby's cheeks
- Nipple sliding in and out of the baby's mouth when the baby sucks or pauses
- Smacking or clicking sounds with sucking
- Blanched, compressed, or misshapen nipple when the baby unlatches
- Nipple pain during and after feedings
- Engorgement (after lactogenesis II)

Problems with Sucking

- Disorganized sucking may result from illness, prematurity, maternal or infant medications, delay in the first nursing at birth, neuromotor dysfunction, variations in oral anatomy, or nipple preference due to artificial nipple use.
- Babies can develop oral aversion after intrusive interventions.
- A baby with sucking or swallowing difficulties may have neurological deficits.
- Passage of time and increased caloric intake resolve most disorganized sucking.
- A baby who is sleepy or not hungry may not suck nutritively.

Consequences of Ineffective Latch or Suck

- Engorgement, ductal narrowing, and mastitis
- Need for milk expression to protect production
- Increased hunger, fussiness, excessive crying, low urine and stool output, jaundice, and inadequate weight gain or weight loss in the infant
- Need for supplementation to ensure adequate nourishment

References

Almeida dos Santos, et al. Nipple shield use in the maternity ward increases risk of exclusive breastfeeding interruption in the first six months of infant's life. *Midwifery*. 2023;128.

Amer F, et al. Knowledge about negative effects of bottle feeding on babies' dental tissues amongst mothers. *Pak J Med Health Sci*. 2022;16(12):238–241.

Azuma D, et al. Individualizing oral feeding assessment and therapies in the newborn. *Res Rep Neonatol*. 2020;10:23–30.

Colson S. *Biological Nurturing: Instinctual Breastfeeding*. 2nd revised and updated ed. Amarillo, TX: Praeclarus Press; 2019.

Cresi F, et al. Effects of a valved infant-bottle with ergonomic teat on the coordination of sucking, swallowing, and respiration in late-preterm infants. The Safe Oral Feeding randomized trial. *Front Pediatr*. 2024;11;12:1309923.

Douglas PS, et al. A brief gestalt intervention changes ultrasound measures of tongue movement during breastfeeding: case series. *BMC Pregnancy Childb*. 2022;22:94.

Felipe de Deus V, et al. Influence of pacifier use on the association between duration of breastfeeding and anterior open bite in primary dentition. *BMC Pregnancy Childb*. 2020;20(1):396.

Floricica CM, et al. The importance of breastfeeding on the development of the mother-child relationship from an emotional point of view. *Technium Soc Sci J*. 2021;23:467.

Fucile S, et al. Enhancing breastfeeding establishment in preterm infants: a randomized clinical trial of two non-nutritive sucking approaches. *Early Hum Dev*. 2021;156.

Geddes DT, et al. 25 years of research in human lactation: from discovery to translation. *Nutrients*, 2021;13(9):1–46.

Genna W. *Supporting Sucking Skills in Infants*. 4th ed. Burlington, MA: Jones & Bartlett Learning; 2022.

Kamity, R., et al. Feeding Problems and Long-Term Outcomes in Preterm Infants—A Systematic Approach to Evaluation and Management. *Children*. 2021;8(12):1158.

Kotowski J, et al. Bottle-feeding an infant feeding modality: an integrative literature review. *Matern Child Nutr*. 2020;16(2):e12939.

LeFort Y, et al. Academy of Breastfeeding Medicine position statement on ankyloglossia in breastfeeding dyads. *Breastfeed Med*. 2021;16(4):278–281.

Lin Y, et al. Factors affecting breast feeding for premature infants in the neonatal intensive care unit. *Int J Clin Exp Med*. 2020;13(6):4588–4597.

McGrath JM, et al. Correlates and trajectories of preterm infant sucking patterns and sucking organization at term age. *Adv Neonatal Care*. 2020;21(2):152–159.

Rocha CR, et al. Pacifier use and breastfeeding: a qualitative study of postpartum mothers. *Breastfeed Med*. 2020;15(1):24–28.

Shandley S, et al. Abnormal nutritive sucking as an indicator of neonatal brain injury. *Front Pediatr*. 2021;8:1–13.

Tolppola O, et al. Pacifier use and breastfeeding in term and preterm newborns—a systematic review and meta-analysis. *Eur J Pediatr*. 2022;181:3421–3428.

Wu X, et al. Modifiable individual factors associated with breastfeeding: a cohort study in China. *Int J Environ Res Public Health*. 2019;16(5):820.

CHAPTER 17

Nursing in the Early Weeks Postpartum

The early weeks with a new baby are a time of great adjustment for families. Some parents adapt with little difficulty, whereas others require help and support. Anticipatory guidance at key times will help parents manage challenges more confidently. During the early weeks of lactation, milk production is established, and parents acquire the skills and confidence needed for nursing. Assistance during this critical time can help prevent a wide range of potential problems, including nipple pain, engorgement, fungal infections, and issues along the mastitis spectrum. Parents will benefit from your guidance and support as they learn how to respond to their babies' needs and navigate the early weeks and challenges of lactation.

KEY TERMS

Alternate massage
Ankyloglossia
Autocrine control
Breast abscess
Breast compression
Candida albicans
Candidiasis
Colostrum
Diabetic mastopathy
Ductal narrowing
Edema
Engorgement
Fat necrosis
Feedback inhibitor of lactation (FIL)
Galactorrhea
Hyperprolactinemia
Iatrogenic
Idiopathic granulomatous mastitis (IGM)
Labial frenum
Lingual frenulum
Mastitis
Mastitis spectrum
Methicillin-resistant *Staphylococcus aureus* (MRSA)
Milk bleb
Milk blister
Milk stasis
Phytoestrogens
Postterm
Raynaud's phenomenon
Recurrent mastitis
Sarcoidosis
Spontaneous lactation
Subclinical mastitis (SCM)
Sublingual
Suppressor peptides
Thrush
Transient nipple soreness
Tuberculosis mastitis
Vancomycin-resistant *Enterococcus* (VRE)
Vancomycin-resistant *Staphylococcus aureus* (VRSA)
Vasospasm
Zuska-Atkin's disease

Commitment to Nursing

Why do some parents nurse for months, some for years, and others wean after a few days or weeks? Why do some parents never nurse or feed their babies human milk? There is a perception in the industrialized world that although nursing is "best," infant formula is equally acceptable and healthy. In most industrialized nations, parents who nurse do so out of choice and often against the cultural norms in their families and communities. This outlook has significant implications for nursing duration. Prenatal intention, a strong desire to nurse express milk for feedings, and a sense of self-efficacy are key determinants of nursing initiation and duration. These factors are seen worldwide and across diverse ethnicities and cultures, as exemplified in studies among the following regions:

- Benin (Kossou et al., 2021)
- China (Guo et al., 2022)
- Denmark (Kronborg et al., 2018)
- Guatemala (Atyeo et al., 2017)
- Gulf Cooperation Countries (Al-Nuaimi et al., 2017)
- Iran (Mirghafourvand et al., 2018)
- Ireland (O'Sullivan et al., 2019)
- Japan (Hitomi et al., 2021)
- Korea (Park et al., 2018)
- Nigeria (Lawal & Idemudia, 2017)
- Portugal (Brandão et al., 2018)
- Saudi Arabia (Khresheh & Ahmad, 2018)
- Spain (Baño-Piñero et al., 2018)
- Sweden (Wahlstrom Henriksson & Rubertsson, 2021)
- Turkey (Gökçeoğlu & Küçükoğlu, 2017)
- United Kingdom (Burton et al. 2022)

When seemingly acceptable alternatives exist, confidence and commitment to nursing can easily be eroded in the absence of support, encouragement, and positive role models. Nursing has been conceptualized as a fundamental reproductive right that needs reclaiming so that women and gender-diverse persons can honor and validate their experiences as nursing parents (Wahlstrom Henriksson & Rubertsson, 2021). Parents who are poor, young, less educated, non-White, trans, and/or gender-diverse find it most difficult to overcome barriers to lactation and nursing (American College of Obstetricians and Gynecologists [ACOG], 2018).

Social, cultural, and economic forces structure most people's daily lives and intimate decisions, including infant feeding choices. Social media is a powerful platform for sharing experiences, information, and opinions on all forms of infant feeding, including nursing (Oyebode et al., 2021). Recognizing the factors that influence true "choice," including class privilege, will help both healthcare providers and parents identify ways to challenge the status quo and take back the practice of nursing.

Persevering Despite Challenges

A parent who says, "I will try to nurse" or "I might try it," is quite different from one who says, "I will nurse my baby." A commitment to nursing increases the likelihood of persevering through challenges that may arise. Confident parents are better able to overcome common challenges and seek support. Those who persevere despite obstacles demonstrate self-efficacy. They try multiple approaches and view problems as challenges that can be overcome, in part because they believe that they can. They are also more likely to turn to healthcare professionals and peers for support (Feenstra et al., 2018; Rocha et al., 2018; Vieira et al., 2018). An "existential security" with nursing is an underlying factor in this confidence.

Parents who wean earlier than planned often express feelings of guilt, failure, inadequacy, and isolation (Oyebode et al., 2021). Most nursing difficulties can be overcome with appropriate and accessible supports. Early infant contact and unrestricted nursing are key factors that influence how long nursing continues. Furthermore, parents benefit from encouragement and guidance tailored to their individual needs. A parent-centered approach supports parents' feelings of self-efficacy and empowerment in their nursing.

Parents who observe their babies grow, gain weight, rarely become ill, settle easily by nursing, and fall asleep during or after nursing are likely to persevere despite challenges. Satisfaction is higher when nursing is comfortable and when any painful phases are short-lived. Conversely, reasons for quitting within the first year reveal a lack of self-confidence in the nursing process and a lack of confidence in a parent's own body's ability to provide sufficient milk for their baby.

The perception that the baby is not satisfied with human milk alone is one of the top reasons for non-medically indicated supplementation with formula and early weaning. It takes time for parents to get to know their babies as individuals and to recognize that the baby's satisfaction is not totally the parent's responsibility. The infant's sucking competence, alertness, stamina, and abilities to self-regulate and respond to soothing also influence the child's satisfaction with nursing.

Increasing Parents' Commitment to Nursing

An important part of empowering new parents is boosting their confidence. Prenatal parenting support and postpartum visits increase the likelihood that families will initiate and continue nursing. A parent's confidence with nursing is affected by caregivers and the consistency of their messages. Self-efficacy and confidence improve when parents know how to recognize, understand, and respond to their baby's cues and states. The key is to help parents learn to understand their baby's behaviors as age appropriate, normal, and communicative, rather than to perceive their baby as helpless or manipulative.

You can help parents prioritize their baby's needs and reinforce areas where they are doing well with comments such as "Your baby is growing so fast!" or "Your baby looks so healthy!" Point out their abilities as well: "You're so nurturing with your baby!" or "You pick up on your baby's cues really well." Help parents recognize and respond to their baby's body language and hunger cues. Emphasize that they know their baby better than anyone else. Validate parents' concerns and their wide range of emotions as a normal part of parenting. Helping parents understand how lactation works, learn practical management techniques, and discover what nursing means to them will help them remain committed to nursing (Cortelo et al., 2018).

Misconceptions That Interfere with Nursing

Misconceptions about what to expect with nursing can undermine parent's commitment when their experience is not what they expected. Some parents worry that they do not have enough milk if their baby wants to nurse frequently. Help them recognize that babies nurse for many reasons other than hunger and that this behavior is normal. Their baby may be uncomfortable and need to suck to relieve the discomfort. They may need to pass gas or have a bowel movement. They may be getting sick or teething. They may be experiencing a growth spurt and are temporarily nursing more frequently to increase milk production. They may simply want the nurturing closeness of nursing. The parents may simply need to learn how to know their baby is getting enough to eat. Parents and caregivers alike are vulnerable to the numerous unfounded and confusing beliefs and myths about nursing. The suggestions in **Table 17-1** will help debunk these misconceptions.

Establishing Milk Production

Milk, in the form of **colostrum**, is present from approximately the fourth month of pregnancy onward. At birth, the delivery of the placenta triggers a reduction in progesterone levels, which are extremely high during pregnancy. Progesterone inhibits prolactin, which is also elevated during pregnancy. As progesterone levels fall precipitously after birth, prolactin release becomes uninhibited, leading to copious milk production (lactogenesis II). Increased amounts of blood and lymph fluid provide the nutrients needed for the milk. The breasts become fuller, heavier, and sometimes tender. This normal fullness diminishes with regular, frequent milk removal. By about 2 weeks postpartum, when lactation is well established, the breasts become comfortably soft and pliable, even when they are filled with milk. Regular, frequent feedings will help avoid **engorgement**.

Table 17-1 Common Misconceptions About Nursing

Misconception About Human Milk	Discussion
The best way to tell that a baby is getting enough milk is that they sleep for several hours after nursing.	Sleeping does not mean that the baby received enough milk. The more calorically deprived a baby is, the more the baby may sleep. Parents need to monitor the number of wet diapers and bowel movements, the baby's disposition during and between feedings, and other growth indicators (**Chapter 14**).
It is important to wait at least 2 to 3 hours between feedings so that the breast can refill and the baby does not use nursing as a pacifier.	The breast is never empty. As the baby removes milk, more is produced. The shorter the period between feedings, the higher the fat content of the milk. Waiting a specified period between feedings can decrease milk production and lessen the amount of fat the baby receives (**Chapter 7**). Additionally, sucking is soothing to the baby. Babies should be pacified at the breast rather than on a rubber nipple—the breast is for nurture in addition to nutrition.
It's not possible to make enough milk for more than one baby.	Most parents make more milk than their baby requires and can regulate production to their singleton's needs. Exclusive nursing of twins is common and exclusive nursing of triplets or higher-order multiples is biologically feasible (**Chapter 15**).
Weaning is recommended when a parent is taking medication.	Most medications do not require weaning (**Chapter 11**). Refer to information in *Hale's Medications & Mothers' Milk 2025–2026* (Hale & Krutsch, 2024) for specific drug information, also available in mobile apps.

(continues)

Table 17-1 Common Misconceptions About Nursing (*continued*)

Misconception About Feedings	Discussion
Nursing requires more of the provider's time than bottle feeding.	Parents who room in with the baby assume more care, thereby freeing up hospital staff to perform other tasks (**Chapter 13**). Anticipatory guidance and appropriate teaching result in fewer visits with the healthcare provider (**Chapter 2**).
Nursing time needs to be limited in the early days to prevent nipple damage.	Poor positioning is the major cause of nipple pain, not the amount of time a baby nurses. Early, frequent, and unlimited feedings maintain milk production.
Most nursing parents will experience nipple pain.	The typically brief moments of latch tenderness when nursing begins disappears within a few days. Nipples should be pain-free within a few minutes after latching and between feedings.
Nursing doesn't need to start until the milk "comes in."	Colostrum is the first milk and sustains the baby until full milk production begins. Babies need to nurse within 1 hour of birth, followed by unrestricted feedings.
Newborns typically need to eat every 4 hours.	Nursing babies may want to feed as frequently as every 1 to 2 hours in the early days. They will exhibit hunger cues when they want to nurse (**Chapter 14**). Parents should be alert to their baby's hunger cues.
After milk production is established, the baby will usually take most of the milk in the first 5 to 7 minutes.	Healthy babies know when they are full and will end a feeding when satiated. The baby should decide when a feeding ends rather than imposing arbitrary time limits (**Chapter 15**).
Sucking time should be limited on the first side so that the baby will nurse on the second side.	Babies should be allowed to end feeding on each side on their own. If a feeding on one side ends before the baby receives hindmilk, the baby may ingest large amounts of foremilk and develop colic-like behavior or poor weight gain. Encouraging the baby to nurse on the second side after ending independently on the first side stimulates milk production on both sides.
Misconception About Formula	**Discussion**
Infant formula is just as healthy as human milk.	Cow's milk is healthiest for cows, just as human milk is healthiest for humans. Infant formula is inherently inferior to human milk for human babies (**Chapter 9**).
Human milk and nursing are essentially alternatives to formula feeding.	Nursing is much more than the delivery of milk. It is a dynamic bonding process that reinforces the biological relationship between parents and their babies (**Chapter 3**).
Misconception About Supplementation	**Discussion**
Bottles given to nursing babies do not interfere with nursing or lactation.	Any artificial nipple given to an infant in the early weeks of nursing has the potential to create a preference for the artificial nipple and negatively affect milk production (**Chapter 22**). Bottles should be delayed until lactation is well established.
Water supplementation will help prevent or reduce jaundice in nursing infants.	A jaundiced baby needs the increased stooling facilitated by the consumption of colostrum. The correct response to jaundice is to increase the number and effectiveness of feedings. Water supplementation can decrease the amount of milk a baby consumes, which can increase bilirubin levels and result in weight loss (**Chapter 23**). Water reduces the baby's calorie consumption and ability to self-regulate intake.
Formula supplementation is necessary when milk production is low.	Most times, low milk production responds to increased feeding frequency and ensuring effective positioning and latch (**Chapter 19** and **Chapter 26**). Formula exposes infants to a greater risk of disease and sensitizes them to cow's milk protein (**Chapter 10**). Nursing babies should receive no infant formula unless medically indicated.

Ongoing milk production requires a functioning letdown, nipple stimulation, and regular milk removal. The process of milk production occurs through local **autocrine control** after the initial endocrine-controlled postpartum period. When a baby nurses frequently and effectively, there is more nipple stimulation, more milk is removed, and consequently, milk production increases. Thus, to ensure ample milk, it is important to avoid missing feedings, especially in the early days while still establishing stable milk production.

A newborn's intake per feeding ranges from 2 to 10 mL on the first day of life, 5 to 15 mL on day 2, 15 to 30 mL on day 3, and 30 to 60 mL on day 4 of life (Academy of Breastfeeding Medicine [ABM], 2022). During the first month of life, babies establish patterns of milk intake that will continue through the first year. Parents need to avoid strict schedules and allow their baby to lead feedings. This flexibility supports the individual nature of infant needs and each parent's rate of milk synthesis and storage capacity. Each baby's feeding pattern reflects their internal rhythm.

One Side or Both?

Feedings may last only 10 to 15 minutes in the first few days of life. During early feedings, it is common for babies to nurse on only one side and then drift off to sleep. They may be too drowsy or too full to nurse on the second side. This drowsiness is due in part to the release of peptide hormones in the baby's system during sucking. These gastrointestinal hormones enhance digestion and sedation and induce a feeling of satiation and well-being (Huang et al., 2019). The levels rise and fall and may help explain why a baby rouses to eat again when put down. **Chapter 9** discusses peptide hormones and other human milk components.

Copious milk production begins within 3 to 5 days postpartum as the transitional milk comes in. The increase in milk production coincides with the baby becoming more alert and more likely to nurse on both sides in the same feeding. Encourage parents to remain flexible, especially in the early days while they and their baby are establishing themselves as partners in this new venture. When milk production is plentiful and the baby is gaining weight, there is no need for concern about nursing on only one side at a feeding. This pattern is common in the early days and may persist for many weeks. In fact, some babies never feed on both sides and thrive. Beginning the next feeding on the side that is fuller will avoid engorgement. Parents who experience discomfort may wish to pump or hand-relieve fullness.

Duration of Feedings

In general, the baby's needs should determine feeding length. When milk flow diminishes, the sucking rate will move from long, drawing nutritive sucks to a faster, gentler suck. The baby's eyes will close, their fists will relax, and their hands will fall away from their face. Often, the baby spontaneously releases the nipple. When this occurs at the end of a long period of nutritive sucking, it usually signals that the baby is finished. Allowing babies to end the feeding helps ensure that they receive the high-fat hindmilk needed for optimal growth. The other side can then be offered until the baby ends the feeding, either by detaching or drifting off to sleep.

If the baby tends to "linger" at a feeding, the parent can watch for a change from nutritive to nonnutritive sucking. Nonnutritive sucking after a lengthy, robust feeding may signal that the baby has finished. Continuing to suck at this point does not necessarily provide the stimulation necessary for increasing milk production. The parent can end the feeding without significantly affecting milk quantity. Even so, parents should be encouraged to follow their baby's cues. Some babies need to spend more nonnutritive sucking for comfort than others.

No Time Limits

Postpartum practices that restrict feeding frequency and duration are detrimental to establishing nursing. Unlimited sucking time, beginning directly after birth, increases nursing duration. Limiting nursing time does not prevent nipple pain. New parents may be told that early feedings should be 10 or 15 minutes per side. They may hear this as "only" 10 or 15 minutes per side and end a feeding even though the baby may cue that they are not ready. Encourage parents to trust their babies to determine the length of feedings. When the baby is sucking robustly, there is no need to end a feeding. Teach parents to watch for ineffective, weak sucking because these babies might nurse for a long time with little or no milk transfer.

After lactogenesis II occurs, restricted feeding lengths can result in the baby's receiving foremilk from both breasts and becoming too full to obtain a significant amount of hindmilk. This type of high-volume, low-fat feeding can result in poor weight gain and colic-like symptoms. As babies mature, they become more efficient at extracting milk, and the time spent nursing usually decreases. Flexibility will accommodate variations in a baby's nursing style, hunger, temperament, and developmental stage.

Frequency of Feedings

During the baby's first month, feeding frequency for a healthy term baby may range from 8 to 14 or more feedings daily. Most babies require at least 8 to 10 feedings per day. A baby who feeds more frequently may feed as often as every 1 to 2 hours, with nighttime feedings spaced further apart. Babies should be aroused to feed if 4 hours have elapsed since the beginning of the previous feeding. Parents can stop initiating night feedings when the baby is gaining weight within normal limits for age, is stooling and voiding normally for age, and is nursing at least eight times during a 24-hour period.

It is common for a baby to nurse as often as every hour or hour and a half during the day or several times at night. Considering the baby's feeding pattern over the course of a day will help parents determine whether they are meeting their baby's requirements. For example, a baby has gained weight well and has nursed 10 times during the day for 10 or more minutes per side with six clear, heavy, wet diapers and three to five ample, seedy, yellow stools. The parents can relax if the baby sleeps longer that night and can enjoy the extra rest!

Contrast this with a lethargic baby who must be awakened to nurse and has fed fitfully only four times in 24 hours for a few minutes at a time. They had only one small stool or no stool and three very yellow, strong voids. This baby is in trouble and needs immediate medical care. Help parents learn to key into their babies rather than clocks while being cognizant of feeding effectiveness.

By 8 to 12 weeks of age, babies usually nurse every 2 to 4 hours, sometimes less often during the night. A longer nighttime stretch may alternate with a period of almost constant wakefulness and sucking at some other time of the day, generally the early evening. These patterns are referred to as *clustered* or *bunched feedings* and are common during growth spurts.

As babies mature and become more efficient nursers, they obtain more milk in a shorter period and may begin to space feedings further apart. Their needs and reasons for nursing also change as they develop. Babies typically feed more frequently when they are going through a growth spurt, teething, getting sick, or about to achieve a new developmental milestone (e.g., rolling over, sitting up, or crawling).

Increases in Frequency

Preparing parents for increases in feeding frequency before they occur will avoid undermining their confidence or causing them to question if they have enough milk for their baby. As babies experience spurts of growth during their early months, they react by feeding more frequently. Such periods of increased feeds usually last only a few days. When babies nurse in response to their hunger cues, parents may not even notice growth spurts. Often, however, parents are aware of fussiness in a previously contented baby, a baby who wants to nurse more frequently than usual, or a baby who has suddenly begun to suck more vigorously. Reassurance, support, and a listening ear can be pivotal to parents who find themselves with a fussy baby who requires a lot of attention. Encourage them to respond to their baby's needs during this time of growth. Reassure them that this is normal behavior for the baby's age and developmental stage.

Although growth spurts can occur at any time, they tend to take place the first days home, between 10 days and 2–3 weeks old, around 6 weeks old, around 3 months old, and around 6 months old. Robust milk production from frequent nursing in the early postpartum days can carry through during these times until the growth spurt has passed. Parents who understand growth spurts are less likely to suspect low milk production and begin supplementation in response. Anticipatory guidance about normal increases in appetite related to growth spurts can help reassure parents who are concerned that the increase in feeding means they don't have enough milk for their baby.

First Days Home. Babies whose feedings were restricted during the hospital stay may nurse more frequently when allowed to establish their own routine. At home, infants may feel overstimulated by eager parents or siblings and nurse for comfort. They may react to the dramatic difference between the hospital environment (the first extrauterine experience) and the home, particularly at night. Even with home births, babies can still feel overstimulated by excited family members. Conversely, some babies may cope with overstimulation by sleeping, thereby missing feedings. Lowering excessive noise, lights, and distractions will provide a soothing environment for the newborn.

Ten to Fourteen Days. Babies experience a growth spurt approximately 10 to 14 days after birth and will want to nurse more often during this period. It is also around this time that initial breast fullness decreases. Uninformed parents may worry that the combination of increased feedings and smaller breasts indicates low milk production. In some countries, samples of infant formula predictably arrive on parents' doorsteps during the early weeks home with a new baby. Formula manufacturers obtain information about expectant and new parents from direct marketing firms and mailing lists sold to them by retail stores, online shopping, social media use, and other sources.

Three to Six Weeks. In addition to a growth spurt at around 3 to 6 weeks after birth, the baby may nurse more often in response to an increase in the parent's activity level at this time. By 6 weeks postpartum, many parents resume their prepregnancy activities, including a return to work or school. This increase in activity may result in fewer feedings and reduced milk production. The baby's response to changes in nursing patterns may be to nurse more frequently to rebuild milk production. The baby may also nurse more often for reassurance and comfort.

Three and Six Months. As the baby continues to grow, feeding frequency increases periodically to meet changing caloric needs. These growth spurts typically occur at about 3 and 6 months. Parents may incorrectly interpret increased feedings around 3 months as a sign of their baby's readiness to begin solid foods. Anticipatory guidance helps educate them that increased feeding frequency around 3 months does not signal a need for other foods. Most babies are ready to begin solid foods at around 6 months of age. **Chapter 18** discusses complementary foods and weaning.

Other Increases in Feedings. Babies nurse for comfort as well as for nutrition. Illness, overstimulation, emotional upsets, or physical discomfort may cause a baby to nurse for security and comfort. Nursing is the only time in parents' lives when they will be able to protect their baby in this unique way. Studies have shown that nursing relieves pain in infants, including the pain associated with medical procedures (Filippa et al., 2019; Friedrichsdorf et al., 2018). Nursing is more effective for reducing infant pain than dextrose, kangaroo care, or topical numbing creams (Soltani et al., 2018).

Decreases in Frequency

Parents often become concerned when their baby begins dropping feedings, especially if they have not started solid foods or other supplements. They may worry that their baby is not getting enough milk if daily frequency suddenly drops from eight or nine to six or seven feedings. This decrease is common when a baby reaches about 3–4 months of age. As babies grow, they obtain a greater amount of milk in a shorter period and may go longer between feedings.

Encourage parents to observe their baby's overall disposition and health. There is no cause for worry if the baby appears content, is alert and engaged, is voiding and stooling appropriately, is gaining weight and height, is meeting developmental milestones, and has good skin tone. If, however, decreased feedings occur when the baby is ill, appears lethargic, or has inadequate growth or any concerning behavior changes, they may need a feeding assessment. Urge them to contact the baby's healthcare provider immediately.

Signs of Sufficient Milk

Although there are several ways to tell when a baby is receiving enough milk, wet and soiled diapers are the best indicators. Babies should soak at least three or more regular diapers by day 3 postpartum and six or more wet diapers a day from day 5 onward. The urine should be clear to pale yellow, with no strong odor (although some medications can cause urine to smell). If superabsorbent diapers are used, the number of diapers may be fewer; a tissue placed in the diaper will tell if the baby has voided.

On day 1 postpartum, babies should pass one stool minimum. Some babies pass meconium as they are born (known as "terminal mec"), and this can be considered a first postbirth stool. By day 2, babies should pass two stools in a 24-hour period, and by day 3 through the first month, the baby should stool three or more times daily. More frequent stooling is also normal.

Parents should consult their baby's healthcare provider anytime in the first month if their baby does not produce at least three yellow, seedy stools larger than a tablespoon (about 15 g) per day (**Color Plate 28**). They should also call the provider if the baby produces dark-yellow voids; urea crystals (brick dust); or fewer than six clear, wet diapers per day after day 4. These are all signs of dehydration.

The baby's appearance and behavior also indicate when they are well nourished. Regular intervals of wakefulness, sleep, and feeding can reassure parents that their baby is satisfied. Healthy skin tone and color, alertness, engagement, and sustained eye contact are other signs of adequate intake. Meeting age-appropriate growth patterns indicates that the baby is thriving. The most obvious signs of a thriving baby are fat creases in the arms and legs, outgrowing clothing, increases in length and head size, and regular weight gain.

Weight Loss

Weight loss of as much as 7% of birth weight during the first week of life is common. Weight loss should not continue past the first week, and the baby should return to birth weight by about day 10. Babies who nurse with unrestricted frequency and duration from birth usually experience less initial weight loss and more rapid weight gain. Frequent and effective feeding usually creates the right amount of milk for the baby. Recognizing the signs of adequate milk production and transfer will ease parents' minds when this initial fluctuation in weight occurs.

Parents whose baby has lost 10% of birth weight in the first week of life will likely be advised to supplement feedings. Encourage parents to pump to increase production and to supplement feedings with the expressed milk. In addition, the baby's feeding ability needs to be assessed to identify the reason for the weight loss. For example, intravenous (IV) fluid intake of at least 1500 mL during vaginal and cesarean births has been associated with rapid weight loss in newborns, as much as 8–10% (Giudicelli et al., 2022).

A complete feeding assessment will help determine the cause of a baby's weight loss. Learn whether feedings are too infrequent or if milk transfer is not effective. Explore possible impaired or delayed onset of milk production. If there is ample milk production and the baby transfers milk but is losing weight, an infection or other organic problem could be the cause of weight loss. Report this condition to the baby's healthcare provider immediately. **Chapter 19** discusses problems and treatment of low milk production in more detail.

Leaking

Leaking milk is common during the early weeks of nursing and is a normal part of lactation. The range of leaking is extremely variable. Failure to leak milk is not an indication that milk production is low. It may simply indicate adequate feeding frequency and duration. In most cases, leaking will subside as harmony develops between the baby's needs and milk production, usually by 6 weeks postpartum. Although leaking can be a nuisance, it is a normal part of lactation, and parents can learn ways to plan for and control it. Assure them that this phase of lactation passes quickly. Many parents consider leaking to be an encouraging sign of plentiful milk production and a functioning letdown reflex. **Figure 17-1** presents techniques to control leaking.

- Press the heel of the hand over the breast, or cross both arms and press them over the breasts.
- Wear absorbent breast pads and change them often.
- Nurse before sexual intercourse and use absorbent towels over bedding.
- Decrease pressure on the breast and elastic in the bra cup; loosen the bra or wear a larger size.
- Express milk when it is necessary to miss or delay a feeding.
- Wear dark, patterned clothing. Keep a sweater handy to conceal wet spots.
- Check for the use of medications or herbs that stimulate milk production. Discontinue their use if the parent's milk production is overly abundant.

Figure 17-1 Techniques to control leaking.

Causes of Leaking

In most cases, leaking results from breast fullness or the milk letting down. It can occur during a feeding from the opposite breast, directly before a feeding when the breasts are full, or if a feeding is late or missed entirely. Leaking can be triggered by sexual stimulation and orgasm, excessive milk expression, clothing that rubs against the nipples, overproduction of milk, or hormone imbalances. It may result from psychological conditioning of the milk-ejection reflex, which is triggered by oxytocin release. It may occur in response to hearing a baby cry, picking up the baby to nurse, or simply thinking about nursing or the baby.

Excessive or Inappropriate Leaking

Occasionally, leaking is excessive or may continue beyond the early weeks of establishing nursing. Any unexplainable excessive milk flow during lactation or milk production that continues beyond 3 to 6 months after the baby weans is not normal. If this occurs, a complete physical examination is appropriate. Excessive leaking can be a sign of an imbalance in other body functions. Sometimes milk production greatly exceeds the baby's needs. Other times, leaking continues after the baby weans or occurs at times unrelated to pregnancy, birth, or nursing. Such nonlactational milk production is termed **galactorrhea**, or **spontaneous lactation**.

Inappropriate milk production in a nonlactating breast may result from the use of thyrotropin-releasing hormones, theophyllines, amphetamines, opioids, psychiatric medications (including gabapentin and palmitate paliperidone), or tranquilizers (Mancano et al., 2019). Even proton pump inhibitors (esomeprazole), used to treat reflux, can result in galactorrhea (Pipaliya et al., 2016). Chest or breast surgery, a fibrocystic breast, or herpes zoster may stimulate nerves enough to induce milk production significantly. In some cases, there may be sensitivity to normal levels of prolactin. Abnormal lactation can also occur in connection with surgery and stress related to the illness. If no underlying disorder is found, a decrease in breast stimulation may help resolve spontaneous leaking.

Galactorrhea is a symptom, not a disease. It may indicate an underlying health problem that causes elevated prolactin levels (**hyperprolactinemia**). Possible causes of hyperprolactinemia include untreated thyroid conditions, including hypothyroidism and hyperthyroidism. Chronic renal failure, as well as pituitary, uterine, and ovarian tumors, may also cause galactorrhea (Huang & Molitch, 2021). Infrequently, parents may use medications to suppress lactation, but these medications are often only temporary measures. Generally, treatment of galactorrhea requires addressing the underlying cause.

Nipple Pain

Although nipple pain occurs with relative frequency, it is not an inevitable part of nursing. Initial tenderness, or **transient nipple soreness**, is part of the typical postpartum course for most parents. The Infant Feeding Practices Study II reported that 73% of nursing parents reported experiencing pain on the first day postpartum, and 86% reported pain in the second week (Centers for Disease Control and Prevention [CDC], 2017).

Tenderness is common with the initial latch and first few sucks. The peak period of nipple tenderness occurs in the first week postpartum, particularly between the third and sixth days after birth. This period of tenderness may be associated with the nipples adjusting to the frequency of use in nursing. It may also be caused by hormonal changes—akin to the breast tenderness felt during the menstrual cycle.

Generally, pain is a sign that something is not right within the body—and this applies to pain during nursing as well. Nipple pain requires investigation if it occurs beyond the transient soreness of the first week or lasts after the first few minutes following latch. Such pain is a common reason for early weaning and constitutes a nursing emergency. Nursing on a damaged nipple is like painful friction on a scraped knee or knuckle. If left untreated, nipple pain can develop into a crack. Open sores allow entry of bacteria and yeast that are present on the skin surface and may lead to infection. In addition, the increased severity of pain when untreated can decrease the desire to nurse. This in turn can lead to engorgement, reduced milk production, and premature weaning.

It is important that complaints of nipple pain be neither minimized nor discounted. To downplay the possibility of nipple pain or say that there will be no pain if they are "doing it right" does a disservice to parents. Perceptions of pain vary widely, and what might not be noticeable to one parent may be excruciating to another. Asking parents to quantify the pain on a scale of 0 to 10 can help determine whether it is transient or symptomatic of latch and sucking problems.

Causes of Nipple Pain

Numerous myths abound regarding the cause of nipple pain. One long-held belief is that a baby left too long on the breast will cause damage; we now know this to be untrue. "Toughening" the nipples prenatally was once recommended as a means of avoiding pain—an unpleasant and unnecessary practice that damages nipple skin. There is also a widely held belief that being fair-skinned increases the incidence of nipple pain, yet there is no conclusive evidence to support this belief. Nipple pain is mostly caused by positioning, latch, or sucking mechanics during nursing.

Positioning and Latch

The most common cause of nipple pain is the way the baby latches. Nursing is difficult when babies do not face the breast and must swallow with their head turned to the side, flexed down to the chest, or tipped too far back. The nipple also experiences extra tension and negative pressure when ineffective positioning is used. A nursing position that places the baby's body facing the nipple to ensure a deep latch avoids damage. In addition, an asymmetrical latch with the baby slightly off-center on the nipple may help achieve a deep latch (refer to Figure 16-5 in **Chapter 16**). Parents need to know these aspects of latch and positioning assessment.

The early introduction of an artificial nipple from a bottle or pacifier can lead to an ineffective latch. Babies suck on a bottle nipple very differently than they do when nursing. When nursing, the baby's sucking controls milk flow unless letdown is strong. With bottle feeding, the rate of flow is much faster, even with "slow-flow" nipples. In addition, milk flows from the bottle until the caregiver stops it. Bottle use during the time that nursing is being established it may produce an unenthusiastic and ineffective suck when the baby nurses. Artificial nipples should be avoided in the early days of nursing unless a nipple is used therapeutically or if a bottle is the only alternative feeding device parents will accept with required supplementation. **Chapter 22** discusses therapeutic uses of artificial nipples, including bottle teats and pacifiers.

Sucking Mechanics

Sometimes nipple pain may result from anomalies in the infant's oral structure that create difficulty with sucking. **Ankyloglossia**, short tongue, and high or bubble palate are discussed in **Chapter 14**. If milk letdown is strong, the baby may clamp down and compress the nipple and areola to stop the overwhelming release of milk. Clenching and compressing the nipple are also common with late-preterm, small-for-gestational-age (SGA), low-birth-weight (LBW), and **postterm** babies because of their generally thin cheeks and sparse buccal fat pads. Also, an eager nurser combined with minimal milk flow in the first day or two may lead to pain, as can ending a feeding without first breaking suction.

Strong pain from sucking pressure beyond the first 4 or 5 days after birth, when mature milk should be established, might indicate low milk flow. In such circumstances, the baby increases sucking intensity to obtain milk. The center of the nipple will often appear to have a bruise or "hickey" when this increased pressure occurs. Measurements of vacuum pressure in babies' mouths have revealed that babies of parents with continued nipple pain had much higher baseline negative pressure and significantly lower milk intake despite professional help with positioning and latch. The reasons for the higher vacuum pressure are unclear.

Other Factors

Abnormal tongue movement during nursing, including restricted movement, is found when nursing is continuously painful (ABM, 2023). Nipple pain may also result from factors related to nipple shape, engorgement, or improper use of breast pumps or nipple shields. Breast and nipple skin can be tender from **thrush** (**Color Plate 29**). Bacterial infection may be the cause of deep, shooting breast pain associated with *Candida* (Mediano et al., 2017). In addition, impetigo, eczema, Paget's disease (**Color Plate 30**), psoriasis (**Color Plate 31**), herpes (**Color Plate 32**), and poison ivy (**Color Plate 33**) can damage the skin. Bacterial infection of the breast is common in the presence of nipple trauma or fissuring. Sensitivity to topical ointments can also occur.

Assessment of Nipple Pain

Nipple pain requires in-person assessment to determine the cause and appropriate measures. Note the baby's age, when the pain began, any chronic health conditions, and medication usage. Ask about the use of soaps, creams, lotions, laundry products, and perfumes, especially recent product changes. Explore milestones such as teething, menstruation, use of hormonal contraceptives, and possible pregnancy. A detailed description of the pain and the times when it feels a certain way can yield clues to the cause. Asking open-ended questions will help elicit descriptive adjectives. "Burning" pain may indicate thrush; "throbbing" may indicate **mastitis**. Pain on exposure to cold may indicate a **vasospasm** or **Raynaud's phenomenon**.

Physical assessment of nipple damage should note the appearance of the nipple before a feeding. If you observe signs of infection (angry, red streaks; swelling; pus), immediate referral to the healthcare provider is important. Having the baby nurse briefly will help you assess latch and positioning. Observe the baby's alignment and proximity to the nipple, the parent's position, and the mouth–breast connection, as described in **Chapter 15**. After a few minutes, ask the parent to end the feeding and observe the technique. Unlatching without breaking suction can cause nipple pain and skin damage. Examine the nipple for blanching or flattening of the nipple, which would indicate an ineffective latch, as does the nipple appearing rounded at the top and flattened at the base, like an "orthodontic" bottle teat.

Visually assess the baby's oral structure, paying close attention to the tongue, palate, **labial frenum**, and **lingual frenulum**. If no obvious cause can be determined by observing the feeding, with the parents' consent, perform a digital exam of the baby's oral structure. Explain each step to the parents as you do it, both to educate them and to reassure them of the purpose (**Chapter 22**). Also explain the reasons for allowing the baby to end feedings.

Degree of Nipple Damage

Terms such as "cracked," "macerated," and "abraded" are common descriptors for nipple damage. **Table 17-2** outlines a grading scale for identifying the severity of nipple trauma, similar to terms used in the medical field for other types of wounds. The stages of nipple trauma range from a superficial and intact nipple to one with deep damage throughout the dermis. These descriptors help to quantify the severity of nipple damage consistently with a common definition. They clarify whether the skin is broken and, if so, how deep the damage goes. **Color Plates 34** to **37** illustrate each stage in this grading scale.

Table 17-2 Scale of Nipple Pain and Trauma

Stage I	Superficial intact	Color Plate 42	■ Pain or irritation with no skin breakdown ■ Could include redness (erythema), bruising (ecchymosis), red spots (petechiae), edema (swelling)
Stage II	Superficial with tissue breakdown	Color Plate 43	■ Pain reported ■ Could include abrasion, shallow crack or fissure, compression stripe, hematoma, shallow ulceration
Stage III	Partial-thickness erosion	Color Plate 44	■ Skin breakdown includes the destruction of the epidermis to the lower layers of the dermis ■ Could include deep fissure, blister, deep ulceration with more advanced erosion
Stage IV	Full-thickness erosion	Color Plate 45	■ Deeper damage through the dermis ■ Could include full erosion of some parts of the nipple

Printed with permission of Ameda.

Cracked Nipples

When nipple damage persists, a crack or fissure can develop either crosswise or lengthwise along the nipple (**Color Plate 38**). Infrequently, a nipple may fold over, causing a stress point at the fold. Bleeding may result from the baby stretching the nipple to twice its resting length. A significant amount of blood may cause vomiting or produce black stools. The baby's provider may want to interrupt nursing for a short time to rule out internal bleeding. If the baby has black stools or vomits blood because of the fissures, the symptoms will cease when the baby stops nursing.

When the integrity of the nipple skin has been compromised, the open wound serves as a pathway for bacteria and allows for the development of mastitis (breast inflammation or infection—discussed later in this chapter). When there is an open wound, it is important to cleanse the nipple and allow time for it to be left open to air. Use of an antibacterial ointment may help, just as in the case of a scraped knee or other open sore. These ointments are compatible with nursing (Hale & Krutsch, 2024). Applying the ointment sparingly after nursing allows it to be fully absorbed before the next feeding. Parents concerned about the baby ingesting the ointment can gently wipe off any residue before the next feeding.

Figure 17-2 presents the formula for a compounded ointment for treatment of cracked nipples that is widely used in Canada and the United States. The ointment is commonly referred to as *all-purpose nipple ointment*, or APNO. Most compounding pharmacies have become proficient in preparing this ointment, which is available by prescription (Newman, 2021a). If other healing methods prove ineffective, interrupting nursing for a day or two may help the nipples heal (expressing milk during that time to protect production). **Table 17-3** summarizes the treatment options for cracked nipples.

> Mupirocin 2 percent ointment (not cream): 15 grams.
> Betamethasone 0.1 percent ointment (not cream): 15 grams.
> Add miconazole powder so that the final concentration is 2 percent miconazole.
> May also add ibuprofen powder, so that the final concentration of ibuprofen is 2 percent.

Figure 17-2 Dr. Jack Newman's all-purpose nipple ointment.

Resolving Nipple Pain

Determining the cause of nipple pain will identify how to make the necessary adjustments in nursing management or respond to other factors. Resolution of the pain may be a simple matter of altering the position of the parent or baby during feedings or ensuring that the baby gets a deep latch. Corrections may be needed in other aspects of the way the parent manages feedings. Resolution may require examining the nipples for evidence of vasospasm or the baby's oral structure for anomalies.

Correct Positioning

If positioning appears to be the cause of nipple pain, help the parent make the necessary adjustments. Ensure that the baby is level with and facing the nipple and that the baby's body and head are aligned. If the baby has been held in only one position to feed, a different position may provide relief to the sore area.

Table 17-3 Causes and Treatment of Cracked Nipples

Causes	Actions to Take
All causes of nipple pain carried to extreme	■ Consult healthcare provider about using ibuprofen, acetaminophen, or other analgesic. ■ Increase protein, vitamin C, and zinc in the diet. ■ Refer to actions for nipple pain.
Nipple folds over (crack may appear at fold)	■ Air-dry nipples after feeding. Breast shells or hydrogel pads may prevent chafing.
Local infection (baby with *Staphylococcus* or other organism may have infected the nipples)	■ Have healthcare provider check nipples, culture baby's throat and parent's nipples, and treat accordingly.
Baby overly eager at feedings	■ Respond to feeding cues promptly. ■ Break the latch before baby stops sucking, to prevent chomping. ■ Limit feedings to 10–15 minutes per side until nipple heals. ■ Pre-express milk to hasten letdown. ■ Nurse in a position that does not aggravate crack.

The parent's body position and postural support for the baby's weight are also important. If their arms tire during a feeding, the baby may not remain level with the nipple. The baby could slip down and exert more pressure on the nipple or slide to the nipple base. While exploring possible causes for the pain, ask what has already been done for relief. Explore all possible causes before suggesting treatment.

Correct Latch

The baby must latch effectively for milk transfer to occur and to ensure the parent's comfort. The baby's mouth should open wide and optimally slightly off-center from the nipple. Because only the lower jaw moves, positioning the mouth so that the baby takes in more of the underside of the areola will help compress the ducts most effectively. Babies mimic the facial expressions of others, so the parent can demonstrate a wide-open mouth and repeatedly say, "o … p … e … n" as the baby works to latch. This is useful for babies who appear to "chew" their way onto the nipple.

The baby's lips should flange outward, and the mouth should have a wide angle when the baby begins sucking. Parents need to be mindful of lip placement and can help the baby flange one or both lips when needed. Working with the baby to establish a deep latch can avoid this. Helpful video clips demonstrating latch techniques can be found on many reputable websites. Babies who bite during nursing often respond well to prone positioning, with the baby self-latching and with chin support or **sublingual** pressure (gentle pressure under the chin) provided.

Alter Nursing Technique

Changing the way feedings are managed may provide relief from nipple pain. Starting a feeding with the least sore side may avoid the stronger sucking that often occurs at the beginning of a feeding. Pumping for a few minutes to initiate milk ejection before feeding will make milk readily available and reduce the stronger sucking. Eliminating prolonged nonnutritive (comfort) sucking will reduce the amount of irritation and allow longer periods between feedings for the nipples to rest. If necessary, **alternate massage** may help sustain sucking and swallowing and relieve long periods of negative pressure. In this technique, massage and compress the breast each time the baby pauses during a feeding. Use of a nipple shield can reduce the friction of a baby sliding back and forth on the nipple. Select the size closest to the nipple size and ensure that the shield is applied correctly. Refer to **Chapter 22** for more information on appropriate use of nipple shields and monitoring milk transfer.

Using a variety of nursing positions can help alleviate pain during sucking. Keeping the baby's chin, and thus the tongue, away from that area will avoid further irritation to a sore spot. Visualizing the breast as a clock can help determine the location of the pain and find a position that will minimize irritation. **Figure 17-3** illustrates the relationship between some common nursing positions and the resulting sore spots. Unusual positions, such as lying down with the baby's feet pointing above the parent's head, may also provide pain relief and distribute stress more evenly.Refer to **Chapter 15** for discussion of various nursing positions.

If dried milk adheres to a bra or breast pad, moistening the fabric before removing it can avoid nipple damage. A parent who has been ending feedings without releasing suction can learn to break suction with a finger between the baby's gums before removing the baby. When the pain is resolved, the baby should be

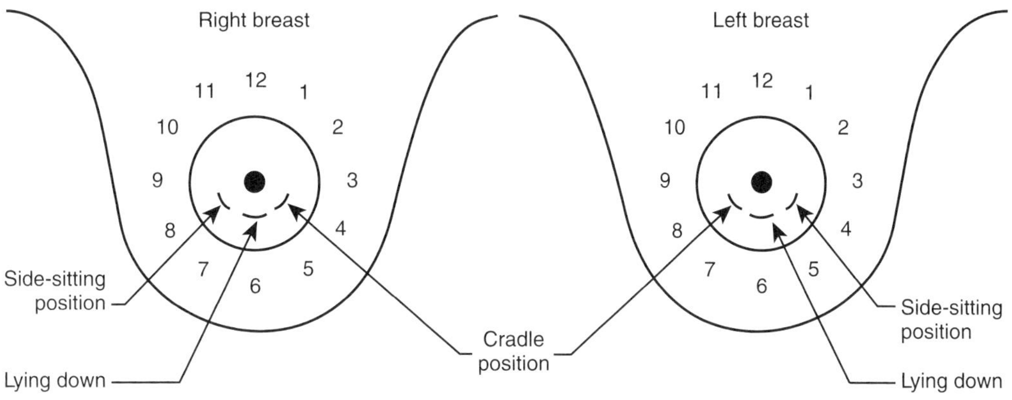

Figure 17-3 Location of nipple sore related to positioning.

allowed to determine when to end the feeding. Pain connected to a retracted or inverted nipple may find relief from techniques that gently evert the nipple, as described in **Chapter 7**.

Address Physical Causes

Vasospasms (constriction of blood vessels) of the nipple create a Raynaud's-like phenomenon, with the pain described as stinging, tingling, burning, very painful, and persisting after the feeding. A triphasic color change occurs, with the nipple turning white (blanching), then purple or blue (cyanotic), and then red (rubor). Vasospasm pain may occur when the nipples are exposed to cold, which is a marker for Raynaud's phenomenon. Vasospasms may result from the baby's jaw clenching and compressing the breast so tightly that it interrupts blood flow to the nipple. Addressing the latch or cause for the compression may resolve the problem.

Treatment for vasospasm includes avoiding cold and applying heat after feedings. Caffeine and nicotine constrict blood vessels and can increase the severity of Raynaud's-related pain. Thus, avoiding caffeine may bring relief. Increasing intake of vitamin B_6 may also help. Use caution when recommending supplementation with this vitamin, however, because high doses (e.g., 600 mg) are associated with lower milk production. Additionally, vitamin B_6 passes readily into the milk, and too much could harm the baby. Consumption of vitamin B_6 should be limited to no more than 25 mg per day (Hale & Krutsch, 2024). Calcium-channel blockers such as nifedipine are also frequently prescribed and have been helpful (Jansen & Sampene, 2019). Often, the validation that continual nipple pain is abnormal and has a cause is a big relief to new parents. Consult **Chapter 26** for further discussion of Raynaud's phenomenon.

Ankyloglossia, or tongue-tie, is a common cause of nipple pain (**Color Plate 23**). If a tight lingual frenulum restricts the tongue's normal range of motion, releasing the frenulum may provide relief. A tight labial frenum on the upper lip (**Color Plate 24**) could also interfere with latch. There is a variance in terminology for tethered oral tissues, with labial frenum also called *labial frenulum*. Refer parents to a provider experienced in assessment of this condition for evaluation and a frenulotomy or frenectomy with a laser or sterile scissors, if appropriate (O'Shea et al., 2017). Refer to **Chapter 14** for more information on oral anomalies.

Pain Management

An anti-inflammatory medication such as ibuprofen or naproxen may be helpful if it is approved for use by the caregiver. Applying ice in a wet cloth to the nipple before the baby latches may provide temporary relief. If this technique is used, the ice should not be placed directly on the skin. An ointment or gel pad may also provide comfort. An allergic reaction to a topical remedy could prevent the nipples from healing and be the cause of continued pain. **Table 17-4** summarizes the treatment options for nipple pain.

Heal the Nipple

Over the centuries, every culture has developed its own comfort measures for nipple pain. Ask the families in your care which healing agents are typically used in their culture and demonstrate respect for their practices. Moist wound healing is the most effective treatment for healing damaged skin. Many practitioners recommend applying expressed milk to the sore area and air-drying the nipple. Properties in human milk protect against tissue damage and help stimulate the immune function and growth of tissue (Vieira et al., 2017). In most cases expressed milk is

Table 17-4 Causes and Treatment of Nipple Pain

Causes	Actions to Take
Soreness from newborn sucking	■ Ensure baby latches and unlatches properly. ■ Ensure nipple is back far enough in baby's mouth. ■ Hold baby closely during nursing so that nipple is not being pulled. ■ Use pure anhydrous lanolin or hydrogel pad as temporary comfort measures.
Dried colostrum or milk causing nipple to adhere to bra or breast pad	■ Moisten bra or pad before removing it.
Poor positioning	■ Hold baby closely during nursing so that nipple is not being pulled. ■ Ensure baby has a big mouthful of breast tissue.
Baby chewing or nuzzling on nipple	■ Form nipple for baby. ■ Encourage rooting reflex so that baby self-latches.
Baby nursing on end of nipple	■ Ensure baby is positioned properly. ■ Check for oral structure anomalies. ■ Check for inverted nipples. ■ Check for engorgement.
Baby chewing their way off nipple or nipple being pulled out of baby's mouth at end of feeding	■ Place a finger between baby's gums to break suction. ■ End feeding when baby's sucking slows, before baby begins to chew on nipple.
Baby overly eager to nurse	■ Respond to feeding cues promptly. ■ Pre-express milk to hasten letdown and avoid vigorous sucking.
Inadequate letdown	■ Use massage and relaxation before feedings. ■ Condition letdown by setting up routine for baby to latch.
Nipples not allowed to dry	■ Check for leaking milk. ■ Remove plastic liners in breast pads. ■ Wear cotton or cotton blends, not synthetic fabrics. ■ Air-dry nipples after feedings. ■ Change breast pads frequently.
Improper use of nipple shield	■ Have baby latch onto nipple after shield draws it out. ■ Avoid shields with inner ridges that irritate nipples.
Inadequate milk production; baby tugging or sucking to encourage milk flow	■ Nurse more frequently (every 1 to 1½ hours). ■ Nurse long enough to facilitate good milk production.
Nipple skin not resistant to stress	■ Improve nutrition, especially by adding fresh fruits and vegetables and vitamin supplements. ■ Eliminate or decrease sugary foods, alcohol, caffeine, and cigarettes. ■ Check for use of cleansing or drying agents.
Natural oils removed or keratin layers broken down by drying agents such as soap, alcohol, shampoo, or deodorant	■ Eliminate irritants. ■ Wash nipples with water only. ■ Use lanolin or hydrogel pads after air-drying.
Nipple irritated by not wearing a bra under rough clothing or by rubbing against bra during vigorous exercise	■ Wear a bra or change to one with more support (e.g., sports bra). ■ Try wearing different fabrics.
Residue of laundry products present on clothing	■ Use less detergent, and rinse laundry twice. ■ Try different laundry products.

Causes	Actions to Take
Teething causes increased feedings, chomping down on nipple, irritation by a change in baby's saliva or medication used for baby's gums	■ Wash nipples after every feeding in plain warm water to remove baby's saliva or other irritants. ■ Use soothing techniques instead of nursing to comfort baby. ■ Stop feeding after the first incident of biting and resume when baby is hungrier. ■ Keep finger ready to break suction, and stop feeding when sucking pattern changes.
Baby falls asleep and clamps down on nipple	■ End the feeding before the baby falls asleep.
Teeth marks on breast (not usually cause for pain, but it may be described as biting)	■ Alternate nursing positions.
Irritation from food particles in toddler's mouth	■ Check toddler's mouth before feedings. ■ Offer toddler a sip of water or wipe their mouth with clean, moist cloth before nursing. ■ Nurse before offering solid foods.
Menstruation or pregnancy	■ If menstruating, discomfort will last only a few days. ■ If pregnant, discuss plans for continued nursing or weaning.
Thrush (*Candida* infection)	■ Have healthcare provider check and prescribe medication for both parent and baby. ■ Discard or boil any items the baby puts in their mouth.

the most convenient option to help with healing and has no adverse side effects for the parent or infant. Many parents use topical applications to treat nipple pain. Make sure they avoid any applications that need to be removed before a feeding. Rubbing to remove topical agents can further aggravate nipple damage. Consult **Chapter 22** for more information on nipple ointments. It may sometimes be necessary to remove dead tissue from the skin—referred to as *debriding*—by gently blotting it with a tissue or peeling off the dead tissue, not scrubbing.

With continued nipple pain, stopping nursing for several feedings or even a few days may preserve long-term nursing. Nursing can resume with every second or third feeding, gradually increasing to full nursing as the nipples heal and latch and suck improve. A lot of skin-to-skin contact during this time will help the baby associate the parent's smell and skin with nurture and nourishment.

Whenever nursing is interrupted, milk must be expressed frequently to maintain milk production. The type of expression used depends on the stage of lactation. A hospital-grade pump is recommended during the early postpartum period to help establish milk production. Hand expression or a personal consumer pump may be sufficient after milk production is well established. If pumping exclusively, parents can double pump for approximately 15 minutes per session, 8 to 12 times in 24 hours, or pumping to match the baby's feeding frequency as closely as possible. A small amount of olive oil dabbed on the flange before pumping lessens the pulling on the areola and makes pumping more comfortable. The pump should be set at the lowest suction level at the beginning of pumping to avoid increased pain. As the condition improves, the suction setting can be increased, although stronger suction does not necessarily produce better results. Refer to **Chapter 22** for further discussion of breast pumps.

Candidiasis

Nipple pain could be caused by *Candida*, also called ***Candida albicans***. *Candida* is a fungus that is typically found in small amounts in the mouth, skin, intestines, and vagina. Under normal conditions, the body's flora keeps its growth in check. When *Candida* is off-balance, the yeast overgrows and causes infection (**candidiasis**). Obesity or excessive sweating provides consistently warm, moist areas in which *Candida* can thrive. Diabetes, illness, pregnancy, oral contraceptives, poor diet, antibiotic therapy, steroid therapy, and immunosuppression can disturb the normal flora and lead to yeast infection (Genovese et al., 2019).

Yeast infection on the nipples is associated with nipple damage early in lactation, mastitis, recent use of antibiotics in the postpartum period, long-term antibiotic use before pregnancy, and vaginal yeast infection. A baby may contract oral yeast while passing through the birth canal during delivery and then transfer the infection to the nipples when nursing. *Candida* infection can be fatal to high-risk populations, such as infants in the neonatal intensive care unit.

Identifying a Candida Infection

The most obvious symptoms of a *Candida* infection are usually breast and nipple pain. When severely sore nipples occur after a period of pain-free nursing, a yeast infection may be the cause. Candida pain is often described as an intense burning sensation deep within the breast during or after feedings. The areola may have a shiny, pinkish cast, which is easily detected with a small flashlight or other focused beam of light. There may be white patches or redness on the nipple (**Color Plate 29**) and slight **edema** in the areola. There may also be a break in the skin similar to a positional compression stripe at the base of the nipple shank, where the nipple joins the areola.

A *Candida* infection can also be present in the baby's mouth—called *thrush*. Thrush presents as white patches that look like milk curds, as presented in **Color Plate 25**. The patches cannot be wiped off, which distinguishes them from the common milk coating on the baby's tongue. In the diaper area, yeast may present as a raised, very red area with a sharply defined border. Symptoms of vaginal yeast are usually difficult to miss. The vaginal area and vulva are tender and very red, with intense itching. There may also be a cheesy, white vaginal discharge. Babies with a yeast infection often seem to be gassy and fussy.

A *Candida* infection does not always present with visual symptoms, making identification challenging. Yeast can also be mistaken for other conditions, most notably vasospasms. These need to be ruled out before treating for yeast, including improving the latch and warming nipples following a feed (International Breastfeeding Centre [IBC], 2021).

Candida and Nursing

Candida infections are more prevalent in infants who are predominantly nursed than in those who are bottle fed. *Candida* is also found more frequently on the nipples of lactating parents than on nonlactating parents. Debate continues over whether yeast can reside within the breast ducts. A prospective study to detect *Candida* in the milk of women with severe nipple and deep breast pain found no significant difference between the control group and the group with pain, leading the researchers to question the existence of ductal yeast (Hale et al., 2009).

Another prospective study proposed that *Candida* and *Staphylococcus aureus* (*S. aureus*) act independently, despite often coexisting. The researchers isolated *Candida* in milk samples from 33% of the women studied (Amir et al., 2013). Other researchers, like Hale, did not determine reliable results (Kaski & Kvist, 2018; Mutschlechner et al., 2016). One group stated that yeasts in breast and nipple pain are marginal, if any, and that staphylococci and streptococci are likely responsible for breast pain (Jiménez et al., 2017).

Treating a Candida Infection

When *Candida* is present on the nipples, the baby often has oral thrush, and the reverse is also true. For this reason, simultaneous treatment of the nipples and the baby is imperative regardless of whether there are symptoms in both. Any other infection sites need treatment as well, including the diaper area and vagina, and family members who harbor the infection. A *Candida* infection recurs very easily, so it is important to follow the full course of treatment even after symptoms subside. The *Candida* strain on the nipples and in the baby's mouth can be different from that found in a diaper rash. Unfortunately, many strains of *Candida* are resistant to the most used medications.

Antifungal topical agents used to treat *Candida* on nipples include nystatin, clotrimazole, miconazole nitrate, ketoconazole, ciclopirox, and naftifine hydrochloride. Although nystatin is often the first treatment suggested, the other topical agents are reportedly more effective. Clotrimazole and miconazole are typically available as over-the-counter products, whereas the other agents may require a prescription. The first-line treatment for *Candida* in the baby's mouth is typically nystatin, an oral antifungal agent.

To treat an oral infection, rinse the baby's mouth with water after feeding, shake and pour nystatin into a cup, and apply it to all surfaces of the baby's mouth with a cotton swab. The swab should never be dipped back into the original vial of nystatin. To treat the nipples, rinse them with a solution made from 1 cup of plain, tepid water mixed with 1 tablespoon of vinegar and air-dry them. Apply an antifungal cream sparingly so that it soaks in by the time the baby is ready to nurse again. The cream does not need to be washed off the nipple, although breast pads should be changed at every feeding. Air-drying and brief exposure to sunlight or artificial light may be helpful, given that yeast thrives in dark, moist environments.

Gentian violet has been used historically to treat both oral and nipple *Candida* infections. However, it has been banned for both human and veterinary uses in some countries, including Australia, England, France, and Canada, because of concerns over toxicity and potential links to cancers (Drugs and Lactation Database, 2024). Gentian violet is available as an over-the-counter solution in many countries, and parents must be informed of the research on the potential risks before using gentian violet as a treatment for thrush. Ulcerations of the mucous membranes in the baby's mouth may result from excessive use or from use of gentian violet at strengths greater than 0.5% (Health Canada, 2019). Use of gentian violet for oral and nipple yeast infection is discouraged.

When discussing treatment options with parents, it is helpful to describe the treatments for *Candida* as a continuum. The lowest level of treatment includes home remedies, such as rinsing the nipples and exposing them to sunlight. The next level includes over-the-counter options such as topical antifungals. Further along on the continuum are the powerful, systemic antifungal treatments such as fluconazole and ketoconazole, which require prescriptions. Encourage parents to discuss treatment options with their healthcare providers, particularly in the event of persistent cases that do not respond to conventional topical medications. If the nipple pain persists, referral to a dermatologist may be appropriate.

Stopping the Spread of Candida

Family hygiene is critical to stopping the spread of *Candida*. This includes good handwashing before and after diapering, using the toilet, or nursing. Any item that contacts nipples needs to be boiled once a day for at least 20 minutes. Bras, breast shells, and breast pump parts are vehicles for reinfection, and boiling kills the *Candida* spores. Items that go in the baby's mouth, such as bottle nipples, pacifiers, and teethers, should be discarded. Toys should be cleaned thoroughly with hot, soapy water, and the family's clothing should be laundered in very hot water.

The parent's diet may be a factor in a persistent *Candida* infection. DNA assay studies of the gut microbiome link high-fat and high-carbohydrate diets to increased *Candida* colonization (Hallen-Adams & Suhr, 2017; Li et al., 2019). Diets high in amino acids, protein, and fatty acids reduce *Candida* colonies. Decreasing or omitting sugars and saturated fats while increasing the intake of probiotics, garlic, zinc, and B vitamins may help. Probiotics have reduced candidiasis in a variety of infections (Kumar & Singhi, 2016; Oncel et al., 2015).

Fresh expressed milk can be fed to the baby during a *Candida* infection. However, there is debate among clinicians as to whether giving previously frozen milk with *Candida* in it will reinfect a healthy baby. There appear to be no studies that definitively settle this question. Freezing does not kill *Candida*, so it is recommended that the frozen milk be pasteurized or discarded. To pasteurize the milk, heat it for approximately 20 minutes at a simmer (62.5°C [144.5°F]) in a double boiler or steamer to prevent direct contact with the water (Peila et al., 2016). Label any milk expressed during the yeast infection so that the milk can be pasteurized before feeding.

Milk Blister or Milk Bleb

Occasionally, milk can clog a nipple pore (**Color Plate 41**). When the site is open, it is referred to as a **milk bleb** or blocked nipple pore. When skin closes over the pore and forms a blister, it is referred to as a *nipple blister* or **milk blister**. Many healthcare providers use these terms interchangeably. Milk blisters and blebs are intensely painful because milk cannot flow from the duct. This is different from the sucking blisters babies can cause in the early days after birth. Some specialists believe that nipple blisters lead to ductal narrowing. Others believe that ductal narrowing actually causes the blisters (Newman, 2021b). These conditions are extremely painful and can lead to mastitis because of milk stasis.

One method for removing a blister is to soak the nipple with a warm, wet compress or in a comfortably hot bowl of water. Sometimes, very gentle rubbing with a soft cloth will remove the pore covering. The hardened plug of dried or crystallized milk may come out. Or the suction of the baby's nursing may remove the plug. There is usually instant relief when the backed-up milk is removed. Soreness may remain for a few days. Encourage nursing on demand to avoid mastitis.

A topical antibiotic ointment can be used to prevent infection of a blister. In addition, choline present in lecithin supplements has anti-inflammatory properties. Inflammation associated with blebs and blisters may respond to oral lecithin and topical steroid ointment. Steroids should be wiped off before the baby nurses. Opening a bleb—called unroofing—with a needle is not recommended because this causes trauma and further luminal narrowing. For further information, refer to general recommendations for mastitis spectrum disorders (ABM, 2022).

Engorgement

An increase in breast fullness occurs as part of the normal physiological process as colostrum transitions to full milk production. Delivery of the placenta at birth triggers a precipitous drop in progesterone (from 55 to 200 ng per mL or more, down to 0 ng per mL). This enables the high prolactin levels to initiate full milk production. Increased blood and lymph are the source of the nutrients needed for milk production. Enlarged blood vessels are often visible beneath the skin. The fluid present in these veins increases breast fullness, weight, and sometimes tenderness. This is *not* engorgement. **Figure 17-4** shows a normally full breast. With unlimited, exclusive nursing, this normal initial fullness diminishes. By about 10 days postpartum, when lactation is fully established, the breasts become comfortably soft and pliable even when they are full of milk. **Table 17-5** compares these and other breast conditions discussed in this section.

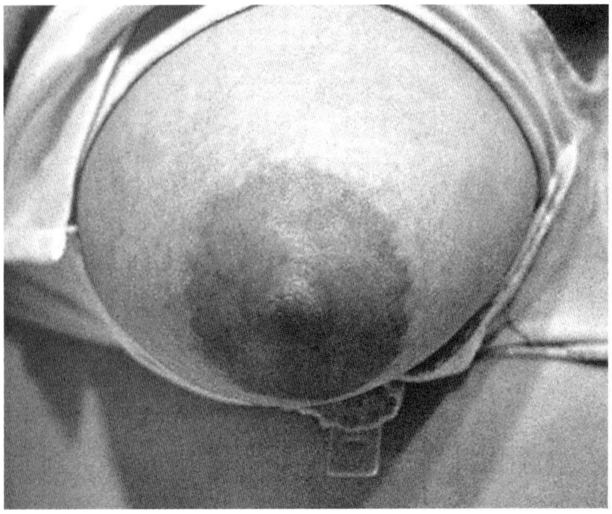

Figure 17-4 A normal full breast.

Printed with permission of Linda Kutner.

Engorgement describes the painful swelling that occurs when fluid accumulates in the breasts from failure to remove milk adequately. Increased pressure on the alveoli and milk ducts causes the breasts to feel firm, hard, tender, and warm or hot to the touch. The skin may appear shiny and transparent, as depicted in **Figure 17-5**. The nipples may flatten and, in extreme cases, may become indistinguishable from the rest of the breast. **Table 17-6** characterizes four stages of breast fullness when describing engorgement.

Causes of Engorgement

Postpartum engorgement can be **iatrogenic**, caused by medical interference with the natural process in the form of inappropriate regulations, schedules, and poor management of lactation. For example, it can result from intravenous (IV) fluids received during labor. Edema may be evident in the breasts, as well as in the feet and ankles (Figure 13-3 in **Chapter 13**). Edema occurs most commonly when nursing is beginning and feeding patterns are irregular. It may also occur when the baby begins sleeping through the night and when feedings are missed. Engorgement is a risk during the weaning process, especially if rapid weaning occurs. Encourage parents to nurse or express milk whenever they have a feeling of fullness, before they become uncomfortable. **Figure 17-6** illustrates the causes and results of engorgement.

Table 17-5 Comparison of Breast Conditions

Condition	Breast Fullness	Engorgement	Blocked Duct	Galactocele	Mastitis	Breast Abscess
Description	Firm, heavy, and full of milk; milk flows readily with sucking or pumping	Hard, enlarged, and shiny; venous and lymphatic drainage is obstructed, impeding milk flow with sucking or pumping	Single lumpy area of localized milk stasis	Smooth, rounded swelling in a localized area with a milk-retention cyst	Hard, inflamed area that is red, hot, and tender to the touch	Swollen lump in a localized area of infection that has formed a barrier of granulation tissue

Condition	Breast Fullness	Engorgement	Blocked Duct	Galactocele	Mastitis	Breast Abscess
Erythema	No	Bilateral	Often over a palpable lump	No	Usually but not always	Yes
Skin Temperature	Occasionally increased	Generalized warmth	Little or no heat	No	Warm to hot	Hot
Edema	No	Yes	No	No	Yes	Yes
Systemic Symptoms	No	There may be chills, feeling unwell, and mild fever	Unlikely	No	Usually flu-like symptoms	Usually flu-like symptoms, nausea, extreme fatigue, and aching muscles
Fever	No	Occasionally <38.4°C	Occasionally <38.4°C	No	Mild <37.5°C Acute <38.5°C Severe: >38°C	>38°C
Pain	No	Generalized	Tender or localized pain	No	Localized	Severe
One or both breasts	Usually bilateral	Usually bilateral	Usually unilateral	Usually unilateral	Usually unilateral	Often unilateral but may be bilateral
Considerations	Occurs 3–5 days postpartum as milk production increases	Often confused with normal fullness	May occur with a painful white bleb	Thought to result from ductal narrowing; compression of the cyst may cause milky fluid to exude from the nipple	Results from unresolved ductal narrowing and inflammation and/or colonization with pathogenic bacteria; requires oral antibiotic treatment Note: Methicillin-resistant *Staphylococcus aureus* may require intravenous antibiotic treatment	Forms from an infection that has no opening for drainage; in neglected cases, the skin may be discolored with necrosis; requires antibiotic treatment, drainage, or aspiration. May require surgery

Data from Academy of Breastfeeding Medicine. ABM clinical protocol #36: the mastitis spectrum, revised 2022. *Breastfeed Med*. 2022;17(5):1–17; Centers for Disease Control and Prevention. Methicillin-resistant *Staphylococcus aureus*. July 19, 2019. https://www.cdc.gov/breastfeeding/breastfeeding-special-circumstances/maternal-or-infant-illnesses/mrsa.html.

Consequences of Engorgement

When milk remains in the breast for extended periods, the suppressor peptide—**feedback inhibitor of lactation (FIL)**—in human milk has a negative effect on milk production. Breast tissue elasticity allows milk storage for as long as 48 hours before milk production and secretion begin to decrease rapidly. **Suppressor peptides** bring about the cessation of milk secretion during **milk stasis** and engorgement. Because unrelieved severe engorgement can result in lowered milk

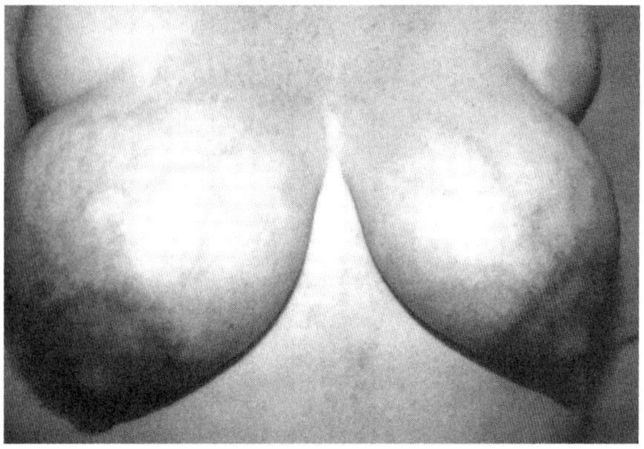

Figure 17-5 Engorged breasts.

Printed with permission of Debi Bocar.

Table 17-6 Four Stages of Breast Fullness

Stage	Definition
+1	Breasts are soft. Milk flows freely.
+2	Breasts are firm and non-tender. Milk flows freely.
+3	Breasts are firm and tender. Milk flows slowly with quick relief.
+4	Breasts are hard and painful. Milk flows slowly with slow relief.

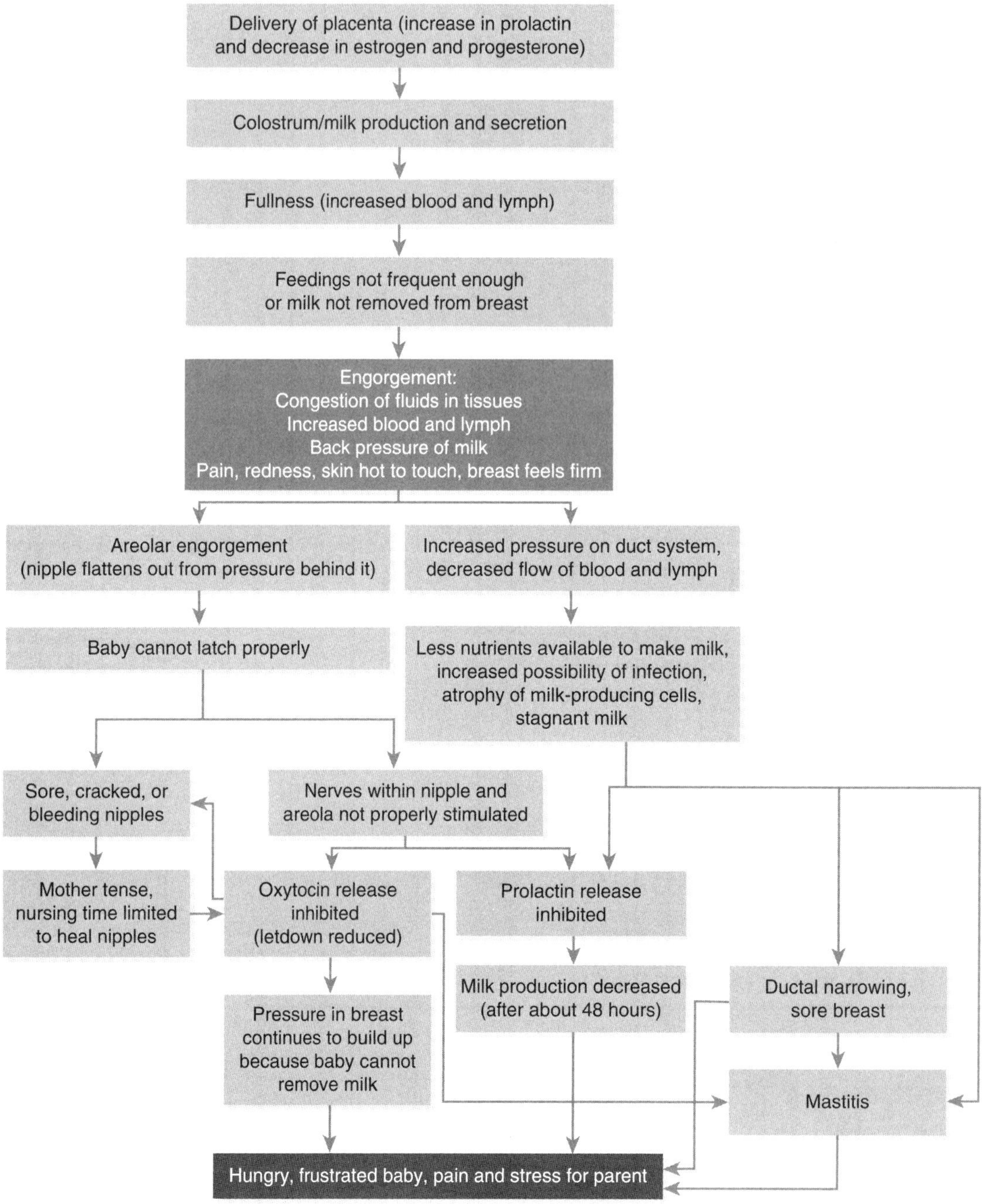

Figure 17-6 Progression of engorgement.

production, both the parent and the baby need close follow-up.

A flattened nipple resulting from engorgement becomes difficult for the baby to grasp and can adversely affect letdown. The resulting shallow latch fails to stimulate the nipple and areola nerves sufficiently, thus increasing the likelihood of impaired letdown. Without letdown, the baby cannot remove milk efficiently, and pressure in the ducts further increases. Engorgement can result in the baby latching onto the end of the nipple, damaging the nipple and further inhibiting letdown.

With severe engorgement, the pressure on alveoli and ducts decreases blood and lymph flow (**Figure 17-7** illustrates the lymphatic system). The slower flow increases the possibility of infection because the lymphatic system cannot remove bacteria at a normal rate. The increased milk pressure can cause alveolar cells and myoepithelial cells to shrink and die off. This atrophy of milk-producing cells can permanently compromise milk-producing ability.

Preventing Engorgement

Initiating nursing within the first hour of life helps prevent engorgement, as do other practices to protect lactation identified in **Chapter 13**. When parents and babies remain together, parents get to know their babies' hunger cues and learn to respond to them. Frequent, unrestricted feedings throughout the day and night will help minimize engorgement. Any time breast fullness increases, the parent can either wake the baby to nurse or express milk to comfort. All lactating parents need to know how to express their milk, an especially important tool for when the baby is sleepy and not nursing adequately.

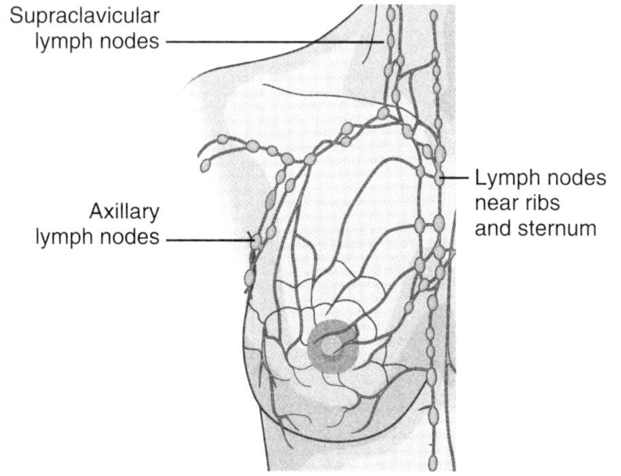

Figure 17-7 Lymphatic system in the breast.

Lymph massage helps prevent and relieve engorgement. Lymphatic massage has been used historically to treat lymphedema in postsurgical patients, including breast surgeries. Manual lymph drainage uses effleurage, a light massage technique. The skin is moved in certain directions based on the structure of the lymphatic system to help fluid drain through the normal lymph channels (Dugdale, 2019). Learning who the practitioners in your area are will enable you to provide a list of providers for this type of help. Self-massage instructional techniques are also available online.

Relieving Engorgement

Engorgement can be anxiety provoking and uncomfortable. It is helpful for parents to know that engorgement is temporary and usually resolves within 24 to 48 hours with proper management. If feeding frequency or duration has been limited, encourage unrestricted feedings—at least every 2 hours—sooner if the baby desires—and for as long as the baby needs. After engorgement resolves, encourage parents to be mindful of the baby's hunger cues and ensure at least eight feedings in every 24-hour period. In addition, gentle **breast compression** during feedings helps drain the breast more completely.

If nursing alone does not reduce the engorgement, it may be necessary to express milk to comfort between feedings. If engorgement prevents the baby from latching, expressing milk before feeding may soften the areola and facilitate latch. It may be relaxing to express milk in a comfortably hot shower. Softening the areolar tissue (also referred to as *reverse-pressure softening*), as illustrated in **Chapter 22**, is another technique that can help the baby latch. Therapeutic breast massage, which combines gentle massage and hand expression, can also facilitate latch and increase comfort for the parent.

Milk Expression for Engorgement

Milk expression will help relieve engorgement and also preserve production. Pumping is usually necessary for only 24 to 48 hours to relieve the discomfort. Continuing to pump beyond that time could maintain milk production at a level that is higher than needed. Briefly massaging and hand expressing milk before using the pump can increase flow significantly (Morton, 2019). Prefeed pumping should end as soon as possible, with pumping after nursing only when necessary. Pumping after feeding can remove remaining milk if needed.

If milk transfers easily and there is audible swallowing, pumping can end when the milk stops flowing quickly. If swallowing is periodic and not sustained, pumping for at least 10 minutes after the feeding is prudent. If the milk continues to flow quickly at the end of 10 minutes, pumping can continue until the flow slows.

If engorgement occurs in only one breast, the unaffected breast does not require pumping. When pumping only one breast at a time, massaging the breast will increase milk flow. Single pumping is appropriate when +2 or +3 engorgement is present and the baby can transfer milk. Consult Table 17-6 for definitions of these levels.

Cabbage for Engorgement

There have been positive results from the use of cabbage for reducing edema in breast engorgement. The use of fresh green cabbage leaves to treat engorgement was described in 1896 in *The Glory of Woman*. An article by Rosier (1988) was instrumental in reviving this ancient remedy for swelling. It may be that **phytoestrogens** in cabbage contribute to reducing swelling in the tissues (Mahmoud et al., 2022). Prolonged applications of cabbage can also be used to wean or to suppress lactation. Folklore suggests that farmers are careful to keep their dairy cows out of the cabbage patch because consumption of cabbage decreases milk production. There are no reports of negative effects from cabbage use. Cabbage is useful for reducing the swelling from ankle sprains and strains as well!

The procedure for applying cabbage is simple. After discarding the outer leaves, pull off several leaves, wash them, pat them dry, and crush them slightly to break up the veins. The remainder of the cabbage can be stored in the refrigerator for later use. Place the leaves on the breasts and hold them in place with a bra (**Color Plate 39**). Apply fresh leaves about every 2 hours for approximately 20 minutes. After a short time, the breast may feel "different"—sometimes described as tingly and cool. The cabbage can be removed when this sensation occurs, when milk begins to leak, or when softening of breast tissue becomes apparent. For sudden weaning or suppressing lactation, cabbage can be worn day and night, changing the leaves as needed until milk production ceases.

The amount of relief experienced from cabbage treatment varies. Relief may occur in as little as 20 to 30 minutes, or the cabbage may be needed over 24 hours. With severe engorgement, the cabbage may wilt from the heat of the skin. In some cases, the decrease of edema is so pronounced that the milk ducts will stand out in bold relief after the cabbage is removed.

Other Treatments for Engorgement

The parent lying flat on their back will elevate the breasts and can help reduce swelling. Cold compresses applied to the breasts between feedings may help decrease discomfort. A small bag of crushed ice or a frozen pack of vegetables (e.g., peas or corn) conforms nicely to the shape of the breast. Refreezing the vegetables for reuse makes it an easy and affordable compress. Herbal compresses and poultices, including hollyhock leaf, have been used to treat engorgement (Ketsuwan et al., 2018; Khosravan et al., 2017). The use of cold gel packs promotes pain relief and reduction in breast hardness, though cold cabbage leaves are reportedly preferred over gel packs (Wong et al., 2017).

The use of a nonsteroidal anti-inflammatory drug (NSAID), such as ibuprofen or naproxen, may reduce some of the inflammation. Acupuncture, proteolytic enzymes, and scraping therapy (Gua-Sha) may also be promising for engorgement. However, there is insufficient evidence to warrant their extensive use (Mangesi & Zakarija-Grkovic, 2016). Ask the families in your care what practices and treatments are typically used in their culture to resolve engorgement. **Table 17-7** summarizes the treatment options for engorgement.

Mastitis Spectrum

The most current Academy of Breastfeeding Medicine (ABM) Clinical Protocol #36 (2022), "The Mastitis Spectrum" asserts that mastitis encompasses a spectrum of conditions resulting from ductal inflammation and edema. The protocol identifies several conditions that fall within the **mastitis spectrum** including **ductal narrowing**, inflammatory mastitis, bacterial mastitis, phlegmon, abscess, galactocele, and subacute mastitis. Galactoceles are discussed in **Chapter 7**.

Ductal Narrowing

The term *ductal narrowing* in the new ABM protocol identifies what was previously referred to as a *plugged duct* or a *blocked duct*. Contrary to older belief, plugs do not form in a single microscopic duct. The plug is actually microscopic narrowing and inflammation, which is linked to congested breast tissue and causes

Table 17-7 Treatment Options for Engorgement

Causes	Actions to Take
Missed or infrequent feedings	■ Room in with baby in the hospital. ■ Nurse 10–12 times day and night every 24 hours, or more if baby is willing. ■ Be alert to baby's hunger cues and respond to them. ■ Use rousing techniques for sleepy baby. ■ Increase skin-to-skin contact to encourage baby to nurse. ■ Express milk anytime baby is unable to nurse.
Milk removal not adequate at feedings	■ Check that latch and position are appropriate. ■ Stop the use of all artificial nipples. ■ Increase skin-to-skin contact during feedings. ■ Do breast compression during feedings to encourage baby to suck. ■ Express milk after the feeding to remove the milk that flows quickly and easily. ■ Pump for comfort between feedings, if necessary, as long as the milk flows quickly and easily.
Inadequate letdown from edema and pain	■ Relax in warm shower with water running over back, avoiding the breasts, and express to relieve fullness. ■ Use reverse-pressure softening to displace edema and soften the areolae enough for baby to latch. ■ Nurse after the breast is soft enough for baby to latch. ■ Use relaxation techniques and gentle breast massage during feedings. ■ Lie flat on back between feedings to elevate breasts. ■ Apply cool packs to the breasts and underarms. ■ Apply green cabbage leaves to breasts.

localized pain and swelling. The blockage created by the ductal narrowing can produce a galactocele, a benign cyst that should resolve on its own without intervention.

Ductal narrowing can resolve on its own. Unrestricted nursing and the use of anti-inflammatories are recommended as a first course of treatment. The relief of pain associated with the inflamed ducts when the baby nurses is from the lessening of alveolar distention. Contrary to popular belief, excess milk removal can worsen the inflammation and narrowing of the ducts. In addition, squeezing the area or breast massage to "clear the duct" worsens the inflammation and can lead to tissue trauma.

Consuming lecithin, a natural fat emulsifier, and reducing the amount of saturated fats in the diet may help prevent recurring ductal narrowing (ABM, 2022). Lecithin is most concentrated in organ meats, red meats, and eggs—foods whose consumption tends to be limited in modern diets. The choline in lecithin supplements may provide an anti-inflammatory effect as well (McGuire, 2015). The recommended dosage of lecithin is 1 tablespoon three or four times daily or 1 to 2 capsules (1200 mg each) three or four times daily. Ultrasound is also used to treat ductal narrowing. Newman (2021b) recommends a maximum of two treatments on two consecutive days, noting that ultrasound seems to prevent the ductal inflammation that occurs in the same part of the breast. The recommended dosage is 2 watts per cm^{-2} continuously for 5 minutes to the affected area, once daily for up to two doses.

Advise parents to call their healthcare provider if the ductal narrowing and inflammation do not respond to treatment or if there are signs of infection, including fever or tachycardia that lasts 24 hours or longer (ABM, 2022). If ductal narrowing persists, increased inflammation can occur and develop into inflammatory mastitis, discussed in the next section. **Figure 17-10** at the end of the mastitis discussion presents management and treatment of mastitis spectrum disorders, which includes ductal narrowing and inflammation.

Mastitis

Mastitis is inflammation of the breast. It can be classified on the mastitis spectrum as either inflammatory or bacterial. Inflammatory mastitis begins as ductal narrowing, leading to an inflamed area that is red, hot, and tender to the touch (**Color Plate 43**). It is usually accompanied by fever and flu-like symptoms. Bacterial mastitis occurs when inflammatory mastitis progresses to include a bacterial infection and presents as cellulitis, often with fever or tachycardia lasting more than 24 hours (ABM, 2022). When there is a history of mastitis or symptoms of mastitis without accompanying fever, **subclinical mastitis (SCM)** may be present. This condition is linked to lactation failure, suboptimal growth in early infancy, and as with clinical mastitis, an increased risk of parent-to-child transmission of HIV via human milk (Schaub et al., 2018; Wren-Atilola et al., 2018). Nonlactational mastitis can also occur, sometimes even during pregnancy. Rarely, infants can have mastitis.

Open-ended questions will help identify the presence of mastitis. **Figure 17-8** presents a sample discussion. Signs of inflammatory mastitis include increasing redness, swelling, and pain, which may be accompanied by fever, chills, and tachycardia (ABM, 2022). If a parent reports that their baby will not nurse on one side, mastitis may be present. Sometimes, babies will reject the infected breast, possibly because of a salty taste resulting from increased sodium and chloride levels in the milk. If the baby will not nurse on that breast, the parent should express milk to comfort only.

Mastitis is of particular concern for parents who are HIV positive. It can lead to an increased risk of parent-to-child transmission of HIV via human milk as a result of an increased viral load (Schaub et al., 2018; Wren-Atilola et al., 2018). Improving postpartum health care, with an emphasis on managing maternal infections, is key to preventing breast disorders and infection along the mastitis spectrum.

Causes of Mastitis

Nipple damage, overactive milk production, nipple shield use, and the presence of *S. aureus* on the nipple or in the milk are risk factors for disorders on the mastitis spectrum. The underlying immunological processes remain largely unknown. Although most instances of mastitis occur in the first 6 weeks postpartum, mastitis can occur at any time during lactation. Mastitis commonly occurs during the newborn period, when parental fatigue is common and when immunity has been lowered by pregnancy. Evidence suggests inflammatory mastitis is triggered or perpetuated in large part by psychosocial stress. An infection can develop when the parent's time and energy become overextended, such as by returning to work or school, holidays, vacations, houseguests, family crises, or infant/other child illness. In addition, while

This parent has come to see the lactation consultant (LC) as an outpatient in a pediatric practice. The baby is 8 weeks old, and the parent is complaining of pain.

LC:	How is nursing going for you and Chloe?
Parent:	Not so good. It hurts.
LC:	I'm sorry to hear that. What hurts?
Parent:	My breast.
LC:	Which part of your breast hurts?
Parent:	Well, it hurts on the inside.
LC:	It hurts on the inside of your breast. When does it hurt?
Parent:	It hurts all the time, but especially after the baby nurses and at night.
LC:	How would you describe your pain on a scale of 0 to 10, with 0 being no pain and 10 being the worst pain you've ever felt?
Parent:	I would say it is a 1 all the time and a 2 or 3 at night.
LC:	How do your nipples feel?
Parent:	My nipples are fine. This is my third baby. I am sure Chloe is latching well. She's gaining weight and pooping a lot.
LC:	How can you best describe your pain—is it dull, aching, throbbing, burning, itching?
Parent:	It's a dull ache most of the time, like bruising. But there's no redness or hard lump. If my other children hug me, it hurts more. If Chloe bumps me while I'm holding her, it hurts, too.
LC:	How is your stress level?
Parent:	It's pretty high. My partner lost his job 2 weeks ago, and we may have to move. One of my parents was just diagnosed with cancer at only 55. I may have to go back to work full-time.
LC:	Wow, that's a lot to deal with. It sounds quite overwhelming. How are you taking care of yourself through all this?
Parent:	I can barely take care of everyone else, much less myself.
LC:	How is your postpartum health besides the breast pain?
Parent:	Well, I had mastitis 3 weeks ago. My doctor called in an antibiotic, so I must be okay now. I haven't had any fever. And I don't have any redness or streaking.
LC:	Which antibiotic was used, and for how long?
Mother:	I think it was ampicillin. I took it for about 5 days and then I felt better. But this pain seems different.

Figure 17-8 Problem-solving to identify mastitis.

a parent is establishing lactation, any interruption or change in nursing pattern can cause milk to remain in the ducts and lead to mastitis.

Mastitis can also develop when a crack in the nipple skin exposes a pathway for *Staphylococcus* and other invasive organisms. The infection probably came from bacteria in the baby's mouth or the home environment. Therefore, the milk is likely to contain

- Damaged nipple, especially if colonized with *S. aureus*
- Infrequent feedings, scheduled feedings, or limited duration of feedings
- Missed feedings
- Poor latch or weak or uncoordinated sucking leading to inefficient milk removal
- Illness in parent or baby
- Overproduction of milk
- Rapid weaning
- Pressure on the breast (e.g., tight bra or car seatbelt)
- Bleb or nipple blister (also called milk blister)
- *Candida* infection
- Plugged or blocked milk duct
- Malnutrition in the parent (evidence of specific dietary risk factors in humans has not been identified)

Figure 17-9 Events that may lead to mastitis.

Data from Academy of Breastfeeding Medicine (ABM). ABM clinical protocol #36: The mastitis spectrum. Revised 2022. www.bfmed.org

antibodies to the infectious organism. It is considered best practice for the baby to continue to nurse through an infection. The breast needs to continue to be drained, and the baby's sucking usually removes milk more effectively than either a pump or hand expression. Additionally, frequent feedings can prevent milk stasis from developing. **Figure 17-9** describes events that may lead to mastitis (although evidence for some is inconclusive).

Treatment of Mastitis

Many parents may self-treat a breast infection and not seek medical treatment. Advise them to call their healthcare provider if signs of an infection are present, including fever or tachycardia, and last 24 hours or longer. Inflammatory mastitis can progress to bacterial mastitis, presenting as cellulitis in the affected area(s) of the breast. This requires immediate medical attention and antibiotics or probiotics to resolve (ABM, 2022).

Treatments for disorders on the mastitis spectrum include efficient milk removal by unrestricted nursing, cold compresses on the site of inflammation, and anti-inflammatory medication. If the infection has progressed to bacterial mastitis, antibiotics and probiotics may be required. When mastitis develops, a feeding assessment will help ensure that the baby is latching and feeding effectively. Rest will help fight the infection. If employed, this may require taking time off work. Relatives and friends can help with meals, grocery shopping, and caring for other children so that the parent can rest and recuperate.

Table 17-8 Causes and Treatment of Mastitis

Causes	Actions to Take
Milk stasis: Poor milk removal	■ Nurse as long as the baby desires and express milk after the feed as needed for relief.
Milk stasis: Missed feedings, irregular nursing pattern, or engorgement	■ Avoid missed or delayed feedings. ■ When feedings are delayed, express to remove milk. ■ Only pump if the baby cannot latch.
Overwork	■ Rearrange priorities and daily schedule.
Low resistance to infection from anemia, poor diet	■ Get help with tasks. ■ Improve diet. ■ Exercise. ■ Reduce stress.
Lack of adequate sleep; fatigue	■ Take daytime naps or rest periods to rebuild the immune system. ■ Nurse lying down. ■ Take baby to bed at night.
Ductal narrowing and inflammation	■ Avoid massage and vibration. ■ Have baby nurse with chin pointed toward inflammation. ■ May require lymphatic drainage.
Infection via cracked nipple	■ Eliminate nonnutritive sucking. ■ Briefly soak nipples in saline solution (¼ tsp salt in 8 oz water) after feeding and air dry.
Infection passed from baby or other family member	■ Treat primary infection in conjunction with mastitis.

When mastitis is suspected, the primary healthcare provider needs to be contacted immediately. If a temperature higher than 100°F (37.8C) is present and symptoms do not resolve within 24 hours, the caregiver will likely prescribe antibiotic therapy for 10 to 14 days. In the absence of a fever, the healthcare provider may wait a few days to determine whether other measures are appropriate.

As with engorgement, some clinicians have found relief from cabbage leaves on the breast until the inflammation resolves. Anecdotal reports suggest that acupuncture and chiropractic care are effective for both ductal narrowing and mastitis. **Table 17-8** lists treatment suggestions relative to specific causes of mastitis. ABM recommendations for management and

- Heat: Apply warm, moist compresses to the inflamed area before and during feedings.
- Cold: Apply cold packs to reduce pain and edema in the affected area after nursing or pumping.
- Rest: Get as much bed rest as possible.
- Remove milk: Nurse in a position that points the baby's chin toward the inflamed area.
- Nurse as often as possible: Use of breast compression and massage may help drain the breast more effectively.
- Contact the caregiver for an antibiotic: Follow the entire regimen, even if the infection seems to clear quickly.
- Express to drain the milk if the baby does not nurse or if separated from baby.
- Use caregiver approved over-the-counter anti-inflammatory pain relievers such as ibuprofen, naproxen, aspirin, or acetaminophen to reduce inflammation and discomfort.

Figure 17-10 Measures to treat mastitis.

treatment of mastitis spectrum disorders are incorporated into **Figure 17-10**.

Recurrent Mastitis

Some parents have **recurrent mastitis** that requires investigation for the source of the infection. Explore potential causes within the family, such as stress, financial stress, fatigue from a new baby, and older children. There may have been a bout of mastitis that was not treated. Prescribed medication may have ended before completing the entire prescription.

Parents who are prone to recurring bouts of mastitis should be taught how to assess regularly for signs of infection. They will want to be especially vigilant in removing milk regularly and routinely express milk whenever a feeding is missed. They should practice self-care, including getting enough rest and having support systems in place. At the first sign of recurrent mastitis, applying cold compresses, nursing frequently, and getting rest will help shorten the length of the infection. If infection recurs within 2 months of a previous infection, refer the parent to their healthcare provider for medication.

Parental Factors

Parents who are prone to recurrent mastitis should evaluate their diet, rest, and exercise. They might consider reducing daily activities and commitments and soliciting help from family and other support networks. Parents who are isolated with young children may need help locating sources of support. Learning about the family's support needs will help identify community supports for those who are at risk for isolation. Peer counselors, breastfeeding support groups, churches, and other nonprofit groups can assist families in ways that go far beyond nursing support. Many communities offer meals for postpartum families and support groups for new or lone parents. Learn which private and government resources are available in your community so that you can refer families who need help.

Anemia or other health deficiencies predispose some individuals to recurrent mastitis. Familial history is a risk factor (Mediano et al., 2014). Recurring infection may also occur if the parent does not complete the entire course of treatment to fully clear the infection. Recurring episodes can occur when a particular antibiotic does not provide relief. If the bacteria are resistant to the antibiotic, as discussed in the next section, a broader-spectrum antibiotic may be necessary.

Antibiotic-Resistant Bacteria

Antibiotic-resistant strains of *S. aureus* are increasingly found in mastitis and **breast abscesses**. *Staphylococcus* strains appear to be the most frequent cause of lactational mastitis (Jiménez et al., 2017). This condition could result from a bacterial species usually present in human milk growing (Staphylococci) while others (Lactobacilli or Lactococci) disappear. Lactoferrin, a constituent of human milk, has a weak antibacterial effect when used alone but appears more effective when administered at a low concentration in combination with several antibiotics. Because lactoferrin in combination with other medicines can penetrate bacteria biofilms, it holds promise as a treatment for matitis (Lepanto et al., 2019).

Culturing the milk, nipple, and the baby's throat before beginning treatment may help determine an appropriate antibiotic. Culturing milk to identify the specific pathogen may be problematic, however, because studies show mixed results. The ability to use RNA sequencing holds great promise. Combining the use of culturing with molecular techniques allows for better characterization of the bacterial diversity in milk from individuals experiencing symptoms of infectious mastitis.

Determining the type of bacteria present in recurrent infections is important, given the increase in antibiotic-resistant bacteria (Angelopoulou et al., 2018). Bacteria are especially resistant to penicillin-based antibiotics. **Methicillin-resistant *Staphylococcus aureus* (MRSA)** requires much stronger antibiotics than those usually used to treat a *Staphylococcus* infection. MRSA occurs commonly in healthcare facilities and communities. It is associated with recent antibiotic use, sharing contaminated items, having active skin diseases, and living in crowded settings (CDC, 2019).

Local resistance patterns for MRSA should be considered when choosing an antibiotic for unresponsive cases of mastitis while culture results are pending (ABM, 2022). Two of the antibiotics used to treat MRSA—vancomycin and teicoplanin—may be toxic and must be administered by IV infusion, typically while admitted to the hospital. Vancomycin-resistant strains of bacteria, including **vancomycin-resistant *S. aureus* (VRSA)** and **vancomycin-resistant Enterococcus (VRE)**, have increased, especially in hospital settings (Narayanan et al., 2019).

Nonlactational Mastitis or Breast Disease

Lactation is somewhat of a "red herring" in women's health. Healthcare providers may discount or ignore symptoms associated with non–lactation-related conditions when a client is nursing. Providers who work with nursing families need to be familiar with various types of nonlactational mastitis or inflammatory breast disorders. Parents may develop these conditions before or during pregnancy, while nursing, after weaning, or between pregnancies.

Idiopathic Granulomatous Mastitis (IGM)

Idiopathic granulomatous mastitis (IGM) mimics breast cancer. It is most common in women of childbearing age who have given birth within the previous 5 years and nursed for 3 to 36 months. A small subset of women who restricted nursing to one breast developed IGM in the nonlactating breast (Pluguez-Turull et al., 2018). This condition can develop within 6 months to 2 years after weaning, is difficult to treat, and recurs frequently.

Treatments include steroids; antibiotics; anti-inflammatory compounds; and surgery, including mastectomy (Alrayes et al., 2019; Barreto et al., 2018; Tan et al., 2019; Vanovcanova et al., 2019). Although usually not cancerous, granulomatous mastitis can occur concurrently with breast cancer (Oddó et al., 2019) and rarely occurs in males. A lactating parent with a painful, irregular breast mass or skin lesion needs referral to their primary caregiver or a breast specialist.

Diabetic Mastopathy

Diabetic mastopathy is associated with long-standing type 1 insulin-dependent diabetes. It presents as a hard, painless lump. There may be multiple masses in one or both breasts. Imaging cannot distinguish between diabetic mastopathy and breast carcinoma. Thus, the masses must be biopsied to rule out cancer (Li & Erickson, 2018; Ng et al., 2019). Diabetic mastopathy masses do not respond to standard treatments for disorders along the mastitis spectrum. If symptoms do not resolve with standard treatment, the parent needs to be referred to a breast specialist.

Fat Necrosis

Fat necrosis is an inflammatory process of adipose tissue. It can occur after trauma, surgery, biopsy, reconstruction, fat grafting, radiotherapy, infection, or duct ectasia, among other conditions (Tayyab et al., 2018). The resulting scarred tissue may appear as a palpable lump, skin tethering, thickening and hardening, and occasionally axillary lymphadenopathy. The lesion may be inflamed or fibrous. Careful examination by a specialist is warranted to rule out cancer (Genova et al., 2019; Vasei et al., 2019).

Sarcoidosis

Sarcoidosis is the growth of inflammatory cells and usually presents as lumps or masses in the lymph nodes or lungs. There may be a genetic predisposition—triggered by bacteria, viruses, dust, or chemicals—that causes an autoimmune response that produces granulomas. Sarcoidosis of the breast is rare but can occur (Reis et al., 2021).

Tuberculosis Mastitis

Tuberculosis mastitis presents with masses that can mimic malignant tumors or IGM. Although rare in industrialized countries, tuberculosis mastitis comprises 0.1% of examined breast lesions and about 3 to 4.5% of breast diseases treated with surgery in low-income nations (Thimmappa et al., 2015). Tuberculosis mastitis can occur simultaneously with breast cancer and is challenging to diagnose (Qiao et al., 2018).

Zuska-Atkin's Disease

Zuska-Atkin's disease is a chronically oozing lesion on or near the areola and underlying ducts. Variations of this condition are known as a *periductal fistula*, a *mammary duct fistula*, or a *lactiferous mammary fistula*. Abscesses frequently occur as a result of reinfection through the fistula tract from the nipple to the abscess. This condition occurs more frequently in women who smoke (Taffurelli et al., 2016). Surgery is a common treatment (Zhang et al., 2018).

Breast Abscess

An abscess is a localized collection of pus that forms from an infection that has no opening for drainage. An abscess in the breast usually forms from bacterial mastitis or phlegmon (inflammation of the soft tissue) that either did not respond to treatment or was left untreated (ABM, 2022). Breast abscesses occur in under 1% of nonlactating women and in 11% of women experiencing lactational mastitis (Russell et al., 2020).

Symptoms of an abscess are the same as for mastitis—fever, flu-like symptoms, nausea, extreme fatigue, and aching muscles. The infection site becomes red, swollen, and tender (**Color Plate 44**). Symptoms may be less severe than with mastitis because the abscess is isolated from the rest of the breast. Occasionally, an abscess can occur in the absence of any systemic symptoms.

Abscesses can be prevented with appropriate lactation management and immediate treatment of mastitis. If treatment for what appears to be ductal narrowing does not resolve within 48 hours, an abscess needs to be ruled out. If improperly treated, an abscess can lead to serious bacterial infections. An increased rate of MRSA infection has been seen in lactating parents with breast abscesses compared with non-lactational breast abscesses (Lodhi et al., 2018). Prompt treatment of mastitis can avoid the progression of a MRSA infection to a breast abscess.

Treatment of an Abscess

An abscess requires immediate assessment and treatment by a healthcare provider. A breast abscess is typically lanced and drained (**Color Plate 45**), and antibiotic medication is prescribed for the infection. A milk fistula forms in 5% to 12% of incisions for deep, large abscesses (Larson & Valente, 2016). Ultrasound-guided percutaneous needle aspiration is a less invasive treatment and more protective of continued nursing (Colin et al., 2019). A treatment option that is less disruptive to nursing is the use of a vacuum-assisted biopsy system that provides the drainage necessary in larger masses (Chen et al., 2019).

Nursing with an Abscess

Nursing may be possible, depending on the size and location of the abscess, the associated pain, and the type of treatment (Boakes et al., 2018). The suggestions for treating mastitis in Table 17-8 will facilitate continuing to nurse on the affected breast. If nursing is not possible, milk expression from the affected breast will maintain production until the abscess heals. One-sided nursing can provide sufficient milk for the baby. The parent may choose to wean from the affected breast only or to totally wean. Reducing milk production slowly will help avoid another infection.

Summary

Nursing families need information, education, reassurance, and assistance in the early weeks following delivery. Discussing their expectations and reinforcing what is normal can ease new parents through this time. Having support and guidance when difficulties arise will help them persevere. Anticipatory guidance in the early days and weeks after birth will help to reduce concerns, especially those based on myths and misconceptions. Educating parents about prevention and treatment of nipple pain, engorgement, *Candida*, and the disorders along the mastitis spectrum is crucial to reducing the occurrence of these common issues.

What You Learned—At a Glance

Conversation Starters with Parents

- What is your baby's nursing pattern?
- How many dirty diapers does your baby have each day?
- How is your breast fullness before and after nursing?
- How much leaking do you experience?
- How do your nipples look and feel during and after nursing?

Confidence to Nurse

- Pointing out positive things about nursing and the baby will boost confidence and encourage continuance.
- Dispelling misconceptions will help increase long-term nursing.
- Boosting confidence will help avoid the likelihood of weaning when obstacles arise.
- Parents' confidence is affected by caregivers and the consistency of their messages.

Milk Production

- Signs of sufficient milk include three wet diapers per day by day 3 and six per day after day 5; three or more stools per day from day 3 through the first month; and regular intervals of wakefulness, sleep, and feeding.
- Nursing on one side can provide adequate nutrition.
- Feedings need to be long enough to ensure the baby receives sufficient hindmilk.
- Regular, frequent feedings will maintain milk production.
- Babies may nurse every 1 to 2 hours (8–14 feedings) in the early days.
- By 8 to 12 weeks of age, babies usually nurse every 2 to 4 hours.
- Feeding frequency typically increases at about 10 days, 2–3 weeks, 6 weeks, 12 weeks, and 6 months of age.
- Illness, overstimulation, emotional upsets, or physical discomfort may increase feeding frequency.
- At about 3 months, babies obtain more milk in a shorter time and may go longer between feedings.

Causes of Leaking

- Breast fullness or milk ejection
- Nipple stimulation
- Overproduction of milk
- Hormone imbalance
- Hearing a baby cry
- Nonlactational milk production (galactorrhea)

Nipple Pain

- Tenderness with the initial latch and first few sucks is common.
- Nipple pain typically occurs at 3 to 6 days, especially when the baby has a strong suck.
- Ineffective latch is the major cause of nipple pain; limiting duration does not prevent it.
- Nipple trauma ranges from superficial and intact to deep damage throughout the dermis.
- Ankyloglossia, short tongue, high or bubble palate, or other oral structure anomaly can cause nipple pain.
- Sore nipples respond to a variety of treatments, including ointments and hydrogel dressings.
- A yeast infection requires treating the baby and nipples simultaneously.
- A *Candida* infection does not always present with visual symptoms.
- Repeated *Candida* infections require measures to stop the spread of the infection.
- A milk blister or bleb can be removed with a warm, wet compress and gentle rubbing.

Engorgement

- Engorgement is most common early in lactation when feeding patterns are irregular.
- Engorgement occurs from failure to remove milk adequately or frequently enough.
- Engorgement can compromise milk production and lead to mastitis.
- Engorged breasts feel firm, hard, tender, and warm or hot to the touch.
- Hand expression and gentle compression help drain milk and soften the areola.
- Cold compresses help decrease discomfort; cabbage leaves may reduce swelling.

Ductal Narrowing

- Ductal narrowing and inflammation cause localized soreness, swelling, lumpiness, or slight pain.
- Ductal narrowing is part of the mastitis spectrum.
- Feeding on demand, NSAIDs, analgesics, and cold compresses help decrease inflammation.
- Reduced intake of saturated fats and use of lecithin supplements may reduce recurrence.
- Ultrasound therapy may help recurring cases.

Mastitis

- Mastitis is part of the mastitis spectrum and may be inflammatory or bacterial.
- The area becomes red, hot, and tender to the touch.
- Fever and flu-like symptoms are common.
- A salty taste from increased sodium and chloride in the milk may cause the baby to reject the infected breast.
- Treatment includes efficient milk removal, cold compresses, anti-inflammatory medication, a full course of antibiotics (for bacterial mastitis), and rest.
- Untreated mastitis can lead to an abscess, which requires prompt medical treatment.
- Nursing may continue with an abscess, depending on location, size, and treatment.
- Nonlactational mastitis and abscesses can mimic breast cancer.

References

Academy of Breastfeeding Medicine. ABM clinical protocol #36: the mastitis spectrum, revised 2022. *Breastfeed Med.* 2022;17(5):1–17.

Academy of Breastfeeding Medicine. ABM clinical protocol #26: persistent pain with breastfeeding. *Breastfeed Med.* 2016;11(2): 46-53.

Al-Nuaimi N, et al. Breastfeeding trends and determinants: implications and recommendations for Gulf Cooperation Council countries. *Sultan Qaboos Univ Med J.* 2017;17(2):e155–e161.

Alrayes A, et al. Surgical treatment of granulomatous mastitis: our experience in Bahrain. *Breast J.* 2019;25(5):958–962.

American College of Obstetricians and Gynecologists. ACOG committee opinion no. 756: optimizing support for breastfeeding as part of obstetric practice. *Obstet Gynecol.* 2018;132(4):e187–e196.

Amir LH, et al. Does *Candida* and/or *Staphylococcus* play a role in nipple and breast pain in lactation? A cohort study in Melbourne, Australia. *BMJ Open.* 2013;3(3).

Angelopoulou A, et al. The microbiology and treatment of human mastitis. *Med Microbiol Immunol.* 2018;207(2):83–94.

Atyeo NN, et al. Early initiation of breastfeeding among Maya mothers in the western highlands of Guatemala: practices and beliefs. *J Hum Lact.* 2017;33(4):781–789.

Baño-Piñero I, et al. Impact of support networks for breastfeeding: a multicenter study. *Women Birth.* 2018;31(4):e239–e244.

Barreto DS, et al. Granulomatous mastitis: etiology, imaging, pathology, treatment, and clinical findings. *Breast Cancer Res Treat.* 2018;171(3):527–534.

Boakes E, et al. Breast infection: a review of diagnosis and management practices. *Eur J Breast Health.* 2018;14(3):136–143.

Brandão S, et al. The Breastfeeding Self-Efficacy Scale-Short Form: psychometric characteristics in Portuguese pregnant women. *Midwifery.* 2018;66:49–55.

Burton AE, et al. A photo-elicitation exploration of UK mothers' experiences of extended breastfeeding. *Appetite.* 2022;168:1–15.

Centers for Disease Control and Prevention. Infant Feeding Practices Study II and its year six follow up: results. Updated December 5, 2017. https://www.cdc.gov/breastfeeding-data/studies/methods-results-ifps.html?CDC_AAref_Val=https://www.cdc.gov/breastfeeding/data/ifps/results.htm

Centers for Disease Control and Prevention. Methicillin-resistant *Staphylococcus aureus* (MRSA) infections: general information about MRSA in the community. February 1, 2019. https://www.cdc.gov/mrsa/about/?CDC_AAref_Val=https://www.cdc.gov/mrsa/community

Chen C, et al. Surgical drainage of lactational breast abscess with ultrasound-guided Encor vacuum-assisted breast biopsy system. *Breast J.* 2019;25(5):889–897.

Colin C, et al. Breast abscesses in lactating women: evidences for ultrasound-guided percutaneous drainage to avoid surgery. *Emerg Radiol.* 2019;26(5):507–514.

Cortelo FM, et al. Women's sense of coherence and its association with early weaning. *J Pediatr (Rio J).* 2018;94(6):624–629.

Drugs and Lactation Database (LactMed) [Internet]. Gentian Violet [Updated August 15, 2024]. Bethesda, MD: National Institute of Child Health and Human Development; 2006-. https://www.ncbi.nlm.nih.gov/sites/books/NBK501869/

Dugdale D. Lymphatic obstruction. *MedlinePlus.* January 10, 2019. medlineplus.gov/ency/article/001117.htm

Feenstra MM, et al. Early breastfeeding problems: a mixed method study of mothers' experiences. *Sex Reprod Healthc.* 2018;16:167–174.

Filippa M, et al. Pain, parental involvement, and oxytocin in the neonatal intensive care unit. *Front Psychol.* 2019;10:715.

Friedrichsdorf SJ, et al. A hospital-wide initiative to eliminate or reduce needle pain in children using lean methodology. *Pain Rep.* 2018;3(suppl 1):e671.

Genova R, et al. Breast fat necrosis. In: *StatPearls*. Treasure Island, FL: StatPearls Publishing; June 2, 2019.

Genovese C, et al. Combined systemic (fluconazole) and topical (metronidazole + clotrimazole) therapy for a new approach to the treatment and prophylaxis of recurrent candidiasis. *Minerva Ginecol.* 2019;71(4):321–328.

Giudicelli M, et al. Influence of intrapartum maternal fluids on weight loss in breastfed newborns. *J Matern Fetal Med.* 2022;35(4);692–698.

Gökçeoğlu E, Küçükoğlu S. The relationship between insufficient milk perception and breastfeeding self-efficacy among Turkish mothers. *Glob Health Promot.* 2017;24(4):53–61

Guo H, et al. The use of Kumpfer's resilience framework in understanding the breastfeeding experience of employed mothers after returning to work: a qualitative study in China. *Int Breastfeed J.* 2022;17(13):1–15.

Hale T, et al. The absence of *Candida albicans* in milk samples of women with clinical symptoms of ductal candidiasis. *Breastfeed Med.* 2009;4(2):57–61.

Hale T, Krutsch K. *Hale's Medications & Mothers' Milk 2025–2026: A Manual of Lactational Pharmacology*. 21st ed. New York, NY: Springer Publishing Company; 2024.

Hallen-Adams HE, Suhr MJ. Fungi in the healthy human gastrointestinal tract. *Virulence.* 2017;8(3):352–358.

Health Canada. Health Canada warns of potential cancer risk associated with gentian violet. 2019. https://recalls-rappels.canada.ca/en/alert-recall/health-canada-warns-canadians-potential-cancer-risk-associated-gentian-violet

Hitomi I, et al. Factors influencing exclusive breastfeeding rates until 6 months postpartum: the Japan Environment and Children's Study. *Sci Rep.* 2021;11(1):1–11.

Huang MS, et al. Most commensally bacterial strains in human milk of healthy mothers display multiple antibiotic resistance. *Microbiologyopen.* 2019;8(1):e00618.

Huang W, Molitch ME. Prolactin and other pituitary disorders in kidney disease. *Semin Nephrol.* 2021;41(2):156–167.

International Breastfeeding Centre. *Candida* Protocol. Updated 2021. https://ibconline.ca/information-sheets/candida-protocol/

Jansen S, Sampene K. Raynaud phenomenon of the nipple: an under-recognized condition. *Obstet Gynecol.* 2019; 133(5): 975–977.

Jiménez E, et al. Mammary candidiasis: a medical condition without scientific evidence? *PLoS One.* 2017;12(7):e0181071.

Kaski K, Kvist LJ. Deep breast pain during lactation: a case-control study in Sweden investigating the role of *Candida albicans*. *Int Breastfeed J.* 2018;13:21.

Ketsuwan S, et al. Effect of herbal compresses for maternal breast engorgement at postpartum: a randomized controlled trial. *Breastfeed Med.* 2018;13(5):361–365.

Khosravan S, et al. The effect of hollyhock (*Althaea officinalis* l) leaf compresses combined with warm and cold compress on breast engorgement in lactating women: a randomized clinical trial. *J Evid Based Complementary Altern Med.* 2017;22(1):25–30.

Khresheh RM, Ahmad NM. Breastfeeding self efficacy among pregnant women in Saudi Arabia. *Saudi Med J.* 2018;39(11): 1116–1122.

Kossou J, et al. Factors influencing exclusive breastfeeding practices in rural areas in south Benin. *E3S Web Conf*. 2021;319:1–5.

Kronborg H, et al. The role of intention and self-efficacy on the association between breastfeeding of first and second child, a Danish cohort study. *BMC Pregnancy Childbirth*. 2018;18(1):454.

Kumar S, Singhi S. Role of probiotics in prevention of *Candida* colonization and invasive candidiasis. *J Matern Fetal Neonatal Med*. 2016;29(5):818–819.

Larson KE, Valente SA. Milk fistula: diagnosis, prevention, and treatment. *Breast J*. 2016;22(1):111–112.

Lawal AM, Idemudia ES. Examining maternal age, breastfeeding self-efficacy and health locus of control in psychological wellbeing of mothers. *Psychol Health Med*. 2017;22(10):1230–1238.

Lepanto MS, et al. Lactoferrin in aseptic and septic inflammation. *Molecules*. 2019;24(7).

Li AM, Erickson LA. Diabetic mastopathy. *Mayo Clin Proc*. 2018;93(9):1334–1335.

Li XV, et al. Gut mycobiota in immunity and inflammatory disease. *Immunity*. 2019;50(6):1365–1379.

Lodhi N, et al. Is our choice of empirical antibiotics appropriate for patients with methicillin resistant *Staphylococcus aureus* in breast abscess? *Iran J Microbiol*. 2018;10(6):348–353.

Mahmoud M, et al. The natural isoflavone biochanin-A synergizes 5-fluorouracil anticancer activity in vitro and in vivo in Ehrlich solid-phase carcinoma model. *Phytother Res*. 2022;36(3):1310–1325.

Mancano MA, et al. ISMP adverse drug reactions: longitudinal thumbnail fissures due to erlotinib priapism associated with the use of ExtenZe blindness from a nevirapine-based HAART regimen hyperprolactinemia and galactorrhea due to aripiprazole trypophobia associated with gabapentin coadministered linezolid and methadone cause serotonin syndrome. *Hosp Pharm*. 2019;54(2):88–92.

Mangesi L, Zakarija-Grkovic I. Treatments for breast engorgement during lactation. *Cochrane Database Syst Rev*. 2016;28(6): CD006946.

McGuire E. Case study: white spot and lecithin. *Breastfeed Rev*. 2015;23(1):23–25.

Mediano P, et al. Case-control study of risk factors for infectious mastitis in Spanish breastfeeding women. *BMC Pregnancy Childbirth*. 2014;14:195.

Mediano P, et al. Microbial diversity in milk of women with mastitis: potential role of coagulase-negative staphylococci, viridans group streptococci, and corynebacteria. *J Hum Lact*. 2017;33(2):309–318.

Mirghafourvand M, et al. Relationship of breastfeeding self-efficacy with quality of life in Iranian breastfeeding mothers. *J Matern Fetal Neonatal Med*. 2018;31(20):2721–2728.

Morton J. Hands-on or hands-off when first milk matters most? *Breastfeed Med*. 2019;14(5):295–297.

Mutschlechner W, et al. Mammary candidiasis: molecular-based detection of *Candida* species in human milk samples. *Eur J Clin Microbiol Infect Dis*. 2016;35(8):1309–1313.

Narayanan N, et al. Comparison of linezolid and daptomycin for the treatment of vancomycin-resistant enterococcal bacteremia. *Ther Adv Infect Dis*. 2019;6:2049936119828964.

Newman J. All purpose nipple ointment (APNO). Updated September 2021a. ibconline.ca/information-sheets/all-purpose-nipple-ointment-apno/

Newman J. Blocked ducts and mastitis. Updated 2021b. ibconline.ca/information-sheets/blocked-ducts-mastitis/

Ng WK, et al. Diabetic mastopathy: a breast carcinoma mimic. *Hong Kong Med J*. 2019;25(3):251.e1–251.e3.

Oyebode O, et al. Health, psychosocial, and social issues emanating from the COVID-19 pandemic based on social media comments: text mining and thematic analysis approach. *JMIR Med Inform*. 2021;9:1-27.

Oddó D, et al. Coryneform bacteria in granulomatous lobular mastitis: morphological diagnosis in breast biopsies. *Int J Surg Pathol*. 2019;27(4):380–386.

O'Shea JE, et al. Frenotomy for tongue-tie in newborn infants. *Cochrane Database Syst Rev*. 2017;3(3):CD011065.

O'Sullivan EJ, et al. Antenatal breastfeeding self-efficacy and breastfeeding outcomes among mothers participating in a feasibility breastfeeding-support intervention. *Ir J Med Sci*. 2019;188(2):569–578.

Oncel MY, et al. Comparison of *Lactobacillus reuteri* and nystatin prophylaxis on *Candida* colonization and infection in very low birth weight infants. *J Matern Fetal Neonatal Med*. 2015;28(15):1790–1794.

Park HW, et al. Positive effect of Baby-Friendly Hospital Initiatives on improving mothers' intention for successful breastfeeding in Korea. *J Korean Med Sci*. 2018;33(43):e272.

Peila C, et al. The effect of Holder pasteurization on nutrients and biologically-active components in donor human milk: a review. *Nutrients*. 2016;8(8):477.

Pipaliya N, et al. Esomeprazole induced galactorrhea: a novel side effect. *Clin J Gastroenterol*. 2016;9(1):13–16.

Pluguez-Turull CW, et al. Idiopathic granulomatous mastitis: manifestations at multimodality imaging and pitfalls. *Radiographics*. 2018;38(2):330–356.

Qiao Y, et al. Tuberculosis mastitis presenting as bilateral breast masses. *Clin Imaging*. 2018;52:28–31.

Reis J, et al. Breast sarcoidosis: clinical features, imaging, and histological findings. *Breast J*. 2021;27:44–48.

Rocha IS, et al. Influence of maternal confidence on exclusive breastfeeding until six months of age: a systematic review. *Cien Saude Colet*. 2018;23(11):3609–3619.

Rosier W. Cool cabbage compresses. *Breastfeed Rev*. 1988;1(12):28–31.

Russell SP, et al. Breast infections—microbiology and treatment in an era of antibiotic resistance. *Surgeon*. 2020;18(1):1–7.

Schaub R, et al. The immune response to sub-clinical mastitis is impaired in HIV-infected women. *J Transl Med*. 2018;16(1):296.

Soltani S, et al. Comparison of the effectiveness of breastfeeding, oral 25% dextrose, kangaroo-mother care method, and EMLA cream on pain score level following heal pick sampling in newborns: a randomized clinical trial. *Electron Physician*. 2018;10(5):6741–6748.

Spaeth A, et al. Baby-Friendly Hospital designation has a sustained impact on continued breastfeeding. *Matern Child Nutr*. 2018;14(1):e12497.

Taffurelli M, et al. Recurrent periductal mastitis: surgical treatment. *Surgery*. 2016;160(6):1689–1692.

Tan QT, et al. Granulomatous mastitis and factors associated with recurrence: an 11-year single-centre study of 113 patients in Singapore. *World J Surg*. 2019;43(7):1737–1745.

Tayyab SJ, et al. A pictorial review: multimodality imaging of benign and suspicious features of fat necrosis in the breast. *Br J Radiol*. 2018;91(1092):20180213.

Thimmappa D, et al. Breast tuberculosis. *Indian J Surg*. 2015;77(suppl 3):1378–1384.

Vanovcanova L, et al. Idiopathic granulomatous mastitis—a new approach in diagnostics and treatment. *Neoplasma*. 2019;66(4):661–668.

Vasei N, et al. Fat necrosis in the breast: a systematic review of clinical. *Lipids Health Dis*. 2019;18(1):139.

Vieira ES, et al. Breastfeeding self-efficacy and postpartum depression: a cohort study. *Rev Lat Am Enfermagem.* 2018;26:e3035.

Vieira F, et al. Effects of anhydrous lanolin versus breast milk combined with a breast shell for the treatment of nipple trauma and pain during breastfeeding: a randomized clinical trial. *J Midwifery Women's Health.* 2017;62(5):572–579.

Wahlstrom Henriksson H, Rubertsson C. Bodies get in the way: breastfeeding and gender equality in Swedish handbooks for new parents. *NORA.* 2021;29(4):330–342.

Wong BB, et al. Application of cabbage leaves compared to gel packs for mothers with breast engorgement: randomised controlled trial. *Int J Nurs Stud.* 2017;76:92–99.

Wren-Atilola HM, et al. Infant growth faltering linked to subclinical mastitis, maternal faecal-oral contamination, and breastfeeding. *Matern Child Nutr.* 2019;15(3):e12756.

Zhang Y, et al. Clinical characteristics, classification and surgical treatment of periductal mastitis. *J Thorac Dis.* 2018;10(4): 2420–2427.

CHAPTER 18

Nursing Beyond the First Month

As babies mature beyond their first month, their nursing needs will change in response to rapid periods of growth and development. Babies of this age are awake for longer periods and are more interactive with their environment. This is crucial for their physical and social development. Parents will learn to adapt to accommodate new nursing patterns. They will learn to navigate feeding in public, traveling with a nursing baby, returning to work or school, and adjusting to new feeding routines as their baby grows.

Over time, parents will learn their baby's unique means of communication. Waking and sleeping patterns, crying, cooing, smiling, and frowning will elicit parental responses and readjustments. Babies will progress through teething, crawling, standing, separation anxiety, experimenting with vocabulary sounds, and self-feeding. Parents will face the challenges of nursing a toddler and, ultimately, weaning. You can help parents appreciate these developmental milestones as they nurture and celebrate their growing child.

KEY TERMS

Allergen
Bauer crawling reflex
Body length
Complementary feeding
Food intolerance
Head circumference
Hematocrit
Minimal nursing
Moro reflex
Nursing strike
Palmar grasp
Parent-led weaning (mother-led weaning)
Pincer grasp
Prone
Reflexes
Soporific
Tonic neck reflex

Patterns of Growth in a Nursing Baby

The World Health Organization (WHO) growth charts are the premier global reference for infant and young child growth. They provide best practices in child growth assessment and establish the nursing infant as the norm against which to assess growth potential. **Table 18-1** depicts infant weight range from birth to 12 months for boys and girls. Researchers have observed differences in growth rates by country (Garzón et al., 2019). For accuracy and consistency, it is important that caregivers use the WHO charts to measure growth for the first 5 years of life (Centers for Disease Control and Prevention [CDC], 2022). Older charts from the CDC and National Health and Nutrition Examination Survey were based on mixed and formula feeding and primarily Caucasian infants. Because these charts were based on formula fed infants, some nursing infants appeared to falter in growth around 3 to 4 months. It is important to be aware that these older charts are still in print and available online.

Table 18-1 Infant Weight Ranges

Girls (kg)	Boys (kg)	Month	Girls (pounds/oz)	Boys (pounds/oz)
2.3–4.4	2.3–4.6	Birth	5.1–9.11	5.1–10.1
3.0–5.7	3.2–6.0	1	6.9–12.9	7.1–13.3
3.8–6.9	4.1–7.4	2	8.6–15.3	9.0–16.4
4.4–7.8	4.8–8.3	3	9.11–17.3	10.9–18.4
4.8–8.6	5.4–9.1	4	10.9–19	11.14–20.1
5.2–9.2	5.8–9.7	5	11.8–20.4	12.12–21.6
5.5–9.7	6.1–10.2	6	12.1–21.6	13.8–22.8
5.8–10.2	6.4–10.7	7	12.12–22.8	14.1–23.9
6.0–10.6	6.7–11.1	8	13.3–23.6	14.12–24.8
6.2–11.0	6.9–11.4	9	13.11–24.4	15.3–25.1
6.4–11.3	7.1–11.8	10	14.1–24.14	15.11–26.0
6.6–11.7	7.3–12.1	11	14.9–25.12	16.1–26.11
6.8–12.0	7.5–12.4	12	15.0–26.8	16.5–27.3

Reproduced from World Health Organization. *The WHO Child Growth Standards*. Geneva, Switzerland: World Health Organization; 2006. https://www.who.int/publications/i/item/924154693X. Printed with permission of the International Lactation Consultant Association.

Nursing babies typically gain weight quickly during the first 3 to 4 months of life, after which their rate of growth slows. They double their birth weight by 5 to 6 months of age and triple it by 1 year. In the first few months after birth, nursing babies generally grow at about the same rate as their formula-fed counterparts. After this time, formula-fed infants typically begin to exceed nursing infants in weight, whereas human milk–fed infants tend to gain more **body length**. Body length and head circumference are indicators of appropriate growth. At 1 year of age, a baby's length is typically about 1½ times the newborn's length at birth. Brain growth is quite rapid in the first year of life, with **head circumference** increasing approximately 7.6 cm (3 inches) by 1 year of age.

Like adults, babies come in all shapes and sizes, and there is great variance in the range of normal weight gain. If the parents of a petite, wiry infant are petite or slim-framed, chances are that their baby will be, too. Sometimes nursing babies are chubby, and parents wonder if they are overweight. Some research reports that formula-fed infants are heavier than nursing infants because of higher energy intake (Pattison et al., 2019). Formula-fed infants have been found to be less energy efficient, taking in more milk and using nutrients less effectively than infants who are nursed. Growth outcomes of infants fed with infant formula with relatively low protein/energy ratios have been found to be comparable to those of infants fed on human milk (Kouwenhoven et al., 2022; Ren et al., 2022).

Weight gain in nursing infants can be higher than normal, with no known adverse effects. Chubby nursing babies usually slim down in toddlerhood. Help from a lactation consultant can avoid overfeeding. Rarely, an infant who seems insatiable may need to be assessed by an endocrinologist to rule out growth disorders, including Sotos, Beckwith–Wiedemann, Marfan, and Simpson–Golabi–Behmel syndromes (Barisic et al., 2018; Plachý et al., 2018; Zhao et al., 2018). Feeding difficulty is one of many markers for these syndromes.

Infant Development

Parents begin to get to know their newborn's unique personality in the first few hours and days after birth. As they become familiar with waking and sleeping patterns, crying and cooing, and smiling and frowning, parents learn how to adapt their responses and parenting to meet their baby's specific needs. Despite each baby's individuality, there are developmental patterns that all babies exhibit at roughly the same age range as their cognitive, social, emotional, and physical functions mature. Given this commonality, caregivers who have experience with many babies at different ages are able to identify those who do not exhibit age-appropriate **reflexes** and developmental milestones. Babies develop as individuals within certain universal parameters. Parents need to be aware of developmental milestones and communicate with their healthcare provider if their baby is not meeting the milestones appropriate for their age.

Infant Development in the First Year

There is a wide range of normal variation in infant development. Babies grow and develop at their own rate. Humans develop progressively from head to foot and from the center of the body or torso out to the extremities. Parents usually look forward to experiencing their baby's new abilities with each milestone. Awareness of normal stages of gross motor, fine motor, cognitive, social, communication, and emotional development can help them anticipate and respond appropriately to their baby. Providing anticipatory guidance on what to expect as their baby changes and grows can be reassuring to parents.

Reflexes

Newborn reflexes remain in place until babies develop more mature fine and gross motor skills to replace them. These early reflexes are necessary for survival. Reflexes such as rooting, sucking, grasping, and swallowing enable babies to obtain food. The gag reflex protects infants from choking while they learn to take in food. Newborns exhibit the **Moro reflex**, startling in response to sudden noise. The **palmar grasp** enables them to grasp objects such as their parents' fingers.

Until 3 or 4 months of age, infants exhibit the **tonic neck reflex**, also referred to as the *fencer position*. When they lie on their backs, they extend the arm and leg on the side of the body opposite to the direction in which the head is turned. This prevents them from rolling over until adequate neurological and motor development occurs.

Pressure on the soles of a baby's feet will elicit the **Bauer crawling reflex**, with movements similar to crawling or kicking. This reflex is exhibited when babies are given the opportunity to move up the parent's abdomen to find the nipple and latch after birth. This reflex disappears when the baby is around 6 weeks old and reappears when learning to crawl. Moro, palmar grasp, and tonic neck reflexes disappear by about 6 months of age. Rooting and sucking reflexes continue to about 9 months. **Chapter 15** provides more information on the baby's innate feeding abilities.

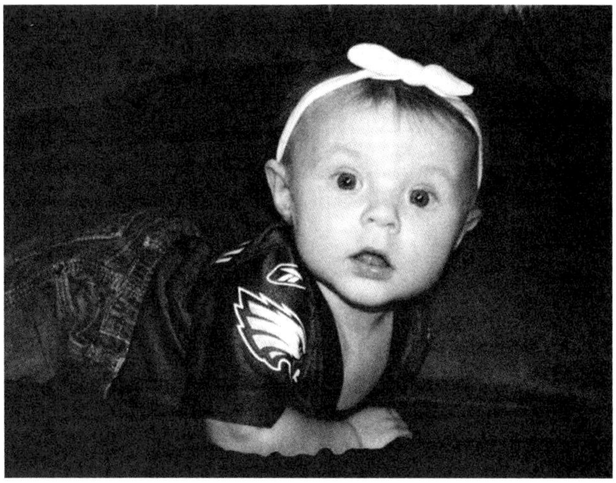

Figure 18-1 Baby at 3 months holding head up.

Printed with permission of Judith Lauwers.

Head and Body Control

Newborns can raise their heads purposefully from birth. At about 3 months of age, a baby can support their upper body with their arms when lying on their stomach and begin to raise their head from a **prone** position more consistently (**Figure 18-1**).

By 4 to 5 months, as the infant gains head and neck strength, they can raise their head higher and hold it for longer periods. They also become more alert and turn their head toward voices or movement. During this same period, they begin to rest on their forearms as the torso becomes stronger.

By 6 months, large muscle motor development enables babies to roll over. The torso strengthens as they prepare for crawling. By 7 months, babies can roll over in either direction and can pull themselves to a standing position. Babies need to regularly spend supervised time on their tummies to achieve these developmental milestones.

Hand Movement

At 1 month, most babies bring their hands near their faces and keep them in tight fists. By 3 months, they open and shut their hands and bring them to their mouths. During this period, they start using their hands and eyes in coordination and will grab and shake toys. At 4 to 5 months, infants can control hand movements and begin to play with their fingers. They are fascinated by movement and will wave and bat at objects.

By 6 months, the infant masters visually directed reaching. They can grasp desired items and pull them toward their mouth. Tongue movement allows them to take in solid foods and begin to learn the social art of eating. Many babies at this age begin reaching for food at family meals. Watching family members eat and grabbing food are some of the signs of developmental readiness to begin complementary foods. These babies are signaling that they are interested in self-feeding, the developmental stage of readiness to feed themselves.

By 7 months, babies' hands and arms are more developed. They learn to wave goodbye and can transfer objects from hand to hand. They struggle to get objects that are out of reach and explore objects with their hands and mouths. They begin to use their thumb and forefinger to pick up objects, in what is called the **pincer grasp**, by about 8 to 9 months of age.

Sitting

Sitting upright is one of the first gross motor milestones achieved by infants. At 4 months, the baby's back is rounded, and the head is erect when held in a sitting position (see **Figure 18-2**). By 5 months, the body will be erect when supported. At 6 months, increased head and neck control make it possible to pull the infant to a sitting position. By this age, most babies can sit when propped. By 7 months, they can sit without being propped. By 9 months, they can sit well in a chair and pull themselves into a sitting position.

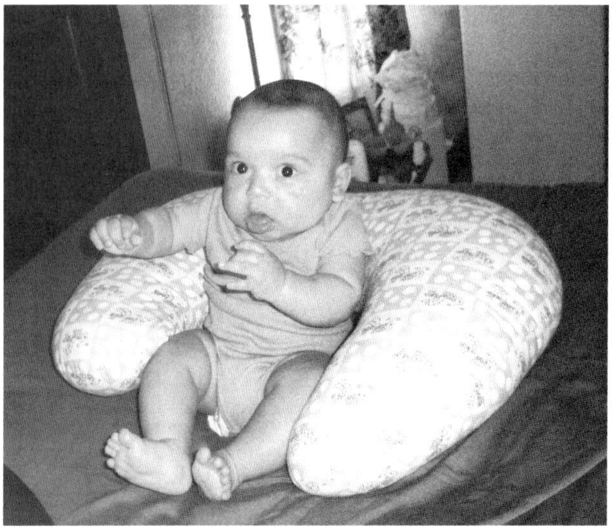

Figure 18-2 Baby at 4 months sitting with support.

Printed with permission of Anna Swisher.

Crawling and Walking

By 7 months, babies are more active. This is a time when they expand their world through physical movements. Many babies begin the early stages of crawling at about 6 to 8 months, raising themselves onto their hands and knees and rocking back and forth (**Figure 18-3**).

By 10 to 12 months, babies are able to more fully explore their environment with increasing locomotion. This is an expansive age for infants as they enthusiastically practice many new motor skills while avidly exploring the environment. They learn to cruise by using tables and chairs for balance as they learn to walk (**Figure 18-4**). Babies progress from cruising to walking, typically between 9 and 17 months of age. Because experience is a stronger predictor than age for skill improvement, babies need lots of safe opportunities for floor play and time for practice.

By 1 year, babies are interested in everything around them and show their pleasure and displeasure easily. Because they can reach many items that pose a danger, parents need to examine their house for potential hazards. Freedom to move safely within the home is important to satisfying babies' strong desire to explore and learn about their world.

As early as 10 months, they can crawl up a set of stairs, but they cannot crawl down them. Children typically master stair ascent at about 11 months, several months after learning to crawl. They learn to descend stairs a month or two later. Parents in homes with stairs will want to teach their child to ascend and descend stairs safely and install safety gates at both ends of the stairs. Babies should never be left alone near or on stairs.

When baby-proofing a home, parents can get on the floor and crawl around at the same level as a baby. Many hazards that are easy to miss from a standing

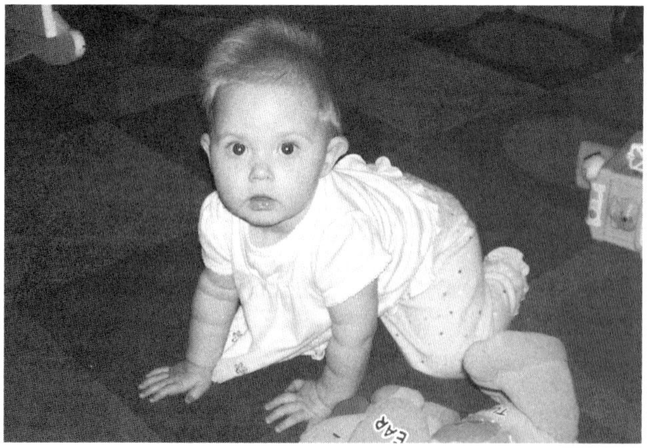

Figure 18-3 Baby at 6 months starting to crawl.

Printed with permission of Judith Lauwers.

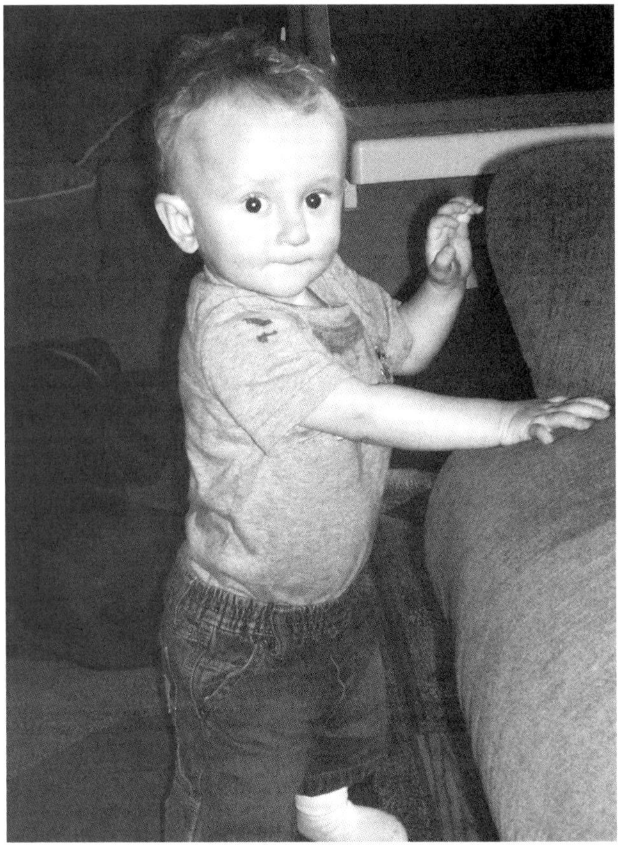

Figure 18-4 Baby cruising at 1 year with support of furniture.

position become apparent at eye level. Objects such as cords, curtains, window blinds, and electrical outlets can be dangerous to curious young explorers. Water should never be heated on the front burner of a stove, and pot handles should be turned to the back of the stove so that they cannot be reached. Reliable child safety information is available online. Many businesses and community organizations provide child safety assessments and child-proofing services. Providing a list of those in your area may be helpful to new families.

Sleeping

Physical development determines when an infant can sleep through the night. The ability to sleep for longer periods increases as the baby's central nervous system develops. Close contact with the parent and lighting/darkening cues may help the infant's circadian rhythm development (McKenna & Reiss, 2018). Nursing dyads develop sleep synchronicity, with the infant adapting to the parent's circadian rhythm (Kikuchi et al., 2020).

Some of the components of milk produced at night may contribute to this development (Schneider et al., 2018). Research shows that nursing parents contribute more to their baby's circadian rhythm than mixed-feeding or nonnursing parents (Kikuchi et al., 2020). These findings confirm that nursing enhances the maturation of the infant's sleep–wake cycles and the central nervous system.

Babies' sleep–wake cycles shorten by about 3 months of age. Daytime cycles become shorter than the nighttime ones, with a pattern of one longer rest period at night and several naps during the day. Personality may determine the part of the 24-hour cycle when a baby sleeps for a longer period. The cycle can be adjusted by initiating feedings more frequently during the day. When changes in the baby's sleep pattern occur, the parent's breasts may become fuller or engorged. Nursing directly before going to bed for the evening will promote the longest nighttime sleep period, with perhaps 5 or 6 hours of uninterrupted sleep.

At around 8 months of age, a baby may experience separation anxiety on waking during the night without the parents nearby. Even after developing the ability to sleep for longer periods, a baby may experience disturbed sleep because of dreams. The need to nurse can also cause disturbed sleep. This sort of disruption is common during periods of rapid physical and mental growth, increased activity during the day, and teething. In the second year of age, the child may still need close physical contact to fall asleep. Reassure parents that this is normal.

Social Development

For the first 3 months, babies experience the nursing parent–baby dyad as a single entity. Their reliance on the nursing parent, usually the primary caregiver, as the person who responds to their needs is absolute. It is normal for parents to have ambivalent feelings about the baby's seemingly constant demands on their time. It is also normal for parents to enjoy the early baby period because they feel important and useful to their baby. Some parents may miss the personal time they had for relaxation and recreation. It takes time for new parents to settle into their new roles. Each dyad and family will require support tailored to their unique needs and circumstances.

Interaction. By 3 months, babies respond more purposefully to stimuli and become highly social. They begin to focus on objects around them and actively interact with their parents and the environment (**Figure 18-5**). Visual acuity becomes clearer, and they will bat at objects to touch and move them. They will

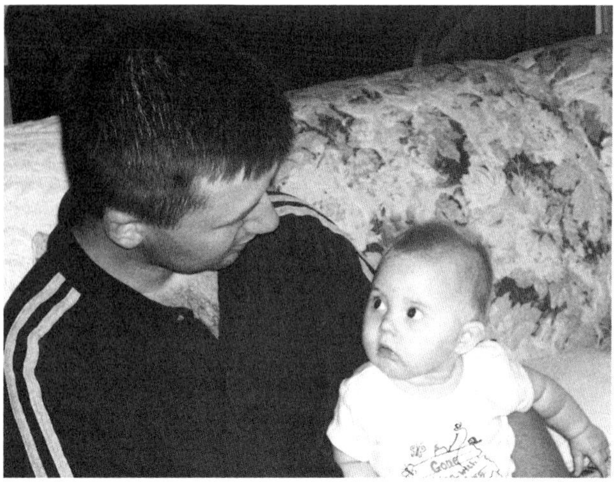

Figure 18-5 Baby at 3 months interacting with parent.

Printed with permission of Judith Lauwers.

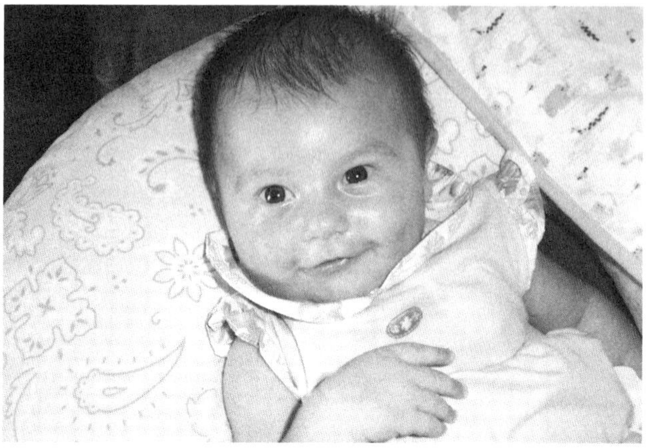

Figure 18-6 Baby at 2 months responding with a smile.

Printed with permission of Judith Lauwers.

respond more readily to high-pitched voices. They may show more interest in children than in adults, which encourages siblings to entertain and interact with the infant.

By 3 months, the baby will be awake for more hours each day, and more alert and responsive to interaction. Parents begin to interact with their babies in ways other than nursing, exposing them to everyday household sounds and activities. Babies begin to enjoy bright, colorful toys and decorations. Varying positions and the environment during the day can provide the stimulation needed for physical and mental growth. Encouraging daily tummy time promotes muscle development and helps prevent positional plagiocephaly (the baby's head developing flat areas) because of long periods of time lying on their back.

By 10 to 12 months, most babies are eager to participate in family activities. Mealtime becomes a time of discovery and interaction. When parents offer finger foods that they can study, touch, turn over, and taste, babies can participate in the feeding process and experience the independence they crave. As their mobility increases, babies discriminate more between self and others. Children at this age freely move away from parents to explore their environment while continually checking back for assurance that the parent will be there when the child returns.

Disposition. Social smiles typically begin at around 2 months (**Figure 18-6**), although many infants smile much earlier. Smiling is detected in utero by the early second trimester. Big social smiles are evident by 3 months. Infants learn to express unhappiness, delight, and excitement during this time. They may show a preference for their parents, especially the primary caregiver, and will fuss when others provide care. They can sense tension in a caregiver and will respond with tension and fussiness, quieting down when held in a calm and relaxed manner. Their eating and sleeping patterns will become more predictable.

By 4 months, babies have mastered the art of laughing aloud, to the delight of everyone around them. By this time, most parents have adapted their lives to the needs of their new baby and feel more confident in their parenting abilities. The hours of patience, understanding, and love are rewarded by babies' responsiveness and development of elementary skills. They begin to use their motor skills to amuse themselves for short periods of time, and their demands on the parents decrease accordingly.

At about 9 months, babies' awareness of the parent's absence may bring on separation anxiety when a loved one leaves the room. As a result, they may cry in anticipation that the parent will leave, as well as during the parent's absence. They may wake during the night and cry out for reassurance that the parents are nearby. Although they have learned that parents are important, they do not have the awareness that their parents will return. This anxiety is a normal stage in a baby's development.

At 9 months, it is common for babies to prefer their nursing parent to the other parent or family members. Their increased awareness of differences in people may cause them to react fearfully to strangers and to need contact with the nursing parent for reassurance. These fearful reactions to strangers are normal. Parents do not need to protect infants from exposure to new people. Meeting new people in a safe manner is important for social development.

At 10 to 12 months, babies may become overwhelmed by outside stresses such as contact with strangers, separation from their primary caregiver, and changes in schedule. They may react with shyness or fear or begin clinging like a much younger baby. They may climb into their parents' lap to escape stresses and to refuel emotionally. Infants of this age need several periods of rest from active exploration each day to renew their energy.

Vocalization. During the first year of life, early spontaneous facial movements undergo significant changes necessary for speech. Parents talking to their babies, even in utero, promotes speech and language development and healthy social development. By 4 to 5 months, babies begin to imitate sounds. By 6 months, babbling, cooing, and squealing mark the beginning of expressive language. Babbling represents babies learning vowel–consonant combinations.

This is a highly active and social period for babies. As they experiment with language, infants need to interact with those around them. Parental response to these language efforts is essential for their speech and language development. At 10 to 12 months, the amount of receptive vocabulary (words they understand and respond to) increases noticeably. Babies begin experimenting with vocabulary sounds, which is the beginning of expressive speech.

Developmental Delays. Well-baby checkups typically occur at about 2, 4, 6, 9, and 12 months of age and include early vaccinations. The baby's healthcare provider will check that the baby is meeting developmental milestones and will monitor for signs of potential developmental delays. Signs of developmental delays at each of these stages are described in **Figure 18-7**. Be aware that feeding difficulties can be symptoms of underlying developmental issues. Mobile apps are available to help track developmental milestones, including one at no cost from the CDC (2023a).

Babies typically cut their first tooth between 6 and 8 months of age, although teething can occur at any time between 4 and 14 months. As a tooth erupts, it causes gum swelling and irritation. When the baby sucks, blood rushes to the gums, adding to the swelling that is already present and causing immediate discomfort. Thus, when beginning to nurse, the baby may quickly pull away from the breast and cry out with pain. Other signs of teething include irritability, a slight fever, increased drooling, unexplained spit-up, loose stools, and waking at night to seek comfort.

Two months:
- Doesn't respond to loud sounds
- Doesn't watch things as they move
- Doesn't smile at people
- Doesn't bring hands to mouth
- Can't hold head up when pushing up when on tummy

Four months:
- Doesn't watch things as they move
- Doesn't smile at people
- Can't hold head steady
- Doesn't coo or make sounds
- Doesn't bring things to mouth
- Doesn't push down with legs when feet are placed on a hard surface
- Has trouble moving one or both eyes in all directions

Six months:
- Doesn't try to get things that are in reach
- Shows no affection for caregivers
- Doesn't respond to sounds
- Has difficulty getting things to mouth
- Doesn't make vowel sounds ("ah", "eh", "oh")
- Doesn't roll over in either direction
- Doesn't laugh or make squealing sounds
- Seems very stiff, with tight muscles
- Seems very floppy, like a rag doll

Nine months:
- Doesn't bear weight on legs with support
- Doesn't sit with help
- Doesn't babble ("mama", "baba", "dada")
- Doesn't play any games involving back-and-forth play
- Doesn't respond to own name
- Doesn't seem to recognize familiar people
- Doesn't look where you point
- Doesn't transfer toys from one hand to the other

Twelve months:
- Doesn't crawl
- Can't stand when supported
- Doesn't search for things they see you hide
- Doesn't say single words like "mama" or "dada"
- Doesn't learn gestures like waving or shaking head
- Doesn't point to things
- Loses skills he once had

Figure 18-7 Signs of developmental delays.

Data from Centers for Disease Control and Prevention. Developmental Milestones. November 8, 2023. https://www.cdc.gov/ncbddd/actearly/milestones/index.html. Learn the Signs. Act Early. November 8, 2023. https://www.cdc.gov/ncbddd/actearly/index.html. Teething and Biting

Overcoming Teething Pain. Because the nerves to the teeth branch out to the face, cheek, and outer ear, the baby may rub their jaw or pull on an ear to relieve the discomfort from teething. Babies discover that chewing and rubbing their gums help reduce the pain. A cooled teething ring or rubbing ice or a cold cloth on the gums before nursing can relieve the soreness long enough for the baby to nurse comfortably. Hard foods, such as toast for the baby to chew on, also helps relieve the pain and promote tooth eruption. Over-the-counter pain relievers can help with the pain also. Parents can consult their pharmacist for medications and dosages. They will want to consult the baby's caregiver before using locally acting over-the-counter preparations that temporarily numb gum tissue.

Discouraging Biting. Teething may cause the baby to clamp down on the nipple during feeding. Parents need to be alert for signs that a feeding is ending and unlatch the baby when the suck–swallow rhythm slows. If biting occurs in the middle of a feeding, parents can remove the baby immediately and say, "No." They can wait a few minutes before resuming the feeding. If the baby bites again, they can end the feeding promptly and gently repeat, "No." Remaining consistent with these responses will help deter this behavior. When a baby bites for the first time, a common reaction is an outcry and a startled jerk away from the baby. This may scare the baby, and they may reject nursing at subsequent feedings. Biting can usually be overcome and does not need to lead to weaning.

Because of the sucking mechanics involved during nursing, it is difficult for a baby to suck and bite at the same time. Clamping down tightly will interfere with the tongue compressing the nipple. A baby who bites may not be hungry enough to nurse at that time. The parent can end the feeding and try again later when the baby's hunger returns. If teething pain is suspected as the cause of biting, parents can try some comfort measures and then resume nursing.

Biting may occur at the end of a feeding as the baby falls asleep and the jaw closes. Such clamping down on the nipple may be prevented by removing the nipple when it appears that the baby is nearly finished. Inserting a finger between the baby's gums and withdrawing it slowly will break suction and avoid discomfort. Alternately, pushing the baby's head into the breast will interrupt their natural nose breathing and cause the baby to open their mouth to breathe.

Nursing Behavior

Nursing patterns evolve naturally over the first several weeks after birth. Practices in the early days that support nursing help to establish these natural rhythms. Nursing immediately after birth is recommended, although many babies do not actively feed during this early period. Some babies may be sleepy after delivery or simply need time to explore how to suck and latch or how to lick and nuzzle the nipple. A healthy, unmedicated, full-term baby who is allowed to self-latch will usually progress to effective nursing with minimal interventions. In the days and weeks that follow, nursing behavior will continue to evolve as the baby matures and lactation is established.

One Month. By 1 month, infants are efficient at sucking and will actively nurse for 15 minutes or longer at a feeding. They typically establish a pattern ranging between 8 and 16 feedings per day. Periods of increased appetite and growth can occur at any time. Babies typically experience appetite spurts at about 2 weeks, 6 weeks, 3 months, and 6 months of age. During these times, they nurse more frequently, in spurts that can last 2 to 3 days. These frequent feedings associated with periods of rapid growth are sometimes called *cluster feeds*. Encourage parents to nurse frequently, snuggle with their baby, and provide lots of skin-to-skin contact.

Two to Three Months. By 2 to 3 months, babies will typically spend less time at each feeding and may use methods other than nursing for self-comforting. Some parents may perceive this change as a declining interest in nursing. Additionally, normal hormonal changes during this period cause the breasts to lose fullness. This combination of events can cause apprehension and worry about adequate milk production.

You can help families anticipate these changes as normal parts of nursing. Encourage them to focus on the baby's disposition, appearance, number of voids and stools, weight gain, interactions, and vigor. These signs will reassure parents that their baby is growing and thriving. Open-ended questions, positive feedback, and descriptive statements can help increase their confidence that they and their baby are working in harmony and there is no cause for concern. Their continued symbiotic relationship provides the baby with the precise amount of milk to support optimal growth.

Regular separations of the nursing parent and baby may begin around 3 months. A return to work may occur as early as 4 to 6 weeks after birth. Make sure parents know how to express milk for use when they are away from their baby. Explore a variety of feeding options in the event that their baby will not feed from a bottle. For example, nursing babies often find the transition to a cup easier than a move to a bottle. **Chapter 22** discusses expressing and feeding milk to the baby in more detail.

Four to Six Months. By 4 months, most babies are noticeably more efficient at nursing. Feedings are shorter and may be less frequent. The baby may shorten or miss some feedings because they are curious about everything in their environment and become easily distracted. Between 4 and 6 months, babies who have been sleeping through the night commonly begin waking to nurse. Nursing at night enables them to receive the calories they miss during their active day. Reassure parents that this is normal.

Protein levels in human milk fluctuate throughout the day, and night nursing may be important for protein intake (Khan et al., 2013). Safe cosleeping or keeping the baby in the same room enables parents to nurse frequently, maintains milk production, and provides the baby with a sense of security. Nighttime intake may account for as much as 20% of their total 24-hour intake.

By 4 to 5 months, babies may pat or stroke the breast and strain their body away during feeding to have a better look at the parent or to scan the environment. Reassure parents that distractions are normal and not a sign that their baby is losing interest in nursing. This tendency toward distraction is a step forward in the baby's development. It shows that they are reaching out to learn more about their world.

Nursing usually continues easily during this expansive time as babies internalize their new knowledge and gain confidence. For roughly 25% of babies, an apparent disinterest in nursing leads to what is referred to as a "**nursing strike**." This describes a baby who suddenly becomes unhappy and fussy during feedings. Despite being hungry, the baby resists latching, pulls off, and cries. In some instances, the baby may not cry but still pushes away. **Chapter 23** discusses how to manage a baby resisting nursing.

By 6 months, the frequency of feedings usually continues to diminish. The longest feeding usually occurs before the baby is put to bed for the night. Complementary foods will begin around this time, and the baby may wake more often during the night to nurse. Parents may consider beginning complementary foods earlier than 6 months, perhaps because their baby seems old enough, seems hungry, or wants the food the family is eating. They may want their baby to receive more than milk or believe that additional foods will help promote nighttime sleep. In some cases, the family's healthcare provider may have recommended that the baby begin eating solid food. Formula-fed infants are more likely to start complementary foods early than those who are exclusively nursed or receive mixed feedings. You can remind parents that a baby's swallowing mechanism and gastrointestinal tract are too immature to handle solid foods until about 6 months of age. Assure them that their milk is the ideal food to support their baby's growth through the first 6 months of life.

Teething will begin soon, which can result in increased nursing for comfort. Babies may drool, suck on their fingers, or chew on objects. Sucking can induce pain in tender gums and may cause the baby to pull away abruptly when nursing. Fluctuations in nursing patterns may decrease milk removal and lead to engorgement, ductal narrowing, or mastitis. Regular milk removal and breast care will help maintain milk production and prevent overfullness.

Seven to Twelve Months. By 7 to 9 months of age, most babies will be teething and eating a healthy variety of foods. They may actively seek to nurse anytime and anywhere, pulling at the parent's clothing or attempting to unbutton a shirt. They may hold the breast with one or both hands while nursing. Over the next couple of months, they may become distracted easily and will need quiet locations for uninterrupted feedings.

By 10 to 12 months, babies master motor skills and establish regular meal patterns. Newfound freedom can result in further changes in nursing patterns. Some babies increase feeding frequency and duration as new events and experiences prompt a need for reassurance and closeness. Parents who anticipated their baby weaning soon may be discouraged by an apparent lack of progress toward independence. You can assure them that satisfying a child's emotional needs during this time is important for healthy mental growth and the development of self-reliance and independence later in childhood.

By 12 months, most babies are eating solid foods at regular mealtimes with their family. It may seem that they are outgrowing nursing and when coupled with outside pressure parents may consider weaning. You can assure parents that most babies at this age still need the security and comfort of nursing as a stabilizing factor in their lives. Moreover, solid foods do not usually contain the special fatty acids needed for continued brain growth that are present in human milk. Furthermore, human milk contains the immune factors and antibodies specific to the baby's environment.

There is a prevalent myth in many cultures that infants do not need human milk after their first year. Globally, the recommendation that babies nurse for the first year and beyond is often not met. For example, less than 36% of babies in the United States receive any human milk at 12 months of age (CDC, 2018; Meeks & Noble, 2022). Less than 1% of babies in the United Kingdom still receive any human milk at 6 months of age (Fallon et al., 2019).

You can help parents recognize the continuing nutrition and protection afforded by their milk through the baby's second year of life. Parents who nurse an older baby, especially those in a culture where bottle feeding prevails, need support and encouragement to overcome obstacles and validate their choice. Factors related to nursing an older baby appear later in this chapter.

Overfeeding a Nursing Baby. Some parents may worry that frequent and lengthy feedings will lead to their baby receiving too much milk and being overfed. This worry could stem from a baby who appears to be overweight or who spits up milk. Babies are considered overweight if they are approximately two categories above the weight-for-height standard, as determined by standard height and weight charts. A normal weight gain is 1 to 2 pounds per month for the first 4 or 5 months of life. This rapid weight gain does not typically continue into the second half of the first year.

Some families have heavier babies who slim down in the second year, regardless of whether they are nursed or formula fed. If the baby is significantly heavier than other family members were at that age, the child may be getting too much milk. An older baby who often spits up or vomits from an overly distended stomach may be overfed. In such a case, milk production may be overly abundant. The parent can shorten or decrease feedings and substitute other activities for nursing until the spitting up diminishes. **Chapter 15** offers additional suggestions for dealing with overactive milk production.

Overfeeding can occur when a baby nurses frequently for comfort or has a great sucking need. You can suggest other ways to comfort the baby so that nursing is not used as a response to every cue. Help parents learn ways to interact with their baby through activities other than nursing. These activities will expand the child's world in the direction of optimal physical, mental, emotional, and social development. **Figure 18-8** presents tips to avoid overfeeding.

- Let the baby suck on their thumb or finger.
- Nurse on one side per feeding and allow the baby to continue sucking on the less full side.
- Learn other ways to interact with the baby—rock, carry, and keep the baby within view of the parent; talk to the baby; change their position; play with and sing to the baby.
- Interest the baby in other activities—a stroll, toys, baby exercises, and so on.

Figure 18-8 Tips to avoid overfeeding.

Infant Development Beyond 1 Year

Early in the baby's first year, a fear of strangers may reemerge and a reluctance to be away from the parents, especially the primary caregiver. Over time, the child learns that the parents always return, which minimizes separation anxiety. Working parents may notice these regressions more than those who stay at home. Optimally, the baby's caretaker will provide the attention and nurturing the child needs to develop emotional stability in the parents' absence.

As babies progress to toddlerhood, nursing patterns reflect changes in their social, emotional, and physical development. Overstimulation during the day or separation anxiety may cause a baby to wake at night to nurse. They may nurse less frequently when they are busy experimenting with new skills or more frequently because of an increased need for security or attention. Many toddlers continue to nurse into their second or third year or beyond. Others wean themselves and never seem to miss nursing. Both patterns are normal. Providing anticipatory guidance to parents will relieve concerns and help them enjoy this stage of their children's lives.

As babies grow older, communication and play become increasingly important. The child's world extends to increase interaction with the nonnursing parent and extended family members. These relatives present the novelty of other personalities with different ideas and responses. When the baby begins to develop a close relationship with another person, the nursing parent may worry that their role is diminishing. Reassure them that babies continue to need them as they develop relationships with others. Developing new relationships is a positive step in a child's development and leads to the ability to pursue their own interests as autonomous human beings. Allowing safe opportunities for the child to become self-reliant at a comfortable pace is an important part of healthy emotional and social development.

Accommodating a Nursing Baby

Each family's nursing experience is influenced by their attitudes, preferences, and philosophies. Some parents prefer nursing only in the privacy of their homes. They may be uncomfortable nursing in the presence of other people or worry that others will disapprove. Some are comfortable nursing in the homes of friends and family or in public places. Parents may need guidance for nursing in public places and traveling with a nursing child.

Nursing in Public

Many families enjoy taking their babies along with them everywhere they go and are comfortable feeding in public places (**Figure 18-9**). Parents can gain confidence in nursing in public by watching other parents nurse their babies, observing practical methods and other people's reactions. Nursing in front of a mirror or another person may develop more self-assurance. A family member is often a great "mirror" for giving candid comments about what others might see. Another excellent place to develop confident public nursing is within support groups, where parents can learn from each other.

Wearing clothing that easily accommodates discreet nursing will facilitate feeding in public. Loose-fitting clothes allow easy access for feedings. A sweater, jacket, or similar garment worn over the shoulders can restrict the side view. A baby sling will provide support and extra cover, as well as ease in mobility. Beginning a feeding before the baby becomes overly hungry and starts to fuss will avoid attracting attention. Allowing extra time for nursing during shopping or running errands will also help make feeding in public more comfortable.

With forethought and planning, parents can choose a time and location for nursing in which they can be relaxed and comfortable. A spot that is out of the way of aisles and walkways will provide privacy and be less distracting for the baby. Out-of-the-way spaces like a corner table or booth in a restaurant, a bench next to a wall, sitting next to a family member or friend, a dressing room or lounge, or a parked car are good for nursing highly distractable babies.

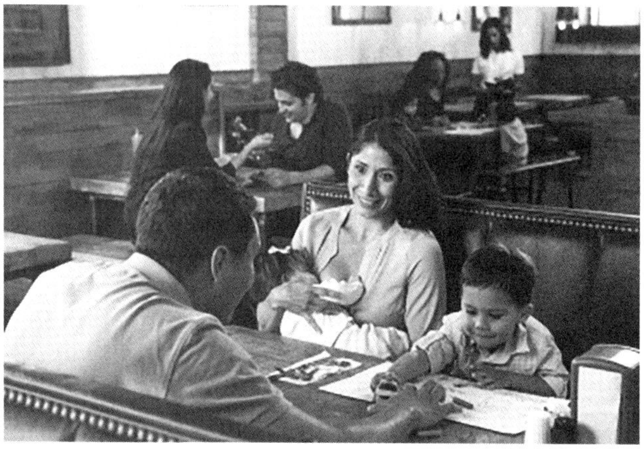

Figure 18-9 Nursing in public.

Courtesy of U.S. Department of Agriculture's Food and Nutrition Service.

No parent should ever have to nurse in a restroom or any place where they feel uncomfortable or unsafe. Confidence increases as parents learn they can nurse in public and that few people even notice. Public nursing has gained more acceptance as people recognize the importance of human milk for lifelong health. In many places around the world, nursing in public is considered normal. The United States, Puerto Rico, and the Virgin Islands have laws that protect nursing in any public.

Traveling with a Nursing Baby

Traveling with a baby avoids the apprehension parents may feel about being apart from their baby. Although it is more cumbersome than traveling alone, careful planning and preparation can help make it both convenient and enjoyable. A nursing baby between 6 weeks and 6 months of age is usually an ideal traveler. They have a predictable routine, do not yet eat other foods, and are not very mobile. Babies at this age often sleep through the monotony of an automobile, train, bus, or plane ride, making the trip easier and more enjoyable.

To avoid overburdening themselves when they travel, parents can limit baby care items to those that are essential. Nursing eliminates the need for supplemental foods or formula, as well as the equipment necessary to prepare and transport them. It also eliminates the worry about safe water to reconstitute powdered formula. Parents can purchase disposable diapers along the way, limiting the number that need to be packed. Several changes of baby clothing in the diaper bag will decrease the need to open suitcases in search of clothing while en route. A lightweight diaper bag can also double as a purse.

Traveling by Foot

A baby sling or other mode of baby wearing is convenient for walking with a baby. It is more versatile than a stroller, especially in crowded shops, on stairways, on hiking trails, and in the sand. The comfortable position and motion associated with a sling often lull an infant to sleep. A lightweight cloth sling fits easily into a diaper bag, ready to use at any time. For added protection in cold weather, parents can place the baby in the carrier under their coat. Caution them to always wear their baby safely, ensuring that the baby's face is visible and not pressed tightly against the wearer.

Traveling by Vehicle

A baby should always be strapped securely into an approved infant car seat when traveling by vehicle. Infant car seats are also effective for other modes of travel and are more comfortable for the baby than adult seats. Parents should never hold their baby in a moving vehicle. A sudden stop could result in the parent losing hold and hurling the baby from the car or against the car's interior. Likewise, caution parents against carrying their baby in a sling or baby carrier while riding in the car. The force of the parent's body could cause serious injury to the baby in the event of a sudden stop.

For safety reasons, nursing during a car ride should be discouraged. Leaning over the baby to nurse could crush or suffocate the baby in the event of a crash, even when both the baby and parent are secured by seat belts. Some parents find that leaving early in the morning gives them a few hours' drive time before the baby awakens. Others prefer driving at night when the baby, especially an older baby, may sleep longer.

Safety experts recommend frequent stops during long trips for driver safety and alertness Parents can plan to stop about every 2 hours or when the baby wakes to allow for nursing, diaper changes, and for the baby to move around freely. Long periods of travel without frequent stops can result in a crying, fussy baby. If it is not possible to stop and the baby is not yet eating other foods or cannot be otherwise distracted, a bottle of expressed milk can help stretch nursing times. Allowing extra time for frequent stops will help meet everyone's needs.

Traveling by Air

When planning a trip by air, parents can request a roomier seat behind the bulkhead. Babies should be placed in their car seats strapped into a regular seat if parents can afford a ticket for the baby. Otherwise, the baby must be held on the parent's lap. Parents should check the airline rules before traveling. They can check strollers and other baby equipment with the luggage and carry their baby and personal items during the flight. Airlines typically allow parents with small children to board the plane before other passengers so that they can get settled and avoid waiting in line. Nursing can help minimize the baby's discomfort when changes in cabin pressure during takeoff and landing affect their ears. If the baby is too stimulated or fussy, a bottle of expressed milk or a pacifier may help soothe the baby.

Nursing Beyond the First Year

Each society defines the term "older baby" differently when used in the context of nursing. You can help families who want to nurse for the recommended 2 years and beyond by providing evidence-based information and support. With loving patience from their parents, children outgrow their need to nurse and move on to more independence.

Human milk continues to provide significant calories, vitamins and minerals, and immunity to illness after the first year of life. The composition of the milk responds to changes in the baby's nursing pattern. Milk in the second year has a higher concentration of lactoferrin, serum albumin, and immunoglobulins, including secretory immunoglobulin A (IgA) (Verd et al., 2018). These properties help protect young children who put their hands into their mouths as they explore the world and build their immune system. Milk composition at 18 months postpartum shows increased fat and protein content, with decreased carbohydrates. Fats are the main calorie source in human milk for older nurslings, compared with carbohydrates in the first year (Czosnykowska-Łukacka et al., 2018).

Continued nursing provides toddlers with about 33% of their daily energy needs, 43% of their protein, 75% of their vitamin A, 60% of their vitamin C, 76% of their folate, 94% of their vitamin B_{12}, and nearly a third of their calcium requirements (Australian Breastfeeding Association [ABA], 2023; CDC, 2023b; WHO, 2023a). Extended nursing also plays a role in helping to prevent childhood obesity through early programing of healthy appetite regulation (Bruun et al., 2018; Gridneva et al., 2018; Shrivastava & Jain, 2023).

Nursing a Toddler

Families may not expect to continue nursing into the toddler years, and simply respond to their babies' needs as a natural part of parenting. Framing nursing a toddler as an extension of their bond with their child will help parents view this stage positively. Parents who continue nursing into toddlerhood often need reassurance that it is natural and normal to do so. Support from the parent's social circle is important, especially the emotional and practical support of other parents who have nursed toddlers. It is also important to have support from informed healthcare professionals who can answer their questions.

Nursing a toddler can fit comfortably into family routines, sometimes in creative ways (**Figure 18-10**). As a toddler becomes more alert and more easily distracted, nursing in a quiet place will limit distractions and interruptions. When adding other foods to the baby's diet, parents should nurse first and then offer the other food. The frequency and duration of nursing will continue to diminish as the child receives increased amounts of solid foods. Parents can continue to respond to the toddler's desire to nurse, reducing the number of feedings gradually and naturally while providing sufficient complementary foods. There are many online resources for parents who nurse older children. You can guide parents to reputable evidence-based sites by staying current regarding professional online resources.

Continuing to nurse into toddlerhood can be a source of great comfort and stability to a child who is stressed, injured, has hurt feelings, feels shy, or is in a new environment. Nursing provides a comforting way for an active child to connect with the parent between periods of exploration. It also offers a reassuring way for parents to communicate their love at times when they and their child may be at odds over the child's behavior. A child who communicates verbally can bring parents great joy by expressing their feelings about nursing. There can be love and humor in this relationship, with both parent and child being the giver and the receiver.

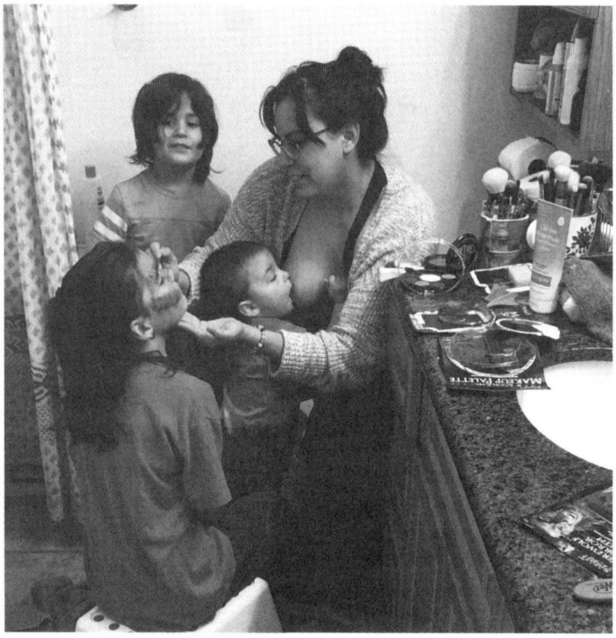

Figure 18-10 A toddler nursing.

Printed with permission of TR Andrew.

Challenges to Nursing a Toddler

Nursing a toddler can produce challenges that rival those of the newborn period. A toddler may not wish to be held and will assume a position that allows them to conveniently view the room, including standing or straddling. Developing teeth may leave pressure marks on the areola until the toddler learns to hold the breast with the lips. Crumbs or food particles in the child's mouth may irritate the nipples.

Although there is much debate about whether nursing beyond 12 months increases the risk of dental caries (Branger et al., 2019), recent research confirms that extended nursing is not a cause of cavities (Canadian Dental Association [CDA], 2023; Devenish et al., 2020). Practicing good dental hygiene when a baby begins teething and wiping their teeth with a clean, wet cloth after feeding helps reduce the risk of developing cavities regardless of the method of feeding (CDA, 2023).

Some parents find they are nursing beyond the point when they anticipated weaning would occur. They may consider weaning because they feel they have lost control of their bodies. The child may insist on nursing at inconvenient or embarrassing moments, tugging at clothing and exposing the breasts. The toddler may fondle the parent's body, which embarrasses them when others notice. Parents can prevent feeling trapped and resentful by providing boundaries to nursing, just as they provide guidance and age-appropriate boundaries for other aspects of the child's life, such as eating, sleeping, and playing.

Consistent boundaries help keep nursing positive for both the parent and child. If touching the other breast while nursing is unpleasant, the toddler can be told, "No." Perhaps nursing can take place only at certain times and places that coincide with the parent's needs so that nursing continues to be a source of pleasure. Parents can arrange signals with the child or adopt a special name for nursing to avoid embarrassment from the child asking to nurse while in public. Rather than arguing with the child at ill-timed requests to nurse, distraction and redirection may work. The toddler may, for example, be satisfied with a drink or a snack just before the usual time for nursing. Fun activities like playing a game or going for a walk may also help redirect the child from nursing.

Encourage parents to remain flexible and to adjust their approach if it causes undue stress for the child. The concept of waiting for an appropriate time is often difficult for a child to comprehend. Instead, nursing can be linked to a special location. For example, "Let's nurse when we get home in our special chair." Being consistent in restricting nursing to a particular place can be the key to making this phase in their relationship mutually satisfying for both parent and toddler. Peer support from local groups or reputable online communities can provide practical advice and help normalize extended nursing.

Opposition from Others

Sometimes, the nonnursing parent or another family member may consider it inappropriate to nurse an older child. They may believe the child is too dependent or may worry about the social stigma or sexual nature of nursing an older child. You can help parents explore these concerns. It may help to discuss the baby's physical and emotional needs at this stage of development and reasons to continue nursing. Seeing other children continue to nurse, as in a support group or play group, may help normalize nursing an older child. Parents who continue to nurse despite objections will benefit from your support, online resources, and other reading. **Chapter 21** presents suggestions for handling criticism about nursing toddlers.

Complementary Feeding

Nutritional decisions during pregnancy and lactation may influence a child's later nutritional choices through early flavor exposure and prime the child's palate to eat the foods commonly eaten in their home. Infant food preferences may begin prenatally as infants are exposed to different flavors in the amniotic fluid (Spahn, 2019). Preference continues to evolve after birth as nursing infants consume a variety of flavors in the milk. This early flavor exposure may influence food preferences for life. Nursing introduces the baby to the taste of a variety of foods through the parent's milk. Food preferences continue to develop when the baby is exposed to new foods.

The introduction of complementary foods expands a baby's diet and complements human milk during weaning. **Complementary feeding** refers to the addition of new foods to the growing nursing infant's diet that are intended to meet the energy and nutrient needs no longer met by human milk alone. The introduction of complementary foods begins to establish eating patterns that will last a lifetime.

Counseling Implications

You can be a valuable source of information for parents about introducing complementary foods to their baby. Parents often feel pressure from baby food manufacturers, social media, family, and friends to start solid foods before their baby is ready. They need encouragement and a high level of self-efficacy to nurse exclusively to 6 months despite pressure to start complementary foods before then. You can be an active force in helping parents delay complementary foods until their baby is developmentally ready. Provide them with clear, accurate, well-documented facts to eliminate possible confusion resulting from contradictory advice.

Sometimes, the baby's healthcare provider may suggest beginning complementary foods when it does not seem appropriate or before the parent wishes. You can help parents recall what the healthcare provider said, clarifying whether they said the baby *may* begin complementary foods if desired or whether they recommended them for a specific reason. Empower parents to talk openly with their healthcare providers. They can reinforce their nursing goals and discuss how their baby's health factors into their wish to nurse exclusively to 6 months of age.

Reinforce with parents that their milk is adequate to meet their child's needs through 6 months. Reassure them that their baby looks and acts healthy and is well nourished through exclusive nursing. Human milk serves as "nutritional insurance" as babies grow and begin other foods. Continuing to nurse allows parents to introduce complementary foods as a socialization measure, knowing that their milk continues to provide the bulk of the baby's nutritional needs through 1 year.

Choosing the Appropriate Time

Beginning complementary foods before 6 months or in response to early appetite spurts can seriously compromise milk production. Help parents understand that introducing complementary food into the baby's diet is the first step toward weaning. In general, the ideal time for complementary food falls between when the baby's system is mature enough to handle foods and when the child needs more nutrients than can be obtained solely from human milk. Babies of average birth weight with adequate fetal stores of fat and iron do well on human milk alone until about 6 months of age. Thus, an exclusive diet of human milk is ideal nutrition and sufficient to support optimal growth and development for the first 6 months after birth. Human milk provides all the calories, vitamins, and minerals in the proper proportions needed by the baby. Introducing other foods before the baby is physiologically mature enough for them can lead to frequent digestive upsets, increased upper respiratory infections, poor nutrient absorption, and excessive weight gain due to increased calorie consumption.

Sleeping Through the Night

The advice to start complementary foods before the baby is ready often occurs in relation to sleep issues. Parents are sometimes told that a baby needs cereal before going to bed to fill them up and help them sleep. Warm milk contains a **soporific** (sleep-inducing) agent that helps people fall asleep. Thus, human milk is the ideal food for encouraging a baby to sleep. Because human milk is digested more quickly than cow's milk, it is reasonable that a nursing baby would wake up hungry in the middle of the night. Sleeping through the night is related to developmental factors, not necessarily hunger.

Lowered Risk of Obesity

The introduction of complementary foods before the baby is four months of age and/or developmentally ready has been found to correlate with obesity later in childhood (Pluymen et al., 2018). Excessive weight gain in infancy can lead to lifelong obesity, underscoring the importance of extended exclusive nursing to 6 months. Nursing helps establish healthy early appetite self-regulation for babies (Shrivastava & Jain, 2023). Continuing to nurse after beginning complementary foods increases a parent's responsiveness to the child's hunger and satiety cues as the child transitions to table foods. They are less likely to feel pressured to feed the child more food than needed and they are reinforcing the child's natural satiety cues.

Signs of the Baby's Readiness

Babies display outward signs that they are ready for complementary foods when their internal functions have matured to the point where they can handle a diverse diet. Neuromuscular development at 6 months of age allows for chewing and swallowing of nonliquid foods. Intestinal maturation promotes digestion and absorption of a variety of foods. This enables a baby's body to handle the waste products from solid foods. The immune system has also matured to the point that the infant no longer depends solely on the protection provided by human milk.

Other signs of a baby's readiness for additional foods include the ability to sit up with support, the disappearance of the tongue extrusion reflex, improved eye–hand coordination, and the ability to grasp objects with the thumb and forefinger. The most obvious sign of readiness is the baby's behavior when others are eating. The baby may watch family members intently, imitate their chewing, and reach for food while loudly vocalizing a desire for it. An intensified demand to nurse that is not satisfied after several days of increased nursing may be an additional clue that it is time to begin complementary foods.

Introducing Complementary Foods

Beginning complementary foods should be a pleasurable experience for both parents and baby. A gradual and pressure-free approach will prevent the baby from feeling overwhelmed by this new experience. The infant's digestive system will also have a chance to adjust to each new change in diet. Ideally, culturally appropriate complementary feeding will begin at a relaxed pace with no pressure on the parent or baby. A complementary food can be given every 1 or 2 days when the baby is still hungry after nursing. Giving complementary foods after, rather than before, nursing will help maintain milk production.

Often, the afternoon and early evening hours are times when the baby may accept additional foods more readily. This period usually coincides with the time when parents are most tired and busy with other tasks. The other parent or family member can feed the child and give the nursing parent a break from baby care. Working parents can nurse exclusively when they are with the baby and the caregiver can feed the complementary foods in the parents' absence.

The WHO (2023b) universal guidelines for the introduction of solid foods are that the foods are timely, adequate, safe, and properly fed. *Timely* means introducing the foods when the need for energy and nutrients exceeds what can be provided through human milk. The foods need to provide *adequate* energy, protein, and micronutrients to meet the baby's nutritional needs for healthy development. The foods need to be stored and prepared in a *safe* manner, being hygienically stored and prepared, and fed with clean utensils (not bottles and teats) by a caregiver with, clean hands. *Properly fed* means the food is offered in response to the baby's hunger and satiety cues (WHO, 2023b).

Age of the Baby

Babies are ready for complementary foods at different ages. Despite global recommendations, not all babies can wait until 6 months of age to start complementary foods. Babies who begin nursing constantly at 4 or 5 months and never seem to be satisfied may be biologically ready for additional nourishment. Parents can be alert for their baby's signs of developmental readiness and discuss starting healthy, culturally appropriate complementary foods with the healthcare provider.

By age 7 to 9 months, one or two complementary feedings a day with regular nursing will satisfy the baby's nutritional needs. By 9 to 12 months, the child becomes an active participant in family meals, with three meals a day. They will still require nutritious snacks several times a day, in addition to several nursing sessions. Nursing should be allowed to naturally decrease slowly until solid foods become the primary source of nutrition. Human milk continues to meet three-fourths of a baby's nutrient needs during the second 6 months of life. Even during the baby's second year, human milk continues to be nutritionally valuable and provides a significant source of energy.

Texture of Food

Food texture needs to be compatible with the baby's ability to chew and swallow. Initial foods should be extremely small (to avoid choking) and possibly diluted with liquid (e.g., expressed milk). New textures can be added as the baby becomes accustomed to eating solid foods. Eating will slowly transition to chunky foods, finger foods, and finally, table foods. **Table 18-2** presents developmental skills and recommended sequences for solid foods. The average baby will begin eating small, chunky finger foods at about 9 months. By 1 year of age, they will be eating regular table food, cut into age-appropriate sizes, along with the rest of the family.

Some families follow the principles of "baby-led" weaning for introducing complementary foods. They bypass offering pureed food and spoon feeding by offering soft finger foods and allowing the baby to self-feed (Fangupo et al., 2016; Rapley & Murkett, 2009; Solid Starts, 2023). The food is soft, large enough to hold, and easy to squish to decrease the risk of choking. As with all methods of offering solid foods, the baby should always be supervised while eating (Rapley & Murkett, 2009).

Type of Food

The type of food the child receives depends on their age and food preferences, the family's cultural practices, and recommendations from the healthcare provider (Canadian Pediatric Society [CPS], 2023). Global recommendations on how to start complementary foods have changed in the past decade in response to current research and evidence around nutritional needs for young children and best practices related to food allergies. Current research supports starting foods that are common allergens (e.g., peanut products and eggs) by 6 months of age asserting that the early introduction of these foods into a baby's diet lowers the risk of developing food allergies (Australasian Society of Clinical Immunology and Allergy [ASCIA, 2023]; Food Allergy Canada [FAC], 2023).

Starting with a single-ingredient food and adding a new food every 3–5 days provides an opportunity to identify potential **food intolerance** or allergies (American Academy of Pediatrics [AAP], 2022; ASCIA, 2023). If the baby were to consume several foods together, it would be difficult to identify which one causes a reaction. When a single food is offered and food sensitivity occurs, the food can be discontinued and reintroduced later. Some babies may tolerate small amounts of a food, whereas larger amounts will cause reactions. Allergy considerations are discussed in more detail later in this chapter.

As long as the consistency of the food is appropriate to the child's developmental stage and not a choking hazard, almost any healthy food the family enjoys can be offered from 6 months onward (AAP, 2022; ASCIA, 2023; CPS, 2023; FAC, 2023). There are a few exceptions. Honey should not be given until the child is at least 1 year of age because of the risk of botulism spores. Hot dogs, whole nuts, and whole grapes pose a choking hazard. Babies under 12 months of age should not be given juice because of risk of dental decay (AAP, 2022). After 12 months, 100% fruit juice can be given in a cup, limited to no more than 4 oz per day (AAP, 2022).

The first recommended foods are iron-rich meats or meat alternatives and/or iron-fortified infant cereals (CPS, 2023; Dieticians of Canada, 2023; Meeks & Noble, 2022). If giving processed baby foods, careful reading of labels can avoid added sugars or salt. By 12 months of age, the baby needs a variety of foods, including human milk, meats, vegetables, tofu, eggs, fish, legumes, fruits, and grains (AAP, 2022; ASCIA, 2023; CPS, 2023).

In the second year of life, a child will be eating the same foods as the rest of the family, simply with smaller portions and being aware of choking hazards. Avoiding excessive salt, cutting food into appropriate-sized pieces, and serving food at a moderate temperature will help transition the toddler to family

Table 18-2 Sample Food Ideas: 6 Months to 24 Months

Age	Suggested Foods	Eating Methods	Developmental Stages
6 months	Iron-rich foods, including meat, legumes, iron-fortified cereals, scrambled eggs, tofu, any fruit or vegetable, shredded cheese, full-fat yogurt, 2% milk, and cottage and ricotta cheese Human milk and/or iron-fortified infant formula	■ Soft, lumpy, tender cooked foods ■ Purees or mashed soft foods ■ Iron-fortified cereals in a bowl (not a bottle) ■ Fingertip, spoon, or self-feeding ■ Human milk via nursing ■ Formula via feeding device	■ Tongue-thrust and gag reflexes lessen ■ Interested in foods the family is eating ■ Willingly accepts foods ■ Can sit up unassisted ■ Teething may begin
7 to 9 months	New foods, including whole-grain rice, pasta, toast, small pieces of cheese, and nut butters on bite-sized toast Mixed-grain cereals Human milk and/or formula	■ Soft, lumpy, tender cooked foods ■ Purees or mashed soft food ■ Finger foods ■ May be able to drink liquids from a cup ■ Human milk via nursing ■ Formula via feeding device	■ Begins to drink from an open cup (spilling is normal) ■ Can pick up small pieces of food ■ Puts everything in mouth (be alert for choking hazards) ■ Reaches for food and utensils, then drops or flings them ■ Munches food
9 to 12 months	Finger foods, including whole-grain bagels, rice cakes, and pasta, and continue with all nutritious foods eaten by the family Human milk and/or formula Can slowly introduce cow's milk at 12 months once a wide variety of food is being eaten	■ Family foods that are grated, finely chopped, or in small pieces or strips ■ Finger foods ■ Melt-in-mouth foods ■ Water and other liquids in a cup ■ Continued nursing ■ Formula or cow's milk via feeding device	■ More adept at self-feeding ■ More adept at holding bottle and cup ■ Enjoys playing with food ■ More active in highchair ■ May try using utensils
12 to 18 months	All nutritious family foods	■ Eats with the family at mealtimes ■ Weans from a bottle if one is used ■ Family foods in small pieces or strips ■ Begins eating on own with utensils ■ Liquids by cup ■ Continued nursing if desired	■ Longer attention span ■ Increased desire to "do it myself" ■ Better control with cup, spilling less ■ Better utensil control ■ Active and unable to sit still for long ■ Enjoys trying other people's food
18 to 24 months	Toddler food in small portion sizes to make food fun and relaxed: avocado boats, fun-shaped sandwiches, cooked carrot wheels, cheese blocks, broccoli trees, O-shaped cereal, toast sticks, cookie-cutter cheese melts, and sailboat salads	■ Eats small amounts often, sometimes called *grazing* ■ May be a "picky eater" ■ Drinks water from a cup ■ Uses utensils ■ Continues nursing if desired	■ Begins chewing food well when molars erupt ■ Uses utensils without much spilling ■ Uses words for food and eating, can sign for "more," "all done," and "please" if taught signing ■ Eats on the run and needs creative feeding to hold attention ■ Erratic eating habits

Data from Unlock Foods- Dieticians of Canada (DC), 2023 https://www.unlockfood.ca/en/articles/breastfeeding-infant-feeding/introducing-solid-food-to-your-baby.aspx and Ottawa Public Health (2018) Feeding your baby: What you need to know about starting solids https://www.parentinginottawa.ca/en/babies-and-toddlers/resources/documents/Feeding-Baby-Brochure-Starting-Solids-2018-01-EN.pdf meals. If the baby rejects a particular food, it can be withheld for several weeks before offering it again. The experience of trying new foods should be pleasant for the baby. Parents should not force them to eat a food they do not want and should avoid starting new foods when the child is ill or has recently had an immunization.

Amount of Food

Parents often wonder how much food they should feed their babies. To avoid waste, they can begin with a teaspoon or so of creamy-consistency food and then work up to a few tablespoons at a rate led by the baby's appetite. Too often, babies are overfed because parents expect them to consume an entire jar of commercially prepared baby food in one sitting. Parents need to allow their babies to exercise control over their intake and follow their cues to recognize when their baby has had enough.

At first, parents can expect to see more food running down the sides of the baby's mouth than being swallowed. Messiness is a normal, and sometimes amusing, part of this new experience with food. There will be less mess as the newly developed swallowing mechanism matures. The mess will return when the baby starts self-feeding. Some babies are not interested in solid foods until they can handle the food themselves and control their intake. A young baby's mechanism for determining hunger is by food volume. Caution parents not to overfeed an eager baby. Overfeeding can manifest itself as constipation, spitting up, excessive weight gain, or a rapid decrease in nursing frequency.

Vitamin and Mineral Supplements

The average healthy, full-term nursing baby generally does not need vitamin and mineral supplements. For the most part, healthy food selection by the parent or when complementary foods begin can provide the nutrients that human milk lacks.

Vitamin D

Nursing infants need an additional 400 IU per day of vitamin D from birth to 12 months of age (CPS, 2023). An alternative to infant supplementation is for the nursing parent to consume 4000 IU of vitamin D_2 daily. This will potentially transfer 400 IU to the exclusively human milk–fed infant. The amount transferred is based on the baseline vitamin D status of the lactating parent and the infant's milk intake (Jullien, 2021). For nursing babies in far northern regions, who have darker skin, whose skin is covered by clothing or sunscreen most of the time, or who live in communities where vitamin D deficiency is common, 800 IU per day of vitamin D is recommended (CPS, 2023).

Vitamin A

Approximately 190 million preschool-age children worldwide are vitamin A deficient, with the largest numbers in South East Asia and Africa (WHO, 2023a). Foods rich in vitamin A (including leafy greens, eggs, and orange and yellow vegetables) should begin at about 6 months of age and continue throughout childhood.

Vitamin B12

Vitamin B_{12} supports brain development and the production of blood cells. Vitamin B_{12} deficiency in infants can lead to brain damage (CDC, 2023b). Parents with adequate B_{12} levels typically do not need to supplement their nursing infant. If they are vitamin B_{12} deficient, they should supplement their infants, and once they start solids, offer vitamin B_{12}–rich foods (CDC, 2023b). Foods rich in vitamin B_{12} are primarily derived from animals and include poultry, fish, eggs, dairy products, clams, and beef liver. Nursing parents who consume a vegetarian or vegan diet are at increased risk of vitamin B_{12} deficiency and should consult their healthcare provider about vitamin B_{12} supplements for their nursing infant.

Iron

In healthy full-term infants, human milk typically supplies sufficient iron until the second half of the first year. Preterm infants and infants of anemic parents will need iron supplementation when a **hematocrit** (hemoglobin blood test) determines that iron stores are low. When complementary foods are introduced, adding iron-rich food to the infant's diet is important (CDC, 2023b). Iron-rich foods include seeds, legumes, red meats (including wild game), egg yolks, fish and shellfish, dark-green vegetables, and whole grains (Health Canada [HC], 2023).

Vegetarian Diet

Most families who follow a vegetarian diet are well educated about their dietary choices and know how to prevent nutritional deficiencies. A well-planned vegetarian diet can be safe during pregnancy, lactation, infancy, childhood, and adolescence. Extremely restrictive vegetarian diets, such as fruitarian and raw food diets, are not appropriate for infants. Children who consume vegan diets may require micronutrient and macronutrient supplements to support healthy growth and development (Fewtrell et al., 2017).

Research-based dietary tools for vegetarian meal planning for all age groups are available online (Academy of Nutrition and Dietetics, 2019). Infant growth is normal when adequate human milk is provided and the maternal diet contains good sources of energy, iron, vitamin B_{12}, and vitamin D. Guidelines for the introduction of solid foods are the same as for other infants. Protein-rich foods include tofu, legumes, soy or dairy yogurt, cooked egg yolks, and cottage cheese. Foods rich in energy and nutrients include legumes, tofu, and avocado.

The primary concern with vegetarian diets is obtaining enough vitamin B_{12}. Severe vitamin B_{12} deficiency produces neurological symptoms in infants, including irritability, faltering growth, apathy, anorexia, and developmental regression (Wolffenbuttel et al., 2019). Vitamin B_{12} deficiency can also result in skin pigmentation changes, atrophic glossitis, brittle or matted hair, skin lesions, and diaper dermatitis. Anemia is also a risk (Falcone et al., 2018; Kaur & Goraya, 2018). Because vitamin B_{12} is one of the vitamins in human milk whose quantity depends on the parent's diet, it is imperative that parents eating a vegetarian diet take vitamin B_{12} supplements while nursing.

Allergy Considerations

When babies nurse exclusively, components in the milk coat the intestinal tract to prevent foreign proteins from entering the baby's system and causing allergic reactions. Eventually, the baby's body develops the ability to protect itself. Children of parents with a history of allergies appear to have a more prolonged dependence on the protective factors in human milk. These children may have an increased susceptibility to ingested food proteins. The hereditary risk of food allergy seems to be lower when a baby nurses exclusively for several months. For more detailed information on allergies consult **Chapters 9** and **10**.

Signs of Food Intolerance

The degree of infant responses to foreign proteins varies widely. Some babies exhibit sudden and clear-cut allergic reactions, whereas others appear only slightly fussy or irritable. The signs of food reactions that may help parents to recognize intolerance in their baby are presented in **Figure 18-11**. Food reactions may be mistaken for signs of illness or drug reactions, and vice versa. If symptoms persist, parents should contact their healthcare provider to rule out illness in the baby.

- Runny nose, stuffiness, and constant cold-type symptoms
- Skin rashes, eczema, hives, especially around the mouth and diaper area
- Wheezing or asthma
- Ear infections
- Intestinal cramping, pain, or gassiness
- Diarrhea
- Spitting up
- Vomiting
- Fussiness, irritability, and excessive crying
- Poor weight gain due to malabsorption of food
- Red itchy eyes, swollen eyelids, dark circles under the eyes, constant tearing, and gelatin-like fluid in the eyes

Figure 18-11 Signs of food intolerance in the infant.

Family History of Allergies

Parents with a family history of allergies should notify their healthcare provider when they suspect an allergic response in their baby to something they consumed. If a particular food results in repeated symptoms after the baby nurses, that food may be the cause. The parent may need to remove a food from their diet to eliminate a reaction entirely. By experimenting with known allergens, the offending foods can be identified and eliminated. The healthcare provider can help parents identify the **allergen** and create a plan to eliminate the offending food from the diet.

When a food is eliminated from the parent's diet, another food or supplement can be added to obtain the necessary nutrients to support lactation. For example, cow's milk, which is high in protein and calcium, can be replaced with foods high in those nutrients. Parents should discuss food substitutes with their healthcare provider or a nutritionist to ensure a balanced, nutritious diet. Foods do not need to be eliminated unless they are suspected as the cause of an issue with the nursing baby. When there is a family history of severe allergies, parents need to introduce one food at a time and wait at least a full week for a possible reaction before introducing the next new food.

Weaning

Cultural practices often set the standards for weaning without regard for the baby's biological and emotional needs. Within social groups where early weaning is common, parents may feel pressured by a lack of acceptance and misinformation about nursing an older baby. Pressure to wean intensifies as families continue to nurse beyond their culture's accepted normal period. Parents who practice extended nursing describe facing negative attitudes and criticism from others. Given accurate information on nursing and normal infant growth, development, and behavior, parents can make informed decisions about when to wean their baby. This will allow them to be confident that they are basing their decision on the baby's physical and emotional needs. Parents will then be less likely to allow misconceptions or pressure from others to cause them to initiate weaning before they or their baby is ready.

Biological Self-Weaning

The biologically normal method for weaning is for the baby to slowly drop nursing sessions as table foods become a regular part of their diet. When parents are content and relaxed with nursing and are not pressured to wean prematurely, their baby will naturally drop feedings gradually, based on hunger. Normal biological self-weaning responds to the baby's developmental needs. It nurtures eventual independence, with the baby determining readiness to move to the next stage of development.

Biological weaning commonly occurs between 2 and 4 years of age. Parents can trust their baby to naturally lead the weaning process by following their hunger cues and neither denying nor initiating nursing. As babies mature, they may become more self-reliant and go for long stretches without nursing, perhaps accepting a drink or snack as a substitute. The baby may be easily distracted while nursing, spend less time at feedings, frequently reject nursing, and show a greater interest in solid foods. These are signs that the baby may be physically and psychologically ready to wean.

Parents who are unprepared when self-weaning occurs may respond by trying to entice the child to nurse more frequently. You can help parents learn to appreciate the child's maturity by stressing new achievements and showing them new ways to interact and maintain closeness with their baby. If parents overlook their baby's signs of readiness to wean they may initiate feedings that could have been eliminated, such as keeping the child quiet while engaged in other activities. Parents who wish to change these patterns can read stories, offer a snack, or provide toys and activities to occupy the child. Rocking, cuddling, singing, and holding can effectively replace the coziness and comfort of nursing.

Parent-Led Weaning

Weaning is a transitional period during which it is important to ensure the baby's needs are met. **Parent-led weaning**, also called **mother-led weaning**, describes a parent's effort to end nursing before the baby shows signs of readiness. You can help parents explore their goals and how to continue to meet their baby's needs. When parents raise the topic of weaning, help them explore the reasons why they are considering it. They may have outside pressure or misconceptions about nursing an older baby. They may believe they must wean when they return to work. They may sense that the baby is no longer satisfied with nursing. Some parents simply become impatient for their baby to wean. If feelings of resentment emerge, it may be time to wean.

Parent-led weaning of an older child who is not ready to give up nursing may be challenging, at times even including bargaining with the child to establish acceptable substitute activities. Parents who initiate weaning may approach it with hesitation because of the promotion of extended nursing. Be sensitive to their cues and let them know that you will help them whether they decide to wean or to continue nursing. A nonjudgmental approach will encourage parents to express concerns freely and ask questions that will allow them to understand weaning and do what is best for their family.

Gradual Weaning

The family and baby both adjust better when weaning is gradual and tailored to the baby's needs. Parents can eliminate the least preferred feeding first, allowing at least 2 days for the baby and milk production to adjust to the dropped feeding. A drink, snack, cuddling, or favorite activity can substitute for the dropped feeding. When dropping an early-morning feeding, for example, the baby can have breakfast after awakening. When dropping a late-night feeding, alternative ways of helping the child fall asleep can be explored. Perhaps the partner or other family member can put the child to bed with stories or rocking. As the dyad adjusts to each new substitution, another feeding can be dropped, continuing in this manner for several weeks or months. The child may wish to continue a preferred feeding and may decrease feeding frequency to once every few days until nursing ends.

If weaning proceeds too quickly, the baby may demand more attention; want to nurse more frequently; or exhibit physical changes such as allergic reactions, stomach upsets, or constipation. Weaning too quickly may also cause the breasts to become uncomfortably full. Expressing milk to comfort will help. It will be important to watch for any symptoms of mastitis and to wear a supportive bra that is not binding. Anti-inflammatory pain relievers, ice packs, or cabbage leaves may provide relief. A patient and gradual approach to weaning over several months helps to minimize physical and emotional discomfort for both the child and the parent.

Miscues That Can Lead to Early Weaning

Weaning sometimes results from misconceptions, outside pressure, or a change in personal circumstances. When this happens, parents may feel anger, resentment, or guilt because of being unable to continue nursing. Common misconceptions and miscues that lead to untimely weaning include crying, teething, biting, illness, nighttime feedings, changes in the family, and social pressure.

Crying. A family with a baby who cries a lot may doubt that nursing is satisfying the child's hunger. Stress from the worry may cause parents to consider weaning. You can help them explore the reason for the baby's crying, which may be allergies, pain, distress, sensory integration issues, or hunger. Teach them comfort measures, and if needed, explore ways to increase milk production. Make sure they know how to respond to hunger cues and monitor their baby's output to confirm that their baby is getting enough milk. Helping them feel good about their parenting will increase their confidence in nursing.

Teething, Biting, or Illness. When teething, biting, or illness occurs, parents may become frustrated with trying to simultaneously manage nursing and comforting their baby. The idea of someone else feeding the baby may seem like a good solution to a tired parent. You can help parents understand that these occurrences are temporary and that nursing provides comfort to an uncomfortable baby and immune support for an ill baby. Switching to formula will likely not improve the situation for either the parent or baby. Furthermore, weaning can create additional issues with engorgement and the inconvenience of trying to decrease milk production. In times of stress, nursing provides the closeness and reassurance the baby needs.

Nighttime Feedings. Continued nighttime feedings may create so much fatigue from lack of sleep that it is difficult for parents to function well during the day. If the baby is older, weaning may seem to be the answer. Sometimes, the simplest solution is to drop night feedings. Help parents explore the possible reasons for their baby's wakefulness. It may be from separation anxiety, habit, insufficient daytime feedings to satisfy hunger, or a need for attention. Napping during the day, safely cosleeping with the baby at night, or having other family members help put the wakeful baby back to sleep may help them get more rest.

Changes in the Family. Family life can become complicated with events like moving, job changes, illness, divorce, emotional upsets, and other stressful situations. Although it might appear that weaning would make life simpler, the baby's needs for security and continuity are even greater when significant changes occur. Ending nursing at this time could lead to fussiness, illness, or increased demands for attention. You can guide families to develop ways to integrate nursing into their lifestyle so that stress is reduced.

A parent may consider weaning because they want to start or resume taking oral contraceptives. You can provide them with information about methods of contraception that are compatible with lactation and encourage them to discuss these options with their healthcare provider. Chapter 20 discusses contraceptives.

A nursing baby sometimes becomes a point of contention between parents who are involved in a divorce or separation. Some parents feel pressured to wean to allow extended visitation between the nonnursing parent and the child. Perhaps they can arrange visitation in a way that accommodates nursing. Information on nursing in the context of family law and the best interest of the child is available on various legal and nursing support websites. Get to know the culturally appropriate resources available to support parents in your region.

Social Pressure. Well-meaning family members or friends can often be a source of pressure to wean before the parent or the child is ready. Sometimes the nonnursing parent feels left out because of the closeness of the nursing relationship. They may miss evenings out with their partner or simply would like more of their attention. Encourage parents to plan time together as a couple and to share feedings using expressed milk when the nursing parent is away from home. If a parent decides to wean to maintain harmony in the home, your role is to support that decision.

If family or friends criticize the decision to nurse an older baby, help parents develop strategies to deal with the criticism. For example, they might refrain from nursing in front of those who disapprove or keep a toy or snack ready as a distraction to postpone feedings. They can share with them the nutritional advantages that human milk has for a toddler and that the immunological benefits continue for as long as the child nurses. Furthermore, the emotional security of nursing can be a stabilizing factor in a child's life and a valuable tool to calm an upset toddler. Linking parents with other families who are nursing older babies can help them build confidence and provide a supportive social network. Public awareness of extended nursing has grown exponentially. Social media provides support groups and forums for families who nurse older babies.

Untimely Weaning

It is sometimes necessary to wean abruptly, with no time for preparation or forethought. In these cases, weaning can begin with dropping every other feeding on the first day and replacing the dropped feeding with limited milk expression to relieve discomfort but not stimulate further production. The remainder of the feedings can be eliminated in this manner, ensuring that the baby receives extra nurturing and attention.

Emergency Weaning. If weaning must occur immediately, there may be 24 to 48 hours of painful engorgement. The extent of engorgement will depend on the level of milk production and how often the baby had been nursing. Engorgement will subside gradually. Wrapping the breasts in cabbage leaves may reduce swelling. **Chapter 17** presents guidelines for applying cabbage to engorged breasts. An anti-inflammatory medication can relieve pain and help reduce swelling. The parent's healthcare provider may prescribe medication to lower milk production, avoiding antihistamines with pseudoephedrine, drugs in the ergot family, and oral contraceptives with estrogen.

Placing ice wrapped in a towel on the breasts may help reduce the swelling and pain associated with engorgement. Heat should be avoided because it increases blood flow and swelling. Breast issues along the mastitis spectrum may occur with emergency weaning. **Chapter 17** provides more information on the mastitis spectrum.

Your attention and availability will be critical during this stressful period. Outdated medical literature and older relatives may recommend breast binding, that is, wrapping a stretchable elastic bandage tightly around the breasts. This practice can lead to mastitis-related complications and intensify the pain or illness. Parents should never bind their breasts.

Unintentional Weaning. Sometimes, parents inadvertently wean despite wanting to continue nursing. Perhaps they started giving occasional bottles of formula, which led to diminished milk production. For some families, the hectic pace of holidays or travel can cause missed feedings and lead to a menstrual cycle, reduced milk production, increased infant fussiness, and supplementation. When the regular routine resumes, the baby has begun weaning much sooner than the parent had planned.

These parents may feel that nursing has slipped away to the extent that they are unable or unwilling to turn back. They will especially need your acceptance and support to help them through their disappointment. If they ask about relactating, you can discuss the issues related to relactation, as covered in **Chapter 25**. Weaning before the parent or baby is ready can shake a parent's confidence in their parenting abilities. Encourage them to continue giving their baby the same nurturing and attention they provided when nursing.

Unavoidable Weaning. Circumstances outside the family's control can lead to weaning. Parents may have a serious illness or require medication that would pass through the milk and harm the baby (although most medications are compatible with nursing). Perhaps they must return to work or school and find it difficult to continue to nurse. The baby may suddenly reject nursing. The parent may become pregnant, and a history of miscarriage or preterm birth leads their healthcare provider to advise against continuing nursing. Furthermore, nipple pain during pregnancy, coupled with a decrease in milk production, may suppress any desire to continue nursing.

After forced weaning, parents may feel guilty or question their parenting ability. Validating their feelings will help them work through this personal loss. You can discuss the differences between guilt and regret, as covered in **Chapter 3**. Be present, be mindful, and hold space while parents, and possibly other family members, process the feelings associated with an unavoidable weaning. As appropriate, you may stress the benefits the baby received from nursing. Encourage the parents to focus on other parenting behaviors that provide the closeness that nursing did.

Minimal Nursing

Some families practice **minimal nursing** as a compromise to total weaning. Minimal nursing describes a pattern of nursing one to three times per day, with complementary foods providing the baby's remaining nourishment. This practice may be an option when the parents and baby are separated for regular periods, such as during a return to work or school. Nursing one to three times per day can help continue the special relationship between the baby and the parent. It maintains a useful tool to comfort the child when they are upset, in pain, or ill. Minimal nursing for an extended period can provide a comfortable transition to eventual weaning.

After Weaning

Parents commonly feel some regret or sadness when nursing ends, even if they wanted to wean. They will benefit from support and understanding from those close to them as they work through those feelings. You can help parents recognize that new skills for comforting their child will replace nursing, without minimizing or discounting their sadness at the end of nursing. Help them recognize weaning as another step in their child's development and encourage them to look forward to new stages. You can praise the family for having met their child's need for both nutrition and nurturing.

Physical Changes with Weaning

Anticipatory guidance will prepare parents for physical adjustments after weaning. To avoid gaining weight, diet modification can eliminate the extra calories that were needed during lactation. There may be a sudden weight loss of a few pounds resulting from a loss of fluid and fat from the body's fat stores. If menstruation had not resumed before weaning, menstrual cycles may be somewhat irregular for a few months, with intermittent bleeding, light flow, or spotting. The hormonal changes related to weaning can cause nausea or fatigue in some parents, as well as emotional changes, including mood swings, anxiety, weepiness, and even depressive moods.

The breasts may become soft, flat, or droopy for a few months after weaning. Breasts usually return to their prepregnancy size gradually. Sometimes they remain larger than they were before pregnancy. Some breasts never fully regain the fatty layer that was present before conception. The Montgomery glands recede, and the areola may remain darker than before pregnancy. Stretch marks may become apparent on the breasts.

Continued Milk Secretion

The total cessation of milk secretion varies greatly and may occur over several weeks or as long as 1 year after weaning. Continued secretion longer than 6 months after weaning may be from holding the baby against the chest, wearing clothing that rubs against the nipples, or sexual activity that involves the breasts. Parents who work with infants report continuing to be able to express drops of milk years after weaning their own children. Perhaps it is the effect of working in an oxytocin-rich environment!

After milk secretion has stopped completely, any nipple discharge should be reported to the healthcare provider to determine the cause. Sometimes, old milk works its way out; other times, fluid may result from an infection or growth. Review the discussion in **Chapter 17** if it seems appropriate to investigate whether there is an underlying medical reason for the continued milk secretion.

Summary

Anticipatory guidance helps parents recognize what to expect as their babies develop throughout infancy and toddlerhood. Over time, the baby's world expands as they develop both physically and socially. Babies develop cues that elicit responses from the parents. They may cry, coo, smile, or frown, depending on their needs. They become increasingly aware of others and of their environment. Motor skills develop further as the infant begins to crawl and then walk. Teething, shorter feedings, separation anxiety, experimenting with vocabulary sounds, and self-feeding evolve gradually. Parents find creative ways to nurse their toddler and eventually manage weaning. This expansive time can be both exhilarating and challenging for parents. Your advice and support can help them transition to their new role and to meet their baby's changing needs.

What You Learned—At a Glance

Conversation Starters with Parents

- How are your baby's weight and sleep patterns?
- What changes have you noticed with the frequency and length of feedings?
- How comfortable are you nursing in front of others?
- What other foods is your baby receiving?
- How will you know when it is time to stop nursing?

Reflexes

- Innate reflexes of rooting, sucking, grasping, swallowing, and gagging enable babies to obtain food.
- The Moro reflex causes the baby to startle in response to sudden noise.
- The palmar grasp enables babies to grasp objects such as their parents' fingers.
- The tonic neck reflex prevents babies from rolling over.
- The Bauer crawling reflex elicits movements similar to crawling or kicking.

Infant Growth and Development

- Nursing babies typically double their birth weight by 5 to 6 months of age.
- Head and body control, hand movement, sitting, crawling, walking, and socialization all progress at different stages during the first year of life.
- Babies sleep for longer periods as the central nervous system develops, with one longer rest period and several naps daily at about 3 months.

Nursing Behavior

- Increases in appetite occur at about 2 weeks, 6 weeks, 3 months, and 6 months of age.
- By 1 month, expect 8 to 14 feedings per day.
- By 2 to 3 months, babies spend less time at feedings.
- By 4 to 6 months, feeding frequency decreases; some babies fuss or appear to lose interest.
- By 6 months, frequency continues to diminish, and complementary foods begin.
- By 7 to 9 months, babies actively seek to nurse and may be distracted during feedings.
- By 10 to 12 months, separation anxiety may increase frequency and duration.

Nursing an Older Baby

- Babies typically double birth weight by 6 months and triple birth weight by 1 year.
- Human milk provides significant calories, vitamins and minerals, and immunity to illness throughout the second year and beyond.
- Nursing in public and traveling with a nursing baby create new challenges.
- Teething occurs between 4 and 14 months and may cause pain while nursing.
- Nursing frequency diminishes as the baby consumes more complementary foods.
- Children typically outgrow their need to nurse by 2 to 4 years of age.

Complementary Feeding

- Complementary foods should begin when the baby is developmentally ready, usually around 6 months of age.
- Human milk meets three-fourths of the baby's nutrient needs from 6 to 12 months.
- Neuromuscular development at 6 months enables chewing and swallowing of foods.
- Ability to sit up, disappearance of tongue extrusion reflex, improved eye–hand coordination, and ability to grasp objects with the thumb and forefinger indicate readiness for complementary foods.
- It is normal for babies to watch adults eat, imitate chewing, and reach for food.
- Parents should begin with small amounts of one new food weekly. This should be very soft, small, nutrient dense, and relatively high in protein, and it can be softened with fluid.

Weaning

- Biological weaning responds to the baby's developmental needs.
- Parent-led weaning should eliminate the least preferred feeding first and allow at least 2 days before dropping another feeding.
- Crying and teething may be miscues that a baby is ready to wean.
- Minimal nursing with increased complementary foods is a low-pressure alternative to weaning.

References

Academy of Nutrition and Dietetics, Vegetarian Nutrition Dietetic Practice Group. Vegetarian nutrition. 2019. https://vegetariannutrition.net/

American Academy of Pediatrics. Starting solid foods. 2022. https://www.healthychildren.org/English/ages-stages/baby/feeding-nutrition/Pages/Starting-Solid-Foods.aspx

Australasian Society of Clinical Immunology and Allergy. How to introduce solids foods: FAQ. 2023. https://www.allergy.org.au/images/pcc/ASCIA_PCC_How_to _introduce_Solid_Foods_FAQ_202.pdf

Australian Breastfeeding Association. Breastfeeding your toddler. November 9, 2023. https://www.breastfeeding.asn.au/resources/breastfeeding-toddler

Barisic I, et al. Beckwith Wiedemann syndrome: a population-based study on prevalence, prenatal diagnosis, associated anomalies and survival in Europe. *Eur J Med Genet.* 2018;61(9):499–507.

Branger B, et al. Breastfeeding and early childhood caries. Review of the literature, recommendations, and prevention. *Arch Pediatr*. 2019;26(8):497–503.

Bruun S, et al. Satiety factors oleoylethanolamide, stearoylethanolamide, and palmitoylethanolamide in mother's milk are strongly associated with infant weight at four months of age—data from the Odense Child Cohort. *Nutrients*. 2018;10(11).

Canadian Dental Association. 2023 CDA position on infant feeding and healthy dental development. 2023. https://www.cda-adc.ca/en/about/position_statements/breastfeeding/

Canadian Pediatric Society. Caring for kids: vitamin D. November 12, 2023. https://caringforkids.cps.ca/handouts/pregnancy-and-babies/vitamin_d

Centers for Disease Control and Prevention. Breastfeeding report card United States, 2018. August 20, 2018. https://www.cdc.gov/breastfeeding/data/reportcard.htm

Centers for Disease Control and Prevention. Growth chart training: using the WHO growth charts. February 3, 2022. https://www.cdc.gov/nccdphp/dnpao/growthcharts/who/breastfeeding/index.htm#:~:text=Healthy%20breastfed%20infants%20typically%20put,the%20first%20year%20of%20life.&text=Formula%2Dfed%20infants%20typically%20gain,after%20complimentary%20foods%20are%20introduced

Centers for Disease Control and Prevention. CDC's milestone tracker app. November 10, 2023a. https://www.cdc.gov/ncbddd /actearly/milestones-app.html

Centers for Disease Control and Prevention. Vitamin B_{12} and breastfeeding. Accessed November 12, 2023b. https://www.cdc.gov/breastfeeding/breastfeeding-special-circumstances/diet-and-micronutrients/vitamin-b12.html

Czosnykowska-Łukacka M, et al. Breast milk macronutrient components in prolonged lactation. *Nutrients*. 2018;10(12).

Devenish G, et al. Early childhood feeding practices and dental caries among Australian preschoolers. *Am J Clin Nutr*. 2020;111(4):821–828.

Dieticians of Canada. Introducing solid food to your baby. 2023. https://www.unlockfood.ca/en/articles/breastfeeding-infant-feeding/introducing-solid-food-to-your-baby.aspx

Falcone V, et al. Pregnancy after bariatric surgery: a narrative literature review and discussion of impact on pregnancy management and outcome. *BMC Pregnancy Childbirth*. 2018;18(1):507.

Fallon VM, et al. The impact of the UK Baby Friendly Initiative on maternal and infant health outcomes: a mixed-methods systematic review. *Matern Child Nutr*. 2019;15(3):e12778.

Fangupo L, et al. A baby-led approach to eating solids and risk of choking. *Pediatrics*. 2016:138(4).

Fewtrell M, et al. Complementary feeding: a position paper by the European Society for Paediatric Gastroenterology, Hepatology, and Nutrition (ESPGHAN) Committee on Nutrition. *J Pediatr Gastroenterol Nutr*. 2017;64(1):119–132.

Food Allergy Canada. Preventing food allergies in babies. 2023. https://foodallergycanada.ca/living-with-allergies/ongoing-allergy-management/parents-and-caregivers/early-introduction/

Garzón M, et al. Comparison of growth curve estimates of infants in São Tomé Island, Africa, with the WHO growth standards: a birth cohort study. *Int J Environ Res Public Health*. 2019;16(10).

Gridneva Z, et al. Human milk adiponectin and leptin and infant body composition over the first 12 months of lactation. *Nutrients*. 2018;10(8).

Health Canada. Canada's Food Guide-Resources for Professionals. Applying Canada's Dietary Guidelines: examples of nutritious foods that provide iron, calcium or that contain mostly unsaturated fat. 2023. https://food-guide.canada.ca/en/applying-guidelines/examples-nutritious-foods-iron-calcium-unsaturated-fat/

Jullien S. Vitamin D prophylaxis in infancy. *BMC Pediatr*. 2021:8(1)(suppl 1):319.

Kaur S, Goraya JS. Dermatologic findings of vitamin B(12) deficiency in infants. *Pediatr Dermatol*. 2018;35(6):796–799.

Khan S, et al. Variation in fat, lactose, and protein composition in breast milk over 24 hours: associations with infant feeding patterns. *J Human Lact*. 2013;29(1):81–89.

Kikuchi S, et al. The influence of feeding method on a mother's circadian rhythm and on the development of her infant's circadian rest-activity rhythm. *Early Human Development*. 2020;145:1–6.

Kouwenhoven SMP, et al. Low-protein infant formula and obesity risk. *Nutrients*. 2022;14(13):1–12.

McKenna H, Reiss IKM. The case for a chronobiological approach to neonatal care. *Early Hum Dev*. 2018;126:1–5.

Meeks JY, Noble L. The American Academy of Pediatrics. Policy statement: breastfeeding and the use of human milk. *Pediatrics*. 2022;150(1):e2022057988.

National Conference of State Legislatures. Breastfeeding state laws. April 30, 2019. https://www.ncsl.org/research/health/breastfeeding-state-laws.aspx

Pattison KL, et al. Breastfeeding initiation and duration and child health outcomes in the first baby study. *Prev Med*. 2019;118:1–6.

Plachý L, et al. For debate: the significance of etiologic diagnosis in neonates with overgrowth syndromes. Lesson learned from the Simpson-Golabi-Behmel syndrome. *Pediatr Endocrinol Rev*. 2018;16(1):171–177.

Pluymen LPM, et al. Early introduction of complementary foods and childhood overweight in breastfed and formula-fed infants in the Netherlands: the PIAMA birth cohort study. *Eur J Nutr*. 2018;57(5):1985–1993.

Rapley G, Murkett T. *Baby-Led Weaning: The Essential Guide to Introducing Solid Foods and Helping Your Baby to Grow Up a Happy and Confident Eater*. London: Random House; 2009.

Ren Q, et al. The association of formula protein content and growth in early infancy: a systematic review and meta-analysis. *Nutrients*. 2022;14(11):2255.

Schneider N, et al. Diet and nutrients in the modulation of infant sleep: a review of the literature. *Nutr Neurosci*. 2018;21(3):151–161.

Shrivastava A, Jain S. Appetite self-regulation in infancy—the role of direct breastfeeding. *World Nutr*. 2023;14(1):22–27.

Solid Starts. What is baby-led weaning? 2023. https://solidstarts.com/baby-led-weaning/

Spahn J. Influence of maternal diet on flavor transfer to amniotic fluid and breast milk and children's responses: a systematic review (P11-029-19). *Curr Dev Nutr*. 2019;3(suppl 1).

Verd S, et al. Variation in the protein composition of human milk during extended lactation: a narrative review. *Nutrients*. 2018;10(8).

Wolffenbuttel BHR, et al. The many faces of cobalamin (Vitamin B_{12}) deficiency. *Mayo Clin Proc Innov Qual Outcomes*. 2019;3(2):200–214.

World Health Organization. Vitamin A supplementation in infants 1–5 months of age. 2023a. https://www.who.int/tools/elena/interventions/vitamina-infants

World Health Organization. WHO complementary feeding. 2023b. https://www.who.int/health-topics/complementary-feeding#tab=tab_1

Zhao M. Clinical phenotypes and a genetic analysis of patients with Sotos syndrome. *Zhongguo Dang Dai Er Ke Za Zhi*. 2018;20(6):481–484 [in Chinese].

CHAPTER 19

Problems with Milk Production and Transfer

Some parents experience problems with producing sufficient milk to sustain their babies. Other parents may lack confidence in their ability to produce enough milk despite having a healthy, thriving baby. In addition, some babies have difficulty transferring milk despite ample volume. The information presented in this chapter will assist you in helping parents recognize when milk production is truly a concern. You will learn to recognize when newborns are receiving enough milk, as well as measures for increasing milk production and efficient transfer. With appropriate teaching and follow-up, you can help parents maximize their capacity for adequate milk production and transfer of sufficient milk for their baby to thrive.

KEY TERMS

Digital baby weight scale
Donor milk
Galactagogues (also spelled *galactogogues*)
Growth faltering
Poor weight gain
Slow weight gain

Perception of Insufficient Milk Production

There are several reasons parents might perceive a problem their milk production. They may believe it is not rich or satisfying enough. They may worry that their milk is causing an allergic response or excessive gas in the baby. By far, the most common worry is that the amount of milk is not sufficient for the baby. The perception of insufficient milk is the most common reason for early weaning (Academy of Breastfeeding Medicine [ABM], 2018; Tawfik et al., 2019). It is a universal belief that transcends nationalities and cultures and leads to early weaning and unnecessary use of formula.

If a parent voices a concern about having enough milk, you first need to determine the reason for concern. Although low milk production may be possible, the belief could stem from a lack of confidence or a lack of knowledge about typical newborn behavior. Misconceptions about the normal intake of nursing babies are common, especially if friends or family fed their children formula. Helping parents identify whether there actually is a problem and reassuring them when production is good can have a tremendous influence on both nursing exclusivity and duration.

Reasons for Perceived Milk Insufficiency

There are differences between parents who perceive they have insufficient milk and those who are confident in their ability to produce milk for their baby. Recognizing these differences will enable you to give parents the support and information they need. Parents' perceptions are significantly related to their nursing self-efficacy after birth. High self-confidence and self-efficacy go hand in hand with a belief in sufficient milk production (Li et al., 2019). This underscores the importance of sending parents home from the birth facility feeling confident in their ability to sustain a nursing baby.

Parents who perceive their milk production to be insufficient often worry that their baby does not seem satisfied and is fussy after feeding. They may not understand normal newborn behavior and when to be concerned. They may not understand or recognize early hunger cues. They may view crying as a symptom of insufficient milk intake. Some parents are concerned about infant weight gain and the perception that their baby nurses too frequently. The small volume of colostrum during the first few days postpartum can cause parents to doubt that their infants are getting enough milk. You can help parents recognize that frequent nursing patterns in the early weeks of life are normal and critical to long-term nursing.

Some parents lack confidence in their body's ability to function as nature intended. The medical profession's use of negative terminology in women's health may be a contributing factor. Terms such as "elderly primigravida," "hysterectomy," "lactation failure," "failure to progress," and "incompetent cervix" may subconsciously undermine new parents' self-confidence and self-esteem at a time when they are vulnerable to negative talk and disempowering labels.

Many new parents do not live near their extended family, and may lack a strong support system and positive role models for birthing and parenting. Parents who nurse in a culture saturated with messages that bottle-feeding formula is best face many societal challenges. Friends and relatives may have formula fed their babies. The expectations of society and the media are that babies are fed by bottles. Healthcare providers may lack correct information regarding nursing care or are noncommittal in an attempt to avoid causing parents to "feel guilty" if they formula feed.

Ironically, nursing and formula-feeding parents alike can encounter judgment from their community and healthcare providers. Formula-feeding parents report feelings of guilt and blame for not nursing their babies. Nursing parents report feeling embarrassment and isolation when feeding their babies around others. Parents who do not achieve their nursing goals and switch to formula report feelings of personal crisis, anxiety, failure, shame, body mistrust, confusion, and grief (Ayton et al., 2019).

Parents want to know they are doing the best for their baby. The stress of becoming a new parent can feed into worries about overall competence. Parents in small families may have had little or no experience in caring for small infants. Misconceptions about the realities of parenthood can cause parents to question their choices and doubt their parenting abilities. Preconceived notions of a perfect baby may not match the reality of their baby's needs. Lack of familiarity with normal infant behavior and development can create anxieties in inexperienced parents. They may incorrectly blame nursing as the cause of fussiness, wakefulness, or other typical newborn behaviors.

Recognizing Sufficient Milk Production

It is important that parents feel secure in their ability to nurse and confident that they can produce the milk their baby needs. Parents have fewer worries about their milk production when they understand the basic premise that frequent milk removal triggers further milk production. Three factors influence nursing frequency: breast storage capacity (the milk available for the infant when the breast is full), infant stomach capacity, and the infant's gastric emptying time. These rates and capacities differ for each parent and baby.

Recognizing normal newborn behavior reassures parents that they are meeting their babies' needs. Knowing the signs that their baby is receiving sufficient nourishment from exclusive nursing can prevent unnecessary supplementation and early weaning. Nursing exclusively helps ensure babies have adequate energy intake and normal growth. Having appropriate support helps parents feel more confident in their nursing abilities. Refer to **Figure 19-1** for signs that nursing is going well.

Healthcare providers can help ensure appropriate newborn nourishment. If hospital discharge occurs within 48 hours after delivery, an appointment with the baby's primary caregiver needs to occur within 2 days after going home. A second visit should occur at about 2 weeks for a physical assessment (well-baby check) and another weight check. The second visit should be sooner if the baby's condition warrants it, especially if there are concerns about milk production or intake. These safeguards help to ensure healthy babies and confident parents.

As a baby's nursing pattern changes and the breasts become softer, some parents may feel that their milk production has declined. This is often

- By day 4 the baby has at least six wet diapers in each 24-hour period.
- The baby has pale, diluted urine.
- By day 4 the baby has three or more ample stools that are yellow or at least are turning yellow.
- The baby continues to have at least three stools in each 24-hour period until they are about 5 to 6 weeks old.
- The baby routinely nurses at least 8 to 12 times in each 24-hour period.
- The breasts feel softer after a feeding (although some parents feel no dramatic change).
- The nipples are not painful during or after feedings.
- The baby regains birth weight by 10 to 14 days.
- The baby gains 4 to 8 ounces a week.
- During a feeding the baby's sucking rhythm changes and slows as they obtain milk; the parent may notice swallowing or gulping.
- The baby is alert and active.
- The baby is content between feedings, usually rests for 1 to 2 hours, wakes on their own, and signals to nurse again (although well-fed infants may be fussy for other reasons).

Figure 19-1 Signs that nursing is going well.

because the baby is more efficient at milk removal. You can assure parents that these changes in nursing behavior are normal and healthy. When parents have regular separations from their infant, such as when returning to work or school, regular pumping will protect long-term milk production. **Chapter 25** discusses maintaining milk production during regular separation.

Risks for Low Milk Production

The occurrence of insufficient milk production is growing, partly because of advanced maternal age, hormonal imbalances and complex health conditions. The protein phosphatase is essential for normal lactation function. Lack of this protein delays the onset of lactogenesis. The highest amount of protein is present in colostrum and tapers off in mature milk. Another protein, seipin, also appears to be required for normal lactation function (El Zowalaty et al., 2018). In addition, nursing parents with genetic defects in the ability to transport and use zinc may be at risk for low milk production (Lee et al., 2018). These findings may further our understanding of true insufficiency and lead to more effective treatments targeted to specific causes.

Globally, low milk production continues to be a common cause of early weaning. Most cases of insufficient milk production result from ineffective nursing. This can usually be corrected if not too much time has passed. The *inability* to produce adequate amounts of milk is quite different from the lack of *opportunity* to produce milk or the inability of the baby to transfer milk. Some feeding-related causes of low milk production are the baby's inability to suck well, ineffective positioning, and limited time on each side, leading to milk downregulation.

Delayed onset of lactogenesis II (secretory activation) differs from low milk production. About 12–55% of nursing parents experience a delay in lactogenesis II, often leading to a shorter duration of nursing (Lian et al., 2022). Lactogenesis can be delayed by cesarean delivery or preterm birth. Other risk factors include antidepressants taken during pregnancy, primiparity (perhaps because of low prolactin receptors), stress, and birth interventions. Milk production can also diminish when the baby receives supplemental or complementary feedings. A specific cause may not always be apparent. As nursing becomes more established, problems that cause low milk production often diminish if volume has not been downregulated beyond rescue. **Chapter 26** discusses causes of insufficient milk production.

Measures to Increase Milk Production

A need to increase milk production can occur at any time in the early days of lactation. A concern about milk production surfaces most often because of **poor weight gain** in the baby. Therefore, while taking measures to increase milk production, the baby needs sufficient nourishment. The cause of reduced production may be the supplements the baby receives. Paradoxically, those supplements need to continue until milk production increases sufficiently to provide total nourishment.

Your assistance will help parents increase milk production in a manner that is both safe for the baby and supportive of nursing. The degree to which milk production increases depends on the baby's age, medical condition, and willingness and ability to nurse. The amount and length of time of any supplements the baby may have received are factors in the degree of any possible breast involution. Success also depends on the parent's motivation to devote the necessary time and energy to the task. The baby needs to nurse at least 10 to 12 times or more in 24 hours. If the baby is unable to nurse robustly or is not hungry that frequently, adding pumping to the feeding

Table 19-1 Measures to Increase Milk Production

Actions to take	Rest as much as possible and relax when nursing to promote milk flow. Spend uninterrupted time with baby for 48 hours, increasing feedings and resting. Get help with other tasks. Hold baby skin to skin in laid-back/reclined position to elicit feeding instincts. Ensure a deep latch to preserve nipple health. Use galactogogues (foods, drinks, or herbs) to increase milk production. Record feedings (nursing sessions and formula). As nursing increases, decrease supplements. Use a hospital-grade electric breast pump to ensure maximum milk removal and stimulate production. Pump for 5 or 10 minutes after nursing, with massage and breast compression to maximize milk removal. Improve diet with more protein, fresh fruits and vegetables, and B vitamins to reduce fatigue. Drink noncaffeinated beverages based on thirst.
Management of feedings	Use relaxation techniques to encourage letdown. Maximize skin-to-skin contact. Wear baby with a sling or front carrier. Rouse or soothe baby as necessary before nursing. Ensure a deep latch for effective sucking. Nurse on both sides at a feeding, several times each, to increase stimulation. Encourage the baby to feed more frequently and longer, both day and night. Nurse long enough for the baby to receive hindmilk. Nurse for comfort if the baby is fussy. Avoid pacifier use until feeding problems resolve. Resume night feedings if they were dropped. Use paced feeding for supplements. Help baby self-regulate intake, register satiety, and minimize negative feeding experiences.

regimen will mimic the nursing frequency needed to stimulate production.

Table 19-1 presents suggestions for increasing milk production. Many parents can simply alter their pattern of feedings and increase the number of times they nurse daily. Several measures can be considered when developing a plan to increase milk production. Be careful not to overwhelm parents with too many suggestions or with measures that are not realistically achievable. Although every parent will have different support and information needs, all parents will benefit from close contact and support from you, especially in the early days when they are trying to find effective methods.

Herbal Galactagogues

Galactagogues are foods, drinks, medications, or herbs that are believed to increase milk production. It is important to target any herb or medicine to the core reason behind low milk production. For example, the traditional herb fenugreek is thought to raise a parent's prolactin levels, but in some cases, it can reduce milk production (Marasco & West, 2019). Notably, if prolactin levels are normal, neither fenugreek nor medications that raise prolactin will be effective. Hormonal screening—done by testing serum levels of prolactin, progesterone, testosterone, and thyroid hormones—can help determine whether hormonal factors are the cause of low milk production (refer to **Chapter 26**).

Other herbs for galactogogues include fennel (*Foeniculum vulgare*), alfalfa (*Medicago sativa*), blessed thistle (*Cnicus benedictus*), shatavari (*Asparagus racemosus*), goat's rue (*Galega*), and nettle (Marasco & West, 2019). Some studies support using *Moringa oleifera* as an herbal galactogogue (Fungtammasan & Phupong, 2022). Some galactogogues contain phytoestrogens, which may stimulate prolactin naturally to increase production (Marasco & West, 2019). More research is needed on the effects of herbal galactagogues. Online resources such as https://www.lowmilksupply.org may be helpful to parents seeking an herbal approach. You can refer interested parents to herbalists or naturopathic practitioners for more information.

Domperidone

Domperidone is a drug used to treat gastroesophageal reflux disease that also increases the amount of prolactin secreted by the pituitary gland (Ou et al., 2021). It is widely prescribed in many countries and is available as an over-the-counter medication in some countries.

Domperidone is only available in the United States from a compounding pharmacy and via the internet.

The U.S. Food and Drug Administration (FDA) cautions that use of domperidone to stimulate milk production may cause serious adverse effects (FDA, 2023). Therefore, due to the lack of FDA approval, many providers are hesitant to prescribe this drug to lactating parents. Because of concerns about arrhythmias and sudden cardiac death with use of the drug, the European Medicines Agency recommends limiting the daily dose to 30 mg per day for no more than 1 week (McBride et al., 2023). Despite these concerns, some lactation experts believe that domperidone has an excellent effectiveness rate for increasing milk production. Efforts to obtain "orphan status" for domperidone in the United States (a designation for a drug used to treat a rare disease or condition) have not been successful.

Metoclopramide

Metoclopramide is a prescription medication used to treat nausea, gastroesophageal reflux, and other gastrointestinal problems (multiple trade names, including Reglan, Maxolon, Afipran). It has been prescribed off-label for many years as a galactagogue. Metoclopramide increases milk production by raising prolactin levels (Grzeskowiak et al., 2019). It passes through the blood–brain barrier, and side effects can include fatigue, irritability, depression, and dystonia (Hale & Krutsch, 2024). These side effects are least common when used for gastrointestinal problems but are reported more in the postpartum period. Because of the potential for causing or exacerbating depression, domperidone is preferred by clinicians over metoclopramide. However, as discussed, domperidone can be difficult to obtain.

Oxytocin

Oxytocin prepared in the form of a nasal spray has been used for many years as a galactagogue. It is no longer marketed in the United States but is available from some compounding pharmacies. Oxytocin is still used worldwide (under the trade name Syntocinon), and studies report differing levels of efficacy (Axelsson et al., 2014; Marcacine et al., 2018). Lactation consultants have observed that oxytocin spray can be helpful for nursing parents with breast surgeries or chest injuries that affect letdown. However, oxytocin is not as commonly used as domperidone and metoclopramide for parents with low milk production.

Metformin

Metformin is a prescription drug that lowers the body's resistance to insulin. Metformin therapy is sometimes used for people with prediabetes, in hopes of preventing type 2 diabetes from developing (American Diabetes Association, 2024). Candidates include individuals with prior gestational diabetes mellitus. Metformin is also used to treat the symptoms of individuals with polycystic ovarian syndrome (PCOS). Clinicians have empirically observed that some lactating parent treated with metformin for gestational diabetes, type 2 diabetes, or PCOS experience increased milk production. Additionally, metformin is sometimes used as a galactagogue in nursing parents with reduced milk production; however, little evidence supports this (Newman et al., 2023).

Other Medications

Several other medications have been used as galactagogues in various countries. There is a paucity of research demonstrating their efficacy, and newer studies are needed. Studies report that milk production increases with some agents (Grzeskowiak et al., 2019):

- Chlorpromazine: an antipsychotic that raises prolactin levels
- Sulpiride: an antipsychotic that raises prolactin levels
- Human growth hormone: mechanism of action not understood
- Recombinant human prolactin: hormone that raises prolactin levels
- Thyrotropin-releasing hormone: thyroid hormone that raises thyroid-stimulating hormone and prolactin levels
- Medroxyprogesterone: a progesterone derivative, mechanism of action not understood

Medication should not be the first approach to correcting nursing difficulties. Most researchers believe that medication use is appropriate only after exploring all other factors that might result in insufficient milk production and responding appropriately. However, some researchers hypothesize that with prenatally known conditions (e.g., breast surgery, PCOS, previous low milk production), immediate postpartum use may be more successful (Nommsen-Rivers et al., 2019). Problem-solving should include correcting any issues with the baby's latch or sucking. Breast compression during feedings and milk expression after feedings may also help to increase production. More research is needed to support lactating parents.

Concerns About Infant Growth

Several factors contribute to the total picture of adequate infant growth. Birth weight in a healthy, full-term baby typically doubles by 6 months and triples by 12 months. Body length is a significant indicator of growth, and the baby should increase in length by 50 percent at 12 months. Head circumference, which indicates brain growth, should increase by 3 inches (7.6 cm) at 1 year. Other signs of healthy growth are adequate voids and stools, which are frequent in the first month and less frequent thereafter. Bright eyes, an alert manner, and good muscle and skin tone also indicate a healthy baby. Family history of small stature or **slow weight gain** in children are important factors when assessing weight. Refer to **Figure 14-5** in **Chapter 14**) for the World Health Organization (WHO) growth charts (WHO, 2006) for normal growth in a baby's weight, height, and head circumference.

To ensure the health of every infant in your care, be alert to weight gain and to the factors that could contribute to low milk production. Understand each dyad's feeding pattern to help assess adequate growth. Consider all growth indicators and possible causes of poor growth as you work with parents to develop a plan for improvement. Communicating about issues with infant growth with parents can lead to a variety of emotions, such as fear, disappointment, guilt, and failure. Be aware that how you communicate about infant weight and possible formula use may have unintended consequences, including the termination of nursing. It is imperative that you exhibit sensitivity and tactfulness when exploring these issues with families.

Newborn Dehydration

A baby who does not receive enough fluids can become dehydrated. This can occur when a nursing baby is not receiving an adequate amount of milk. Parents with short hospital stays are not in the hospital long enough to experience secretory activation (lactogenesis II) before discharge. Furthermore, these dyads may leave the hospital before someone who is knowledgeable about nursing has evaluated their nursing competency. Consequently, some parents may not have established sound feeding practices before they go home.

Early follow-up after discharge is imperative with a short hospital stay. Babies born at home or in a free-standing birth center also need early follow-up, often provided by a midwife throughout the first 2 weeks. Appropriate care and sound feeding management will prevent a healthy newborn from progressing to the point of dehydration. Recognizing the symptoms of dehydration will help you identify infants at risk (refer to **Figure 19-2**).

- Few or no stools
- Scant urinary output
- Dark, strong-smelling urine
- Infant sleeps at feedings
- Infrequent feedings
- Weight loss greater than 10 to 15 percent of birth weight
- Lethargy
- Weak cry
- Dry mucous membranes
- Lack of tearing
- Poor skin turgor
- Sunken fontanels

Figure 19-2 Symptoms of dehydration in the infant.

Weight-Gain Issues

Before lactogenesis II establishes mature milk production, it is often difficult to ascertain whether effective nursing has been established at the time of discharge. The number of feedings, voids, stools, and normal weight loss are the key markers for adequate intake. Observing a baby's jaw moving up and down is not by itself a sign of milk transfer. Hospital staff need to teach patients how to recognize effective latching and sucking. It is also important that parents know what is appropriate weight loss after birth and when weight gain begins.

A follow-up visit to the healthcare provider's office or health clinic within 1 to 2 days after hospital discharge should include a review of the number of feedings, stools, and voids. A diary to document feedings, stools, and voids helps parents monitor their baby's intake and output. Many parents use mobile apps on their smartphones to document these markers. Most of these applications are free. Some are provided by formula companies with biased, pro-formula messaging and should be avoided.

Concerns about the baby's weight usually surface during the first month. Inadequate intake, low weight gain, or vomiting can have organic or nonorganic causes or a mix of both. Organic causes include gastroesophageal reflux disease (GERD), milk allergy, and idiopathic or nutritional malnutrition. These organic conditions require some form of medication or nutritional therapy for improvement. Inadequate weight gain in a nursing infant that begins after the first month is likely to have an organic cause.

Weight loss beyond 7 percent in the first week warrants an evaluation and assistance with nursing, as discussed in **Chapter 14**. There should be no further weight loss after the third day for full-term infants. Weight gain should begin by day 4, with the onset of full milk production. The baby should be back to birth weight by 10 to 14 days. In unfavorable environments, babies' energy requirements may be higher than usual. Thus, rather than low milk production or intake, the baby's environment could explain the growth differences. This may be an issue for babies who live in high-poverty areas. Babies who lack restful sleep or who have multiple care providers may also have increased caloric needs.

Nursing infants grow at different rates compared to formula-fed infants. Formula-fed infants are at risk of being overfed. They sleep longer, digest their food slower, have high energy expenditure, and have more of an increased heart rate. Because of the difference in growth patterns between exclusively nursed infants and those fed formula, healthcare providers should replace outdated growth charts with the WHO growth charts based on children who are nursed (WHO, 2006). **Chapter 14** discusses normal milk intake and growth rates for nursing infants.

Slow Weight Gain

All children develop at their own rate. Some adolescents can experience a growth spurt and grow 6 inches in 1 year. Differences in growth rate are true for babies as well. Some babies naturally gain weight more slowly than others. It is important to distinguish between a baby who is not gaining weight adequately and one who is gaining weight slowly. A slow-gaining infant demonstrates slow and steady growth over time and grows proportionally for weight, length, and head circumference. Development will be age appropriate. Infants who are born small for gestational age usually gain weight faster, whereas infants who are born large for gestational age will gain weight at a slower rate.

In the absence of other risk factors, minimal intervention, if any, is required for a pattern of slow growth. You can observe nursing to evaluate the parent's technique. Ask about the baby's feeding pattern and suggest any necessary changes if indicated. Some parents believe they should nurse on only one side at a feeding. Simply changing to both sides can produce a significant improvement in weight. Avoiding the use of pacifiers or bottles ensures adequate sucking time through nursing. Also confirm that the parents are not restricting feeding frequency or limiting their baby's time nursing. Review hunger cues with the parents to be sure that they respond to their baby at appropriate times. If there are concerns, suggest checking the baby's weight weekly to monitor growth. These may be all the measures that are necessary for a slow-gaining infant.

Signs of Inadequate Weight Gain

You need to recognize signs that alert you to problems related to inadequate infant weight gain or low milk production. Babies who are not gaining adequately frequently sleep for long periods to conserve energy. Some parents may say they are nursing "all the time" and cannot put the baby down without the baby fussing. The baby may fuss when the parent ends a feeding and then go back to sleep as soon as the parent attempts to resume feeding. Other parents may describe a "good" baby who sleeps a lot and nurses infrequently. Poorly nourished infants may sleep through the night and have few periods of alertness and engagement.

A baby with inadequate weight gain often appears worried or anxious, maintaining a flexed fetal position to preserve temperature. A baby who has lost a large amount of weight will have hanging folds of skin on the thighs and buttocks. Crying may be high-pitched, like the "mew" of a cat. Urinary output may decrease, or the baby may pass dark, concentrated urine. In an older baby, urine may smell strongly of ammonia. Babies younger than 6 weeks of age should stool on average 1-3 times per day. Less frequent stooling might indicate low milk intake. Meconium will have completely passed by day 4 of life for an infant with adequate intake.

Assessing Inadequate Weight Gain

If you question the adequacy of an infant's weight gain, evaluation of feeding practices will help determine the cause. This applies to a newborn who has not regained birth weight by 14 days, as well as an older baby who is not gaining or who is gaining less than 4 oz per week in the first 3 to 4 months of life. Confirm whether the baby receives a minimum of 8 to 12 feedings per day around the clock and an appropriate number of complementary foods if the baby is 6 months or older. Non-nutritive sucking on a pacifier should be avoided so that the baby nurses nutritively increase caloric intake. The baby should be able to sustain sucking bursts without tiring. Audible swallowing usually indicates milk transfer, though some babies who swallow are just swallowing their saliva, with little intake. On the other hand, many babies feed robustly and transfer milk well without audible swallowing. The breasts should feel softer after feeding as an indication of milk transfer.

An intake assessment with pre- and postfeeding weights is warranted anytime weight gain is a concern. Use of a calibrated, accurate, quality **digital baby weight scale** will help assess milk transfer during a feeding (**Figure 19-3**). Most digital scales are calibrated in both grams and ounces; gram weights are more precise. When obtaining these measurements, first weigh the baby naked to determine the baby's weight gain pattern between visits. Obtain the prefeed weight by weighing the baby before nursing wearing only a diaper. Weigh the baby after the feeding for the post-feed weight. The difference in weight will indicate the amount of milk transfer. Most electronic scales automatically calculate the intake amount. Weighing the baby between feeding on the first and second side can help assess any marked difference in milk production between sides. The weighing process may also waken a sleepy baby to take the second side.

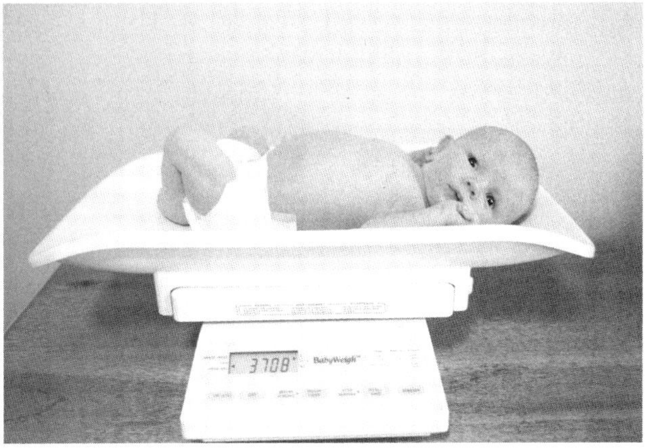

Figure 19-3 Baby being weighed on a digital scale.
Printed with permission of Anna Swisher.

Ask the parent to pump after the feeding and measure the amount of residual milk remaining. This will help distinguish between ineffective milk transfer and low milk production. Feed the baby any pumped milk and use formula, if necessary, to achieve the needed supplementation amount. If the parents use a bottle to feed the expressed milk, teach them paced feeding (described in **Chapter 22**) to slow the flow rate and prevent overfeeding. Intake assessment and supplementation are discussed further in this chapter under Growth Faltering.

Managing Inadequate Weight Gain

The top priority in managing inadequate weight gain is to feed the baby sufficient calories to increase weight. It may be necessary to weigh the baby twice per week to monitor weight changes. If milk production is low, the baby needs to receive supplemental **donor milk** or formula. If the baby was born preterm or has health problems, donor milk may be available by prescription. Parents can check with their insurance providers about covering the cost of donor milk.

The second goal in inadequate weight gain is to increase milk production to a level that can sustain the infant. This must be achieved before discontinuing supplements. Supplementing the baby through a tube while nursing may help accomplish both goals at the same time. The parent receives stimulation for milk production, and the baby receives necessary nourishment if the baby can transfer milk effectively. Expressing milk with a hospital-grade electric breast pump immediately after feedings will further increase production until the baby can more effectively transfer milk.

It is important that the baby's healthcare provider be informed about any feeding plan developed with the parents. They also need to be involved if milk production is impaired. Send a report of your consultation to both caregivers or call them with your evaluation and suggestions as appropriate. Encourage the parents to stay in close contact with you and the healthcare team until the cause of the baby's weight has been resolved. The amount of supplementation can decrease slowly when the baby begins to gain weight and transfers more milk. Caregivers should monitor weight with the growth chart and ensure that the infant does not progress to growth faltering.

Growth Faltering

For many years, the term failure to thrive (FTT) identified an infant with a weight significantly below that of other infants of similar age and sex. FTT has been defined as continuing to lose weight after 10 days of life, not regaining birth weight by 3 weeks of age, or having a weight gain below the 10th percentile beyond 1 month of age. Further, in older infants, weight that is 2 standard deviations or more below where it should be on a standard growth chart has been an indication of FTT. More recent criteria for FTT include weight for age under the 5th percentile on standard growth charts, a reduced weight percentile of more than 2 major percentile lines, and less than the 80th percentile of weight for height/length ratio (Smith et al., 2023).

The term "failure to thrive" has been replaced with **growth faltering** to better capture the symptoms of inadequate nutrition. This abnormal growth pattern occurs in 5–10% of children in the outpatient primary care setting (Lezo et al., 2020). Plotting the baby's predictable growth curve using the WHO growth charts based on human milk–fed babies helps assess whether their growth is within established guidelines. Symptoms in a baby experiencing growth faltering may include the following:

- Lack of appropriate weight gain
- Irritability
- Easily fatigued
- Excessive sleepiness
- Lack of age-appropriate social response (e.g., smile)
- Lack of vocal sounds
- Delayed motor development (Johns Hopkins Medicine, 2019)

Causes of Growth Faltering

Causes of growth faltering have historically been categorized as either organic (intrinsic medical) or nonorganic (externally caused illness, social or environmental). In many cases, aspects of both categories exist, and growth faltering may develop from the interaction between these factors (Kliegman et al., 2020; Mazze et al., 2019). Inadequate caloric intake is the most common cause of growth faltering.

A framework for assessing growth faltering considers medical issues, nutrition, feeding skills, and psychosocial characteristics (Goday et al., 2019). Lactation consultants can assess for caloric inadequacy and notify the primary care provider if intake volumes are normal. This would suggest that the baby is burning more calories, perhaps because of infection, or may have malabsorption problems. The baby's compromised status could relate to the baby's or parent's physical condition. If you encounter a baby who is not gaining weight despite ample milk intake, an undetected afebrile infection or disorder may be present. The baby needs immediate medical assessment and should be referred to the appropriate provider for evaluation.

The risk factors for growth faltering vary depending on demographics. Infectious diseases, poverty, and inadequate nutrition are the main risk factors for infants in low-income settings. Preterm birth and psychosocial factors (including family dysfunction) are primary risk factors for infants in high-income areas. **Table 19-2** identifies potential parent and infant causes of growth faltering. It is important to realize that even a baby who appears to be satisfied can have faltered growth. Easy, placid babies are vulnerable to growth faltering because they may not display sufficient hunger cues. Feeding problems are an early marker for babies with inadequate nutrition. (Mazze et al., 2019).

Exploring the Cause of Growth Faltering

The answer to a baby's faltered growth is not merely to supplement with formula or to cease nursing. The underlying cause of the growth faltering must be identified and treated. The use of open-ended questions and complete maternal and infant histories will help identify possible causes of the baby's compromised status. Learning how much weight the parent gained during pregnancy may provide a clue to the possibility of an eating disorder or low-fat content in the milk. Asking about breast changes during pregnancy can help determine whether there is sufficient functional tissue. A history of infertility or miscarriage can be a marker for hormonal or thyroid disorders.

Ask about medications the parent is taking, including contraception to prevent another pregnancy. Estrogen-containing forms of contraception can lower milk production. Learn if there was excessive blood loss or if synthetic oxytocin (Pitocin) or intravenous fluids were used during labor and delivery. Hemorrhage or edema can delay the onset of milk production. Furthermore, hemorrhage may be treated with methylergonovine (Methergine), which belongs to a class of drugs called *ergot alkaloids*. The ergot family includes bromocriptine and cabergoline, which can inhibit milk production.

Ask about the parent's general health and diet to learn about their overall eating pattern. Ask about cigarette smoking, including how many per day. Smoking has been associated with low milk production, although studies are conflicting (Hale & Krutsch, 2024). Learning about the parent's alcohol or

Table 19-2 Causes of Growth Faltering

Causes related to the nursing parent:
- Previous breast surgery, including reduction, lift, augmentation, or breast trauma
- Back or thoracic surgery
- History of infertility
- Low prolactin levels (hypoprolactinemia)
- Anatomic position of the ducts
- Insufficient glandular tissue
- Hormonal disorders, including untreated hypothyroidism and polycystic ovary syndrome (PCOS)
- Sheehan's syndrome
- Disrupted neurohormonal pathways
- Inappropriate use of a nipple shield
- Retained placental fragments
- Gestational theca lutein cyst
- Use of medications that inhibit lactation, including ergot/alkaloids, estrogen, progestin, corticosteroids
- Scheduling or restricting feedings
- Psychosocial issues, including mental health, neglect, and abuse

Infant causes that affect nursing:
- Preterm birth, intrauterine growth restriction, or small for gestational age
- Difference between infant's oral structure and breast shape and size
- Inability to latch or suck effectively
- Oral anomaly, such as tongue-tie, short tongue, high palate, submucosal clefts
- Cleft lip, palate, or both
- Disorganized suck
- Lack of hunger cues

Other causes related to the infant:
- Neurodevelopmental disorders
- Illness or infection, including gastrointestinal, respiratory, and urinary
- Endocrine disorders
- Genetic disorders, especially inborn errors of metabolism
- Gastrointestinal disorders, including gastroesophageal reflux disease (GERD) and eosinophilic esophagitis
- Childhood cancers
- Immunodeficiency disorders
- Cardiac disease/defects

cannabis use helps to rule these drugs out as a cause. Alcohol is associated with a reduction in letdown, infant intake, infant sleep, and impaired immune function in the infant. The use of cannabis (marijuana) has grown in popularity with increased legalization in many regions. Cannabis use is associated with low birth weight, cognitive deficits, poor sucking, and delayed growth in the nursing infant (Navarrete et al., 2020). **Chapter 11** discusses the transfer of drugs into human milk.

Learn about any previous surgery that would compromise milk ducts, such as a biopsy, cyst removal, augmentation, or reduction. Ask specifically about any injury to the chest area, which may not come to mind when you inquire about breast procedures. **Color Plate 46** displays a scar from a childhood injury which was deep enough to have damaged milk ducts.

Explore issues related to lactation. Ask about any breast engorgement or mastitis, including severity and treatment course. Pathologic engorgement can lead to the loss of milk-producing cells. Inflammatory mediators activated during mastitis can reduce milk production during the infection. Explore the parent's nursing routine, including frequency, duration, and whether the baby nurses on one or both sides at a feeding. If feeding length or frequency is restricted, milk production may have downregulated. Ask how many voids and stools the baby had in the previous 24 hours and their color and size. Scant or no stooling is a marker for inadequate intake. Green stools could indicate a lactose overload, which is usually consistent with overproduction.

Finally, explore issues related to parenting practices. Learn whether the baby receives a pacifier, the reasons why, and the frequency. Although pacifiers are useful tools in the right circumstances, inappropriate use is linked with fewer feedings and reduced nursing duration. **Chapter 16** discusses pacifier use. Similarly, ask how much time the baby spends in a swing or other pacifying apparatus. Use of such devices to delay or avoid feedings can contribute to underfeeding. Asking an open-ended question such as, "What parenting books or apps are you using with your baby?" will identify whether the parents use a parenting program that restricts the frequency or length of feedings. Programs that place rigid restrictions on feeding length and frequency are associated with low weight gain, growth faltering, and reduced milk production. **Chapter 20** discusses these programs.

Managing Growth Faltering

If growth faltering is suspected, measures must begin immediately to reverse the trend of inadequate weight gain or weight loss. Interventions may be required for a long time, so help parents form realistic expectations. They may be expressing milk to increase production and supplement nursing, using infant formula as a supplement, increasing feeding frequency, and monitoring their baby's weight. As a baby's condition begins to improve, caution parents to proceed slowly with decreasing the amount of supplement and frequency of milk expression. Depending on the cause, interventions may be required for the entire time the baby is nursing or until they start complementary foods.

Assess the baby's latch, sucking technique, and positioning at feedings. If oral anomalies are noted or if you cannot determine why the baby fails to transfer milk, the baby will need to be referred to an appropriate specialist. Submucosal clefts and other subtle oral anomalies can easily be missed during assessment. Babies with oral structure anomalies may be referred to ear, nose, and throat specialists or to pediatric dentists for assessment and treatment. Babies with ineffective or disordered sucking may be referred to an occupational therapist or a speech-language pathologist for assessment and therapy.

Assess milk transfer with pre- and postfeeding weights on a quality, calibrated, digital baby weight scale. If the baby does not transfer at least 60 mL or more and the parent is able to express that amount, refer the baby to the healthcare provider for assessment. If the baby transfers milk adequately, increasing the frequency and duration of feedings may be sufficient. Clinical test weights are a *core component* of a comprehensive feeding assessment for lactation consultants when there are concerns about infant growth and milk transfer. Accurate weight is especially crucial in abnormal feeding situations, such as a preterm or compromised infant and parents with insufficient milk.

Explore any adjustments that are needed in the nursing routine. Encourage nursing a minimum of 8 to 12 times in 24 hours around the clock until there are three stools per 24 hours for 3 days in a row. Suggest switching sides when the baby's sucking pattern changes and swallowing ceases so that more time is spent transferring milk from the fuller side. In addition, use of alternate breast compression during the feeding increases milk flow. Limiting feedings to 40 minutes per session—regardless of which combination of feeding methods is used—helps prevent fatigue and stress for both the baby and the parent.

Expressing milk immediately after nursing will help increase production. Massage and hand expression before pumping have been found to increase milk production significantly. Use of a hospital-grade electric breast pump and double pumping for 10 to 15 minutes or until milk stops flowing helps stimulate milk production. Turning the pump off, massaging the breasts, and then pumping again for a few more minutes may be helpful as well.

Protecting the baby's health is a priority when managing growth faltering. It is essential to meet the baby's caloric needs with frequent feedings and provide supplements if recommended by the baby's healthcare provider. Assess the baby's feeding and growth regularly and follow the provider's guidelines for supplementation until the baby is gaining well. Keep the provider apprised of any increased ability to transfer milk by direct nursing as well as any increase in milk production. Monitor the baby's weight and growth closely, and confirm that the baby visits the healthcare provider frequently. Urge the parents to stay in close contact with you and their baby's healthcare provider.

The stress of having a compromised baby can negatively affect a parent's mental health and well-being. Parents may need help coping with the stress and pressure associated with a feeding plan for their baby, as well as support for their own mental health. As the situation improves, you can help parents identify the intervention(s) that are causing them the most stress and work to eliminate or modify that aspect of the feeding plan. For example, parents frequently ask to discontinue nighttime supplements when things improve. Reminding them that nursing at least once during the night capitalizes on higher nighttime maternal prolactin levels may help them remain committed to that.

Counseling the Family

It is extremely common for parents of an infant with faltered growth to feel highly stressed. The baby's compromised state plays into parents' fears and insecurities about inadequacies, including the ability to nurse. It is important that you approach the family with sensitivity, offering validation and reassurance. Close contact with you or another source of support will help to provide the encouragement and objectivity they need. Lack of familiarity with infant development and a lack of follow-up support with the healthcare system are factors in many cases of growth faltering.

Chapter 26 discusses biologically insufficient milk and ways to help those parents to optimize their nursing. Some parents will need to come to terms with impaired milk production and the need for continued supplementation. The loss of exclusive nursing can cause lingering grief and feelings of failure. It may be helpful for these parents to reframe their concept of nursing as a family practice, including the nonnursing parent or other family members as part of the experience. This inclusive approach may help them to negotiate and sustain nursing and come to terms with nursing grief (Ayton et al., 2019).

Supplementing the Baby

Adequate nourishment of the baby is critical whenever there is a concern about weight. If milk production does not provide sufficient calories with expressed milk, donor milk or formula will be needed. Generally, encourage nursing first, followed by the supplement. However, babies who are frantic to eat may nurse better by first receiving a small amount of supplement (15 mL or a half ounce) before nursing. Pumping after feedings provides further stimulation for milk production, and the pumped milk can be fed to the baby. As milk production improves, supplements can decrease slowly if the baby is nursing effectively and frequently enough.

Amount to Supplement

Providing supplements in measured amounts avoids the baby receiving so much supplement that it causes a lack of interest in nursing. Standard instructions to "nurse first and supplement afterward" may be misleading. Some babies nurse as few as six times a day, whereas others nurse as many as 12 or more times. A baby who nurses frequently and receives supplementation after every feeding could consume so much formula or donor milk that nursing may never resume. Likewise, a baby who nurses infrequently may not receive sufficient supplementation.

Suggest a plan for the number of milliliters or ounces to feed the baby during a 24-hour period. Quantifying the amount of supplement guides parents in dividing the supplement over the number of their baby's feedings per day. Each dyad is different and requires careful assessment to create an individualized feeding plan to meet their unique needs.

You can work collaboratively with parents and their healthcare provider to determine an appropriate amount of supplement for their baby per day. The baby can receive supplements through a tube at the breast while nursing. If the baby does not finish the entire amount at one feeding, it may be that the amount of daily supplement is more than the baby needs. On the other hand, the baby may need the remaining amount sometime later within that 24-hour period. Urge parents to monitor the amounts of supplement consumed at each feeding and to watch their baby carefully for signs of hunger so that they can respond accordingly. The ABM (2017) recommends that supplemental feedings be given according to infant satiety cues.

Intake Assessment

An intake assessment with pre- and post-weights will determine the amount of supplement the baby needs. Optimally, the baby will not have been nursed immediately prior to the assessment. However, let parents know not to hold the baby off for the assessment. A frantic, overly hungry baby can be difficult to calm sufficiently to nurse. Additionally, crying stresses parents and care providers alike. Delay expressing milk until after the feeding assessment as well.

Weighing the baby before and after a feeding establishes how much milk is consumed by directly nursing. Pumping after feeding will measure the amount of residual milk. The amount of milk the baby consumed added to the amount of residual milk gives an estimate of milk production over the preceding 2 or 3 hours. More than one ac/pc weight may be needed if you doubt whether the transfer amount represents average intake and if you are dealing with growth faltering or other serious weight loss. Additional test weights over a couple of days provide a clearer picture of the baby's ability to transfer milk adequately.

Knowing the amount of milk the baby consumed from nursing compared with normal intake will give you and the parents an accurate measurement of the amount of supplement their baby requires. Infants typically take about 2.5 oz (75 mL) of milk per day for every pound (435 g) of body weight. Using this information, you can calculate how much supplementation is needed (American Academy of Pediatrics [AAP], 2022). Mobile apps are available for these calculations as well.

The infant's age is also a factor in considering the amount to supplement. On average, babies will take in about 1–2 oz (30–60 mL) of milk in the first week of life. The volume per feeding will increase by an ounce (30 mL) each week in the first month of life. After that, babies typically take about 25–30 oz (750–900 mL) in a 24-hour period (ABM, 2017; Centers for Disease Control and Prevention [CDC], 2023). When assessing intake needs for a baby with faltered growth, it is important to recognize that babies differ greatly in the amounts of milk they consume. There is a wide range in what is "normal." Refer to **Chapter 9** for a more in-depth discussion.

Weaning from Supplementation

The process of eliminating supplementation and increasing milk production to replace it can take several days to weeks of concentrated effort. Encourage parents to watch for small daily successes. They can keep a record of the amount of supplements, that the baby receives, as well as the number of direct nursing sessions, wet diapers, and stools. They can also record the type of supplement, whether it is expressed milk, donor milk, or formula.

The baby needs enough supplements to provide nourishment for adequate growth. At the same time, sufficient nipple stimulation and effective milk removal are needed to increase milk production. Any reduction in supplement needs to be based on confidence that milk production has increased sufficiently to warrant it. Caution parents to decrease the amount of supplementation slowly, with frequent weight checks to monitor the baby's continued growth. A parent should never dilute formula to cut back on supplements because this can lead to insufficient caloric and nutritional intake for the baby.

Summary

Giving families the information and support they need for nursing increases parents' confidence in their ability to provide sufficient milk to their baby. A parent who is physically unable to establish adequate milk production or an infant who is physically unable to achieve milk transfer is uncommon in the general population. However, concerns about milk production and transfer constitute a large part of lactation consultations beyond the immediate postpartum period. These problems may stem from ineffective nursing technique, or from numerous complex maternal or infant factors. Identifying the cause and taking appropriate action is crucial to preventing serious consequences for the baby. No nursing baby should reach the point of dehydration or growth faltering. Be alert to significant barriers to adequate milk production or effective milk transfer.

What You Learned—At a Glance

Conversation Starters with Parents

- How many wet and soiled diapers does your baby have each day?
- How can you tell that your baby is receiving milk during a feeding?
- What is your baby's behavior between feedings?
- How comfortable are you with expressing your milk?
- How can you tell that your baby is gaining weight well?

Signs of Sufficient Milk Production

- Baby passes 6 voids per day by day 4 with pale, diluted urine.
- Baby passes 3 or more yellow stools per day from day 4 to 5 to 6 weeks.
- Baby nurses at least 8 to 12 times per day.
- Breasts feel softer after feeding.
- Nipples are not painful during or after feedings.
- Baby regains birth weight by 10 to 14 days and gains 4–8 oz (114–227 g) per week for the first 3 months.
- Sucking rhythm slows, and parents may notice swallowing or gulping, indicating milk transfer.
- Baby is alert, active, and content between feedings.
- Baby rests for 1 to 2 hours, wakes, and signals to feed.

Measures to Increase Milk Production

- Rest as much as possible and relax during feedings to lower stress and help milk flow.
- Hold the baby skin to skin for 48 uninterrupted hours, feeding and resting.
- Nurse in a reclined position to elicit feeding instincts.
- Use herbal or medicinal galactagogues, if appropriate.
- Record nursing sessions and supplements; decrease supplements as nursing increases.
- Use a hospital-grade electric breast pump with breast massage and compression to increase milk removal and production.
- Eat protein, fresh fruits and vegetables, and B vitamins to reduce fatigue.
- Encourage the baby to nurse more frequently and longer, both day and night.
- Alternate sides several times at feedings to increase stimulation.
- Use alternate breast compression during the feeding to increase milk flow.

Symptoms of Dehydration

- Few or no stools
- Scant, dark, strong-smelling urine
- Infant sleeping at feedings
- Infrequent feedings
- Weight loss greater than 10% to 15% of birth weight

- Lethargy and weak cry
- Dry mucous membranes and lack of tearing
- Poor skin turgor and sunken fontanels

Infant Signs of Inadequate Weight Gain

- Sleeps for long periods to conserve energy, with few periods of quiet, alert time.
- Flexed in a fetal position and appears worried or anxious.
- Passing meconium after day 4.

Managing Inadequate Weight Gain

- Supplement the baby to provide calories.
- Pump to increase milk production until supplements can be decreased and discontinued.
- Assess for hormonal factors, and target galactagogues if appropriate.
- Assess milk transfer with prefeed and postfeed weights on a sensitive digital scale twice weekly.
- Assess nursing technique and management.

References

Academy of Breastfeeding Medicine. ABM clinical protocol #3: supplementary feedings in the healthy term breastfed neonate, revised 2017. *Breastfeed Med.* 2017;12(9):575–576.

Academy of Breastfeeding Medicine. ABM clinical protocol #9: use of galactogogues in initiating or augmenting maternal milk production, second revision. *Breastfeed Med.* 2018;13(5):307–314.

American Academy of Pediatrics. Amount and schedule of baby formula feedings. May 16, 2022. https://www.healthychildren.org/English/ages-stages/baby/formula-feeding/Pages/amount-and-schedule-of-formula-feedings.aspx#:~:text=On%20average%2C%20your%20baby%20should,when%20they've%20had%20enough

American Diabetes Association. Consumer guide: metformin. 2024. https://consumerguide.diabetes.org/products/metformin

Axelsson PB, et al. Treatment of insufficient lactation is often not evidence-based. *Dan Med J.* 2014;61(7):A4869.

Ayton JE, et al. Women's experiences of ceasing to breastfeed: Australian qualitative study. *BMJ Open.* 2019;9(5):e026234.

Centers for Disease Control and Prevention. How much and how often to feed infant formula. June 29, 2023. https://www.cdc.gov/nutrition/infantandtoddlernutrition/formula-feeding/how-much-how-often.html

El Zowalaty AE, et al. Seipin deficiency leads to increased endoplasmic reticulum stress and apoptosis in mammary gland alveolar epithelial cells during lactation. *Biol Reprod.* 2018;98(4):570–578.

Fungtammasan S, Phupong V. The effect of *Moringa oleifera* capsule in increasing breast milk volume in early postpartum patients: a double-blind, randomized controlled trial. *Eur J Obstet Gynecol Reprod Biol.* 2022;16:100171.

Goday PS, et al. Pediatric feeding disorder: consensus definition and conceptual framework. *J Pediatr Gastroenterol Nutr.* 2019;68(1):124–129.

Grzeskowiak LE, et al. What evidence do we have for pharmaceutical galactagogues in the treatment of lactation insufficiency?—a narrative review. *Nutrients.* 2019;11(5).

Hale T, Krutsch K. Hale's *Medications & Mothers' Milk 2025–2026: A Manual of Lactational Pharmacology*. 21st ed. New York, NY: Springer Publishing Company; 2024.

Johns Hopkins Medicine. Failure to thrive. *Health Library*. 2019. https://www.hopkinsmedicine.org/healthlibrary/conditions/pediatrics/failure_to_thrive_90,P02297/

Kliegman RM, et al. *Nelson Textbook of Pediatrics, 2-Volume Set.* 21st ed. Philadelphia, PA: Elsevier; 2020.

Lee S, et al. A genetic variant in SLC30A2 causes breast dysfunction during lactation by inducing ER stress, oxidative stress and epithelial barrier defects. *Sci Rep.* 2018;8(1):3542.

Lezo A, et al. Failure to thrive in the outpatient clinic: a new insight. *Nutrients.* 2020;12(8):2202.

Li T, et al. Breastfeeding self-efficacy among parturient women in Shanghai: a cross-sectional study. *J Hum Lact.* 2019;35(3):583–591.

Lian W, et al. Determinants of delayed onset of lactogenesis II among women who delivered via Cesarean section at a tertiary hospital in China: a prospective cohort study. *Int Nurs J.* 2022;17(1):81.

Marasco L, West D. *Making More Milk: The Breastfeeding Guide to Increasing Your Milk Production.* 2nd ed. New York, NY: McGraw-Hill Education; 2019.

Marcacine KO, et al. Factors associated to breast implants and breastfeeding. *Rev Esc Enferm USP.* 2018;52:e03363.

Mazze N, et al. Biopsychosocial factors in children referred with failure to thrive: modern characterization for multidisciplinary care. *Glob Pediatr Health.* 2019;6:2333794X19858526.

McBride G, et al. Women's experiences with using domperidone as a galactagogue to increase breast milk supply: an Australian cross-sectional survey. *Int Breastfeed J.* 2023;18:1.

Navarrete F, et al. Cannabis use in pregnant and breastfeeding women: behavioral and neurobiological consequences. *Front in Psychiatry.* 2020;11:586447.

Newman C, et al. Focus on metformin: its role and safety in pregnancy and beyond. *Drugs.* 2023;83:985–999.

Nommsen-Rivers L, et al. Feasibility and acceptability of metformin to augment low milk supply: a pilot randomized controlled trial. *J Hum Lact.* 2019;35(2):261–271.

Ou LB, et al. Domperidone and the risks of sudden cardiac death and ventricular arrhythmia: a systematic review and meta-analysis of observational studies. *Br J Clin Pharmacol.* 2021;87(10):3649–3658.

Smith AE, et al. Failure to thrive. In: *StatPearls*. Treasure Island, FL: StatPearls Publishing; November 12, 2023. https://www.ncbi.nlm.nih.gov/books/NBK459287/

Tawfik S, et al. Formula feeding and associated factors among a group of Egyptian mothers. *Open Access Maced J Med Sci.* 2019;7(11):1854–1859.

U.S. Food Drug Administration. Information about domperidone. December 12, 2023. https://www.fda.gov/drugs/information-drug-class/information-about-domperidone

World Health Organization, Multicentre Growth Reference Study Group. *The WHO child growth standards*. Geneva, Switzerland: World Health Organization; 2006. https://www.who.int/childgrowth/standards/en

PART 4

Special Care

CHAPTER 20

Family Dynamics in Lactation

Family routines, roles, and relationships all take on new dimensions when a baby enters the picture. As couples merge into their parental roles, they undergo adjustments with one another and with their baby. If other children are at home, siblings' adjustments to the new baby present further challenges. The family will benefit from assistance and support as they settle into newly defined roles and relationships. While acknowledging that non-female parents can nurse and that some couples share the same gender, this chapter primarily focuses on distinguishing between the traditional roles associated with mothers and fathers.

KEY TERMS

Adverse childhood experiences (ACE)
Amenorrhea
Anovulatory
Anticipatory stage
Baby blues
Barrier methods
Contraception
Edinburgh Postnatal Depression Scale (EPDS)
Engrossment
Formal stage
Implants
Informal stage
Injectables
Intimate partner violence (IPV)
Intrauterine device (IUD)
Lactational amenorrhea method (LAM)
Lochia
Luteinizing hormone
Menses
Natural family planning
Perineum
Personal stage
Postpartum depression
Postpartum psychosis
Posttraumatic stress disorder
Reciprocity
Reproductive coercion
Sexual abuse
Sleep training
Transdermal patch
Tubal ligation
Vaginal ring

Acquiring the Parental Role

Many people enter parenthood with no family support system for everyday parenting. Thus, they are on their own as they use trial and error to establish themselves in their new role. Realistic expectations can help parents maintain a positive perspective and facilitate their transition. New parents may not feel prepared for the reality that caring for a baby is a constant responsibility and that their lives have changed forever. Newborns have the capacity to engage in social exchange, known as **reciprocity**. Bonding with the baby by both parents in the first hours and days of life enhances the couple's parental roles and their attachment to the baby (**Figure 20-1**).

Parenthood can create conflict in the balance between work and family, including the division of household responsibilities (Shapiro et al., 2020; Van Rijn-Van Gelderen et al., 2020). Although family transitions can strain relationships, they also provide

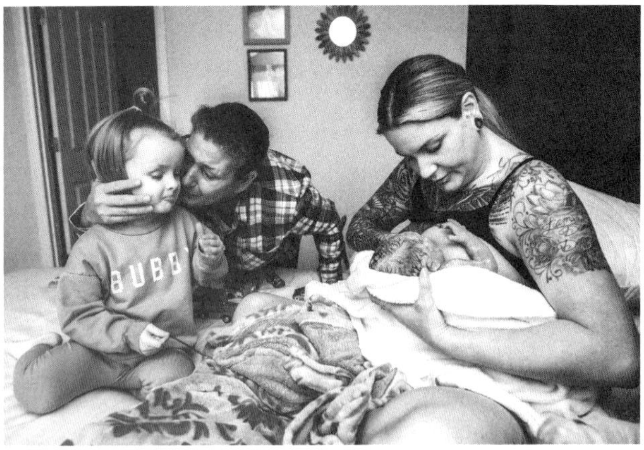

Figure 20-1 A family enjoying their new baby.

Courtesy of Tiarra Doherty.

opportunities to strengthen a partnership and achieve a more closely united relationship. The quality of a couple's relationship affects the degree to which parents support each other's level of involvement in parenting (Han et al., 2023; Le et al., 2021; Liekmeier et al., 2023).

Stages of Role Acquisition

Parents typically progress through predictable stages as they prepare for and care for their first child. The four classic stages of role acquisition are anticipatory, formal, informal, and personal. Each parent's role will grow and change in response to their baby's needs, their family backgrounds, and the couple's interactions. Both parents define their roles gradually through experience. Open communication enhances the process, makes it more enjoyable, and helps the couple relax with each child.

In the **anticipatory stage**, parents begin to learn about their new roles. They may take classes; read books; and browse parenting blogs, forums, and other social media. They often ask questions of their own parents and other families or friends with children. As they enter the **formal stage**, they begin to view their roles more personally. They strive for perfection, with a goal of doing everything "just right." The frustration of trying to achieve perfection and the realization that "just right" is individual leads the parents into the **informal stage**. They will modify, blend, and individualize their roles to fit their unique family. As they become more comfortable in their parenting, they move into the **personal stage**. Their style of parenting evolves to be consistent with their personalities to develop parenting that fits their lifestyle.

Learning About Parenting

Novice parents typically turn to outside resources for guidance and support for their parenting. Parents today possess continual, seamless online connectivity for many aspects of parenting (Huang et al., 2024; Spencer et al., 2020; Tuntipuchitanon et al., 2024). They turn to social media for feelings of community or acceptance, parenting guidance, emotional support, and practical and experiential advice (Chee et al., 2023). In addition, many healthcare providers reach out to parents through interactive classes, health texts, telehealth, and postpartum support (Chirumamilla & Gulati, 2021; Farsi, 2021; Forgie et al., 2021).

Parents who lack knowledge about infant physiology and the daily care of a baby can have unrealistic expectations of life with a new baby. A goal for many parents is to have their babies sleep through the night. In this pursuit, they may be attracted to parenting programs that train babies to sleep. **Sleep training** is an umbrella term that refers to a variety of approaches to help babies learn to fall asleep by themselves and to sleep for long stretches. These teachings recommend that parents schedule their babies' feedings and allow them to cry. Sleep training is not realistic or compatible with lactation, especially for babies who are exclusively nursing. Any parenting program that advocates scheduled feedings contradicts the recommended cue-based feeding for nursing infants. Scheduled feedings can downregulate milk production and cause low infant weight gain. The parenting approaches of these programs appeal to couples in demanding careers who seek full nights of uninterrupted sleep. Parents who ascribe to these programs may receive support in a peer group with other like-minded parents. They may find it difficult to move beyond the formal stage of learning to mature in their parenting style.

Adjustments for Nursing Parents

Although individuals respond to parenthood in their own ways, they often have one characteristic in common: They have little or no idea of what to expect in their babies' behavior and development! They may have formed opinions on infant care, only to find that much of what they know does not work with their baby. They may have had preconceived ideas about types of personalities and demeanors and find that their baby is another type entirely. Parents eventually develop their own parenting style. Their competence and confidence grow with practice, experimentation, observation, and self-education.

Postpartum care is often perceived as focusing on the baby postdelivery, with little attention to the birthing parent's physical and mental health care (Adams et al., 2023). Psychosocial distress, medical recovery, breast health, available support, pain, physical function, sleep, parenting experience, fatigue, sexual function, and cognition can all affect adjustments to parenthood (Sultan & Carvalho, 2021). Parenthood requires reestablishing relationships and behaviors as the couple works together to meet the physical and emotional needs of the infant and other family members. They need psychological support, sharing of experiences, practical and material support, and knowledge of how to turn the challenges of this period into an opportunity for growth (Asadi et al., 2022; Slomian et al., 2021). Social support, self-efficacy, positive coping strategies, and realistic expectations will help in achieving these goals.

Changing Priorities

As energy returns, parents who tend to overexert may need a reminder about moderation and avoiding strenuous activities in the early weeks after delivery. Making rest a priority in the first 6 weeks after giving birth will aid in the parent's physical recovery. Insufficient rest can cause excessive bleeding, exhaustion, dizziness, or weak pelvic floor muscles. Discouraging visitors from staying too long, napping when the baby naps, and nursing lying down can help parents catch up on needed rest.

An overactive lifestyle or physical activity can affect milk production and cause fussiness in the baby. It can also lead to mastitis. Parents may need to relax their standards and priorities concerning household chores and other obligations. They can resume obligations slowly and cut back on activities when possible. Many parents will return to full- or part-time work, school, or volunteer work, in addition to caring for older children. Arranging compromises or trade-offs will allow time for the baby and for self-care. Parents can also avoid missed feedings by participating in activities where the baby is welcome.

Emotional Adjustments

New parents experience dramatic hormonal shifts within the first 24 hours after giving birth. Their emotions are subject to biochemical, psychological, and societal influences. The birth experience may have been exhilarating, confusing, exhausting, or disappointing. Ideas and expectations about parenting, the baby, and family may not reflect reality. Furthermore, the transition to parenthood can create a loss of a sense of self as well as body changes that affect self-image (Serrano Drozdowskyj et al., 2020). Staff and family support, information, follow-up, and access to resources are all integral to a postnatal sense of security, control, and confidence (Werner-Bierwisch et al., 2018).

Parenthood is an ever-present responsibility that can feel overwhelming. A baby may be continually fussy, rarely sleep, and fail to live up to parents' expectations of a happy and responsive baby. The birth may have been unpleasant or may have resulted from an unintended pregnancy. Poor nutrition and lack of rest can cause emotional distress, especially when coupled with the many adjustments to a new baby. Ambivalence about being a parent, fear of judgment, compromised self-care, and relationship changes can hinder adjustments to parenthood (Young et al., 2022). A positive postnatal experience helps parents adapt to a new self-identity and develop a sense of confidence and competence. They are better able to adjust to changes in family relationships and navigate physical and emotional challenges (Finlayson et al., 2020).

Some new parents need do no more than make room for their baby as they adjust to parenthood. It is also common for couples to feel unprepared for their new role as parents, regardless of their status or lifestyle. They may lack personal experience in caring for a baby and may not have family close by to support them in the early weeks. Uncertainty may occur as a specific concern or worry, such as a fussy baby or low milk production. Quitting work to stay at home with the baby causes a loss of income, status, and adult interaction. This decreased contact with adults can create feelings of isolation and loneliness.

Many parents have a few rough days of despondency balanced by high moments. These **baby blues** frequently appear around the third day postpartum and could last for a couple of weeks. There may be bouts of tearfulness and sadness, mingled with happiness and excitement. Such emotions are more common when parents have their first baby. A positive birth experience and an abundance of emotional support and practical help following the birth help to minimize baby blues. Childbirth and parenting education can significantly increase parenting self-confidence and reduce depression, anxiety, and stress (Baldwin et al., 2022; Shorey et al., 2019).

Postpartum Depression

Loss of control is a significant emotion experienced after the birth of a baby. Effective education helps parents and other family members understand the difference between baby blues and postpartum depression. **Postpartum depression** is a common illness and is treatable, like any other biological illness. When this is understood, obstacles around diagnosis and treatment are less likely, and parents seek help more readily.

Physical and psychological stress increase the risk of postpartum depression by upregulating proinflammatory cytokines, thus increasing inflammation. Postpartum depression occurs in an estimated 10% to 15% of births (Kroska & Stowe, 2020; Shorey et al., 2018). It creates extensive mood changes, loss of pleasure, poor concentration, low self-esteem, guilt at failing as a parent, sleep disturbances, fatigue, and a flat affect in voice tone. Episodes of depression typically last for 1 to 6 weeks postpartum. In some cases, postpartum depression can turn into clinical depression and last for several months, requiring professional help.

Parents who experience postpartum depression may not answer the phone or may stay away from home to keep busy. They may have a low tolerance for other family members and feel detached from their baby. Postpartum depression is associated with impaired bonding with the infant (Kasamatsu et al., 2020; Śliwerski et al., 2020; Vanwalleghem et al., 2023). One red flag for postpartum depression is not referring to the baby by name or failing to bond with the baby. The effectiveness of attachment between parents and children is closely related to the parent's mood. Thus, mood stability is important for secure attachment (Slomian et al., 2019).

Symptoms of postpartum depression make it difficult, to experience genuine pleasure and joy. Depressed parents may cope with their baby and with household tasks, but their enjoyment of life is seriously affected. These parents generally feel unable to cope with life and worry that something is not "right." They may even entertain occasional thoughts of harming themselves or the baby. This requires an urgent evaluation by a psychiatrist, preferably one who has a special interest in antenatal and postpartum care. These psychiatrists are more likely to accommodate lactation in their treatment plan.

Identifying Risk Factors

Most parents at risk for postpartum depression can be identified before delivery based on psychiatric history, symptoms during pregnancy, and any recent psychosocial stressors (Kroska & Stowe, 2020). The rate of postpartum depression is higher when there is a history of depression (Liu et al., 2022; Qi et al., 2021). Pregnant and postpartum adolescents are at a greater risk for experiencing depressive symptoms than pregnant and postpartum adults (Dinwiddie et al., 2018; Ladores & Corcoran, 2019). Immigrants have a higher risk of postpartum depression than native-born parents (Daoud et al., 2019; Johansson et al., 2023; Marcos-Nájera et al., 2020; Xiong & Deng, 2020). Physical and psychological stress increases the risk of postpartum depression by upregulating proinflammatory cytokines, thus increasing inflammation. Lifetime exposure to **intimate partner violence (IPV)** (Ankerstjerne et al., 2022; Wei et al., 2024) or psychological trauma, including a negative birth experience (Rosseland et al., 2020; Yakupova & Suarez, 2021) may be factors.

Distress during the transition to parenthood places first-time parents at risk for depression and anxiety (Adina et al., 2021; Johansson et al., 2020). Stressful life events, adversity, and low income can increase anxiety in new parents and lead to depression. Parents of very-low-birth-weight (VLBW) infants and late-preterm infants are vulnerable partly because of the stress associated with early lactation challenges (Barkmann et al., 2018; Premji et al., 2018). Depression is a greater risk for parents who want to nurse and are unable to or when challenges lead to early introduction of formula or early weaning (Bauman et al., 2020; Brown, 2018; Stuebe et al., 2019).

Healthcare providers who interact with young parents are pivotal in the early identification and treatment of postpartum mood disorders. Because emotional stress increases inflammation, it is important to address pain as a potential symptom (Beurel et al., 2020). Worrisome interactions with the baby may warrant a social service consultation. Emotionally distressed parents may need a referral to a behavioral health specialist. In addition to counseling, treatment may involve medications, most of which are compatible with lactation.

Measuring the Risk for Depression

The **Edinburgh Postnatal Depression Scale (EPDS)** helps health professionals detect parents experiencing postnatal depression. The EPDS is an easy self-rating depression scale that indicates the normal range of postpartum emotions and degree of danger for depression (Cox et al., 1987). Responses to 10 short statements that describe feelings during the past week identify the likelihood of a depressive illness. The EPDS score should not override clinical judgment or careful clinical assessment to confirm diagnosis. The scale will not detect anxiety neuroses, phobias, or personality disorders. Although not tailored to postpartum depression, another helpful screening tool is the Beck Depression Inventory. This 21-question test is widely used to measure the severity and depth of depressive symptoms (Bulteau et al., 2021; Ranney et al., 2021). Both screening tools are available online at no cost.

Postpartum Psychosis

Postpartum psychosis involves symptoms far more serious than those of baby blues or postpartum depression. Symptoms may progress beyond insomnia, fatigue, and depression. Postpartum psychosis occurs on a much more intense level than postpartum depression. It can lead to a loss of control and social functioning, as well as overwhelming delusions and hallucinations triggered by irrational thoughts. Postpartum psychosis typically develops within 90 days of delivery in 1 to 2 of 1000 births (Friedman et al., 2023; Perry et al., 2021).

Postpartum psychosis places parents at high risk of harming themselves, their baby, and other children. Parents who take the life of a child display clear depressive symptoms, such as severely depressed mood with crying spells, insomnia, fatigue, anxiety, and preoccupation with worries about the baby's well-being and their own ability to care for their baby. Their conditions can rapidly deteriorate to suicidal or psychotic thoughts. The priority is to keep the parent and child safe and to begin effective treatment immediately.

Lactation and Postpartum Depression

Many studies report reduced risks of postpartum depression among nursing parents (Mikšić et al., 2020; Slomian et al., 2019; Toledo et al., 2022; Xia et al., 2022). Lactation downregulates inflammatory and stress responses and upregulates oxytocin. Nursing helps regulate sleep, improves self-efficacy, and promotes positive interaction with the child (McKenna, 2020). Longer nursing duration is also protective against depressive symptoms. Parents who nurse 8 weeks or longer report less general anxiety and depressive symptoms than parents who never nursed or who stop sooner than 8 weeks (Bauman et al., 2020; Dagla et al., 2021; Ritchie-Ewing et al., 2019). Those who nurse exclusively have the lowest rates of postpartum depression (Alimi et al., 2022; Figueiredo et al., 2021; Shimao et al., 2021).

Individuals who are anxious or depressed during pregnancy are at risk for early cessation of exclusive nursing (Cato et al., 2019; Coo et al., 2020; Horsley et al., 2019). Early lactation difficulties and early weaning increase the likelihood of postpartum depression (Cooklin et al., 2018; Silva et al., 2017; Woolhouse et al., 2016). Thus, empowering parents with the skills and knowledge they need for lactation reduces the risk of postpartum depression.

Postpartum mood disorders can undermine lactation and have a negative impact on both parents and babies (Kendall-Tackett, 2016; Wouk et al., 2017). Postpartum depression and anxiety disorders are associated with lower numbers of feedings and early weaning (Sha et al., 2019; Stuebe et al., 2019). They can lower oxytocin, resulting in feelings of being overwhelmed, stressed, and less happy (Roschina et al., 2021; Serati et al., 2021; Tsai et al., 2019). Depressive symptoms may increase the lack of confidence in the ability to nurse (Avilla et al., 2020; Mercan & Tari Selcuk, 2021).

Survivors of Trauma

Trauma can affect relationships, health care, and coping ability. How a trauma survivor reacts depends on their resilience and the protective factors they have developed. Depression is common for trauma survivors during pregnancy and the postpartum period. The risk for anxiety and **posttraumatic stress disorder** (PTSD) is also increased (Kendall-Tackett, 2022). PTSD, which can result from childbirth trauma, decreases lactation self-efficacy (Türkmen et al., 2020), as well as initiation and duration (Cook et al., 2018; Garthus-Niegel et al., 2018).

A parent's behavior may be adaptive responses to trauma they experienced. Trauma may cause parents to be hypervigilant, be easily startled, have difficulty paying attention or concentrating, or demonstrate avoidance behavior. They may feel guilt or blame or have negative thoughts about themselves or the world. They may have negative coping skills and find it difficult to trust and form attachments. They may have chronic pain, poor health, or poor hygiene habits.

The healthcare world can be scary for someone who has experienced trauma and it can cause retraumatization. The feeling of being out of control or losing autonomy is difficult. The perinatal period can be especially vulnerable, overwhelming, and frightening for someone whose background includes trauma. Trauma can significantly affect pregnancy, labor, birth, infant bonding, lactation, and parenting. Many routine birth practices violate a person's bodily autonomy and dignity. Seemingly harmless events such as childbirth and lactation have the potential to cause further trauma or trigger memories of abuse. Infertility, illness, high-risk pregnancy, traumatic birth, high-risk infant, lactation difficulties, and exhaustion are additional stressors.

Some adults who are overcoming abusive backgrounds received emotional support during childhood from a nonabusive adult and have participated in therapy and education (Chamberlain et al., 2019). They have helped to equip themselves to have a healthy, stable, and emotionally supportive relationship with their mate (Kendall-Tackett, 2016). Aspects of resiliency and recovery for survivors include becoming aware of and accepting the reality of the abuse and how it has affected their lives and ability to parent. They will navigate typical parenting challenges as they develop balance in their parental roles.

Intimate Partner Violence

Globally, women are disproportionately victims of IPV. The risk increases during pregnancy, affecting about one-quarter of women globally (Román-Gálvez et al., 2021a). Having experienced IPV before pregnancy is associated with negative attitudes during pregnancy and an inability to bond with the baby (Kita et al., 2019). The prevalence of psychological violence during pregnancy is higher when partners consume alcohol, refuse to use condoms, do not work, and are not the infant's biological father (Silva & Leite, 2020). Because refusal to use condoms is higher in relation to IPV, there is an increased likelihood of an unintended pregnancy (Flaathen et al., 2021).

IPV during pregnancy can result in preterm delivery, a low-birth-weight infant, stillbirth, or death of the abused parent (Belay et al., 2022; Da Thi Tran et al., 2022; Drexler et al., 2022; Gebreslasie et al., 2020; Román-Gálvez et al., 2021b; Yaya et al., 2021). Perinatal death may be about three times more likely (Pastor-Moreno et al., 2020). Individuals of ethnic groups exposed to violence are at increased risk of adverse outcomes (Greely et al., 2022). The incidence of homicide resulting from IPV is more than threefold higher for Black people than for White people or Hispanic people (Kivisto et al., 2022). Partner involvement and social support are two important factors that might help reduce IPV related to pregnancy and childbirth (Chan et al., 2022).

IPV that occurs during pregnancy typically continues into the postpartum period. It is estimated that one in five parents experiences psychological IPV (Martin-de-Las-Heras et al., 2019). IPV can significantly affect stress, mental disorders, substance use, and nutritional intake (Murray et al., 2020). It increases the odds of postpartum depression and decreases nursing in the year after birth (Ankerstjerne et al., 2022; Tran et al., 2022). Studies find lower rates of initiation and duration of nursing in relationships involving domestic abuse (Ribeiro et al., 2021; Tran et al., 2022; Wallenborn et al., 2018).

Adverse Childhood Experiences

Adverse childhood experiences (ACEs) affect lifelong health and behavior. Victims of ACE may experience violence, neglect, discrimination, and poverty, as well as emotional, sexual, and/or physical abuse. In a cross-sectional study of 306 nursing parents, 83% had experienced emotional or verbal abuse, and 78% had lived with someone who was depressed, mentally ill, or suicidal. Sexual abuse was reported by 46%, and 51% had experienced physical abuse as children (McCloskey & Pei, 2022).

Lactation initiation is reportedly higher among parents with two or more ACEs (Watson et al., 2021). This may reflect a greater effort to nurse and develop a strong attachment to their child or an attempt to compensate for past traumas by doing what is best for their baby. Exclusivity and duration are lower among abuse survivors (Kendall-Tackett, 2022). Some parents find it difficult to be touched and also struggle to manage the power differential with their healthcare providers (Channell Doig et al., 2020).

Sexual Abuse

A history of **sexual abuse** or assault is common among new parents (Kendall-Tackett, 2016). Physical sexual abuse involves intercourse and other forms of unwanted touch. Psychological sexual abuse can be just as devastating, with the victim being forced to view something sexual or the perpetrator taking inappropriate interest in the victim's sexual development. Verbal sexual abuse with erotic talk or innuendo also occurs.

Globally, 1 in every 20 girls aged 15 to 19 (around 13 million) has experienced forced sex during their lifetime (United Nations Children's Fund [UNICEF], 2020). The majority of sexual abuse survivors have never disclosed their history to a healthcare provider. They may feel comfortable discussing their abuse when caregivers create a safe space to listen to their concerns. Assisting parents with such an intimate topic requires listening intently with warmth and caring and regarding them with openness and acceptance.

Sexual abuse is a major risk factor for psychiatric disorders and suicide. Characteristics among survivors include depression, anxiety disorders, smoking, alcohol and drug abuse, aggression and violence, risky sexual behavior, and posttraumatic stress. Physical abuse in childhood is associated with sexual revictimization in the future (Mazzarello et al., 2022; Munroe & Shumway, 2022). There is a greater likelihood of revictimization by the adult survivor's partner and fear of abandonment (Webermann & Murphy, 2019; Zerubavel et al., 2018).

Marriage, pregnancy, birth, and lactation are common triggers for individuals who have suppressed the memory of abuse. These events can facilitate healing from the effects of childhood sexual abuse when a sense of safety and well-being is restored through nurturing, supportive relationships with others (Chamberlain et al., 2019). Another trigger for remembering abuse may be when a child reaches the age when the parent's abuse had occurred. Media coverage of others who were abused or who disclose abuse by the same perpetrator can also be a trigger. Memories may be triggered by the sounds or feelings of giving birth, the tactile sensation of nursing, the loss of control felt in the early days of parenting, or even the sight of milk during letdown. Times of stress, such as surgery, death of a loved one or the perpetrator, and quitting smoking, are triggers as well. These flashbacks can make nursing uncomfortable.

Some warning signs that may indicate a history of sexual abuse are late prenatal care, substance abuse, mental health concerns, eating disorders, poor compliance with self-care, and sexual dysfunction. Rates of teen pregnancy, prostitution, and promiscuity are higher among sexual abuse survivors. Other markers are being a high achiever, having dysfunctional relationships, fear of medical procedures, discomfort with touch, and morbid obesity. Mistrust of authority figures, fear of being out of control or dependent, and gender preference for baby and caregiver are also common. Parents who were sexually abused as children need to be approached in a way that offers a sense of safety, acceptance, sensitivity, and believability.

Survivors of sexual abuse have similar lactation rates to those of parents who have not been abused (Coles et al., 2016). The most stressful time in lactation for a survivor is during the early postpartum period, when stress, fatigue, and vulnerability are highest. Because of the intimate nature of nursing, past sexual abuse may cause a disruption in nursing. Memories, flashbacks, and feelings from the abuse may interfere with the ability to nurse directly, preferring to feed expressed milk to the baby with a bottle. The parent may appear uncomfortable positioning themselves for feeding, holding the baby, or discussing nursing.

Because sexual assault tends to occur at night or at bedtime, nighttime feedings can be especially difficult. Having someone feed expressed milk to the baby for nighttime feedings may help. When the baby gets older and becomes more playful, it may be uncomfortable to continue to nurse. Reviewing normal infant behaviors may be reassuring and help extend nursing longer. Some parents find nursing to be healing. Others find it too uncomfortable to continue and will need compassionate support with weaning.

Adjustments for Partners

Partners experience social, emotional, and behavioral adjustments as they redefine themselves as parents. As they adapt to a changed relationship with their mate, they will experience changes brought about by a new family member—a newborn baby who poses a serious responsibility (**Figure 20-2**). Their role expands to one of supporter and helpmate to the nursing parent and protector of and provider for their newborn infant. This represents a remarkable responsibility for many partners, and each will adjust in their own way as they define their new role.

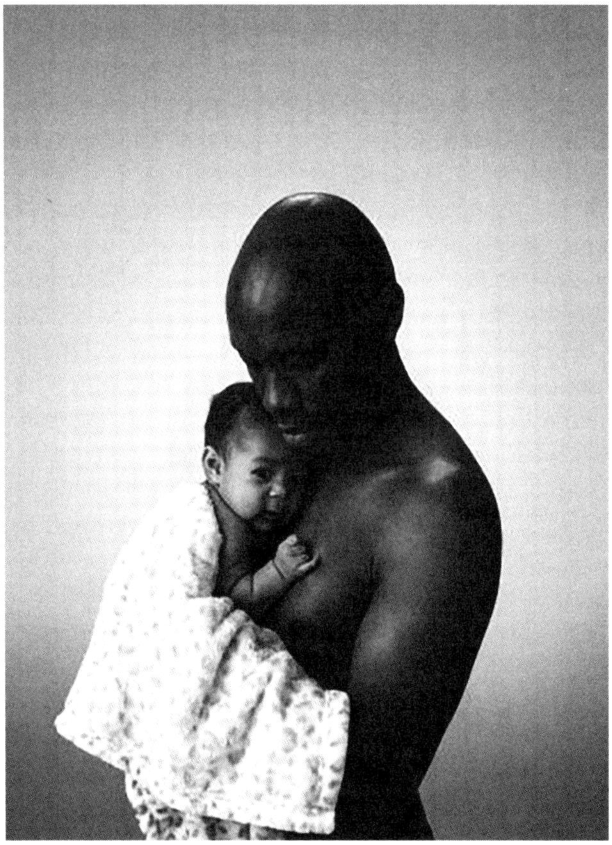

Figure 20-2 New father bonding with baby.

Courtesy of USDA's Food and Nutrition Service.

Learning the Parental Role

Early parenting is physically and emotionally intense, regardless of whether the baby is nursing. Expectant couples frequently seek prenatal classes to prepare for life with a baby. Learning what to anticipate as a couple and how to cope lowers stress and helps both parents ease into their roles. Including partners in learning about lactation strengthens their involvement and validates their reactions in the early postpartum period. Partners often express concern that nursing will limit their initial opportunity to develop a relationship with their children. With the nursing parent seemingly immersed in the care of the new baby, partners may feel as though they have lost their mate. They may also feel inadequate in their parenting abilities.

Emotional Reactions to Parenthood

Partners can experience emotional adjustments, such as feelings of abandonment and postpartum depression. Masculine norms of self-reliance and primacy of work are related to depression in male partners (Short et al., 2023). Fathers often lack support networks and have no one to turn to other than their mate and work colleagues. They may find it difficult to share emotions and feelings with other men about their new status. Although it is normal to have fears and concerns about parenthood, high rates of negative thoughts are associated with increased depression and lower perceived competency as a parent (Wroe et al., 2019).

Approximately 1 in 10 new fathers experiences postpartum depression (Bruno et al., 2020; Rao et al., 2020). Younger fathers are at increased risk for depression (Henshaw et al., 2023; Philpott et al., 2022). Depression also tends to be higher in nontraditional family structures. There is a moderate correlation between depression in both partners. Fathers are more likely to be depressed if the mother is depressed (Ansari et al., 2021; Nishigori et al., 2020; Thiel et al., 2020; Wang et al., 2021). Paternal postpartum depression increases in the first 3 to 6 months postpartum (Da Costa et al., 2019; Dennis et al., 2022).

Depression is associated with worry about parenting competence, the quality of infant temperament and interactions, sleep disturbances, and the quality of the marital relationship (Atif et al., 2022; Philpott et al., 2022). Anxiety can negatively affect partners' mental and physical well-being, social relationships, and parenting abilities. This, in turn, contributes to stress, depression, fatigue, and reduced self-efficacy. Lower education and income levels, lower coparenting and social support, and conflicts with work and family are among the factors that contribute to this anxiety.

Negotiating their role change to being parents creates tension in the couple and contributes to depression. Partner depression can decrease positive attitudes toward sex, satisfaction with the couple's relationship, and positive attitudes toward the pregnancy and the baby (Pinto et al., 2020). The child's temperament can contribute as well. Some researchers advocate assessing all new parents for their adjustment to parenting (Walsh et al., 2020).

Partners and Lactation

The lactation experience is much more rewarding and fulfilling when shared by the entire family in a positive and accepting atmosphere. Partners' views about lactation are complex and change as infants grow and partners mature in their role. When lactation problems occur, the entire family is affected, not just the nursing dyad (Hansen et al., 2018). Discussing plans for nursing enables couples to share their opinions and concerns and arrive at mutual decisions.

Counseling couples together could facilitate their support for each other in optimizing health postpartum (Benedict et al., 2018). Peer and professional support, lactation consultant service, and education can all increase support. Although attitudes can support nursing, they do not necessarily influence duration. However, involving partners could significantly increase the rates of exclusive nursing in the infant's first 6 months of life (Rempel et al., 2017).

The partner's presence affects nursing exclusivity and duration (Chan et al., 2023). Infants are more likely to be nursed if the partner has paid leave from work or is able to be home during the infant's first year (Grandahl et al., 2020). The likelihood of exclusive nursing to 6 months is higher in two-parent homes than in a single-parent home (Odar Stough et al., 2019). Babies whose parents agree on lactation are more likely to be nursed for over 6 months (Dogan et al., 2023; Marks et al., 2018).

Partner Education About Nursing

Partners who attend prenatal classes are better able to assist with feedings in tangible ways, fill in forgotten pieces of information, and provide encouragement. Prenatal classes expose partners to the normalcy of lactation and its importance to babies. Partners learn practicalities such as the ease of nighttime feedings, decrease in health issues, economic benefits, and overall convenience of nursing. These influences may further cement their support for nursing. **Table 20-1** lists

Table 20-1 Partner Education Topics

The Partner's Role	Adjusting to Living with a Baby
■ Benefits of partner involvement ■ Components of the partner's role ■ How to be engaged ■ Partner role models ■ Expectations for partners	■ Stressors: fatigue, baby crying, work/family balance ■ Relationship changes for couples ■ Emotions and concerns for the couple
Caring for the Baby	**Sharing of Partner Experiences**
■ Baby care ■ Age-appropriate toys ■ Baby carriers ■ Swaddling and baby wearing ■ Home security	■ Guests: new partners with their babies ■ Pregnancy, birth, early months with baby ■ Learning baby language: hunger, fatigue, need for calm or stimulation, crying, sleep

Data from Bourget M, Héon M, Aita M, Michaud M. An Educational Intervention to Support the Development of a Sense of Mastery of the Anticipated Paternal Role in Expectant Fathers: A Clinical Project. *J Perinat Educ.* 2017;26(1):23-36.

possible topics in teaching sessions for partners. Varied teaching strategies using videos, lectures, demonstrations, games, case studies, discussion, and invited guests will keep sessions interesting and relevant.

Partner Reaction to Nursing

Partners' ethnicity, country of origin, education level, and socioeconomic status all contribute to norms and expectations about lactation. Some partners may view the nursing parent as the main parent and feel excluded (Martínez-Plascencia et al., 2017; Sihota et al., 2019). Some may consider the process of not feeding the baby until complementary foods begin as a significant issue. Perceptions of nursing as a sexual activity may present obstacles to support. Also, attitudes about public images of nursing oftentimes influence the choice of whether to nurse exclusively (Magnusson et al., 2017). Opportunities to witness babies nursing may increase acceptance and reduce concerns that public nursing will involve excessive exposure and attract attention.

Partner's Practical Support

Entry into parenthood creates new responsibilities and changes family dynamics. A partner's support can range from caring for the baby to helping with household chores to providing strong philosophical support. Primary roles for partners are learning about, encouraging, and assisting with feedings, as well as sharing housework and child care. Involvement in caregiving, generous parental leave, and interaction-based parenting promote sensitive responsiveness in partners (Bakermans-Kranenburg & van Ijzendoorn, 2023). Shared strategies for feedings and parenting problem-solving can lower anxiety and increase partner support (Charandabi et al., 2017; Srisopa & Lucas, 2021). Partner involvement in prenatal care can reduce the incidence of postpartum blues and increase the couple's intimacy (Dehshiri et al., 2023).

Accurate and consistent information about nursing and postnatal support will enhance partner support (Baldwin et al., 2018, 2019, 2021). Learning about lactation and how to be involved enables partners to provide practical help (Leng et al., 2019; Ngoenthong et al., 2020). Participants in one study largely attributed their nursing success to the support they received from their partners (Dogan et al., 2023).

Interaction with the Baby

Partners choose their own level of comfort in the care and nurturing of their baby. Being actively involved in the pregnancy and birth enhances their participation. Partners benefit from learning about infant cues and responsiveness so that they can recognize what is normal and how to interact with their young infants. Researchers continue to study the role of hormonal changes during the transition to fatherhood in predicting father–infant interactions. Paternal oxytocin levels increase with father–infant contact, especially during skin-to-skin contact. The higher oxytocin levels are predictive of fathers' increased responsiveness and bonding with their infants (Morris et al., 2021; Scatliffe et al., 2019). Decreased paternal testosterone levels may also predict fathers' postpartum involvement and bonding (Bakermans-Kranenburg et al., 2022; Gettler et al., 2021). Men in committed relationships have lower testosterone than single men, and fathers have lower testosterone than men without children (Grebe et al., 2019).

Because partners typically spend less time with the baby than nursing parents do, they need patience and encouragement to learn their new role. This is a time of **engrossment** as they find unique ways to interact with their baby. When partners are encouraged in their role, they often become avid supporters and outspoken advocates of lactation. Partners may be further encouraged by the fact that they are the first person who teaches the baby that food and love must not always come from the same person.

Partners who participate in the birth process can begin to bond with the baby immediately after birth. Their help is invaluable in the postpartum period and beyond. They can help soothe a fussy baby through walking, rocking, singing, and cooing. They can share in the baby's care and provide the nursing parent some free time alone. Partners can bond with the baby through infant care tasks like bathing, burping, and diapering. They can transport the baby for nighttime feedings, help with positioning at feedings, carry the baby in a sling, and hold the baby skin to skin.

Babies initially indicate a preference for the nursing parent in the early postpartum period. Partners need time alone with the baby to develop their own parenting style and to learn how to interact and bond. Many partners increase their involvement as the baby gets older and responds to their attention. Whatever type of interaction partners choose, their efforts need to be accepted and encouraged without criticism or judgment. Although they may do things differently, their way may be satisfying for them and for the baby. If a certain practice might be harmful to the baby, instructive guidance can be offered without criticism (e.g., pointing out the need to support the baby's head when being held or carried).

A partner's involvement in nurturing a baby correlates with many positive outcomes for the child. Greater father–infant engagement can improve children's cognitive and socioemotional development (Garcia et al., 2022; Henry et al., 2020; Rollè et al., 2019). Babies whose fathers interact with them continually and consistently display an eagerness for learning. They are more likely to have a sense of humor and a longer attention span, a more positive self-image and exhibit more confidence in relating to males. On the other hand, disengaged and remote interactions between fathers and their infants can affect the child's social adaptation (Bureau et al., 2017; Chang et al., 2024).

Changes in Family Relationships

Changes inevitably occur in a couple's relationship as they transition to parenthood. The sense of responsibility that accompanies parenthood presents a major adjustment. Both partners may feel inadequacies and need support in establishing their new roles. Parenthood increases work/family conflict and triggers a redivision of housework (Zhang et al., 2020). New parents may react strongly to the ways in which each partner performs their role. They may find it difficult for the baby to receive a lot of the affection and intimacy previously shared only between them. At times, they may resent the disruption in their lives and their loss of freedom. Such ambivalence is normal and is often balanced by deep feelings of affection and love for their infant. If there are siblings in the family, the parents will also need to help them adjust to a new baby joining the family.

Sexual Adjustments

The need for sexual adjustment is common to most new parents. Their relationship adjustments occur during a vulnerable period for sexuality and well-being (Rosen et al., 2022). Becoming parents can initially contribute to reduced sexual desire; changes in marital relationships; and lifestyle changes, especially regarding baby care (Serrano Drozdowskyj et al., 2020). Declines in relationship quality are associated with declines in sexual satisfaction and increases in sexual distress (Tavares et al., 2024).

As parents settle into their new role, they can boost their energy by napping when the baby naps and nursing lying down. They can also explore ways to prioritize household tasks and seek help to maximize their time. Open communication between the couple and the passage of time will help in reestablishing enjoyable sexual relations. Some nursing parents report improved intimate relationships with their partners (Papp, 2012).

Resuming Sexual Intercourse

Caregivers typically advise delaying resumption of sexual intercourse until after the 6-week checkup or after **lochia** discharge has completely stopped. The 6-week checkup indicates how postpartum recovery is progressing and whether any complications exist. Some couples resume sexual intimacy before this checkup. Multiparous and younger parents report earlier resumption of sex and better satisfaction, as do those who give birth vaginally as opposed to parents who undergo cesarean birth.

Low estrogen levels while lactating result in decreased vaginal lubrication. This can cause painful intercourse, the most prevalent postpartum sexual complaint. Intercourse may also be uncomfortable because of a vaginal tear, episiotomy, abdominal incision, or internal injury from the use of forceps during delivery (Gutzeit et al., 2019; Sayed Ahmed et al., 2017). Adjustments in positioning at feedings can help alleviate the discomfort.

It is common to leak milk during intercourse as a result of the oxytocin released during orgasm. Nursing the baby before intercourse will decrease breast fullness and potential leaking. A towel can absorb dampness, and an adjustment in positioning can alleviate pressure on the breasts. Breasts may be overly sensitive during foreplay, or at the other extreme, there may be no sensual response to touch. Responses usually return to normal within several months after delivery, although this change can continue throughout lactation.

Either partner may be reluctant to engage in foreplay that involves the breasts for fear of passing on germs. If the skin is healthy and unbroken, the chances of transmitting an infection are minimal. Antibodies to the partner's germs pass through the milk and protect the baby from infection. Showering or washing the breasts before nursing the baby after sex will provide further protection.

Sexual Responsiveness

It can sometimes take several months to regain sexual desire or for responses to return to normal after giving birth. For some parents, the affection and emotional gratification received from the baby may diminish the need for further intimacy. On the other hand, the hormones associated with lactation may increase their libido. Both responses are normal. A feeling of increased sensuality or sexual arousal when nursing the baby is common. The sensation is a result of the hormone oxytocin released during both lactation and sexual orgasm.

Although sexual desire and frequency of intercourse are lower among nursing parents, the level of satisfaction appears similar to that of nonnursing parents (Alp Yılmaz et al., 2019). Parents who are depressed or exclusively nursing have an increased likelihood of problems with sexual functioning (Matthies et al., 2019; Szöllősi & Szabó, 2021). Postpartum sexual health is influenced by a partner's understanding of the changes in the female body and sexual responses after giving birth. This support may be more important than the factors of nursing, pain, stress, body image, or social support (Fuentealba-Torres et al., 2019).

Menstruation and Fertility

A phase of **amenorrhea** (absence of menstruation) occurs in the initial postpartum period and for several months thereafter. The early establishment of frequent and strong sucking is the single most important factor in suppressing ovulation during lactation (Academy of Breastfeeding Medicine [ABM], 2015). The baby's sucking and other stimuli alter the release of hormones and disrupt the cycle of ovulation and menstruation. Various hormones are involved, with links between levels of gonadotropin-releasing hormone, **luteinizing hormone**, follicle-stimulating hormone, prolactin, and estrogen.

Menstruation may resume at any time during lactation and greatly depends on overall feeding patterns. The length of amenorrhea and infertility is linked to nursing frequency, short intervals between feedings, duration of feedings, the presence of nighttime feedings, and the absence of supplemental foods in the baby's diet. The menstrual cycle can be delayed for several months, followed by a period of resumed menstrual cycles that may be **anovulatory** (producing an inadequate ovum).

Menstruation could resume as early as 6 to 12 weeks or after lactation has totally ceased. Scanty bleeding may occur before full menstrual cycles resume. Bleeding during the second month postpartum can signal an end to lochial discharge or may reflect a change in activity level. If other bleeding occurs or bleeding is accompanied by lactation difficulties, immediate healthcare advice is recommended.

Babies can continue to nurse during menstrual cycling. Menstruation causes no significant changes in the composition of the milk. Hormonal changes may alter the taste of the milk, which can cause fussiness during a feeding or a refusal to nurse. The baby's reaction may also result from heightened tension in the parent or swelling in the breast caused by menstrual edema and hormones. Any of these factors can affect letdown.

Contraception

Many options for **contraception** are compatible with lactation. The World Health Organization (WHO) offers comprehensive information about contraceptive choices worldwide. A mobile application, Medical Eligibility Criteria for Contraceptive Use, is available for smartphones. This free app from the WHO (2019) reviews the medical eligibility criteria for use of contraception, as well as the safety of various methods. The WHO recommendations are based on systematic reviews of available clinical and epidemiologic research and are updated regularly.

Lactational Amenorrhea Method

Lactation can delay the return of fertility during the postpartum period. When babies nurse fully (i.e., frequently, day and night) and menstrual cycling has not resumed, the rate of contraceptive protection from pregnancy for 6 months after birth is 98% (Calik-Ksepka et al., 2022). This protection is called the **lactational amenorrhea method (LAM)**

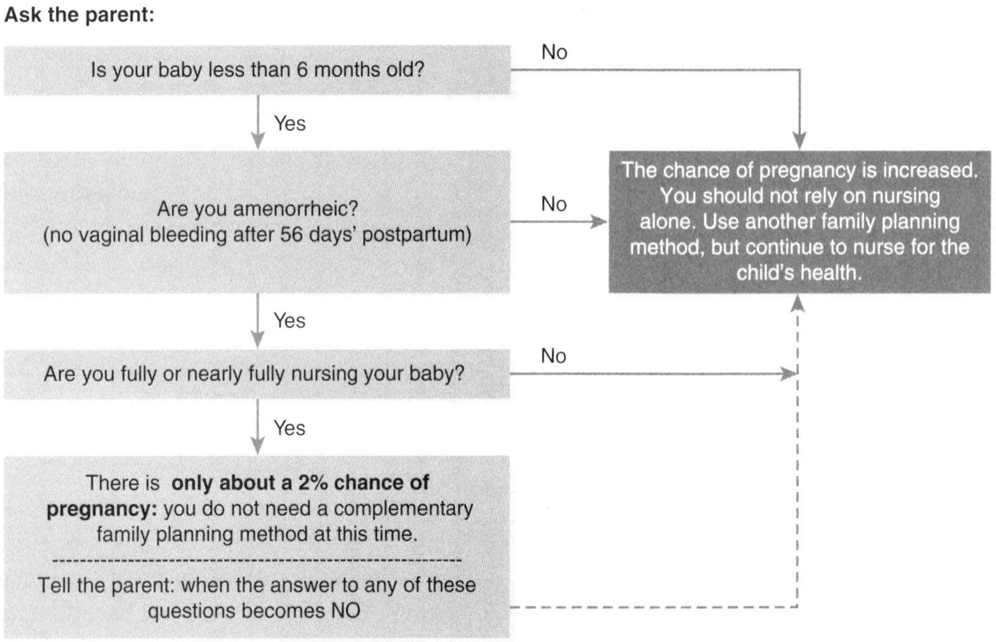

Figure 20-3 Lactational amenorrhea method.

Reprinted with permission of the institute for international studies in natural family planning from guidelines for breastfeeding in family planning and child survivial programs, Washington DC, Georgetown University, Labbok M, Koniz-Booher P, Cooney K, Shelton J, and Krasovack K (eds); Jan 1990.

of contraception (**Figure 20-3**). LAM requires that **menses** has not returned, the baby nurses around the clock without significant amounts of other foods, and the baby is younger than 6 months of age.

Parents are often unaware of nursing's effects on menses and fertility and have no knowledge of LAM as a contraceptive method (Eticha et al., 2023; Hoyt-Austin et al., 2023). Awareness is especially low among adolescents (Birabwa et al., 2022; Figaroa et al., 2020). A Cochrane review found no clear differences in pregnancy rates between parents using LAM and fully nursing amenorrheic parents not using any method (Van der Wijden & Manion, 2015).

If any one of the three conditions for LAM is not met, there is an increased risk of pregnancy, requiring another contraceptive method to ensure adequate protection. To be most effective, it is recommended that the baby nurse soon after birth and continue to nurse exclusively, day and night, for 6 months. The use of artificial nipples, such as a bottle or pacifier, interferes with the frequency and duration of sucking during feedings and should be avoided. Contraceptive protection from LAM decreases as soon as there is a decline in nursing, either because complementary foods or supplements have begun or the baby is nursing less often. An online educational tool can help with the transition from amenorrhea to ovulation, lowering unintended pregnancies to 2% at 12 months (Fehring et al., 2017).

Natural Family Planning

Periodic abstinence, or **natural family planning**, is a contraceptive method that involves charting the basal body temperature (temperature taken on waking, at around the same time each day) or checking vaginal secretions. It requires keeping a careful calendar record of menstrual periods to predict fertile days. Typical effectiveness for natural family planning in preventing pregnancy is estimated at 76%. The couple's motivation and commitment to the method are necessary to achieve a higher rate of effectiveness. When used exactly as intended under perfect conditions, natural family planning is estimated to be 95% effective (Berglund Scherwitzl et al., 2017).

In natural family planning, changes in cervical mucus before ovulation help signal the beginning of the fertile days. These signs can be quite different during lactation. Cervical mucus patterns in the first few months postpartum may be less clearly defined than after regular cycles have resumed. Mucus changes from a scant semisolid white or yellowish matter to an abundant thin, clear, watery, and slippery fluid that allows the sperm to penetrate the canal of the cervix easily. Fluctuations in basal body temperature help predict fertile periods. Basal body temperature is at its lowest during menses and up to ovulation. After ovulation, the temperature rises and levels off until just before the onset of menses.

Monitoring mucus and temperature changes identifies the 5 to 7 days per month when pregnancy can occur. Websites and electronic apps are available to predict fertile windows for natural family planning (Simmons et al., 2017). However, most are generally inaccurate, with wide variability in the range of the fertility window (Ali et al., 2020; Ford et al., 2022; Manhart & Duane, 2022; Worsfold et al., 2021).

Oral Contraceptives

High-quality research on hormonal methods for contraception related to lactation and neonatal growth outcomes is limited. Nonhormonal and progestin-only oral contraceptives are preferred over combination oral contraceptives (Spencer et al., 2022). There is variability in individual sensitivity to the effects of progesterone and estrogen on milk production. If estrogen-containing contraception is used, the lowest estrogen dosage appropriate is recommended, along with monitoring of milk production. Caution is advised when there are problems with milk production and when nursing a child 1 year old or older (Infant Risk Center, 2019).

Combination oral contraceptives contain the hormones estrogen and progesterone, and estrogen can lower milk production. They appear to cause the most difficulty before lactation is well established. The timing of beginning contraception and sensitivity to estrogenic effects appear to be highly variable. As noted in **Table 20-2**, use of a combination pill is not recommended until after 21 days postpartum because of an increased risk of thromboembolism postdelivery (Centers for Disease Control and Prevention [CDC], 2016; Peragallo Urrutia et al., 2018; Trussell et al., 2018).

Progestin-only oral contraceptives (the mini-pill) do not appear to interfere with milk production and are therefore considered acceptable during lactation. Generally, this method should be delayed until 6 weeks postpartum. There are numerous anecdotal reports of drops in milk production after starting the progesterone-only pill. Milk production recovers when the pill is discontinued. In a study of parents intending to nurse for at least 4 months, those using progestin-only pills were the most likely to achieve their feeding goals. Parents using combination estrogen/progestin pills were the least likely to reach their goals (Goulding et al., 2018).

Contraceptive Devices and Procedures

A variety of devices and procedures are available for contraception. Long-acting reversible contraceptives (LARCs) are popular as first-line contraceptive methods. They are inserted by healthcare providers and offer the most available form of contraception that is reversible. The primary ones are intrauterine devices (IUDs), vaginal rings, and hormone-emitting subdermal **implants**. Once inserted, the devices can remain in place for 3 to 10 years (CDC, 2023). **Barrier methods** and sterilization are other options.

Intrauterine Device. An **intrauterine device (IUD)** is a copper or hormonal device placed into the uterus. The copper IUD prevents a fertilized egg from implanting on the lining of the uterus. This nonhormonal IUD does not seem to have any effect on lactation. Hormonal IUDs slowly release progesterone which thickens the cervical mucus. They act as a barrier to the entry of sperm into the uterus, thereby preventing implantation of a fertilized egg. Mean time to lactogenesis and lactation rates are similar between immediate and delayed insertion of progesterone-emitting IUDs (Levi et al., 2018; Stanton & Blumenthal, 2019).

Complication rates are low in both copper and hormonal IUDs. The risk of uterine perforation may be greater in the postpartum period, especially during lactation (Barnett et al., 2017; Heinemann et al., 2017; Reed et al., 2022). The WHO and reproductive health experts caution that use of the general acronym *IUD* fails to clarify whether the device releases a hormone. They recommend the nomenclature be replaced with the terms *nonhormonal IUD* and *hormonal IUD* to better describe each type for a broad global audience (Creinin et al., 2022; WHO, 2021).

Vaginal Ring. The progesterone-releasing **vaginal ring** can be self-inserted and has similar effectiveness rates during lactation as a copper IUD. The ability to self-insert this device makes it easier to use and reduces reliance on healthcare providers for placement. It is designed for 3-month use, and must be renewed every 3 months as long as nursing continues. Vaginal ring users maintain lactational amenorrhea significantly longer than IUD users (Roy et al., 2020).

Transdermal Patch. A **transdermal patch** contains estrogen and progesterone. It is applied once weekly for 3 weeks, followed by a patch-free week. Contraceptive effectiveness appears to be similar to that of a combined oral contraceptive. Effectiveness is lower for individuals who are obese (Nelson et al., 2021). Breakthrough bleeding and spotting are less common with the patch than with oral contraceptives.

Implants. Levonorgestrel is an implant made of a small plastic rod inserted surgically under the skin of the upper arm. The rod slowly releases progesterone

Table 20-2 Recommendations and Risk Classifications for Contraceptive Methods Postpartum

Condition	CHC	POP	DMPA	Implants	LNG-IUD	Cu-IUD
Postpartum (nonnursing)						
a. <21 days	4	1	1	1		
b. 21 days to 42 days						
• With other risk factors for VTE	3*	1	1	1		
• Without other risk factors for VTE	2	1	1	1		
c. >42 days	1	1	1	1		
Postpartum (nursing)						
a. <21 days	4	2	2	2		
b. 21 to <30 days						
• With other risk factors for VTE	3*	2	2	2		
• Without other risk factors for VTE	3	2	2	2		
c. 30–42 days						
• With other risk factors for VTE	3*	1	1	1		
• Without other risk factors for VTE	2	1	1	1		
d. >42 days	2	1	1	1		
Postpartum (nursing or nonnursing including post-cesarean delivery)						
a. <10 min after delivery of the placenta					2	1
b. 10 min after delivery of the placenta to <4 wk					2	2
c. ≥4 wk					1	1
d. Puerperal sepsis					4	4

BMI = body mass index; CHC = combined hormonal contraceptives (oral, patch, ring); Cu-IUD = copper- containing intrauterine device; DMPA = depot medroxyprogesterone acetate; LNG-IUD = levonorgestrel-releasing intrauterine device; POP = progestin-only pill; VTE = venous thromboembolism.

Categories: 1 = there is no restriction for the use of the contraceptive method; 2 = the advantages of using the method generally outweigh the theoretical or proven risks; 3 = the theoretical or proven risks usually outweigh the advantages of using the method; 4 = there is an unacceptable health risk if the contraceptive method is used.

*Note: With other risk factors for VTE (such as age ≥35 years, previous VTE, thrombophilia, immobility, transfusion at delivery, BMI ≥30 kg/m^2, postpartum hemorrhage, post-cesarean delivery, preeclampsia, or smoking) the classification may increase to a 4.

Data from CDC's U.S. Medical Eligibility Criteria for Contraceptive Use, 2020. https://www.cdc.gov/reproductivehealth/contraception/pdf/summary-chart-us-medical-eligibility-criteria_508tagged.pdf

into the body for up to 3 years. Levonorgestrel can also be implanted in the uterus for up to 5 years. Randomized controlled studies found that immediate postpartum implants did not affect infant growth or lactation (Averbach et al., 2019; Turok et al., 2017).

Injectables. Medroxyprogesterone depot injections given every 3 months include the trade names Depo-Provera and NET-EN. Infertility may last up to 1 year or longer after the depot subsides. Lactation consultants have noted impaired milk production with the administration of **injectables** immediately postpartum. The ABM recommends delaying the use of progesterone injectables until lactation is well established.

Barrier Methods. Barrier methods include condoms, diaphragms, cervical caps, and the use of a spermicide with or without physical barriers. Spermicides destroy sperm before they can reach and fertilize an egg. A male condom is a thin latex or silicone sheath that covers the penis. A female condom is a thin polyurethane sheath with soft rings at each end. One ring is covered with polyurethane and fits over the cervix to act as an anchor. A larger, open ring stays outside the vagina, covering part of the **perineum** and labia during intercourse. The diaphragm and cervical cap are dome-shaped devices that cover the cervix to stop sperm from entering the uterus. The diaphragm covers a larger area of the vagina, whereas the cervical cap covers only the cervix. Spermicides used without a physical barrier average 28% failure rates for typical users. Male condoms have about a 13% failure rate and female condoms about 21%. Diaphragms average 17% failure rates (CDC, 2023).

Sterilization. Female sterilization is the most common method of contraception worldwide (Christin-Maitre, 2022). Bilateral **tubal ligation** ties the fallopian tubes to prevent released eggs from reaching the ovaries and to block sperm from accessing the egg. Many women undergo tubal ligations following a vaginal or cesarean delivery, known as a *postpartum ligation*. Male vasectomies are typically easier to perform and less invasive than tubal ligation. The surgery snips the vas deferens, the main duct in the penis through which sperm travel during ejaculation. Sterilization is a permanent decision, although a vasectomy may be reversed.

Reproductive Coercion

There is an established link between reproductive health and IPV (Bauleni et al., 2018; Mandal et al., 2018). Women who experience IPV, who are in underrepresented racial/ethnic groups, and who are of lower socioeconomic status are more likely to experience **reproductive coercion** (Rosenfeld et al., 2018). The incidence is almost one in eight adolescent females (Hill et al., 2019).

Reproductive coercion interferes with decision-making related to reproductive health. It involves behavior intended to maintain power and control in a relationship (Capasso et al., 2019; Kusunoki & Barber, 2019). Behaviors include attempts to impregnate a partner against their will, control pregnancy outcome, coerce a partner into having unprotected sex, and interfere with contraceptive methods (American College of Obstetricians and Gynecologists [ACOG], 2019). Interventions for clients who experience reproductive and sexual coercion include educating them about the symptoms and outcomes of coercive behaviors, counseling on harm-reduction strategies, and offering long-acting methods of contraception that are less detectable to partners (ACOG, 2019).

Sibling Reactions and Adjustments

Welcoming a new baby can range from a smooth adjustment to a distant or demanding attitude by siblings (**Figure 20-4**). Reactions can depend on the child's age and the length of separation following the birth of the new baby. The nursing parent may be engrossed with the baby and feel less close to their other children for a while. This can cause the children to appear distant and display jealousy. They may develop a closer relationship with their other parent or another relative in the early weeks and appear distant with the nursing parent. Relationships will mend as all family members learn to bond with the baby in their own way.

Parents can begin preparing their children for the baby's arrival by sharing the events of pregnancy with them. They can explain how a baby develops, visits to the caregiver, and what will happen in the hospital. They can read books or share media with their children depicting a new baby in the family. Children can participate by helping with baby clothes and equipment and preparing for the hospital stay. Any changes in the child's sleeping arrangements should occur early and in such a way that the older child does not feel crowded out by the new baby.

Parents can create a booklet with pictures about what it is like in the hospital, coming home, at home with the baby (bathing, sleeping, nursing, crying), and the new family. Reviewing the family's current baby pictures and videos can be fun, too. Parents can prepare the child for what new babies do, such

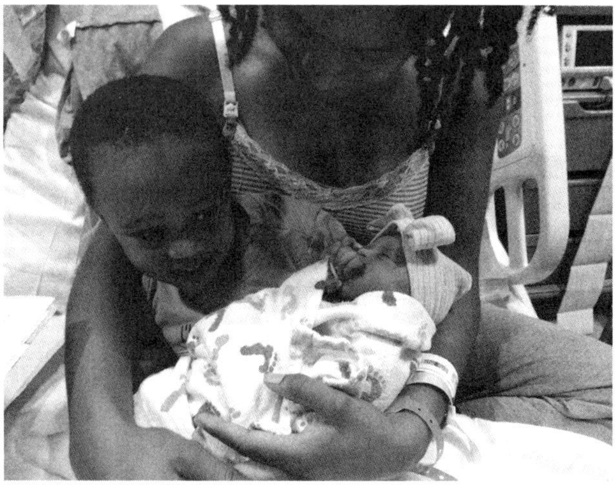

Figure 20-4 Sibling enjoying time with the new baby.

Printed with permission of Anna Swisher.

as nursing, sleeping, and crying, and the fact that they are not yet able to play. They can explain any changes that will take place in usual family activities and the reasons for the changes. They can involve the child in caring for the new baby, enlisting help with bringing diapers and clothes, holding and talking to the baby, and encouraging the baby to smile. Siblings can visit a family with a new baby to observe how a baby appears and sounds and how it has changed their family.

Adjusting to the New Baby

Whenever a new baby joins a family, the role of each family member is redefined and expanded. An older child who previously had been the "baby of the family" is no longer the center of attention. Older children may assume responsibility for tasks previously performed by their parents. Parents may expect them to dress themselves, help with household chores, and generally fend for themselves instead of always relying on someone to help them. The ease with which they do this will depend on their age, their personality, and their sense of security.

Each child needs time and understanding when assuming a new role in the family. Parents can help the child feel special in new ways. They can foster the older child's emotional growth by giving them undivided attention the first time they are together after the birth of the baby. Another adult can hold the baby while they renew contact and express love with the older child. After the family is settled, parents can create situations in which each child can interact with and hold the baby.

Some young children display regressive behaviors when a new baby arrives. Reactions can include whining, baby talk, bed-wetting or accidents in a previously toilet-trained child, waking during the night, clinging to the parent, or hitting the baby. Such behavior may be the child's way of seeking attention and reassurance. They may enjoy cuddling and talking to the baby but, at the same time, find it difficult to share the parent's attention. Spending focused time with each parent can help alleviate an older child's feelings of displacement and ease the adjustment to being the older sibling.

Sibling Behavior During Feedings

A sibling may want to be included in the closeness and interaction during feedings. Parents can accommodate this by nursing the baby where there is ample room for all family members, such as on the bed, couch, or floor. They can plan activities to share with the toddler during nursing times, such as reading books, playing simple games ("I spy something red"), and activities (paper and crayons, tea party, puzzles, board games, selective use of electronic games and media, or playing music).

If a toddler who had weaned asks to nurse again, the parent's awareness of the child's needs and their willingness to respond favorably are reassuring to the child. The child may want only to taste the milk, in which case some expressed milk in a cup may satisfy their curiosity. This renewed interest in nursing is usually temporary. Occasionally, a toddler resumes nursing on a regular basis, and these parents will benefit from support for tandem nursing, discussed in **Chapter 15**.

Summary

Support for couples will encourage them as they mature into the parental role. Understanding typical postpartum adjustments can help parents avoid needless worry. Learning about the differences between baby blues, postpartum depression, and postpartum psychosis is crucial. Partners have their own unique adjustments as they provide support to the nursing parent and learn how to interact with their new baby. Parents will experience changes in their sexual relationship and will need to learn about contraceptive options that are compatible with nursing and fit their lifestyle. Siblings benefit from preparation for the birth, as well as extra patience, love, and understanding as they adjust to the new baby. This is an exciting time for the family as they welcome a new baby into their home and learn to respond to one another in new ways.

What You Learned–At a Glance

Conversation Starters with Parents

- What are your sources for information about infant feeding?
- How many of your friends and family members nurse their babies?
- How are you and your partner adjusting to life with a nursing baby?
- What are your plans for contraception?
- How are your other children adjusting to your new baby?

Becoming Parents

- Parents seek information and support on the internet and through parenting programs.
- Parents progress through anticipatory, formal, informal, and personal stages in their role acquisition.
- Parents need to know the danger of sleep training programs for lactation and the baby.

Adjustments for the Nursing Parent

- Encourage parents to express their feelings.
- Encourage friendships with other new parents.
- Help parents recognize that not all problems with the baby are related to nursing.
- Recognize when baby blues progress to depression or psychosis.
- Recognize characteristics of survivors of sexual abuse.
- Help parents anticipate their physical recovery and emotional adjustments after birth.

Adjustments for the Partner

- Partners experience social, emotional, and behavioral adjustments.
- Fathers may experience postpartum depression.
- Learning about lactation to help the nursing parent, interacting with the baby, and sharing housework and child care are primary roles for partners.
- A partner's involvement with their baby correlates with positive outcomes for the child.

Sexual Adjustment

- The need for sexual adjustment is common to new parents.
- Nursing parents are fatigued and may not desire intimacy.
- The breasts are sensitive and may leak during sex.
- Lactation hormones decrease vaginal lubrication.
- Incisions from birth may cause discomfort during sex.
- Sensitivity and adjustments in routine will help parents through this time.

Menstruation and Fertility

- Amenorrhea (lack of menstruation) depends on feeding frequency, duration, nighttime feeds, and absence of other foods or pacifier use.
- Menstruation may resume at any time during lactation.
- Lactational amenorrhea contraception requires no return of menses, exclusive nursing, and a baby younger than 6 months.
- Nonhormonal and progestin-only contraceptives are preferred over combination oral contraceptives.

Sibling Adjustments

- Involving siblings in preparing for the baby will help them welcome the baby.
- Preparing children for the parents' absence during birth will ease the separation.
- Older children need to adjust to a new role in the family.
- Siblings may express a desire to resume nursing.

References

Academy of Breastfeeding Medicine. ABM clinical protocol #13: contraception during breastfeeding, revised 2015. *Breastfeed Med.* 2015;10:3–12.

Adams YJ, et al. Postpartum care needs assessment: women's understanding of postpartum care, practices, barriers, and educational needs. *BMC Pregnancy Childbirth.* 2023;23(1):502.

Adina J, et al. Effect of parenting interventions on perinatal depression and implications for infant developmental outcomes: a systematic review and meta-analysis. *Clin Child Fam Psychol Rev.* 2022;25(2):316–338.

Ali R, et al. Do fertility tracking applications offer women useful information about their fertile window? *Reprod Biomed Online.* 2020:S1472-6483(20)30509-5.

Alimi R, et al. The association of breastfeeding with a reduced risk of postpartum depression: a systematic review and meta-analysis. *Breastfeed Med.* 2022;17(4):290–296.

Alp Yılmaz F, et al. Breastfeeding and sexual activity and sexual quality in postpartum women. *Breastfeed Med.* 2019;14(8):587–591.

American College of Obstetricians and Gynecologists. ACOG Committee opinion no. 554: reproductive and sexual coercion. Reaffirmed 2019. https://www.acog.org/Clinical-Guidance-and-Publications/Committee-Opinions/Committee-on-Health-Care-for-Underserved-Women/Reproductive-and-Sexual-Coercion

Ankerstjerne LBS, et al. Landscaping the evidence of intimate partner violence and postpartum depression: a systematic review. *BMJ Open.* 2022;12(5):e051426.

Ansari NS, et al. Risk factors for postpartum depressive symptoms among fathers: a systematic review and meta-analysis. *Acta Obstet Gynecol Scand.* 2021;100(7):1186–1199.

Asadi M, et al. Identifying women's needs to adjust to postpartum changes: a qualitative study in Iran. *BMC Pregnancy Childbirth.* 2022;22(1):115.

Atif M, et al. Risk factors of paternal postnatal depression in Pakistan: findings from an urban sample. *Nurs Health Sci.* 2022;24(3): 618–624.

Averbach S, et al. The effect of immediate postpartum levonorgestrel contraceptive implant use on breastfeeding and infant growth: a randomized controlled trial. *Contraception.* 2019;99(2): 87–93.

Avilla JC, et al. Association between maternal satisfaction with breastfeeding and postpartum depression symptoms. *PLoS One.* 2020;15(11):e0242333.

Bakermans-Kranenburg MJ, van Ijzendoorn MH. Sensitive responsiveness in expectant and new fathers. *Curr Opin Psychol.* 2023;50:101580.

Bakermans-Kranenburg MJ, et al. Is paternal oxytocin an oxymoron? Oxytocin, vasopressin, testosterone, oestradiol and cortisol in emerging fatherhood. *Philos Trans R Soc Lond B Biol Sci.* 2022;377(1858):20210060.

Baldwin A, et al. Transition to parenthood: antenatal education promotes perinatal mental health when collaboratively delivered by midwives, mental health peer workers and perinatal and infant mental health professionals. *J Perinat Educ.* 2022;31(2):104–110.

Baldwin S, et al. Mental health and wellbeing during the transition to fatherhood: a systematic review of first-time fathers' experiences. *JBI Database of Systematic Reviews and Implementation Reports.* 2018;16:2118–2191.

Baldwin S, et al. A qualitative exploratory study of UK first-time fathers' experiences, mental health and wellbeing needs during their transition to fatherhood. *BMJ Open 9.* 2019;13;9(9): E030792. https://bmjopen.bmj.com/content/9/9/e030792.info

Baldwin S, et al. A mixed-methods feasibility study of an intervention to improve men's mental health and wellbeing during their transition to fatherhood. *BMC Public Health.* 2021;21:1813.

Barkmann C, et al. Is very low infant birth weight a predictor for a five-year course of depression in parents? A latent growth curve model. *J Affect Disord.* 2018;229:415–420.

Barnett C, et al. Perforation risk and intra-uterine devices: results of the EURAS-IUD 5-year extension study. *Eur J Contracept Reprod Health Care.* 2017;22(6):424–428.

Bauleni EM, et al. Intimate-partner violence and reproductive decision-making by women attending Victorian maternal- and child-health services: a cross-sectional study. *Aust J Prim Health.* 2018;24(5):422–427.

Bauman BL, et al. Vital signs: postpartum depressive symptoms and provider discussions about perinatal depression—United States, 2018. *MMWR Morb Mortal Wkly Rep.* 2020; 69(19):575–581.

Belay HG, et al. Intimate partner violence during pregnancy and adverse birth outcomes in Ethiopia: a systematic review and meta-analysis. *PLoS One.* 2022;17(12):e0275836.

Benedict RK, et al. Effectiveness of programmes and interventions to support optimal breastfeeding among children 0-23 months, South Asia: a scoping review. *Matern Child Nutr.* 2018; 14(suppl 4):e12697.

Berglund Scherwitzl E, et al. Perfect-use and typical-use Pearl Index of a contraceptive mobile app. *Contraception.* 2017;96(6): 420–425.

Beurel E, et al. The bidirectional relationship of depression and inflammation: double trouble. *Neuron.* 2020;107(2):234–256.

Birabwa C, et al. Knowledge and use of lactational amenorrhoea as a family planning method among adolescent mothers in Uganda: a secondary analysis of demographic and health surveys between 2006 and 2016. *BMJ Open.* 2022;12(2):e054609.

Brown AE. What do women lose if they are prevented from meeting their breastfeeding goals? *Clin Lact (Amarillo).* 2018; 9(4):200–207.

Bruno A, et al. When fathers begin to falter: a comprehensive review on paternal perinatal depression. *Int J Environ Res Public Health.* 2020;17(4):1139.

Bulteau S, et al. Higher negative self-reference level in patients with personality disorders and suicide attempt(s) history during biological treatment for major depressive disorder: clinical implications. *Front Psychol.* 2021;12:631614.

Bureau JF, et al. Correlates of child-father and child-mother attachment in the preschool years. *Attach Hum Dev.* 2017;19(2): 130–150.

Calik-Ksepka A, et al. Lactational amenorrhea: neuroendocrine pathways controlling fertility and bone turnover. *Int J Mol Sci.* 2022;23(3):1633.

Capasso A, et al. Pregnancy coercion as a risk factor for HIV and other sexually transmitted infections among young African American women. *J Acquir Immune Defic Syndr.* 2019;82(suppl 2):S155–S161.

Cato K, et al. Antenatal depressive symptoms and early initiation of breastfeeding in association with exclusive breastfeeding six weeks postpartum: a longitudinal population-based study. *BMC Pregnancy Childbirth.* 2019;19(1):49.

Centers for Disease Control and Prevention. CDC's U.S. medical eligibility criteria for contraceptive use. 2016. https://www.cdc.gov/reproductivehealth/contraception/mmwr/mec/summary.html

Centers for Disease Control and Prevention. Reproductive health. Contraception. Birth control methods. May 1, 2023. https://www.cdc.gov/reproductivehealth/contraception/index.htm

Chamberlain C, et al. Parenting after a history of childhood maltreatment: a scoping review and map of evidence in the perinatal period. *PLoS One.* 2019;14(3):e0213460.

Chan K, et al. Breastfeeding in Canada: predictors of initiation, exclusivity, and continuation from the 2017–2018 Canadian Community Health Survey. *Appl Physiol Nutr Metab.* 2023;48(3): 256–269.

Chan KL, et al. Intimate partner violence before pregnancy, during pregnancy, and after childbirth: a new conceptualization highlighting individual changes in violence against pregnant women over time. *J Interpers Violence.* 2022;37(13–14): NP12111–NP12132.

Chang R, et al. Associations of father absence and limited access to books and toys with early childhood development among children aged 0–6 years in a rural county lifted out of poverty in China. *Child Care Health Dev.* 2024;50(1):e13145.

Channell Doig A, et al. Breastfeeding among mothers who have experienced childhood maltreatment: a review. *J Hum Lact.* 2020;36(4):710–722.

Charandabi SM, et al. The effect of life style based education on the fathers' anxiety and depression during pregnancy and postpartum periods: a randomized controlled trial. *Community Ment Health J.* 2017;53(4):482–489.

Chee RM, et al. The impact of social media influencers on pregnancy, birth, and early parenting experiences: a systematic review. *Midwifery.* 2023;120:103623.

Chirumamilla S, Gulati M. Patient education and engagement through social media. *Curr Cardiol Rev.* 2021;17(2): 137–143.

Christin-Maitre S. La contraception à travers le monde [Worldwide contraception]. *Med Sci (Paris).* 2022;38(5):457–463. French.

Coles J, et al. Breastfeeding duration after childhood sexual abuse: an Australian cohort study. *J Hum Lact.* 2016;32(3):NP28–NP35.

Coo S, et al. The role of perinatal anxiety and depression in breastfeeding practices. *Breastfeed Med.* 2020;15(8):495–500.

Cook N, et al. Maternal posttraumatic stress disorder during the perinatal period and child outcomes: a systematic review. *J Affect Disord.* 2018;225:18–31.

Cooklin AR, et al. Physical health, breastfeeding problems and maternal mood in the early postpartum: a prospective cohort study. *Arch Women's Ment Health.* 2018;21(3):365–374.

Cox L, et al. Edinburgh Postnatal Depression Scale (EPDS). *Br J Psychiatry.* 1987;150:782–786.

Creinin M, et al. Society of Family Planning Committee statement on IUD nomenclature. *Contraception.* 2022;106:1–2.

Da Costa D, et al. A prospective study of postnatal depressive symptoms and associated risk factors in first-time fathers. *J Affect Disord.* 2019;249:371–377.

Dagla M, et al. Women's mental health as a factor associated with exclusive breastfeeding and breastfeeding duration: data from a longitudinal study in Greece. *Children (Basel).* 2021;8(2):150.

Daoud N, et al. Postpartum depression prevalence and risk factors among Indigenous, non-Indigenous and immigrant women in Canada. *Can J Public Health.* 2019;110(4):440–452.

Da Thi Tran T, et al. Intimate partner violence during pregnancy and maternal and child health outcomes: a scoping review of the literature from low-and-middle income countries from 2016–2021. *BMC Pregnancy Childbirth.* 2022;22(1):315.

Dehshiri M, et al. Effects of husband involvement in prenatal care on couples' intimacy and postpartum blues in primiparous women: a quasi-experimental study. *Int J Community Based Nurs Midwifery.* 2023;11(3):179–189.

Dennis CL, et al. Paternal prevalence and risk factors for comorbid depression and anxiety across the first 2 years postpartum: a nationwide Canadian cohort study. *Depress Anxiety.* 2022; 39(3):233–245.

Dinwiddie KJ, et al. Postpartum depression in adolescent mothers. *J Psychosom Obstet Gynaecol.* 2018;39(3):168–175.

Dogan J, et al. "Don't feel like you have to do this all on your own": exploring perceived partner support of breastfeeding among black women in Kentucky. *J Hum Lact.* 2023;39(1): 134–145.

Drexler KA, et al. Intimate partner violence and trauma-informed care in pregnancy. *Am J Obstet Gynecol MFM.* 2022;4(2): 100542.

Eticha TG, et al. Knowledge of lactation amenorrhea method among postpartum women in Ethiopia: a facility-based cross-sectional study. *Sci Rep.* 2023;13(1):14916.

Farsi D. Social media and health care, part I: literature review of social media use by health care providers. *J Med Internet Res.* 2021;23(4):e23205.

Fehring RJ, et al. Effectiveness of an online natural family planning program for breastfeeding women. *J Obstet Gynecol Neonatal Nurs.* 2017;46(4):e129–e137.

Figaroa MNS, et al. Lactational amenorrhoea among adolescent girls in low-income and middle-income countries: a systematic scoping review. *BMJ Glob Health.* 2020;5(10):e002492.

Figueiredo B, et al. Exclusive breastfeeding moderates the association between prenatal and postpartum depression. *J Hum Lact.* 2021;37(4):784–794.

Finlayson K, et al. What matters to women in the postnatal period: a meta-synthesis of qualitative studies. *PLoS One.* 2020;15(4):e0231415.

Flaathen EME, et al. Intimate partner violence and the association of pregnancy intendedness—a cross-sectional study in southeastern Norway. *Sex Reprod Healthc.* 2021;29:100651.

Ford EA, et al. A scoping review of the information provided by fertility smartphone applications. *Hum Fertil (Camb).* 2022;25(4): 625–639.

Forgie EME, et al. Social media and the transformation of the physician-patient relationship: viewpoint. *J Med Internet Res.* 2021;23(12):e25230.

Friedman SH, et al. Postpartum psychosis. *Curr Psychiatry Rep.* 2023;25(2):65–72.

Fuentealba-Torres M, et al. What are the prevalence and factors associated with sexual dysfunction in breastfeeding women? A Brazilian cross-sectional analytical study. *BMJ Open.* 2019;9(4): e025833.

Garcia IL, et al. Father involvement and early child development in a low-resource setting. *Soc Sci Med.* 2022;302:114933.

Garthus-Niegel S, et al. The influence of postpartum PTSD on breastfeeding: a longitudinal population-based study. *Birth.* 2018;45(2):193–201.

Gebreslasie KZ, et al. Intimate partner violence during pregnancy and risk of still birth in hospitals of Tigray region Ethiopia. *Ital J Pediatr.* 2020;46(1):107.

Gettler LT, et al. Fathers' oxytocin responses to first holding their newborns: interactions with testosterone reactivity to predict later parenting behavior and father-infant bonds. *Dev Psychobiol.* 2021;63(5):1384–1398.

Goulding AN, et al. Contraception and breastfeeding at 4 months postpartum among women intending to breastfeed. *Breastfeed Med.* 2018;13(1):75–80.

Grandahl M, et al. Longer shared parental leave is associated with longer duration of breastfeeding: a cross-sectional study among Swedish mothers and their partners. *BMC Pediatr.* 2020; 20(1):159.

Grebe NM, et al. Pair-bonding, fatherhood, and the role of testosterone: a meta-analytic review. *Neurosci Biobehav Rev.* 2019;98: 221–233.

Greely JT, et al. Violence against pregnant women and adverse maternal/ fetal outcomes in the United States: racial/ethnic disparities. *Women Health.* 2022;62(6):513–521.

Gutzeit O, et al. Postpartum female sexual function: risk factors for postpartum sexual dysfunction. *Sex Med.* 2019;8(1):8–13.

Han G, et al. Variation in coparenting quality in relation to child age: links to coparents' relationship satisfaction and education. *Scand J Psychol.* 2023;64(5):632–643.

Hansen E, et al. "They're born to get breastfed"—how fathers view breastfeeding: a mixed method study. *BMC Pregnancy Childbirth.* 2018;18(1):238.

Heinemann K, et al. IUD use among parous women and risk of uterine perforation: a secondary analysis. *Contraception.* 2017; 95(6):605–607.

Henry JB, et al. Fatherhood matters: an integrative review of fatherhood intervention research. *J School Nursing.* 2020;36: 19–32.

Henshaw JE, et al. Psychosocial predictors of early postpartum depressive and anxious symptoms in primiparous women and their partners. *BMC Pregnancy Childbirth.* 2023:27;23(1):209.

Hill AL, et al. Reproductive coercion and relationship abuse among adolescents and young women seeking care at school health centers. *Obstet Gynecol.* 2019;134(2):351–359.

Horsley K, et al. The association between pregnancy-specific anxiety and exclusive breastfeeding status early in the postpartum period. *J Hum Lact.* 2019;35(4):729–736.

Hoyt-Austin A, et al. Understanding of lactational amenorrhea as a contraceptive method among U.S. pregnant women. *Breastfeed Med.* 2023;18(8):621–625.

Huang L, et al. Effects of an online family-focused parenting support intervention on preterm infants' physical development and parents' sense of competence and care ability: a randomized controlled trial. *Int J Nurs Stud*. 2024;149:104625.

Infant Risk Center. Safe use of birth control while breastfeeding. November 4, 2019. https://www.infantrisk.com/content/safe-use-birth-control-while-breastfeeding

Johansson M, et al. Mothers' and fathers' lived experiences of postpartum depression and parental stress after childbirth: a qualitative study. *Int J Qual Stud Health Well-Being*. 2020;15(1):1722564.

Johansson M, et al. Postpartum depression and life experiences of mothers with an immigrant background living in the south of Sweden. *Int J Qual Stud Health Well-Being*. 2023;18(1):2187333.

Kasamatsu H, et al. Understanding the relationship between postpartum depression one month and six months after delivery and mother-infant bonding failure one-year after birth: results from the Japan Environment and Children's study (JECS). *Psychol Med*. 2020;50:161–169.

Kendall-Tackett K. Psychological trauma and breastfeeding: what we know so far. *Medical Research Archives*. 2022;10(10). https://www.researchgate.net/publication/365940647_Psychological_Trauma_and_Breastfeeding_What_We_Know_So_Far

Kendall-Tackett KA. *Depression in New Mothers*. 3rd ed. Abington, UK: Routledge; 2016.

Kita S, et al. Intimate partner violence, negative attitudes toward pregnancy, and mother-to-fetus bonding failure among Japanese pregnant women. *Violence Vict*. 2019;34(3):536–547.

Kivisto AJ, et al. Racial disparities in pregnancy-associated intimate partner homicide. *J Interpers Violence*. 2022;37(13–14):NP10938-NP10961.

Kroska EB, Stowe ZN. Postpartum depression: identification and treatment in the clinic setting. *Obstet Gynecol Clin North Am*. 2020;47(3):409–419.

Kusunoki Y, Barber JS. Intimate relationship dynamics and women's expected control over sex and contraception. *Contraception*. 2019;100(6):484–491.

Ladores S, Corcoran J. Investigating postpartum depression in the adolescent mother using 3 potential qualitative approaches. *Clin Med Insights Pediatr*. 2019;13:1179556519884042.

Le Y, et al. Coparenting and parenting outcomes of online relationship interventions for low-income couples. *J Fam Psychol*. 2021;35(7):1033–1039.

Leng RNW, et al. Fathers' involvement in their wives'/partners' breastfeeding: a descriptive correlational study. *J Hum Lact*. 2019;35(4):801–812.

Levi EE, et al. Placement of levonorgestrel intrauterine device at the time of cesarean delivery and the effect on breastfeeding duration. *Breastfeed Med*. 2018;13(10).

Liekmeier E, et al. Coparenting change after couple therapy using self-reports and observational data. *J Marital Fam Ther*. 2023;49(3):675–691.

Liu X, et al. Prevalence and risk factors of postpartum depression in women: a systematic review and meta-analysis. *J Clin Nurs*. 2022;31(19–20):2665–2677.

Magnusson BM, et al. Perceptions of public breastfeeding images and their association with breastfeeding knowledge and attitudes among an internet panel of men ages 21–44 in the United States. *J Hum Lact*. 2017;33(1):157–164.

Mandal SK, et al. Partner violence and postnatal mental health: cross-sectional analysis of factors associated with depression and anxiety in new mothers. *Aust J Prim Health*. 2018;24(5):434–440.

Manhart MD, Duane M. A comparison of app-defined fertile days from two fertility tracking apps using identical cycle data. *Contraception*. 2022;115:12–16.

Marcos-Nájera R, et al. The prevalence and risk factors for antenatal depression among pregnant immigrant and native women in Spain. *J Transcult Nurs*. 2020;31(6):564–575.

Marks EJ, et al. Agreement between future parents on infant feeding intentions and its association with breastfeeding duration: results from the growing up in New Zealand cohort study. *Int J Environ Res Public Health*. 2018;15(6).

Martin-de-Las-Heras S, et al. Breastfeeding avoidance following psychological intimate partner violence during pregnancy: a cohort study and multivariate analysis. *BJOG*. 2019;126(6):778–783.

Martínez-Plascencia U, et al. Maternal breastfeeding, alone or as a couple? A study on the experiences of reconfiguration of bodies, roles, and daily routines in Mexican mothers and fathers. *Cad Saude Publica*. 2017;33(9):e00109616.

Matthies LM, et al. The influence of partnership quality and breastfeeding on postpartum female sexual function. *Arch Gynecol Obstet*. 2019;299(1):69–77.

Mazzarello O, et al. Risk factors for sexual revictimization and dating violence in young adults with a history of child sexual abuse. *J Child Adolesc Trauma*. 2022;15(4):1113–1125.

McCloskey RJ, Pei F. Associations between mothers' adverse childhood experiences, material hardship, and breastfeeding challenges in the United States. *J Hum Lact*. 2022;38(4):651–660.

McKenna J. *Safe Infant Sleep: Expert Answers to Your Cosleeping Questions*. Washington, DC: Platypus Media; 2020.

Mercan Y, Tari Selcuk K. Association between postpartum depression level, social support level and breastfeeding attitude and breastfeeding self-efficacy in early postpartum women. *PLoS One*. 2021;16(4):e0249538.

Mikšić Š, et al. Positive effect of breastfeeding on child development, anxiety, and postpartum depression. *Int J Environ Res Public Health*. 2020;17(8):2725.

Morris AR, et al. Physical touch during father-infant interactions is associated with paternal oxytocin levels. *Infant Behav Dev*. 2021;64:101613.

Munroe C, Shumway M. Female-perpetrated sexual violence: a survey of survivors of female-perpetrated childhood sexual abuse and adult sexual assault. *J Interpers Violence*. 2022;37(9–10):NP6655–NP6675.

Murray AL, et al. The intergenerational effects of intimate partner violence in pregnancy: mediating pathways and implications for prevention. *Trauma Violence Abuse*. 2020;21(5):964–976.

Nelson AL, et al. Efficacy, safety, and tolerability of a levonorgestrel/ethinyl estradiol transdermal delivery system: phase 3 clinical trial results. *Contraception*. 2021;103(3):137–143.

Ngoenthong P, et al. Integrative review of fathers' perspectives on breastfeeding support. *J Obstet Gynecol Neonatal Nurs*. 2020;49(1):16–26.

Nishigori H, et al. The prevalence and risk factors for postpartum depression symptoms of fathers at one and 6 months postpartum: an adjunct study of the Japan Environment & Children's Study. *J Matern Fetal Neonatal Med*. 2020;33(16):2797–2804.

Odar Stough C, et al. Predictors of exclusive breastfeeding for 6 months in a national sample of US children. *Am J Health Promot*. 2019;33(1):48–56.

Papp LM. The longitudinal role of breastfeeding in mothers' and fathers' relationship quality trajectories. *Breastfeed Med*. 2012;7(4):241–247.

Pastor-Moreno G, et al. Intimate partner violence during pregnancy and risk of fetal and neonatal death: a meta-analysis with socioeconomic context indicators. *Am J Obstet Gynecol.* 2020;222(2):123–133.e5.

Peragallo UR, et al. Effectiveness of fertility awareness-based methods for pregnancy prevention: a systematic review. *Obstet Gynecol.* 2018;132:591–604.

Perry A, et al. Phenomenology, epidemiology and aetiology of postpartum psychosis: a review. *Brain Sci.* 2021;11(1):47.

Philpott LF, et al. Prevalence and associated factors of paternal stress, anxiety, and depression symptoms in the early postnatal period. *Glob Ment Health.* 2022;1–16.

Pinto TM, et al. Depression and paternal adjustment and attitudes during the transition to parenthood. *J Reprod Infant Psychol.* 2020;38(3):281–296.

Premji SS, et al. Mother's level of confidence in caring for her late preterm infant: a mixed methods study. *J Clin Nurs.* 2018; 27(5-6):e1120–e1133.

Qi W, et al. Psychosocial risk factors for postpartum depression in Chinese women: a meta-analysis. *BMC Pregnancy Childbirth.* 2021;21(1):174.

Ranney RM, et al. Effortful control moderates relationships between worry and symptoms of depression and anxious arousal. *Br J Clin Psychol.* 2021;60(3):400–413.

Rao W-W, et al. Prevalence of prenatal and postpartum depression in fathers: a comprehensive meta-analysis of observational surveys. *J Affect Disord.* 2020;263:491–499.

Reed SD, et al. Intrauterine device-related uterine perforation incidence and risk (APEX-IUD): a large multisite cohort study. *Lancet.* 2022;399(10341):2103–2112.

Rempel LA, et al. Relationships between types of father breastfeeding support and breastfeeding outcomes. *Matern Child Nutr.* 2017;13(3).

Ribeiro MRC, et al. Recurrent violence, violence with complications, and intimate partner violence against pregnant women and breastfeeding duration. *J Womens Health (Larchmt).* 2021;30(7): 979–989.

Ritchie-Ewing G, et al. Associations of maternal beliefs and distress in pregnancy and postpartum with breastfeeding initiation and early cessation. *J Hum Lact.* 2019;35(1):49–58.

Rollè L, et al. Father involvement and cognitive development in early and middle childhood: a systematic review. *Front Psychol.* 2019;10:2405.

Román-Gálvez RM, et al. Prevalence of intimate partner violence in pregnancy: an umbrella review. *Int J Environ Res Public Health.* 2021a;18(2):707.

Román-Gálvez RM, et al. Worldwide prevalence of intimate partner violence in pregnancy. a systematic review and meta-analysis. *Front Public Health.* 2021b;9:738459.

Roschina OV, et al. Beta-endorphin and oxytocin in patients with alcohol use disorder and comorbid depression. *J Clin Med.* 2021;10(23):5696.

Rosen NO, et al. Unmet and exceeded expectations for sexual concerns across the transition to parenthood. *J Sex Res.* 2022:1–12.

Rosenfeld EA, et al. Male partner reproductive coercion among women veterans. *Am J Obstet Gynecol.* 2018;218(2):239.e1–239.e8.

Rosseland LA, et al. Are labor pain and birth experience associated with persistent pain and postpartum depression? a prospective cohort study. *Scand J Pain.* 2020;20(3):591–602.

Roy M, et al. Progesterone vaginal ring as a new contraceptive option for lactating mothers: evidence from a multicenter non-randomized comparative clinical trial in India. *Contraception.* 2020;102(3):159–167.

Sayed Ahmed WA, et al. Female sexual function following different degrees of perineal tears. *Int Urogynecol J.* 2017;28(6):917–921.

Scatliffe N, et al. Oxytocin and early parent-infant interactions: a systematic review. *Int J Nurs Sci.* 2019;6(4):445–453.

Serati M, et al. Is there an association between oxytocin levels in plasma and pregnant women's mental health? *J Am Psychiatr Nurses Assoc.* 2021;27:222–230.

Serrano Drozdowskyj E, et al. Factors influencing couples' sexuality in the puerperium: a systematic review. *Sex Med Rev.* 2020;8(1):38–47.

Sha T, et al. A prospective study of maternal postnatal depressive symptoms with infant-feeding practices in a Chinese birth cohort. *BMC Pregnancy Childbirth.* 2019;19(1):388.

Shapiro AF, et al. Father's involvement when bringing baby home: efficacy testing of a couple-focused transition to parenthood intervention for promoting father involvement. *Psychol Rep.* 2020;123(3):806–824.

Shimao M, et al. Influence of infants' feeding patterns and duration on mothers' postpartum depression: a nationwide birth cohort—the Japan Environment and Children's Study (JECS). *J Affect Disord.* 2021;285:152–159.

Shorey S, et al. Prevalence and incidence of postpartum depression among healthy mothers: a systematic review and meta-analysis. *J Psychiatr Res.* 2018;104:235–248.

Shorey S, et al. Effectiveness of a technology-based supportive educational parenting program on parental outcomes (part 1): randomized controlled trial. *J Med Internet Res.* 2019;21(2): e10816.

Short S, et al. An exploration of masculinity, social support and depression in new and experienced fathers. *Midwifery.* 2023;123: 103715.

Sihota H, et al. Fathers' experiences and perspectives of breastfeeding: a scoping review. *Am J Mens Health.* 2019;13(3): 1557988319851616.

Silva CS, et al. Association between postpartum depression and the practice of exclusive breastfeeding in the first three months of life. *J Pediatr (Rio J).* 2017;93(4):356–364.

Silva RP, Leite FMC. Intimate partner violence during pregnancy: prevalence and associated factors. *Rev Saude Publica.* 2020;54:97.

Simmons RG, et al. Assessing the efficacy of an app-based method of family planning: the dot study protocol. *JMIR Res Protoc.* 2017;6(1):e5.

Śliwerski A, et al. The effect of maternal depression on infant attachment: a systematic review. *Int J Environ Res Public Health.* 2020;17(8):2675.

Slomian J, et al. Consequences of maternal postpartum depression: a systematic review of maternal and infant outcomes. *Women's Health (Lond).* 2019;15.

Slomian J, et al. Identifying maternal needs following childbirth: comparison between pregnant women and recent mothers. *BMC Pregnancy Childbirth.* 2021;21(1):405.

Spencer CM, et al Do online parenting programs create change?: a meta-analysis. *J Fam Psychol.* 2020;34(3):364-374.

Spencer JP, et al. Medication safety in breastfeeding. *Am Fam Physician.* 2022;106(6):638–644.

Srisopa P, Lucas R. Maternal perception of paternal breastfeeding support: a secondary qualitative analysis. *Midwifery.* 2021;102:103067.

Stanton TA, Blumenthal PD. Postpartum hormonal contraception in breastfeeding women. *Randomize Obstet Gynecol.* 2019; 31(6):441–446.

Stuebe AM, et al. The mood, mother, and infant study: associations between maternal mood in pregnancy and breastfeeding outcome. *Breastfeed Med.* 2019;14(8):551–559.

Sultan P, Carvalho B. Postpartum recovery: what does it take to get back to a baseline? *Curr Opin Obstet Gynecol.* 2021;33(2):86–93.

Szöllősi K, Szabó L. The association between infant feeding methods and female sexual dysfunctions. *Breastfeed Med.* 2021;16(1):93–99.

Tavares IM, et al. Longitudinal associations between relational and sexual well-being in couples transitioning to parenthood. *Fam Process.* 2024;63(1):192–209.

Thiel F, et al. The relationship between paternal and maternal depression during the perinatal period: a systematic review and meta-analysis. *Front Psychiatry.* 2020;11:563287.

Toledo C, et al. The significance of breastfeeding practices on postpartum depression risk. *Public Health Nurs.* 2022;39(1):15–23.

Tran TDT, et al. Intimate partner violence during pregnancy and maternal and child health outcomes: a scoping review of the literature from low-and-middle income countries from 2016–2021. *BMC Pregnancy Childbirth.* 2022;22(1):315.

Trussell J, et al. Efficacy, safety, and personal considerations. In Hatcher RA, et al. (eds.), *Contraceptive Technology*. 21st ed. New York: Ayer Company Publishers, Inc.; 2018.

Tsai TY, et al. The interaction of oxytocin and social support, loneliness, and cortisol level in major depression. *Clin Psychopharmacol Neurosci.* 2019;17(4):487–494.

Tuntipuchitanon S, et al. Online positive parenting programme for promoting parenting competencies and skills: randomised controlled trial. *Sci Rep.* 2024;14(1):20001.

Türkmen H, et al. The effect of labor comfort on traumatic childbirth perception, post-traumatic stress disorder, and breastfeeding. *Breastfeed Med.* 2020;15(12):779–788.

Turok DK, et al. Immediate postpartum levonorgestrel intrauterine device insertion and breast-feeding outcomes: a noninferiority randomized controlled trial. *Am J Obstet Gynecol.* 2017; 217(6):665.e1–665.e8.

United Nations Children's Fund. A new era for girls: taking stock of 25 years of progress. UN Women and Plan International. New York, 2020.

Van der Wijden C, Manion C. Lactational amenorrhoea method for family planning. *Cochrane Database Syst Rev.* 2015;12(10): CD001329.

Van Rijn-Van Gelderen L, et al. Determinants of non-paid task division in gay-, lesbian-, and heterosexual-parent families with infants conceived using artificial reproductive techniques. *Front Psychol.* 2020;11:914.

Vanwalleghem S, et al. Maternal attachment networks and mother-infant bonding disturbances among mothers with postpartum major depression. *Int J Environ Res Public Health.* 2023;16;20(12):6155.

Wallenborn JT, et al. Association between intimate partner violence and breastfeeding duration: results from the 2004–2014 Pregnancy Risk Assessment Monitoring System. *J Hum Lact.* 2018;34(2):233–241.

Walsh TB, et al. A call to action: screening fathers for perinatal depression. *Pediatrics.* 2020;145(1):e20191193.

Wang D, et al. Factors influencing paternal postpartum depression: a systematic review and meta-analysis. *J Affect Disord.* 2021;293:51–63.

Watson C, et al. Adverse childhood experiences and early and continued breastfeeding: findings from an integrated health care delivery system. *J Womens Health (Larchmt).* 2021;30(3): 367–376.

Webermann AR, Murphy CM. Childhood trauma and dissociative intimate partner violence. *Violence Against Women.* 2019; 25(2):148–166.

Wei X, et al. The impacts of intimate partner violence on postpartum depression: an updated meta-analysis. *Trauma Violence Abuse.* 2024;25(2):1531–1550.

Werner-Bierwisch T, et al. Mothers' and fathers' sense of security in the context of pregnancy, childbirth and the postnatal period: an integrative literature review. *BMC Pregnancy Childbirth.* 2018;18:473.

Woolhouse H, et al. Maternal depressive symptoms at three months postpartum and breastfeeding rates at six months postpartum: implications for primary care in a prospective cohort study of primiparous women in Australia. *Women Birth.* 2016;29(4):381–387.

World Health Organization. New app for WHO's medical eligibility criteria for contraceptive use. 2019. https://www.who.int/reproductivehealth/mec-app/en/

World Health Organization. WHO statement on levonorgestrel-releasing intrauterine device nomenclature. 2021. https://www.who.int/publications/i/item/9789240021730

Worsfold L, et al. Period tracker applications: what menstrual cycle information are they giving women? *Womens Health (Lond).* 2021;17:17455065211049905.

Wouk K, et al. Postpartum mental health and breastfeeding practices: an analysis using the 2010–2011 Pregnancy Risk Assessment monitoring system. *Maternal Child Health J.* 2017; 21:636–647.

Wroe J, et al. "What am I thinking? Is this normal?" A cross-sectional study investigating the nature of negative thoughts, parental self-efficacy and psychological distress in new fathers. *Midwifery.* 2019;79:102527.

Xiong R, Deng A. Prevalence and associated factors of postpartum depression among immigrant women in Guangzhou, China. *BMC Pregnancy Childbirth.* 2020;20(1):247.

Yakupova VA, Suarez A. Postpartum depression and birth experience in Russia. *Psychol Russ.* 2021;14(1):28–38.

Yaya S, et al. Association between intimate partner violence during pregnancy and risk of preterm birth. *BMC Public Health.* 2021;21(1):1610.

Young C, et al. Hindering resilience in the transition to parenthood: a thematic analysis of parents' perspectives. *J Reprod Infant Psychol.* 2022;40(1):62–75.

Zerubavel N, et al. Childhood sexual abuse and fear of abandonment moderate the relation of intimate partner violence to severity of dissociation. *J Trauma Dissociation.* 2018;19(1): 9–24.

Zhang S, et al. A work-life conflict perspective on telework. *Transp Res Part A Policy Pract.* 2020;141:51–68.

CHAPTER 21

Special Counseling Circumstances

Family circumstances can present unique challenges that require special counseling approaches. Families can range from marginalized and underrepresented backgrounds, low income, and non-native-speaking to wealthy or highly educated professionals. Some parents may encounter negative reactions from significant people in their lives. Families in resource-poor communities may have challenges with access to health care. Nursing parents who are solely responsible for their baby's care may face challenges. A teen parent is often coping with single parenthood combined with normal adolescent changes and development. Additionally, working with same-sex couples calls for an awareness of and sensitivity to their practices and personal preferences. Recognizing these differences and learning about trends in the community can help meet families' individual needs.

KEY TERMS

Cisgender
Gender assignment
Gender dysphoria
Gender expression
Gender identity
Lesbian, gay, bisexual, transgender, queer, questioning, plus (LGBTQ+)
Nonbinary

Opposition to Nursing

Despite the strong endorsement of lactation by governments and major health organizations, parents often receive questions and comments that prompt them to explain and defend their feeding choice. Negative remarks can undermine self-confidence and create doubt about their decision or their capability to nurse. It is especially difficult to cope with objections from people close to them. Many people who comment do not truly oppose nursing but simply do not understand it. Parents who are confident in their feeding decision may be able to educate some of these people and familiarize them with the characteristics of a nursing baby.

Opposition to nursing often manifests itself as the subtle undermining of parents' efforts rather than blatant remarks. Healthcare professionals and lay persons alike, quick to state that human milk is "the best" infant food, may point to nursing as the cause when the baby cries or when parents express concern. Parents benefit from education and support to guide them through challenging times when doubts surface that undermine their confidence.

Strangers

It is common for parents to encounter strangers in public who convey negative reactions to a baby nursing. Parents who are confident in their feeding choice are less likely to yield to the opinions or glances from a stranger. They may feel more confident if they are discreet when they nurse in public. They can wear clothing that allows easy access for feeding while still providing coverage. Practicing nursing in front of a mirror will help them become confident with techniques that work for them. Discreet nursing does not mean disguising the fact that they are feeding their baby. Nursing in public normalizes it and helps increase cultural acceptance. Knowing the local laws regarding public protections can increase the nursing parent's confidence. **Chapter 18** discusses nursing in public.

Friends

Opposition from friends may prove more difficult for parents to handle. Depending on the nature of the friendship, it may be possible to educate a friend and help them understand how important it is to the parent and baby. Developing friendships with others who nurse or support nursing can help them feel more confident. Parents also benefit from social networking through the internet, especially those who live in small towns or rural communities that lack support systems.

Employer

When nursing parents return to work, employers play a critical role in their success. Employment is the most common reason parents express milk. The time required for it may create tension at work. Parents can increase support by speaking frankly with their employer about their plans to nurse and ensuring that milk expression does not interfere with their job performance. Employers who have positive experiences with nursing employees are more likely to recognize and appreciate the importance of workplace accommodations. Many employees are uncomfortable approaching their employer, especially if they work in a male-dominated profession or lack job security. These employees may find websites, forums, books, and other media for nursing employees helpful.

In some cases, an employee may be unable to resolve a lack of employer support. This may require reevaluating priorities, changing jobs, or supplementing the baby because of lowered milk production. Sometimes, the employee may feel pressured to wean. Employees can refer unreasonable and unfair treatment by an employer to the human resources department, local labor relations board, or national employment commission (e.g., the U.S. Equal Employment Opportunity Commission). **Chapter 25** discusses combining lactation and employment or schooling.

Healthcare Providers

Parents value healthcare providers' opinions and trust their judgments about their family's health care. A perceived lack of support by a healthcare provider may stem from a lack of knowledge about or experience with lactation. A provider who asserts a commitment to lactation may appear unsupportive and unintentionally give misinformation. Well-meaning healthcare providers may not realize how their remarks to parents can undermine self-confidence. Parents need to be open with providers about their concerns and perceptions so that they may resolve differences about nursing.

Parents with an unsupportive healthcare provider need extra contact and confidence building. Providing scholarly research to share with their provider can reinforce their efforts and raise the provider's awareness of evidence-based practice for lactation care. If differences continue, parents may consider whether this relationship is best for their baby. **Chapter 2** discusses the relationship between healthcare providers and parents.

Grandparents and Other Relatives

Support from a parent's immediate family plays an important role in their feeding decision. New parents often turn to their own mothers for encouragement and wisdom as they begin parenting. Throughout the world, grandmothers are central figures in lactation support. They may either support nursing or discourage it with contrary opinions and inadequate guidance (Angelo et al., 2020). In some cultures, the paternal grandmother is the relative who exerts influence on childcare decisions. Optimal lactation practices are higher in families where grandmothers have correct lactation knowledge (Ferreira et al., 2018; Karmacharya et al., 2017).

Grandparents who did not nurse may not understand the sleep and feeding patterns of nursing babies. They may worry that frequent feedings are a sign of inadequate nourishment and thus recommend supplementing with formula. They may misinterpret the normal loose stools of a nursing baby as diarrhea. They may also believe that nursing increases the strains of early parenting, such as lack of sleep, coping with crying, and physical recovery from birth. In addition, grandparents' advice may reflect cultural beliefs and practices that compromise nursing (Vázquez-Vázquez et al., 2022).

Family members may not recognize that voicing concerns can undermine a parent's confidence and come through as unsupportive. It is often difficult for young parents to disregard misguided advice from older adults or to do so without feeling conflicted. Understanding the motivation behind a family member's perceived lack of support will help parents preserve relationships while they meet their feeding goals. They can help their relatives confront misconceptions and learn current lactation practices. There are many internet and media resources for grandparents of nursing babies, including social media sites.

Partners

It is especially difficult for nursing parents to experience opposition from their partners. A partner's preference is typically significant in the infant feeding choice. Thus, their opposition weighs greatly on the decision to initiate or continue nursing. Sharing information with the partner about the importance of nursing provides a springboard for discussing the value of the their support and the need for mutual support. Open communication about parenting may improve the couple's long-term relationship.

A partner's opposition can stem from the same concerns as those of grandparents and other relatives—the health and well-being of the nursing parent and baby. Educating partners that nursing is beneficial to the entire family and that not nursing increases health risks for the parent and baby may increase their support. The financial strain of product costs and increased healthcare costs from artificial feeding may also garner support. If the partner believes nursing interferes with the couple's sex life, it will help to recognize that having a baby changes all parents' sex lives, no matter how they feed their baby.

A previously supportive partner may question continuing to nurse an older baby, stemming from a concern about overdependence on the nursing parent. The parent can remind the partner about the health benefits of continued nursing and that meeting their child's present needs leads to greater independence in the future. **Chapter 20** discusses the partner's role in supporting nursing. Some partners may oppose nursing as a part of control and power dominance in the relationship. This could be a marker for intimate partner violence, discussed in **Chapter 20**.

Low-Income Families

Many families live near or below the poverty level. This is especially true for families encountered in a public health clinic or hospital or a government nutrition program, such as Women, Infants, and Children (WIC) in the United States. They may not attend childbirth classes because of cost, availability, or lack of interest. These families will benefit from programs that assist low-income populations with health services and supplemental foods, discussed in **Chapter 2**.

Low-income families often live in unfavorable conditions. They may face the challenges of overcrowding, rundown housing, crime, and inadequate community services. They may experience physical and mental health problems, broken families, relocation, isolation, alienation, or language differences. They may receive prenatal care in one place and deliver their baby in another. Or they may seek attention for sick children from a clinic or emergency department. Additionally, their healthy children may lack preventive health care.

Poverty is often associated with low self-esteem and limited expectations. Low-income families may feel detached from society and believe they cannot control their lives and surroundings. Inequities prevail in income, child care, education, preventive health services, life span, and security. Families' lives are often saturated with violence, causing them to feel unsafe in their homes. Parents might hold multiple low-paying jobs and have little discretionary time or money. Life can be a series of crises with a sense of despair or stress. Statistically, substance use and alcoholism are high among this population. One study found increased use of marijuana during pregnancy and lactation because of misperceptions about its risk to infants and benefits to users (Cameron et al., 2022).

Infant Feeding Decision

The lack of prenatal childbirth education typical of this population increases the likelihood that a child will not be nursed (Kehinde et al., 2023). Low-income parents may choose not to nurse because of concerns about their lifestyle or the safety of their milk. Nursing may seem to be one more stress in their lives that could result in failure. Low-income parents can be especially susceptible to formula-feeding messages, believing that formula is equally good or perhaps better because it is more "scientific." There may be little family or community support for nursing compared with bottle feeding.

More than in other populations, low-income parents may find that nursing increases their self-confidence and self-esteem. Realizing that nursing contributes to their child's well-being and that they accomplished it through their own resources enhances their self-image. This can improve their nursing and parenting skills and encourage them to share their success with others. Support during the postpartum hospital stay and early weeks at home can be pivotal to lactation. Healthcare personnel, respected for their expertise, can be instrumental in parents continuing to nurse. They can help families strategize and problem-solve regarding the specific barriers they face that can affect nursing, such as childcare or employer challenges.

Lactation Rates

Low income is associated with a lower incidence and shorter duration of lactation. Many low-income parents work in service-oriented industries, which report low lactation rates (Lauer et al., 2019). Rates are also low among the homeless population (Frenoy et al., 2021). Initiation rates in the United States are similar for WIC-eligible participating children compared to WIC-eligible nonparticipating children. Those who do not receive assistance through WIC discontinue nursing sooner. Exclusivity rates in WIC increased when changes were made in the food packages to support full nursing (Li et al., 2019).

It can be difficult for low-income parents to sustain nursing beyond 2 months (Kay et al., 2020). Family socioeconomic risk and food insecurity are associated with a shorter duration (Borger et al., 2021; Frazier et al., 2023; Natale et al., 2021). Low-income parents may resume employment earlier than those who have greater financial security, increasing the likelihood of a shorter duration of nursing. Peer counselor support has a positive effect on lactation initiation, duration, and exclusivity in this population (Chepkirui et al., 2020).

Even when nursing intent and initiation are high, babies in low-income families are likely to receive early formula supplementation (Lewkowitz et al., 2019; Noble et al., 2023). Early introduction of complementary food is common as well (Hornsby et al., 2021; Marks et al., 2023). Low-income parents with late-preterm and early-term infants are reportedly less likely to nurse exclusively and have lower self-efficacy and satisfaction than parents with full-term infants (Ahmed & Rojjanasrirat, 2021).

Lactation rates among low-income parents increase when healthcare clinics include prenatal classes, one-on-one instruction, and peer counselors. Targeted Baby-Friendly Hospital Initiative practices can have a positive impact on lactation among underserved populations (French et al., 2023; Kivlighan et al., 2020; Patterson et al., 2021). In one study, the use of a smartphone app reduced lactation challenges but did not increase rates (Lewkowitz et al., 2021). The app included educational materials, interactive advice and strategies, and hyperlinks to online videos and other resources.

Teaching and Support Strategies

Low-income parents may be isolated, with no support system and no acquaintances who nursed. Discussion groups with parents who face the same challenges can provide the peer support they need. However, participation in breastfeeding support groups may be minimal for these parents, who are often overwhelmed with work, child care, and obtaining the necessities of life. Furthermore, traveling to and from classes creates a challenge for those with no reliable means of transportation.

Location

Reaching out to families through social networks, clinics, and other public places will support them in their neighborhoods. Parents may be more receptive to attending meetings in surroundings they find comfortable, such as a private residence, church, or community center. Those who have access to the internet might enjoy online support groups because they eliminate the need for travel and child care. When parents have a role in planning and organizing such meetings, they feel like part of the process. They can also help plan topics that are most relevant to them. Keeping presentations short and focused and addressing issues that are relevant to parents' needs will make meetings enjoyable. A casual, informal approach encourages discussion.

Literacy Level

Literacy level could impede parents' ability to absorb information. Written materials need to be at an appropriate reading level with visual images to support the message. Text-based messaging, mobile apps, and internet information are helpful for this population. Verbal explanations with visual aids and a checklist of the suggestions you discuss will reinforce learning. Soliciting feedback will indicate that parents understand the message and will likely act on the suggestions.

Home Visits

Because low-income homes are often in high-risk areas, home visits require special planning. Visiting during daylight hours and notifying a colleague or family member of the visit can increase safety. A map,

Global Positioning System (GPS) capabilities, and a cell phone are especially important when visiting a home in an unsafe neighborhood. If circumstances make it unsafe to visit a home alone, including a colleague or meeting with the parent in a different location are options. Being sensitive and tactful when discussing arrangements can avoid unintentionally offending the family.

Single-Parent Families

A parent may have sole responsibility for their baby because of divorce, separation, death of a partner, single by choice, or when their partner is away for extended periods (e.g., work or military deployment). Single parents account for 39.6% of births in the United States, with three-fourths of these being women (Centers for Disease Control and Prevention [CDC], 2019b). Children from marginalized backgrounds are the most affected. In 2021, 64% of non-Hispanic Black children, 49% of Native American children, and 42% of Hispanic children lived in one-parent households (Annie E. Casey Foundation [AECF], 2021).

Single-parent families face greater economic and social disparities than two-parent families. Trying to meet the baby's needs along with those of everyday life can leave little time for self-care. Simple activities such as taking a walk with the baby in a backpack or stroller or exercising with other parents and babies may provide relief.

Living Arrangements

Many single parents juggle one or more jobs, schooling or training, household responsibilities, and parenting. They may live alone or may reside with their own parents or a friend. Each situation presents unique challenges. Living with their parents can provide support and security. At the same time, they may struggle to maintain their identity as an adult and to preserve a separate identity as a family unit with the baby.

It can be difficult for two-family units to live harmoniously in the same home. Single parents may receive criticism about their parenting, and other family members may discipline their child. Lack of privacy can interfere with lactation. Many parents view their return home as a temporary situation until they secure other living arrangements.

Nursing Challenges

Single parents have lower rates of exclusive nursing and are more likely to introduce complementary foods earlier than someone living in a two-parent household (Arora et al., 2020; Odar Stough et al., 2019; Yasuda et al., 2022). When a parent's single status has resulted from divorce or the death of a spouse, emotional stress and other demands of the aftermath can result in missed feedings and lowered milk production. Babies may tune in to this emotional state and want to nurse more frequently. Nursing can provide comfort in such times of stress, and the increased frequency helps maintain milk production.

Support System

Single parents may lack support among friends and family and have no one with whom to share concerns or parenting responsibilities. Other single parents may provide a good support system. There are support groups specifically for parents who are single by choice. Single parents may also benefit from a local organization, such as Parents Without Partners or other support groups. Many religious and community service organizations offer food assistance, free vehicle care, parenting classes, financial education, and childcare services to single parents.

Teen Parents

Teens seem to be less sexually active, and more of those who are sexually active use birth control than in the past. Although teen birth rates have declined globally, the United States continues to have the highest rate of teen pregnancy among industrialized nations. The rate of births to U.S. parents aged 15 to 19 in 2021 was 14.4%, down 6% from 2020 (Hamilton et al., 2022). Among that age group, 75% of pregnancies are unplanned, and 30% end in abortion (Guttmacher Institute, 2024). Teen birth rates have declined for most racial groups in the United States (Martin et al., 2018). Racial/ethnic and geographic disparities persist (Nandi et al., 2019; Sutton et al., 2019; Thacker et al., 2022).

Many teen parents lack active guidance from their parents and other adults. They may be less likely to convey or advocate for their needs and may have little help or support for nursing at home. Others in the family may not have nursed, and peers are much less likely to have nursed. Interactions between teens and their parents may or may not be positive. They may be in disfavor with their family because of their pregnancy. Most pregnant teens do not marry the father of the baby because they do not feel pressured socially to have a mate or a father for the baby.

They are more likely to:

- Be born at low birth weight
- Have lower school achievement (e.g., lower scores on measures of kindergarten readiness; lower vocabulary, math, and reading scores)
- Exhibit behavior problems
- Experience abuse/neglect
- Rely more heavily on public-sector health care
- Enter the foster care system
- Have chronic medical conditions
- Be raised in single parent families
- Be incarcerated at some time during adolescence
- Drop out of high school
- Be nine times more likely to be poor (if parent didn't finish high school and is unmarried)
- Give birth as a teenager
- Be unemployed or underemployed as a young adult

Figure 21-1 Challenges facing children of teen parents.

Data from Aizer A, et al. Why children of teen mothers do worse in life. December 22, 2018. Vox, Centre for Economic Policy Research (CEPR) Policy Portal. voxeu.org; Centers for Disease Control and Prevention (CDC). About teen pregnancy March 1, 2019a. www.cdc.gov/teenpregnancy/about/index.htm; Hendrick CE, Maslowsky J. Teen mothers' educational attainment and their children's risk for teenage childbearing. *Dev Psychol*. 2019;55(6):1259–1273.

Increased risks to adolescent parents (compared to adults):

- Eclampsia
- Puerperal endometritis
- Systemic infection
- Emotional, social, psychiatric needs
- Stigma or rejection by peers/family
- Intimate partner violence
- Rapid repeat pregnancies, increasing morbidity
- Education drop out rates, resulting in fewer skills and long-term economic disparities

Increased risks to infants of adolescents:

- Low birthweight
- Preterm birth
- Severe neonatal complications, including long-term health conditions

Figure 21-2 Health risks to pregnant teens and their infants.

Data from World Health Organization (WHO). Adolescent pregnancy. Key Facts. February 23, 2018. www.who.int/news-room/fact-sheets/detail/adolescent-pregnancy.

Teen parents may not complete high school because of the demands on their time. They may be unable to care for their baby because they lack the skill or income. They often have no job skills and are financially dependent on their families and society. They are at higher risk for depression, substance use, and socioeconomic disadvantage (Wong et al., 2020). These circumstances can adversely affect parenting and behavioral outcomes for their offspring. Teens typically live in less healthy environments, and their children face significant challenges. Refer to **Figure 21-1** for attributes of children of teens. This is an opportune time to link adolescents to family planning, lactation clinics, and life skills education (Hunter-Adams et al., 2022; Namutebi et al., 2022).

Prenatal Issues

There is a frequent pattern of inadequate prenatal care and poor nutrition among pregnant teens that is associated with poverty, lower educational level, and inadequate family support. Pregnant adolescents are at risk for low weight gain, anemia, and pregnancy-induced hypertension. Some teens attempt to hide or deny their pregnancy in the early months. Consequently, they begin prenatal care late, many times as late as the end of the second trimester. A baby born to a teen is at higher risk for preterm birth, low birth weight, other serious health problems, and demise than a baby born to an older parent (World Health Organization, 2018).

Pregnant teens may be fearful and unhappy about the physical changes that occur with their body during pregnancy. They may feel apprehensive about the impending labor and delivery. They may be concerned about the reactions of family, friends, teachers, and the baby's father. Depending on the degree of their emotional adjustment to pregnancy, teens could doubt their self-worth and have a poor self-image.

Good nutrition is especially important for the developing fetus, as well as the teen's own body. Pregnancy compromises the health of a teen, whose growth needs compete with those of the baby. Teens who are reluctant to gain weight can be encouraged and praised for the weight they gain and its benefit to the baby. They may need to consume more food than adults and would benefit from ongoing individualized advice regarding their diet. Teens who recently experienced puberty may require even more calories to support the rapid growth that follows. Those who live with their parents may have limited influence on meal planning. Nutrition education is a primary achievement for all pregnant teens. **Figure 21-2** identifies the increased health risks of teen pregnancy to both parent and baby.

Postpartum Issues

Teen parents often feel threatened and overwhelmed by the hospital environment. They may be reluctant to ask for anything from the nursing staff. Consequently, they may be less likely to arrange for immediate or prolonged contact with their babies after birth. Teens may not recognize the importance of early contact for bonding and may prioritize the social aspect of visitors. Childbirth is a time of vulnerability for all new parents. For a teen parent, whose confidence is highly fragile, it may be the first realization of the parenting responsibility ahead. Hospital personnel can be sensitive to a teen's fragility and invite interaction with the baby.

After taking the baby home from the hospital, teens may question their adequacy as parents and have difficulty coping with the daily responsibilities of parenthood. In some cases, relatives raise the baby, with the parent having little to do with the baby's care. Maturity and attitude are significant factors in how teens cope with parenthood and lactation. Less mature teens may have difficulty devoting love and attention to the baby at a time when their own need for nurturing is so great. Other teens are ready to accept the responsibilities of parenthood and respond in much the same way as older parents.

Decision to Nurse

Because the greatest proliferation of mammary ducts occurs during pregnancy, teens have the same potential for milk production as adults. Many teens nurse, although rates are lower for teens than for adults. Attitudes about nursing begin forming in the preadolescent to adolescent years. In one study, the intention to nurse among secondary students increased immediately after an educational program. However, 6 months after the education, their intentions were less positive (Čatipović et al., 2021). Continuous educational programs for secondary school students would help maintain their intention to nurse.

Younger, single teens in school with little exposure to lactation need the most outreach and encouragement. Older, married adolescents with higher education are more likely to have knowledge of lactation practices (Kumar et al., 2021). Living with the baby's father increases the odds of lactation initiation (Corsack et al., 2022).

Some teens nurse to establish control, perceiving it as the one thing that only they can do for their baby. They may nurse to limit the biological father's involvement in the baby's care for as long as possible. Some teens find themselves in a power struggle with their parents over the care of the baby. They may want to assert themselves as the parent and demonstrate that they are not too young to care for a baby. Coaching teens with accurate information on baby care prenatally and throughout the hospital stay, as well as follow-up through home visitation, may help decrease misgivings.

Professional, partner, family, and peer support are critical for teens to persevere with nursing. Teens often feel judged for their feeding decisions, including use of a bottle and nursing in public (Buckland et al., 2022). They experience multiple overlapping stigmas, including competing norms for infant feeding and good parenting and mixed support from peers (Chopel et al., 2019; SmithBattle et al., 2020). They may lack futuristic thinking and the ability to anticipate the consequences of their actions and understand that a problem can be resolved "in the moment." Some teens have an excellent support system and nurse for the same amount of time as adults.

Lactation Management

Teens are less likely to exclusively nurse or to nurse for a long duration (Buckland et al., 2020; CDC, 2018, 2019b). Longer-term lactation (up to 24 months) among teens associated with infants not receiving pacifiers (Muelbert & Giugliani, 2018). Teens may abandon exclusive nursing because of a perception of having poor-quality milk or an increase in pacifier use (Hernández & Riesco, 2022). Many who wean have not used available professional help and rely on their network of peers, friends, and family. Thus, when significant others and family members are supportive, their encouragement is especially helpful. If they are negative, they represent a barrier (Academy of Breastfeeding Medicine [ABM] et al. 2015; Godbout et al., 2016).

Problem Solving with Teens

Multidisciplinary interventions for teen parents are valuable for reducing the long-term negative outcomes for both parents and offspring. Teens who encounter difficulties are less likely than adults to overcome them and continue nursing (Barbosa et al., 2017). They may have more difficulties initiating lactation and maintaining milk production than older parents do. The low amount of milk may be from not nursing often enough to establish ample milk production. Asking open-ended questions helps teens learn to quantify their feeding patterns and clarify their needs. Questions may include the following:

- How many times did your baby nurse over the past 24 hours?
- How many minutes did your baby nurse on each side?
- How many times does your baby pee and poop each day?
- How many bottles of formula do you give your baby each day?
- How much formula is in each bottle?

Clarifying teen responses is helpful in understanding their experiences. When a teen says that the baby cries "all day long," asking for a measurement of what that means will help to quantify it. Cradling the baby in a sling or snuggly carrier can reduce the baby's crying. Learning infant hunger cues will help them begin a feeding before the baby starts crying. If they say the baby "never sleeps," they can keep a notepad handy or use a mobile app to record sleep times. If they say that the baby "is always hungry," they can count the number and length of feedings in a 24-hour period. They may find that the baby's patterns of eating and sleeping are perfectly normal. Whereas this tracking might be tedious for an older parent with a better grasp of time, it may help a teen parent learn to modulate, analyze, and describe the baby's behaviors more observantly.

Interactions with Teen Parents

Teen parents usually have a great need for one-to-one relationships with people who care about them and understand their needs. Approaching them sensitively and respectfully can empower them to take ownership of their lives, transition to parenthood, and advocate for their babies. It is important to get to know them as individuals and not just as parents. Ask how they are adjusting, how the birth went, how they feel, and what their needs are. Demonstrating interest in them as a person builds rapport and develops trust in the relationship.

Adolescents wish to be treated as adults and do not respond well to lecturing, being told what to do, or patronizing tones that suggest an adult–child relationship. They need caregivers to be open to their concerns and respond as they would with an older parent. Teen parents want explanations, to have their questions answered, and to receive consistent information. Providing privacy, treating them with respect, and exhibiting calmness can help meet their needs.

Teaching Teens

Teen parents are learning to think abstractly, so it is normal for their adolescent focus to be self-centered. Teaching the benefits of nursing for them (or the risks of not nursing) may carry more weight than information about the baby's health. Learning what they already know about lactation and what they would like to learn will help meet their needs. This can be challenging because teens often fear peer ridicule and may not volunteer information or ask questions. Asking them to write out their questions or concerns anonymously encourages them to think about the situation while still protecting their privacy. Teens can use dolls to practice holding their babies. Marbles and ping-pong balls can illustrate the size of a newborn's stomach over time. When teaching teens in a group setting, time needs to be incorporated to talk with them individually as well.

Because teens may not attend every educational offering or appointment, it helps to review lactation basics whenever possible. New information needs to be simple, in clear terms that do not overwhelm them. Teens typically lose interest after 15 minutes of new information. Interjecting humor with teaching and encouraging nonthreatening participation can lead to meaningful interactions.

Teens relate to downloading lactation apps and finding lactation resources online. Apps abound in most countries for pregnancy, childbirth, the postpartum period, infant care, and lactation. Teens respond well to e-health resources that are visually appealing, engaging, and informative (Abbass-Dick et al., 2021). Interactive websites that depict other nursing teens and concrete, interactive teaching tools invite participation.

LGBTQ+ Families

The **lesbian, gay, bisexual, transgender/transsexual, queer/questioning, plus (LGBTQ+)** community is diverse. The culture can vary widely from one geographic area to another based on the degree of acceptance. The term used for this community varies by country. LGBTQ+ is the term used in the United States. Because there is such identity diversity, there is great diversity in the couples themselves (refer to **Figure 21-3**). Both parents in the couple may identify as female, or both may identify as male. One or both partners may identify as nonbinary, or one or both may identify as transgender. There is no

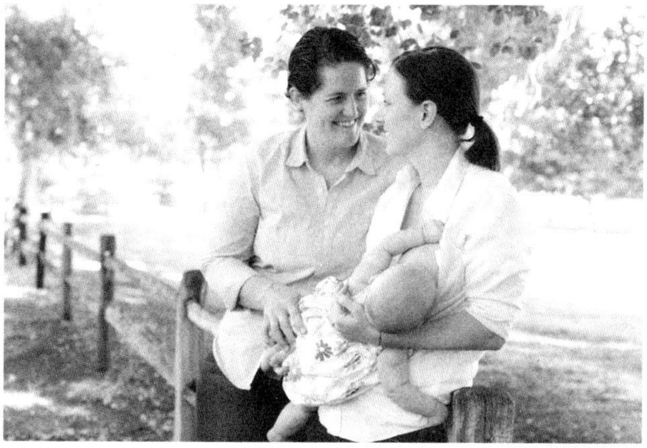

Figure 21-3 Same-sex couple with their child.

Printed with permission of Jaye Simpson and Patricia Berg-Drazin.

traditional relationship arrangement as there is with some heterosexual couples.

Members of the LGBTQ+ community may be more likely to delay care or report negative effects of disclosure to their provider compared with **cisgender** people, whose gender identity corresponds with their birth sex (Macapagal et al., 2016). Individuals who are gender nonconforming have reported a fear of being judged or of feeling invisible to healthcare providers (Landry & Kensler, 2019). Healthcare settings that are not inclusive can affect the quality of care delivered or whether care is pursued at all (Ruud, 2018). Inadequate education and preparation of healthcare providers can contribute to not meeting health needs within the LGBTQ+ community. Creating safe, accepting, affirming, inclusive, and welcoming environments for all parents will reduce the health disparities LGBTQ+ parents face (Kuzma et al., 2019).

Counseling Considerations

If you are unfamiliar with working with LGBTQ+ families, let them know, and ask questions about how the couple would like their care to be handled and how they would like to be addressed as parents. Do not assume that one parent will fulfill the "fathering" role and the other the "mothering" role. Sensitivity to roles within the family will be appreciated.

Individuals who identify as LGBTQ+ may have high rates of anxiety and depression (Rafferty et al., 2018). Affirmative care can help to decrease those feelings, especially around lactation and nursing. LGBTQ+ parents also have higher rates of miscarriage, preterm birth, and stillbirth. They are more likely to utilize alternative fertility treatments, which increases the risk (Croll et al., 2022). These risks can exacerbate the couple's anxiety and stress about pregnancy and lactation.

Gender-affirming care demonstrates compassion and understanding in a nonjudgmental way. It can increase feelings of self-worth and creates a safe space for learning, especially with teen parents who identify as LGBTQ+. The following information about counseling parents in the LGBTQ+ community was provided by Jaye (Janet) Haleryn and Patricia A. Berg. **Chapter 3** discusses cultural humility in your approach to families.

Gender-Neutral Language

By paying attention to our language, we can avoid incorrectly assigning gender to or offending families with whom we work. Using gender-neutral terminology allows inclusion of all sexes, genders, and identities. For example, using the term *parent* rather than *mother* or *father* includes all parents regardless of gender. Likewise, rather than using a gendered pronoun such as *he* or *she*, we can use the neutral term *they*. Asking parents for their preferred pronouns demonstrates recognition of their lifestyle.

The terms sex, gender, identity, gender expression, and sexual orientation are not synonymous. Sex is genetics, a person's reproductive organs. Natal sex is the **gender assignment** of a baby at birth, which may be male, female, or intersex (which can result from any number of conditions). **Gender identity** is a person's internal sense of self and their gender, who they feel they are. **Gender expression** is how a person presents their gender externally (e.g., through clothing, hair, interests, and other physical forms of expression). Transgender describes a person who is genetically female but feels like a male in the wrong body, or vice versa.

Some people are genetically one sex but feel they are neither—neutral or **nonbinary**. Others feel they are genetically one sex, but their gender is fluid—as in feeling masculine at some times and feminine at other times. Some people have no firm gender identity. Identity reflects who a person identifies as, which may include cisgender, transgender, or nonbinary. Sexual orientation reflects how a person views romantic and emotional relationships, which may include lesbian, gay, bisexual, asexual, queer, or heterosexual relationships. Understanding these differences enhances recognition of people as more than just their genetic sex or the gender they appear.

Counseling Dynamics

The assistance LGBTQ+ couples need with pregnancy, birth, lactation, and parenting differ from that of heterosexual parents. It can be difficult for LGBTQ+ parents to find a supportive care provider who knows how to work with LGBTQ+ couples. Many in the LGBTQ+ community have been openly discriminated against and may have been denied treatment or treated rudely. These couples need providers in whose care they will feel safe and supported.

Relationship dynamics vary widely within the LGBTQ+ community. Treating the nonbirth female parent of a same-sex couple the same as a father in a heterosexual couple unfairly and incorrectly stereotypes the relationship. The nonbirth parent may, in fact, be the biological parent. Transgender men who carry and birth a baby may be able to chestfeed, and a transgender woman can induce lactation and nurse. Same-sex female couples may co-nurse their baby. These variations are often unfamiliar to many lactation professionals and require sensitivity and awareness in meeting the family's needs.

Pregnancy and Genetics

Accidental pregnancies are rare among LGBTQ+ couples. Pregnancy is generally planned and often involves fertility assistance and invasive procedures. The parent who carries the pregnancy may not be the biological/genetic parent (also called bio-parent). Many couples harvest one partner's eggs, fertilize them with donor (or the partner's) sperm, and implant the embryos into the other partner who carries the pregnancy. Other couples use donor eggs/embryos and birth a child who is genetically unrelated to either parent.

Learning the history of how the baby was conceived will help rule out fertility and hormonal issues related to milk production. Understanding appropriate terminology and the various genetic roles will help healthcare providers approach couples with sensitivity to their individual circumstances. Understanding that LGBTQ+ parents have worse pregnancy outcomes clarifies the history of the family and how to help them achieve their goals.

Parental Role

In the heterosexual world, the term *mother* or *mom* is assigned to female parents and *father* or *dad* to male parents. LGBTQ+ couples may struggle with parental labels because of gender identity. Female parents may identify as a father role, and male parents may identify as a mother role. In same-sex female couples, there is no commonly agreed-upon language for the nonbirth parent. Terminology such as *co-mom*, *second parent*, or *the other mother* tends to sound negative or place the nonbirth parent in a second-class status. It is important that healthcare professionals validate the nonbirth parent's place and importance in the family.

Parental terminology can vary widely and take on both traditional and nontraditional forms. Some couples choose a name for themselves with variations of mother or father, whereas others use their first names, such as Mama Liz or Daddy Dave. Other couples let their children choose their own names for the parents as they grow. Avoiding labels in your work with these parents demonstrates that they are respected for who they are and not who society thinks they should be. Asking questions such as "What will you have the baby call you?" gives parents an opportunity to identify themselves rather than having their identity chosen for them.

Co-nursing Parents

Female same-sex couples may opt for both parents to nurse the baby. Asking the couple if they are both interested in nursing may introduce an option they did not realize was available to them. In some cases, the birth parent may not wish to share nursing, but the partner may want to. Conversely, the birth parent may wish to share nursing, and the partner may not be interested. It is also possible that the birth parent may not want to nurse and prefers to express their milk while the nonbirth parent nurses with a supplementer. Another variation is that the birth parent will not nurse or pump, and the nonbirth parent will induce lactation to nurse the baby. If the couple wishes to induce lactation, discussing it prior to the birth will enable lactation induction to begin early. Presenting couples with information, education, and support will help them consider their options.

Welcoming the Partner

Just as with heterosexual couples, it is important to include and engage both parents in lactation education and support. LGBTQ+ partners need to know they will be accepted and welcomed at lactation visits. Simply stating, "Your partner is welcome to attend our visit, and I encourage them to do so!" will help them feel comfortable participating. Be mindful to engage both parents equally in teaching and conversation and not focus only on the baby and the nursing parent. If there is a question about privacy for the nursing parent, simply ask, "May I share your personal information with your partner?"

Transgender Parents

Gender dysphoria describes an individual whose gender identity and genetic sex are not in concordance. Transgender people feel they are in the wrong body, that parts of their body do not match their gender identity. This often causes emotional distress, anxiety, and depression. In some cultures, transgender people are accepted, appreciated, and honored members of the community. For others, being a transgender person can be highly dangerous, depending on the part of the world in which they live. Transgender people often face discrimination, misunderstandings, and a lack of acceptance. Finding safe providers for medical, birth, and lactation care can be extremely challenging. Both transgender men and transgender women can lactate—sometimes fully, sometimes partially.

Transgender Women. A transgender woman is genetically a male and identifies as and lives as a female. Transgender women often undergo hormone replacement therapy to stimulate breast and glandular tissue growth, as well as other feminization changes in the body. Breast glandular development takes years, and the amount of glandular tissue growth varies. Many transgender women have breast augmentation surgery, which has the potential to interfere with lactation.

A transgender woman may induce lactation using hormonal therapy or simply feed with a supplementer at the breast. As with any induced lactation, pharmaceuticals, herbs, homeopathy, acupuncture, or essential oils may assist with milk production. They should discuss these options with their healthcare provider. Although transgender women can produce a significant amount of milk, supplementation may be necessary. Focusing on the nursing relationship is a priority.

Transgender Men. A transgender man is genetically a female and identifies as and lives as a male. Many transgender men keep their female reproductive organs and thus have the option to carry a pregnancy. A transgender man may have surgery to remove breast tissue and contour the chest wall to facilitate male gender identity and create a male-appearing chest. Depending on the amount of glandular tissue remaining, some degree of lactation may be possible. Transgender men often take testosterone to induce masculine changes to the body. They will discontinue it to become pregnant.

Some transgender men elect to chestfeed, a term used for the male version of nursing. Those who do chestfeed often use a supplementer to ensure sufficient intake for their baby. There may be minimal chest tissue for the baby to latch on to, posing challenges in positioning and latch.

There is an increased risk of postpartum depression for transgender men. Experiencing pregnancy, birth, and lactation may create emotional challenges stemming from feeling in the wrong body. Using female organs while living as a male can be confusing and emotionally difficult. Chestfeeding may trigger feelings of gender dysphoria in some individuals, causing anxiety or depression. Although this does not happen with all transgender men, it is important to keep in mind if you work with the transgender community. Transgender men need to be counseled to do what will help them be happy and healthy parents.

Lactation in the LGBTQ+ Community

Induction of lactation in a non-gestational parent enables individuals within the LGBTQ+ population to nurse their babies. Emphasizing the nonnutritive and nutritional benefits of nursing will help parents navigate the variable rates of milk production inherent in induced lactation. LGBTQ+ parents are resourceful in educating themselves about inducing lactation (Juntereal & Spatz, 2020). Induced lactation is discussed in **Chapter 23**. Variations in lactation for these parents include co-nursing, chestfeeding, and use a supplemental device.

Breast development from estrogen-based gender-affirming hormone therapy can produce milk with adequate nutrient content for infant growth, with possible supplementation (Weimer, 2023). One transgender parent who had a significant increase in breast size and fullness at 1 month postpartum produced up to 3 to 5 ounces of milk per day (Wamboldt, 2021). Better social and family support is needed to improve chestfeeding by transgender parents.

Improving LGBTQ+ access to peer support is an important priority for lactation and maternity care providers. A gender-affirming perinatal environment can minimize feelings of invisibility, isolation, and loneliness among pregnant and birthing transgender parents (Rafferty et al., 2018). Effective support can improve health outcomes for both the lactating parents and their infants (Farrow, 2015). This is especially important, given that many in this community experience barriers to and stresses in obtaining health care (Dearing & Hequembourg, 2014). The ABM provides a protocol to guide practitioners who work with families in the LGBTQ+ community (Ferri et al., 2020).

Summary

Sensitivity to the characteristics of families in various lifestyles can help tailor counseling to meet their needs. Parents who experience opposition to nursing will benefit from strategies for garnering support from family, friends, employers, and others close to them. Low-income families have many societal challenges to overcome as they navigate parenting and lactation. Single parents often face economic and social disparities as they take on parenting responsibilities with limited support. Teen parents transition into parenthood while also experiencing normal adolescent changes and development. Parents in the LGBTQ+ community need gender-affirming care and support for inducing lactation. These lifestyles all present challenges in supporting parents throughout nursing.

What You Learned—At a Glance

Conversation Starters with Parents

- How do your partner and other family members feel about your nursing?
- How secure is your access to food for your family?
- How are you adjusting to being a new parent?
- What lifestyle challenges affect your parenting?
- What pronouns do you use?

Family Influence on Lactation

- Help parents cope with opposition to nursing.
- Educate an unsupportive partner about health risks associated with not nursing.
- Avoid placing yourself in the middle of conflicts with an unsupportive family member.
- Build parents' confidence with positive feedback.

Low-Income or Single Parents

- Give practical suggestions, not general advice.
- Use visual aids, including electronic and social media, to reinforce verbal explanations.
- Provide educational materials at an appropriate literacy level.
- Reach out to families in their own neighborhoods.
- Help families access supplemental food programs.
- Support choices determined by lifestyle restrictions.

Teen Parents

- Need sound prenatal care and nutrition
- May feel inadequate as parents
- May experience opposition or support from family, friends, and partner
- May not nurse enough for robust milk production
- Need one-to-one, supportive relationships
- Need to be treated as adults
- Need concrete, simple suggestions and information

LGBTQ+ Families

- Gender-neutral terminology allows inclusion of all sexes or genders.
- Parents may have difficulty finding sensitive, emotionally supportive health care.
- There are varied relationship dynamics of couples.
- There is no commonly agreed-upon language for a nonbirth parent.
- Parents may co-nurse, chestfeed, induce lactation, or use a supplemental device.

References

Abbass-Dick J, et al. Designing an ehealth breastfeeding resource with young mothers using a participatory design. *J Transcult Nurs*. 2021;32(3):295–303.

Academy of Breastfeeding Medicine, et al. ABM clinical protocol #19: breastfeeding promotion in the prenatal setting, revision 2015. *Breastfeed Med*. 2015;10(10):451–457.

Ahmed AH, Rojjanasrirat W. Breastfeeding outcomes, self-efficacy, and satisfaction among low-income women with late-preterm, early-term, and full-term infants. *J Obstet Gynecol Neonatal Nurs*. 2021;50(5):583–596. https://cepr.org/voxeu/columns/why-children-teen-mothers-do-worse-life

Angelo BHB, et al. Knowledge, attitudes and practices of grandmothers related to breastfeeding: a meta-synthesis. *Rev Lat Am Enfermagem*. 2020;28:e3214.

Annie E. Casey Foundation. *Kids Count. 2021 Data Book: 2021 State Trends in Child Wellbeing*. Baltimore, MD: Annie E. Casey Foundation; 2021. https://datacenter.aecf.org/data/tables/107-children-in-single-parent-families-by-race-and-ethnicity#detailed/1/any/false/2048/10,9,12,13/432,431

Arora A, et al. Determinants for early introduction of complementary foods in Australian infants: findings from the HSHK birth cohort study. *Nutr J*. 2020;19(1):16.

Barbosa GEF, et al. Initial breastfeeding difficulties and association with breast disorders among postpartum women. *Rev Paul Pediatr*. 2017;35(3):265–272.

Borger C, et al. Prenatal and postnatal experiences predict breastfeeding patterns in the WIC Infant and Toddler Feeding Practices Study-2. *Breastfeed Med*. 2021;16(11):869–877.

Buckland C, et al. Interventions to promote exclusive breastfeeding among young mothers: a systematic review and meta-analysis. *Int Breastfeed J*. 2020;15(1):102.

Buckland C, et al. Experiences of young Australian mothers with infant feeding. *BMC Pregnancy Childbirth*. 2022;22(1):489.

Cameron LD, et al. Beliefs about marijuana use during pregnancy and breastfeeding held by residents of a Latino-majority, rural region of California. *J Behav Med*. 2022;45(4):544–557.

Čatipović M, et al. Effects of a breastfeeding educational intervention on secondary school students after 6 months. *Acta Clin Croat*. 2021;60(4):569–578.

Centers for Disease Control and Prevention. Breastfeeding report card 2018. August 20, 2018. https://www.cdc.gov/breastfeeding/data/reportcard.htm

Centers for Disease Control and Prevention. Births and natality. Births: final data for 2018. 2019b. https://www.cdc.gov/nchs/fastats/births.htm

Chepkirui D, et al. A scoping review of breastfeeding peer support models applied in hospital settings. *Int Breastfeed J*. 2020;15(1):95.

Chopel A, et al. Multilevel factors influencing young mothers' breastfeeding: a qualitative CBPR study. *J Hum Lact*. 2019;35(2):301–317.

Corsack C, et al. Parental cohabitation and breastfeeding outcomes among United States adolescent mothers. *Breastfeed Med*. 2022;17(1):72–78.

Croll J, et al. LGBTQ+ individuals and pregnancy outcomes: a commentary. *BJOG*. 2022;129(10):1625–1629.

Dearing RL, Hequembourg AL. Culturally (in)competent? Dismantling health care barriers for sexual minority women. *Soc Work Health Care*. 2014;53(8):739–761.

Farrow A. Lactation support and the LGBTQI community. *J Hum Lact*. 2015;31(1):26–28.

Ferreira TDM, et al. Influence of grandmothers on exclusive breastfeeding: cross-sectional study. *Einstein (Sao Paulo)*. 2018;16(4): eAO4293.

Ferri RL, et al. ABM Clinical Protocol #33: Lactation care for lesbian, gay, bisexual, transgender, queer, questioning, plus patients. *Breastfeed Med*. 2020;15(5):284–293.

Frazier CM, et al. Breastfeeding: how is it related to food insecurity and other factors among low-income mothers? *Health Care Women Int*. 2023;44(3):234–245.

French CD, et al. Perinatal hospital practices are associated with breastfeeding through 5 months postpartum among women and infants from low-income households. *J Nutr*. 2023;153(1):322–330.

Frenoy P, et al. Demographic, socioeconomic, and sociocultural factors associated with any breastfeeding in homeless mothers. *Matern Child Nutr*. 2021;17(3):e13167.

Godbout JM, et al. Factors associated with infant feeding choices in the adolescent population. *J Hum Lact*. 2016;32(4):642–647.

Guttmacher Institute. Teen pregnancy. 2024. https://www.guttmacher.org/united-states/teens/teen-pregnancy

Hamilton BE, et al. *Births: Provisional Data for 2021*. Vital Statistics Rapid Release No. 20. Hyattsville, MD: National Center for Health Statistics; May 2022.

Hernández MIN, Riesco ML. Exclusive breastfeeding abandonment in adolescent mothers: a cohort study within health primary services. *Rev Lat Am Enfermagem*. 2022;30(spe):e3786.

Hornsby PP, et al. Timing of introduction of complementary foods and beverages to infants of low-income women. *Breastfeed Med*. 2021;16(7):547–552.

Hunter-Adams J, et al. Investigating the disjoint between education and health policy for infant feeding among teenage mothers in South Africa: a case for intersectoral work. *BMC Public Health*. 2022;22(1):16.

Juntereal NA, Spatz DL. Breastfeeding experiences of same-sex mothers. *Birth*. 2020;47(1):21–28.

Karmacharya C, et al. Grandmothers' knowledge positively influences maternal knowledge and infant and young child feeding practices. *Public Health Nutr*. 2017;20(12):2114–2123.

Kay MC, et al. Are low-income, diverse mothers able to meet breastfeeding intentions after 2 months of breastfeeding? *Breastfeed Med*. 2020;15(7):435–442.

Kehinde J, et al. The effectiveness of prenatal breastfeeding education on breastfeeding uptake postpartum: a systematic review. *Midwifery*. 2023;118:103579.

Kivlighan KT, et al. Improved breastfeeding duration with Baby Friendly Hospital Initiative implementation in a diverse and underserved population. *Birth*. 2020;47(1):135–143.

Kumar P, et al. What predicts the knowledge of breastfeeding practices among late adolescent girls? Evidence from a cross-sectional analysis. *PLoS One*. 2021;16(10):e0258347.

Kuzma EK, et al. Lesbian, gay, bisexual, and transgender health: creating safe spaces and caring for patients with cultural humility. *J Am Assoc Nurse Pract*. 2019;31(3):167–174.

Landry J, Kensler P. Providing culturally sensitive care to women who are in the sexual minority or are gender nonconforming. *Nurs Women's Health*. 2019;23(2):163–171.

Lauer EA, et al. Identifying barriers and supports to breastfeeding in the workplace experienced by mothers in the New Hampshire Special Supplemental Nutrition Program for Women, Infants, and Children utilizing the total worker health framework. *Int J Environ Res Public Health*. 2019;16(4):529.

Lewkowitz AK, et al. Infant feeding practices and perceived optimal breastfeeding interventions among low-income women delivering at a Baby-Friendly Hospital. *Am J Perinatol*. 2019;36(7):669–677.

Lewkowitz AK, et al. Effect of a novel smartphone application on breastfeeding rates among low-income, first-time mothers intending to exclusively breastfeed: secondary analysis of a randomized controlled trial. *Breastfeed Med*. 2021;16(1):59–67.

Li K, et al. WIC participation and breastfeeding after the 2009 WIC revision: a propensity score approach. *Int J Environ Res Public Health*. 2019;16(15):2645.

Macapagal K, et al. Differences in healthcare access, use, and experiences within a community sample of racially diverse lesbian, gay, bisexual, transgender, and questioning emerging adults. *LGBT Health*. 2016;3(6):434–442.

Marks KJ, et al. Early introduction of complementary foods/drinks and milk feeding type in the Special Supplemental Nutrition Program for Women, Infants and Children (WIC). *Matern Child Nutr*. 2023;19(4):e13541.

Martin JA, et al. Births: final data for 2017. National vital statistics reports from the Centers for Disease Control and Prevention, National Center for Health Statistics. *Natl Vital Stat Rep*. 2018;67(8):1–50. https://www.cdc.gov/nchs/data/nvsr/nvsr67/nvsr67_08-508.pdf

Muelbert M, Giugliani ERJ. Factors associated with the maintenance of breastfeeding for 6, 12, and 24 months in adolescent mothers. *BMC Public Health*. 2018;18(1):675.

Namutebi M, et al. Teenage first-time mothers' perceptions about their health care needs in the immediate and early postpartum period in Uganda. *BMC Pregnancy Childbirth*. 2022;22(1):743.

Nandi P, et al. Changing disparities in teen birth rates and repeat birth rates in Georgia: implications for teen pregnancy prevention. *Contraception*. 2019;99(3):175–178.

Natale BN, et al. Duration of breastfeeding mediates the association between early socioeconomic risk and child vocabulary at age 4. *J Dev Behav Pediatr*. 2021;42(6):472–480.

Noble L, et al. The effect of breastfeeding in the first hour and rooming-in of low-income, multi-ethnic mothers on in-hospital, one and three month high breastfeeding intensity. *Children (Basel)*. 2023;10(2):313.

Odar Stough C, et al. Predictors of exclusive breastfeeding for 6 months in a national sample of US children. *Am J Health Promot*. 2019;33(1):48–56.

Patterson JA, et al. Differences in exclusive breastfeeding rates in US hospitals according to Baby-Friendly Hospital Initiative designation and Area Deprivation Index category. *Breastfeed Med*. 2021;16(10):799–806.

Rafferty et al. Ensuring comprehensive care and support for transgender and gender-diverse children and adolescents. *Pediatrics*. 2018;142(4):e20182162.

Ruud M. Cultural humility in the care of individuals who are lesbian, gay, bisexual, transgender, or queer. *Nurs Women's Health*. 2018;22(3):255–263.

SmithBattle L, et al. Navigating a minefield: meta-synthesis of teen mothers' breastfeeding experience. *MCN Am J Matern Child Nurs*. 2020;45(3):145–154.

Sutton A, et al. Rural-urban disparities in pregnancy intentions, births, and abortions among US adolescent and young women, 1995–2017. *Am J Public Health.* 2019;109(12):1762–1769.

Thacker K, et al. Swimming upstream: addressing racial disparities in teen births in North Carolina. *N C Med J.* 2022;83(4): 249–252.

Vázquez-Vázquez ADP, et al. Do maternal grandmothers influence breastfeeding duration and infant nutrition? Evidence from Merida, Mexico. *Am J Biol Anthropol.* 2022;179(3):444–459.

Wamboldt R, et al. Lactation induction in a transgender woman wanting to breastfeed: case report. *J Clin Endocrinol Metab.* 2021;106(5):e2047–e2052.

Weimer AK. Lactation induction in a transgender woman: macronutrient analysis and patient perspectives. *J Hum Lact.* 2023; 39(3):488–494.

Wong SPW, et al. Risk factors and birth outcomes associated with teenage pregnancy: a Canadian sample. *J Pediatr Adolesc Gynecol.* 2020;33(2):153–159.

World Health Organization. Adolescent pregnancy. Key facts. February 23, 2018. https://www.who.int/news-room/fact-sheets/detail/adolescent-pregnancy

Yasuda S, et al. Risk factors for discontinuation of exclusive breast feeding within 1 month: a retrospective cohort study in Japan. *Int Breastfeed J.* 2022;17(1):20.

CHAPTER 22

Nursing Techniques and Tools

Humans are fascinated with the use of technology, and lactating parents are no exception. A wide variety of tools and technologies are marketed to expectant and nursing families. It is important that caregivers and parents alike consider what families really need for nursing. Moreover, what do parents really need to care for their infant? Advertisements for baby care items often focus on separation of parents and babies, giving the impression that separation is the desired norm. This trend is evident in nursing tools as well, with the use of a breast pump often reflecting an assumption that the parents and baby will be apart during feedings. Appropriate and conservative use of nursing and lactation tools increases your effectiveness with parents. Overuse of tools can overwhelm new parents and make nursing seem tedious. Teaching parents to nurse with only the tools they truly need increases their self-efficacy.

KEY TERMS

Alternate feeding method
Breast massage
Breast pump
C-hold
Cup feeding
Dancer hand position
Digital techniques
Disorganized suck
Exclusively pump
Finger feeding
Holder pasteurization
Human milk bank
Inverted nipple
Manual expression
Nil per os (NPO)
Nipple shield
Nursing supplementer
Paced feeding
Paladai
Pinch test
Pooled milk
Reverse pressure softening

Nursing Techniques

Teaching parents some simple skills to help with nursing is useful prenatally and in the early weeks postpartum. Performing a **pinch test**, for example, helps to determine whether the nipples will evert for feedings. Learning how to massage the breasts and how to soften the area around the nipple helps with latch and facilitates milk expression. Supporting the breast during feedings can help the baby maintain a good latch during the early days of nursing.

Testing for Nipple Eversion

Babies need the nipple to evert sufficiently to latch for feeding. The pinch test can be used prenatally to assess the ability of the nipples to evert. **Figure 22-1** illustrates a nipple before testing it for inversion. The parent grasps the base of the nipple with their forefinger and thumb and presses them together several times around the base. If the nipple moves outward, it everts normally and needs no intervention. Stimulating the nipple by rolling it can also cause it to evert more prominently.

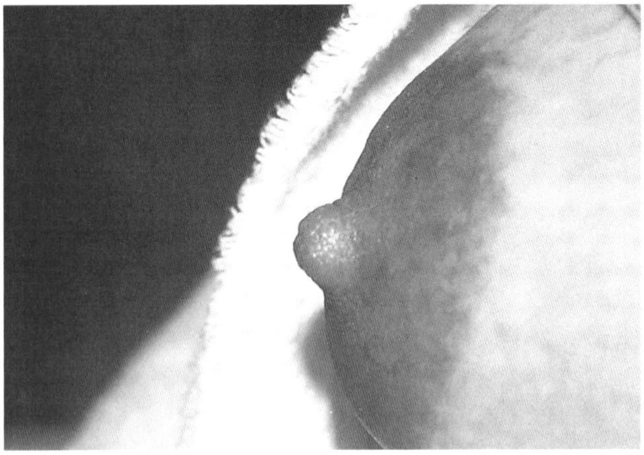

Figure 22-1 Pinch test: nipple at rest.

Courtesy of B. Wilson-Clay/K. Hoover.

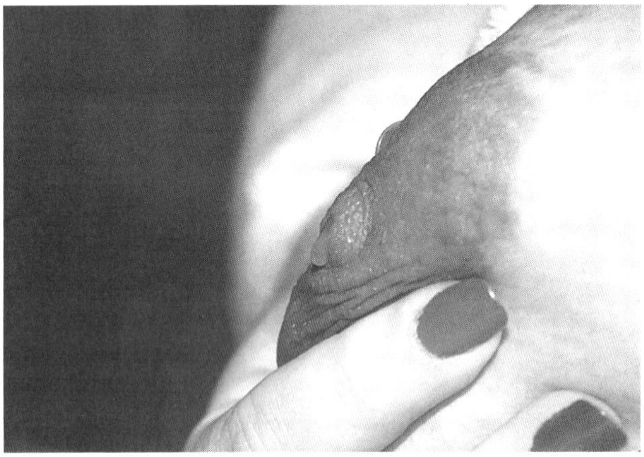

Figure 22-2 Pinch test: nipple retracts after compression.

Courtesy of B. Wilson-Clay/K. Hoover.

A retracting nipple moves inward rather than outward when tested, as depicted in **Figure 22-2**. A parent who learns they have retracted or **inverted nipples** near the end of the pregnancy can begin manipulating their nipples to help increase protraction. After the baby is born, a nipple that retracts may benefit from the use of a nipple eversion tool or a **breast pump**.

Be aware that a nipple may appear to be inverted on visual inspection and then evert when pinched. Although this type of nipple may need shaping before latching the baby, it will most likely not interfere with nursing. A completely inverted nipple appears inverted on visual inspection and does not respond to stimulation. This type of nipple may improve with manipulation. Chapter 7 discusses differences in nipples.

Breast Massage and Compression

Any form of massage encourages relaxation. **Breast massage** and breast compression can be helpful for nursing in a variety of situations. Touch causes myoepithelial cells to contract. Thus, massaging and compressing the breast helps stimulate letdown. Massage works in combination with oxytocin and the myoepithelial cells to help "push" the milk down the ducts so that it is available for the baby to remove or for expression. Squeezing increases positive pressure inside the breast, facilitating the movement of milk from an area of high pressure to an area of low pressure (the baby's mouth).

Breast massage will help stimulate letdown just before a feeding or milk expression. Combining breast massage with other relaxation techniques, such as deep breathing and visualization, will further enhance letdown. Initiating letdown through breast massage can be especially useful when attempting to relactate or to initiate lactation when nursing without birthing. It is useful for any baby who seems impatient for milk flow to begin.

Combining breast massage with gentle compression during a feeding stimulates milk flow and encourages sustained sucking. Intermittent massage also increases fat content with pumping (Orovou et al., 2022). This may be helpful with a preterm, sleepy, or nonrobust baby. During breast massage, oxytocin levels increase and remain high throughout the massage, resulting in more milk production (Orovou et al., 2022).

Parents often instinctively massage and compress the breast while nursing. You can point out these behaviors and praise them for naturally knowing what to do. Affirming their intuitive behavior helps build their confidence in themselves and their bodies. Breast compression can be used to squeeze milk into the baby's mouth when sucking is no longer nutritive. The compression simulates a letdown, often triggering another sucking burst. This can be repeated throughout a feeding whenever the baby stops sucking nutritively.

Breast Massage Technique

Breast massage is a useful technique to teach and easy for parents to learn (**Figure 22-3**). The parent can begin by exerting gentle pressure on the breast with the palm of the hand or fist, massaging in a circular and oscillating motion from the chest wall toward the nipple. They can also gently tap the breast with their fingertips. Massage continues in this manner, rotating around the breast. Parents should focus on the areas of greatest milk duct development, which are under the breast and along the side under the arm. Parents with large breasts can support the breast with the opposite hand while they massage one side at a time.

Although there are cultural variations in breast massage, they all accomplish the same thing. Oketani

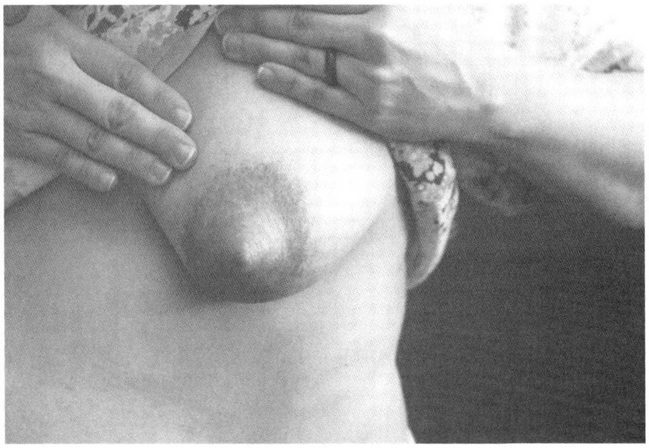

Figure 22-3 Breast massage.

Photo courtesy of Regina Maria Roig-Romero.

breast massage is popular in Asian countries for stimulating milk production. This technique focuses on the tissues that connect the chest muscles to the breast. It involves all breast muscles, affecting lymph and blood flow and decreasing milk stasis. Oketani breast massage reduces the pain associated with engorgement and stimulates oxytocin levels (Mahdizadeh-Shahri et al., 2021). The massager's finger motions simulate the baby's sucking, and the increased pressure helps move the fats and other solids that adhere to the alveoli through the ducts. Massaging the breast tissue before and during a feeding could help to increase the fat content transferred to the infant.

Reverse Pressure Softening

Parents who receive intravenous fluids during childbirth can experience edema in their breasts, resulting in flattening of the areola similar to engorgement. A **reverse pressure softening** technique helps move the fluid away from the areola so that the baby can latch. **Table 22-1** illustrates this procedure, with instructions and alternative positions for finger placement. The procedure is helpful in relieving engorgement and triggering the letdown reflex.

Supporting the Breast

There are a variety of ways to form and support the breast to help the baby latch in the early days. Parents who are uncomfortable touching and handling their breasts may need verbal encouragement and, with their permission, "hands-on" assistance. Not all parents need to support the breast to assist with latch. The need for breast support also depends on the position in which the parent holds the baby for feeding. For example, in a laid-back or side-lying position, there is little need for breast support. The **C-hold** and **Dancer hand position** are two methods for supporting the breast.

C-Hold

The C-hold cups the breast with one hand in the shape of the letter *C* to form the breast and nipple to help the baby latch. The parent can cup the breast in their hand, placing their thumb on top and their fingers below (refer to **Figure 15-5** in **Chapter 15**). Make sure the hand is well behind the nipple so that the fingers do not interfere with latch. They can avoid touching the baby's chin, jaw, or lips by moving the hand back toward the chest wall.

Depending on the baby's position, the fingers and thumb can slightly compress the breast to match the plane of the baby's mouth and help form it for the baby. Describing this as a "breast sandwich" will help parents visualize how to shape the breast. **Figure 16-9** in **Chapter 16** illustrates the sandwich hold. Many babies need this assistance only for the initial latch, until they settle into the feeding. If the baby has difficulty maintaining latch, continuing this support throughout the feeding can prevent the nipple from slipping out of the baby's mouth.

Dancer Hand Position

A slight variation of the C-hold is useful with preterm infants and babies who have weak muscle development and find it difficult to hold their jaw steady while they suck. The Dancer hand position, named for Sarah Danner and Ed Cerruti, begins in the C-hold position. The parent supports the baby's chin in the crook of their hand between the thumb and index finger and supports the breast with the remaining three fingers (refer to **Figure 15-6** in **Chapter 15**).

Bending the index finger slightly enables the parent to gently hold the baby's cheek on one side, with their thumb holding the other cheek. This hold helps decrease the available space in the baby's mouth and increases negative pressure. The use of steady, equal pressure while holding the baby's cheeks avoids interfering with the rooting reflex. As the baby's muscle tone begins to improve, the parent can move their thumb back on top of the breast, with their index finger supporting the baby's chin.

Digital Techniques

The use of **digital techniques** in the baby's mouth ranges from inserting a finger to calm a baby, to assessing the oral cavity, to improving a baby's suck. Many parents use a finger to calm a fussy baby or help

Table 22-1 Reverse Pressure Softening Technique

1. One-handed "flower hold." Fingernails short, fingertips curved, placed where baby's tongue will go.

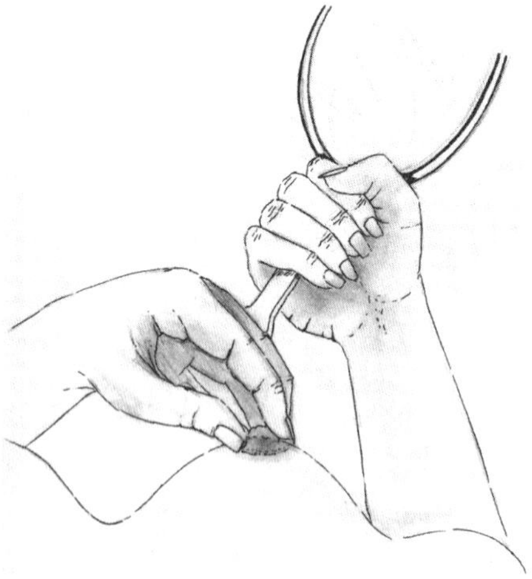

2. Two-handed, one-step method. Fingernails short, fingertips curved, each one touching the side of nipple.

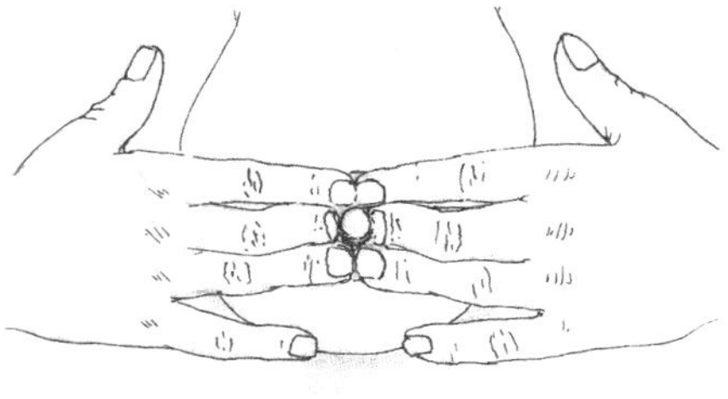

3. You may ask someone to help press by placing fingers or thumbs on top of yours.

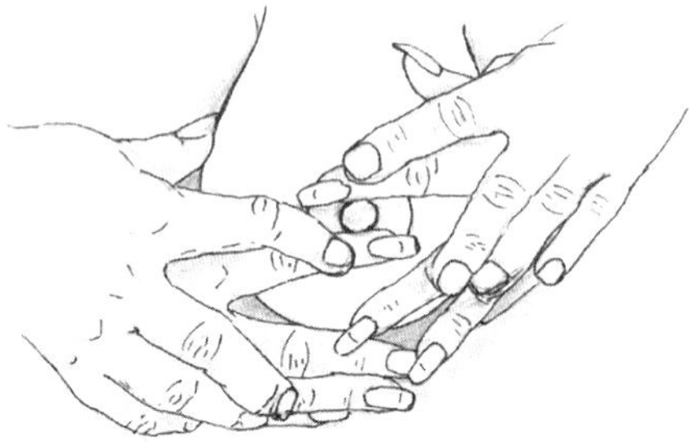

4. Two-step method, two hands, using two or three straight fingers on each side, first knuckles touching nipple. Move ¼ turn, repeat above and below nipple.

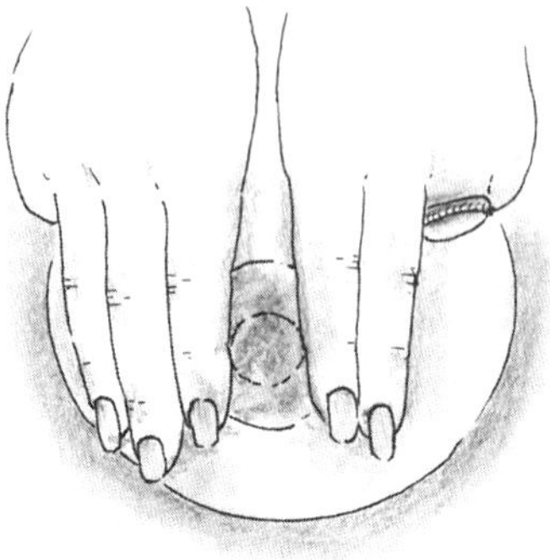

5. Two-step method, two hands, using straight thumbs, base of thumbnail even with side of nipple. Move ¼ turn, repeat, thumbs above and below nipple.

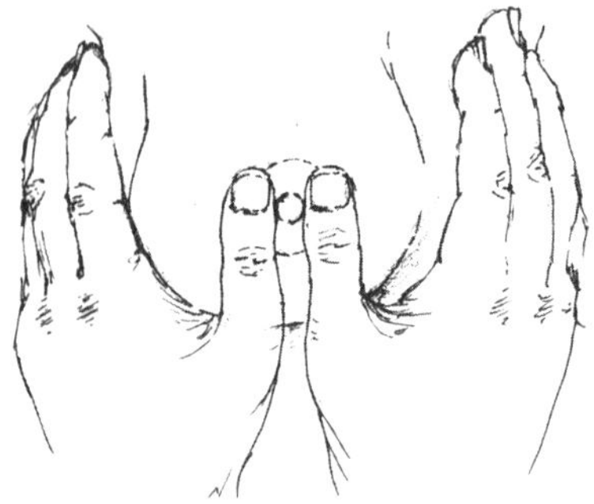

6. Soft ring method. Cut off bottom half of an artificial nipple to place on areola to press with fingers.

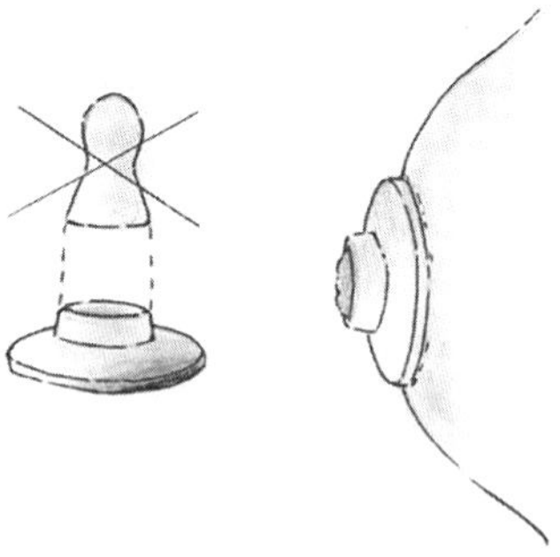

the baby organize sucking before nursing. Clinicians often assess aspects of a baby's sucking competency with a gloved finger (Genna, 2023). The baby's oral cavity is extremely sensitive and contains many nerve fibers and impulses, calling for judicious use of oral assessment. **Chapter 16** discusses digital techniques.

Nursing Tools

In some circumstances specific tools may be needed to manage feedings or to care for breast tissue. Careful assessment will enable you to make appropriate suggestions. Starting with the least invasive, yet effective, methods generally leads to fewer complications. Parents who use nursing tools often need special counseling suggestions and close follow-up. No tool is perfect or appropriate for every situation. It is important to be familiar with several options and collaborate with the parent on their use.

Lubricants and Ointments

Montgomery glands within the areola normally keep the nipple area soft and pliable. An artificial lubricant is necessary only if this natural lubrication is insufficient and needs to be replaced. A lubricant or ointment may be necessary if dry skin or a skin condition requires more moisture. Ointments, also called *balms* and *butters*, might help soothe damaged nipples. Some parents rub expressed milk into the nipple skin to promote healthy tissue. Once the milk has dried, a topical lubricant or ointment can be applied as needed. Research varies on the effect of breast lubricants (refer to the discussion on nipple pain in this chapter and in **Chapter 17**). Parents who use a breast pump may find that lubrication decreases irritation from the friction between the breast tissue and pump flange.

Lubricants to Avoid

The choice of lubricant must take into consideration its potential effects on the health of both the skin and the baby. Avoid any lubricant that contains petroleum because it inhibits skin respiration and can worsen nipple damage. Petroleum-based products include baby oil, petroleum jelly, cocoa butter, A and D ointment, and dimethicone. Additionally, parents should avoid products that contain alcohol, which is drying to the skin. Essential oils should also be avoided because they are unsafe if ingested by the infant.

When there is a family history of allergies, parents should avoid exposing the baby to a potential allergen, such as peanut oil or massé cream. Parents with a family history of wool allergy should avoid lubricants that contain lanolin, which is a wool derivative. Any product that must be washed off can further irritate damaged nipples from rubbing the nipple with a washcloth. Parents receive a variety of breast creams in the hospital that also are available in most pharmacies. Although these products do no harm, they are generally ineffective in preventing nipple pain and may delay families from seeking early help.

Acceptable Topical Treatments

There is no substitute for clinical judgment and experience when managing nipple pain. You should first address the root cause of the pain and determine whether correcting the latch and positioning will provide relief. If pain persists despite adjustments, topical creams or gel pads may help resolve transient pain and extend nursing duration. Some parents massage a small amount of their milk onto the nipples at the end of each feeding until their nipples heal. This may be all that is needed in treating damaged nipple tissue (Peric et al., 2023).

Although there are many nipple ointments on the market, lanolin is one of the most prevalent. Hypoallergenic, medical-grade, anhydrous lanolin may help severely dry or damaged nipples. This form of lanolin does not contain the concerning levels of pesticides or alcohols that contribute to allergic response and is therefore less of a risk in individuals with allergies. A small amount massaged gently onto the nipple and areola is sufficient. When applied after a feeding, the skin absorbs the lubricant before the next feeding. Research reports mixed results on the efficacy of lanolin for preventing tissue damage and promoting healing (Douglas et al., 2022; Peric et al., 2023).

Water-based hydrogel pads can be worn between feedings to keep the skin moist. Wound care gel pads are typically square and can be cut into four pieces. Circular gel pads designed for breast use are typically available two to a package. Storing them in the refrigerator provides the additional comfort of coolness. Some gel pads can be washed and reused. Their use should be discontinued if nipple pain increases or if any sign of infection occurs. When using gel pads, some lactation consultants recommend air-drying the nipple before feeding. Although hydrogel pads are commonly recommended, study results vary regarding their efficacy in wound healing (Douglas et al., 2022). The inconsistent evidence highlights the need for healthcare providers to educate their clients on proper latch and positioning and provide clinical assessment of any skin breakdown.

Silver caps are medical caps impregnated with silver and worn over the nipple inside the bra. Silver has antibacterial properties and can penetrate and destroy bacteria and fungi by producing hydrogen peroxide. The caps are worn continuously when not nursing, providing a barrier to the wound. Silver caps are reportedly more effective than rubbing expressed milk over the area in reducing and healing nipple pain (Niazi et al., 2018). These caps vary in price and are easily available online.

Peppermint, in the form of oils, gels, and water, is also used for damaged nipples. Peppermint, a main active agent of menthol, has antimicrobial properties. Caution is advised when applying peppermint or menthol to nipples because peppermint has the potential to suppress milk production (Suzuki et al., 2020). Nipple wounds reportedly heal faster with peppermint oil or peppermint water than with the use of expressed milk alone. Other herbs and oils, including aloe vera, coconut oil, olive oil, and tea tree oil, are also found to be helpful (Lin & Lu, 2023; Niazi et al., 2018; Sag˘lık & Kısacık, 2021; Şahin et al., 2023).

All-purpose nipple ointment (APNO), or "triple nipple" ointment, is commonly used to treat nipple trauma. It is a mixture of an antibiotic ointment, an antifungal cream, and a steroid (refer to **Figure 17-2**). Careful consideration should be given before using APNO. Most situations do not require all three of these medications to be used. One study found that APNO was not superior to lanolin in the treatment of nipple pain (Niazi et al., 2018). Nipple treatment is discussed more in **Chapter 17**.

Tools for Flat or Inverted Nipples

Several tools are available to help draw out a flat or inverted nipple. It is important to educate parents on their options for nipple eversion so that they can make an informed choice. Suction from a breast pump before a feeding may evert the nipple sufficiently to improve latch. Used after a feeding it can promote long-term nipple protrusion. Some clinicians have used an inverted syringe to evert a flat or inverted nipple. However, because nipple eversion is not the intended use for a syringe, a commercial tool designed for everting nipples is a better option.

Several commercial eversion products are available to help draw out a flat or inverted nipple. One commercial eversion product is a syringe with a soft, flexible tip made of silicone. Applying suction with the syringe helps nipples protrude for easier latch. Another type resembles a miniature bicycle horn and is used by squeezing the bulb. This tool needs to be washed thoroughly with hot, soapy water and many hot water rinses to prevent bacteria from growing in the bulb section.

A nipple everter can be used two or three times a day prenatally for inversion when there is no risk of early labor. After birth, the tool can help evert the nipple before feedings for babies who have difficulty latching. To begin a feeding, the parent applies suction for 30 seconds two or three times, releasing the suction in between. Some parents may find it cumbersome to use this tool before every feeding.

It is important that the parent controls the everter and not the caregiver. Parents can assess their comfort level as they apply appropriate pressure. They should never pull hard enough to cause pain or color changes in the nipple. If they experience pain, they should stop the procedure. After each use, the everter should be washed in hot, soapy water and then rinsed and air-dried for the next use. Several small studies report success with use of a nipple everter (Nabulsi et al., 2022; Kaya et al., 2024 Kaya et al., 2024).

Breast Shells

Plastic breast shells are worn against the breast inside the bra for a variety of purposes. Increasing bra size to accommodate the shell will avoid pressing it too tightly against the breast. Selecting shells with several openings for air circulation will keep the breast skin healthy. Caution parents not to wear breast shells while they sleep and not to use them excessively.

Breast shells are sometimes worn prenatally to place gentle pressure on the areola, which stretches and pushes the nipple forward. There is no clear research to support the premise that wearing breast shells prenatally everts nipples. However, anecdotally, parents have reported good results.

Wearing breast shells between, or for short periods before, feedings can help shape a flat or inverted nipple to improve latch. They might also prevent nipple pain, by promoting nipple eversion and reducing tissue engorgement (Cecilio et al., 2022). Breast shells can protect a damaged nipple between feedings and prevent rubbing against clothing that could irritate the skin further. Combining shell use with an ointment or expressed milk on the nipples may help with healing.

Some parents use breast shells to relieve engorgement, keeping them in place for about 20 minutes before feedings. One study reported a delay in engorgement in the first 5 days postpartum when breast shells were worn daily for most waking hours (Cecilio et al., 2022).

Some parents wear breast shells to protect clothes from milk that leaks between feedings. Milk that accumulates in a breast shell worn between feedings should not be saved because of possible bacterial growth. However, when worn on the opposite side during a feeding, the collected milk may be saved. When saving the drip milk, the shell needs to be clean and put in place immediately before the feeding, with the milk collected as soon as the feeding ends.

Nipple Shield

A **nipple shield** is an artificial nipple placed over the nipple to begin a feeding so that the baby latches on to

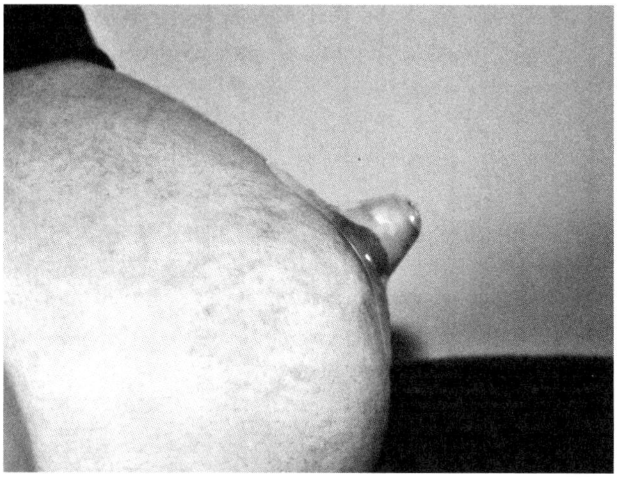

Figure 22-4 Nipple shield on the breast to attach the baby.

Printed with permission of Anna Swisher.

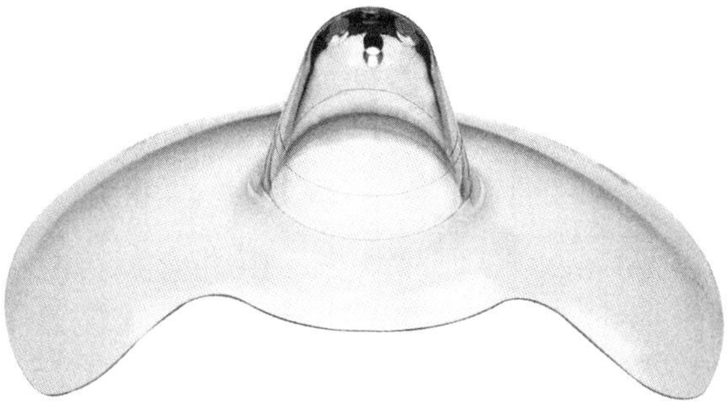

Figure 22-5 Contact nipple shield.

© Medela, Inc.

the nipple shield to nurse (**Figure 22-4**). Several holes on the tip of the nipple shield, like those on a bottle nipple, allow milk to flow when the infant sucks. Most modern nipple shields are made of thin silicone, some with cutouts to allow the baby's nose and chin to remain in contact with the breast (**Figure 22-5**). Nipple shields made of rubber or latex can significantly decrease milk transfer and should not be used. A baby bottle nipple should never be used as a nipple shield.

Nipple shields are widely available online and in retail stores. Parents often purchase them based on recommendations from friends, relatives, or social networks. It is common for parents to bring nipple shields to the hospital when they arrive to have their baby. Considerations when purchasing a nipple shield include comfort and selection of the correct size and material (silicone). Cautions about nipple shield use include the potential for the infant's preference for the artificial nipple, possible breast tissue damage, and incorrect placement during feeding.

Concern has been expressed about the impact of the use of a nipple shield on milk production and transfer. However, studies suggest that neither is negatively affected by the use of a nipple shield (Coentro et al., 2020; Coentro et al., 2021a, 2021b, 2022). Professional support and frequent monitoring can assess adequate milk production and transfer. Your clinical judgment will help you determine the best intervention for each nursing dyad. Optimally, nipple shields should be used under the care of a skilled lactation consultant to ensure appropriate use.

Appropriate Use of a Nipple Shield

A nipple shield can be a useful tool for nursing when used appropriately. It should not be the first intervention for difficulties with latch or sucking. Other techniques need to be tried first, such as a change in positioning, forming the breast tissue to assist latch, reducing breast fullness, and nipple eversion techniques. Nipple shields can help improve latch in the case of flat or inverted nipples or a baby with a persistent shallow latch. They also appear to help preterm and small-for-gestational-age babies with low tone sustain suction within the oral cavity by holding the nipple in their mouth. A nipple shield may compensate for the lack of fat buccal pads and weak suck common in these babies.

Nipple shields are used for babies with a short tongue, tight frenulum, or high palate. They may help reduce excessive milk flow for an infant who has difficulty controlling milk flow as well as to reduce pain caused by an infant's strong suction. A shield can also aid the transition to direct nursing when a baby has been bottle fed and rejects direct nursing. If a parent is considering weaning because of nursing difficulties, a shield can buy time to work through the challenges and preserve nursing (Coentro et al., 2022).

Method for Using a Nipple Shield

Nipple shields are typically available in 16-, 20-, 21-, 24-, 25-, and 26-mm sizes. Selecting the smallest shield possible that accommodates both the baby's mouth and the nipple enables the baby to obtain a deep latch. Parents should never force a large, prominent nipple into a small shield. With the appropriately sized shield, ensure the parent understands how to apply it for the best fit. Moistening the edges of the shield will help it adhere to the skin. Folding it back so that it is almost inside out will ensure snug placement over the nipple. With the nipple centered in the shield, the parent can then smooth the shield over the nipple.

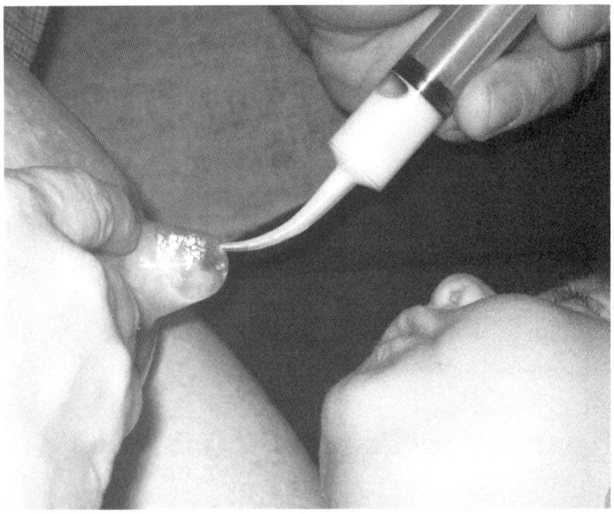

Figure 22-6 Filling nipple shield with milk to entice baby to suck.

Printed with permission of Catherine Watson Genna, BS, IBCLC.

The baby's sucking draws the nipple into the shield. Inserting expressed milk into the shield with a periodontal syringe can encourage the baby to suck (**Figure 22-6**). Sometimes, simply smoothing the shield over the breast draws the nipple into the shield. The nipple shield should optimally remain in place for only a few minutes at the beginning of the feeding. The baby can suck for several minutes to draw the nipple into the shield. After a few more minutes, the parent can unlatch the baby, remove the shield, and relatch the baby to continue feeding without the shield. A preterm or low-birth-weight infant may need the shield in place for the entire feeding to transfer milk.

Monitoring and Follow-up

The need for a nipple shield is a symptom of an underlying problem. Parents will need close follow-up with a lactation consultant or other healthcare provider (Coentro et al., 2022; Maastrup et al., 2019). They will need to monitor the baby's intake and output carefully with a daily record of feedings, voids, and stools until ample milk production is established. Periodic prefeed and postfeed weight checks will determine whether the baby is transferring milk adequately.

Some parents need to pump when they are using a nipple shield to maintain sufficient milk production. If a baby is transferring milk effectively with the nipple shield, excessive pumping in the early days could result in overactive milk production. On the other hand, a parent with a preterm or late-preterm baby needs to pump to establish and maintain milk production while their infant develops adequate suck skills and gains weight. Every nursing couplet's case is unique and requires a feeding plan tailored to their individual needs.

Encourage parents to consider a nipple shield as a bridge to work through a nursing difficulty and to wean from the shield as soon as it is practical to do so. Most infants who need to mature and gain weight can transition easily to direct nursing when they can latch effectively without a shield in place. In the case of severely inverted nipples that will not evert or uncommon infant anomalies such as a submucosal cleft, a nipple shield may be needed for the entire duration of lactation. Provide these parents with lots of praise and affirmation for persevering and help them feel positive about their experience. Many parents nurse with a nipple shield for their entire duration of nursing with no adverse effects.

Weaning the Baby from the Shield

When weaning from the shield, parents can watch for cues that their baby might accept direct nursing and latch the baby without it. Increased skin-to-skin contact aids in discontinuing use of the shield. Some babies are more receptive after the initial fullness at the beginning of a feeding has decreased. A sleepy baby is less likely to resist removal of the shield and will often continue to suck. The parent can try slipping the shield off near the end of a feeding when the baby is in a satiated sleeping state. They might also try to remove the shield after the milk lets down and is flowing. Some babies can be encouraged to nurse directly when co-bathing. A past recommendation of trimming the shield gradually is not advisable because the trimmed edges could lacerate the baby's mouth or the nipple.

Pacifiers

There is debate on the use of pacifiers with nursing babies. Pacifiers help meet the sucking needs of a bottle-fed baby. They can also potentially help nursing babies in limited circumstances. Some parents use a pacifier to help calm their fussy baby and to help their baby fall asleep. The American Academy of Pediatrics (AAP) recommends the use of pacifiers while sleeping after there are sufficient milk production, effective latch, adequate milk transfer, and appropriate infant weight gain (Meek et al., 2022). Pacifier use when the baby is sleeping reduces the risk of sudden infant death syndrome (SIDS) (Moon et al., 2022). If the baby releases the pacifier when they fall asleep, the pacifier does not need to be put back in place.

Although most parents consider pacifiers as a useful tool, they may worry about nipple confusion, lower milk production, and dental issues for their child later in life (Rocha et al., 2020). You can share the benefits and risks of pacifier use with your clients.

Inappropriate use of pacifiers is often a source of difficulty for a nursing baby. Using a pacifier in place of needed time nursing compromises milk production and the baby's growth. Sucking on a pacifier provides no nutritional benefit, expends calories, and can contribute to slowed growth. Pacifiers can also contribute to changes in the baby's dental arch and tooth position and lead to malocclusion (Lima et al., 2017). The American Academy of Pediatric Dentistry (AAPD) supports the use of a pacifier based on the infant's needs and parental preference. They caution that pacifier use after 12–18 months can increase the risk of otitis media and orofacial developmental issues (AAPD, 2022).

Appropriate Use of a Pacifier

Because pacifier use is so prevalent, parents need to receive instructions on safe use, beginning with selection. **Figure 22-7** depicts two types of pacifier designs. The first type, with an "orthodontic" shape, elicits a different sucking pattern from other nipples. The pacifier design (orthodontic, conventional, or physiologic) affects the use and determines the choice of type and brand of pacifier. A pacifier with multiple parts can harbor bacteria, thrush, and mold. A pacifier made from a solid piece of molded silicone with no separate parts is a safer choice.

The pacifier's material is another consideration. Avoiding latex pacifiers will minimize future latex allergy risks. Despite government restrictions, some pacifiers still contain phthalates, industrial chemicals that are suspected endocrine disruptors or hormone-altering agents. If the baby has a medical or therapeutic need for a pacifier, parents can work with their occupational therapist to select one that is best for their baby's particular needs.

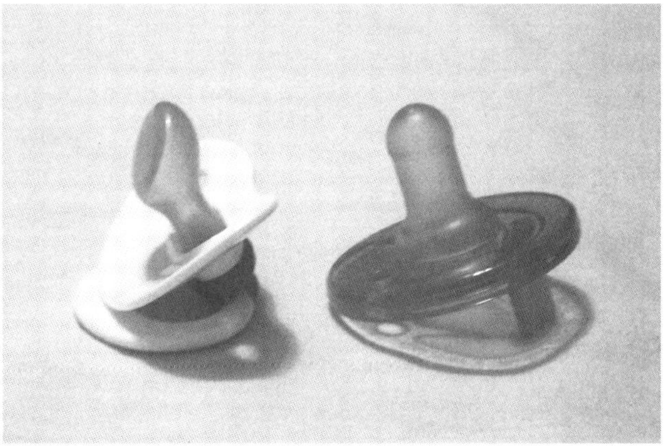

Figure 22-7 Two types of pacifiers.

Printed with permission of Anna Swisher.

Safety guidelines from the U.S. Consumer Product Safety Commission (2020) state that a pacifier should have the following characteristics:

- Not be so small or flexible that it can be sucked completely into a child's mouth
- Not have handles or other protrusions that are long enough to force the pacifier into the child's mouth if they fall or lie face down
- Be labeled to warn caregivers not to tie the pacifier around the child's neck
- Not have the potential to break into small parts

Preterm Infants

Preterm infants separated from their nursing parent while in a special care nursery are at risk of losing their sucking reflex. Infants have two primary sucking patterns, nonnutritive sucking (NNS) and nutritive sucking (NS). Pacifier use for preterm infants provides NNS during gavage feeding (Say et al., 2018). Accelerated maturation of the sucking reflex, decreased intestinal transit time, and increased rates of weight gain are all positive effects of pacifier use in these infants.

Pacifier use for preterm infants lowers the risk of SIDS, provides comfort after invasive procedures, and helps stabilize infants (Orovou et al., 2022). Infants also may transition to nipple feeding sooner and have better weight gain and earlier hospital discharge (Kaya & Aytekin, 2017). Minimizing pacifier use during the transition to nursing is associated with earlier exclusive nursing when parents are admitted to the neonatal intensive care unit (NICU) with their babies (Maastrup et al., 2019). However, extended rooming-in is not a realistic option in many facilities.

Alleviating Pain

A pacifier helps to calm infants who undergo painful procedures (Mangat et al., 2018). There is increasing evidence that the synergistic effect of sucrose and NNS is more effective than the effect of sucrose or NNS alone (Liu et al., 2017). Fussy term babies in NICUs may benefit from a pacifier when feedings are restricted or when they are **nil per os (NPO)** (Latin term meaning "nothing by mouth") for medical reasons. Pacifier use for these babies avoids excessive crying, thus preventing increases in blood pressure, heart rate, and calorie expenditure.

Impact of Pacifier Use on Nursing

Excessive pacifier use interferes with the symbiotic relationship of the baby increasing milk production through sucking. A pacifier should not replace sufficient nursing, interaction, or skin contact with the parent. Pacifier use may indicate problems with the nursing dyad rather than being the cause of problems (Tolppola et al., 2022). A randomized controlled trial determined that the use of pacifiers in the first 2 weeks postpartum does not appear to affect nursing outcomes at 6 months (Hermanson & Åstrand, 2020).

Educating your clients on hunger cues, nursing frequency, and strategies to calm a fussy baby can help to decrease dependence on pacifier use. Pacifiers should be used only after the baby's needs for food, comfort, and human contact are fully met. A baby who settles when being held may simply have needed comfort. A baby who remains unsettled and roots should nurse before being given a pacifier. Rather than using a pacifier in response to crying, encourage parents to respond to early hunger cues and help them learn other ways to comfort their baby (refer to the discussion of crying in **Chapter 14**). A pacifier may be appropriate for a baby who does not want to nurse and continues to demonstrate a need to suck.

Milk Expression

There are times during lactation when parents need to express their milk. Regardless of the method of milk expression used, expression cannot remove milk as effectively as the sucking of a robust baby. The baby combines suction, negative pressure, and rhythmic gum compression of the areola. A parent may express several times before they become proficient and can obtain the desired amount of milk. Gentle breast massage can help them relax so that more milk can be expressed.

Manual Expression

Being independent and nursing without a need for tools can instill self-confidence in parents. Knowing how to perform **manual expression** promotes self-reliance and confidence that milk can be removed no matter what circumstances arise during lactation. Manual expression is convenient during a brief separation despite a broken pump, power failure, natural disaster, or low pump battery. It is free and discreet, and it places the parent in full control to express milk anytime and anywhere.

All parents should be taught to manually express their milk within the first 1–2 hours of the birth. Some studies report that manual expression is especially effective in the first few days of nursing when milk volume is low (Whitburn, 2022). Another study found no difference in the output of colostrum between manual expression and an electric pump (Dhanawat et al., 2022). Parents of preterm babies are encouraged to combine manual expression with use of a breast pump.

Technique for Manual Expression

To begin expressing, the parent can lean slightly forward with the nipple aimed at the collection container, as illustrated in **Figure 22-8**. **Figure 22-9** illustrates the steps in milk expression. The parent's fingers should be placed behind the nipple base and moved forward in a rolling motion toward the nipple. Initially, it may take several attempts until milk begins to drip. Milk will spray out with greater force after the milk lets down. Caution parents not to pinch or tug on the nipple. Such actions have little or no benefit in expressing milk and can irritate the breast tissue.

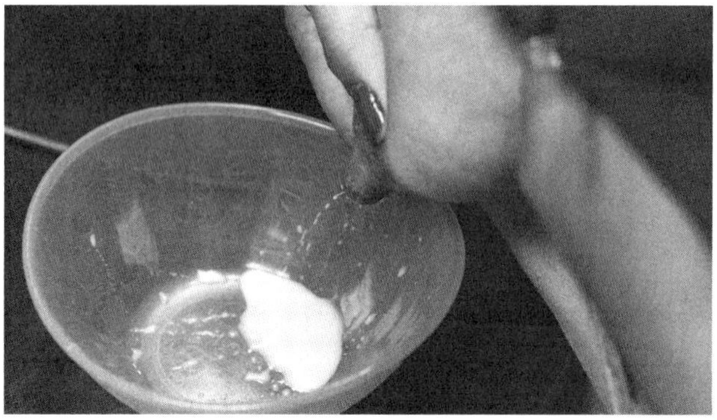

Figure 22-8 Manually expressing milk.

Photo by Every Mother, Inc. and Regina Maria Roig-Romero.

1. Gently massage the breast in circles toward the areola.
2. Support the breast with your fingers below and your thumb on top behind the areola, forming the letter C as in the C-hold.
3. Position a clean container beneath the nipple with your opposite hand to collect the expressed milk.
4. Gently press your thumb and fingers back toward the chest wall without pulling or sliding along the skin.
5. Compress your breast and then release the pressure, repeating several times.
6. Reposition your hand and repeat the compressions as you move around the breast to compress all the ducts.

Figure 22-9 Steps in milk expression.

A demonstration of manual expression is available online from the Stanford School of Medicine (2020a).

Gently massaging the breast and applying a warm, moist cloth for several minutes before milk expression can help promote milk flow. Massaging the breast throughout the expressing session will continue to promote milk flow. Massage includes rolling the breast between two hands or kneading gently with the backs of the parent's fists. Directing the strokes away from the areola and toward the axillae facilitates lymph drainage. Fingertip massage is also helpful.

Many parents find a variation of manual expression that works best for them. Encourage them to experiment with various hand positions until they find what works best for them. For example, they may cup the breast with the C-hold, gently massaging and applying pressure on the ducts. Just as with many other techniques, there is no single correct way to express milk. Honor individual choices by not commenting negatively or insisting on a particular technique. Practice and adaptation are keys to successful manual expression. When mastered, it can be as fast and efficient as a breast pump. The more comfortable a parent becomes with massage and manual expression, the more comfortable they become in all areas of their parenting.

Use of a Breast Pump

Breast pumps are used to increase or maintain milk production when the nursing dyad is separated or when they are working through nursing issues. Breast pumps help to establish milk production in the hospital when nursing cannot begin immediately after birth. They are an efficient means to express milk for preterm infants, sick infants, or infants with impairment. Other conditions associated with pumping are engorgement, flat/inverted nipples, and c-section delivery. Breast pumps also facilitate continuing nursing after returning to work or school. Parents may pump to build a supply of milk prior to their return to use while they are away from the baby. Breast pumps are often a main feature of worksite support programs for nursing employees.

Appropriate Use of Pumps

Pumping is prevalent because of the increased availability of pumping products and a general acceptance of pumping by parents as an important part of their infant feeding experience. Breast pump use is especially popular in parts of the world where enthusiasm for technology and gadgets to "fix" things is high. In many cultures, breast pumps are a standard gift for new parents. Thus, many parents who plan to nurse own a breast pump before they know whether they will need one. In several Western cultures, parents of healthy, term infants pump at least occasionally during the first 2 weeks postpartum (Dietrich Leurer et al., 2020). There is concern that the wide availability of pumps, and the perception that they are required for lactation, contributes to the medicalization of nursing.

Some breast pump advertisements imply that pumping is equivalent to nursing (Dietrich Leurer et al., 2020). For parents using a pump provides "evidence" of how much milk the baby is getting and reassures them that nursing is "working." Teaching clients how to recognize signs of milk transfer and an infant's hunger and satiety cues can provide proof that nursing is going well without relying on a breast pump.

It is important to provide accurate information for appropriate pump use and to not promote pumping to the detriment of nursing. Important differences exist between the act of nursing compared with human milk feeding. Parents demonstrate more sensitivity to their infants' cues when nursing than when bottle-feeding their pumped milk (Whitfield & Ventura, 2019). Aside from the bonding and nurturing aspects, research suggests that babies bottle-fed human milk may be at risk for overfeeding in the same way as their formula-fed counterparts (Kotowski et al., 2020).

Education on pumping is not routinely given in infant feeding classes. Unless an infant is in the NICU, pumping is not usually discussed in the hospital setting. In one study, parents reported receiving no education on how to use a breast pump or that the information they received was inconsistent (Dietrich Leurer et al., 2020). Parents need to learn about pumping from healthcare professionals and not from friends or the internet. Teach them the appropriate use of a pump, how to set it up, pumping regimens, and milk storage guidelines.

Exclusively Pumping

Increasing numbers of parents choose to **exclusively pump** their milk to feed their babies rather than to directly nurse. Over 89% of parents who exclusively pump their milk do so after unsuccessful attempts at direct nursing (Rosenbaum, 2022). For example, they might pump to maintain milk production and decrease nipple pain early in the postpartum period while their infant's sucking skills mature. If they are unable to establish nursing, they may exclusively pump their milk to feed their baby. Some parents may exclusively pump without planning to nurse directly, perhaps because they are uncomfortable with the physical act of nursing. Although not always the case, this could result from previous sexual abuse. Regardless of the reason, the decision to exclusively pump highlights the understanding of the health benefits of human milk for infants and enables parents to provide the best nutrition for their baby.

Discussing exclusive pumping as an option with clients who struggle with nursing might be a solution to their infant feeding dilemmas. These parents have unique needs and often turn to other parents who exclusively pump or to social media for support (Strauch et al., 2019). You can help them grieve the loss of their original nursing goals and incorporate an exclusive pumping regime into their daily life. You might consider facilitating a support group for your exclusively pumping clients.

Selecting a Breast Pump

In selecting a breast pump, parents should consider the baby's age and condition, the reason for pumping, and how long they will need to pump. If they will pump at work or school, they should consider the amount of time available for pumping, facilities for pumping and storage, affordability, and personal preference. A handheld pump may be sufficient for occasional absences at feeding times. Pumping for regular absence of direct nursing will require an efficient electric pump to establish and maintain sufficient milk production. **Figure 22-10** presents criteria parents can consider when selecting a breast pump.

1. Does it cycle quickly, similar to the rhythm of the baby's suck? Or can the parent self-cycle at a rate that is comfortable?
2. Is the flange shape comfortable and an appropriate size for the nipple and areola?
3. Are smaller and larger flanges available?
4. Are inserts available for the flanges for very small areolas and nipples?
5. Are the pump parts dishwasher safe?
6. Is the pump easy to assemble, with few parts?
7. Is the pump easy and comfortable to use with the type of hand or arm motion required?
8. If the pump is electric, is the power source adequate (i.e., type of outlet–two or three prongs–and amount of voltage)?
9. Is the pump quiet?
10. Is the pump easy to transport?
11. Is the pump affordable for the length of time it is required?
12. Are quick service and overnight replacement available?
13. What period and what parts does the warranty cover?
14. Are written instructions provided that are easy to understand?
15. Is there someone at the company who is knowledgeable in nursing to answer questions and resolve problems?
16. Is there a toll-free number to call with questions?
17. Is there an up-to-date website?

Figure 22-10 Criteria for selecting a breast pump.

Familiarize yourself with the many types of available breast pumps and how parents can obtain them. Provide practical information, such as descriptions and prices, how various pumps are used, and their advantages and disadvantages. Because breast pumps manufactured by companies that sell infant formula have a conflicting market agenda, their pumps may not be the best choice. You can encourage parents to select a pump manufactured by a company with a good manufacturing and customer service record whose primary mission is assisting with nursing.

Flange Size. The flange is the part of the pump that rests over the nipple and areola. Many pumps have flange size recommendations and provide a downloadable ruler to measure the diameter of the nipple. Lack of a standard for sizing pump flanges leads to many parents using the wrong size. The size of the flange needs to allow the nipple to move freely inside the tunnel without contacting the sides of the tunnel during suction. Because the nipple expands during pumping, the parent should add 1–3 mm to the measurement of the widest part of the nipple and match that to the flange size. Nipples should not be measured during pregnancy because the nipple continues to expand in size up until the birth.

Flange size ranges from 15 to 40 mm. Current literature recommends using the smallest flange size that is comfortable to yield greater milk output (Higgins, 2022). Many pumps come with specific size flanges, so clients may need to purchase an appropriately sized flange separately. Angled breast pump flanges, as depicted in **Figure 22-11**, can be used on a variety of pumps. Special inserts that rest inside the flange will help small nipples and areolae achieve the proper fit. However, the inserts causes breast or nipple pain in some parents. Assisting parents with flange sizing can increase their success in pumping, regardless of

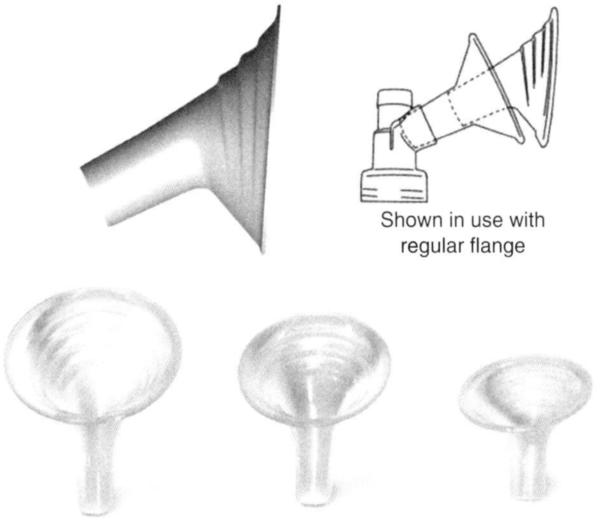

Figure 22-11 Angled breast pump flanges.

Reprinted with permission from Pump N Pal.

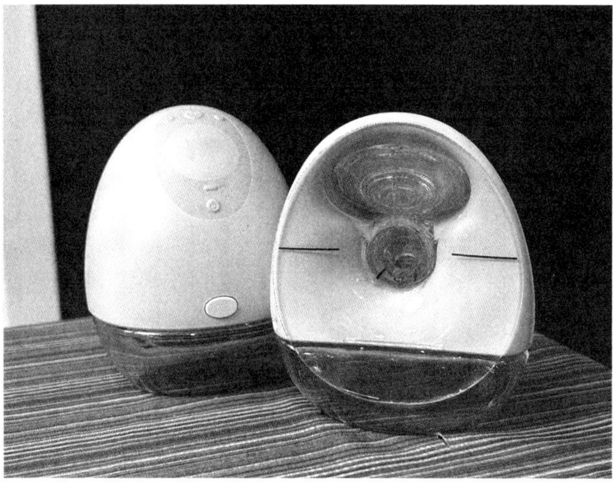

Figure 22-12 Hands-free breast pump.

Used with permission fom Kristina Chamberlain.

why they pump and the duration of their pumping experience.

Handheld Breast Pump. A handheld breast pump is useful as an occasional substitute to nursing or to relieve engorgement in the early postpartum period. A handheld pump consists of a collecting bottle and flange that fits over the nipple and areola. A piston, trigger, or motor provides the suction. Handheld pumps may be manual, battery driven, or electric. Various styles at different prices are available.

A manual pump that uses natural movements will be the most comfortable. Some motorized hand pumps have a control button to regulate suction pressure. Others have an autocycling motor that controls the suction. Foot pedal models are also available. The "bicycle horn" pump was an early handheld breast pump that is still found in some stores. (The name derives from its resemblance to the horn on a bicycle.) This pump can damage nipples and harbors bacteria that could be dangerous to the baby. Parents should not use hand pumps that use a bulb to generate suction.

Battery-Operated Wearable Pump. Wearable breast pumps are battery-operated, fit inside a bra, and allow hands-free pumping (**Figure 22-12**). They are convenient, mobile, quiet, discreet, and easy to clean. Parents can pump while working, driving, or walking. However, wearable pumps are expensive, must be charged regularly, and tend to have weaker suction than electric breast pumps (Carrane, 2021). If a parent uses a wearable pump to increase or maintain milk production, be sure to educate them on signs that milk volume is decreasing and offer follow-up visits.

Electric Breast Pump. Electric breast pumps are the most efficient for expressing milk. They provide the stimulation and milk removal necessary to maintain milk production without the fatigue of manual expression or a manual pump. Heavy-duty double electric breast pumps are produced for both hospital and consumer use. They offer the option of pumping both breasts at the same time, as depicted in **Figure 22-13**, thus saving time and increasing breast stimulation. Leading breast pump manufacturers provide automatic cycling and others require that the parent release the suction manually. Caution users to avoid long periods of uninterrupted vacuum that could damage breast tissue. There are bras designed to provide hands-free operation of electric breast pumps. Low-cost hands-free bras can be created by cutting vertical slits in an inexpensive sports bra.

Hospital-grade electric breast pumps are recommended when the nursing dyad is separated regularly. They are also used with ill babies, preterm or late-preterm babies, multiples (who are usually preterm), and babies with a weak suck. Because these pumps are expensive to purchase, they are usually rented for use at home. Disinfecting and cleaning multiuse hospital-grade pumps between rentals will prevent cross-contamination. Each user purchases a personal pump kit, which should be used only by the purchaser.

Consumer double electric pumps are popular with worksite nursing programs. They provide the most efficient pumping for an employee who is regularly separated from their baby at feeding times.

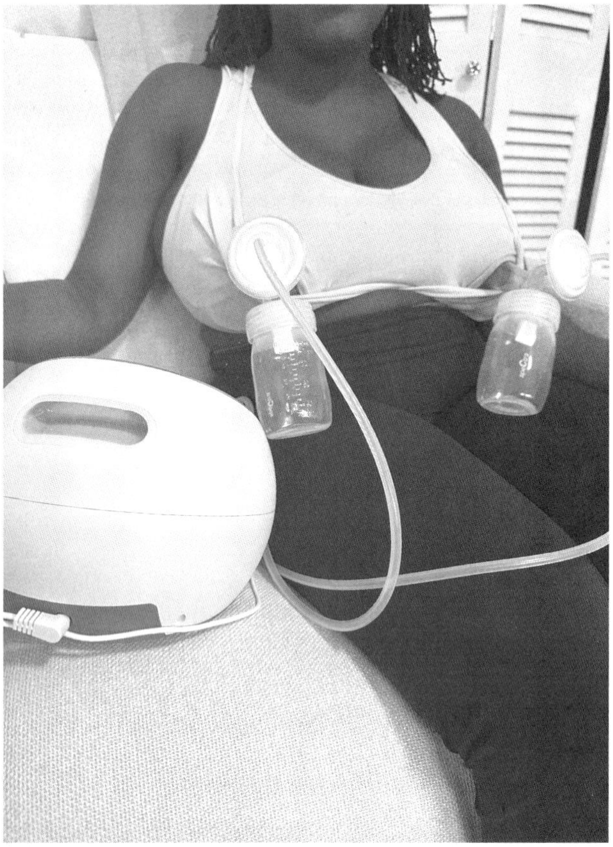

Figure 22-13 Electric double breast pump.
Photo by Kristina Chamberlain.

Consumer pumps are intended for single-person use. The motor and diaphragm parts on consumer pumps are not conducive to multiple use, and the pressure may be lower than needed. Multiuse of consumer pumps could theoretically cause cross-contamination. However, many parents trade, borrow, or purchase previously used consumer pumps. You can encourage parents to research the risks of used pumps. If a parent uses a previously owned pump, suggest that they obtain a new pump kit and that they have the pressure checked.

Pumping Guidelines

Parents need written instructions of proper use of the pump with a demonstration and return demonstration. Because the use of a breast pump accompanies an interruption in nursing, the parent may need specialized counseling as well. For this reason, many lactation consultants have pumps and accompanying equipment readily available for demonstration and hands-on teaching. Trying different pumps and flange sizes will help in finding one that works best. A sterilized, autoclaved kit can be used solely for test pumping.

Conditioning Letdown for Pumping. The stimulation of the baby's sucking on the nipple triggers milk to let down. Milk expression does not provide the same degree of stimulation as that of a robust baby. Massaging the breasts briefly and expressing a few drops of milk by hand helps the milk let down and often yields faster results. The parent's emotional state may also be a factor in the ability to achieve letdown. They can prepare mentally for pumping and arrange to pump at times when they feel rested and unhurried. An atmosphere that is conducive to pumping includes privacy, a comfortable chair, a picture of the baby, and perhaps a recording of the baby's sounds to listen to while pumping. Techniques for establishing letdown appear in **Chapter 7**.

A parent who has difficulty initiating letdown while pumping may become tense, agitated, and upset, possibly inhibiting the letdown even further. First confirm that they are using a quality pump with the correct pressure and using good technique. Mechanical issues should always be ruled out first. Correctly fitting breast flanges help provide the stimulation and comfort needed for their milk to let down. You can then encourage them to continue pumping to obtain the readily available milk. Often, establishing a regular pumping routine helps parents relax and patiently work toward increasing their milk production.

Pumping Technique. A pumping session should begin with handwashing and getting comfortable. Moistening the pump flange with drops of expressed milk or olive oil can help form a tight seal and decrease skin friction. A rolled towel under the breasts can provide support for parents with large breasts. Centering the nipple in the flange ensures contact with the full circumference of the breast to create a vacuum. Suction should increase slowly as needed to maintain milk flow throughout the pumping session. The parent should begin with the suction on the lowest setting and gradually increase suction strength as necessary. Adding intermittent massage and breast compression will further promote milk flow.

Pumping for 10 to 20 minutes may be sufficient when double pumping. When single pumping, alternating between sides several times throughout the pumping session will capitalize on the multiple letdowns that occur. The parent can pump 5 to 7 minutes on one side and then switch to the other side for another 5 to 7 minutes. They can then return to the first side for another 3 to 5 minutes and repeat that time on the second side. They can finish on the first side for 2 to 3 minutes and then the second side for another 2 to 3 minutes until milk flow ceases. Increasing the time of each pumping session too much can create tissue damage and does not necessarily result in more milk output. Parents who pump long term have found that massaging their breasts after the milk stops flowing and resuming for a few minutes yields more milk and better drainage (Stanford School of Medicine, 2020b).

Pumping times can be tailored to specific needs and circumstances. Milk yield can vary on different days and at different times of the day. If the baby nurses some or most of the time, pumping can be adapted to the feeding schedule. Pumping can occur in place of a missed feeding, between feedings, or on one side while nursing the baby on the other side. Some parents "triple feed"—nursing, pumping, and supplementing at each feeding session. For this scenario, it is more effective to pump right after the nursing session. This will help to stimulate milk production and save time. Experimenting will help each nursing dyad find which arrangement best suits their needs.

Pumping for a Hospitalized Baby. Parents of a baby who is hospitalized and unable to nurse need to begin pumping as soon as possible after the birth. Initiating regular milk removal helps build and maintain milk production and establishes long-term lactation. Parents should pump at least 8 to 12 times every 24 hours, regardless of the amount of milk they obtain. Those who need to collect large volumes of milk can pump more frequently and try to reduce stress and get sufficient rest. Stress reduction strategies can include pumping while enjoying music or meditation, having someone massage their back before pumping, and delegating stressful duties. While one side may produce more milk and achieve letdown more easily than the other, both sides need regular milk removal.

Because prolactin levels are highest at nighttime, pumping at that time may produce larger quantities of milk. Parents can pump during the night whenever they wake naturally and can drink extra fluids just before bedtime to facilitate waking. As the time grows closer for the baby to come home, they can begin to pump more regularly at night. A 4- or 5-hour stretch of sleep can help parents maintain their energy.

Many countries have public assistance programs to help with the cost of renting an electric pump for a preterm or ill infant. For example, U.S. government programs—including Medicaid and Women, Infants, and Children (WIC) clinics—provide hospital-grade electric pumps for parents of preterm and ill babies. If a parent has financial constraints, encourage them to explore these avenues. Although hospital NICUs provide electric pumps for use in the hospital, parents also need access to an electric pump for home use. Some hospitals have loaner hospital-grade pumps available through grants and donations. Get to know where your clients can obtain financial aid for hospital-grade electric pumps in your area.

Need for Support and Follow-Up

When a breast pump is used, close contact with a lactation consultant helps identify any difficulties with pumping or maintaining milk production. A parent's needs are especially great when they are using a mechanical tool to drain their breasts without the emotional gratification of nursing. It is common when pumping for preterm babies for parents' emotions to vacillate. Reactions may range from fear of possible pain to embarrassment, irritation, passive acceptance, or gratitude and relief.

If the need for a pump resulted from a problem with the baby's health, parents may be anxious and want to share their concerns with someone. If pumping for an extended time, they may experience periods of discouragement and will benefit from your reassurance and support. Encourage parents to regard pumping as protecting the potential to nurse and something that only they can do for their baby. At a time when they may be able to do little else, pumping can help a parent to feel involved and essential.

A parent who is preoccupied with the situation requiring that they pump may not pay close attention to the information you provide. Make a special effort to offer clear written instructions and explanations. You may need to repeat instructions multiple times before parents absorb the information. The Stanford School of Medicine website (2020b) has a video on maximizing milk production. Although created for NICU parents, it is applicable to any parent needing to pump.

Considerations for Obtaining a Pump

Some lactation consultants rent or sell breast pumps as a convenience to their clients. The International Board of Lactation Consultant Examiners (IBLCE) Code of Professional Conduct (IBLCE, 2022) provides guidance for lactation consultants who do this. Some lactation advocates question the ethics of breast pump sales and rentals through a healthcare facility or private practice. Many choose not to lease or sell pumps to avoid the controversy. Others feel that parents who plan to use a pump need expert help in its selection and use.

In many countries, the cost of breast pumps is covered by public or private health insurance plans. Pumps are often shipped to the subscriber, or vouchers are given toward purchase either at a retail store or online. This can result in the use of pumps with flanges that do not fit, resulting in possible injury and impaired milk removal. Some insurance companies provide quality, name-brand pumps with long track records of dependability. Others send pumps that are new on the market, with little or no performance history. Be sure to know what is covered by insurance for parents where you practice.

Collecting and Storing Expressed Milk

Parents collect and freeze their milk for emergencies and for regular separation, such as working or attending school. They may also store it for a short-term separation, such as a shopping trip or a social event. Preterm infants, infants with a physical disability, and ill infants may need expressed milk for an extended period. Some parents collect their milk exclusively rather than nursing directly. Many parents, especially those with overly ample production, donate their extra milk to **human milk banks** for the use of other babies or children and, rarely, sick adults.

When dual pumping for a healthy baby, milk can be combined from both containers for storage. It can also be combined from different pumping sessions, with the label stating the date and time of the earliest pumping. Newly pumped milk can be added to refrigerated milk after first cooling the newly pumped milk.

Milk expressed to relieve fullness or drip milk collected during a feeding can be saved for later use. Milk that accumulates in a breast shell worn between feedings may have bacterial growth and should not be saved. Parents taking a medication proven to be harmful to babies should not give their milk to the baby. Data are conflicting about whether milk pumped during a yeast infection harbors enough *Candida* to reinfect the baby. Yeast can be present in the milk even when symptoms of a yeast infection are not present (Azevedo et al., 2023; Heisel et al., 2019). The yeast can pass from parent to infant, whether directly nursing or feeding pumped milk. No *Candida* were found in milk cultured from parents with breast pain, although the milk did not seem to inhibit the growth of *Candida* in samples (Hale et al., 2009). If the parent is directly nursing their baby during a *Candida* outbreak, the baby is getting the same milk and theoretical *Candida* load as with pumped milk.

Storage Container

The storage container may be glass or plastic. Glass containers do not absorb the milk's antibodies or other proteins and are the best choice for milk storage. Glass is easy to clean and offers protection against contamination. A hard plastic (polypropylene) container is the next best storage choice. However, the interior surface can scratch and make cleaning difficult. Soft plastic (polyethylene) baby bottle liners are not recommended for storing milk. Certain antibodies in the milk reduce in concentration when it is stored in soft plastic containers. Additionally, soft plastics are difficult to seal and may puncture easily. Many plastic bottles are made with bisphenol A (BPA), a chemical correlated with health hazards. Thus, parents should be sure any older bottles are BPA-free.

Milk must be stored in a manner that preserves its quality and prevents spoiling. Collection containers and any pump parts that have contact with the milk should be cleaned after every use. They can be washed in hot, soapy water and then thoroughly rinsed and air-dried or cycled through a dishwasher. Microwave-safe steam bags allow the parts to be steam-cleaned in the microwave. Although expensive, some parents find them convenient.

The amount of milk stored in each container varies according to the amount the baby needs. Initially storing milk in small amounts—about 28 to 60 mL (1–2 oz)—will minimize waste. As the baby starts consuming more at a feeding, small amounts are useful for topping off when the baby is still hungry. If the milk is to be frozen, leaving space at the top will allow for expansion during freezing.

The container should be labeled with a waterproof marker to include the date and time the milk was expressed. If the milk is to be given to the baby by a caregiver with multiple children, the label should contain the parent's and baby's full names. The baby's last name is important because babies and parents often have different last names. Transporting the milk in a container that is ready for feeding will reduce the possibility of contamination or waste when pouring. Parents can review safety issues regarding milk storage with the childcare provider. You can assist them by providing up-to-date guidelines and educating the childcare staff if needed.

Storage Time

Storage times vary, depending on how soon the baby will receive the expressed milk. A protocol for storing milk for healthy full-term infants is available from the Academy of Breastfeeding Medicine (ABM, 2017). **Figure 22-14** presents milk storage guidelines for term and older babies from the Human Milk Banking Association of North America (HMBANA, 2024b). Milk can be stored in a freezer for up to 1 year, depending on the type of freezer. To avoid extremes of temperature, the milk should not be stored in the refrigerator or freezer door or near the freezer's defrosting unit. Caution parents not to store their milk near an automatic ice maker, where temperature variance can affect the milk.

Some infants will reject the smell and taste of milk that has been frozen. An odor may be caused by the breakdown of fatty acids in the milk, not because of high levels of lipase as previously thought (Eglash et al., 2017). Freezing milk in small amounts will avoid wasting milk rejected by the baby. If the baby rejects the milk because of its taste or smell, parents can gently warm the milk before freezing (never to the point of boiling). Although warming the milk lowers some of the immunoglobulins, it eliminates the need to discard the milk. Expressed milk is always a better option for the baby than artificial milk.

Special NICU Guidelines

Parents who are collecting milk for a baby in the NICU must follow stricter collection and storage guidelines to ensure the baby's safety. NICU staff will provide these instructions. Guidelines may vary from one hospital to another. If your hospital does not offer neonatal intensive care, parents will need guidelines from the NICU that cares for their baby. Make sure parents receive this information before they leave the hospital.

Ensure that parents know that nursing is still an option when they are separated from their baby. Encourage NICU staff to educate them about early pumping to help maximize their milk production potential. Parents should begin milk expression within the first 6 hours after delivery to provide the stimulation necessary for establishing adequate production. When possible, they should express just before feeding the baby. Milk that will not be used within 1 hour should be refrigerated immediately. Parents who collect milk for a preterm infant need to place milk from each pumping session in a separate storage container to minimize handling and contamination (HMBANA, 2024b). If the baby will not receive the fresh milk within 24 hours, the milk should be frozen.

FRESH MILK

- 6 hours at room temperature (60–85°F or 16–29°C)
- 24 hours in an insulated cooler with frozen gel pack (39°F or 4°C)
- 8 days in the refrigerator (39°F or 4°C)

FROZEN MILK

- 2 weeks in the freezer compartment of a 1-door refrigerator (0°F or –18°C)
- 6 months in the freezer compartment of a 2-door refrigerator (0°F or –18°C)
- 12 months in an upright or chest freezer (0°F or –18°C)

THAWED MILK

- 48 hours in the refrigerator (39°F or 4°C)

Figure 22-14 Milk storage guidelines.

Modified from Human Milk Banking Association of North America. Best Practice for Expressing, Storing and Handling Human Milk in Hospital, Homes, and Child Care Settings. 5th ed. Fort Worth, TX: Human Milk Banking Association of North America Inc; 2024b.

Defrosting and Warming the Milk

Appropriate labeling makes it easy to use milk based on the date it was expressed, using the oldest milk first. A large stock of milk in the freezer can be arranged with the oldest containers toward the front. Milk can be thawed by placing it in the refrigerator overnight or by warming it rapidly in a pan of warm water or under a stream of warm tap water. When expressed milk sits in the refrigerator or freezer, the fat rises to the top of the milk. Gently swirling the milk throughout the warming process mixes the fat. Thawed milk must be used or discarded within 24 hours of thawing to ensure the safety of the milk. It should not be refrozen. A microwave oven should not be used for warming milk. Microwaved liquid may contain hot spots that could burn the baby's mouth. Additionally, microwaving substantially decreases the activity of the anti-infective properties in human milk.

Human Milk Banking

Antibodies in the parent's milk reflect the family environment, making it more appropriate than any alternative feeding choice. When enough milk is not available through either nursing or expression, especially in the case of preterm infants, donor milk is the next best option. Improved laboratory testing and pasteurization techniques have eradicated concerns about disease transmission with donor milk. The safety of human milk banking is becoming better known as more NICUs use it and witness the positive outcomes (HMBANA, 2024a, 2024b). HMBANA, a not-for-profit organization established in 1985, provides uniform standards for human milk banking.

Babies who need donor human milk may be temporarily unable to nurse, intolerant of infant formula, or have digestive disorders or severe diarrhea. Some preterm or ill infants need donor milk until milk production increases to meet their needs. Infants with autoimmune disorders, inborn errors of metabolism, or conditions such as cystic fibrosis benefit from human milk. The condition may not occur up until several weeks or months after birth. If the parent cannot relactate, donor milk will help the baby's chances of survival.

Human Milk Banks

The availability of human milk banks varies dramatically by country. Brazil has the largest network in the world, with 228 human milk banks and 236 collection stations in which 31 countries participate (PAHO, 2023). There are 282 active milk banks operating in Europe (European Milk Bank Association, 2025). Human milk banking resources in other parts of the world are available online (PATH, 2025). There are 32 operating milk banks in North America and more in development. Donor milk can be shipped overnight anywhere in the United States and Canada (HMBANA, 2025).

Regional donation is becoming more convenient for families as new depots open. Some milk banks receive support from an associated hospital. Some label the milk with nutritional content analysis (protein and lipid percentages and calorie content). This enables neonatologists to provide the most fragile babies with the best nutritional match possible. Milk banks also provide human milk from parents on dairy-free diets and fat-free human milk for babies with chylothorax.

Recipients of Donor Milk. Donated milk is processed, pasteurized, and dispensed by prescription to infants, children, and rarely, adults with a medical need. Milk banks dispense milk based on the greatest need, prioritizing hospitalized and the most medically fragile infants. Recipient hospitals cover processing fees and shipping costs for inpatient babies receiving donor milk. Nonprofit milk banks depend on donations and grants. Although recipient families pay a processing fee, the milk bank serves anyone with a medical need.

Donating Milk. Parents who express and save milk for another person's baby find great emotional gratification in knowing they are helping a baby in need. Some donors are bereaved parents whose babies died (refer to the discussion on counseling grieving parents in **Chapter 24**). You can facilitate the use of milk banks by providing information to parents in your care who have plentiful supplies of expressed milk or have experienced a loss. Learn the location of milk banks and their policies regarding milk collection and distribution. When a parent expresses a desire to become a donor, you can provide general information and refer them to their nearest milk bank. Because each one has slightly different procedures, it is best for parents to communicate directly with the milk bank.

Milk donors learn hygienic techniques for milk expression, with appropriate handwashing, cleaning and disinfecting of pump parts, and handling of disinfecting equipment. They learn how to collect, label, and store their milk and how to transport it to the bank. Milk banks provide containers for parents to collect and store their milk for shipping. Donors should collect milk in a sterile container and mark it with their name, collection date, number of ounces, and the name and dosage of any drugs they are taking.

Milk banks typically require that donors freeze their milk, attaching the label to the jar before placing it in the freezer to ensure that it adheres. The milk must be insulated well during transport to prevent thawing so that it stays frozen until it arrives at the milk bank. Milk banks accept excess stockpiled milk if the donor requirements are met. The individual milk bank provides its specific collection and storage guidelines.

Screening Donors. Milk banks screen potential donors thoroughly for lifestyle and medical history risks. Parents who are ill or are taking certain medications may be disqualified from donating milk. They can check with the specific milk bank for exclusions. Donors provide a blood test and a written agreement from their healthcare provider and the baby's healthcare provider that they are a viable donor and that donating poses no detriment to their baby. Most parents commit to donating a certain amount of milk (e.g., 100 oz), although one-time donations are also accepted. Milk banks recognize that donating milk after losing a child is a difficult decision for parents and is part of the healing process. Most milk banks will take any milk donation from a bereaved parent, regardless of the amount or the donor's health.

Followers of the Islamic faith believe in the concept of "milk kinship"— a familial relationship between the baby and the parent who donates the milk. As "milk siblings," the donating mother's children and the recipient infant cannot marry (Ghaly, 2018). These families are often in consultation with their spiritual leaders when deciding if donor milk is acceptable. **Pooled milk** is limited to three milk donors (Subudhi and Sriraman, 2021).

Processing Donated Milk. Frozen donor milk is thawed in a refrigerator at the milk bank and pooled under clean conditions (**Figure 22-15**). The milk then undergoes heat treatment at 62.5°C (**Holder pasteurization**) for 30 minutes to kill HIV and other viruses and bacteria. Heat-treated milk retains most of its immunologic and nutritional properties, although vitamin C is destroyed by heating. The pasteurized milk is rapidly cooled and refrozen. Each batch is cultured for bacteria. Any batch containing bacterial growth is discarded or saved for use in research. The milk bank conducts routine antigen testing like that of blood banks to further rule out the presence of HIV, hepatitis B, hepatitis C, cytomegalovirus, human T-cell lymphotropic virus, and syphilis.

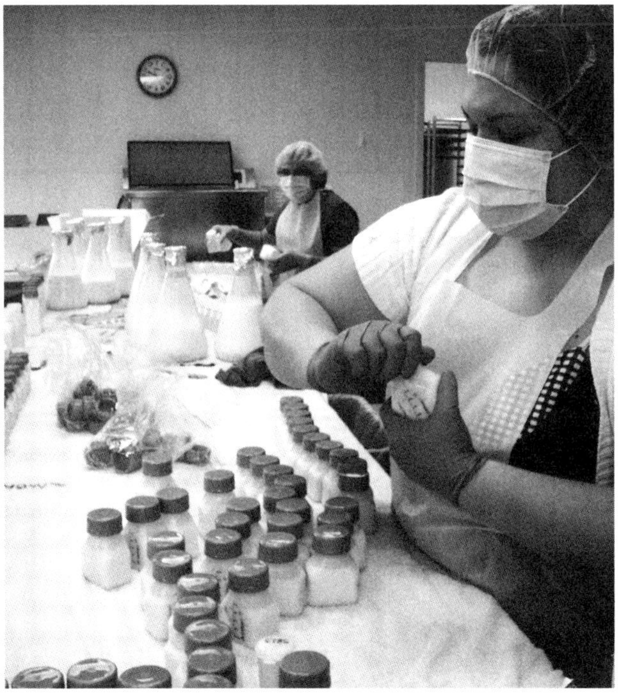

Figure 22-15 Human milk being processed at a milk bank.

Economic Value of Human Milk

For many years, human milk has been considered to be "free." However, it is increasingly recognized that human milk is *not* free. It requires a parent's time, effort, and commitment and has an enormous economic value that has been largely invisible in society. Although farm animal milk is included in a country's gross domestic product (GDP), human milk is not. An analysis of the estimated value (presented in U.S. dollars) of annual human milk production has been reported to be $5 billion in Australia, $1 billion in Norway, and over $60 billion in the United States (Smith et al., 2023). Analysts argue that the invisibility of this value contributes to the financial strength of infant formula manufacturers and ignores the economic contribution lactating parents make to their countries (Smith, 2019).

Milk banking and milk sharing reflect the perception of human milk as a commodity. There are deep ethical considerations inherent in the field of human milk use. Some of these include the following (Thibeau & Ginsberg, 2018):

- Human milk should be reused only with full disclosure and consent of the donating and receiving persons.
- No financial gain should be made by the donor or receiver of human milk.
- Donor milk recipients should receive safe, quality donor milk.
- Human milk should be available to all preterm and medically fragile infants.
- Allocation of human milk should be based on ethical practices.

For-Profit Human Milk Banking

For-profit human milk banking capitalizes the economic value of human milk. Prolacta Bioscience receives milk from unpaid donors, who often believe they are donating to a nonprofit milk bank. The company then sells the processed, patented milk and human milk fortifiers to hospitals (Prolacta Bioscience, 2025). Medolac markets human milk for term babies to hospitals and compensates parents for providing their milk (Medolac, 2020). This practice might motivate low-income parents to donate their milk, withholding it from their own baby and jeopardizing the baby's health. It also objectifies human milk as a product that is separate from nursing. The introduction of the for-profit sale of human milk is complex and fraught with concerns over tampering, dilution, or reducing the biologic child's supply of milk.

Informal Milk Sharing

Parents who cannot obtain donor milk from a milk bank often seek a relative or friend, other parents in the community, or the internet for milk. These parents include those who cannot produce enough milk and nonbinary and adoptive couples. Greater awareness of the importance of human milk has increased the number of parents who share milk informally. Some parents prefer human milk sharing to the potential health risks of infant formula. Contaminated formula scandals have further increased this trend.

Donors cite empathy for recipients and having extra milk they did not want to be wasted as factors in donating. Milk sharing is considered an altruistic act between parents. Many milk-sharing online networks connect donor parents with those who need milk. Two such sites are Human Milk 4 Human Babies, found on social media, and Eats on Feet at https://www.eatsonfeet.org. Eats on Feet (2024) promotes four pillars of safe milk sharing:

- Informed choice: informing parents who may deviate from milk bank standards to maintain cultural or religious beliefs or to suit unique circumstances
- Donor screening: self-exclusion, health and lifestyle communication, and blood testing
- Safe handling: proper handling and accepted guidelines for milk storage
- Home pasteurization: Holder method or flash heating pasteurization, safely and easily done at home

Stigma, concern around milk safety, and the sexualization of breasts are reasons cited against informal milk sharing (Dowling & Grant, 2021). Many parents who donate milk for informal sharing would not be eligible to donate or receive milk from a human milk bank (Peregoy et al., 2022). They often do not meet the stringent health guidelines for milk bank donation. Informal milk sharing reduces the supply of milk available for donor banks who cannot meet the demand for human milk in the NICU. Healthy babies whose parents cannot produce enough milk have little chance of obtaining pasteurized donor milk.

Consumers need information on how to evaluate and manage the risks associated with informal milk sharing and how to make informed decisions. If a family plans to use informally acquired donor milk, you may suggest donor screening, pasteurization, milk testing, and informing their child's caregiver. Home pasteurization is especially important in countries with high rates of HIV infection.

Alternate Feeding Methods

Some parents need tools to help them with lactation. Use of an **alternate feeding method** will enable them to incorporate supplementation into their feeding plan while preserving nursing. Helping parents choose a method that fits best into their lives gives them some control over their feeding. The situation will determine the appropriateness of a method. Options include a cup, a spoon, a syringe, a tube-feeding tool used at the breast, a tube tool used for **finger feeding**, and an artificial nipple and bottle. The cost, care, and cleaning of the tool are factors in selecting what will work.

Parents will need thorough instructions, both verbal and written, with demonstration, encouragement, and close follow-up until the baby can nurse without the supplemental method. Healthcare providers need to be comfortable using any feeding tool before introducing it to parents.

Spoon-Feeding

Spoon-feeding is a common practice for newborns who need a small infusion of calories to get started with nursing. In the early hours or days after birth, some babies are sleepy, hypoglycemic, or have difficulty latching or sustaining a suck for other reasons. Expressing colostrum onto a spoon provides an easy way to get calories into the baby. Spoon-feeding is safe for preterm infants older than 29 weeks' gestation (Genna, 2023).

To feed the baby, place the tip of the spoon gently at the tip of the baby's tongue and ladle the colostrum onto the tongue a few drops at a time (**Figure 22-16**). Most babies find the taste of colostrum appealing and will extend their tongues to lap it up. This small supplement may rouse the baby enough for feeding. Stanford School of Medicine's video on manual expression demonstrates safe spoon-feeding (Stanford School of Medicine, 2020a).

Cup Feeding

When colostrum or early milk becomes more plentiful than what can be accommodated using a spoon, cup feeding offers a baby-led alternative for feedings. **Cup feeding** provides a low level of intervention that is less invasive than finger feeding or the use of an artificial nipple (**Figure 22-17**). Cup feeding is helpful in assisting babies in learning to extend their tongues over the alveolar ridge. Limitations with cup feeding are that it does not encourage sucking and waste occurs from spillage.

Cup feeding avoids bottles until a preterm infant can nurse (Alinezhad Shebilouysofla et al., 2022). The ability to suck and swallow is present at 28 weeks' gestation. Coordination of these abilities develops at 32–34 weeks' gestation. At 30 to 34 weeks, babies lap by protruding their tongues into the cup to obtain small boluses of milk. They often hold the milk in their mouth for some time before swallowing. As the baby matures, a sipping action begins to develop.

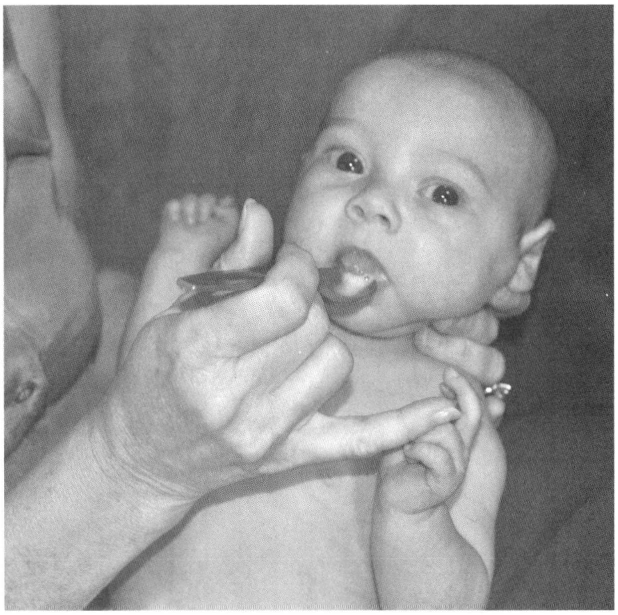

Figure 22-16 A baby being fed by a spoon.

Printed with permission of Anna Swisher.

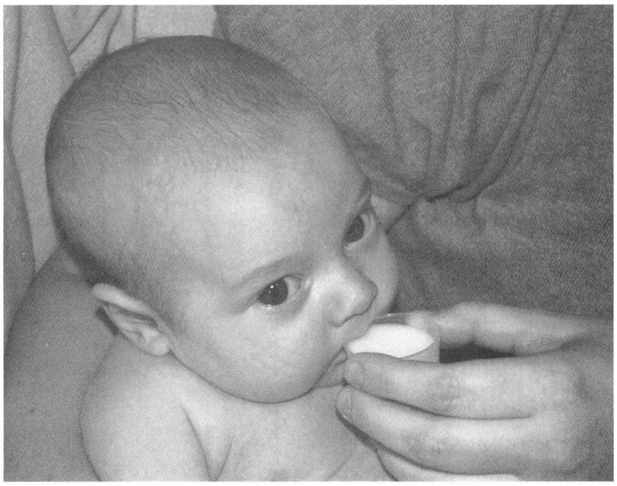

Figure 22-17 A baby being fed by a cup.

Printed with permission of Anna Swisher.

There is debate about whether cup feeding or bottle feeding is more efficient for preterm infants. In addition, a study found no difference in nursing duration between cup feeding, finger feeding, and syringe feeding (Alinezhad Shebilouysofla et al., 2022). Parent satisfaction with cup feeding is high. NICU staff should consider using this method for feeding preterm infants as appropriate. More research is needed.

Procedure for Cup Feeding

Cup feeding is easy for parents and babies to learn. It may take the baby only four or five feedings to master the technique. A small cup with rounded edges works best, such as a medicine cup, hollow-handled medicine spoon, or small disposable paper cup. Parents should avoid using "sippy" cups because the spout does not allow the baby's tongue to form a trough. The spout also makes it difficult for the caregiver to gauge the amount the baby receives. **Figure 22-18** illustrates the steps in cup feeding.

It is important that the baby be in control when cup feeding. To avoid the risk of aspiration, milk should not be poured directly into the baby's mouth. Holding the baby at an upright angle, touch the lip of the cup to the baby's lower lip, with the cup slightly angled so that the milk is at the edge. The baby's tongue will lap the milk from the cup. Slow pacing will avoid aspiration and enable the baby to rest between swallows. If the baby resists the cup, another feeding method may work better.

Paladai

Parents in India have used a small cuplike tool called a **paladai** for centuries (**Figure 22-19**). Recent studies compared the paladai to syringe feeding and cup feeding. The paladai caused more spillage than the syringe

- Fill the cup halfway or less, with about 10 to 15 mL (1/3 to 1/2 oz) of milk.
- Tuck a cloth under the baby's chin to catch spills.
- Hold the baby in a semi-sitting position.
- Bring the cup to the baby's lips and rest the rim of the cup on the lower lip so that it touches the corners of the mouth.
- Tip the cup until the milk touches the baby's lips.
- The baby will begin to lap the milk from the cup. The tongue will form a trough to bring the milk to the back of the throat so that the baby can swallow it.

Figure 22-18 Steps in cup feeding.

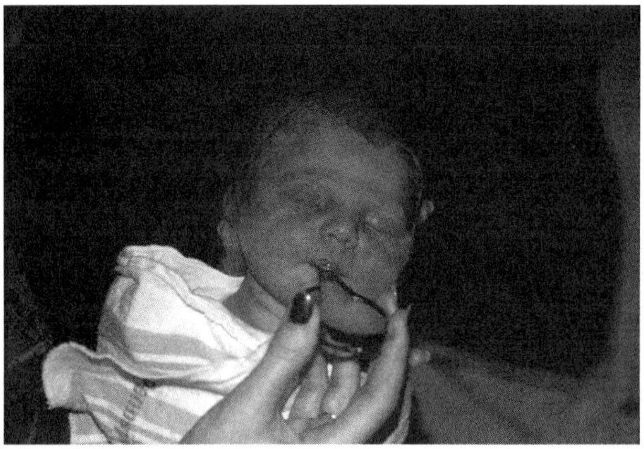

Figure 22-19 Paladai feeding device.

Courtesy of B. Wilson-Clay/K. Hoover.

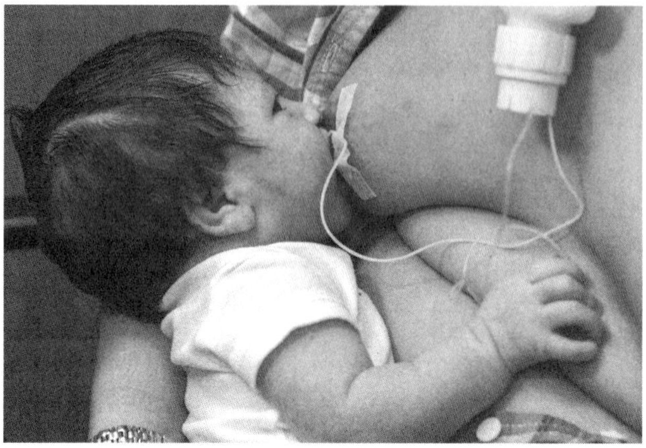

Figure 22-20 Commercial nursing supplementer.

Photo by Every Mother, Inc. and Regina Maria Roig-Romero.

(Thandaveshwara et al., 2022) and was comparable to cup feeding in spillage, duration of feeding, and difficulty of use (McKinney et al., 2020). Successful feedings using the paladai rely in part on the comfort of the user.

Nursing Supplementer

A **nursing supplementer** provides supplemental nutrition while the baby nurses. A commercial supplementer consists of a plastic bag or bottle designed to hold fluid. The parent suspends the supplementer by a cord around their neck or clips it to their clothing at shoulder level so that it rests in the middle of the chest. Thin, flexible tubing leads from the container to the end of the nipple (**Figure 22-20**). A less expensive homemade supplementer can be constructed with the use of a number 5-, 6-, or 8-French oral gastric tube on the end of a syringe or placed in a bottle (**Figure 22-21**). Video clips demonstrating the use of nursing supplementers can be found online and on YouTube.

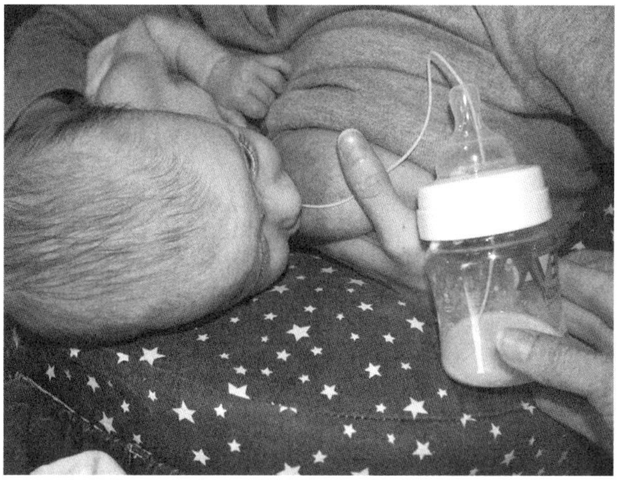

Figure 22-21 Homemade supplementer using a bottle and tubing.

Printed with permission of Anna Swisher.

Deciding to Use a Nursing Supplementer

A nursing supplementer encourages NS at the breast. It can help a parent who has been expressing milk for an ill baby during the transition from bottle feeding to direct nursing. Parents who relactate or induce lactation use this tool to supplement their baby's intake while they increase milk production. Adoptive parents or parents with impaired milk production may use a supplementer for the entire course of nursing.

The flow of milk from the supplementer encourages a baby who has difficulty nursing. The baby grasps the nipple and the tip of the tube simultaneously, and the flow of supplement from the container encourages continued sucking. In this way, the baby receives nourishment at the same time as oral stimulation. For a baby who will latch, a nursing supplementer is the least invasive supplemental method. It avoids the possibility of nipple preference from a bottle nipple and provides nipple stimulation for milk production.

Procedure for a Nursing Supplementer

The substance used in a nursing supplementer can be either expressed milk or infant formula. Some infant formulas are thick and do not flow well through the narrow tubing. Parents may consider powdered formula because of the increased cost of ready-to-feed formula. However, powdered formulas have the potential to clog tubing and prevent the baby from receiving sufficient supplementation. A ready-to-feed formula may be a better option if human milk is not available. If powdered formula is used, it needs to be shaken well to avoid clogging the tubing. Human milk fortifiers can also clog tubing.

Placement of the Tubing

The feeding tube used in a nursing supplementer should extend a few centimeters beyond the end of the nipple. Taping it to the breast keeps it in place. The tape needs to be long enough to prevent it from coming loose in the baby's mouth. Paper tape is the least irritating to the skin. An adhesive bandage can remain on all day, with the tube threaded through the pad part of the bandage. If the supplementer has two tubes, the second tube can be opened as a vent or raised higher to prevent flow, or both tubes can be used on one nipple (Genna, 2023). Parents need to check the roof of their baby's mouth daily to guard against irritation. After every use, the tubing needs to be flushed with cold water, washed with hot and soapy water, and rinsed with clear water.

Position of the Container

Positioning the container level with, above, or below the baby's head will control the rate of flow . The level of the container initially should allow the baby to produce about one suck per swallow. As sucking becomes stronger and milk flow increases, the container can be lowered. Some commercial supplementers have a flow-control valve that responds to the baby's sucking. Other supplementers have various sizes of tubing to adjust flow rate. Compressing the tube manually to control milk flow is unnecessary and can damage the tool or result in the baby expending energy on NNS.

Assisting the Baby

Some babies may initially resist having the tube in their mouths and require time to accept it. Performing alternate breast massage during the feeding increases milk flow and encourages the baby to suck. If the baby is not at risk, the feeding can begin without the supplementer, and it can be added if the baby needs additional nourishment. Some babies become so accustomed to nursing with the tubing that they will not nurse without it. Others may figure out that the milk is coming from the tubing, slide off the nipple, and suck on the tube like a straw. Taping the tubing flush with the nipple or a few centimeters behind it encourages the baby to grab more of the nipple to obtain the milk. Taping the tubing below the nipple may keep the baby from sliding down the tubing.

Amount of Supplement

Pre- and post-test weights will measure the baby's intake of milk and supplement to monitor milk production and determine the amount of milk needed in the supplementer. For example, the supplementer contains 30 mL (1 oz) of expressed milk or formula. The parent weighs the baby, nurses, and then weighs the baby again. If the baby gains 60 mL (2 oz) and there is nothing left in the supplementer, then 30 mL (1 oz) was received from direct nursing and 30 mL (1 oz) from the supplementer. This can guide the amount of supplement needed for the next feeding.

Parents can adjust the nursing supplementer to deliver more fluid when their milk production is low and less fluid as their production increases. When the baby is receiving increasing amounts of milk from direct nursing, the breasts will feel softer and emptier after a feeding, and an increased amount of milk remains in the supplementer. When accompanied by good weight gain, the amount of supplement can be reduced at each feeding.

Reducing the amount of supplement can begin in the morning when milk volume is usually highest. Parents can observe signs of sufficient nourishment, such as wet diapers, ample stooling, good skin turgor, weight gain, and a consistent pattern of eating and sleeping. When they and their baby's healthcare provider are confident that milk production is adequate, supplements can be decreased slowly and finally discontinued.

Finger Feeding

Finger feeding provides supplement to the baby through tubing placed on the end of the caregiver's or parent's finger (**Figure 22-22**). Finger feeding is more invasive than the use of a nursing supplementer. It can be beneficial for a baby who has low muscle tone, who has a **disorganized suck**, or who needs stimulation to elicit sucking. This is common in babies from heavily medicated births where the central nervous system is depressed. Although healthcare providers need to use a glove when demonstrating finger feeding, parents can generally finger feed without gloves. Because of the potential for allergy, latex gloves should not be used. As with any alternative feeding method, theoretically, the baby may come to prefer the finger to direct nursing.

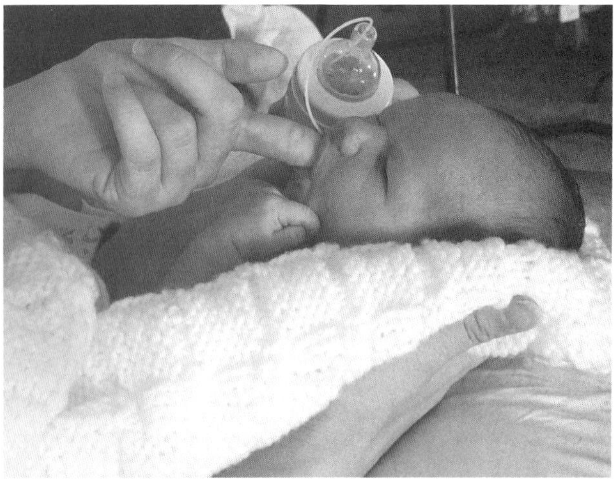

Figure 22-22 Baby being finger fed with tubing attached to the parent's finger.

Procedure for Finger Feeding

Before beginning finger feeding, ensure that the nail of the index finger is short and smooth. A parent with long nails can wear a nonlatex glove to prevent scratching and protect the baby from possible bacteria under their nails. Place a number 5-, 6-, or 8-French oral gastric tubing on the pad of the finger, flush with the end or a few centimeters behind it to prevent the tubing from poking the baby. If desired, the tubing can be taped to the finger to keep it in place.

Gently tickling the baby's lips will encourage them to open their mouth to accept the finger. Caution parents not to push their finger into the baby's mouth. Teach them how to wait until the baby invites them to insert their finger. They can then place the pad of their finger with the tube on it into the baby's mouth against the hard palate (the fingernail will be against the baby's tongue). The baby should be allowed to pull the finger back near the juncture of the hard and soft palates (Genna, 2023).

The baby's condition and the indication for finger feeding determine the number of times this technique is used and the amount of milk the baby receives. Holding the baby against the parent's chest as for nursing, at a 45° angle, keeps milk from getting into the baby's ears. The goal is to elicit one suck per swallow, as with nursing. More than four sucks per swallow may be tiring to the baby. Pace the feeding so that the baby receives a comfortable flow.

Monitoring the Use of Finger Feeding

Evaluating the baby's actions during finger feeding can be a helpful diagnostic tool. Finger feeding is not a useful feeding method if the baby does not respond to the finger by sucking, cannot sustain sucking bursts, or cannot take three or four sucks to form a bolus big enough to swallow. A baby who does not suck may need to be fed by syringe, or possibly gavage fed, to increase caloric intake and develop more effective sucking. Encourage parents to check the roof of the baby's mouth several times daily for possible irritation. After every use, the tubing needs to be flushed out with cold water, washed with hot and soapy water, and rinsed with clear water. Water can be siphoned through the tube by sucking on the other end if necessary.

Syringe Feeding

A standard syringe or periodontal syringe with a curved tip can be used with either finger feeding or direct nursing. Depressing the plunger at the end of the syringe delivers the milk to the baby. Syringe feeding is typically used for very short periods of time, usually in the hospital at early feedings. It can also be helpful for feeding an infant with a cleft palate, holding the infant in a prone position.

Feeding a baby with a syringe places the caregiver in control of milk transfer rather than the baby. Teach parents to deliver the milk bolus in small amounts and not to squirt the milk into the baby's mouth. Squirting the milk could cause aspiration, especially when done by someone who is inexperienced with the technique.

A standard oral syringe can be placed forward in the middle of the baby's mouth, avoiding poking the baby's tongue, gums, or palate. A periodontal syringe can be placed in the corner of the baby's mouth while the baby sucks on a finger (**Figure 22-23**). Placing a

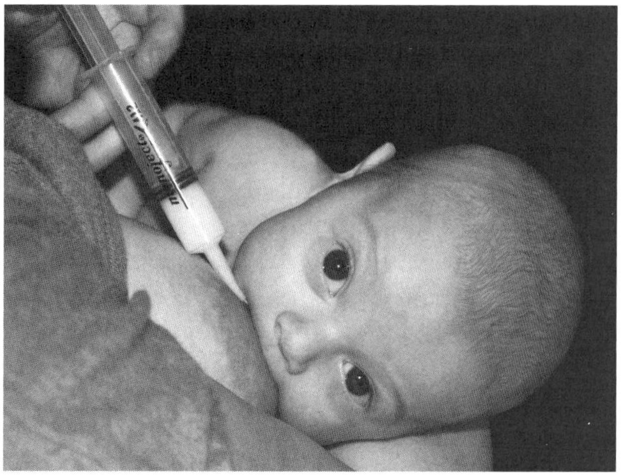

Figure 22-23 Baby being fed by syringe.

small amount of milk toward the front third of the tongue encourages the baby to extend the tongue outward. A periodontal syringe can also be used during direct nursing with the syringe placed along the side of the nipple.

A newborn's typical swallow is 0.6 mL, so the bolus of milk should be between 0.25 and 0.5 mL (Lawrence & Lawrence, 2016). Some babies quickly become proficient at sucking with a syringe and learn to pace themselves. When sucking begins or improves, the parent can remove the syringe and transfer the baby to nurse directly.

Bottle Feeding

Feeding infants with baby bottles was the cultural norm for several generations in Western countries. In many regions, it still is. When prior generations bottle-fed their infants, parents may lack support for the use of any other feeding tool. Some parents are only comfortable with the use of a bottle. Others may try another feeding method for some time and then switch to a bottle. Bottles are usually the method of choice when parents are separated regularly from their babies during feedings, as with a return to work or school. Parents who bottle-feed frequently tend to encourage the baby to finish the bottle even after the baby demonstrates satiety. You can encourage the appropriate use of a bottle by helping parents recognize their baby's hunger and full cues.

No bottle and nipple can mimic baby-led feeding with nursing. In nursing, the baby's entire oral cavity fills with breast tissue, not just with the nipple. Milk flow responds to the baby's sucking, and flow stops when the baby stops sucking. No artificial nipple can conform to the individual shape of the baby's mouth as the breast does. A bottle provides a continuous flow of fluid, and the baby must clamp the nipple to stop the flow. The baby's action changes to one of protecting the airway. Some babies have difficulty adjusting to the different sucking mechanisms when switching between nursing and bottle-feeding. They may develop a preference for the artificial nipple and reject nursing (Batista et al., 2019). **Chapter 15** discusses sucking differences between nursing and bottle feeding.

Parents who use bottles for feeding need appropriate guidelines to minimize risks to their baby. Learning this information from healthcare professionals prenatally assists parents as they make their infant feeding choice. Postpartum healthcare providers need to include complete and correct information for bottle-feeding parents. A baby with low tone who cannot sustain a suck on the bottle, whose mouth leaks milk, or who elicits no "pop" sound when the bottle is pulled out needs to be referred to a healthcare provider for a possible physical or neurologic problem.

Selecting a Bottle Nipple

Most bottle nipples are made of latex rubber or silicone. Latex nipples are cheaper and are available in more shapes than those made of silicone. However, they do not last as long and can become gummy, particularly after boiling. There is also concern that boiling latex can release nitrates, which are potentially carcinogenic. Many people are latex allergic, and using latex products could lead to future latex allergies. Although silicone nipples are firmer and more expensive, they withstand boiling better than latex and thus last considerably longer.

Flow rate of the bottle nipple needs to match the baby's ability to suck, swallow, and breathe. Hole size determines flow rate, which can range from 2 to 85 mL per minute (Pados et al., 2015). Bottle feeding with a fast-flow nipple with an unlimited volume of milk can lead to excessive weight gain and increased gastroesophageal reflux (GER) (Hernandez & Bianchini, 2019). Even "slow-flow" nipples continue to drip when the bottle is turned upside down and can squirt milk when barely compressed. There are no standards to define flow rate of bottle nipples (McGrattan et al., 2017).

Another factor in the choice of a bottle nipple is the size and shape of the nipple base. Parents who combine nursing and bottle feeding may want to avoid a bottle nipple with a small base (**Figure 22-24**). Babies who suck on this type of nipple tend to purse their lips, and may repeat the action when nursing. A nipple with a large base and a short teat encourages the baby's mouth to open wide (**Figure 22-25**). The wide base may help minimize latch difficulties when switching back and forth between bottle feeding and direct nursing.

Some babies have difficulty pulling a nipple with a large base back far enough into the mouth to flange their lips on the wide part of the base. Instead, they slide down and purse their lips around the narrow part of the nipple. A few bottles on the market have a shorter teat, illustrated by the nipple on the left in **Figure 22-25**. A parent who hears smacking or clicking when the baby drinks from a bottle can try a different nipple, ideally finding one that does not cause the baby to purse their lips.

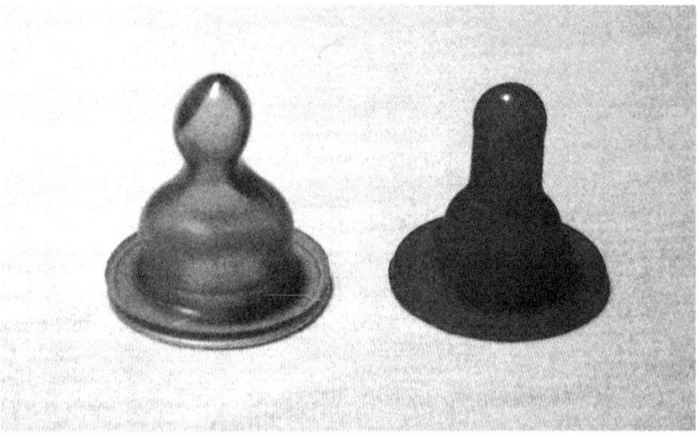

Figure 22-24 Artificial nipples with small bases.

Printed with permission of Anna Swisher.

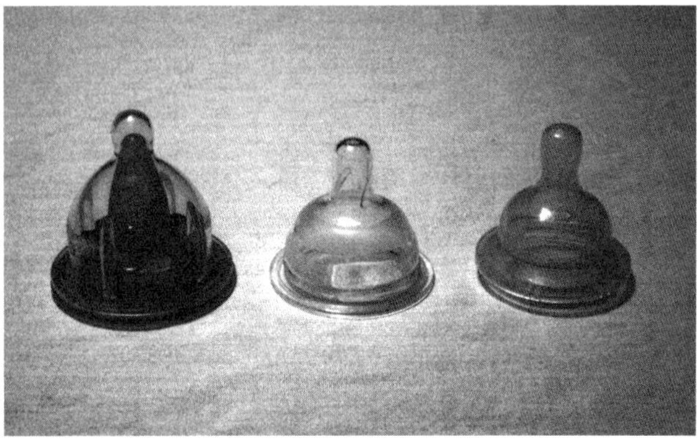

Figure 22-25 Artificial nipples with large bases.

Printed with permission of Anna Swisher.

Table 22-2 Infant Cues During Bottle Feeding

Signs of Stability in Bottle Feeding
- Smooth, regular respirations
- Hand activity near face, with good and consistent postural control
- Organized and calm, with optimal color and oxygen saturation
- Focused and alert
- Good coordination of suck, swallow, breathe
- Sustained awake behavior

Signs of Disorganized Bottle Feeding
- Sucking bursts that vary in length, usually consisting of 5–10 sucks each
- Flaring of nose; uncoordinated suck, swallow, breathing
- Worried appearance
- Extraneous movement of upper extremities
- Head turning
- Irregular, jerky jaw excursions
- Lack of response to nipple insertion
- Rapid deterioration of normal sucking pattern that denotes potential aversion to the nipple
- Difficulty latching or initiating sucking

Signs of Dysfunctional Bottle Feeding
- Lack of role change between nonnutritive and nutritive suck
- Excessively wide jaw excursions
- Restricted range of motion at temporal mandible joint with jaw clenching
- Flaccid or retracted tongue with absence of tongue groove
- Hyperactive gag

Reprinted with permission from Seton Healthcare Network.

Selecting a Feeding Bottle

The feeding bottle may be either glass or plastic. Concerns about bisphenol A (BPA) in plastic bottles increased the popularity of glass bottles, which had previously all but disappeared from store shelves in many countries. BPA is a chemical used in the manufacture of polycarbonate plastic that is found in many plastic baby bottles. BPA can increase reproductive risks in men and women. BPA-free plastic bottles are now available.

The feeding bottle needs to be thoroughly washed with a bottle brush that can reach into crevices. Elongated 0-shaped bottles designed for easy holding by the baby cannot be cleaned as easily as a plain bottle. An angled bottle may give the baby more control, especially when feeding in an upright or semi-upright position. Baby bottles come in many themes and colors, including soft drink brands. This cuteness factor perpetuates the bottle as an icon of babyhood and raises questions about ethical marketing.

Responding to the Baby's Hunger Cues

A bottle delivers milk without much effort from the baby. Parents need to be alert to cues that their baby is responding favorably to the feeding and is sucking on the nipple appropriately. **Table 22-2** presents the signs of stability, disorganization, and dysfunction in bottle feeding. In addition to watching the baby's responses, parents can optimize their method of bottle feeding using the techniques in **Figure 22-26**. This is often referred to as **paced feeding**, discussed later in this section.

Stress Cues During Bottle Feeding

Inexperienced parents tend to ascribe cognitive behaviors to newborns that are not age appropriate. Help parents recognize that their baby's aversive behaviors convey stress or discomfort. Stress cues are avoidance behaviors that indicate something is bothering the baby. They include frowning, wrinkling the brow, squinting, and closed eyes as if in pain. The baby may appear tense and may flail or have clenched

- Touch the corner of the baby's mouth to stimulate sucking.
- Allow the baby to root for the nipple.
- Insert the nipple into the baby's mouth and over the tongue.
- Position the baby in a flexed position so the baby's head is above the stomach and midline.
- Hold the bottle at a horizontal angle to prevent a rapid rate of flow (it is okay for baby to take in some air).
- Pace the feeding by removing the bottle after every two or three sucks, so the baby can order their suck-swallow-breathing, slow the feeding, and better emulate nursing.
- Avoid a rocking motion while feeding to avoid overstimulation.
- Avoid constantly moving the nipple in the baby's mouth, which may cause stress.
- Observe the baby for signs of stress.

Figure 22-26 Optimizing bottle-feeding method.

fists. Milk may spill out of the baby's mouth. The baby may stop sucking and gag, choke, or sputter or may become stiff with an arched back. Teach parents to watch for stress cues in their baby during bottle feeding, presented in **Figure 22-27**.

- Color change
- Tachypnea, or nasal flaring
- Shallow breathing
- High-pitched crowing noise
- Drooling
- Gulping
- Coughing
- Choking
- Changes in oxygen needs
- Squirming
- Arching
- Yawning
- Hiccuping
- Finger splaying
- Increased fussiness
- Saluting sign
- Covering face with hands
- Looking away from caretaker
- Tongue extension
- Falling asleep
- Changes in vital signs
- Hypertonicity or motor flaccidity

Figure 22-27 Signs of infant stress during bottle feeding.

Paced Feeding to Mimic Nursing

Babies can be overwhelmed by the amount of fluid and the rate of delivery with bottle feeding. Although babies can suck and breathe simultaneously, when they attempt to swallow and breathe at the same time, they can aspirate milk into their lungs and nasal cavity (Genna, 2023). A baby who gulps a full bottle quickly is attempting to breathe. Paced feeding slows bottle feeding to mimic nursing and helps the baby coordinate sucking with breathing. Pacing encourages the baby to suck, swallow, and breathe in a rhythm like that in nursing.

Paced feeding is a gentle and healthy way to bottle-feed any baby. It helps a frantic, worried baby become calm, with the hands relaxing, the brow smoothening, and the eyes opening. The baby learns that feeding does not have to be an aversive experience. A few minutes of slow-paced feeding can raise the trust level of a baby who is unenthusiastic about nursing. Point out this stress-free composure and alertness to parents and teach them what to anticipate. Paced feeding can be a tool to calm the baby enough to switch to direct nursing.

Figure 22-28 describes how to use paced feeding. In a variation, the bottle can be held horizontally in the baby's mouth so that a limited amount of milk enters the nipple. Infants who are in the NICU might benefit from this slower milk flow. Swallowing fluids too rapidly is a greater concern than swallowing air because it can lead to apnea, bradycardia, and fatigue aspiration. Although the baby takes in more air with this method, the slower delivery rate allows the baby to breathe between swallows. Frequent burping can help decrease any discomfort caused by swallowing air.

- Hold the baby at a 45-degree angle or greater. Provide postural support to the neck, shoulders, back, and torso. Some babies calm better if they are swaddled. This may be helpful in preventing the baby's arms from flailing. Other babies transition better to nursing by being held on the parent's bare chest, with the bottle near the breast.
- Tickle the baby's upper lip, just as the parent would with their nipple. When the mouth opens, let the baby pull the bottle nipple in; do not force the bottle into the baby's mouth.
- Hold the bottle at an angle that is as close as possible to the angle of the breast, so the baby's neck angles slightly up at its most open position, providing a clear airway.
- Allow the baby three or four sucks, then remove the bottle and rest the nipple on the baby's upper lip. Observe what the baby does. Most babies swallow, then breathe, and then open their mouths and root for the nipple.
- Put the bottle back to the baby's mouth for three or four sucks and remove the bottle again. Continue in this pattern for the rest of the feeding.

Figure 22-28 Instructions for paced bottle feeding.

Bottle Feeding the "Nursing Way"

The advantages of nursing for parents and babies extend far beyond the nutritional and immunologic properties of human milk. Nursing provides a method of communication between a parent and their infant. A parent who bottle-feeds can provide some of the advantages of nursing. Babies nursed from both the right and the left sides of the parent's body receive a different visual perspective when they change sides. Bottle-fed babies can receive this same advantage by being cuddled in the right arm for one feeding and in the left arm for the next feeding.

Likewise, nursing involves continuous skin-to-skin contact with the parent throughout a feeding. Bottle-feeding parents can provide frequent skin-to-skin contact with their babies and hold their babies for feedings rather than propping the bottle. Holding the baby also avoids the risk of choking or aspirating milk. Nursing parents instinctively "groom" their babies during feedings by stroking, patting, and otherwise touching them with their free hand. This is a bit more difficult to do while bottle-feeding. Parents who bottle-feed can snuggle and hold their baby for at least 15 to 20 minutes after a feeding and carry their baby in a sling or baby carrier.

A bottle-fed baby is unable to suck nonnutritively on a bottle because any mouth movement results in milk flow. Regular use of a pacifier can provide the nonnutritive sucking that nursing babies typically enjoy at the end of a feeding. Nursing babies often cuddle in bed with the parent during feedings. Lying down with the bottle-fed baby after feeding provides this special time.

Knowing When to Use a Nursing Tool or Technique

Your clinical judgment will help you identify the nursing tool or technique that is appropriate for a particular situation. Practitioners should recommend them only when there is a clear need. Inappropriate use can negatively affect nursing. Begin with the least invasive method appropriate to the situation to minimize interference. **Table 22-3** summarizes the appropriate uses of tools and techniques used with nursing.

Table 22-3 Nursing Tools and Techniques and When to Use Them

Tool/Technique	Appropriate Use
Breast Massage/Compression	Relaxes parents before nursing Elicits letdown and encourages milk flow Shapes breast tissue and/or everts nipple for nursing
Reverse Pressure Softening	Removes fluid away from areola to allow deeper latch Use when parent has had excessive intravenous fluids
Dancer Hand Position	Helps infants with poor muscle tone to latch
Lubricants and Ointments	Protect the integrity of nipple tissue Make pump flanges more comfortable against the skin
Nipple Everter	Draws out flat or inverted nipples Must have prenatal provider approval for use during pregnancy
Breast Shells	Protect damaged breast tissue Relieve engorgement Collect leaking milk
Nipple Shield	Assists with latch, especially in the presence of short frenulum, flat/inverted nipples, or excessive milk flow Often used with preterm infants
Pacifiers	Reduce risk of sudden infant death syndrome (SIDS) when used while infant is sleeping Facilitate nonnutritive sucking in preterm infants Comfort infants after procedures Help to stabilize infants
Manual Expression	Removes milk, especially colostrum Increases parent's nursing self-efficacy

Tool/Technique	Appropriate Use
Breast Pump	Removes milk when parent and infant are separated Initiates and maintains milk production
Spoon/Cup/Paladai	Provides supplemental milk, often when milk volume is low
Nursing Supplementer	Provides supplemental milk when nursing Used for finger feeding
Bottle	Used to feed baby when nursing is not an option

Summary

Teach parents techniques to assist with latch and milk transfer, and to soothe nipple discomfort. Help them understand the appropriate use of a pacifier for a nursing baby. Teach them how to manually express and pump their milk for when they are away from their babies during feedings. Make sure they know the proper collection and storage techniques for preserving the nutritional quality of their milk. When parents need to supplement their milk, help them find a human milk bank for donor milk. Discourage the use of for-profit milk banks, purchasing milk on the internet, and informal milk sharing. Help parents select alternate feeding methods that work best for them. Provide guidance, support, and follow-up to ensure the proper use of any tool. Serve as an advocate for the nursing dyad remaining together with minimal interventions. Incorporate special aids into care plans only when necessary.

What You Learned–At a Glance

Conversation Starters with Parents

- How can you increase milk flow during a feeding?
- How do you help your baby stay latched?
- How often does your baby suck on a pacifier or bottle nipple?
- How is milk expression going for you?
- How do you collect, store, and thaw your frozen milk?
- What tools do you use to feed your baby?

Nursing Techniques

- The pinch test helps determine nipple eversion.
- Breast massage helps with relaxation, stimulates milk flow, and increases fat in the milk.
- Breast compression squeezes milk into the baby's mouth to encourage sucking.
- Reverse pressure softening of areolar tissue promotes latch.
- The C-hold supports the breast when needed.
- The Dancer hand position supports the breast and the infant's chin for babies born preterm or with weak muscle development.
- A baby can be calmed by inserting a finger into their mouth.

Nursing Tools

- Lubricants are needed only if Montgomery gland secretions are disturbed or there is nipple damage; avoid petroleum-based products and allergens.
- Tools to draw out a flat or inverted nipple can improve latch.
- Breast shells worn inside the bra help evert the nipple, protect damaged nipples, and catch leaking milk; they should not be worn when sleeping or for prolonged periods.
- Nipple shields assist with latch; they require careful instructions, monitoring, and assistance with discontinuing use.
- Pacifier use should not replace needed nursing time and may interfere with hunger cues.
- Pacifier use can reduce SIDS and may help preterm infants during gavage feeding.

Milk Expression

- Breast massage helps promote letdown before and during milk expression.
- Parents need to know how to manually remove milk from their breasts.
- Manual and battery-operated breast pumps are useful for occasional milk expression.
- Double-pumping electric breast pumps are the most efficient for promoting milk production.
- Proper pump flange size and placement prevent friction and ensure efficient milk expression.

- A double electric pump may drain the breasts in 10 to 20 minutes.
- Alternating single pumping several times between breasts increases milk output.

Milk Collection and Storage

- Glass containers are the best choice for milk storage; hard plastic (polypropylene) is the next best choice.
- Storing milk in small amounts reduces waste.
- Labeling containers facilitates using the oldest milk first.
- Fresh milk can remain at room temperature for 6 hours or in an insulated cooler for 24 hours.
- Milk can be refrigerated for up to 8 days and frozen for 6 months in a freezer compartment or 12 months in a separate freezer.
- Milk can be thawed in the refrigerator or in warm water.
- Thawed milk can remain in the refrigerator for 24 hours.
- Expressed milk for an infant in the NICU requires special guidelines.

Donor Milk

- Non-profit human milk banks provide donated milk at no cost to babies with a medical need.
- For-profit human milk banks pay donors and charge users a fee.
- Donors are screened and donated milk is processed, pasteurized, and dispensed by prescription.
- There are potential safety and ethical concerns with informal sharing and internet purchasing of human milk.

Alternate Feeding Methods

- Spoon-feeding can feed small amounts of colostrum or milk for calories or to encourage latch and sucking.
- Cups can feed larger amounts of milk to initiate or supplement nursing.
- A nursing supplementer provides nutrition while the baby sucks at the breast.
- Finger feeding with tubing elicits sucking for babies with low muscle tone or a disorganized suck.
- A syringe at the nipple or tip of the finger delivers milk and elicits sucking.
- A bottle provides a continuous flow of fluid, and the baby must stop the flow with the tongue or jaw.
- Paced bottle feeding puts the baby in control and allows monitoring for stress.

References

Academy of Breastfeeding Medicine. ABM clinical protocol number #8: human milk storage information for home use for full-term infants, revised 2017. *Breastfeed Med.* 2017;12(7):390–395.

Alinezhad Shebilouysofla P, et al. Effect of cup, syringe, and finger feeding on time of oral feeding of preterm neonate's: a randomized controlled clinical trial. *J Health Popul Nutr.* 2022;1(1):52.

American Academy of Pediatric Dentistry. Policy on pacifiers. In *The Reference Manual of Pediatric Dentistry*. Chicago, IL: American Academy of Pediatric Dentistry; 2022:86–89.

Azevedo MJ, et al. Vertical transmission and antifungal susceptibility profile of yeast isolates from the oral cavity, gut, and breastmilk of mother-child pairs in early life. *Int J Mol Sci*. 2023;24(2):1449.

Batista CLC, et al. Nutritive and non-nutritive sucking patterns associated with pacifier use and bottle-feeding in full-term infants. *Early Hum Dev.* 2019;132:18–23.

Carrane L. Pros and cons of wearable breast pumps. January 25, 2021. https://www.nebmedical.com/blog/pros-and-cons-of-wearable-breast-pumps/

Cecilio JO, et al. Breast shells for pain and nipple injury prevention: a non-randomized clinical trial. *PEC Innov*. 2022;1:100101.

Coentro VS, et al. Effect of nipple shield use on milk removal: a mechanistic study. *BMC Pregnancy Childbirth*. 2020;20(1):516.

Coentro VS, et al. Impact of nipple shield use on milk transfer and maternal nipple pain. *Breastfeed Med.* 2021a;16(3):222–229.

Coentro VS, et al. Nipple shield use does not impact sucking dynamics in breastfeeding infants of mothers with nipple pain. *Eur J Pediatr*. 2021b;180(5):1537–1543.

Coentro VS, et al. Breast milk production in women who use nipple shields for persistent nipple pain. *J Obstet Gynecol Neonatal Nurs*. 2022;51(1):73–82.

Dhanawat A, et al. Manual method vs breast pump for breast milk expression in mothers of preterm babies during first postnatal week: a randomized controlled trial. *Indian Pediatr.* 2022; 59(8):608–612.

Dietrich Leurer M, et al. "We just kind of had to figure it out": a qualitative exploration of the information needs of mothers who express human milk. *J Hum Lact*. 2020;36(2):273–282.

Douglas P. Re-thinking lactation-related nipple pain and damage. *Womens Health (Lond)*. 2022;18:17455057221087865.

Dowling S, Grant A. An "incredible community" or "disgusting" and "weird"? Representations of breastmilk sharing in worldwide news media. *Matern Child Nutr.* 2021;17(3): e13139.

Eats on Feet. The four pillars of safe breast milk sharing. 2024. http://www.eatsonfeets.org/4pillars

Eglash, A, et al., ABM Clinical Protocol #8: human milk storage information for home use for full term infants, revised 2017. *Breastfeeding Med*. 2017;12(7).

European Milk Bank Association. Welcome! 2025. https://europeanmilkbanking.com/

Genna CW. *Supporting Sucking Skills in Breastfeeding Infants*. 4th ed. Burlington, MA: Jones & Bartlett Learning; 2023:19–302.

Ghaly M. Human milk-based industry in the Muslim world: religioethical challenges. *Breastfeed Med*. 2018;13(S1):S28–S29.

Hale T, et al. The absence of *Candida albicans* in milk samples of women with clinical symptoms of ductal candidiasis. *Breastfeed Med*. 2009;4:57–61.

Heisel T, et al. Breastmilk and NICU surfaces are potential sources of fungi for infant mycobiomes. *Fungal Genet Biol*. 2019;128:29–35.

Hermanson Å, Åstrand LL. The effects of early pacifier use on breastfeeding: a randomised controlled trial. *Women Birth*. 2020;33(5):e473–e482.

Hernandez AM, Bianchini EMG. Swallowing analyses of neonates and infants in breastfeeding and bottle-feeding: impact on videofluoroscopy swallow studies. *Int Arch Otorhinolaryngol*. 2019;23(3):e343–e353.

Higgins AF. Flange sizing recommendations for frequent breast pump use. *Clinical Lactation*. 2022;13(3):159–169.

Human Milk Banking Association of North America. HMBANA Standards for Donor Human Milk Banking. Fort Worth, TX: Human Milk Banking Association of North America; 2024a. https://www.hmbana.org/file_download/inline/c4bd9e2e-4257-4441-a93a-94cc7647b304

Human Milk Banking Association of North America. *Best Practice for Expressing, Storing and Handling Human Milk in Hospitals, Homes, and Child Care Settings*. 5th ed. Fort Worth, TX: Human Milk Banking Association of North America; 2024b.

Human Milk Banking Association of North America. Find a Milk Bank. 2025. https://www.hmbana.org/find-a-milk-bank/overview.html

International Board of Lactation Consultant Examiners. *Code of Professional Conduct: International Board Certified Lactation Consultants*. Falls Church, VA: International Board of Lactation Consultant Examiners; 2011. Updated September 2022. https://iblce.org/wp-content/uploads/2022/08/2022_August_17_Code-of-Professional-Conduct_FINAL.pdf

Kaya V, Aytekin A. Effects of pacifier use on transition to full breastfeeding and sucking skills in preterm infants: a randomised controlled trial. *J Clin Nurs*. 2017;26(13–14):2055–2063.

Kaya O, et al. The effect of interventions on flat and inverted nipple on breastfeeding: a systemic review. *J Pediatr Nurs*. 2024:S0882–5963.

Kotowski J, et al. Bottle-feeding an infant feeding modality: an integrative literature review. *Matern Child Nutr*. 2020:16(2):e12939.

Lawrence R, Lawrence R. Chapter 8: Breastfeeding: a guide for the medical profession. In *Practical Management of the Mother-Infant Nursing Couple*. 8th ed. Philadelphia, PA: Elsevier, Inc.; 2016:230–284.

Lima AA, et al. Effects of conventional and orthodontic pacifiers on the dental occlusion of children aged 24–36 months old. *Int J Paediatr Dent*. 2017;27(2):108–119.

Lin CX, Lu YY. Comparative effectiveness of olive oil and breast milk on nipple soreness in breastfeeding mothers. *Breastfeed Med*. 2023;18(10):779–784.

Liu Y, et al. Effects of combined oral sucrose and nonnutritive sucking (NNS) on procedural pain of NICU newborns, 2001 to 2016: a PRISMA-compliant systematic review and meta-analysis. *Medicine (Baltimore)*. 2017;96(6):e6108.

Maastrup R, et al. Nipple shield use in preterm infants: prevalence, motives for use and association with exclusive breastfeeding—results from a national cohort study. *PLoS One*. 2019;14(9):e0222811.mangat

Mahdizadeh-Shahri M, et al. The effect of Oketani breast massage on successful breastfeeding, mothers' need for breastfeeding support, and breastfeeding self-efficacy: an experimental study. *Int J Ther Massage Bodywork*. 2021;14(3):4–14.

Mangat AK, et al. A review of non-pharmacological treatments for pain management in newborn infants. *Children (Basel)*. 2018;5(10):130.

McGrattan KE, et al. Effect of single-use, laser-cut, slow-flow nipples on respiration and milk ingestion in preterm Infants. *Am J Speech Lang Pathol*. 2017;26(3):832–839.

McKinney C, et al. A comparative study of two infant feeding tools: the nifty cup and the paladai. *Indian J Pediatr*. 2020;87(7):505–511.

Medolac. FAQs. 2020. https://www.medolac.com/faq/#:~:text=Members%20are%20compensated%20for%20providing%20their%20surplus,designated%20for%20compassionate%20use%20at%20no%20charge).&text=Additional%20information%20about%20the%20Mothers%20Milk%20Cooperative,be%20found%20on%20their%20website:%20http://www.mothersmilk.coop/donor_faq%20.

Meek J, et al. Policy statement: breastfeeding and the use of human milk. *Pediatrics*. 2022;150(1):e2022057988.

Moon RY, et al. The Task Force on Sudden Infant Death Syndrome and the Committee on Fetus and Newborn; evidence base for 2022 updated recommendations for a safe infant sleeping environment to reduce the risk of sleep-related infant deaths. *Pediatrics*. 2022;150(1):e2022057991.

Nabulsi M, et al. The inverted syringe technique for management of inverted nipples in breastfeeding women: a pilot randomized controlled trial. *Int Breastfeed J*. 2022;17(1):9.

Niazi A, et al. A systematic review on prevention and treatment of nipple pain and fissure: are they curable? *J Pharmacopuncture*. 2018;21(3):139–150.

Orovou E, et al. Correlation between pacifier use in preterm neonates and breastfeeding in infancy: a systematic review. *Children (Basel)*. 2022;9(10):1585.

Pados BF, et al. Milk flow rates from bottle nipples used for feeding infants who are hospitalized. *Am J Speech Lang Pathol*. 2015;24(4):671–679.

Pan American Health Organization (PAHO). Human Milk Banks in the Americas. 2023. https://www.paho.org/en/partnerships/instituto-fernandes-figueirafiocruz-human-milk-banks-americas

PATH. Increasing access and intake of human milk. 2025. https://www.path.org/who-we-are/programs/maternal-newborn-child-health-and-nutrition/newborn-nutrition-resources-page/

Peregoy JA, et al. Human milk-sharing practices and infant-feeding behaviours: a comparison of donors and recipients. *Matern Child Nutr*. 2022;18(4):e13389.

Peric O, et al. Comparison of lanolin and human milk treatment of painful and damaged nipples: a randomized control trial. *J Hum Lact*. 2023;39(2):236–244.

Prolacta Bioscience. Home page. 2025. http://www.prolacta.com

Rocha CR, et al. Pacifier use and breastfeeding: a qualitative study of postpartum mothers. *Breastfeed Med*. 2020;15(1):24–28.

Rosenbaum KA. Exclusive breastmilk pumping: a concept analysis. *Nurs Forum*. 2022;57(5):946–953.

Sağlık DK, Kısacık ÖG. Comparison of the effects of olive oil and breast milk on the prevention of nipple problems in primiparous breastfeeding women: a randomized controlled trial. *Health Care Women Int*. 2021;42(4–6):877–894.

Şahin E, et al. Effect of tea tree oil and coconut oil on nipple crack formation in the early postpartum period. *Breastfeed Med.* 2023;18(3):226–232.

Say B, et al. Effects of pacifier use on transition time from gavage to breastfeeding in preterm infants: a randomized controlled trial. *Breastfeed Med.* 2018;13(6):433–437.

Smith JP. Counting the cost of not breastfeeding is now easier, but women's unpaid health care work remains invisible. *Health Policy Plan.* 2019;34(6):479–481.

Smith JP, et al. The volume and monetary value of human milk produced by the world's breastfeeding mothers: results from a new tool. *Front Public Health.* 2023;11:1152659.

Stanford School of Medicine. Newborn nursery at LPCH. Hand expression of breastmilk. 2020a. https://med.stanford.edu/newborns/professional-education/breastfeeding/hand-expressing-milk.html

Stanford School of Medicine. Newborn nursery at LPCH. Maximizing milk production with hands on pumping. 2020b. https://med.stanford.edu/newborns/professional-education/breastfeeding/maximizing-milk-production.html

Strauch L, et al. Mechanisms of support for exclusive breastmilk expressers in the community: a scoping review. *BMC Pregnancy Childbirth.* 2019;19(1):511.

Subudhi S, Sriraman N. Islamic beliefs about milk kinship and donor human milk in the United States. *Pediatrics.* 2021;147(2): e20200441.

Suzuki N, et al. Menthol from *Mentha piperita* suppresses the milk production of lactating mammary epithelial cells in vivo and in vitro. *Mol Nutr Food Res.* 2020:e2000853.

Thandaveshwara D, et al. Comparison of efficacy between paladai and syringe feeding in stable preterm neonates—a randomized control trial. *Breastfeed Med.* 2022;17(3):247–251.

Thibeau S, Ginsberg HG. Bioethics in practice: the ethics surrounding the use of donor milk. *Ochsner J.* 2018;18(1): 17–19.

Tolppola O, et al. Pacifier use and breastfeeding in term and preterm newborns—a systematic review and meta-analysis. *Eur J Pediatr.* 2022;181(9):3421–3428.

U.S. Consumer Product Safety Commission. Pacifiers business guidance. What requirements apply to my product? 2020. https://www.cpsc.gov/Business--Manufacturing/Business-Education/Business-Guidance/Pacifiers-Business-Guidance

U.S. Department of Health and Human Services. Health benefits & coverage. Breastfeeding benefits. 2020. https://www.healthcare.gov/coverage/breast-feeding -benefits/

Whitburn S. Breastfeeding: expressing and supplementing. *Aust J Gen Pract.* 2022;51(3):112–115.

Whitfield KC, Ventura AK. Exploration of responsive feeding during breastfeeding versus bottle feeding of human milk: a within-subject pilot study. *Breastfeed Med.* 2019;14(7): 482–486.

CHAPTER 23

Temporary Nursing Situations

A temporary interruption in nursing requires extra encouragement and suggestions. Jaundice, for example, is common in the early days, and understanding its relationship to lactation practices helps parents reduce its incidence and severity. Hypoglycemia can occur in the hours or early days after birth and interfere with nursing. Later in lactation, some babies seem to resist nursing or may prefer one side to the other. Parents who experience a delay in initiating nursing or who wish to resume or initiate lactation will benefit from advice and support. Nonbiologic, nonbinary, and adoptive parents may need assistance initiating nursing. Caregiver guidance and support will help parents through these temporary nursing situations.

KEY TERMS

Acute bilirubin encephalopathy (ABE)
Albumin
Bili-bed
Bili-light
Bilirubin
Blood incompatibility
Breast compression
Breastfeeding-associated jaundice
Breastmilk jaundice
Conjugation
Coombs' test
Edema
Exchange transfusion
Fiber-optic blanket (bili-blanket or bili-wrap)
Hemoglobin
Hemolysis
Hyperbilirubinemia
Hypoglycemia
Induced lactation
Involution
Jaundice
Kernicterus
Lactogenesis
Late-preterm (LPT)
Normal newborn jaundice
Nursing supplementer
Pathologic jaundice
Phototherapy
Physiologic jaundice
Prolactin receptor cells
Rebirthing
Relactation
Remedial co-bathing
Respiratory distress syndrome
Transcutaneous bilirubin (TcB) measurement systems
Unconjugated

Hyperbilirubinemia (Jaundice)

Clinically, **hyperbilirubinemia (jaundice)** is the most commonly treated medical condition in healthy newborns. More than 80% of newborns develop elevated **bilirubin** levels within several days of birth (Academy of Breastfeeding Medicine [ABM], 2017; Flaherman et al., 2017; Kemper et al., 2022; Sukkar et al., 2023). The risk increases with each additional week less than 40 weeks' gestation. Most jaundice is physiologically normal and clears up spontaneously within a few days with no intervention and no ill effects. Prolonged jaundice can be dangerous when bilirubin levels rise too high or when other risk factors are present. **Figure 23-1** describes risk factors for jaundice.

Jaundice is traditionally identified by a progressive yellow coloring of the skin and the whites of the eyes (sclera). Although the yellow pigmentation is

- Bruising (e.g., cephalohematoma, shoulder dystocia, forceps- or vacuum-assisted delivery)
- Hemolysis (prevalent in ABO incompatibility or Rh incompatibility)
- Direct antiglobulin titer (DAT) positive
- Glucose-6-phosphate dehydrogenase (G6PD) deficiency (an enzyme deficiency)
- Congenital spherocytosis
- Pyruvate kinase deficiency
- Galactosemia
- Crigler–Najjar syndrome
- Ingested maternal blood
- Preterm 36 to < 38 weeks
- Preterm < 36 weeks
- Infection
- Maternal diabetes
- Jaundice in the first 24 hours of life
- Family history of Gilbert's Syndrome
- East Asian ethnicity
- Family history of neonatal jaundice
- Sibling treated with phototherapy
- Sibling treated with exchange transfusion
- Delayed passage of meconium
- Poor feeding (breast or formula)
- Weight loss > 10 percent of birth weight

Figure 23-1 Risk factors for jaundice.

apparent in pale skin, dark-skinned babies rarely appear yellow. The sclera can be yellow in nearly all skin types. In addition, the infant may exhibit sleepiness and loss of appetite. All jaundice warrants investigation and follow-up.

Testing is required to differentiate between normal and abnormal jaundice patterns. Jaundice becomes clinically significant when it develops within the first 24 hours of the baby's life. There is concern when bilirubin rates increase rapidly, when levels become exaggerated, or when the condition is prolonged beyond 2 weeks in term babies and beyond 3 weeks in preterm babies. Infants of Southeast and East Asian descent have higher bilirubin levels, as do American First Nation peoples and Inuits (Bentz et al., 2018; Thielemans et al., 2021). Jaundice rates are also higher in babies who live at higher elevations. It may be that the decrease in oxygen levels leads to an increase in **hemoglobin** and the number of red blood cells (Martinez-Torres et al., 2023).

Types of Jaundice

A healthy newborn's bilirubin level at birth has historically been measured as 1.5 mg per dL or less. Bilirubin levels change hourly in a newborn and typically peak at approximately 6.5 mg per dL by 4 days postpartum. Bilirubin then returns to a normal level of less than 1.5 mg per dL by around the 10th day of life (Kemper et al., 2022). This natural rise and fall of the newborn's bilirubin is referred to as **physiologic jaundice**, also called **normal newborn jaundice**. Prolonged physiologic jaundice—also called *late-onset jaundice* is referred to as **breastmilk jaundice**. High bilirubin levels can also result from mismanagement of lactation, referred to as **breastfeeding-associated jaundice**. Jaundice is considered nonphysiologic when the bilirubin level exceeds 12 mg per dL and the jaundice has no identifiable cause. The term **pathologic jaundice** applies when a disease process causes elevated bilirubin.

Physiologic Jaundice

In utero, the fetus produces large amounts of red blood cells, which transport oxygen to the fetus from the parent's blood via the placenta. This is the baby's only source of oxygen until they leave the womb and draws in oxygen through the lungs. The hemoglobin (a protein) portion of the body's red blood cells transports oxygen. Newborns have more hemoglobin than adults do, and healthy, full-term infants are born with both fetal and adult hemoglobin. Although fetal hemoglobin is efficient in handling oxygen in utero, only adult hemoglobin is efficient after birth.

Because the newborn does not need fetal hemoglobin, their body breaks it down, separates it, and reuses the globin portion. The heme portion undergoes many changes, the final by-product of which is bilirubin. Bilirubin acts as a powerful antioxidant and may provide protection against free radical cellular damage after birth. Thus, the low bilirubin levels of physiologically normal newborn jaundice may play a protective role for infants (Duvigneau et al., 2019; Itoh et al., 2023).

Every infant is born with an increased concentration of bilirubin. However, not all infants have the high concentrations that result in the visible yellow coloring associated with jaundice. An estimated 20% to 30% of predominantly nursing newborns have mild physiologic jaundice (bilirubin levels at ≥ 5 mg per dL) at age 3 to 4 weeks. In infants with mild jaundice, the yellow coloring may be difficult to detect visually under artificial light. It is normal for physiologic jaundice to last longer in healthy, nursing babies.

Conjugated Bilirubin. Under normal conditions, the baby's bilirubin becomes bound chemically to proteins, such as **albumin**, which transport it to

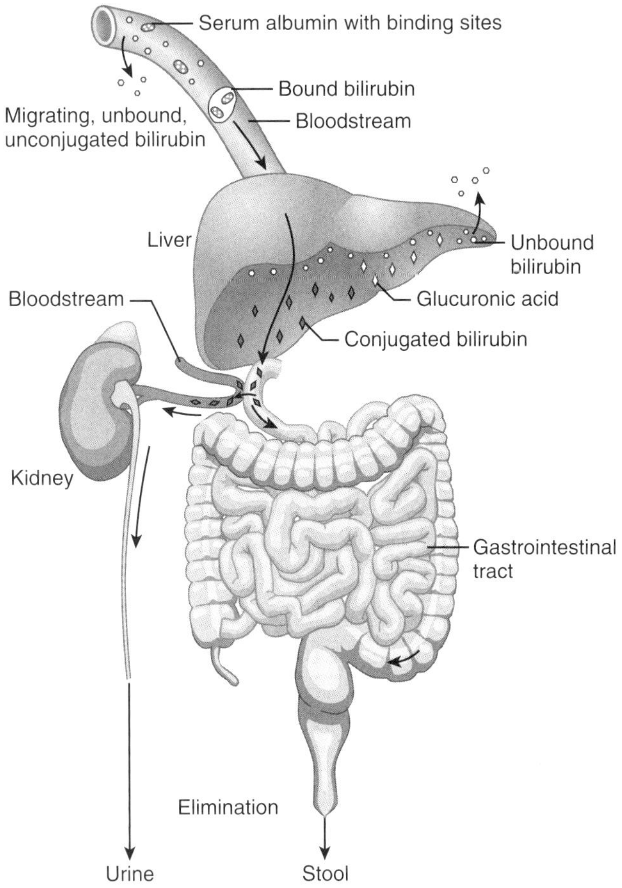

Figure 23-2 How the body handles bilirubin.

the liver. The liver converts the bilirubin through a process of **conjugation** into a form that can pass through the bile to the intestine. In the intestine, it undergoes further changes that enable the baby's stools and, to a much lesser extent, urine, to excrete it. Many infants dispose of bilirubin through this physiologic process. Bilirubin that is conjugated, or bound (attached to albumin) remains in the bloodstream and is not harmful to the baby.

Unconjugated, Unbound Bilirubin. Frequently, a newborn's red blood cells break down more quickly than their immature liver can process. This results in a temporary buildup of bilirubin leading to physiologic jaundice. Bilirubin levels will gradually decline as the excess hemoglobin breaks down, bacteria colonize the intestines, and the transition from fetal to adult hemoglobin occurs. The decreased rate of bilirubin conjugation in physiologic jaundice allows unbound, **unconjugated** bilirubin to circulate freely in the bloodstream. The unbound bilirubin can migrate to other parts of the body with high fat content, such as the brain, skin, muscle tissue, and mucous membranes, where it deposits (**Figure 23-2**).

Kernicterus. Elevated bilirubin has a toxic effect on brain and nerve cells and can result in bilirubin encephalopathy, or **kernicterus**. Kernicterus risks long-term neurologic damage and even death (Gazzin et al., 2023). Conditions such as preterm birth, asphyxia, starvation, and hemolytic disease can disrupt the blood–brain barrier. This allows bilirubin to pass the blood–brain barrier and deposit in nerve cells in the brain. The term **acute bilirubin encephalopathy (ABE)** describes the acute phase of bilirubin toxicity associated with brain damage.

Consequences of kernicterus include hearing loss; cognitive impairment (mental retardation); muscle rigidity (including cerebral palsy); speech impairment; seizures; and movement disorders, including impaired upward gaze. There is a spectrum of debility associated with kernicterus, sometimes called *bilirubin-induced neurologic dysfunction* (BIND). BIND is a syndrome of subtle bilirubin neurotoxic disorders that present as deficits in auditory, cognitive, and motor processing (Bahr et al., 2019; Mosallam et al., 2019).

The bilirubin level at which ABE occurs varies with the infant's gestational and postnatal ages, birth weight, the presence of other disease, and the availability of albumin-binding sites. Statistically, infants most at risk for kernicterus are those born at 35 to 38 weeks' gestation, male, and Asian. A preterm infant can progress quickly to bilirubin encephalopathy and to the chronic stage of kernicterus at lower bilirubin levels than a full-term infant (Kasirer et al., 2023). A review of all recorded kernicterus cases in Denmark from 2000 to 2015 identified ABO hemolytic disease as the most common cause (Donneborg et al., 2020).

Special Health Conditions. Conditions such as hepatitis, galactosemia, biliary atresia, and sepsis cause abnormal excretion or reabsorption of bilirubin. Bruising, **blood incompatibility**, lack of enzymes, or antibodies against the baby's red blood cells can create a rapid rise in bilirubin level. In addition, diseases and drugs can lead to the production of autoantibodies, which destroy red blood cells and may cause anemia (Buhari et al., 2023). The direct **Coombs' test** is used to detect the presence of these autoantibodies and to help diagnose the cause of anemia, jaundice, or red blood cell abnormalities.

Glucose-6-phosphate dehydrogenase (G6PD) deficiency, is the most prevalent enzyme deficiency. It is estimated to affect an average of 8% of people worldwide, with great variance in regional and ethnic distribution. This deficiency is a hereditary genetic defect that causes newborn hyperbilirubinemia and chronic hemolytic (red blood cell destruction) anemia. Certain drugs or infections can cause acute **hemolysis** (Kaplan et al., 2023).

Breastfeeding-Associated Jaundice

Breastfeeding-associated jaundice occurs because of inadequate milk intake (Scott & Kirkland, 2023). Elevated bilirubin levels in breastfeeding-associated jaundice result from from caloric deprivation and the resultant decreased stooling. It occurs because of such iatrogenic causes as scheduled feedings, routine separation of nursing parents and babies, unnecessary formula supplements, and pacifier use. A parent unfamiliar with nursing may fail to nurse frequently enough for adequate nourishment. The use of labor medications may result in sleepy babies who have difficulty nursing.

Breastfeeding-associated jaundice is usually preventable through appropriate nursing practices. Treatment includes increasing the number and quality of feedings, observing the baby's positioning and latch, listening for swallowing, and taking pre- and postfeed test weights. Rooming-in and frequent skin-to-skin contact can increase the number of feeding opportunities. Implementing care guidelines that protect lactation significantly decreases the number of hyperbilirubinemia cases (Hui et al., 2024). Frequent cases of exaggerated jaundice in a hospital or community of nursing babies may indicate a need to improve lactation policies and support.

A baby who is an effective feeder can be given unlimited access, with no restrictions on frequency or duration. However, unlimited sucking is not productive for a baby with an ineffective suck, which is common in preterm babies. Intermittent **breast compression** during feedings can help increase milk flow for a baby with a weak and ineffective suck (Wight et al., 2023). In addition, hand-expressed colostrum can be fed to the baby with a spoon or syringe, as discussed in **Chapter 22**.

Prolonged Physiologic Jaundice (Breastmilk Jaundice)

Breastmilk jaundice typically occurs between the fourth and seventh days of life when mature milk begins to replace colostrum. Some research suggests that gene variations play a role in the development of breastmilk jaundice. The enzyme beta-glucuronidase in human milk deconjugates conjugated bilirubin in the intestines and increases intestinal absorption, contributing to this type of jaundice (Huang et al., 2023). This type of jaundice may persist through the sixth week of life, even up to 15 weeks. Bilirubin reaches a maximum concentration by the second or third week. This type of prolonged physiologic jaundice is usually self-limiting and benign. The baby is lively and does not appear to be sick.

Most cases of breastmilk jaundice require no interruption in nursing. Just as with newborn physiologic jaundice, it can be treated with increased feedings. In addition to avoiding jaundice, frequent and effective nursing beginning soon after delivery minimizes weight loss and helps the baby gain weight. Continuation of jaundice into the later weeks of life in a healthy nursing newborn may be a normal extension of physiologic jaundice.

Because sunlight breaks down bilirubin, exposure to sunlight has been a treatment historically to reduce jaundice levels. Babies were placed near a sunny window because bilirubin breaks down when exposed to sunlight or its equivalent. If parents state they plan to use sunlight exposure, encourage them to ask their care provider for guidelines. The American Academy of Pediatrics (AAP) does not recommend sun exposure because of cancer risk (refer to the discussion on vitamin D in **Chapter 8**).

Pathologic Jaundice

Pathologic jaundice occurs in 6% to 10% of newborns and requires intervention (Sandhya et al., 2023). This type of jaundice in an infant can result from conditions such as infections in the blood or liver, diseases of the liver, obstructions in the gastrointestinal system, and interference with the binding of bilirubin in the bloodstream. Many of these circumstances are also associated with jaundice in an adult. These situations require treatment of both the disease and the jaundice. Because of its diverse nature, pathologic jaundice can appear at any time after birth, making diagnosis relatively difficult.

Blood incompatibility and certain drugs can also result in pathologic jaundice. A nursing parent and baby should discontinue any drugs that contribute to the buildup of bilirubin. Blood incompatibility occurs when the baby of a birth parent with blood type O has blood type A, B, or AB. The parent's blood contains naturally occurring antibodies to type A and B which can cross the placenta and destroy (hemolyze) the baby's red blood cells. Rhesus (Rh) incompatibility occurs when a birth parent with Rh-negative blood creates antibodies to an Rh-positive baby. G6PD enzyme deficiency and more than 50 known red cell enzyme deficiencies are associated with newborn jaundice (Zakerihamidi et al., 2023). There is also an association between urinary tract infections and jaundice, especially within the first 2 weeks of life (Özcan et al., 2017; Tola et al., 2018). Therefore, culturing urine for infection is recommended when a baby develops jaundice after the first week or has prolonged jaundice.

Parents whose infants have pathologic jaundice need the reassurance that nothing is wrong with their milk. Prepare them for a long period of resolution if the baby's skin remains yellow after the second week. If a family's previous baby experienced jaundice, you can prepare them for the possibility that this baby may develop it as well.

Detection of Jaundice

Jaundice is visible when the bilirubin level reaches 5 to 7 mg per dL. Among babies with visible jaundice, 15% have a bilirubin level of 10 mg per dL or higher. Approximately 3% of these babies have exaggerated or prolonged bilirubin levels because of a normal development process in their ability to conjugate and excrete bilirubin. The safe level for bilirubin is lower for an ill, preterm, or **late-preterm (LPT)** infant. The resulting jaundice requires quicker treatment and close monitoring.

Multiple factors can limit or delay detection of dangerously high bilirubin levels after hospital discharge. An infant may be discharged early without follow-up, a family may have minimal knowledge, or there may be conflicting cultural practices or traditional home treatments for jaundice. The incidence of dangerous bilirubin levels is associated with disjointed care during the first week after the baby's birth. Taking steps in the early postpartum period can reduce the incidence and severity of jaundice by increasing effective feedings. An appointment with a healthcare provider for all babies within 3 to 5 days of age is important for detecting jaundice. Infants discharged before 48 hours of age need a provider visit within 24 to 48 hours after discharge. This visit should include a weight and color check for early detection of nursing problems and significant jaundice levels.

Progression of Yellowing

Historically, bilirubin levels have been described as corresponding to the visual jaundicing of the baby's body. As jaundice levels increase, the body's yellowing progresses from the head down to the chest; to the knees, lower legs, and arms; and finally, to the hands and feet. Visual assessment correlates to the following estimated serum bilirubin values (Dzulkifli et al., 2018):

- Head and neck: 4 to 8 mg per dL
- Upper trunk above umbilicus: 5 to 12 mg per dL
- Lower trunk and thighs below umbilicus: 8 to 16 mg per dL
- Arms and lower legs: 11 to 18 mg per dL
- Palms and soles: greater than or equal to 18 mg per dL

Testing Bilirubin Levels

Blood types of both the parent and baby are evaluated at birth to rule out blood incompatibility as a risk factor for jaundice. The Coombs' test performed at birth checks for antiglobulins in the baby's blood. **Transcutaneous bilirubin (TcB) measurement systems** are noninvasive handheld devices similar to a small calculator or flashlight held over the baby's skin to indicate the bilirubin level. Although TcB measurements provide a good estimate of the total serum bilirubin (TSB) level, they are not a substitute for TSB values.

Depending on the bilirubin level indicated by the TcB meter, the baby may have a serum bilirubin drawn, usually via a heel stick. A TSB level should always be obtained when therapeutic intervention is being considered. Performing the TSB test at the same time as the newborn blood type screening will minimize heel sticks. A baby with high bilirubin typically receives multiple heel sticks throughout the course of treatment. Nursing has been found to be analgesic for infants when undergoing a painful procedure such as this (Shah et al., 2023). Parents can request to nurse during heel sticks to reduce their babies' pain level.

Treatment of Jaundice

In most cases, bilirubin values rise slowly (less than a 5-mg per dL increase in 24 hours). Bilirubin reaches a noticeable level by the third day of life and remains slightly elevated for several days. It then falls by the end of the first week. Increasing the frequency and effectiveness of feedings in the early days helps to reduce bilirubin levels in the infant. Active treatment is rarely required as long as levels remain within a safe range.

Several types of treatment are appropriate when a bilirubin level is significant, based on the baby's condition. For mild jaundice, regular visual observation and periodic testing of bilirubin levels may be sufficient. Physiologic jaundice is usually mild and causes no known lasting effects in a healthy full-term infant. Other treatments include **phototherapy** and, when jaundice is severe, blood **exchange transfusion**. Keeping abreast of current recommendations enables you to help parents persevere in nursing through the temporary challenges jaundice presents.

Increased Feeding

The incidence of jaundice decreases when meconium, which is laden with bilirubin, is passed quickly. Because colostrum has a laxative effect on the baby, early and frequent nursing helps prevent jaundice by eliminating bilirubin from the gut. Additionally, frequent feedings help establish milk production, thus increasing the baby's milk intake in the early weeks. Water supplementation is not recommended in the treatment of jaundice because it causes a baby to void, not stool.

Jaundice can cause the baby to have sluggish responses and a noticeably weak sucking reflex. More frequent and shorter feedings and supplementation with expressed milk can improve the baby's feeding behavior. However, these symptoms may also be a sign of something more serious. Encourage parents to observe the baby's feeding behavior during treatment, while nursing, and when given supplementation and to report any changes to the healthcare team. If the baby is not nursing well or if there was a delay in the onset of mature milk, the baby can be supplemented with expressed milk. If sufficient expressed milk is not available, donor milk or infant formula can be considered.

Phototherapy

When bilirubin approaches a level that requires more aggressive treatment, the baby may be placed under a special fluorescent **bili-light** for phototherapy. A bili-light works in the same way as sunlight to break down bilirubin, forming products that can be excreted without conjugation. The following bilirubin levels are those at which the AAP recommends phototherapy based on the baby's age. The ranges reflect gestation from 35 to 40 weeks (Espinosa & Brown, 2023).

- 25 to 48 hours of life: 10 to 17 mg per dL or above
- 49 to 72 hours of life: 14 to 22 mg per dL or above
- Greater than 72 hours of life: 22 mg per dL or above

Types of Phototherapy. Maximum skin exposure is desirable for traditional phototherapy conducted in the hospital. Traditional treatment equipment uses an overhead bili-light. The infant is placed under the lights with their eyes covered for protection (**Figure 23-3**). The infant usually remains under the bili-light continuously except for brief feeding periods. This type of phototherapy using overhead bili-lights increases separation of parents and infants and may thus have a negative impact on nursing.

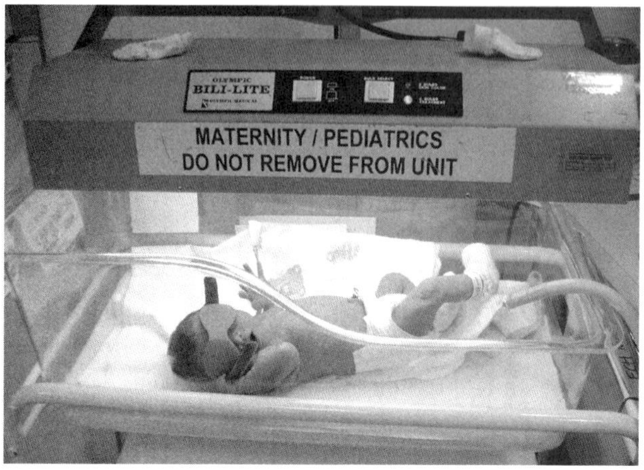

Figure 23-3 Baby receiving treatment under a bili-light.
Reprinted with permission of Jeremy Kemp.

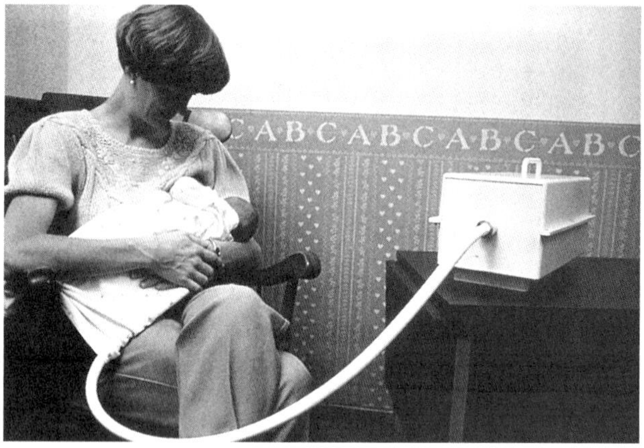

Figure 23-4 Fiber-optic blanket for treating jaundice.
© Medela, Inc. 2010.

Newer phototherapy options include a **bili-bed** or a **bili-blanket** (also called **fiber-optic blanket** or **bili-wrap**). Depicted in **Figures 23-4** and **23-5**, these treatments can take place in the client's room. A bili-bed provides light underneath the baby, allowing the baby to lie in an open bed. No eye patches are needed, and parents can hold their baby's hand, stroke their body, and make eye contact.

A fiber-optic blanket enables parents to nurse during treatment. A receiving blanket placed over the bili-blanket keeps the baby warm. Eye patches are unnecessary, and treatment can take place at home with the family's support system around them. Compliance with home phototherapy and ongoing follow-up may be a challenge for some families. Home phototherapy should not be used for infants with risk factors (DeZure, 2023; Flaherman et al., 2017; Kemper et al., 2022).

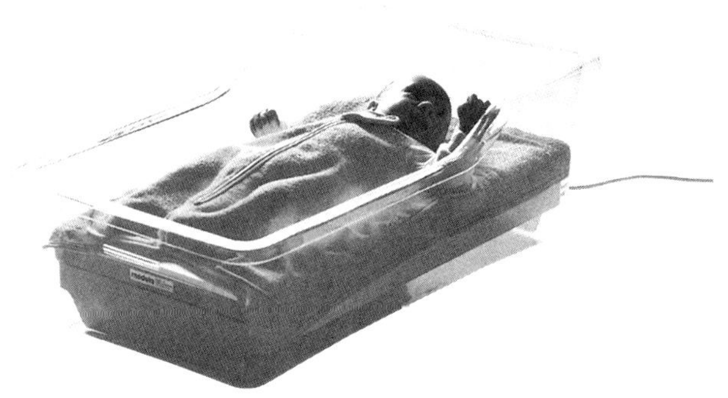

Figure 23-5 Bili-bed for treating jaundice.

Exchange Transfusion

A baby whose bilirubin levels fail to drop after phototherapy or whose bilirubin levels continue to rise may require a blood exchange transfusion (Kemper et al., 2022). Babies with dangerously high bilirubin levels receive a combination of exchange transfusion and intensive phototherapy. Fortunately, babies rarely need blood exchange transfusions. With the advent of RhoGAM, Rh-negative birth parents can be prevented from making antibodies to their baby's Rh-positive blood. Preventing jaundice from reaching levels high enough to warrant an exchange transfusion is imperative; an exchange transfusion should be the treatment of last resort.

Jaundice in a Preterm Infant

Jaundice that is not truly physiologic occurs more frequently in preterm infants and may last for up to 3 or 4 weeks. The preterm infant's liver is smaller than a full-term infant's and is less able to conjugate and eliminate bilirubin efficiently. In addition, the infant's brain is especially sensitive to bilirubin. Permissible bilirubin levels in the preterm infant are inversely related to the degree of prematurity. Jaundice is also more common in LPT and early term infants (Boies & Vaucher, 2016).

Experience with preterm infants demonstrates that neurologic impairment can occur with physiologic jaundice, even at lower bilirubin levels. Bilirubin encephalopathy is reported in extremely preterm infants (born at 22–27 weeks' gestation). These infants often have prolonged unbound bilirubinemia beyond the first week of life (Hirayama et al., 2023). Because other factors may cause the rise in bilirubin levels, preterm infants may be put on intravenous (IV) fluids and receive nothing by mouth while tests are run. If direct nursing is suspended temporarily, milk expression will help protect production. Staff in the neonatal intensive care unit (NICU) can help parents with collection and storage guidelines.

Milk expression, in addition to direct nursing, may be necessary for LPT infants, as discussed in **Chapter 24**. There is a strong correlation between lower gestational age and risk for jaundice. Babies born at 37 weeks' gestation are much more likely to develop a serum bilirubin level of 13 mg per dL or higher than those born at 40 weeks' gestation. Practitioners are urged not to treat LPT newborns as term newborns in the management of hyperbilirubinemia. LPT infants are at an increased risk of developing significant jaundice compared with infants of 38 to 42 weeks' gestation (Karnati et al., 2020).

Parental Concerns About Jaundice

Because newborn jaundice is common, it is helpful for all expectant parents to learn about the condition prenatally. Let parents know that jaundice is a common newborn condition that can be evaluated and treated without compromising nursing. Encourage them to focus on ways they can ensure continued close contact with their baby if jaundice requires treatment.

Optimal Birth Practices

When parents learn about the factors associated with jaundice, they can take action to minimize its occurrence. This includes avoiding unnecessary drugs during pregnancy and planning a birthing environment that promotes early, uninterrupted nursing. Home births or birthing center births reduce unnecessary interventions. If they deliver in a hospital, they can arrange to nurse immediately after birth and frequently in the early days postpartum.

Expectant parents are encouraged to avoid elective induction performed solely for convenience and without medical need. A parent who goes into labor spontaneously receives a reduced amount of IV fluids during delivery. Laboring and birthing without routine IV administration helps avoid **edema** (which affects latch), delayed **lactogenesis** II, and greater-than-normal newborn weight loss (Kearney et al., 2024; Lothian, 2019). Avoiding elective induction for nonmedical need may also lower the risk of a cesarean delivery (Tarimo et al., 2020). Cesarean deliveries with increased IV fluid requirements are associated with delayed onset of milk production and newborn weight loss (Rich et al., 2023).

Interventions that delay milk production increase the likelihood of jaundice.

Concerns About the Baby

Parents can reduce emotional stress by arranging to be with their jaundiced baby whenever possible. They can request treatment at the bedside with intervals of interaction for holding, bonding, and nursing. If the baby must remain hospitalized when the parent is discharged, the parent can request to remain in the hospital to stay with the baby. If the baby is readmitted to the hospital, parents can ask whether rooming-in is available. Family-centered care may be better facilitated at a children's hospital or larger birthing facility. Insurance coverage may determine where the baby is treated and limit the parents' options.

To eliminate an extended hospital stay, parents can explore home phototherapy if it is economically feasible and appropriate (e.g., no risk factors as listed in **Figure 23-1**). You can reassure them that nursing is the most important thing they can do while their baby receives treatment and that most jaundice resolves with standard phototherapy treatment. If nursing is interrupted, you can assist with pumping and a return to exclusive nursing as soon as cleared to do so by the baby's caregiver.

Vulnerable Child Syndrome

Although newborn jaundice is common, it can be worrisome for parents. Vulnerable child syndrome is a psychological condition in which parents regard their child as being vulnerable to illness and become hypervigilant. It usually follows a child's serious illness, hospitalization (including for preterm birth), or survival of a life-threatening event (Hoge et al., 2021). Internet resources and improved caregiver education and parental support may alleviate this phenomenon.

Anticipatory guidance can empower parents to be proactive, prudent, and effective advocates in caring for their baby. Family-centered care validates parents' concerns and distress, empowers them, and includes them in caring for their child as much as possible. This partnership can forge a strong alliance between the parents and their healthcare providers. Asking for the parents' input and providing reassurance throughout the treatment period will help maintain lactation and encourage parents to anticipate resolution. Treatment for physiologic jaundice is typically brief—only a day or two. Attentive, collaborative care may reduce the parents' feelings of powerlessness or victimization. This in turn may help to reduce the incidence of perceiving their child as unusually vulnerable or fragile.

Working with the Baby's Caregiver

Encourage parents to stay well informed of their baby's condition and treatment and to discuss concerns with their baby's caregiver. Parents of a jaundiced baby can work with their baby's healthcare provider to develop a care plan that allows them easy access for frequent feedings. Understanding the cause and treatment of their baby's jaundice will help them recognize that it will most likely resolve within a few days or weeks. They can remain in close communication with the caregiver to learn which screening tool will be used for detecting bilirubin levels, the results of the tests, and any further testing that will be needed.

Parents can discuss options and criteria for home phototherapy and express their desire for a treatment plan that allows their baby to nurse during the procedure (e.g., a bili-blanket). If the baby will receive treatment under a bili-light, they can ask how often they can remove the baby to nurse and how frequently they can hold their baby. If nursing is interrupted, they can ask about the rationale for the decision and the criteria for when nursing can resume. **Table 23-1** provides further suggestions for counseling parents of a jaundiced baby.

Hypoglycemia

Temporary low blood glucose, or **hypoglycemia**, is normal for a healthy newborn. Hypoglycemia occurs when the baby's blood sugar level is lower than the standard range. Because of the transient nature, universal screening in newborns is not recommended. In fact, unnecessary testing can interfere with the initial bonding between the parent and infant and the establishment of successful feeding patterns.

Typically, a blood glucose level of 45 mg per dL or lower is considered low for a newborn. Transitional newborn hypoglycemia usually resolves within 48 hours after birth. Continued hypoglycemia beyond 48 hours may be pathologic. There is consensus in the neonatology community that blood glucose should be measured for infants who are at risk for significant hypoglycemia. These infants include those born to parents with diabetes and large-for-gestational age (LGA), small-for-gestational age (SGA), and LPT infants (Hubbard & Hay, 2021).

Treatments for hypoglycemia depends on the severity of the blood glucose levels. The ABM's protocol

Table 23-1 Counseling the Parents of a Jaundiced Baby

Parents' Concern	Suggestions
Parents feel bewildered by procedures and other caregivers	Discuss questions and other aspects of baby care with the baby's healthcare provider. Research available information.
Separation from baby	Arrange for bedside treatment of baby, if possible, using portable bili-blanket or bili-bed. Arrange for regular intervals of interaction for eye and skin contact.
Treatment interfere with nursing	Arrange for fiber-optic blanket for phototherapy. Arrange for regular contact with baby and frequent feedings. Use relaxation techniques to promote letdown. Arrange for uninterrupted feedings.
Baby has sluggish responses and a weak sucking reflex	Nurse more frequently, using breast compression to encourage sucking. Use a tube-feeding device to augment nursing. Use cup, spoon, or syringe feedings if latch is poor.
Healthcare provider is considering interruption in nursing	Ask for recheck of bilirubin level after baby nurses or receives a supplement. Ask for frequent checks of the baby's bilirubin level.
Nursing must be interrupted	Begin expressing milk as soon as possible to establish and maintain milk production.
Prevention of jaundice	Avoid prenatal exposure to chemicals. Avoid jaundice-producing drugs during labor and delivery. Nurse within 1 hour after birth and frequently thereafter.

protects the establishment and maintenance of nursing while providing appropriate interventions and treatment (Wight & ABM, 2021). Among the recommendations are early, frequent, and exclusive nursing; expressing and supplementing the baby with colostrum; using donor human milk; and using dextrose buccal gel. The oral use of dextrose gel has reduced the need for IV glucose and is more widely used in order to avoid formula supplementation. Dextrose gel plus nursing is considered the first line oral treatment of hypoglycemic newborns (Parappil et al., 2023).

Delayed Nursing

At times, circumstances do not permit nursing immediately after birth. A short-term delay can last from a few hours to a couple of days. It may be caused by the baby being born with a low body temperature, aspirating meconium at birth, low Apgar scores, or symptoms of infection. Such conditions may necessitate the separation of the dyad because of admission to the NICU until the condition stabilizes. Some hospitals isolate parents and babies together to avoid a separation when an infection is suspected. Preterm birth, **respiratory distress syndrome**, and other birth complications can require several days, weeks, or even months of hospitalization. Although nursing can usually begin at some point during the hospitalization, it may not be possible in the early days.

Human milk will aid in the recovery of babies who are born with health problems. **Chapter 24** discusses preterm and ill babies. Some parents who intend to nurse abandon their plan when they are separated from their infant or when nursing is delayed for another reason. Caregivers involved with these parents and babies can reassure them that a temporary delay does not preclude nursing. The parents will need a great deal of encouragement, support, and information on how to establish and maintain milk production until they can nurse.

Expressing Milk to Maintain Production

When a delay occurs in nursing, milk expression needs to begin as soon as possible and continue regularly to establish and maintain milk production. Even if the baby's prognosis is poor, parents can be comforted knowing that they are providing milk for their baby. If the baby is not yet able to receive the milk,

milk expression provides parents with the opportunity to be involved in a nurturing role. Suggest milk expression at least 8 to 10 times every 24 hours until lactation is well established. Drinking fluids before bedtime increases the likelihood of waking during the night to urinate and creates an opportunity to express milk when prolactin levels are highest.

Sleep and rest will be at a premium during this time. Parents who cannot room-in or stay nearby if the baby remains hospitalized will need to travel to and from the hospital to visit the baby. A routine of expressing milk and trying to recover physically from childbirth can add to worry and exhaustion. Other children at home may need attention. Depending on the length of the baby's hospitalization, parents may need to return to work or school before the baby is discharged.

Establishing letdown may be difficult for parents who are worried about a sick baby and must rely on a breast pump to establish and maintain milk production. Having a picture of the baby handy and playing a recording of the baby's sounds while expressing can promote letdown and output. Milk expression may also be more successful at the hospital near the baby.

In the absence of nursing, high-quality hospital-grade electric double pumps usually provide the best yield. In some cases, milk production decreases over time, whereas sometimes it exceeds the baby's needs. Milk production may correspond to the baby's condition, with worry causing volume to decrease when the baby's condition worsens. You can reassure parents that stimulating the production of **prolactin receptor cells** with frequent pumping will help milk production rebound after the baby begins nursing. **Chapter 22** discusses various types of milk expression.

An electric pump is convenient for maintaining milk production on a long-term basis. A hand pump is useful when an electric pump is inaccessible. Many parents express milk manually or with a hand pump and do not use an electric pump. Knowing how to hand express ensures that parents are not reliant on the availability of a pump. Combining hand expression several times a day before pumping can increase milk production significantly. Chapter 22 presents guidelines on expressing, storing, and transporting milk for a hospitalized baby.

Transition to Nursing

Parents may need help when transitioning from milk expression to nursing. Ideally, the first feeding takes place in the hospital as the baby's condition improves.

- Express milk onto a breast pad and place it near the baby.
- Place a picture of the parent in the baby's view.
- Provide frequent skin-to-skin contact.
- Shape and hold the breast for the baby with the Dancer hand position.
- Express milk into the baby's mouth.
- Consider use of a nipple shield, especially for babies who have been bottle feeding.
- Use a tube-feeding device for feedings.

Figure 23-6 Conditioning the baby to nurse.

The outcome for transitioning a preterm infant to direct nursing as they mature can be reassuring. NICU staff can provide a privacy screen for nursing the baby and can assist with feedings. For some babies, the first direct nursing may not occur until after the baby is home.

The baby's first feeding can be stressful because of insecurity about how to nurse and doubt about the adequacy of milk production. The baby may be confused about how to suck and may have a poor sucking reflex. Some babies may initially appear to be uninterested in nursing. Milk production may need to increase and adjust to the difference between the pump and the baby's sucking pattern. These are all issues parents can work through with varying degrees of success, depending on the baby's condition. Parents will benefit from your support and guidance until the transition is complete.

It may take several days or even months to transition to exclusive nursing. When a baby is unable to nurse every 2 or 3 hours, milk expression and supplementation will need to continue to maintain production. A baby who is nursing frequently and not transferring milk adequately may need to be supplemented with expressed milk or infant formula until milk transfer improves. Encourage parents to concentrate on enjoying their baby and to manage one day at a time. **Figure 23-6** provides guidelines on helping the baby make the transition to nursing.

Parents Who Wean

Because of the health importance of human milk, caregivers strongly urge parents to nurse their ill or preterm babies. Some of these parents may not have planned to nurse and prefer to express their milk. Others may nurse only while it is medically necessary and switch to formula when the baby is out of danger. Even short-term human milk feedings are beneficial. Remember that your role is to support parents in their choices, including guiding them through weaning when it is their wish.

Resuming or Inducing Lactation

Relactation is defined as reestablishing milk production in a person who has either greatly reduced milk production or who has stopped nursing. A parent who had a previous pregnancy is considered to be relactating, even if they never gave birth or nursed. A perception that milk production is inadequate and lack of education are associated with a lack of awareness that relactation is an option (Cevik & Yasar, 2023). A parent who has never been pregnant and is attempting to produce milk is considered to be inducing lactation. With **induced lactation** the parent has not experienced the mammary growth associated with pregnancy.

Realistic Expectations

Parents' expectations will largely determine their feeling of success with resuming or inducing lactation. They may not be able to nourish their baby entirely on their milk. Encourage them to regard nursing as a means of nurturing their baby and not just as a feeding method. Help them measure success in terms of bonding with their baby rather than the amount of milk they produce or the length of time they nurse. Parents who begin nursing with a goal of exclusivity may feel unsuccessful and disappointed if they must supplement. If the goal is an emotionally gratifying experience and an opportunity for a warm and loving bond with their baby, they will find greater satisfaction in their feeding plan.

Candid, sensitive discussion with parents will help assess their motivation and perseverance. You can help them explore how they define success and how they will react if their milk production does not fully meet their baby's needs. Parents whose decision is at another person's urging or is based solely on cognitive knowledge may lack the motivation to persevere. Parents who are highly motivated and enthusiastic are likely to be more successful. Factors affecting success include education, partner involvement and support, and avoiding artificial nipples.

Sources of Support

Encourage parents to determine their sources of support and gauge how others in their household feel about the process. Parents who experience opposition to their plans will need to consider how to proceed despite the lack of support. You can help them identify people in their life who support their efforts, such as a peer counselor, nutritionist, or a relative or friend. Parents who do not produce enough milk for the baby's total nourishment will need extra support and encouragement. These parents benefit from problem-solving, coaching, and support from groups and online resources, such as nursing after breast surgery (e.g., https://www.bfar.org) and adoptive breastfeeding groups. Breastfeeding support websites and social networks provide helpful suggestions and support.

Simplifying their life and other demands can optimize parents' quest to relactate. Encourage them to rest as much as possible; to eat nutritiously; and to accept offers from family and friends to perform errands, care for other children, and prepare meals. A young teen or retired neighbor may be willing to help for part of the day. The religious community may have volunteers to help new parents as well. A postpartum doula or maid service can help with household chores, if affordable and available.

Enticing the Baby to Nurse

Recreating the birth experience helps some parents encourage their babies to nurse. **Rebirthing**, or **remedial co-bathing**, simulates the birth experience by having both parent and infant spend gentle, calming time together in warm bathwater. After some time, the parent can recline and place the baby on their abdomen. The baby may then crawl unassisted to root and latch. This technique is similar to the self-attachment process used in laid-back feeding. **Chapter 15** and **Chapter 16** provide suggestions on encouraging the baby to nurse and increasing milk production.

Frequent and continuous skin-to-skin contact in a relaxed, unpressured atmosphere may entice the baby to latch. A baby who is drowsy or in a light sleep state may be encouraged to latch with skin-to-skin contact and some expressed milk or formula on the end of the nipple. If the baby is unable to suck, pumping with a double electric breast pump can match the frequency to the baby's feeding pattern. The baby may become more interested in sucking when milk is available, so breast massage and compression can also help.

Promoting Milk Production

Milk production for resuming or initiating lactation is dependent on the amount of stimulation the breast receives, which in turn depends on the baby's willingness to suck. The baby's frequent sucking is by far the most efficient way to increase milk production, so the amount of milk produced will increase more rapidly after the baby begins sucking. The baby's age is a factor, with babies younger than 3 months more likely to suck.

Regular milk removal is necessary for continued milk production. If the baby will latch and suck, supplementing at the breast provides simultaneous stimulation and nourishment for the baby. Hand expression before nursing, intermittent massage, and alternating sides several times during a feeding will help increase milk production. Cosleeping so that the baby can suck sleepily for comfort throughout the night may enhance milk production as well. Back rubs and breast massage several times daily can also help. These approaches will help increase blood circulation to and within the breast. Expressing milk between feedings provides further stimulation to increase milk production.

Parents can also discontinue possible milk-reducing substances, such as hormonal contraceptives, nicotine, antihistamines, or herbs like peppermint and sage (Mehta et al., 2018). Make sure they know that alcohol is not a galactagogue and can inhibit milk yield. Galactagogues are discussed in **Chapter 19**.

Decision to Relactate

Understanding why parents discontinue or do not initiate nursing, and their reasons for wanting to relactate, will help you assist them in achieving their goals. Possible reasons include the following:

- Baby's allergic reaction to formula
- Separation because of hospitalization
- Regret for weaning because of misinformation
- Being in an abusive relationship or coerced into formula feeding or weaning
- Milk production downregulated or never established
- Baby rejected or sucked was unable to establish nursing
- Healthcare provider recommendation, family pressure, or guilt
- Using nursing as a factor in a divorce or custody dispute

Understanding parents' motivations without judgment will enable you to determine the best counseling approach. Some parents may not know that resuming lactation is possible. Because of the emotional and physical demands involved, the topic needs to be approached sensitively and tactfully. If the baby is in the NICU or readmitted to the hospital for illness, you can make parents aware of this option and give them more information if they seem interested.

Before devising a feeding plan, you will want to explore the parent's lactation history and reasons for nursing or not nursing other children. Weaning may have resulted from a perception of inadequate milk production, especially if older children were formula fed. Review and confirm that parents understand the basics of milk production and biologically normal infant behaviors. Discuss skin-to-skin contact, feeding frequency, clustered feedings, growth spurts, and sleep patterns.

Success in Relactating

Estrogen concentrations fall rapidly immediately after birth, and prolactin levels drop to normal by about 3 weeks in the absence of nursing. The degree of postpartum breast **involution** is a factor in successful relactation. The time that elapsed since weaning or since the baby's birth is also a factor, with the least time being best. Effective milk removal within the first few weeks postpartum continues the proliferation of prolactin receptors that began during pregnancy and early lactation. The process of involution seems to vary, and there may be a narrow window of opportunity for prolactin receptor multiplication. Therefore, if nursing did not begin at birth, too few receptor cells may have been triggered before involution. On the other hand, if nursing began and was interrupted, there may be enough functional prolactin receptors. Factors influencing relactation success include the following:

- Amount of time since milk was removed
- Feeding method since weaning
- Initial feeding pattern (e.g., time of initiation, frequency, and length of feedings)
- Whether weaning was sudden or gradual

Caregiver sensitivity and empathy, as well as ongoing, positive support from family members make a difference in relactation success. In one study, complete relactation was reported in 85% of parents under 25 years old and those with infants under 6 weeks of age. Bottle feeding and longer formula duration lowered the ability to relactate (Mehta et al., 2018). A parent whose 14-week-old infant was admitted for severe dehydration successfully relactated by day 10. Relactation success for parents of infants hospitalized for more than 10 days with acute respiratory infections or diarrhea ranged from 15 to 40 days (Amat Camacho et al., 2023). Relactating to feed abandoned and orphaned infants or when a parent is too sick to nurse is an age-old tradition in many cultures. Two nonpregnant, nonnursing caregivers who previously had nursed were successful in reestablishing full milk production for refugee infants (Sujon et al., 2024).

Inducing Lactation

Healthcare professionals, adoption case workers, and social service providers need to be knowledgeable about and supportive of nursing nonbiologic babies. Many adoptive parents are not aware that nursing is possible. A parent who wishes to induce lactation requires unique and personalized care. Inducing lactation in the absence of a pregnancy is time-consuming and challenging. Without the estrogen concentrations of pregnancy that prepare the breasts for lactation, prolactin may not sufficiently signal milk secretion. If the inability to conceive has hormonal causes, those same issues can affect inducing lactation.

The age of the child, use of bottles, breast stimulation, and support are important factors in the induction of lactation (Cazorla-Ortiz et al., 2020). Parents can use the same measures as biologic parents for nipple preparation, including avoiding soap and other drying agents and checking for nipple inversion. You can assist parents in locating online resources such as websites, blogs, social networks, and books about nursing nonbiologic babies. Parents may also benefit from attending a support group for nursing or adoptive parents while they wait for the baby's placement.

Often, parents who are adopting receive only a few days' notice before they receive their baby, permitting little time for preparation. Parents who know when the baby's birth is expected can begin pumping to stimulate milk production in the months before placement, pumping several times a day for 10-minute sessions. By the time placement occurs, they should be pumping every 2 to 3 hours throughout the day. A hospital-grade double electric breast pump typically provides the most effective stimulation. It may be some time before pumping produces results, and parents can be encouraged by even the smallest amount of milk they produce. The time it takes for milk to appear and the amount of milk produced will vary.

Various medications and hormones are used to initiate lactation. Some parents use hormonal supplements to mimic the hormones of pregnancy. They begin with combination oral contraceptives, followed by medications such as domperidone to raise prolactin levels. External hormone therapy, use of domperidone as a galactagogue, and pumping can enhance induction of lactation for nonbinary and transgender parents (Gargiulo-Welch et al., 2023; Weimer, 2023).

Feeding the Baby

When resuming or inducing lactation, the baby's health and well-being must always take priority. Infant malnutrition is a main component of relactation-supportive interventions (Amat Camacho et al., 2023). The milk of a relactating parent appears to be a good source of total and bioactive proteins. In one study, the milk had similar or higher levels of total protein, secretory immunoglobulin A, lactoferrin, and lysozyme compared with the mature milk of birth parents (Perrin et al., 2015).

A diary of nursing sessions will help parents monitor their baby's intake and any need for supplemental feedings. They should record nursing frequency and duration as well as the baby's disposition. Encourage frequent visits to the baby's caregiver for weight checks and the monitoring of other signs of growth. Sample pre- and post-feeding weights on an accurate digital scale and a daily weight check at the same time every day will help determine how much supplement the baby may need.

Parents will need to supplement with donor milk or infant formula until they are confident that their milk production reaches a level to serve as the baby's sole form of nourishment. Using a **nursing supplementer** during feedings will provide sucking stimulation to increase milk production. As milk production increases, the amount of supplement the baby receives can be reduced accordingly. Parents should work closely with the baby's caregiver to decrease the supplement in relation to milk production and to monitor the baby's weight closely as the supplement decreases.

Caution parents to proceed slowly with any decrease in supplement, ensuring that the decrease corresponds with the amount of milk the baby receives from nursing. Make sure they understand that they must decrease the supplement rather than dilute it. It is best to limit the decrease to no more than 25 mL per feeding. The baby's growth and output should be monitored for 4 to 7 days before decreasing the supplement further.

Milk production will typically increase slowly and may not be copious enough to sustain the baby's growth. Anecdotally, many nonbiologic parents produce one-third to one-half of their infants' needs. Parents most likely will need to supplement their baby with donor milk or infant formula. Adoptive parents are increasingly turning to donor milk to avoid the risks of infant formula. **Chapter 22** discusses the use of donor milk. **Table 23-2** provides suggestions for counseling parents who are inducing or resuming lactation.

Nursing During Emergencies

Natural disasters and war focus global attention on feeding babies as safely as possible when emergencies

Table 23-2 **Counseling Parents Who Are Relactating or Inducing Lactation**

Concern	Suggestions
Inadequate letdown	Use relaxation techniques.
Establishing milk production	Begin nursing as early as possible and nurse frequently. Use regular supplements and decrease them as milk production increases. Use breast massage. Get sufficient rest and eat a nutritious diet. Keep a diary of nursing and formula feedings.
Baby is reluctant to nurse	Use soothing techniques and increase skin-to-skin contact. Apply expressed milk or a sweet substance to the nipple (not honey). Slowly drop expressed milk into the side of the baby's mouth before attempting a feeding. Use a nursing supplementer during feedings.
Preparation for nursing	Massage the parent's back and breasts. Stimulate the nipples manually. Stimulate milk production with a breast pump. Avoid soap and other drying agents on the breasts.
Low milk production	Supplement with formula. View nursing as a means of nurturing the baby's emotional health. Monitor the baby's weight while replacing formula with nursing.
Baby has a nipple preference	Use a nursing supplementer, cup, spoon, or dropper.
Frustration with partial nursing	Simplify bottle preparation techniques or use a nursing supplementer. Learn to appreciate nursing as a nurturing relationship with the baby.

strike. Tsunamis, hurricanes, cyclones, earthquakes, and global conflict have highlighted the plight of society's most vulnerable population—infants and young children. The Operational Guidance on Infant and Young Child Feeding in Emergencies (IYCF-E) outlines strategies and recommendations for ensuring the nutritional needs of infants and young children are met during emergency situations (Bilgin & Karabayir, 2024).

Guidance for infant feeding in emergencies (IFE) is particularly important when the usual food supplies and healthcare services are disrupted, making infants and young children at higher risk of malnutrition and illness. The guidance emphasizes the importance of providing support to parents attempting relactation. Support includes psychological encouragement, practical advice on stimulating milk production (e.g., frequent nursing or expressing milk), and ensuring adequate nutrition and hydration.

The disruption of healthcare services and the destruction of infrastructure leave many parents without access to essential prenatal and postnatal care. This can severely affect their ability to nurse effectively. The stress and trauma associated with displacement, the necessity of constant movement, malnutrition, and unsanitary living conditions impede nursing efforts. Parents lacking access to their customary postpartum practices and facing difficulties with nursing in a foreign country are more inclined to stop nursing (Tomori, 2023).

Nursing plays a vital role in emergency response worldwide (**Figure 23-7**). The Emergency Nutrition Network (2021), an interagency international agency, provides training and guidance for relief workers. It offers strong guidance to avoid practices that could disrupt lactation, such as distribution of formula and feeding supplies. Many organizations and governments have emergency feeding guidelines to help people continue nursing or relactate. Infant feeding recommendations in emergencies are presented in **Table 23-3**.

Parents, lactation advocates, health professionals, governments, aid agencies, donors, and the media need to learn how to actively support lactation before and during an emergency. You can work with your local community's emergency responders and healthcare facilities to raise awareness that in a disaster, formula donations do more harm than good. They result in an immediate decrease in the rates of nursing and higher rates of diarrhea and death among young children (Hwang et al., 2021).

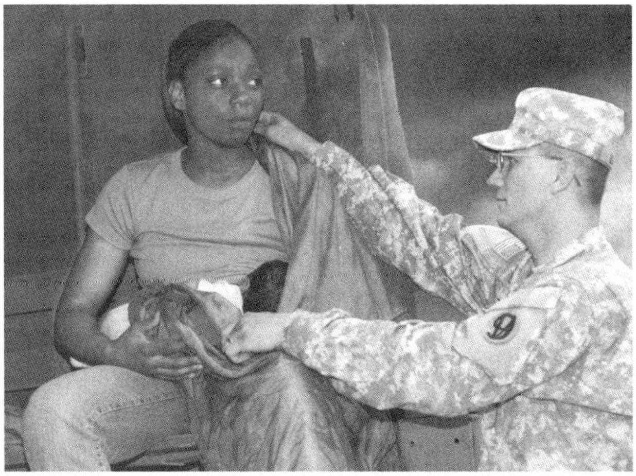

Figure 23-7 Lactation support during a disaster.

Disaster relief camps should consider sociocultural elements, including informal and formal support networks, cultural norms, and beliefs related to spirituality (Hirani et al., 2023). Vulnerable groups need special attention, especially infants, pregnant individuals, and lactating parents. Displaced persons face critical health and nutrition challenges. In addition to nursing support, they need complementary foods that are easy to digest and nutritionally balanced (Masresha, 2023; Saggu et al., 2023). Ensuring adequate medications, improving water supply, and constructing additional sanitation facilities will address health risks and improve living conditions for affected families.

Protecting and promoting nursing saves lives, even more so during emergencies. When greater numbers of babies exclusively nurse, the community is more resilient. This frees up responders to address the needs of infants who are formula fed. In emergency settings, providing critical nutrients and immunity to newborns through nursing is a pronounced lifesaving intervention. Targeted support will ensure that displaced parents have the necessary resources, support, and safe environments to nurse. This safeguards the health and well-being of the youngest and most vulnerable victims of the crisis.

Baby Resists Nursing

Some babies seem to resist nursing as early as 3 or 4 months and most commonly around 7 months of age. The baby may appear happy to nurse and mouth the nipple and then seems disinterested or cries. This phenomenon, is referred to as a *nursing strike* or *refusal*, is marked by resistance to direct nursing. It could happen suddenly, or the baby may gradually decrease the number of feedings. This behavior is common and appears to be a normal part of infant development. It usually lasts only a few days to a week, though some periods of nursing abstinence may continue for several weeks.

Parents might become uncomfortably full or feel emotionally drained from trying to satisfy the baby. They may also feel personally rejected by the baby and grieve the loss of their previously harmonious nursing relationship. Reassure parents that this phase will pass and that the baby will likely return to a regular nursing pattern within several days. Encourage them to relax and be patient as they learn to manage the change in feeding pattern. Expressing milk regularly and cradling the baby frequently without pressure to nurse will help maintain milk production.

This temporary phase of apparent rejection of nursing is not a sign of a desire to wean. A baby who temporarily resists nursing is unhappy, hungry, and unable to settle to nurse. Few infants self-wean before 1 year of age. Toddlers generally are not fussy when they wean. Rather, they are simply ready to move on to their next stage of development.

Developmental Causes

Many times, a lack of interest in nursing occurs during a particular developmental stage and subsides as the baby matures. You can help parents understand their growing baby's changing needs. The baby may simply be more efficient at nursing and obtains more milk in a shorter time. They may be distracted by new objects and people. They can be moved away from the distraction, or the feeding can end and resume when the baby seems more interested. Alternately, a distracted baby can be positioned to face the activity while nursing and allowed to play and nurse intermittently.

A baby who needs the parent's undivided attention while nursing may nurse better late at night when the house is quiet and the baby is too sleepy to be distracted. Extra evening or late-night feedings may make up for missed daytime feedings. Retiring to a quiet, darkened room for these brief periods of nursing can help. Distractions can also be avoided by not talking, reading, using a cell phone or other electronic device, or watching television during feedings. Some babies become uninterested in nursing when their parents manipulate feedings to encourage them to sleep through the night or fit into a schedule. They may reject nursing when their parent fails to respond to hunger cues.

Table 23-3 Guide for Action on Infant and Young Child Feeding in Emergencies

Entity	Emergency Preparedness	On the Ground	Support from Afar
Government/ national policymakers	■ Develop/strengthen national infant and young child feeding policy and emergency preparedness plans/ policies to include IFE. ■ Enact strong national *Code* legislation. ■ Translate key resources. ■ Orient and train key staff on IFE. ■ Coordinate/link to networks of expertise. Make plans to prevent and handle donations of formula, bottles, and teats in emergencies. ■ Give the media clear guidelines on IFE. ■ Include lactation promotion, protection, and support in emergencies for the general public.	■ Ensure that basic support for lactation is integrated across all sectors of emergency response. ■ Prevent/handle donations of BMS, bottles, and teats. ■ Monitor and report *Code* violations.	■ Watch out for appeals for donations of formula, bottles, and teats, and act to stop them.
National lactation advocates/ counselors/ trainers	■ Undertake orientation and further training on infant feeding in emergencies. ■ Identify and network with agencies, local emergency committees, and communities involved in emergency response. ■ Organize a seminar for emergency workers on helping parents and babies in emergencies. ■ Create a network of experienced staff available for training and/or deployment in emergencies. ■ Organize, with government and NGO allies, a press conference or media event on IFE. ■ Update your website with key links to resources.	■ Get involved in early protection and support of lactation, such as training community counselors and emergency relief staff, individual counseling, and person-to-person and phone support. ■ Adapt materials and key messages to the context of the emergency.	■ Identify agencies that support lactation in emergencies and offer them your help. ■ Respond to negative stories and/or appeals for donations in the media.
Aid agencies/ NGOs and United Nations staff	■ Integrate operational guidance on IFE into agency guidance and policies. ■ Orient all emergency response staff on IFE. ■ Identify networks of expertise (e.g., breastfeeding counseling) in countries/regions of operation. ■ Enroll health/nutrition staff in IFE training and communicate a clear plan to all staff on preventing/ handling donations of BMS, bottles, and teats. ■ Lobby the government and donors to include lactation support in emergency action plans.	■ Integrate IFE into minimum response across sectors, including nutrition, health, shelter, and protection. ■ Implement skilled programs to protect, support, and promote lactation. ■ Act to prevent/handle donations of formula, bottles, and teats.	■ Support "on-the-ground" staff by not soliciting or accepting donations of formula. ■ Support fundraising and send money instead of formula.

Entity	Emergency Preparedness	On the Ground	Support from Afar
Health professionals	■ Increase your lactation support skills and follow a breastfeeding counseling training course or, at minimum, an IFE training course for health/nutrition workers in emergencies. ■ Implement the Baby-Friendly Initiative in hospitals and community health services. ■ Advocate for updated training on breastfeeding counseling and HIV and infant feeding counseling at national/local level. ■ Gather information on available support for lactation at national/local level (lactation consultants, peer counselors, support groups). ■ Organize a training/seminar for colleagues on IFE.	■ Ensure that parents and their children are kept together. ■ Implement the 10 Steps to Successful Breastfeeding in appropriate reproductive, maternal-newborn, and child health programs in emergencies. ■ Ensure that skilled lactation and infant feeding support is available antenatally, at delivery, and postnatally for 2 years. ■ Ensure that skilled childbirth attendance is available for pregnant individuals. ■ Ensure that nursing is fully supported for HIV-infected parents unless AFASS conditions for replacement feeding are in place.	■ Be vigilant for local appeals for donations of infant formula, other formula, and bottles/teats to emergencies, and act to stop them.
Parents/ caregivers	■ Exclusively nurse your baby until they are 6 months of age. ■ Continue to nurse your baby to 2 years or beyond. ■ Encourage your local support group(s) to discuss emergency preparedness such as staffing a safe place for parents and providing individual support for nursing if large numbers of people are made homeless. ■ Make contact with local emergency authorities and community groups and tell them about IFE.	■ Offer support to those who are having difficulties or to parents of newborns in an emergency. ■ Consider wet nursing if needs are identified (e.g., orphans, very ill parents). ■ Help organize safe places for individual nursing support.	■ Identify agencies that support nursing in emergencies and fundraise for them.

AFASS = acceptable, feasible, affordable, sustainable, and safe; IFE = infant and young child feeding in emergencies; NGO = nongovernmental organization.
Data from Infant and Young Child Feeding in Emergencies: Operational Guidance for Emergency Relief Staff and Programme Managers. Version 3.0 October 2017. New York: UNICEF; 2017 and Joint Statement: Infant And Young Child Feeding In Emergencies. The Ministry of Health and Child Care, World Health Organization (WHO), UNICEF and World Food Programme (WFP). April 2, 2019.

A baby may reject nursing because their sucking needs are satisfied in another way, such as sucking on a thumb or other object. Parents can attempt a feeding when they observe this behavior. Sometimes receiving solid foods or supplemental bottles causes the baby to become less interested in nursing. If the baby has been receiving supplemental foods, the quantity and frequency can be reviewed with the baby's caregiver to avoid overfeeding.

Discomfort or Pain as a Cause

An ear infection or a head cold with a stuffy nose will create difficulty in nursing. Nursing in an upright position or with the side-sitting hold takes pressure off the baby's ears and facilitates nasal drainage. Breast massage and milk expression before nursing will promote letdown. Performing intermittent breast compression during the feeding will help the baby obtain milk more easily. Encourage parents to consult the baby's caregiver about medications to decrease the baby's mucus production or mechanical methods for removing mucus before nursing.

Babies sometimes reject nursing because they are in pain. Thrush, for example, is painful in adults, and it is fair to expect that it causes discomfort in babies as well. A baby may have an ear infection or other illness, even in the absence of a fever. Teething pain can make sucking uncomfortable and cause the baby to nurse sporadically, fuss, and pull away. Comfort measures to ease gum pain, such as rubbing the gums with a cool washcloth or allowing the baby to bite on a cooled teether, usually renew interest in nursing. Teething is discussed in **Chapter 18**.

If pain causes the baby to bite when nursing, the parent may unintentionally rebuff the baby with an overwhelming reaction and cause the baby to feel rejected. This could result in the baby associating nursing with the parent becoming upset because of the biting and not wanting to risk trying it again. Skin-to-skin contact between the parent and baby helps to reestablish trust. The parent can undress and take the baby to bed or into the bath, hold the baby close, and gently latch for a feeding if the baby seems receptive. Use of a baby sling also provides increased intimacy to build the baby's trust. At home, the baby can be worn in the sling without a shirt, with the baby snuggled against the bare chest.

Resuming Nursing

Parents can examine events in their lives to determine whether their overexertion, tension, eating habits, or fatigue led to the baby's decreased feedings. They can focus on adequate rest, nutrition, exercise, and stress reduction. During menstruation, the taste of the milk and the scent of the secretions on the skin may change slightly. Feedings may then seem less familiar and desirable to the baby. The baby's interest in nursing will be renewed after the end of the menstrual cycle. Any medication such as pseudoephedrine or birth control pills that reduced milk production can be discontinued. If there is a possibility of a pregnancy, the taste of the milk may have changed, or milk production may be reduced.

During the time the baby is not nursing, the parent will need to pump as frequently as the baby was nursing to protect milk production and prevent engorgement. They need to use a method for supplementing the baby, such as cup feeding, that does not interfere with resuming nursing. Discontinuing any pacifier use will ensure that sucking is on the parent's nipple and not an artificial nipple. **Table 23-4** provides measures to encourage the baby to nurse.

Baby Prefers One Side

It is common for a baby to display a preference for one side over the other. Although it is often difficult to determine a cause, one factor may be the parent's hand preference. For example, if the parent is right-handed, the baby may prefer nursing on the left side when held in a cross-cradle position. The parent may also tend to nurse on the left side more often while they use the right hand for other tasks, unconsciously promoting a preference. It may simply feel more natural to hold the baby with the dominant hand. By evaluating feeding patterns, positions can be adjusted so that the baby nurses comfortably on both sides.

It is common for one side to produce more milk than the other. Although both sides have similar storage capacities, there can be wide variance in milk production. In most cases, the greater-producing side is sufficient to meet the needs of one baby. Marked asymmetry or a significant difference in production can alert you to possible hypoplasia, surgery, or injury. A feeding assessment provides appropriate information about production and intake.

A baby may dislike the appearance or feel of one side, perhaps because of a mole, hair, or other difference. If the baby seems to dislike the smell of the skin on one side because of deodorant or perfume, the parent can stop using these products and wash the skin with clear water before nursing. In rare cases, a baby may seem to dislike the taste of the milk on one side. Feeding the milk to the baby with a cup can help rule this out. Refusal may result from a plug of thick milk that has broken loose and is traveling through the ducts and out of the nipple. As soon as the plug clears, usually after one pumping session, regular nursing typically resumes. Refusal to nurse may also occur during bouts of mastitis.

Areolar tissue may be firmer on one side than the other and not allow for a comfortable and productive suck. Hand expressing or pumping to soften the tissue may encourage the baby to nurse on that side. The baby's birth experience may have involved trauma to one side of the face, chin, neck, or shoulder, causing pain when they are held in certain positions. Careful attention to positioning may entice the baby to nurse equally on both sides. After the discomfort is relieved, the baby usually returns to the refused side. If a baby continually rejects one side without a logical reason, a consultation with a breast specialist experienced with lactation can rule out possible causes.

Encouraging the Baby to Feed on Both Sides

To encourage the baby to nurse on both sides the parent can begin feedings on the preferred side to promote letdown. They can then switch the baby to the other side and express milk to entice the baby to latch. Alternatively, they could pre-express milk to achieve

Table 23-4 Encouraging a Baby to Nurse

Issue	Advice
Baby	Check for illness or teething pain and contact the baby's caregiver if necessary. Discontinue any use of pacifiers. Take a warm bath with the baby, with dim lighting, such as candles. The tranquility will relax both the parent and baby. Co-bathing works well for newborns who cannot latch, and it is often effective for older babies who resist nursing.
Nursing parents	Cleanse the breasts with clear water before feedings to remove deodorant, lotions, or other substances. Discontinue the use of any new brand of deodorant or lotion. Get plenty of rest, consume adequate protein and fresh vegetables, and drink sufficient fluids. Express milk between feedings to maintain milk production. Determine if the parent is pregnant or taking any new medications.
Managing feedings	Nurse in a quiet, dark room without distractions. Attempt to nurse when the baby is almost asleep, or when they first fall asleep. Express a little milk onto the nipple or the baby's lips to encourage feeding. Feed the baby using an alternative method for a few minutes and then attempt to feed. Feed the baby in the presence of other nursing babies. Hold the baby in an upright position for easier breathing during feedings. If the baby prefers one side, transfer to the other side by gently sliding the baby over. Use breast compression while the baby is nursing to increase milk flow. If the baby's gums are sore, rub them with ice or a finger before the feeding. Increase skin contact with the baby before feedings. Use relaxation techniques and breast massage before feedings. Increase evening and nighttime feedings. Nurse before offering any supplements and reduce the amount of supplements. Supplement liquids with a cup or other method that avoids an artificial nipple. Attempt to feed when the baby begins sucking on a thumb or other object.

letdown and then begin nursing on the less preferred side. When the baby is sleepy, they may be unaware of being on the less preferred side. Using the side-sitting hold sometimes fools babies into thinking they are on the preferred side, especially if they have an earache or other sensitive ear condition. Sometimes simply placing the baby in a new position will do the trick.

Expressing milk from the less preferred side regularly will relieve any discomfort and maintain milk production. Some parents resort to nursing primarily or totally on one side. One side can produce enough milk for the baby. Although that side may be slightly larger for a time, the size difference can be concealed with loose-fitting clothing.

Summary

Temporary nursing challenges can be overwhelming to parents regardless of the duration. Preserving nursing may involve altering the feeding routine or supplementing with expressed milk or formula while increasing milk production. It may mean promoting milk production for resuming or inducing lactation. It may require maintaining lactation with the use of a breast pump for a period of nursing abstinence. Anticipatory guidance and timely education help achieve satisfying outcomes for nursing families. Your support and suggestions will help parents navigate these challenges.

What You Learned—At a Glance

Conversation Starters with Parents

- Has anyone commented on the color of your baby's skin?
- How much time do you and your baby spend separated?
- How soon did your baby nurse after birth?
- How can you protect your milk production if your baby is not nursing well?
- How do you feel about resuming lactation?
- How do you manage your baby's reluctance to nurse?

Occurrence of Jaundice

- Jaundice occurs in up to 40% of full-term infants and nearly all preterm infants.
- Most jaundice is physiologic and clears up spontaneously within a few days with effective nursing.
- Physiologic jaundice occurs when bilirubin production exceeds the liver's ability to process it.
- Bilirubin has a toxic effect on brain and nerve cells and can result in severe neurologic damage, including kernicterus.
- Breastfeeding-associated jaundice occurs from caloric deprivation and decreased stooling to eliminate bilirubin.
- Breastmilk jaundice occurs between 4 and 7 days of life.

Treatment of Jaundice

- Increase the quality and number of feedings (10–14 times a day).
- Keep dyads together skin to skin.
- Use intermittent breast compression to increase milk flow.
- If phototherapy is needed, request treatment at the bedside when possible.
- Request home phototherapy with a bili-bed or bili-blanket when appropriate and available.
- Parents may perceive their jaundiced newborn as a vulnerable child.

Delayed Nursing

- Begin pumping with a hospital-grade pump immediately when nursing initiation is delayed.
- Pump for 15 minutes 8 to 10 times per day, combined with massage and hand expression, until lactation is well established.
- Keep well informed of the baby's condition and treatment plans.

Resuming or Inducing Lactation

- Measure success in terms of bonding rather than the amount of milk.
- Provide frequent and continuous skin-to-skin contact and co-bathing to encourage latch.
- Feed frequently with a supplementer and pump between feedings to promote milk production.
- Do breast massage and back rubs to increase blood circulation to and within the breast.
- Use hormonal supplements to promote milk production.
- Consider medications and other galactagogues.
- Discuss plans to nurse with the adoption agency.
- Supplement the baby in the absence of full milk production.

Resisting Nursing

- Some babies resist nursing, commonly around 7 months and as early as 3 to 4 months.
- A tube-feeding device at the breast encourages the baby to nurse.
- Undivided time, skin-to-skin contact, and a dark and quiet room will promote latch.
- Expressing milk regularly will maintain production and prevent engorgement until nursing resumes.
- Supplementation needs to decrease slowly as the baby resumes nursing.
- Avoiding bottles and pacifiers ensures that sucking needs are met on the parent's nipple.
- It is common for a baby to prefer one side over the other; one side can produce sufficient milk.

References

Academy of Breastfeeding Medicine, et al. ABM clinical protocol #22: guidelines for management of jaundice in the breastfeeding infant equal to or greater than 35 weeks' gestation, revised 2017. *Breastfeed Med.* 2017;12(5):250–257.

Amat Camacho N, et al. Interventions to support the re-establishment of breastfeeding and their application in humanitarian settings: a systematic review. *Matern Child Nutr.* 2023;19(1):e13440.

Bahr TM, et al. The Neonatal Acute Bilirubin Encephalopathy Registry (NABER): background, aims, and protocol. *Neonatology.* 2019;115(3):242–246.

Bentz MG, et al. Beyond "Asian": specific East and Southeast Asian races or ethnicities associated with jaundice readmission. *Hosp Pediatr.* 2018;8(5):269–273.

Bilgin DD, Karabayır N. Infant and young child feeding in emergencies: a narrative review. *Turk Arch Pediatr.* 2024; 59(2):135.

Boies EG, Vaucher YE. ABM clinical protocol #10: breastfeeding the late preterm (34–36 6/7 weeks of gestation) and early term infants (37–38 6/7 weeks of gestation), second revision 2016. *Breastfeed Med.* 2016;11:494–500.

Buhari HA, et al. Diagnosis and treatment of immune heamolytic aneamia. *NIJBAS*. 2023;4(1):11–16.

Cazorla-Ortiz G, et al. Methods and success factors of induced lactation: a scoping review. *J Hum Lact*. 2020;36(4):739–749.

Cevik E, Yasar O. Interruption of breastfeeding, relactation, relactation awareness, and related factors: a cross-sectional study. *Breastfeed Med*. 2023;18(1):48–58.

DeZure C. Updated clinical practice guidelines for management of hyperbilirubinemia in infants born at 35 weeks or more gestation. *Pediatric Annals*. 2023;52(12):e436–e439.

Donneborg ML, et al. Extreme neonatal hyperbilirubinemia and kernicterus spectrum disorder in Denmark during the years 2000–2015. *J Perinatol*. 2020;40(2):194–202.

Duvigneau JC, et al. Role of heme oxygenase as a modulator of heme-mediated pathways. *Antioxidants (Basel)*. 2019;8(10):1–26.

Dzulkifli FA, et al. Methods for determining bilirubin level in neonatal jaundice screening and monitoring: a literature review. *J Eng Educ Res*. 2018;10:1–10.

Emergency Nutrition Network. Operational guidance on infant feedinginemergencies.2021.https://www.ennonline.net/breast feedingcounsellinginemergencies

Espinosa K, Brown SR. Hyperbilirubinemia in newborns: updated guidelines from the AAP. *Am Fam Physician*. 2023; 107(6), 661–664.

Flaherman VJ, et al. ABM clinical protocol #22: guidelines for management of jaundice in the breastfeeding infant equal to or greater than 35 weeks' gestation, revised 2017. *Breastfeed Med*. 2017;12(5):250–257.

Gargiulo-Welch S, et al. The lactation and chestfeeding/breastfeeding information, care and support needs of trans and non-binary parents: an integrative literature review. *NZ Col Midwives J*. 2023;59:47–55.

Gazzin S, et al. Models of bilirubin neurological damage: lessons learned and new challenges. *Pediatr Res*. 2023;93(7): 1838–1845.

Hirani SAA, et al. Sociocultural factors affecting breastfeeding practices of mothers during natural disasters: a critical ethnography in rural Pakistan. *Glob Qual Nurs Res*. 2023;10.2333393 6221148808.

Hirayama K, et al. Sustained lower bilirubin-binding affinity of albumin in extremely preterm infants. *Pediatr Res*. 2023;94(4): 1400–1407.

Hoge MK, et al. Vulnerable child syndrome in the neonatal intensive care unit: a review and a new preventative intervention with feasibility and parental satisfaction data. *Early Hum Dev*. 2021;154:105283.

Huang H, et al. Breast milk jaundice affects breastfeeding: from the perspective of intestinal flora and SCFAs-GPR41/43. *Front Nutr*. 2023;10:1121213.

Hubbard EM, Hay WW Jr. The term newborn: hypoglycemia. *Clin Perinatol*. 2021;48(3):665–679.

Hui LL, et al. Reducing admissions for neonatal jaundice are needed to maximise benefits of breastfeeding promotion. *Acta Paediatr*. 2024;113(2):362–364.

Hwang CH, et al. Barriers and challenges of infant feeding in disasters in middle- and high-income countries. *Int Breastfeed J*. 2021;16(1):62.

Itoh S, et al. Fetal and neonatal bilirubin metabolism. *Front Pediatr*. 2023;10:1002408.

Kaplan M, et al. Grand rounds hyperbilirubinemia following phototherapy in glucose-6-phosphate dehydrogenase-deficient neonates: not out of the woods. *J Pediatr*. 2023;261:113452.

Karnati S, et al. Late preterm infants—changing trends and continuing challenges. *Int J Pediatr*. 2020;7(1):36–44.

Kasirer Y, et al. Kernicterus on the spectrum. *Neoreviews*. 2023; 24(6):e329–e342.

Kearney L, et al. Evidence-based guidelines for intrapartum maternal hydration assessment and management: a scoping review. *Birth*. 2024;51(2):253–263.

Kemper AR., et al. Clinical practice guideline revision: management of hyperbilirubinemia in the newborn infant 35 or more weeks of gestation. *Pediatrics* 2022;150(3):e2022058859.

Lothian JA. Healthy birth practice #4: avoid interventions unless they are medically necessary. *J Perinat Educ*. 2019;28(2): 94–103.

Martinez-Torres V, et al. Anemia and associated risk factors in pediatric patients. *Pediatr Health Med T*. 2023;14:267–280.

Masresha Y. Disaster emergency response among internally displaced peoples in North Gondar, Ethiopia 2021. *Inter J Infec Dis*. 2023;130:S105.

Mehta A, et al. Relactation in lactation failure and low milk supply. *Sudan J Paediatr*. 2018;18(1):39–47.

Mosallam S, et al. Use of serum bilirubin/albumin ratio for early prediction of bilirubin induced neurological dysfunction. *Gaz Egypt Paediatr Assoc*. 2019;67(1):1–10.

Özcan M, et al. Association between early idiopathic neonatal jaundice and urinary tract infections. *Clin Med Insights Pediatr*. 2017;11:1179556517701118.

Parappil H, et al. Oral dextrose gel use in asymptomatic hypoglycemic newborns decreases NICU admissions and parenteral dextrose therapy: a retrospective study. *J Neonatal Perinatal Med*. 2023;16(1):111–117.

Perrin MT, et al. A pilot study on the protein composition of induced nonpuerperal human milk. *J Hum Lact*. 2015;31(1):166–171.

Rich M, et al. Maternal intrapartum fluids and neonatal weight loss in the breastfed infant. *Br J Midwifery*. 2023;31(6):344–351.

Saggu AK, et al. Consideration of phytonutrients, probiotics and prebiotics for enhanced immunity during disaster relief situation—a review. *Clin Nutr Open Sci*. 2023;47:131–146.

Sandhya J, et al. Cord blood bilirubin and albumin as predictors of neonatal hyperbilirubinemia in healthy term babies. *J Cardiovasc Dis Res*. 2023;14(8):1929–1935.

Scott A, Kirkland T. Rethinking breastfeeding management: a patient-centered approach based on new guidelines. *Nurse Pract*. 2023;48(3):11–19.

Shah PS, et al. Breastfeeding or breast milk for procedural pain in neonates. *CDSR*. 2023;8(8):CD004950.

Sujon H, et al. Non-puerperal adoptive breastfeeding as lactational rescue in the Rohingya refugee camp: 2 case studies. *J Hum Lact*. 2024;40(1):51–56.

Sukkar S, et al. Decreasing bilirubin serum tests in healthy newborns during birth hospitalization. *Pediatrics*. 2023;151(6): e2022059474.

Tarimo CS, et al. Prevalence and risk factors for caesarean delivery following labor induction at a tertiary hospital in North Tanzania: a retrospective cohort study (2000–2015). *BMC Pregnancy Childbirth*. 2020;20(1):173.

Thielemans L, et al. High levels of pathological jaundice in the first 24 hours and neonatal hyperbilirubinaemia in an epidemiological cohort study on the Thailand-Myanmar border. *PLoS One*. 2021;16(10):e0258127.

Tola HH, et al. Prevalence of UTI among Iranian infants with prolonged jaundice, and its main causes: a systematic review and meta-analysis study. *J Pediatr Urol*. 2018;14(2):108–115.

Tomori C. Protecting, promoting and supporting breastfeeding in all policies: reframing the narrative. *Front Pub Health.* 2023; 11: 1149384.

Weimer AK. Lactation induction in a transgender woman: macronutrient analysis and patient perspectives. *J Hum Lact.* 2023;39(3):488–494.

Wight N, Academy of Breastfeeding Medicine. ABM clinical protocol #1: guidelines for blood glucose monitoring and treatment of hypoglycemia in term and late-preterm neonates, revised 2021. *Breastfeed Med.* 2021;16(5):353–365.

Wight N, et al. Outcomes of a breast pump combining compression and vacuum technology in exclusively pumping mothers of VLBW infants in the NICU. *Clin Lactat.* 2023;14(4):184–195.

Zakerihamidi M, et al. Comparison of severity and prognosis of jaundice due to Rh incompatibility and G6PD deficiency. *Transf Apher Sci.* 2023;62(4):103714.

CHAPTER 24

High-Risk Infants

Expectant parents anxiously anticipate giving birth, bringing their baby home, and getting to know this new member of their family. Unfortunately, some parents must leave their baby in the special care of medical personnel and return home alone. Hospitalization of a high-risk infant creates trauma, anxiety, stress, and uncertainty for parents. All parents respond to and cope with this disruption in their own way. The transition from hospital to home can be another stressful and challenging time. Familiarizing parents with what is normal and helping them find ways to cope will aid them in planning for and bringing their baby home. Understanding what these families experience will help you tailor your counseling to meet their unique needs.

KEY TERMS

Adipose tissue
Apnea
Appropriate for gestational age (AGA)
Blood glucose
Bradycardia
Enteral
Extremely low birth weight (ELBW)
Gavage feeding
Glucuronic acid
High-risk infant
Human milk fortifier (HMF)
Hyperalimentation
Hypoxia
Intralipids
Intrauterine growth restriction (IUGR)
Kangaroo care
Lactoengineering
Late preterm
Nasogastric (NG)
Necrotizing enterocolitis (NEC)
Neonatal intensive care unit (NICU)
Nosocomial
Orogastric (OG)
Parenteral
Percutaneous endoscopic gastrostomy (PEG) tube
Postterm
Posttraumatic stress disorder (PTSD)
Preterm
Skin-to-skin care
Small for gestational age (SGA)
Tertiary
Total parenteral nutrition (TPN)

Prolonged Hospitalization of the High-Risk Infant

Parents of a vulnerable infant may have little opportunity to interact with their baby in the first few hours following the birth. Depending on the baby's condition, several days or weeks may pass before they can hold or even touch their baby. It may be several weeks before the baby can nurse directly. In the absence of nursing, milk production will need to be initiated and maintained by milk expression. At the same time, parents must deal with the challenges and emotional trauma of having an infant who is hospitalized. Refer to **Chapter 25** for more information on delayed and interrupted nursing.

Families' Reactions

Care of **high-risk infants** in a **neonatal intensive care unit (NICU)** is delivered in the safest and gentlest way possible. Specialized healthcare providers aim to achieve the best outcomes for the infant medically, nutritionally, and developmentally. The NICU environment can be frightening, even when families know before the birth that their baby will require special

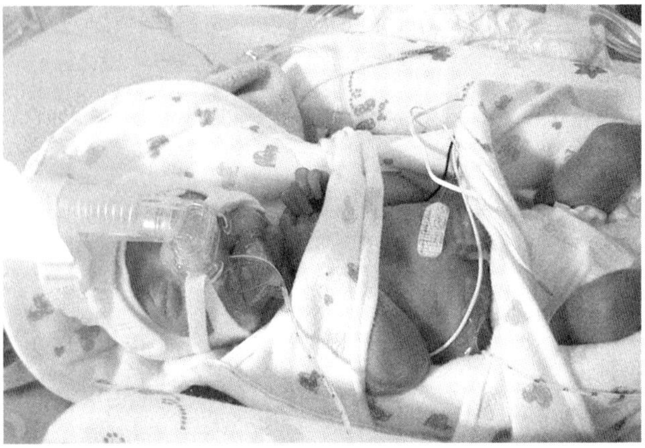

Figure 24-1 The neonatal intensive care unit (NICU) environment can be unsettling to parents.

care. Families' first experience with the NICU will most likely be viewing their infant lying unclothed in an open radiant warmer or an incubator, connected to machinery with tubing (**Figure 24-1**). Some hospitals provide anticipatory care for expectant parents with high-risk pregnancies by providing tours of the NICU ahead of the birth to help ease the fear of the unknown.

Families sometimes find it difficult to focus on their high-risk infant as an individual. Even with a favorable prognosis, they may worry about their baby's survival or potential long-term health concerns. There is a lot of uncertainty for parents of infants in a NICU. They may feel helpless, wanting to do something for their baby and not knowing what or how. They worry about not knowing how soon their baby will be out of danger and disconnected from tubes and monitors. Above all, they wonder when they can take their baby home.

You can support families with hospitalized infants with reassurance, guidance, and information. Parents will benefit from this even if they had anticipated the need for NICU care for their baby or had previous experience with having a child in the NICU. They may be asked to pump and provide their colostrum and later milk for the baby while they are in the NICU. Those who did not plan to nurse or provide their milk will need basic information on lactation. Those who planned to nurse may wonder when their infant will be ready. Your guidance and support will be important no matter what the feeding plan.

The experience in the NICU can resemble arriving in another country where a foreign language is spoken. Knowing common NICU terms (**Table 24-1**) enables you to discuss the baby's care with the parents and healthcare providers. You can help parents formulate questions for their baby's caregivers and ask for explanations and clarification of anything they do not fully understand. New, overwhelmed parents may find it difficult to absorb and process all the information they receive. Consequently, you may find that you need to continually repeat, review, and clarify important points about lactation and providing milk for a vulnerable infant. Provide clear, simple directions along with pertinent handouts at an appropriate literacy level for the family. Instructions and even introductions may need to be repeated frequently because parents are often fatigued and in shock. Be patient and recognize that any inability to remember or process information reflects stress, not lack of interest.

Feelings of Detachment and Grief

Hospitalization of a newborn is highly stressful and overwhelming when a baby is born preterm or in a compromised condition. Parents may feel guilt, loneliness, and anxiety. If the baby is born **preterm**, they may grieve the interruption of the pregnancy and feel that it was incomplete. These parents and their partners are at high risk for depression and **posttraumatic stress disorder (PTSD)** (MacKay et al., 2020).

Parents' trauma is related more to the prolonged uncertainty and alterations in parental role expectations than to the infant's characteristics, such as gestational age, birth weight, Apgar scores, or length of stay in the NICU (Krick et al., 2021). PTSD symptoms can continue for more than a year after parents bring their baby home (Schecter et al., 2020). Thus, providing them with links to long-term counseling services and community support can be highly beneficial.

Parents whose babies are in the NICU may avoid contact with those who have healthy babies. While in the hospital, they may detach themselves from other parents and babies. They may try to avoid involvement with their own baby in an instinctive effort to protect themselves from becoming attached to a child they may lose. Some parents are afraid to touch their child, viewing them as too fragile to handle. These reactions tend to subside when the parents accept their baby's condition.

Parents may not be present during the baby's hospital stay, perhaps because they cannot take time off work or lack child care for older children. Rarely, parents may disconnect to the point that they abandon their baby emotionally, mentally, and even physically. There are many complex barriers, ranging from mental health challenges to addictions to incarceration.

Table 24-1 Neonatal Intensive Care Unit (NICU) Acronyms

A&B	Apnea (pause in regular breathing) and **bradycardia** (slow heart rate)
Bili	Bilirubin (breakdown of red blood cells)
BP	Blood pressure
BPD	Bronchopulmonary dysplasia (lungs and airways [bronchi] are damaged [dysplasia])
cc or mL	Metric measures of liquid; 30 cc (or mL) is 1 oz; 5 cc is ~1 teaspoon
CNS	Central nervous system (brain and spinal cord) or clinical nurse specialist
CPAP	Continuous positive airway pressure (air or oxygen delivered under a small amount of pressure)
CPR	Cardiopulmonary resuscitation (chest compressions with artificial ventilation)
CPT or chest PT	Chest physiotherapy (vibrating or tapping on the chest)
ET	Endotracheal (a tube placed through the mouth or nose to the windpipe)
gms or grams	Metric weight; 450 grams (g) = 1 pound; 1 kilogram (kg) = 1000 g
HMD	Hyaline membrane disease (another name for respiratory distress syndrome)
HI-FI	High-frequency ventilator
ID	Infectious disease or identification
IMV	Intermittent mandatory ventilation (number of breaths per minute by the ventilator)
IV	Intravenous (by vein)
IVH	Intraventricular hemorrhage (bleeding into the ventricles surrounded by the brain)
LP	Lumbar puncture (inserting a needle to get a sample of spinal fluid)
NEC	Necrotizing enterocolitis (inflammation of the intestine leading to bacterial invasion)
NG	Nasogastric (tube going from nose to stomach)
NICU	Neonatal intensive care unit
NPO	Nothing by mouth (*nil per os*)
O2	Oxygen
OG	Orogastric (tube going from mouth to stomach)
OT	Occupational therapist
PDA	Patent ductus arteriosus (opening between the aorta and pulmonary artery)
PICC or PCVL	Peripherally Inserted Central Catheter or Percutaneous Central Venous Line (small tube placed into a vein to give fluids or nutrition)
PT	Physical therapist
PVL	Periventricular leukomalacia (injury to the white matter of the brain)
ROP	Retinopathy of prematurity (abnormal blood vessel growth in the retina)
RDS	Respiratory distress syndrome
SIDS	Sudden infant death syndrome
SIMV	Synchronized intermittent mandatory ventilation (machine breaths timed to baby's)
TPR	Temperature, pulse, and respiration
TTNB	Transient tachypnea of the newborn (mild breathing problem)
TPN or TNA	Total parenteral nutrition (nutrition by vein)
UAC	Umbilical artery catheter
UTI	Urinary tract (kidney or bladder) infection
UVC	Umbilical venous catheter
VS	Vital signs (temperature, pulse, respiration, blood pressure)

Data from 2000-2020 StayWell, 780 Township Line Road, Yardley, PA 19067. Publish Date: September 30, 2017. Retrieved from http://poc.select.kramesstaywell.com/Content/healthsheets-v1/common-terms-and-abbreviations-used-in-the-nicu.

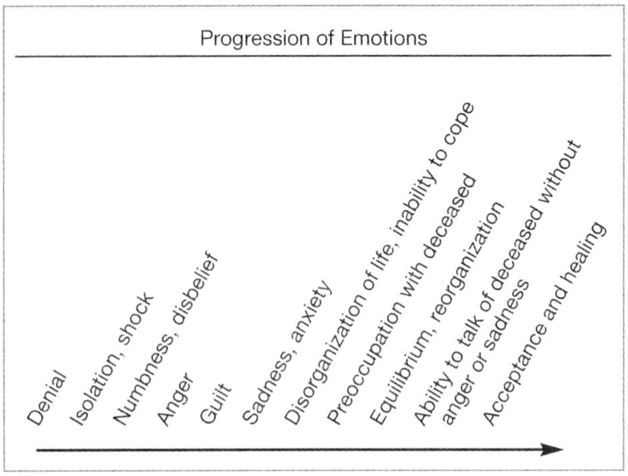

Figure 24-2 Sequence of the grief process.

Be aware of your own distress when working with high-risk families. Pace yourself, especially if you work exclusively in the NICU setting. Mindfulness can be a helpful tool for care providers. Refer to **Chapter 29** for tips to help you avoid stress and burnout as you work within high-acuity settings.

Most parents work through the shock and trauma of an intensive care experience. Regardless of the baby's prognosis, families typically move through stages of grief (**Figure 24-2**) as they mourn the loss of their anticipated healthy baby. After parents have mourned the healthy baby they expected, they can begin to accept the baby they have. Recognize that the stages of grief are not linear and that emotions can swing back and forth. Families may also grieve far longer than is typically described.

It is common for high-risk infants to be transferred from their birth hospital to a facility that provides a higher level of care. The necessity of a transfer underscores the seriousness of the baby's condition. Parents experience real grief when it is necessary to transfer their infant to another facility. They will lose many of the familiar supports and routines they had established in the previous NICU. Furthermore, the new medical and nursing personnel caring for their infant will be complete strangers to them.

Need for Support

A critically ill or preterm infant adds one more stressor to a life that may already be filled with challenges (Govindaswamy et al., 2019). Families may struggle with poverty, job insecurity, isolation, housing insecurity, and systemic racism. Thus, social support and mental health services in the NICU are crucial. Unfortunately, many parents face barriers to frequent visitation and accessing support, including lack of paid work leave, lack of transportation, or lack of help caring for their other children (Hall et al., 2020).

Families of high-risk infants are tired and anxious, which can put a strain on their relationship. Often, a crisis brings out unresolved conflicts in a couple's relationship, with the baby's condition serving as a catalyst for problems rising to the surface (Miller et al., 2021). Thus, disagreements or arguments that you observe in the parents' interactions may be unrelated to the baby's condition. Encourage parents to seek sources of support, both in the hospital and within their community. Most hospitals assign case managers to help families through this type of crisis. Social service workers and chaplains are trained in grief and crisis counseling.

Communicating with other parents who have experienced similar situations can help NICU parents realize that their reactions are common and help them develop healthy coping techniques. Some hospitals have family support groups facilitated by trained staff. Support groups are also available in many communities and through online social networks for parents of high-risk infants. Group discussions and bonding with other parents with similar experiences provide parents the opportunity to share their feelings and concerns. Parents learn that they are not alone and that, despite different medical conditions, families share common and predictable stages in their journey.

Most NICUs have a case manager or nurse navigator to provide help and referrals for the family both during and after the baby's stay. You can also refer parents to resources in their communities of faith, such as a pastor, priest, rabbi, or the hospital chaplaincy. Nonprofit organizations, such as Hand to Hold (2025), provide ongoing education, support, and postdischarge resources for NICU families.

Nursing is more likely to continue when families of vulnerable infants have sources of support (Yang et al., 2019). About a third of parents of infants admitted to a NICU report obstacles to lactation, including difficulty pumping milk and inadequate milk production (Gianni et al., 2018). The duration of lactation after the baby goes home can be influenced by **skin-to-skin care**, prenatal education, milk production during the first week home, knowledge about lactation, and the parent's perception of the adequacy of their milk production to meet their baby's needs (Naja et al., 2022).

Familiarize yourself with available support resources for these parents and make appropriate referrals. Many people do not live near their extended families and need to establish a circle of support. Therefore, inquire about family and friends as support systems. In addition, NICU parents may be low-income, face cultural or language barriers, or have a history of drug use. Consequently, they may have many other social support needs as well.

Because a high-risk infant requires a great deal of attention and care, parents' needs often go unrecognized or unmet. Your sincere interest in parents can encourage them to discuss their labor and delivery experience and express any current concerns and worries about the future. A parent who perceives that their needs are validated is more likely to share their anxieties about their birth, their baby, and their coping abilities. Asking the parent about their rest, their appetite, and their discomfort or postpartum recovery shows concern about them as a person.

Healthcare providers often expect partners to assist the birth parent, and the partner's feelings may receive less consideration. This can influence insecurity in the partner's parenting role (Feenstra et al., 2018). These feelings are exacerbated if the birth parent is severely ill and the partner is the one who first cares for the baby in the NICU. Families will receive information and advice from many sources. Birth parents and their partners will benefit from being listened to in an accepting, objective, and interested manner. Sincere and honest concern is natural. Let families know that you care and that you are there to support them.

Neonatal Intensive Care Unit

The NICU is an overwhelming environment for the infant as well as the family. In the womb, the parent's voice and rhythmic body sounds soothed the fetus The surroundings were dark and comforting, with only subtle variance in diffused light. The fetus was continuously bathed in warm amniotic fluid, constantly fed, and rocked by the parent's movements. In contrast, the NICU can be a noisy environment with many variations and types of noise and harsh mechanical sounds occurring at varied times. The noise level in NICUs often reaches 120 decibels and exceeds the American Academy of Pediatrics (AAP) noise level recommendations more than 90% of the time (Mayhew et al., 2022). Voices are often indistinct, and the constant bright lighting lacks a predictable daily rhythm.

Environmental protection from lights (e.g., eye patches, incubator covers) may result in limited exposure to normal visual stimulation. Overstimulation of the infant's auditory system can trigger **apnea** and fluctuations in heart rate, blood pressure, and oxygen saturation. Preterm infants exposed to prolonged excessive noise are at increased risk for hearing loss, abnormal brain and sensory development, and speech and language problems (Beken et al., 2021).

Need for Special Care

Tremendous medical advances have improved the morbidity and mortality rates of high-risk infants, as evidenced by the multiple levels of neonatal care. Level I nurseries provide routine newborn care. Level II units provide monitoring and care beyond routine newborn care. These babies are typically over 33 weeks of age and need feeding support, tube feedings, and intravenous (IV) therapy such as fluids or medications. Birth facilities typically house these levels of newborn care.

Level III units (**tertiary** care) are high-risk facilities equipped to care for the smallest and sickest babies. They care for infants born at **extremely low birth weight (ELBW)** and full-term infants with severe or potentially life-threatening conditions. They may also care for infants requiring surgical interventions or complex care modalities, such as extracorporeal membrane oxygenation (ECMO) or high-frequency oscillator or jet ventilation. ECMO provides longer-term life support (heart–lung bypass) for babies needing recovery from severe conditions. Although advanced prevention and treatments are available, ECMO is still necessary for certain conditions and surgeries. Some facilities have a level IV subspecialty unit, with specialized staff providing care for the highest-acuity infants.

Maternal conditions may also require special care of the newborn. The prevalence of older birthing parents in many industrialized nations has increased steadily since the 1990s. Moreover, more birthing parents used assisted reproductive technologies (ARTs) to help them get pregnant, resulting in higher rates of multiple births. Preexisting health conditions are also exacerbated during many pregnancies. Prenatal risk factors include medical risk, lifestyle, and psychosocial factors, of which half are related to personal characteristics (Stoll et al., 2023).

Medically complex pregnancies must be managed carefully to protect both the parent's and baby's health. Globally, person-centered perinatal care, particularly midwifery care, has been shown to improve outcomes. There is a need for a systematic method to screen and identify complex medical needs within perinatal care and integrate supportive care structures.

A pregnancy may be identified as high-risk when the unborn baby is diagnosed with a medical condition ranging from mild to severe, including nonviability. Early identification optimally brings a maternal-fetal medicine specialist, or perinatologist, into the family's healthcare team. These specialists manage "un-routine" pregnancies and perform diagnostic tests and prenatal treatments and care, including fetal surgeries (Society for Maternal-Fetal Medicine, 2025). Refer to

Chapter 26 for further discussion of maternal health conditions and effects on lactation.

When a high-risk pregnancy is detected, the parent may deliver in a tertiary care facility that has the means to care for both the birthing parent and baby. These level III facilities care for babies transported from outside the immediate geographical area. Often, the parent of a high-risk infant has had a cesarean delivery and will remain at the birth facility for 2 days or longer. NICU case managers can assist families with information on extended-stay resources, such as Ronald McDonald Houses and Family Rooms (inside the hospital) or other resources specific to the community. Information is available at https://www.rmhc.org. These corporate-sponsored facilities offer free accommodation for parents visiting sick children.

Care of a High-Risk Infant

Initially, a high-risk infant in the NICU experiences touch that is either technical or medical in nature. The baby may thus learn to associate touch with unpleasant events. There is debate among healthcare professionals regarding the degree of appropriate stimulation for a high-risk infant (refer to the discussion on skin-to-skin care later in this chapter). You can suggest ways in which families can nurture their infants through gentle, warm, and loving touch, presence, and voice. Being aware of current research in neonatal special care helps you advocate for a lactation-friendly environment that encompasses the best of high-tech developmental care.

Neo-BFHI Practices

Lactation promotion and staff training in the NICU increase exclusive nursing rates, including a multidisciplinary team, support for the NICU family, family-centered care, skin-to-skin care, and the use of donor human milk (Li et al., 2019). Partial nursing, low maternal education, and longer NICU stays increase the risk of weaning during the first year (Ericson et al., 2018). NICUs affiliated with the Baby-Friendly Hospital Initiative (BFHI) have higher rates of nursing and human milk feeding than those that are not designated as Baby-Friendly (Maastrup et al., 2019; Tambani et al., 2019). An expert group developed three guiding principles and expanded the Ten Steps to Successful Breastfeeding (**Figure 24-3**) to apply to practices in the special care setting (Maastrup et al., 2022).

Massage. Infant massage is an ancient therapeutic technique incorporated into the care regimen for NICU infants. Gentle massage therapy for NICU infants enhances weight gain, reduces pain and length of stay, and improves feeding tolerance and neurodevelopment (Pados & McGlothen-Bell, 2019). In addition, the benefits for parents performing therapeutic

Guiding Principles

1. Staff attitudes toward the mother must focus on the individual mother and her situation.
2. The facility must provide family-centered care, supported by the environment.
3. The healthcare system must ensure continuity of care from pregnancy to after the infant's discharge

Step 1.	Have a written breastfeeding policy that is routinely communicated to all healthcare staff.
Step 2.	Educate and train all staff in the specific knowledge and skills necessary to implement this policy.
Step 3.	Inform all hospitalized pregnant women at risk for preterm delivery or birth of a sick infant about the management of lactation and breastfeeding and benefits of breastfeeding.
Step 4.	Encourage early, continuous, and prolonged mother-infant skin-to-skin contact (kangaroo mother care) without unjustified restrictions. Place babies in skin-to-skin contact with their parents immediately following birth for at least an hour. Encourage parents to recognize when their babies are ready to breastfeed and offer help if needed.
Step 5.	Show parents how to initiate and maintain lactation and establish early breastfeeding with infant stability as the only criterion.
Step 6.	Give newborn infants no food or drink other than breast milk, unless medically indicated.
Step 7.	Enable parents and infants to remain together 24 hours a day.
Step 8.	Encourage demand feeding or, when needed, semi-demand feeding as a transitional strategy for preterm and sick infants.
Step 9.	Use alternatives to bottle-feeding at least until breastfeeding is well established and use pacifiers and nipple shields only for justifiable reasons.
Step 10.	Prepare parents for continued breastfeeding and ensure access to support services/groups after hospital discharge.

Figure 24-3 Neonatal intensive care unit (NICU) Ten Steps.

Reproduced from Nyqvist KH, Maastrup R, Hansen MN, Haggkvist AP, Hannula L, Ezeonodo A, Kylberg E, Frandsen AL, Haiek LN. Neo-BFHI: The Baby-Friendly Hospital Initiative for Neonatal Wards. Core document with recommended standards and criteria. Nordic and Quebec Working Group; 2015.

massage on their infants include a reduction in stress, depression, and anxiety (Pados & McGlothen-Bell, 2019).

Nonnutritive Sucking. Pacifier use in the NICU is therapeutic, especially in the birth parent's absence. Nonnutritive sucking (NNS) is an important skill for the NICU infant, especially before beginning oral feeds. NNS can improve the baby's state regulation and is a comfort measure during lengthy separation from the birth parent, **gavage feeding**, and painful procedures (Wu et al., 2020). NNS is also associated with a faster progression to oral feedings, especially in combination with oral stimulation (John, 2019).

Babies who cannot yet receive human milk feedings in nutritional volumes can receive trophic (minimal) feedings in small volumes of expressed or donor milk. Trophic feeds facilitate protective gut flora, improve passage of meconium, and may decrease rates of necrotizing enterocolitis (NEC). They are also associated with a faster progression to full oral feedings, with a reduced time on **parenteral** nutrition and central line access (Kwok et al., 2019).

Many special care units use colostrum for oral care and refer to it as *oral immune therapy* (OIT) in recognition of its value in supporting the baby's immature, developing immune system and decreasing time to oral feedings (Garofalo & Caplan, 2019). Researchers call for large-scale studies of this treatment, noting nonsignificant associations (Panchal et al., 2019).

NNS on a recently drained breast can provide comfort as well as support prefeeding and early nursing behaviors. This allows the baby to associate nursing with the smell of the milk and practice suck coordination without yet needing to be skilled at coordinating the suck–swallow–breathe pattern. The practice of providing oral stimulation interventions as prefeeding skill development presents an opportunity for lactation consultants to collaborate with an occupational therapist (OT) and speech-language pathologist/therapist (SLP). You can advocate for the stable baby to practice NNS through direct nursing.

Nourishment. A high-risk infant may receive nourishment initially through intravenous **total parenteral nutrition (TPN)**. TPN solutions are tailored to meet individual nutritional needs. They typically include carbohydrates, proteins, fats, vitamins, and minerals. This is also known as parenteral **hyperalimentation** (administration of nutrients by intravenous feeding). **Intralipids** may be added for fats and additional calories if IV nutritional support is expected to be required for more than a few days. As the TPN is reduced, the baby progresses to gavage feedings via **nasogastric (NG)** tubing (passed through the nasal passage down to the stomach) or **orogastric (OG)** tubing (passed through the mouth and down the throat). NG tubing and OG tubing can be used for either continuous or intermittent feeding. OG feeding is also used for a baby with structural nasal anomalies or for a baby receiving continuous positive airway pressure (CPAP) (Isayama, 2019).

After achieving the ability to tolerate **enteral** feedings and growing more clinically stable, the infant can progress to oral feedings, including nursing. They can also be fed via an alternative feeding method such as a cup, spoon, bottle, or dropper. An oral feeding protocol based on infant hunger cues has been instituted in some NICUs. Also known as *infant-driven feeding*, this practice promotes a natural and responsive feeding experience that is especially important for preterm infants.

Feeding readiness cues, not just weight and gestational age, guide the feeding protocol. Feeding on cue rather than based on scheduled, volume-based feedings leads to shorter hospital stays and faster full oral feeds (Samane et al., 2022). Some preterm or sick infants do not demonstrate overt, robust, or predictable hunger cues. Pointing out any subtle cues, such as rooting, that indicate the baby's readiness to feed will help parents know what to anticipate.

Currently, there is no national or international consensus for oral feeding guidelines for preterm infants in a NICU. A global analysis of published NICU feeding guidelines concluded there was no systematic utilization of scientific evidence to support the different recommendations (Bakker et al., 2021). One of the regrets that parents report is that the baby's first oral feeding is given by medical staff and not the parents. Parents can ask to be allowed to observe and participate in their baby's feeding and care as soon as possible.

Because imprinting affects babies' feeding abilities, high-risk infants may develop oral aversions. If the oral aversions cannot be resolved easily or if there is a long period of nonprogressing oral feeding skills, a **percutaneous endoscopic gastrostomy (PEG) tube** may be placed through the skin directly into the baby's stomach. Other medical or surgical conditions may also require PEG tube feedings. The parent can provide skin-to-skin care and access to nursing to aid in overcoming aversion.

Bottle Feeding. Bottle feeding is deeply entrenched in the culture of NICU care in most developed nations (Flint et al., 2016). Caregivers often give the first feeding by bottle because it is a somewhat passive, feeder-controlled process and the NICU staff can monitor the infant's response and intake. Rationale for this practice cites concerns about choking, aspiration, or other stresses with oral feedings. The use of bottles for initiating oral feeding occurs for multiple reasons, including the following:

- Management practices
- Perception that bottle use is faster and easier
- Belief that babies must "prove" themselves on a bottle before nursing
- Familiarity and comfort with bottle feeding
- Lack of knowledge about lactation
- Time constraints to help parents with nursing or expressing milk
- Lack of lactation consultants dedicated to the NICU

Cup and Syringe Feeding. Cup and syringe feeding are helpful tools for transitioning preterm infants from a feeding tube to nursing (Penny et al., 2018). Given the challenges that NICU infants face with nursing, it is beneficial to eliminate any unnecessary obstacles such as feeding bottles. A recent randomized, controlled, single-blinded study evaluated the efficacy of cup, syringe, and bottle feeding with preterm infants. Syringe feeding produced higher mean heart rates and oxygenation and a shorter duration from enteral feeding to nursing (Inal et al., 2023). Cup feeding is associated with stability in heart rate and oxygen saturation and higher rates of nursing at discharge (Çamur & Çetinkaya, 2022; Penny et al., 2018). Cup and syringe feeding can also be used when the birth parent is not present. Appropriate training, support, and guidelines should be established to educate staff on the use of cup and syringe feeding as viable alternatives to bottle feeding in the NICU.

Nursing. You can advocate for evidence-based practices that protect nursing, such as the importance of direct nursing as a first oral feed and limiting pacifiers to appropriate use. You can also advocate for eliminating practices that are not evidence based, such as the introduction of bottle feeding before nursing. A recent retrospective analysis of infants in a Canadian NICU noted no increase in hospitalization days based on the method of oral feeding, maternal age, or first-time nursing status (Wener et al., 2021).

Babies all differ in their capabilities and should be assessed on an individual basis. Many preterm babies are ineffective feeders because of low muscle tone, poor coordination, and limited stamina. However, those who are physiologically stable should be held skin to skin with a chance to nurse directly and progress from NNS to nutritive nursing. Preterm infants with daily skin-to-skin care for 1 month postnatally had higher mean body weight, had higher milk intake, and were nursing at discharge (Kucukoglu et al., 2021). An individual feeding plan helps the baby progress predictably from parenteral feeding through each stage until reaching the ability to nurse directly.

Websites, social networks, blogs, parent forums, and other media resources abound for parents of babies in the NICU. The parent's hospital stay provides an opportunity for caregivers to dispel myths and provide anticipatory guidance on initiating nursing. Many large NICUs have lactation consultants who work exclusively with families of babies in their care. An increase in nursing rates for preterm and **late preterm** infants is associated with NICUs having full-time dedicated lactation support (Sankar et al., 2022). Direct nursing increases human milk use at discharge.

The health benefits of human milk are especially vital for vulnerable infants in the NICU. Human milk diets for preterm infants decrease the risk of sepsis, feeding intolerance, chronic pulmonary disease, retinopathy of prematurity, neurocognitive impairment, and readmission between the ages of 18 and 30 months (Sokou et al., 2022). Despite all these benefits, the rate of infants discharged from the NICU exclusively nursing remains low in many parts of the world. For example, rates are 55% in Australia, 45% in Sweden, 23% in Japan, and 22% in the United States (Maastrup et al., 2021). Parents with lower socioeconomic status and single-parent households are at risk for lower nursing rates in a NICU (Carpay et al., 2021; Sankar et al., 2022). An algorithm was created for parents to attempt to nurse their infants three times a day once oral feedings are allowed and even in tandem with gavage feeding. Results are promising, with a statistical difference in the number of infants discharged and receiving human milk through exclusive nursing (Phillips et al., 2024).

Parenting in the NICU

Parents' hands-on care of their infants in the NICU develops empowerment and self-efficacy. Nursing, skin-to-skin care, and family-centered practices are meaningful to these parents. Although progress is being made toward family-centered care, logistics and the need for a paradigm shift for healthcare providers continue to be a challenge (Benzies, 2019). Developing a partnership between staff and families and allowing unrestricted parental presence and involvement in infant caregiving help parents construct their role as parents and help give them a sense of autonomy and confidence.

Family-Centered Care. Family-centered care with increased parental involvement in caring for their infant results in a collaborative atmosphere. Healthcare providers develop greater awareness of the families' psychosocial situations because of increased interactions. Moreover, healthcare providers shift from being the infant's active caretaker to a facilitator who supports the parents in their caregiving. Family-centered care can differ greatly by country and even by NICU. For example, a NICU in Finland utilizes nursing as an intervention to maintain closeness with the infant, not solely as a means of nutrition (Holdren et al., 2019). As the implementation of family-centered care increases, lactation consultants are valuable to NICU staff.

Close mentorship is crucial when enacting changes that guide the NICU toward this type of care (Toivonen et al., 2019). Family-centered care requires training and educational support for the hospital staff and families. This collaboration provides a mutual partnership and shared decision-making that assist the staff in supporting the families (Toivonen et al., 2020). Accommodating parents' rooming-in with their infants promotes parental confidence and self-efficacy and can reduce the length of the hospital stay (Benzies et al., 2020). In facilities with family-centered care, infants are more likely to be nursing at discharge (Maastrup et al., 2019; Tambani et al., 2019).

It is challenging for parents to embrace the parental role when their baby is in the NICU. Initiating as much meaningful interaction as possible can help parents minimize the impact of early separation from their high-risk infant. The overwhelming nature of the experience can cause parents to feel hesitant or fearful about interacting with their baby. Inquiring about and addressing their concerns can help bridge this gap. Encourage their participation, and provide explanations in simple and concrete terms.

Supporting Parents. Key needs for parents of NICU infants are described in **Figure 24-4**. A welcoming environment with supportive policies and practices will provide emotional and practical support to empower parents. Parent education should provide opportunities to practice new skills through guided participation.

Personalized, culturally appropriate care is crucial for families of infants in the NICU. Caregivers need to use inclusive language, provide relevant information, and provide nonjudgmental support for all families. Same-sex parents may be providing milk from the biologic birth parent. Adoptive parents may want to induce lactation to nurse their baby. Parents with language or other cultural barriers may need medical language translation services, including a language line, if no certified translator is available. Cultural practices surrounding the newborn may include waiting for ceremonies to be completed before naming the baby; tying on small silk bracelets, gold jewelry, and other amulets; or outlining the baby's eyes in kohl. These customs should be honored and respected, barring any safety issues. Refer to **Chapter 21** for additional information about providing culturally sensitive care for families.

- Being positively perceived by the nursery staff
- Therapeutic relationship with the NICU staff
- Family-centered care (in particular, self-defined family/support people)
- Accurate information
- Privacy with infant
- Inclusion in the infant's care
- Individualized, guided practice in providing care for their infant
- Physical comfort care (e.g., food, fluid, place to rest)
- Assistance in grieving for expected pregnancy and baby
- Support in parental role attainment

Figure 24-4 Key needs for parents of infants in the neonatal intensive care unit.

Alterations in their parental role and the infant's appearance are stressors for parents. They cite a need to be involved in decision-making and for accurate and honest information focused on sensitive infant care. Enhancing staff–parent communication better meets parental needs for information and reduces stressors (Govindaswamy et al., 2019). Family-centered practices, including intentional rounding by the healthcare team and focused communication, increase family trust and patient safety. These practices also have the potential to shorten NICU stays, which benefits both families and hospitals (Benzies et al., 2020; Toivonen et al., 2020).

Needs of Non-Birth Parents. Partners frequently feel marginalized in the child-bearing experience, perhaps even more so in a special care setting. During pregnancy, labor, and childbirth, attention is focused on the birthing parent. When NICU care is needed, attention turns to the infant. Partners convey feelings of anxiety, depression, and stress within the first 2 weeks of their compromised babies being admitted to the NICU. They also report engaging in harmful alcohol use behavior (Dickinson et al., 2022).

Partners often feel a lack of control in the NICU experience. Engaging partners in the care of their infant can help them regain a sense of control and transition to their new parental role. This can be a more difficult task than with birth parents, who are the most frequent visitors after the initial postpartum period. Optimally, family care needs should be identified and incorporated into the development of a care plan. Efforts to provide family-focused interventions that include partners, such as psychoeducation and self-care, are recommended (Grunberg et al., 2020).

Not surprisingly, the most stressful part of the NICU experience for partners is juggling their time between work and family needs. Non-birth parents often return to work quickly after the infant's birth and remain primarily focused on work. This may be partly to provide financially for the family and partly to use their work expertise to compensate for their feelings of inadequacy or lack of control in the NICU.

Skin-to-skin contact between non-birth parents and their infants facilitates acquiring the parental role and increases feelings of control despite the stresses and demands of the NICU. The benefits of skin-to-skin care while in the NICU appear to continue after discharge, with partners reporting lowered stress responses and fewer spousal relationship problems (Louis & White, 2023). Partners who participate in skin-to-skin care report feelings of inclusivity, as well as a sense of fairness in their importance in the care of their infant.

Adolescent Parents. Supporting adolescent parents of high-risk infants can be a special challenge. At a time when they are still developing their sense of self and autonomy, they may be able to describe their infant's diagnosis and treatment but may underestimate the seriousness of the baby's condition. They may hesitate to ask for clarification of technical language and may become confused when speaking with a healthcare provider. Their parental knowledge is better when healthcare providers make explicit efforts to communicate with them.

It helps to ask young parents of infants in the NICU to demonstrate understanding of milk expression, pumping, nipple shield use, positioning, and latch. Do not assume that they understand what you are saying when they agree verbally. It is also important to affirm their successes and empower their development and self-efficacy. Adolescent NICU parents respond well to a collaborative, team approach with increased parent engagement and confidence (Orr et al., 2023). Refer to **Chapter 21** for further discussion about working with adolescent parents.

Parent-Infant Interaction. Parents are often not aware of what is normal for their baby in the NICU. They will benefit from resources and teaching about what to expect based on their baby's condition and gestational age. Parents express less concern and more realistic expectations when they recognize their baby's behavioral capabilities. Those who participate regularly in their baby's care have lower anxiety levels and higher competency in problem-solving related to their infant's needs (Ochandorena-Acha et al., 2022). Touching and caring for their baby as much as the baby's condition allows will facilitate competency (**Figure 24-5**).

Eye-to-eye contact between the parents and their baby facilitates early attachment. If eye patches are

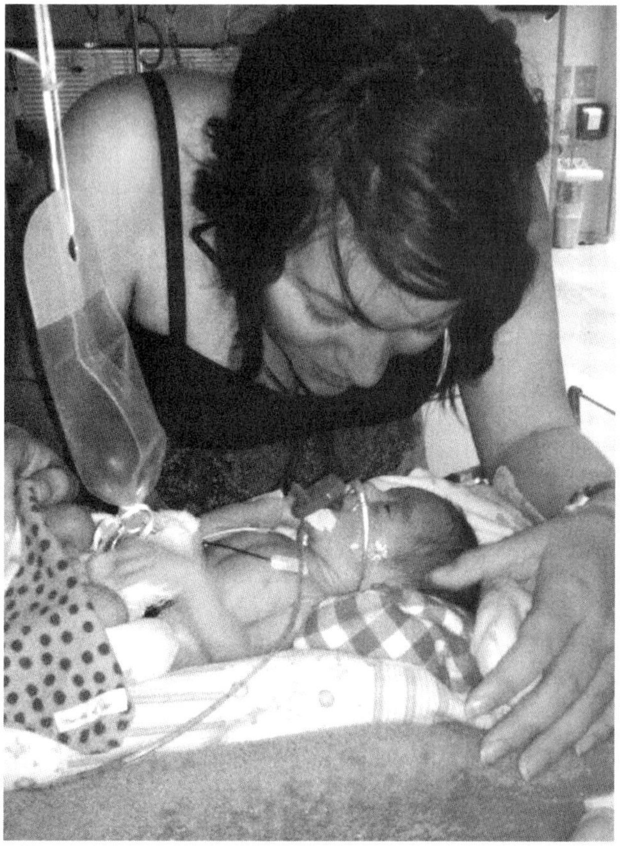

Figure 24-5 Parents visit, touch, and fondle their baby in the NICU.

used, parents can ask for them to be removed when they are with their baby. When the baby is stable enough, they can request time alone with them to interact as a family without the presence of hospital staff. Encourage parents to also take part in caring for their baby with feeding, bathing, and diapering. Many facilitiess actively enable parents to room with their babies in the NICU to facilitate skills acquisition in infant care.

As the baby's discharge nears, parents begin the transition to becoming their infants' primary caregivers. NICU staff can educate and support them to increase their confidence and empowerment. This transition is especially important in the days preceding the baby's discharge. Privacy screens and rooming-in with the baby give parents the chance to solidify the bond with their baby and fully embrace their parental role. Encourage parents to arrange private time whenever the baby's condition permits.

Pressure of Other Demands. Parents who want to spend as much time as possible with their high-risk baby are often pressured by competing demands and a lack of practical support. Logistical constraints such as caring for siblings and transportation to and from the hospital may interfere with their ability to interact with their baby. They should not be made to feel guilty or negligent if they cannot visit their baby as often as you or others consider appropriate.

Time commitments present challenges for the birth parent in achieving adequate rest, expressing milk, and caring for other children or family members. Some parents return to work before the baby's discharge because of financial constraints or lack of employment flexibility. While they may not get needed rest and cannot provide hands-on care during the baby's NICU stay, an early return to work may allow for more time at home after the baby's discharge. Another challenge is that care providers or family members may not be comfortable caring for babies just discharged from the NICU. Group daycare is often not an option for these babies.

Taking the Baby Home

Parents' emotions when taking their fragile baby home can be a mixture of elation, anxiety, caution, and insecurity in their roles as full-time caretakers. Parents are often anxious at the time of discharge and overwhelmed at the thought of caring for their baby full time. Although some parents receive advance notice of the date that their baby will go home, it is not always predictable. Thus, discharge may occur relatively quickly for some parents. The parents are relieved to be finally taking their baby to their home. Yet they will miss the camaraderie and support they experienced from exceptional caregivers. Instead of being enveloped in the NICU "bubble," they will be on their own with a possibly fragile baby. Many parents perceive their baby as needing ongoing special care, and this may be true in some cases.

Baby's Health Status. A high-risk baby must demonstrate normal breathing, oxygenation, voiding, stooling, and body temperature before discharge. They must tolerate feedings by mouth, including coordinated sucking, swallowing, and breathing during feedings. Depending on hospital protocol, the baby may require a car seat study to determine whether apnea is a risk. Discharge commonly occurs when an infant can maintain body temperature in an open crib, gains weight appropriately on full oral feedings, passes the car seat study, and is in stable medical condition. Small infants are discharged much earlier than in the past, and babies are not required to reach a target weight.

Discharge Planning. The Academy of Breastfeeding Medicine (ABM) protocol for the preterm infant's transition from the NICU to home provides postdischarge guidance for nursing families (ABM, 2018). Parents need to understand the baby's feeding plan and any necessary special care procedures or restrictions. If supplements are required, they need to know how much and how often they must feed them to the baby. They also need a clear plan for when and how supplements are to be discontinued.

Before taking the baby home, parents will schedule a postdischarge visit with the baby's primary care healthcare provider. Medically fragile babies may also need specialist follow-up appointments. Parents can also prepare for the baby's homecoming by arranging for household help when possible. Freezing meals for later use, stocking up on grocery items, and other practical preparations will maximize their time with the infant.

At Home with Baby. After parents arrive home with their baby, many issues unrelated to feedings are likely to surface. This can be a challenge in the chaotic environments of many families with fragile babies. Parents often experience an initial phase of excitement, followed by exhaustion and, eventually, a return of enjoyment and self-confidence. They will likely feel drained, both physically and emotionally, while their baby is still recovering. Limiting visitors will allow quiet time with other family members as parents reestablish relationships and integrate their baby into the family.

While most countries offer 10 to 20 weeks of maternity leave, paid maternity leave in the United States may be as brief as 6 weeks. Some parents divide their maternity leave by taking a brief time off after the birth, returning to work while the baby is in the NICU, and then taking the remainder of their leave after the baby is home. After they exhaust their maternity leave, they must arrange for caregivers, with the accompanying emotional, logistical, and financial toll. Resources such as home health services, specialized daycare providers, social assistance programs, employment insurance programs, and respite caregivers may be helpful for these families.

Baby Care and Feeding at Home. You can assist parents through the transition home by providing anticipatory guidance and education. Parents of high-risk infants are concerned about crying, breathing noises, spitting up, and infant behavior, all of which relate to feeding. Those who lack necessary information regarding their babies' care and expected behavior may be more anxious and less confident in caring for their babies. Postdischarge follow-up, assistance, and support can help ease their concern and build their confidence in their baby's transition to home.

The crying behavior of a preterm infant varies according to gestational age. Infant cries may be more frequent, higher-pitched, and uneven than those of a full-term baby. A preterm baby may have a greater incidence of reflux as well. These behaviors can be very trying for parents as they learn how to console their child. Anticipatory guidance helps them learn what to expect and how to cope with crying. Teach parents typical infant responses that indicate overstimulation or stress. These include the baby's finger splay (in the shape of a starfish), color change, variation in muscle tone, state variability, breathing changes, frowning, back arching, arm waving, hiccupping, and avoidance of eye contact. Review the discussion of avoidance cues in **Chapter 14**.

Nursing can be compromised when a baby has multiple health issues that require intensive parental care. Health conditions may require that the infant go home with a heart monitor or apnea monitor. The baby may also have an NG or a PEG tube in place for feedings. Complex congenital issues might require additional surgeries or procedures. Barriers to nursing these infants include other parental responsibilities, previous lack of nursing success, concerns about the emotional and physical costs of nursing and providing human milk, and doubts about adequate milk transfer.

Preterm Infant

Preterm birth is a serious health problem. There are 15 million babies born too early worldwide annually. The rate of preterm birth ranges from 5% to 18% of babies born across 184 countries. Preterm birth is the leading cause of newborn death, affecting almost 1 million babies per year. More than 90% of extremely preterm babies (under 28 weeks) born in low-resource countries die. Less than 10% of these babies die in high-resource areas (World Health Organization [WHO], 2018a). Babies who survive an early birth often face the risk of lifetime health challenges, including respiratory problems and cognitive disabilities. Babies born even a few weeks early have higher rates of disability and mortality than full-term babies (WHO, 2018b).

Most preterm infants weigh less than 5.5 pounds (2500 g). Because health problems increase with lower birth weights, it is important to learn a baby's gestational age and birth weight even if it is months later and the baby appears to be healthy. Suboptimal birth weight and length affect the infant's health immediately after birth. The child also has a propensity to develop chronic diseases in later life (Martín-Calvo et al., 2022; Suzuki, 2018).

If the rate of intrauterine growth is normal, the infant is deemed **appropriate for gestational age (AGA)**. If intrauterine growth was slowed, referred to as **intrauterine growth restriction (IUGR)**, the baby is considered **small for gestational age (SGA)**. The underlying factor in IUGR may be restricted fetal growth followed by rapid postnatal "catch-up growth," as well as maternal health issues, including hypertension and smoking. IUGR is associated with an increased risk of coronary heart disease, stroke, chronic kidney disease, diabetes, and high blood pressure in adult life (Al Salmi & Hannawi, 2020; Sacchi et al., 2020). Refer to **Table 24-2** for a classification of preterm babies by birth weight.

Baby's Appearance and Health Status

Depending on the baby's gestational age at birth, a preterm infant's skin may be loose and wrinkled, with a gelatinous appearance. Because they have little subcutaneous fat, blood vessels and bony structures are

Table 24-2 Classification of Preterm Infants by Birth Weight

LBW	Low birth weight	Under 5 pounds, 8 oz	2500 g
VLBW	Very low birth weight	Under 3 pounds, 5 oz	1500 g
ELBW	Extremely low birth weight	Under 2 pounds, 3 oz	1000 g

visible. Fine, downy hairs may be present on the sides of their face and on their forehead, back, and extremities. Hair on the baby's head is scanty, and there are usually no visible eyebrows. The baby's eyelids may still be fused (**Figure 24-6**). Their ears may fold in many positions, lacking full development of the cartilage needed to support them. Because skull growth is complete before other body growth, the baby's head appears large in proportion to the rest of the body. Preterm infants are at risk for several health conditions, as presented in **Figure 24-7**.

Respiratory Risk

Congenital defects, such as cardiac or intestinal defects, or various syndromes affecting limb and extremity development are common. The preterm infant's heart is usually well developed. However, the lungs and rib cage may not function efficiently at birth because of muscular weakness. This places the infant at risk for respiratory distress syndrome (RDS), chronic lung disease/bronchopulmonary dysplasia (BPD), and respiratory syncytial virus (RSV).

Heat Regulation

Heat regulation is poorly developed in a preterm infant, requiring stabilization and careful monitoring of the baby's body temperature. It is during later gestation that **adipose tissue** is laid down and fat stores accumulate. Therefore, the preterm infant has minimal stores of fat. White fat develops first and provides insulation. Brown fat develops last, providing thermoregulation and rapidly producing large amounts of heat. Preterm birth impairs the utilization of brown fat stores and further predisposes the baby to hypothermia.

Jaundice

Because of immature liver and digestive systems and low levels of **glucuronic acid**, preterm infants tend to have higher rates of physiologic jaundice than full-term infants (refer to **Chapter 23** for an in-depth

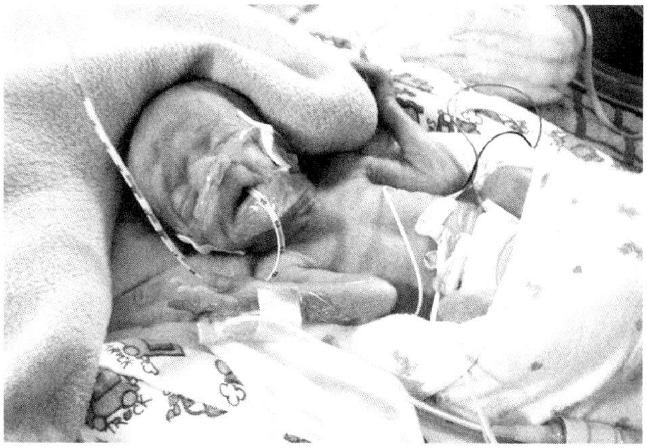

Figure 24-6 Preterm infant's eyelids may still be fused.
Reprinted with permission of Leslie and Brad Jackson.

- Retinopathy of prematurity (ROP)
- Apnea and bradycardia
- Anemia of prematurity (low blood cell count)
- Heart murmurs
- Infection, including necrotizing enterocolitis
- Poor weight gain
- Feeding difficulty

Figure 24-7 Health conditions for which preterm infants are at higher risk.

discussion on jaundice). A 30–60 second delay in cord clamping increases infant iron stores and is considered a safe and effective intervention against iron deficiency even in busy settings (Chaudhary et al., 2023).

Feeding Effectiveness

Gastrointestinal and neuromotor immaturity affect a preterm infant's suck and swallow coordination and feeding tolerance (Hasenstab & Jadcherla, 2022). Because of limited amounts of adipose tissue, SGA or preterm infants also often have problems regulating their **blood glucose** and body temperature. Early feeding problems may require supplementation with expressed milk or donor milk and **human milk fortifier (HMF)** until their condition stabilizes and they begin to gain weight. Preterm infants typically nurse frequently and intermittently. Even with a stable condition, these infants often require frequent feedings (10 or more in 24 hours), as if they are trying to gain the weight they should have gained in utero.

A full-term infant develops a mature sucking pattern during the third trimester in utero. Preterm infants' sucking maturity and coordination peak at different times and rates. The baby's readiness to feed orally depends on a combination of neurologic development, behavioral state organization, and physiologic stability. Although NNS as a single data point is not associated with feeding success, it is a prerequisite skill for oral feeding. Successful feeding at 38 weeks results from small advances in NNS peak pressures on a weekly basis. Preterm infants who receive more supplemental oxygen are more likely to struggle with NNS (Pineda et al., 2019).

Readiness to Nurse

Practices differ for determining a preterm infant's physical ability to nurse. Readiness to nurse begins after the baby is stable. Each preterm infant needs an individual assessment, irrespective of size or ability to suck on a bottle. Withholding nursing until the infant first "proves" the ability to bottle-feed well frequently does not allow infants to progress to complete direct nursing before they go home. In place of scheduled and specific volume feedings, many NICUs now use cue-based feeding to guide the transition to oral and breast feedings (Samane et al., 2022; Tandberg, 2025). Cue-based feedings rely on observing the infant's behaviors, such as awakening, displaying rooting reflexes, sucking on hands and fingers, and turning towards the nipple. Engaging in skin-to-skin contact with the infant provides the birth parent an opportunity to identify these hunger cues (Tandberg, 2025).

Promoting Nursing of the Preterm Infant

Healthcare providers in a NICU can be very influential in promoting nursing and the importance of human milk for preterm and medically fragile infants. Collaborating with a multidisciplinary team of NICU staff will ensure evidence-based care. Understanding the health benefits of human milk to their preterm infant enables parents to make evidence-informed decisions on feeding practices that are best for them and their baby. Protocols need to encompass lactation and nursing education, including skin-to-skin care, NNS, protecting milk production, and unlimited access to nursing. At a time when a birth parent can do little else for their baby, expressing their milk is something they can do that is crucial to their baby's health and development.

Expressing Milk

Most NICUs encourage the use of human milk for all babies. Providing milk enables parents to be physiologically and emotionally connected to their preterm infant in the NICU and reinforces their new identity and role as parents. Parents may feel overwhelmed by the birth of their preterm baby and may need hands-on, individualized lessons and support in establishing lactation. A parent who cannot nurse their preterm infant needs to begin expressing milk as soon as possible, preferably within the first hour or two and no later than 6 hours after delivery. Postpartum staff can help them develop a plan for milk expression until their baby can nurse.

Parents who planned to nurse likely anticipated settling comfortably into nursing and not being separated from their baby. Parents who did not plan to nurse may need time to process the idea of expressing their milk. They may feel pressured to provide milk for their baby and should be counseled respectfully. Be careful not to focus exclusively on managing milk expression while neglecting their other needs. Refer to **Chapter 22** for a discussion on expressing milk for a hospitalized baby.

Volume of Milk Expressed

Initially, milk expression may produce only a few drops of colostrum. A combination of hand expression and pumping may achieve the best results for this small quantity. The initial small volume of colostrum is normal at the beginning of lactation and provides essential health protection for the baby. If oral feedings are tolerated, the expressed colostrum can be fed to the baby or added to an NG or OG tube. Very small amounts of colostrum are used for OIT by swabbing the baby's cheeks, even before enteral feedings begin (Garofalo & Caplan, 2019). This practice may reduce the time to full enteral feedings and provide some immunologic support to the extremely preterm infant.

Frequent milk expression in the early weeks determines the amount of milk that will be produced in the long term. A diary can help keep track of pumping schedules and milk production. It is recommended that milk expression occur as often as possible, at least eight times in 24 hours, in the first few days after birth. One session should occur during the late-evening or early-morning hours. Recommend allowing at least 10 to 15 minutes of expressing time for each side, using a hospital-grade double electric breast pump. Longer pumping sessions do not increase milk yield, although pumping more frequently throughout the 24 hours can increase volume.

Adding hand expression to five out of the eight daily pumpings, along with breast massage during pumping sessions, can lead to faster flow. It may also produce increased amounts, especially after full milk production is established (Stanford School of Medicine, 2020a, 2020b). Milk expression is discussed further in **Chapter 22**.

Stimulating Letdown

Stimulating the milk-ejection reflex helps obtain the greatest amount of milk in the least time. Sensory stimulation through a picture or piece of the baby's clothing and auditory and visual relaxation can help. Some parents find that neck or back massage helps them relax while pumping. Other relaxation techniques described in **Chapter 15** will help parents relax physically and mentally. Pumping comfortably in a quiet location will also help stimulate letdown.

Fluctuations in Milk Production

Milk production may fluctuate in response to the parent's concern about the baby's condition, dropping in volume if the baby experiences a setback. Even if their baby is doing well medically, viewing other babies nearby who have debilitating or terminal conditions can be disheartening and overwhelming to parents. Encourage parents to take frequent breaks for self-care, including fluids, nutrition, pumping, and walking outside the unit.

Decreased frequency of pumping, long intervals between pumping sessions, pumping only when full, or stopping before all the milk is removed are common reasons for decreased milk production. Changes in lifestyle may affect milk production as well, especially for a parent who returns to work while the baby remains in the NICU. Over time, they may notice an unexplained decrease in volume or a longer time for milk to let down. Follow-up is important for parents who encounter problems with milk production, and support is a high priority. One study found that at 3 months of corrected age, the main reason for the discontinuation of nursing was insufficient milk (Dong et al., 2022).

Caution parents about the use of galactagogues such as fenugreek or blessed thistle and prescription medications such as metoclopramide or domperidone (Hale & Krutsch, 2024). Herbs or medicines that are safe for full-term infants could be harmful to an extremely preterm or sick infant. They could also interact with medications the baby is receiving. Encourage parents to discuss any planned galactagogue use with their neonatologist.

Illness in parents of NICU babies can cause a delay in reaching full milk production. Parents who deliver extremely preterm infants may also have delays establishing adequate milk production. Betamethasone, a corticosteroid administered prenatally to hasten preterm lung development and provide neuroprotection, may have a negative impact on lactation. Administering the medication within 3 to 9 days before delivery might negatively affect milk production (National Institute of Child Health and Human Development [NICHHD], 2023). Because the medication is vital to the preterm infant's lung maturity, withholding it is not an option. Be aware of this connection and follow these parents closely.

Significance of Human Milk for the Preterm Infant

Human milk is the ideal food for infants. It is especially vital to the preterm infant, who is at risk for developing a variety of infections. Immunologic properties in human milk can help protect preterm infants. The milk promotes neurodevelopment, immunologic development and protection, and a healthy gut microbiome, especially in preterm infants (Beghetti et al., 2019). The milk of parents who deliver preterm has special properties that are particularly beneficial to the infant. Preterm milk contains higher concentrations of sodium, chloride, and nitrogen, as well as immunoprotective factors. The composition of the milk helps promote maturation of the infant's gastrointestinal tract, in addition to meeting their unique nutritional needs.

Formula fed preterm infants have an increased risk of **necrotizing enterocolitis (NEC)** and infection (Fang et al., 2021). They also have lower neurodevelopment than preterm infants fed human milk (Lapidaire et al., 2022). Preterm infants are born at a time when the growth and development of the nervous system is still occurring in utero. Because of these health concerns, it is recommended that preterm infants receive human milk, regardless of whether the parent had planned to nurse. **Chapter 10** discusses in more detail the increased risks in babies who do not receive human milk.

The WHO (2023) recommends donor milk if the parent's milk is not available for the baby. Refer to **Chapter 9** for more information on the specificity of human milk for human babies and **Chapter 22** for a discussion of human milk banking. Because donor milk is often from parents of older infants, it is not immune-specific to the baby and the NICU environment. It lacks the unique properties of preterm milk but can be combined to provide the targeted protein and calorie rates the baby needs.

Health Importance to the Preterm Infant

Because of the health concerns that accompany preterm birth, human milk is especially important to the baby. Human milk helps establish enteral (through the digestive system) tolerance and allows for an earlier discontinuation of parenteral (IV) nutrition. The laxative effect of the milk, especially colostrum, helps clear meconium. During the initial stages of lactation, preterm milk offers more protein, fat, free amino acids, and sodium, the levels of which decrease over time (Granger et al., 2021).

Neurologic outcomes from receiving human milk, compared with formula, are especially significant for preterm babies. Human milk contains a variety of macronutrients and micronutrients, including immunoglobins, cytokines, growth factors, hormones, antimicrobial agents, immune cells, stem cells, and oligosaccharides (Parker et al., 2021). The human milk oligosaccharides (HMOs) support the infant's immune system, brain development, and cognitive function. They are a family of structurally diverse and complex sugars that are present in human milk and not formula. HMOs are modified depending on the infant's genetics, nutrition and body weight, and the stage of lactation. They vary between preterm and term birthing parents (Granger et al., 2021).

Human milk helps prevent retinopathy of prematurity in preterm infants (Raghuveer & Zackula, 2020). Exclusive human milk feedings may reduce the incidence of bronchopulmonary dysplasia as well (Villamor-Martínez et al., 2019). Long-term cardiovascular concerns for preterm infants continue into adulthood. Human milk has a mitigating effect and supports cardiovascular health (El-Khuffash et al., 2020).

Protection Against Necrotizing Enterocolitis and Sepsis

NEC, an acute gastrointestinal illness, occurs in 5% to 10% of preterm babies with a birth weight of less than 1500 grams (3.3 pounds) (Garg, 2022). NEC is characterized by inflammation of the intestinal wall, often causing the tissue to die. It is frequently associated with preterm birth, respiratory disease, and early enteral feedings of formula and cow's milk-based HMFs in preterm babies. Almost 60% of infants who develop NEC require surgical intervention and will experience long-term health issues.

Among infants who develop NEC, 24% have associated sepsis (Gang et al., 2022). Sepsis is the presence of bacteria, other infectious organisms, or toxins created by infectious organisms in the bloodstream that spreads throughout the body. The three classifications of organisms associated with NEC are gram-positive bacteria, gram-negative bacteria, and *Candida*. The mortality rate for NEC is 25%. Risk factors for NEC include formula feeding, infection, and gut immaturity (Xiong et al., 2020). Human milk reduces the risk of NEC (Altobelli et al., 2020; Lapidaire W, et al., 2022).

Human Milk Fortifiers

A nutritional goal for the preterm infant to match the growth rate of a full-term infant is a challenge. There is concern that human milk may not provide sufficient nutrition for preterm infants, especially those born under 1500 g (3.3 pounds). Moreover, these small babies cannot take in the volume needed for full nutrition from nursing. Because preterm infants require more protein, calories, fatty acids, minerals, and other micronutrients, the parent's milk may be fortified (Adamkin, 2023). Multinutrient HMFs are designed to be added to the parent's milk, especially to donor milk, in which the micronutrient levels are lower than the parent's milk (Parker et al., 2021). HMFs are discussed in detail in **Chapter 10**.

The WHO recommends that HMFs not be used routinely for all preterm or low-birth infants receiving human milk. Instead, multicomponent fortification of the milk may be appropriate for extremely preterm or ELBW infants (Darmstadt et al., 2023). There is a modest increase in in-hospital growth rates with HMF use, but there are insufficient data regarding long-term benefits for growth or neurodevelopment (Adamkin, 2023). There is also concern that some brands of liquid HMF are given in a 1:1 ratio with human milk, which can result in the baby receiving less milk.

Lactoengineering

Researchers have long proposed using specific components of human milk, specifically expressed hindmilk, to increase the calories, carbohydrates, and proteins available to preterm infants. Proteins and calcium in human milk can also be separated and used to fortify expressed milk. This engineering of human milk, referred to as **lactoengineering**, is considered to be a cost-effective feeding strategy (Knake et al., 2020).

A recent study explored the use of expressed hindmilk to supplement preterm infants born at less than 30 weeks of gestation. Hindmilk was defined as the milk collected after the first three minutes of pumping. The fat concentration of hindmilk is two to three times higher than that of foremilk, therefore providing more calories and essential fatty acids to the infant. The results are promising, with higher gains in weight, head circumference, and plasma fatty acid levels (Alshaikh et al., 2023). Further research is needed.

Preserving the Safety of Expressed Milk

The safety of expressed milk is especially critical for a fragile preterm infant. Parents will need verbal and simple written instructions for pumping hygiene and handling and storage of their milk. Individual NICUs will have their own collection and storage guidelines and usually provide the desired containers to parents. Encourage thorough handwashing with soap and drying with disposable paper towels or a clean towel before every pumping session.

Pump parts exposed to the milk should be rinsed immediately with cold water and then washed in hot, soapy water. The milk should be stored in sterile, hard plastic or glass containers that maintain the integrity of the milk's composition. Parents should record the date and time of day the milk was expressed. Milk from each pumping session needs to be stored separately and labeled according to the NICU's specifications.

The hospital will provide instructions on whether expressed milk can be delivered fresh or frozen. Handling should be kept to a minimum because the more often milk is moved and the more surface areas it touches, the greater the potential for fat loss and contamination. Freshly expressed colostrum, transitional milk, and then mature milk are preferred for feedings when the baby is not yet able to nurse directly.

The hospital may request that the milk be frozen if the baby is unable to tolerate oral feedings or if the milk will be fed to the baby more than 24 hours after it was expressed. Placing it in a cold, insulated container helps avoid thawing during transport. The composition of fresh milk is most suitable for the baby, whereas frozen milk loses a portion of its protective properties, especially vitamin C.

Skin-to-Skin Care

Skin-to-skin care, also called **kangaroo care**, places the baby in skin-to-skin contact with the parent in close proximity to the chest. Kangaroo care as a clinically defined process began in the late 1970s in Bogotá, Colombia, where preterm babies had a high mortality rate. It is so named because of its resemblance to baby kangaroos crawling inside their mother's pouch and latching on to a nipple for feeding. Because of its hallmark feature of skin-to-skin contact, most clinicians now refer to it as *skin-to-skin care.*

Skin-to-skin care allows the baby to become gently familiar with a new feeding method and environment after leaving the womb. It is nature's way of stabilizing the baby, especially when incubators are not available. WHO guidelines to improve survival and health outcomes for babies born before 37 weeks of gestation include skin-to-skin contact with a caregiver starting immediately after birth, before any time in an incubator (WHO, 2022). Skin-to-skin care can begin as soon as the baby's condition permits. Stable infants may be held skin to skin even when they are still on a ventilator. Holding the baby skin to skin promotes respiratory stability (Thompson, 2024) and protects against apnea (Montealegre-Pomar et al., 2020).

Skin-to-Skin Care Method

To use this technique, the parent places the baby on their chest, clothed only in a diaper, skin to skin, upright and prone. The baby and parent are then covered or wrapped together to maintain the baby's body temperature (**Figure 24-8**). The parent can be topless or wear an opened button-down shirt and no bra for easy access. To avoid overstimulation, they can hold the baby quietly, with minimal or no talking, singing, stroking, or rocking. Often while being held skin to skin, the baby initially is in a quiet, alert state and then settles down to sleep. As the baby's condition improves, their ability to maintain eye contact will increase.

Benefits of Skin-to-Skin Care

Skin-to-skin care lowers stress for both the preterm baby and the parents. It is an affordable method of providing safe preterm care and is a core component

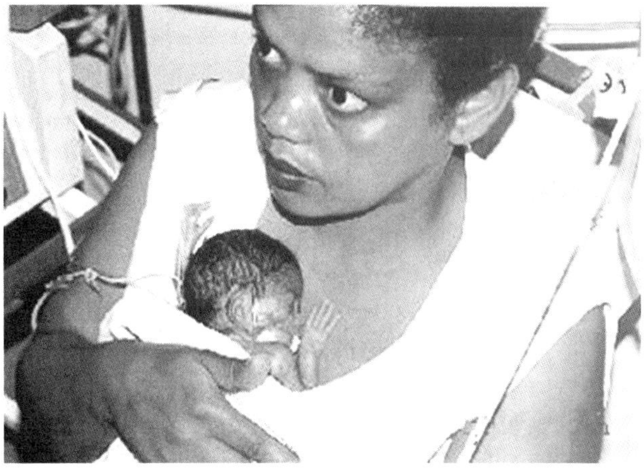

Figure 24-8 Holding the baby skin to skin.

of postpartum care worldwide. Survival for preterm low-birth-weight (LBW) infants is significantly higher for newborns held skin to skin, irrespective of place of birth (Mazumder et al., 2019). The method is associated with a reduced risk of mortality, **nosocomial** infection or sepsis, hypothermia, and length of hospital stay. Increased infant growth, nursing, and parent–infant attachment are associated with this care as well (Mehrpisheh et al., 2022). The parent's partner or other support person can also hold the baby skin to skin and should be encouraged to do so. Families from lower socioeconomic status report receiving less support for holding their babies skin to skin (Brignoni-Pérez et al., 2022).

Transition to Nursing

Parents can contribute to the baby's transition from gavage feeding to nursing directly. Placing a breast pad or cloth with drops of expressed milk in the baby's incubator will increase familiarity with the scent. When parents refresh the scent cloths, they can bring the older cloth home, which now has the baby's scent, to help achieve letdown during milk expression. During gavage feedings, the parent can hold their baby skin to skin on their chest to increase the association with sucking and eating.

A private and supportive environment will help ensure a smoother transition for babies and parents as they begin nursing. Progressive hospitals support family care with single-family rooms in the NICU (O'Callaghan et al., 2019). This helps develop the parent–infant bond and shared awareness with the baby during feeding. It facilitates pumping privacy, creates a sense of ownership and a homey atmosphere, and promotes skin-to-skin care. Lying quietly on the chest—becoming familiar with the scent, sight, and sensations—gradually develops into rooting, licking, and tasting. This is a very important step in the baby's progress toward direct nursing. As the baby becomes stronger and more alert, being held skin to skin facilitates latch and active sucking.

Initial Feedings

It is important to provide parents with reassurance about their progress toward direct nursing. Encourage them to approach feedings in a relaxed and unhurried manner. Initial feedings are characterized by minimal nursing, interspersed with much resting time. Parents can use this time to become acquainted with their baby and practice nursing technique. Ideally, the location for feedings should be quiet and private and near any equipment needed. Parents should avoid unnecessary stimulation from bright lights; loud noises; or stroking, rocking, or talking to the baby. Excessive external stimulation can be overwhelming. Learning the new skill of nursing requires a great deal of the baby's attention.

Nipple shields are often used to help small preterm infants stabilize the nipple in their mouth and maintain latch. Every baby is different, however, so it is important to first observe the baby nursing to determine whether a nipple shield is needed. Practicing nursing, followed by NG or OG feeding, may be a more effective way to feed an extremely preterm baby. Later use of a nursing supplementer may be appropriate for older preterm babies when milk production is low.

Milk Flow

Breast massage before and during a feeding can increase milk flow and encourage the baby to nurse. Some parents express with a breast pump to initiate milk flow before they settle in with the baby. This can also help minimize the gush of a strong letdown or prevent overwhelming the baby with too fast of a flow. If the baby gulps and chokes, an adjustment in positioning can slow milk flow. A position with the back of the baby's throat somewhat higher than the nipple or sitting in a semireclined position may help. Expressing milk in the middle of the feeding may allow the baby to nurse with a less intense milk flow.

Positioning

Holding the baby in the side-sitting (also called *football* or *clutch*) or cross-cradle position enables the parent to view and handle their baby. Laid-back positioning, with the baby's entire body supported against the parent's body, triggers the baby's neonatal reflexes to feed. Parents can begin the feeding by holding the baby level with the nipple and supporting the baby's entire body. Jaw and cheek support with the Dancer hand position will help the baby maintain latch and increase milk intake. This technique supports the baby's jaw while minimizing the weight of the breast in the baby's mouth (refer to **Figure 15-6** in **Chapter 15**).

Monitoring Intake and Weight

Parents who have been pumping were able to quantify their milk production and their baby's intake by tube or bottle. When the baby nurses directly, they may feel uncertain about milk intake. The use of pre- and postfeed weight assessments with sensitive digital electronic scales will help measure the baby's milk intake. Test weights are reassuring and easy to perform. Teaching parents how to perform the pre- and post-feeding test weights can help to increase their confidence and self-efficacy.

Early nursing sessions may require supplementary feedings when weight gain is a concern. For increased calories, the baby can receive the creamy portion of expressed milk that rises to the top or hindmilk expressed after a feed. The neonatologist may recommend continued test weights to determine milk intake from nursing to calculate supplement needs and identify the baby's trends and progression toward exclusive nursing.

Taking the Preterm Infant Home

When a hospitalized baby nears discharge home, parents' emotions can range from excitement and anticipation to apprehension and worry about caring for their fragile baby. Rooming-in with the baby in the hospital for several days before discharge or spending multiple feeding sessions during extended time together eases this transition. Because nighttime care of the infant seems especially daunting to new parents, 24-hour rooming-in in a homelike setting is especially valuable.

Discharge Guidelines

Discharge instructions are tailored to the individual needs of each infant in the NICU. The discharge planning team typically includes clinical nurses, healthcare providers (physician and nurse practitioner), discharge coordinators, social workers, speech pathologists, lactation consultants, and nutritionists. Discharge planning begins early during the infant's stay to provide a holistic treatment plan that will carry the infant through a seamless transition to the home environment. The healthcare provider determines when the infant has met the physiological discharge criteria to ensure a smooth transition home.

Before discharge, the family is instructed on care management, expected infant behaviors and patterns, signs of potential illness, whom to contact in an emergency, and scheduling of follow-up appointments. Mental health services should be made available to the family because of the higher risk of mental health issues following discharge from the NICU environment. Social workers and case managers will determine the family's needs and include community partnerships and referrals for services as appropriate (Gupta et al., 2019; Smith et al., 2022).

Special Care at Home

After the baby's discharge, the parents need to follow the recommendations for follow-up and when to contact their provider with concerns about their baby's progress. They will need resources for ongoing care, especially if their baby has extensive complex medical needs. Early intervention assistance programs through government, schools, and other organizations help identify and provide interventions and treatments that the baby may need. In the United States, the March of Dimes (2025) offers a NICU Family Support program to educate NICU staff and support families.

Encourage parents to access local resources to monitor their baby's growth and development. Healthcare providers use growth charts that are specific for preterm infants. For the first 2 years of life, parents should use the infant's corrected age to track developmental milestones. The corrected age can be calculated by subtracting the weeks preterm from the actual age in weeks. For example, an infant born at 28 weeks' gestation was born 12 weeks (3 months) early. At 6 months of age, the corrected age is 3 months. Therefore, the parent would anticipate the infant reaching the 3-month-old developmental milestones (Healthy Children, 2018).

Test Weights

Preterm infants who do not nurse effectively need close monitoring. Periodic weight checks will help determine adequate growth. If parents do not use in-home scales for test weights, they will need to have frequent weight checks by their baby's healthcare provider until their baby demonstrates the recommended weight gain. Some lactation supporters worry that the use of test weights may suggest to parents that their milk is inadequate. While this can be a legitimate argument for a healthy, full-term baby, a preterm baby needs the growth monitoring these test weights provide.

Nursing at Home

Parents should receive a written, individualized feeding plan before they take their baby home. Recommendations for nursing after discharge should be included, along with progression toward normalization of nursing and any supplementation or fortification needs. The plan should be included in the medical record shared with follow-up care providers. If the hospital provides no outpatient lactation follow-up, parents will need a referral to a community-based lactation consultant who has extensive experience with preterm babies and NICU graduates.

Maintaining hospital routines for the first few days at home can help to ease the transition. Milk expression needs to continue, gradually decreasing pumping time when the baby begins to nurse more frequently and more efficiently. Any supplementation or special devices the baby required at discharge can be discontinued gradually as well. Periodic weight checks should continue as feeding routines change. Follow-up will ease the parents' worries as they settle in with their baby. Remind them that overt hunger cues and other infant expectations do not always apply to preterm infants. Encourage them to regard the baby's gestational age, rather than age from birth, as an indicator of what to expect. **Table 24-3** provides suggestions for counseling parents of a preterm infant.

Initiating and maintaining lactation with a preterm infant is a time-consuming process that has been described as "triple feeding." The term describes the combination of direct nursing, pumping, and feeding the pumped milk to the baby. Anticipatory guidance about what to expect with the baby's feeding behaviors and routine after discharge may increase parents' comfort in making the transition.

Table 24-3 Counseling Parents of a Preterm Infant

Concern	Suggestions
Anxiety about taking a small baby home	■ Continue close medical supervision of the baby.
Anxiety about beginning nursing	■ Keep realistic expectations. ■ Allow a transition period.
The baby tires easily when nursing	■ Rouse the baby frequently during feedings. ■ Stimulate the baby to nurse. ■ Nurse frequently for short periods as long as the baby is sucking and swallowing. ■ Use a nipple shield.
Weak rooting reflex	■ Provide skin-to-skin contact. ■ Turn the baby's head toward the nipple. ■ Help the baby open their mouth. ■ Form the nipple and initiate latch.
Weak suck	■ Use Dancer hand position to increase intraoral negative pressure. ■ Use a nipple shield.
Intermittent sucking and resting during feedings	■ Allow a lengthy time for feedings.
Nipple preference from bottle feeding	■ Express milk until letdown occurs. ■ Avoid artificial nipples. ■ Use an alternate feeding method when not able to nurse.
Difficulty getting the baby interested in nursing	■ Provide frequent skin contact and nuzzling. ■ Familiarize the baby with the smell of the milk.
Difficulty positioning the baby to nurse	■ Use pillows to bring the baby to nipple level. ■ Use the side-sitting hold for positioning and the Dancer hand position under the baby's chin.
Difficulty determining adequate milk intake	■ Determine with NICU staff the number of wet diapers and stools to expect each day. ■ Plan a schedule of follow-up visits with the baby's primary care provider. ■ Determine the minimum feeding frequency to expect and what to do if the baby does not meet the goal. ■ Consider renting an electronic scale for daily weights at home. Plan with baby's provider what weight gain to expect. Learn from NICU staff how to determine accurate weights.

Table 24-4 Factors Influencing the Decision to Exclusively Pump

Perceived Challenges with Nursing	Perceived Benefits of Expressed Milk
■ Not having planned to nurse before the birth ■ Inadequate milk production ■ Feelings of vulnerability and lack of confidence ■ Infants' immature feeding behaviors ■ Lack of commitment to pump and store milk ■ Lack of informational and emotional support	■ Perception of bottle-feeding as more convenient ■ Family members can participate in feedings ■ Not feeling embarrassed feeding in public ■ Able to quantify the baby's intake

Some parents pump their milk for the baby in the NICU and continue to pump after discharge without transitioning to direct nursing. Many can meet all of their babies' nutritional needs with their pumped milk. **Table 24-4** describes factors that influence the choice to pump exclusively rather than nurse directly.

Other Babies Not Born at Term

In addition to prematurity, other extremes of gestational age also require special care at birth. Babies who are born near the early range of gestation, beginning at 34 weeks are referred to as late preterm. Those who are born at the other extreme of 42 weeks are referred to as **postterm** or *postmature*. The length of hospitalization and degree of care needed for these babies depend on their condition and the number of weeks before or after term that birth occurs. You can familiarize parents with the typical characteristics of these babies as well as with the implications for nursing.

Late Preterm Infant

Late preterm birth can result from increased maternal age, obesity, diabetes, poor nutrition, smoking, alcohol use, assisted reproductive technology resulting in multiple births, induction of labor, gestational hypertension resulting in preeclampsia and eclampsia, and cesarean delivery (Karnati et al., 2020). The WHO estimates that most preterm and late preterm births occur in areas with minimal resources (Karnati et al., 2020).

An infant considered to be late preterm is born between the gestational ages of 34 and 36 weeks and 6/7 days. Gestational age is rounded to the nearest completed week. For example, an infant born on the 5th day of the 36th week (35 weeks and 5/7 days) is at a gestational age of 35 weeks (The Joint Commission, 2024). These infants were previously referred to as *near term*. Terminology was changed because of concerns that it conveyed the impression that these infants are "almost term." This misconception can underestimate risk, resulting in insufficient evaluation, monitoring, and follow-up.

Because late preterm infants appear to be healthy and competent, they often receive the same treatment as full-term infants. They are typically cared for in a normal newborn nursery and go home at 48 to 72 hours postpartum. The baby is generally able to maintain body temperature, is at or above 2500 g, and may nurse well in the hospital.

Late preterm infants may have cardiorespiratory instability, poor temperature control, metabolic instability, immunologic and neurologic immaturity, or immature oral motor development. These complications result in limited stamina to do the work of nursing. Late preterm infants are also at increased risk for hypoglycemia, hypothermia, severe hyperbilirubinemia, and dehydration (Karnati et al., 2020). Late preterm infants make up a large percentage of kernicterus events in the United States, as discussed in **Chapter 23**.

Researchers report long-term outcomes for these infants in later life. An infant's central nervous system continues to grow and change until birth. Longer gestation is associated with reduced illness and death. Issues with speech and language development and cognitive issues in school-age children have been documented globally and warrant additional follow-up as the late preterm infant develops (Karnati et al., 2020). **Table 24-5** identifies short- and long-term health conditions for which late preterm infants are at a higher risk than full-term infants.

Taking the Baby Home

Encourage parents to approach taking their infant home with caution and guarded optimism. Late preterm infants will often have a honeymoon of 2 to

Table 24-5 Conditions for Which Late Preterm Infants Are at Higher Risk Than Term Infants

Short Term
Apgar scores under 7 at the 5th minute
Apnea
Cerebral palsy
Feeding difficulties
Hypocalcemia
Hypoglycemia
Hypothermia
Intraventricular hemorrhage
Jaundice requiring phototherapy
Necrotizing enterocolitis
Need for neonatal resuscitation
Neonatal intensive care unit admission
Overall neonatal morbidity
Pneumonia
Pneumothorax
Prolonged hospitalization
Pulmonary hypertension
Rates of readmission to hospital
Respiratory distress syndrome (hyaline membrane disease)
Sepsis
Septicemia
Transient tachypnea
Long Term
Asthma
Attention-deficit hyperactivity disorder
Autism (associated with)
Delayed mental development
Delayed psychomotor development
Diabetes
Higher rates of mortality in the first year of life and again in early adulthood
Inadequate growth at 2 years
Lower preschool/school performance
Lower proportion finishing college
Lower proportion finishing high school
Schizophrenia
Impaired verbal skills
Impaired visual processing

Data from Baron et al., 2009; Ben Amor et al., 2012; Chan et al., 2014; de Jong et al., 2012; Guy et al., 2014; Harris et al., 2013; Hirvonen et al., 2014; Machado et al., 2014; Melamed et al., 2009; Morse et al., 2009; Noble et al., 2012; Talge et al., 2012.

4 days or more when they seem to rise to the challenges, and then they tire out and need assistance. These infants need unlimited, almost continuous skin-to-skin care and careful attention to their needs for nutrition, thermoregulation, and rest. They can move quickly from a hyperalert state to deep sleep, exhibit subtle hunger cues or none at all, and be overstimulated easily.

Late preterm infants may experience poor neurologic organization, with an immature rooting reflex and difficulty coordinating the suck–swallow–breathe cycle. Early delivery results in decreased albumin sites and therefore an increased risk of jaundice. This can lead to sleepiness and difficulty with effective milk transfer. There is a 28.9% risk of readmission to the hospital because of jaundice and/or weight loss (Karnati et al., 2020).

Nursing Precautions

A late preterm infant often has low muscle tone and finds it difficult to initiate and maintain milk production because of poor lip and cheek tone. Because of the early delivery, full development of buccal fat pads and masseter muscles was not accomplished. There may also be anatomic incompatibility, with the nipple too large for the baby's small mouth, making it difficult to maintain a seal and latch.

A tendency to tire quickly can make it difficult for the infant to draw the nipple into their mouth, maintain a good latch, and compress the nipple during sucking. Babies with an immature suck rely more on compression to move milk than full-term babies do. Most milk is moved during the vacuum phase once the baby progresses to more mature suck patterns.

Parents need clear and consistent teaching about what to expect with their late-preterm infant. Ensure that the baby nurses at least eight times in 24 hours. Many of these babies tire easily and do better with shorter, more frequent feedings. They should go no longer than 3 hours between feedings during the day, with a goal of 8 to 12 feedings in 24 hours. Parents need to watch closely for subtle hunger cues and nurse as often as the baby indicates a need. Realizing that hunger cues may be subtle or lacking, gentle waking techniques (e.g., holding the baby upright, wearing the baby, skin-to-skin contact) will help accomplish the appropriate number of feedings (refer to **Figure 24-9**).

Parents need to count voids and stools until the baby has exhibited a pattern of robust weight gain without supplementation. Frequent voids in a baby born early may indicate an immature renal system that can quickly lead to dehydration. Thus, voids alone are not a good indicator of sufficient intake. Stools are a better indicator, especially in babies born early.

Physiologically, a late preterm baby is meant to be in utero, sleeping and growing, not working for nourishment. Because of the baby's compromised condition, parents cannot rely on sucking alone to initiate and maintain sufficient milk production and transfer.

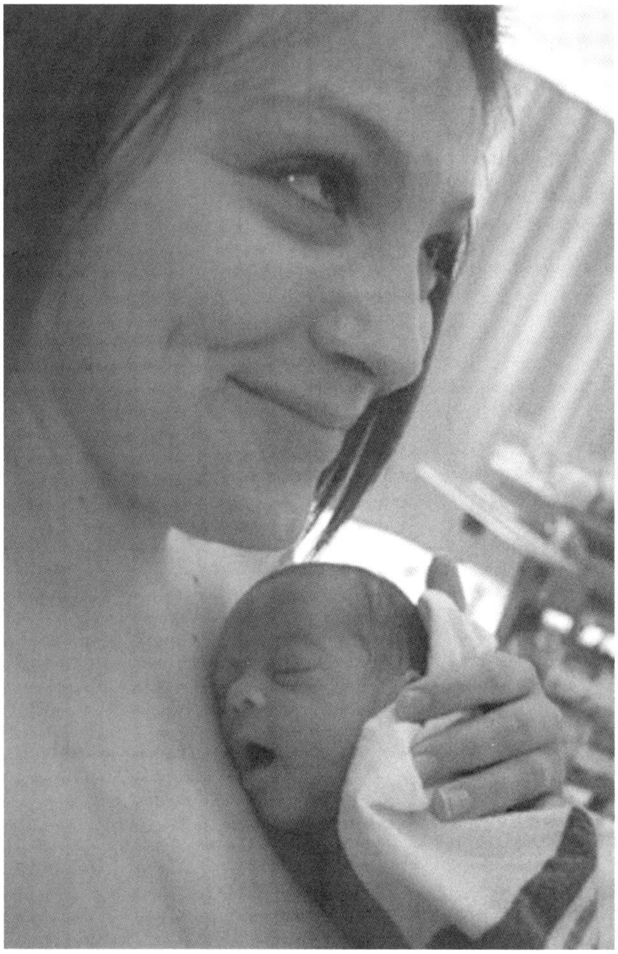

Figure 24-9 Parent with late preterm infant.

Printed with permission of Anna Swisher.

Milk expression with an electric breast pump is required until the baby's due date arrives or until the baby is well over birth weight and milk production is well established. Pumping frequency depends on how effectively the baby is transferring milk. If expression after a feeding produces minimal milk, the baby may be transferring milk well. Alternatively, it may indicate that milk production is low because the baby is not transferring milk and stimulating more milk production.

Careful monitoring will help identify whether there is a problem. For example, a parent who pumps a significant amount of milk after a feeding will need to continue pumping to maintain lactation until the baby's nursing ability matures and milk transfer improves. The baby's weight, stooling, and voiding history should be checked weekly during this time.

Although some parents of late preterm babies find that a nipple shield helps with milk transfer, routine use is not recommended (Carpay et al., 2021). It is important to have adequate follow-up when a nipple shield is used. Typically, these babies nurse well without a shield after they have grown and matured more. It often helps for parents to realize that most late preterm babies seem to "wake up" and begin to nurse like term babies when they reach their due date.

Postterm Infant

An infant considered to be postterm is born after 42 weeks' gestation. Maternal and infant mortality risk increases among this population (Kortekaas et al., 2020). A danger in postmaturity is that the placenta progressively deteriorates and becomes less efficient after the normal gestation period of 40 weeks. Postterm infants may have appropriate body length for gestational age but are often small for gestation because of the progressive decrease in placental function and wasting/weight loss in utero. Fetal oxygenation may be marginal or depressed before labor. The baby has difficulty tolerating the stresses of labor and may struggle to maintain respiration. Delivery may be through labor induction or cesarean section.

Sometimes, a postterm baby passes meconium in utero, which can lead to meconium aspiration syndrome (MAS). MAS occurs when the baby passes meconium while still in the womb and then breathes meconium into their lungs during birth. Meconium can block the infant's airways right after birth, leading to respiratory distress (Kortekaas et al., 2020). Maintenance of blood glucose levels and nervous functioning is also a challenge. These situations are generally manageable. **Table 24-6** describes the postterm infant's appearance and other factors at the time of birth.

Even though born postterm, the baby may initially behave like a preterm baby. They may be sluggish during initial attempts at nursing and may need coaxing and prodding in much the same way as a baby born preterm. The strategies used to nurse a late preterm infant usually work well with these babies. As postterm babies gain weight, their feeding behaviors mature.

Fetal or Infant Death

Caring for parents who have experienced fetal demise (miscarriage), stillbirth, neonatal death, or the death of a nursing child can be distressing. It may be challenging to find the right words and avoid painful remarks while expressing sensitive support. Appropriate counseling techniques, insight into parents' emotions, and sincere empathy enable you to support parents in their grief. Sensitive and appropriate intervention can aid in healing their pain, with the utmost

Table 24-6 Postterm Infant Characteristics

Physical Appearance	Developmental and Health Factors
■ Lean and long, little body fat ■ Cracked, dry, leathery, peeling skin ■ No vernix ■ Yellow-greenish staining of nails and skin from meconium passed in utero ■ Longer hair and longer nails than a term newborn ■ Large, alert eyes	■ More alert than a term newborn ■ Respiratory issues due to meconium passage or **hypoxia** during labor ■ Hypoglycemia ■ Hypothermia ■ Large for gestational age (kept growing in utero) ■ Small for gestational age (growth stalled in utero)

Data from Perry SE, et al. *Maternal Child Nursing Care*. 6th ed. Ch. 25. St. Louis, MO: Elsevier Mosby; 2018.

care to avoid insensitive remarks or minimizing interactions. Bereavement counseling includes validating the family's grief; encouraging the family to tell their stories; providing mementos; and facilitating rituals of remembrance or religious significance, such as baptism or naming. **Figure 24-10** identifies grieving parents' practical, emotional, and spiritual needs.

- The need for privacy
- The need for access to their child
- Opportunities to participate in their child's care
- Self-care such as a place to eat, shower, and sleep
- Physical presence of professional and personal support
- Transfer of child's body to mortuary
- Autopsy questions
- Legacy items (mementos)
- Necessary documentation process
- Making funeral arrangements
- Navigating social media
- Canceling medical appointments, home nursing, etc.
- Disposition of baby items and medical equipment
- Support for lactating parents, including milk donation and supplies
- Accessing the child's health records

Figure 24-10 Practical needs of grieving parents.

Data from Meert K. Exploring parents' environmental needs at the time of a child's death in the pediatric intensive care unit. *Pediatr Crit Care Med*. 2008;9:623-628; October T, et al. Caring for parents after the death of a child. *Pediatr Crit Care Med*.

What to Say to Parents

Every person handles loss of a loved one differently. Having an insight into parents' emotions will help you determine how to best support them. For many parents, bonding and maternal feelings begin the day they learn they are pregnant or when they first hear their baby's heartbeat. Parents need others to acknowledge that their baby was loved before birth and was a person who meant a lot in their lives. Avoid comments such as "At least you can have more children" or "It was for the best." You can acknowledge their grief by asking the baby's name and using it during your discussion.

Be sensitive to parents' signals that they may or may not want to interact or ask questions. Some parents do not wish to converse with caregivers following the loss of their child. If you are uncertain, a gentle opening statement may be "If you would like, I will sit here with you," or "What would you like to ask?" or "I am here for you if you would like to talk." If grieving parents want to communicate, pay attention to them without interruptions or interpretations as they share their experience. Avoid saying, "I know how you must feel" or "I can imagine what you are going through." You cannot know what the parents are feeling. Even if you also lost a child, it is not appropriate to discuss your own loss. Referring to your experience takes the focus off the parents' grief and minimizes it. Instead, saying, "I am so sorry for your loss" validates their pain without taking the focus off them and their baby. In addition, sitting in silence holding space for parents in their time of grief can be just as supportive as any spoken words.

If you have contact with parents beyond the hospital stay, at the appropriate time, you can share that other families who have suffered similar losses find it helpful to discuss their feelings. Their grief could continue unresolved until they share their feelings and work through them. The people closest to them sometimes feel uncomfortable listening to them relate their birth experience and the circumstances surrounding their baby's death. Parents may appreciate being able to turn to you. Let them know you are glad to listen, assuring them that you do not want to invade their privacy (Falkenburg et al., 2018). Many times, it is difficult to be in situations we are powerless to resolve. Become comfortable with being mindfully present and with the reality that you cannot fix this situation.

Grieving for Their Loss

Parents will progress through several stages of grief before their loss is resolved, typically beginning with denial and ending in acceptance. **Figure 24-2** illustrates the range of emotions parents experience between these two extremes. The time it takes to move from denial to acceptance varies greatly, and they may need gentle reminders of resources to support grieving parents. Making sense of the loss is an important predictor of grief intensity (Kochen et al., 2020). Parents never truly "get over" the loss of a child. It is never appropriate to minimize the loss of a child, even after decades have passed. Parents' lives are irrevocably changed, and they hold on to their relationship with their deceased child.

If there are other children in the family, encourage the parents to communicate openly and honestly with them about their sibling dying. Although the baby's life may have been brief, consequences for survivor siblings can be lifelong. Siblings born both before and after the death of an infant may need psychological support. Photos and family rituals help everyone in the family grieve and remember the infant.

Although some grieving parents will require formal and structured psychological support, not everyone will need formal intervention (Boyle et al., 2020). Parent support groups and the peer support of others with similar experiences may be beneficial for some parents. Effective and compassionate communication is critical, as is respect for privacy. Suggestions in **Table 24-7** will help you counsel grieving parents.

Table 24-7 Counseling Grieving Parents

Helpful responses:

- Showing genuine concern and caring
- Conversing and empathizing
- Saying you are sorry about what happened
- Allowing them to express their grief
- Encouraging them to be patient with themselves
- Allowing them to talk about their baby
- Pointing out special qualities of the baby they lost
- Acknowledging the impact of the baby's death
- Reassuring them that they did everything possible for their baby
- Referring to the baby by name
- Showing your sadness and disappointment

Unhelpful responses:

- Allowing your sense of discomfort or helplessness to prevent you from reaching out to them
- Suggesting you know how they feel
- Suggesting they will feel better after some time
- Appearing to indicate what they should feel or do
- Changing the subject when the baby is mentioned
- Trying to find something positive about the baby's death
- Remarking that they can have other children
- Suggesting that they should be grateful for other children they have
- Suggesting that the baby's care was inadequate
- Avoiding use of the baby's name for fear of causing pain
- Appearing overly cheerful or casual

Lactation Concerns

A parent whose baby has died may have concerns specific to lactation. Consistent and adequate information given to grieving parents about the lactation process and their options can help avoid further distress. Parents need at least one lactation-specific visit while in the hospital, regardless of whether they planned to nurse. Some parents may not know that they will produce milk. Anticipatory guidance will help them avoid becoming painfully engorged. Even if nursing did not begin, secretory activation (lactogenesis II) will typically occur a few days after delivery. Expressing milk only until the breasts are soft and comfortable will help avoid stimulating further milk production. Comfort measures for engorgement, as described in **Chapter 17**, will help these parents.

A parent who had been nursing or expressing their milk may have more difficulty ending lactation. They will need to decrease pumping slowly in a weaning pattern to avoid problems associated with abrupt weaning, such as mastitis. Teach them about signs of mastitis and advise them to contact their healthcare provider if symptoms begin. These parents often find comfort in knowing they gave their babies the best possible care, both nutritionally and emotionally. Many bereaved parents donate their milk to a milk bank. Donating milk to help save another baby's life can add to their emotional healing. Caregivers can suggest milk donation to receptive parents and refer them to the nearest milk bank.

The Perinatal Society of Australia and New Zealand and the Australian Stillbirth Center developed guidelines to improve the quality of bereavement care (Boyle et al., 2020). Based on evidence-based practice, the guidelines contain 49 recommendations to address basic goals of care. Becoming familiar with these or similar guidelines will help you provide supportive care for parents experiencing a fetal demise. You can also research resources available for providers and families in your area.

Support for Grieving Parents

Healthcare providers trained in perinatal loss are best able to support healing care. Demonstrating a caring presence through your words and actions can create opportunities for parents to meet their own needs (October et al., 2018). Parents need to stay connected with their deceased child. They need time and privacy with their family to begin grieving for their loss. Parents have the right to hold or view their baby after the demise. If they wish to visit with their baby before discharge, a staff member can bring the baby to their room wrapped in warm blankets. This practice is particularly helpful for parents of a stillborn infant.

Parents benefit from memories and mementos that will bring them comfort in the future. Many hospitals provide memory boxes to hold mementos of the baby's birth. Giving parents their infant's identification bracelet is validation of the importance to them as a family member and a memento of their brief time together. Pictures can help parents put their baby's death into perspective. Offering parents an opportunity to take pictures can provide them with a treasured image of their child. Some hospitals take pictures of the deceased infant for parents to keep. A staff member can cleanse, dress, and swaddle the infant for the pictures. This can be especially important to parents who choose not to view their infant at the time of death and would appreciate a photo of their baby months later.

Encourage parents to seek information about their options with hospital personnel and their baby's caregiver. When requested, hospital chaplains can baptize stillborn infants. In some hospitals, nurses or other staff are authorized to baptize a baby. Hospital staff can also arrange for the baby's transfer to a funeral home. Caregivers, especially the midwife or labor nurse, often attend the funeral. If you have cared for the dyad, your attendance acknowledges the baby's importance and means a lot to families, even if they do not express their appreciation at the time.

Parents who lose a child may find comfort through altruistic acts such as organ donation, volunteer work, and charitable fundraising. Connection with others is important to their spiritual healing. Connecting with parents who experienced a similar loss can encourage them to express their feelings. Becoming involved in a support group can help them heal while they maintain a connection with their baby. They may benefit from professional counseling, available through local clergy and social service organizations. Even after a considerable lapse of time, parents may continue to need to express their loss. They benefit from the ongoing support they receive from other parents and professionals in a support group. Many support groups and organizations provide ongoing care for grieving parents (Camacho Ávila et al., 2020; Fernández-Basanta et al., 2020).

Summary

Members of the healthcare team caring for high-risk infants in the hospital and after discharge can help parents provide milk for their baby and make the transition to nursing. You can support parents as they work through their feelings related to this unexpected outcome. Your support helps parents develop realistic expectations and plan for their baby's nutrition, including expressing and storing their milk. Be available to support early nursing in the hospital and to guide parents through the transition of bringing their baby home. Compassion and experience will help you support parents who experience the loss of their infant, through either miscarriage, stillbirth, or neonatal death. Your participation in the healthcare team is critical in these special circumstances.

What You Learned—At a Glance

Conversation Starters with Parents

- How do you protect your milk production while you and your baby are separated?
- How are you and your partner managing with your baby being hospitalized?
- How are feedings going with your late preterm ... preterm ... postterm baby?
- How are you and your partner doing after your baby's death?
- What emotional support do you have to help you during this period?

Parents' Needs with a Hospitalized Infant

- Initiating and maintaining milk production
- Delay in nursing
- Worry about the baby's survival
- Feelings of guilt, loneliness, and anxiety
- Strain on the couple's relationship
- Desire for privacy and time alone with their baby

Milk for Babies Who Deliver Preterm

- Milk is higher in protein, sodium, chloride, nitrogen, and immunoprotective factors.
- HMFs—protein, calcium, potassium phosphate, carbohydrates, vitamins, and trace minerals—are used to supplement extremely preterm infants.
- Lactoengineering increases calories, carbohydrates, and proteins for preterm infants.
- HMFs made solely from human milk are commercially available for use in extremely preterm infants.

Counseling Preterm Parents in the Hospital

- Ask the baby's caregivers for explanations and clarification.
- Seek out sources of community support and resources.
- Provide gentle, warm, and loving touch.
- Express milk for the baby.
- Participate in feeding, bathing, and diapering the baby.
- Use skin-to-skin care with their infant.
- Encourage NNS on an emptied breast.

Counseling Preterm Parents at Home

- Learn hunger cues and infant responses that show signs of overstimulation.
- Plan for frequent feedings with long periods of rest.
- Stimulate letdown and manage fluctuations in milk production.
- Support the baby's jaw with the Dancer hand position.
- Monitor the baby's intake and weight.
- Base expectations on gestational age rather than age from birth.

Counseling Parents of Late Preterm Babies

- Plan for short, frequent feedings.
- Allow no longer than 3 hours between feedings during the day.
- Watch closely for subtle hunger cues.
- Use gentle waking techniques and plenty of skin-to-skin contact.
- Use a nipple shield as necessary.

Counseling Parents of Postterm Babies

- Baby may exhibit behaviors like a preterm baby.
- Baby may have respiratory issues, hypoglycemia, or hypothermia.
- Strategies for nursing the late preterm baby may work well.

Counseling Parents Who Lose a Baby

- Help them arrange time and privacy with their baby.
- Express your concern and sorrow.
- Use reflective listening and be available.
- Key into their needs and how often they would like to hear from you.
- Help them relieve fullness without stimulating more milk production.
- Refer them to a milk bank if they wish to donate their milk.
- Refer them to a support system and help them learn their rights and options.

References

Academy of Breastfeeding Medicine. ABM clinical protocol #12: transitioning the breastfeeding preterm infant from the neonatal intensive care unit to home, revised 2018. *Breastfeed Med.* 2018;13(4):230–236.

Adamkin DH. Use of human milk and fortification in the NICU. *J Perinatol.* 2023;43(5):551–559.

Al Salmi I, Hannawi S. Birth weight and susceptibility to chronic kidney disease. *Saudi J Kidney Dis Transpl.* 2020;31(4):717–726.

Alshaikh BN, et al. Hindmilk as a rescue therapy in very preterm infants with suboptimal growth velocity. *Nutrients.* 2023;15(4):929.

Altobelli E, et al. The impact of human milk on necrotizing enterocolitis: a systematic review and meta-analysis. *Nutrients.* 2020;12(5):1322.

Bakker L, et al. Oral-feeding guidelines for preterm neonates in the NICU: a scoping review. *J Perinatol.* 2021;41(1):140–149.

Beghetti I, et al. Human milk's hidden gift: implications of the milk microbiome for preterm infants' health. *Nutrients*. 2019;11(12).

Beken S, et al. Negative effects of noise on NICU graduates' cochlear functions. *Fetal Pediatr Pathol*. 2021;40(4):295–230.

Benzies KM. The health care system is making "too much noise" to provide family-centred care in neonatal intensive care units: perspectives of health care providers and hospital administrators. *Intensive Crit Care Nurs*. 2019;50:44–53.

Benzies KM, et al. Effectiveness of Alberta Family Integrated Care on infant length of stay in level II neonatal intensive care units: a cluster randomized controlled trial. *BMC Pediatrics*. 2020;20:1–11.

Boyle FM, et al. Clinical practice guidelines for perinatal bereavement care—an overview. *Women Birth*. 2020;33(2):107–110.

Brignoni-Pérez E, et al. Disparities in kangaroo care for premature infants in the neonatal intensive care unit. *J Dev Behav Pediatr*. 2022;43(5):e304–e311.

Camacho Ávila M, et al. Parents' experiences about support following stillbirth and neonatal death. *Adv Neonatal Care*. 2020;20(2):151–160.

Çamur Z, Çetinkaya B. The effects of oral feeding methods in preterm infants on transition to direct-breastfeeding and discharge time: a retrospective cohort design. *Clin Lact*. 2022;13(2).

Carpay NC, et al. Barriers and facilitators to breastfeeding in moderate and late preterm infants: a systematic review. *Breastfeed Med*. 2021;16(5):370–84.

Chaudhary P, et al. Effects of delayed cord clamping at different time intervals in late preterm and term neonates: a randomized controlled trial. *Eur J Pediatr*. 2023;182(8):3701–3711.

Darmstadt GL, et al. New World Health Organization recommendations for care of preterm or low birth weight infants: health policy. *EClinicalMedicine*. 2023;63:102155.

de Gamarra-Oca LF, et al. Long-term neurodevelopmental outcomes after moderate and late preterm birth: a systematic review. *J Pediatr*. 2021;237:168–176.

Dickinson C, et al. Psychological impact of neonatal intensive care unit admissions on parents: a regional perspective. *Aust J Rur Health*. 2022;30(3):373–384.

Dong D, et al. A prospective cohort study on lactation status and breastfeeding challenges in mothers giving birth to preterm infants. *Int Breastfeed J*. 2022;17:1–13.

El-Khuffash A, et al. Preventing disease in the 21st century: early breast milk exposure and later cardiovascular health in premature infants. *Pediatric Research*. 2020;87(2):385–390.

Ericson J, et al. Breastfeeding and risk for ceasing in birth parents of preterm infants—long-term follow-up. *Matern Child Nutr*. 2018;14(4):e12618.

Falkenburg JL, et al. The importance of parental connectedness and relationships with healthcare professionals in end-of-life care in the PICU. *Pediatr Crit Care Med*. 2018;19(3):e157–e163.

Fang L, et al. Is preterm donor milk better than preterm formula for very-low-birth-weight infants? *Food Nutr Res*. 2021;65.

Feenstra MM, et al. "Dad—a practical guy in the shadow": fathers' experiences of their paternal role as a father during early discharge after birth and readmission of their newborns. *Sex Reprod Healthc*. 2018;15:62–68.

Fernández-Basanta S, et al. Multicultural coping experiences of parents following perinatal loss: a meta-ethnographic synthesis. *J Adv Nurs*. 2020;76(1):9–21.

Flint A, et al. Cup feeding versus other forms of supplemental enteral feeding for newborn infants unable to fully breastfeed. *Cochrane Database Syst Rev*. 2016;(8):CD005092.

Garg PM, et al. Clinical impact of NEC-associated sepsis on outcomes in preterm infants. *Pediatr Res*. 2022;92(6): 1705–1715.

Garofalo NA, Caplan MS. Oropharyngeal birth parent's milk: state of the science and influence on necrotizing enterocolitis. *Clin Perinatol*. 2019;46(1):77–88.

Gianni ML, et al. Maternal views on facilitators of and barriers to breastfeeding preterm infants. *BMC Pediatr*. 2018; 18(1):283.

Govindaswamy P, et al. Needs and stressors of parents of term and near-term infants in the NICU: a systematic review with best practice guidelines. *Early Hum Dev*. 2019;139:104839.

Granger CL, et al. Maternal breastmilk, infant gut microbiome and the impact on preterm infant health. *Acta Paediatrica*. 2021;10(2):450–457.

Grunberg VA, et al. Infant illness severity and family adjustment in the aftermath of NICU hospitalization. *Infant Ment Health J*. 2020;41(3):340–355.

Gupta M, et al. Preparing for discharge from the neonatal intensive care unit. *Pediatrics*, 2019;143(6).

Hale T, Krutsch K. *Hale's Medications & Mothers' Milk 2025–2026: A Manual of Lactational Pharmacology*. 21st ed. New York, NY: Springer Publishing Company; 2024.

Hall EM, et al. Development of postpartum depression interventions for birth parents of premature infants: a call to target low-SES NICU families. *J Perinatol*. 2020;40(1):1–9.

Hall SL, et al. Improving staff knowledge and attitudes toward providing psychosocial support to NICU parents through an online education course. *Adv Neonatal Care*. 2019;19(6):490–499.

Hand to Hold. Fragile babies. Family support. 2025. https://handtohold.org/

Hasenstab KA, Jadcherla, SR. Evidence-based approaches to successful oral feeding in infants with feeding difficulties. *Clinics Perinatol*. 2022;49(2):503–520.

Healthy Children. Corrected age for preemies. 2018. https://www.healthychildren.org/English/ages-stages/baby/preemie/Pages/Corrected-Age-For-Preemies.aspx

Holdren S, et al. A qualitative cross-cultural analysis of NICU care culture and infant feeding in Finland and the U.S. *BMC Pregnancy Childbirth*. 2019;19(1):345.

İnal S, et al. Comparison of effect of feeding premature infants with either cup, bottle, and syringe on transition to breastfeeding, breastfeeding success, weight gain, and duration of hospitalization. *Breastfeed Med*. 2023;18(8):586–595.

Isayama T. The clinical management and outcomes of extremely preterm infants in Japan: past, present, and future. *Transl Pediatr*. 2019;8(3):199–211.

John HB. Nonnutritive Sucking at the mother's breast facilitates oral feeding skills in premature infants: a pilot study. *Adv Neonatal Care*. 2019;19(2):110–117.

Karnati S, et al. Late preterm infants—changing trends and continuing challenges. *Int J Pediatr*. 2020;7(1):38–46.

Knake LA, et al. Optimizing the use of human milk cream supplement in very preterm infants: growth and cost outcomes. *Nutr Clin Pract*. 2020;35(4):689–696.

Kochen EM, et al. When a child dies: a systematic review of well-defined parent-focused bereavement interventions and their alignment with grief-and loss theories. *BMC Palliat Care*. 2020;19(1):28.

Kortekaas JC, et al. Risk of adverse pregnancy outcomes of late- and postterm pregnancies in advanced maternal age: a national cohort study. *AOGS*. 2020;99(8):1022–1030.

Krick JA, et al. Living with the unknown: a qualitative study of parental experience of prognostic uncertainty in the neonatal intensive care unit. *Am J Perinatol.* 2021;38(8):821–827.

Kucukoglu S, et al. The effect of kangaroo care on breastfeeding and development in preterm neonates. *J Pediatr Nurs.* 2021;60:e31–38.

Kwok TC, et al. Early enteral feeding in preterm infants. *Semin Perinatol.* 2019;43(7):151159.

Lapidaire, W, et al. Human milk feeding and cognitive outcome in preterm infants: the role of infection and NEC reduction. *Pediatric Research.* 2022;91(5):1207–1214.

Li XL, et al. Breastfeeding promotion strategies study on preterm infants in the neonatal intensive care unit. *Beijing Da Xue Bao Yi Xue Ban.* 2019;51(4):711–715.

Louis K, White A. Impact of kangaroo care on caregivers in the NICU: an integrative review. *Pediatr Nurs.* 2023;49(4).

Maastrup R, Neo-BFHI Survey Group. Compliance with the "Baby-Friendly Hospital Initiative for neonatal wards" in 36 countries. *Matern Child Nutr.* 2019;15(2):e12690.

Maastrup R, et al. Improved exclusive breastfeeding rates in preterm infants after a neonatal nurse training program focusing on six breastfeeding-supportive clinical practices. *PLoS One.* 2021;16(2):e0245273.

Maastrup R, et al. The Baby-Friendly Hospital Initiative for neonatal wards. A mini review. *Acta Paediatrica.* 2022;111(4):750–755.

Mackay LJ, et al. A scoping review of parental experiences caring for their hospitalised medically fragile infants. *Acta Paediatr.* 2020;109(2):266–275.

March of Dimes. NICU Family Support®. 2025 https://www.marchofdimes.org/our-work/nicu-family-support

Martín-Calvo N, et al. Low birth weight and small for gestational age are associated with complications of childhood and adolescence obesity: systematic review and meta-analysis. *Obes Rev.* 2022;23:e13380.

Mayhew KJ, et al. Elevated sound levels in the neonatal intensive care unit: what is causing the problem? *Adv Neonatal Care.* 2022;22(6):e207–e216.

Mazumder S, et al. Effect of community-initiated kangaroo birth parent care on survival of infants with low birthweight: a randomised controlled trial. *The Lancet*, 2019;394(10210):1724.

Mehrpisheh S, et al. The effectiveness of kangaroo mother care (KMC) on attachment of mothers with premature infants. *Eur J Obstet Gynecol Reprod Biol X.* 2022;15:100149.

Miller J, et al. Clinician-family relationships may impact neonatal intensive care: clinicians' perspectives. *J Perinatol.* 2021;41(9):2208–2216.

Montealegre-Pomar A, et al. Systematic review and meta-analysis suggest that kangaroo position protects against apnoea of prematurity. *Acta Paediatr.* 2020;109(7):1310–1316.

Naja F, et al. Prenatal breastfeeding knowledge, attitude and intention, and their associations with feeding practices during the first six months of life: a cohort study in Lebanon and Qatar. *Int Breastfeed J.* 2022;17(1):15.

National Institute of Child Health and Human Development. Betamethasone. Drugs and Lactation Database (LactMed®). Updated May 15, 2023. https://www.ncbi.nlm.nih.gov/books/NBK501171/

O'Callaghan N, et al. Evidence-based design for neonatal units: a systematic review. *Matern Health Neonatol Perinatol.* 2019;5:6.

Ochandorena-Acha M, et al. Experiences and coping strategies of preterm infants' parents and parental competences after early physiotherapy intervention: qualitative study. *Physiother Theory Pract.* 2022;38(9):1174–1187.

October T, et al. Caring for parents after the death of a child. *Pediatr Crit Care Med.* 2018;19(8S suppl 2):S61–S68.

Orr E, et al. Providers' perspectives of the neonatal intensive care unit context and care provision for adolescent parents: an interpretive description. *BMC Pregnancy Childbirth.* 2023;23(1):259.

Pados BF, McGlothen-Bell K. Benefits of infant massage for infants and parents in the NICU. *WHNP.* 2019;23(3):265–271.

Panchal H, et al. Oropharyngeal colostrum for preterm infants: a systematic review and meta-analysis. *Adv Nutr.* 2019;10(6):1152–1162.

Parker MG, et al. Promoting human milk and breastfeeding for the very low birth weight infant. *Pediatrics.* 2021;148(5).

Penny F, et al. Cup feeding as a supplemental, alternative feeding method for preterm breastfed infants: an integrative review. *Matern Child Health J.* 2018;22:1568–1579.

Phillips R, et al. Breastfeeding Practice Before Bottle-Feeding: An Initiative to increase the rate of breastfeeding for preterm infants at the time of neonatal intensive care unit discharge. *Crit Care Clin.* 2024;36(2):251–260.

Pineda R, et al. Non-nutritive sucking in the preterm infant. *Am J Perinatol.* 2019;36(3):268–276.

Raghuveer TS, Zackula R. Strategies to prevent severe retinopathy of prematurity: a 2020 update and meta-analysis. *Neoreviews.* 2020;21(4):e249–e263.

Sacchi C, et al. Association of intrauterine growth restriction and small for gestational age status with childhood cognitive outcomes: a systematic review and meta-analysis. *JAMA Pediatr.* 2020;174(8):772–781.

Samane S, et al. Cue-based feeding and short-term health outcomes of premature infants in newborn intensive care units: a non-randomized trial. *BMC Pediatr.* 2022;22(1):23.

Sankar MN, et al. Barriers to optimal breast milk provision in the neonatal intensive care unit. *J Perinatol.* 2022;42(8):1076–1082.

Schecter R, et al. Prevalence and Longevity of PTSD symptoms among parents of NICU infants analyzed across gestational age categories. *Clin Pediatr (Phila).* 2020;59(2):163–169.

Sharma D, et al. Late preterm: a new high risk group in neonatology. *J Matern-Fetal Neonatal Med.* 2021;34(16):2717–2730.

Smith VC, et al. NICU discharge preparation and transition planning: guidelines and recommendations. *J Perinatol.* 2022;42(1):7–21.

Society for Maternal-Fetal Health. (2025). Executive actions updates. https://www.smfm.org/#

Sokou R, et al. Breastfeeding in neonates admitted to an NICU: 18-month follow-up. *Nutrients.* 2022;14(18), 3841.

Stanford School of Medicine. Newborn Nursery at LPCH. Early hand expression increases later milk production. *Morton J.* 2020a. http://newborns.stanford.edu/Breastfeeding/Hand Expression.html

Stanford School of Medicine. Newborn Nursery at LPCH. Maximizing milk production with hands-on pumping. *Morton J.* 2020b. http://newborns.stanford.edu/Breastfeeding/Max Production.html

Stoll, K, et al. Beyond medically complex pregnancy: a scoping review to understand how complexity in pregnancy is conceptualized. *JMWH.* 2023;68(1):71–83.

Suzuki K. The developing world of DOHaD. *J Dev Orig Health Dis.* 2018;9(3):266–269.

Tambani E, et al. Exploring the gap between needs and practice in facilitating breastfeeding within the neonatal intensive care setting: an Italian survey on organizational factors. *Front Pediatr.* 2019;7:276.

The Joint Commission. Specification Manual for Joint Commission National Quality Measure (v2024A1). 2024. https://manual.jointcommission.org/releases/TJC2024A1/DataElem0265.html

Thompson MT. Kangaroo care to improve respiratory function in preterm infants: a literature review. *J Neonat Nurs.* 2024;30(3):109–118.

Toivonen M, et al. Key factors supporting implementation of a training program for neonatal family-centered care—a qualitative study. *BMC Health Serv Res.* 2019;19(1):394.

Toivonen M, et al. Close collaboration with parents intervention improves family-centered care in different neonatal unit contexts: a pre–post study. *Pediatr Res.* 2020;88(3):421–428.

Tandberg BS, et al. Practices supporting cue-based breastfeeding of preterm infants in neonatal intensive care units across Europe. *Int Breastfeed J.* 2025;20(1):2.

Villamor-Martinez E, et al. Association of chorioamnionitis with bronchopulmonary dysplasia among preterm infants: a systematic review, meta-analysis, and metaregression. *JAMA Netw Open.* 2019;2(11):e1914611.

Wener E, et al. Evaluation of methods of breast or bottle feeding on length of hospitalization of preterm infants. *Breastfeed Med.* 2021;16(11):899–903.

World Health Organization. Preterm birth. Fact sheet N 363. Updated February 19, 2018a. http://www.who.int /mediacentre/factsheets/fs363/en/

World Health Organization. *Survive and Thrive: Transforming Care for Every Small and Sick Newborn.* Geneva, Switzerland: World Health Organization; 2018b. https://www.who.int/maternal_child_adolescent/documents/care-small-sick-newborns-survive-thrive/en/

World Health Organization. WHO advises immediate skin to skin care for survival of small and preterm infants. 2022. https://www.who.int/news/item/15-11-2022-who-advises-immediate-skin-to-skin-care-for-survival-of-small-and-preterm-babies

World Health Organization. Donor human milk for low-birth-weight infants. Updated August 9, 2023. https://www.who.int/tools/elena/interventions/donormilk-infants

Wu HP, et al. Integration of different sensory interventions from birth parent's breast milk for preterm infant pain during peripheral venipuncture procedures: a prospective randomized controlled trial. *J Nurs Scholarsh.* 2020;52(1):75–84.

Xiong T, et al. An overview of systematic reviews of randomized-controlled trials for preventing necrotizing enterocolitis in preterm infants. *Neonatology.* 2020;17(1):1–11.

Yang Y, et al. Breastfeeding experiences and perspectives on support among Chinese birth parents separated from their hospitalized preterm infants: a qualitative study. *Int Breastfeed J.* 2019;14:45.

CHAPTER 25

When Nursing Is Interrupted

Ideally, nursing parents and babies are together throughout the lactation period. However, the reality for most parents is that at some point while nursing, they will be separated from their baby. A separation may be for a few hours or a few days; it may be temporary or long-term; it may be planned or unexpected. The parent may return to work or school or require hospitalization. Parents may be able to plan the time away around the baby's feeding schedule, or they may need to pump and leave milk for a caregiver. Regardless of the length of the separation or the reason, nursing parents need support and encouragement for managing feedings and maintaining milk production.

KEY TERMS

Antibodies	COVID-19	Reverse-cycle nursing

Managing Nursing During Separations

Separation from their baby can create stress and anxiety for new parents.It is especially stressful when the separation is unexpected, for example, as the result of illness. You can help relieve some of the anxieties by providing information and supporting parents' decisions concerning feedings. Parents who combine nursing with a daily or prolonged separation benefit from information about expressing milk and maintaining milk production. You can help them obtain a pump and offer practical suggestions for its use. A strong sense of commitment and motivation will help them overcome potential difficulties and pressures.

Parents' Needs

Separation from their baby is especially challenging when feedings are missed. Attitudes of family members, childcare arrangements, and time management all factor into finding a comfortable rhythm to their new routine. The greatest needs will be maintaining milk production and feeding the baby during the separation. Milk must be expressed regularly to relieve fullness and maintain production. You can help by ensuring that parents know how to hand express and use a breast pump to remove milk during missed feedings. In addition, parents may need guidance in finding a feeding method their baby will accept for nourishment during the absence.

Parents may experience conflicting emotions about continuing to nurse through the separation.

Effective use of counseling skills will help you listen and respond to their concerns about the cause of the separation, especially if the baby is hospitalized. This time can be challenging and stressful for families. Your support and encouragement are critical to their success.

Timing of the Separation

Parents often have no control over the timing of a separation. For example, limited or no paid leave from their employer may require an early return to work. A parent may need to return to school soon after giving birth. An unexpected hospitalization can occur for either the parent or baby. Ideally, the parent will be able to delay the separation until their milk production is well established. However, this is not always possible.

Barring any interference or health condition, milk production and nursing are well established for most parents by the time the baby is 2 months old. Waiting until this time makes the separation and maintenance of milk production easier to manage. The transition is even smoother if a separation is delayed until about 6 months, when the baby is old enough to begin eating complementary foods. At that time, there is less need for supplemental feedings when the parent is not present.

Maintaining Milk Production

Milk production may diminish somewhat when the separation is substantial. The key to maintaining production at the level that meets the baby's needs is to remove milk to trigger further production. Many parents who are away from their babies on a regular basis manage to establish a pumping routine that fits their schedule, typically at times when the baby would nurse if they were together. Some parents prefer to express only enough milk to relieve discomfort, allowing production to diminish slightly and feeding their babies infant formula rather than expressed milk during their absence. Remember, milk expression cannot remove milk from the breasts as effectively as the sucking of a healthy baby.

Nourishing the Baby

Parents who are away from their baby during feeding times must arrange for the baby's nourishment until they return. If they do not have sufficient expressed milk, the baby may need to be supplemented with donor milk or formula. A baby who is old enough to receive complementary foods (6 months and older) will not need as much expressed milk during the absence.

Practicing alternate feeding methods for at least 2 weeks before a planned separation helps the baby accept a feeding method other than nursing. Ensuring this before the separation helps to decrease stress for both the parents and caregiver. Cup feeding may be a good option for short-term supplementary feedings. Feeding the baby with a cup eliminates the possibility of nipple preference with a bottle. Although it can be more time-consuming than bottle feeding, cup feeding does have advantages if the caregiver is able to spend the extra time.

Bottle feeding is often a more convenient method for feeding the baby when long-term supplementation is required. Parents may need to try more than one type of nipple to learn which works best for their baby. A nipple that encourages the baby's mouth to open wide may accommodate the transitions back and forth from nursing to bottle feeding more easily for a young baby. Many babies accomplish a wide gape with a nipple that has a large base. However, some babies tend to clamp down on the nipple at the narrowest part and do not take the bottle in down to the wide base. The key factor for many babies is the rate of flow rather than the type of nipple. Be aware that even "slow-flow" nipples will drip milk. Slowing down bottle feedings, or paced feeding, will allow the baby to follow their satiety cues, and they will be less likely to overfeed. Refer to **Chapter 22** for more information on nipple selection and paced feeding.

Motivation to Continue Nursing

Anticipating a separation from their baby can cause parents to reevaluate their nursing goals. Some parents believe they must wean when a separation occurs. Motivation and determination are critical factors for continuing to nurse and express milk despite separation from the baby. You can assure parents that lactation is compatible with any length of separation. If a parent's commitment to nursing wavers, they might use the separation as a natural time to wean their baby. If weaning occurs, you can encourage parents to focus on the quality of the nursing relationship and all the benefits the baby received rather than the duration.

Parents who want to continue nursing may feel discouraged or frustrated when faced with a separation. Open-ended questions and reflective listening will help parents explore their situation, identify options, and validate choices. By assessing their motives and tailoring any interventions accordingly, you can help parents achieve their desired outcomes. Whether they decide to continue nursing or to wean, parents who are dealing with separation from their baby benefit from lots of nonjudgmental anticipatory guidance, emotional support, and practical suggestions.

Coping with Difficulties

A separation between parent and baby can create physical consequences related to lactation, as well as emotional tension and anxiety. Milk must be expressed regularly to avoid leaking, engorgement, lowered milk production, and mastitis. Hand expression or pumping does not remove milk as efficiently as the baby does. Thus, despite being diligent in expressing milk, problems may still occur.

If the baby is hospitalized, traveling back and forth to the hospital may tax the parents' energy reserves. Returning to work, school, or other responsibilities can be exhausting as well. Urge parents to pay close attention to self-care, including getting enough rest. This is especially important if the separation is due to the parent's illness. Sometimes parents need "permission" to rest because of the demands on their time. You can encourage them to take regular short, quiet rest periods. Parents need to be mindful of their food intake as well. Skimping nutrition can affect their health as well as milk production. Reminding parents to drink water before or during milk expression serves as a reminder of the importance of remaining well hydrated.

Many parents experience a sense of guilt about a separation, regardless of whether it is planned or optional. At times, a baby may demonstrate a strong desire to remain with the parent. At other times, the baby may appear to reject the parent and seem more attached to the caregiver. This can be either a source of comfort to parents or a source of jealousy and anxiety. You can help parents cope with their feelings by supporting them during the separation as well as when they and the baby reunite and resume nursing.

After the Separation

Milk production varies widely, and some parents are more sensitive to fluctuations in milk removal than others. If a separation results in a decline in milk production, hand expression or pumping can increase production again. Feeding the expressed milk through a tube-feeding device during nursing can further increase production from the sucking stimulation. Galactagogues can help boost milk production as well.

Table 25-1 Counseling Issues When Separated from the Baby

Concern	Suggestions
Overfullness or leaking	■ Express milk during the absence. ■ Wear breast pads when away. ■ Nurse directly before and after the absence.
Low milk production	■ Delay the separation until milk production is well established (around 2 months) if possible. ■ Practice milk expression well in advance of separation to achieve efficiency and know what method works best. ■ Drink to thirst. ■ Nurse frequently when with the baby.
Feeding the baby	■ Have the caregiver feed the baby expressed milk or formula. ■ Use a cup to avoid bottles if nipple preference is a concern. ■ Practice alternate feedings before the separation to make sure the baby will accept the method.

The baby may need supplemental feedings for a while until milk production increases sufficiently. Arranging for help with daily activities can allow more time to focus on nursing and reconnecting with the baby. Refer to the suggestions in **Chapter 22** for getting the baby back to nursing. **Table 25-1** presents counseling suggestions for when the nursing dyad is separated.

Short-Term Separations

Most parents will have short-term separations from their babies during a usual feeding time at some point while nursing. Breaks from the routine and minutiae of baby care can be good for a new parent's mental health. A brief time away can strike a compromise between stay-at-home parenting and attending to outside interests such as schooling, part-time work, volunteer work, sports, exercise classes, or other activities. Other responsibilities may necessitate a short absence as well, such as healthcare provider appointments or attending functions for family members. Parents may wish to plan an evening out, run errands, or spend "adult time" with a friend. They may time outings to avoid missed feedings or take the baby with them. For occasions when the baby stays home, the baby can receive expressed milk.

Some parents express milk in the morning and throughout the day for several days before a planned separation, storing the milk in the refrigerator or freezer. If they become uncomfortably full or experience leaking while away, they can express milk for comfort and to avoid overfullness. They can hand express or carry a handheld pump for that purpose. Many pumps have car adapters for use while on the go. **Table 25-2** offers counseling suggestions for planning a hospitalization.

Table 25-2 Preparing for Hospitalization

Points to Consider	Suggestions
Explore options	■ Learn if there is an alternative to hospitalization. ■ Request a second opinion. ■ Learn if hospitalization can be delayed until the baby is older and milk production is established. ■ Learn whether early discharge is possible if home nursing care is arranged. Explore local home healthcare options.
Be assertive	■ Discuss wishes with healthcare provider to avoid separation or to minimize missed feedings. ■ Examine hospital policies concerning rooming-in and the use of hospital breast pumps.
Become well informed	■ Learn about hospital procedures and factors surrounding hospitalization. ■ Review informed consent, as discussed in **Chapter 4**. ■ Contact local and online resource groups.
Keep clear, organized records	■ Record childcare and travel expenses for income tax deductions, and breast pump rental expense for possible insurance reimbursement. ■ Provide details of your care plan to your healthcare provider and the hospital.
Prepare for transportation to and from the hospital	■ Arrange for someone to drive you to and from the hospital and to remain with you if possible.

When the Nursing Parent Is Ill

When a nursing parent contracts an infection such as a cold, fever, or more serious illness, **antibodies** in their milk help protect their baby. Although some viruses are transmitted through human milk, in most cases, the presence of antibodies offsets any potential harm to the baby. The more likely mechanism of disease transmission from parent to baby is through touching and close face-to-face contact, not through the milk.

When a parent becomes ill, exposure to their baby has already occurred through contact during the most contagious period, often before the parent was symptomatic. Therefore, a parent who develops a cold or fever does not need to worry about infecting their baby through their milk. The most effective treatment is for the baby to continue to nurse while the parent recovers from the illness and, if necessary, takes medications.

Reducing Transmission

Parents can reduce the risk of disease transmission to their baby by washing their hands with soap and water before nursing. If soap and water are not available, they can use an alcohol-based hand sanitizer. They should avoid coughing or sneezing in the baby's face, and if possible, restrict baby care to family members who are healthy. If there is no one else to care for the baby, wearing a face mask will help protect the baby. The parent should cover their mouth and nose when coughing or sneezing. Parents also need to take care of themselves, including getting rest, eating nutritious foods, and following any treatment plan prescribed by their healthcare provider.

Influenza and Other Outbreaks

It is important that parents continue to nurse their babies during seasonal influenza and other outbreaks such as **COVID-19**. The risk of transmission to the newborn is through droplet exposure to the baby's mucosal surfaces during coughing, sneezing, or talking while in close contact, not through the milk. Antibodies in the milk provide immunologic protection to the infant against infection for both seasonal influenza strains and severe acute respiratory syndrome coronavirus 2 (SARS-CoV-2; the virus that causes COVID-19) (American Academy of Pediatricians [AAP], 2023). If the infant does get ill, the respiratory symptoms are less severe for exclusively nursing infants (AAP, 2023).

Current recommendations for infectious diseases spread by droplet transmission during close contact include continuing to nurse or provide expressed milk. In addition, wearing a mask and washing hands with soap and water (or using hand sanitizer when soap and water is not available) before handling the infant are advised (AAP, 2023; CDC, 2024a). Precautions for parents with COVID-19 infections can be discontinued once the parent is fever-free for 48 hours or it has been 10 days since the onset of symptoms (CDC, 2024b). It is important to regularly check for updates on recommendations for nursing and infectious diseases. More information about nursing during an illness can be found in **Chapter 26**.

Hospitalization of the Nursing Parent

In most cases, a nursing parent hospitalized because of illness or injury can continue to feed their baby their milk, provided they are not on medications that could be harmful to the baby. Healthcare providers can refer to LactMed, *Hale's Medications & Mothers' Milk 2025–2026* (Hale & Krutsch, 2024), or InfantRisk.com to determine the safety of a medication. Parents can ask to be assigned to an area of the hospital that accommodates rooming-in with their baby (they may need an adult in the room to help care for the baby). If rooming-in is not possible, they might arrange for someone to bring the baby to the hospital intermittently throughout the day to nurse.

The Parent's Needs

If a parent is physically unable to nurse, hospital staff can be instrumental in helping them maintain milk production. Knowledge about lactation, acceptable medications, and milk expression and storage will enable them to help the parent sustain nursing. Failing to address these needs can lead to mastitis or a breast abscess. If the parent is having a long surgery or is incapacitated afterward, the hospital staff should be trained in the use a breast pump to express the parent's milk. Interdepartmental knowledge; collaboration with perinatal healthcare providers; and support of nursing in areas such as medical, surgical, and emergency departments, provide critical continuity of care. **Figure 25-1** offers suggestions on how staff can assist hospitalized nursing families.

Parents report fear, wanting to know about the baby, worrying about their partner, needing someone to talk to, and feeling unprepared for what to expect in the hospital. They want to be in control and to be together as a family. Healthcare providers need to give continuous updates to the parent about their status, keep them informed about their baby, and enable the family to be together as much as the parent's condition allows. A parent who develops severe mastitis or an abscess and decides to wean should recover from the mastitis before initiating weaning. They will need to continue to express milk during the course of the mastitis (Academy of Breastfeeding Medicine [ABM], 2022).

- Encourage rest, good nutrition, and hydration.
- Support efforts to nurse and reinforce the benefits for the parent and baby.
- Provide privacy as needed.
- Assist the parent with protecting any surgical site during feedings.
- Encourage the parent to take postoperative analgesia to alleviate pain.
- Promote good handwashing, limited contact with the infant's face, and continued nursing as the best ways to prevent transfer of infection from parent to infant.
- Reassure the parent when medications and procedures have been investigated and it is determined that nursing will not harm the infant. If medications are contraindicated, research acceptable alternatives and work with primary caregiver. If the contraindicated medications must be used, help the parent initiate pumping to protect milk production.

Figure 25-1 Staff assistance for hospitalized nursing parents.

Challenges for the Parent

Many parents continue to nurse throughout hospitalizations or chronic illnesses. However, continuing to nurse through a complicated medical situation may not be the best choice for every parent. If nursing would compromise the parent's condition or if they find it difficult to cope, pumping or weaning may be better alternatives. Support families to make the choices that are best for their health and the health of their baby on an individual, family-by-family basis.

Although a medical condition can make nursing or caring for the baby challenging, advance planning, when possible, is helpful. Some parents know in advance of their delivery that they will need surgery soon after having the baby (e.g., gallbladder or appendix removal). Obtaining a preoperative list of the anesthesia and medications they will receive will identify the safety measures to be taken for their baby. Parents benefit from help in planning for the hospitalization, managing nursing or milk expression during the hospital stay, and obtaining support at home.

Hospitalization of the Baby

Having a hospitalized baby is always stressful for parents. A baby may remain hospitalized for a prolonged period after birth or may return to the hospital because of complications, a contagious illness, or injury. Traveling back and forth to the hospital can be exhausting for parents, especially if the hospitalization occurs directly after the birth. If the baby is in a high-risk center, parents can inquire about a transfer to a facility closer to home after the baby's condition has stabilized. This may depend on whether it is allowed by the insurance carrier or the local hospital system or health authorities.

Staying with the Baby

Parents who wish to remain with their babies throughout the hospitalization can inquire about rooming-in policies. Most major hospitals have corporate or charity-sponsored housing available, such as a Ronald McDonald House or family rooms. Hospitals designed with families in mind allow parents to share a room with their child. Most often, it is safe for parents to room-in with the baby, and they can request this option. If the baby has a contagious illness, they may be isolated from other babies in a special isolation room.

Nursing the Baby

Nursing is an effective analgesic for painful procedures, such as heel sticks (Aydin & İnal, 2019). Parents can discuss options with their healthcare provider for nursing during such procedures. A baby who must undergo surgery will benefit from the parent's presence immediately before and after the procedure.

Healthcare providers generally request that nothing be consumed within 8 hours preceding surgery. However, because human milk digests so quickly, a baby may become hungry by the time of surgery if not permitted to feed closer to surgery than formula fed infants are. Babies are often able to continue nursing exclusively without interruption. Guidelines for infants and children recommend allowing clear fluids up to 2 hours before surgery, human milk up to 4 hours before surgery, and formula and solids up to 6 hours before surgery (ASA, 2023).

If the parent needs to pump to maintain milk production, they can ask about using a hospital breast pump so that they can express milk regularly during the baby's stay. If the baby cannot receive the expressed milk, pumping is still important to maintain milk production.

Pain Relief

A pacifier may be used as a comfort measure before surgery. Because pacifiers generate saliva, parents need to discuss this with the anesthesiologist. An alternative measure is to nurse the baby on an emptied breast. However, because some milk is always present, this should also be discussed with the anesthesiologist. Parents can also ask to be with the baby in the recovery room, although hospital policy may preclude this option. The ABM (2012) recommends nursing immediately after a procedure to increase comfort and reduce pain, even following cleft lip and palate repairs.

After the Hospitalization

Parents will benefit from frequent contact and support after they return home with their baby. They may need to increase milk production if nursing was interrupted during the hospitalization. If the separation was for an extended period, they may need to relactate. Even if the baby was able to nurse during the hospitalization, they may need help reestablishing their nursing routine. In addition, the concern about the situation that precipitated the hospitalization does not necessarily subside when they get home. Parents may appreciate having a compassionate, concerned listener to help them talk through their emotions.

Regular Separations

Successfully combining nursing with regular separations is a common concern for families. Many parents face regular separations from their baby because of a return to work. The information in this section may also be modified for use in other situations when parents and babies are separated. For example, a young parent may continue to nurse when they return to school to finish their education. A parent who is incarcerated may wish to nurse or provide their milk for their baby. A parent may be involved in a child custody dispute that affects their ability to nurse without interruption.

Supporting Working Parents

Working parents are challenged with balancing their professional roles with their expanded family roles. They typically put in a double day, fulfilling job requirements and meeting the needs of their children. To compound the issue, women in many parts of the world work in occupations with low pay, long hours, and lack of social or union protection (Snyder et al., 2018).

The number of women in the workforce is increasing throughout the world. Women make up 55% of the global workforce (International Labour Organization [ILO], 2025). Thus, parents are a significant segment of the workforce, and most parents with young children work outside the home. Part-time work, lack of lengthy separations from their babies, supportive work environments, and childcare options can all help parents continue to nurse.

Societal and employer attitudes are pivotal in encouraging and supporting continued nursing for working parents. Healthcare providers have a unique opportunity to help them as well. They can help parents make informed decisions by being knowledgeable and up to date about breast pumps, expression and storage of milk, and local resources to support nursing parents. Employers can ensure a supportive work environment by providing a private lactation space for milk expression, providing time for expressing milk or nursing, and a comprehensive lactation support program.

Lactation Rates for Working Parents

Parents who work outside the home initiate nursing at the same rate as parents who stay at home. However, continuation rates decline sharply (Riaz & Condon, 2019; Tampah-Naah et al., 2019). The likelihood of continuing nursing is higher for parents who hold professional jobs, have graduate degrees, do not have significant nursing problems, and have family or friends who nursed their babies. However even parents who are healthcare professionals and embrace the health importance of nursing and human milk feeding find it hard to continue nursing their own children when they return to work (Pesch et al., 2019). Parents with a parental leave of 6 months or less stop nursing sooner than those who return to work after 6 months or more (Rimes et al., 2019).

Societal Support

Online nonprofit and grassroots organizations such as mothersandmore.org, mops.org, and momsrising.org offer support, validation, and networking for employed parents. Media and online resources can aid nursing parents in advocating for their families and for flexible employment choices. Parents who are most vulnerable to economic discrimination and employer harassment may have low-income, nonnative, or illegal immigration status and may be unaware of resources.

Most countries provide parents a generous amount of time off after the birth of their baby. However, in the United States, only 15% of private industry, state, and local government employees receive paid family leave. Although the Family Medical Leave Act (FMLA) provides up to 12 weeks off for eligible workers, employers are not required to pay them, and most do not (Jagannathan, 2019). Advocacy and education can benefit and empower these parents to nurture their children while achieving more social and economic justice.

It is challenging to combine employment with long-term nursing in a culture that fails to support lactation. For some parents, a return to work is viewed as synonymous with weaning. Nursing needs to be supported in the context of parents' lives, including all their roles and activities. Employee leave of 6 weeks or less fails to provide the support necessary to accommodate lactation. Healthcare providers can advocate for extending paid postpartum leave and flexibility in working conditions.

The disparities and inequities in health care and social support are critical factors in nursing duration. In the United States, Black parents, who have lower nursing rates, are more likely than White parents to wean when they return to work (Johnson et al., 2015a, 2015b; Spencer et al., 2015). Many parents work in minimum-wage jobs without benefits and return to work within 6 weeks after birth. Despite laws that provide time to pump in the United States, many parents fear being terminated from employment or having their work hours reduced if they seek support for nursing or pumping from their employers (Lauer et al., 2019). Cultural support and protective national health policies related to employment, health, and early childhood can increase the rates of nursing in all employed parents, especially those historically underserved.

Maternity Benefits

In 2021, 82 countries failed to meet the ILO standards for the protection of maternity leave and parental rights in the workplace. Approximately 649 million women across the globe do not have adequate maternity benefits or protection (ILO, 2022). Paid maternity leave is provided in only 20 of 41 countries, with some type of leave for fathers in 34 countries. The United States is the only one among 41 nations that does not mandate paid leave for new parents (Livingston & Thomas, 2019). In times of global economic recession, some employees are afraid to take maternity leave for fear of losing their job (de Lauzon-Guillain et al., 2019). Partner presence and support have an important influence on nursing initiation and duration. Expanding employee protections for parental leave to include partners can have significant benefits for maternal and child health.

Employer Support

Awareness of nursing employees' rights and corporate actions to support lactation-friendly workplaces have increased over the past two decades. However, despite advancement and legal protections, many parents across the globe cite employment as a barrier to continuing nursing. Employers most frequently cite monetary reasons such as decreased productivity for not supporting parents to pump at work.

In 2015 the World Breastfeeding Week theme focused on accommodating nursing employees. The initiative called for multidimensional support for families from all sectors and for strengthening national legislation. It urged partnering with specific target groups, such as trade unions, worker rights organizations, and women's and youth groups, to protect the rights of nursing parents in the workplace (World Alliance for Breastfeeding Action, 2015). Two decades later there is still work to be done globally to protect the rights of nursing parents.

Employers play a critical role in employees' success with lactation after returning to work. The quality and level of workplace support have the potential to increase or decrease nursing rates among employees. The U.S. Office on Women's Health hosts an online resource to promote employer support for nursing employees and help them establish worksite lactation programs (U.S. Department of Health and Human Services [USDHHS], 2025).

Employee Awareness and Advocacy

Continuing to nurse after returning to work can be challenging for parents in all types of employment and in all socioeconomic demographics. Employees at all points in the economic spectrum may discover that their return to work is marked by resentment from colleagues or less favorable treatment by supervisors. Negative treatment can take the form of a lower position, job loss, verbal abuse, sexual harassment, or social isolation.

Employee awareness and education are needed among businesses and organizations offering lactation support. Employers need to clearly communicate their policies and services supporting lactation to all of their employees. Employees who plan to nurse need to learn prenatally about the services, including the location for milk expression and policies for working flexible hours and taking breaks to express their milk. All employees need to recognize the importance of accommodating nursing parents' needs while they are at work.

Some human resource departments provide holistic, well-organized leave packages for employees. Lactation support is highlighted among wellness programs, fitness centers, and other work–life balance offerings. These companies and organizations view lactation support as a marketing and competitive edge to attract and retain highly educated and motivated employees (MacMillan Uribe et al., 2019).

Childcare Arrangements

Access to quality child care is a crucial concern for employed parents. Exploring childcare options in their community will help parents make informed choices. Governmental child care is provided in many countries. Many childcare facilities train their staff in the correct handling of human milk and working with nursing families. Examples of innovative staff training materials and resource kits, including those modeled on the Ten Steps to Successful Breastfeeding, can be found on the CDC website (CDC, 2025).

When interviewing caregivers, parents can address the needs of their nursing baby, the care and use of expressed milk, and feeding methods compatible with nursing. It is important that both the parents and substitute caregivers are comfortable with the arrangement. Caution parents that weaning at the same time they begin daycare increases the risk of illness for the baby. Selecting a supportive caregiver will enable parents to continue to protect their baby with their expressed milk.

Feeding Options

You can help parents explore infant feeding options that will work for them. Parents who plan to send expressed milk for their baby while at child care will need information about breast pumps and begin to express and store milk before their baby starts child care (**Figure 25-2**). Some parents limit the amount of

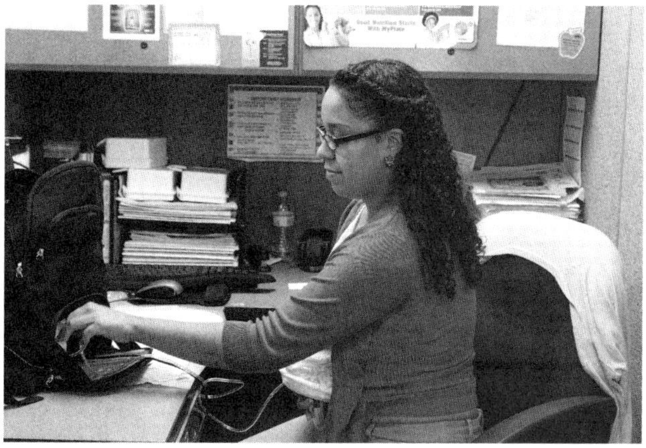

Figure 25-2 Parent pumping while at work.
Photo by Every Mother, Inc. and Regina Maria Roig-Romero.

expressed milk needed during their absence by manipulating their child's nursing cycle to provide most or all feedings at times when they are together. This is referred to as **reverse-cycle nursing**. Others may opt for their baby to receive infant formula during the separation and nurse when they are with their baby. These parents will need anticipatory guidance about mixed feeding.

Parents can provide written instructions related to the care of their milk and the baby's special preferences. They and the care provider can review the baby's feeding method and the importance of watching for signs of hunger so that the baby does not become overly hungry. Parents may want the baby held in the same position for feedings as when they nurse. However, some babies will not accept a bottle in the same position used for nursing and may do better when held in a different position.

When bottles are used, the baby needs to be in charge of drawing in the bottle nipple rather than having the caregiver control it. Parents can teach caregivers paced feeding, as described in **Chapter 22**, to avoid overfeeding and stress. If the feeding method is something other than a bottle, such as cup feeding, the caregiver should be trained and observed in feeding the baby with the alternate method.

Parents and care providers need to communicate closely about the amount of milk consumed at feedings and how the baby handles the feeding method and feedings in general. Avoiding a feeding too close to the time the parent is to arrive ensures that the baby is hungry and eager to nurse. This relieves the parent's breast fullness and facilitates reconnecting with their baby at the end of the day. If the baby seems especially hungry just before the parent's return, the caregiver can provide only a partial feeding. If the baby is cared for outside the home, parents may want a quiet place at the caregiver's to nurse when they arrive. Some parents prefer to drive home immediately to settle in with their baby. Still others prefer the baby to be fed before their arrival and will pump at home. These are all arrangements parents need to discuss with their caregiver.

Tips for Returning to Work or School

It is normal for parents to feel some apprehension when leaving their baby for the first time. Scheduling the first day back to work in the middle of the week may help parents feel less overwhelmed. If the return to work is a bit rocky, they and their baby will have more time to recoup and get ready for a full week the next week. Parents might also explore returning to work on a part-time initially, either in terms of days per week or hours per day, as well as telecommuting or online classes. Parents who return to school may not have much flexibility in the day they return.

Preparing for the Separation

About 2 to 3 weeks before their return, parents can begin planning for the baby's needs while they are separated. Packing a bag for both of them the night before the separation avoids a harried morning start and allows an opportunity to snuggle and nurse before beginning the day. As the parent becomes familiar with breast pump use or manual expression, your assistance can help them learn these techniques and increase their self-confidence. They can begin expressing on the unused side at the end of a feeding or express between feedings. In addition to practicing technique, this enables the parent to begin storing milk for their baby.

Parents can also practice with their chosen feeding method. Enlisting the help of another person familiar to the baby will increase the likelihood that the baby will be receptive to being fed by someone else. That helper can feed the expressed milk to encourage the baby to accept the new method of feeding. If using a bottle with an artificial nipple, warming the nipple to body temperature may make it more appealing to the baby. Occasionally, a baby will refuse any alternative method while the parent is nearby, so the parent may need to leave the room. It is also best not to try a new feeding method when the baby is too hungry to deal with something new and unfamiliar.

As parents become more proficient with expressing milk and the baby is more accepting of the new feeding method, they can do one or more trial runs with the baby's substitute care provider. They can begin to gradually ease into a feeding routine that mimics their work schedule. As they are in the midst of these intense changes, encourage them to keep open communication with those closest to them. Combining caring for a young baby with going to work requires adjustments in many areas. Housework and errands may become less of a priority as parents consider what must be done, what can wait, what can be streamlined for greater efficiency, and who is able to do it best.

Many resources are available for combining nursing with working or school. Online resources include social media sites, forums, and support groups, such as those on Facebook. Local breastfeeding support groups such as La Leche League often accommodate parents with evening, weekend, and virtual (online) meetings. Get to know the resources in your area and keep up to date with online support options.

Milk Expression

Parents will need to express milk regularly while away from the baby to maintain milk production and avoid excessive leaking, engorgement, and issues along the mastitis spectrum. After their return, they will learn where to fit milk expression into their daily routine. Ideally, they can work toward matching their pumping sessions to meet their baby's nutrition needs. At a minimum, they should respond to any uncomfortable fullness in their breasts.

If the baby is still quite young, the parent may find it best to express milk every 3 hours while away from the baby. With a double electric breast pump, about 10 to 15 minutes' pumping time is usually sufficient to stimulate milk production and remove the available milk. If they are using a single pump or hand expression, they will need about 20 minutes for the process. As the baby grows older, the time needed for pumping will decrease.

The parent will need a safe, private, comfortable space to express milk. Breast massage and, if possible, applying moist heat will help them relax and promote letdown before and during pumping. Having something that reminds the parent of their baby helps, too. It could be a recording of the baby's sounds, a picture, or even an article of clothing. Many parents use their smartphones or webcams to Skype with the caregiver, enabling them to see and talk to their baby in real time.

The expressed milk can be stored in quantities the baby will take at one feeding. Although initially this amount may be uncertain, the amount needed at a feeding becomes clearer as the parent and baby settle into their new routines. Freshly expressed milk can remain at room temperature safely for up to 6 hours (HMBANA, 2024). Regardless of the way the milk is stored, keeping it cooled on the commute home will preserve it safely for refrigeration after arriving home. Refer to **Chapter 22** for further discussion of collecting and storing expressed milk.

Comfort and Adjustment

Milk production can fluctuate as parents adjust to their new routine. This change could be a by-product of missed feedings as well as emotional swings associated with being separated from their baby. If they experience delays in expressing milk, their breasts can become uncomfortably full and may leak. Some parents keep a change of clothes with them for when leaking occurs. Prints rather than solid colors help to conceal breast fullness, leaks, or lopsidedness. Parents can also keep a jacket or sweater handy and wear breast pads to absorb leaked milk. Clothing needs to allow easy breast access for pumping, as well as for nursing the baby just before leaving for the day and when reuniting at the end of the day.

Routine At Home

The way parents spend their time at home with their baby is as important as their routine during the separation. Combining employment or education with caring for a young baby presents challenges, regardless of how the baby is fed. Planning quiet time with the baby and self-care as priorities over other demands can help parents deal with the pressures of the multiple demands. Nursing provides a unique and comforting way to reconnect at the beginning and the end of the day. The first feeding when returning home from a busy day provides a special time for the parent and baby to be alone with one another. It can help the parent relax and reconnect with their baby.

Some babies react to separations by increasing the frequency and duration of feedings when with the parent. This can further stimulate milk production. The more frequently a baby nurses when the dyad is together, the less frequently a parent will need to pump to maintain production.

Some parents reduce the need to express milk by encouraging their babies to reverse their nursing cycle so that more of their feedings occur at night. If a baby nurses more at night, keeping the baby close will minimize active wakefulness (i.e., the baby waking, fussing, and progressing to crying before the parent wakes and responds). This will allow the parent to get more rest during nighttime hours.

Interestingly, some parents who experience regular separations from their baby continue to nurse far longer than they originally planned. These parents benefit from the reassurance that extended nursing is a biologic norm, albeit not always a cultural one. You can recommend resources such as toddler nursing groups, social network support groups, and internet resources.

Employer Lactation Program

A concrete way employers can support nursing employees is by developing a coordinated lactation program that provides what the employees need for continuing to nurse. Extended paid maternity leave would allow the employee to remain at home with the baby for as long as possible. The employer can incorporate pumping breaks into the employee's work schedule or give employees the option of bringing the baby to work to avoid missed feedings. They can provide information about child care or, better yet, provide child care at or near the worksite. Some companies offer prenatal and postpartum programs for parents. Employers can also provide appropriate accommodations for employees to nurse or pump, as well as a policy of support among coworkers (**Figure 25-3**). **Table 25-3** describes three levels of support in an employer lactation program.

- Less illness among human milk fed children of employees.
- Reduced absenteeism to care for ill children (half the number of 1-day absences as with parents of infants not human milk fed).
- Higher employee morale and greater loyalty.
- Higher retention rates.
- Estimated return on investment (ROI) of $3 savings for every $1 invested in support of continued lactation.
- Improved employee productivity.
- Improved marketing ability to attract and retain valuable employees.
- Family-friendly, work-life balance, public image.

Figure 25-3 Benefits of workplace lactation programs to employers.

Table 25-3 Components of a Worksite Lactation Support Program

	Adequate	Expanded	Comprehensive
Facilities	Provide a clean or private, comfortable multipurpose space (that not a bathroom) with an electrical outlet for breast pump use, with a table and comfortable chair. Sink, soap, water, and paper towels are available If they are very far from the multipurpose space, extra time is allowed for cleaning hands and equipment. Employees provide their own breast pumps. Employee supplies cold packs for milk storage.	Dedicate a permanent space dedicated as a milk expression room for use only by nursing employees. Improve aesthetics to promote relaxation. Sink, soap, water, and paper towels are available near the milk expression room. Employer provides a multiuser electric breast pump, and employees provide their own collection kits. Provide refrigerator space near the milk expression room.	Dedicate a milk expression room close to employee worksites. Room is large enough to accommodate several users comfortably. Sink, soap, water, and paper towels are available in the milk expression room. Employer provides collection kits and additional multiuser electric pumps if needed. Provide a small refrigerator in the milk expression room.
Written Company Policy	Grant at least a 6-week unpaid maternity leave. Allow creative use of accrued vacation days, personal time, sick days, and holiday pay after childbirth. Allow two breaks and a lunch period during an 8-hour workday for expressing milk or nursing the child.	Grant at least a 12-week unpaid maternity leave. Allow part-time work, job sharing, individualized scheduling of work hours, compressed workweek, or telecommuting. Allow expanded unpaid breaks during the workday for expressing milk or nursing the child.	Offers a 14-week paid maternity leave or more. Allow employee to bring the child to work or caregiver to bring the child to the workplace to nurse; or on-site daycare is available. Count nursing breaks as working time.

(continues)

Table 25-3 Components of a Worksite Breastfeeding Support Program (continued)

	Adequate	Expanded	Comprehensive
Workplace Education	Have a lactation support policy that is communicated to all pregnant employees. Provide a list of community resources for lactation support.	Train new employees, supervisors, and coworkers on the lactation support policy. Contract with skilled lactation care provider on an "as-needed" basis.	Offer lactation education to the partners of employees who are expectant fathers. Hire a skilled lactation care provider to coordinate a lactation support program.

Data from the United States Breastfeeding Committee.

The International Lactation Consultant Association (ILCA, 2025) provides a searchable online directory to help employers locate an International Board Certified Lactation Consultant to set up and tailor a worksite program. Assistance includes supervisor and employee education, one-on-one consultations, classes and support group meetings, advice on breast pump equipment, and educational resources.

Lactation Room

In the United States, the ACA requires most employers to provide reasonable break time and a private place that is shielded from view and free from intrusion from coworkers and the public for an employee to express milk (U.S. Department of Labor, 2025). Workplace break laws are also prevalent in European countries and less commonly in East Asia and the Pacific (Atabay et al., 2015). Increasing numbers of employers are establishing lactation rooms at the worksite. A private room with a lockable door will ensure privacy and safety; a screen inside the door offers additional privacy. Pumping signs are also available to hang on outside doors. Nearby access to a sink for handwashing and washing of pump parts is a necessity. Refer to Table 25-3 for more details on accommodations in a lactation room.

Coworker Support

The support of management is crucial to an employee's ability to balance work with nursing. A positive climate established by management encourages coworkers to support nursing parents in a meaningful way. Company policy needs to incorporate protection of the right to pumping time and intolerance of nonsupport or sexual harassment from other employees. The policy can establish the expectation that coworkers will not question or complain about time away from work to tend to nursing or pumping needs.

Working parents who perceive greater peer and environmental support have higher job satisfaction (Karakaya & Kılı, 2024). Improving workplace accommodations for lactation can improve employees job satisfaction. Workplace lactation support, especially adequate time for milk expression, enhances employees' personal lives and helps them achieve work–life balance (Jantzer et al., 2018).

Summary

It is important to help parents manage times when they are away from their babies and cannot nurse. When a nursing parent or baby is hospitalized, practical ways to protect milk production and the baby's feeding needs are paramount. Your support is a valuable resource to parents throughout the stress of separations. Most separations are for social events, school, or work and may be accommodated by planning. You can help parents recognize their options for providing expressed milk to the baby. Continued assistance after they have implemented their plans helps them find ways to fine-tune pumping, milk storage, use of alternative feeding methods, and other changes in their nursing routine. A corporate lactation program or on-call assistance provides essential support and encouragement to parents as they blend nursing with employment or education.

What You Learned–At a Glance

Conversation Starters with Parents

- How will your baby be fed while you are separated?
- How are you protecting your milk production while you are separated?
- How are you managing regular separations from your baby?
- How long can you remain home before you return to work or school?
- How does your employer/school management support your continued nursing?

Managing a Separation

- Ensure the baby will accept an alternative feeding method during the separation.
- Express milk regularly to relieve fullness and maintain milk production.
- Plan the least disruptive timing for the separation when possible.
- Get adequate rest and nutrition.

Short-Term Illness and Hospitalization

- Pump to maintain milk production.
- Decrease the baby's exposure by careful handwashing before contact.
- Arrange for another adult to stay with the parent to help care for the baby if rooming-in.
- Have the baby brought to the hospital throughout the day to nurse if the parent is physically able.
- Nurse before and after surgery when physically able.

Returning to Work or School

- Recognize stresses of combining parenthood with employment or education.
- Recognize that goals may change after the baby arrives.
- Enlist support from family, friends, and coworkers.
- Explore work, education, and childcare options that protect nursing.
- Nurse uninterruptedly and bond with the baby until the return to work.
- Practice for the separation with the childcare provider and feeding method.
- Plan for milk expression, enhancing letdown, and storage of milk.
- Plan for relieving breast fullness and leaking.
- Plan quiet time for nursing after returning home.
- Discuss plans, needs, and concerns with the employer or school management.
- Educate parents about their legal rights and labor provisions.
- Provide resources for starting a lactation support program if none exists.

Features of Comprehensive Worksite Support

- Dedicate milk expression room that accommodates several users comfortably, is close to employees' worksites, and is clean and safe.
- Equip milk expression room with sink, soap, water, paper towels, small refrigerator, comfortable chair, table for breast pump, and aesthetics to promote relaxation.
- Provide multiuser electric breast pumps and collection kits
- Provide paid maternity leave for at least 6 to 14 weeks.
- Allow employees to bring their child to work, or caregivers to bring the child to the workplace; or provide on-site daycare.
- Have a written company lactation policy that ensures that nursing or pumping breaks are supported by coworkers and counted as work time.
- Train new employees, supervisors, and coworkers on the lactation support policy.
- Offer lactation education to the partners of employees.
- Contract with or hire a skilled lactation care provider to coordinate a lactation support program.

References

Academy of Breastfeeding Medicine. ABM clinical protocol #25: recommendations for preprocedural fasting for the breastfed infant: "NPO" guidelines. *Breastfeed Med*. 2012;7(3):197–202.

Academy of Breastfeeding Medicine. ABM clinical protocol #36: mastitis spectrum. 2022. https://abm.memberclicks.net/assets/DOCUMENTS/PROTOCOLS/36-mitchell-et-al-2022-academy-of-breastfeeding-medicine-clinical-protocol-36-the-mastitis-spectrum-revised-2022.pdf

American Academy of Pediatrics. Healthy Children.Org. Breastfeeding and Covid-19: what parents need to know.

March 7, 2023. https://www.healthychildren.org/English/health-issues/conditions/COVID-19/Pages/Breastfeeding-During-COVID-19.aspx#:~:text=Yes%2C%20babies%20can%20still%20receive,a%20face%20mask%20while%20nursing.

Atabay E, et al. Facilitating working mothers' ability to breastfeed: global trends in guaranteeing breastfeeding breaks at work, 1995–2014. *J Hum Lact.* 2015;31(1):81–88.

Aydin D, İnal S. Effects of breastfeeding and heel warming on pain levels during heel stick in neonates. *Int J Nurs Pract.* 2019;25(3):e12734.

Centers for Disease Control and Prevention. Early care and education (ECE). 2024a. https://www.cdc.gov/early-care-education/php/public-health-strategy/index.html

Centers for Disease Control and Prevention. Covid-19 and Breastfeeding. 2024b. https://www.cdc.gov/breastfeeding-special-circumstances/hcp/illnesses-conditions/covid-19.html

Centers for Disease Control and Prevention. Guidance for the prevention and control of influenza in the peri- and postpartum settings. November 22, 2024. https://www.cdc.gov/flu/professionals/infectioncontrol/peri-post -settings.htm

de Lauzon-Guillain B, et al. Maternity or parental leave and breastfeeding duration: results from the ELFE cohort. *Matern Child Nutr.* 2019;15(4):e12872.

Hale T, Krutsch K. *Hale's Medications & Mothers' Milk 2025–2026: A Manual of Lactational Pharmacology*. 21st ed. New York: Springer Publishing Company; 2024.

Human Milk Banking Association of North America Inc. (HMBANA). *Best Practice for Expressing, Storing and Handling Human Milk in Hospital, Homes and Child Care Settings*. 5th ed. Fort Worth, TX: Human Milk Banking Association of North America Inc; 2024.

International Labour Organization (ILO). Care at work: Investing in care leave and services for a more gender equal world of work. 2022. https://www.ilo.org/sites/default/files/wcmsp5/groups/public/%40dgreports/%40dcomm/documents/publication/wcms_838653.pdf

International Labour Organization (ILO). ILO Modelled Estimates and Projections database (ILOEST). 2025. https://data.worldbank.org/indicator/SL.TLF.ACTI.FE.ZS

International Lactation Consultant Association. Find a lactation consultant directory. 2025. https://portal.ilca.org/i4a/memberDirectory/index.cfm?directory_id=19&pageID=4356

Jagannathan M. The real reason companies like Target are offering paid parental leave and child-care. MarketWatch. June 15, 2019. https://www.marketwatch.com/story/the-real-reason-companies-like-target-are-offering-paid-parental-leave-and-child-care-2019-06-13

Jantzer AM, et al. Breastfeeding support in the workplace: the relationships among breastfeeding support, work-life balance, and job satisfaction. *J Hum Lact.* 2018;34(2):379–385.

Johnson A, et al. Enhancing breastfeeding rates among African American women: a systematic review of current psychosocial interventions. *Breastfeed Med.* 2015a;10(1):45–62.

Johnson AM, et al. Overcoming workplace barriers: a focus group study exploring African American mothers' needs for workplace breastfeeding support. *J Hum Lact.* 2015b;31(3):425–433.

Karakaya N, Kılıç M. The relationship between breastfeeding motivation, workplace breastfeeding support, and job satisfaction among working mothers. *Afr J Reprod Health.* 2024;28(11):141–151.

Lauer EA, et al. Identifying barriers and supports to breastfeeding in the workplace experienced by mothers in the New Hampshire Special Supplemental Nutrition Program for Women, Infants, and Children utilizing the total worker health framework. *Int J Environ Res Public Health.* 2019;16(4).

Livingston G, Thomas D. Among 41 countries, only U.S. lacks paid parental leave. December 16, 2019. https://www.pewresearch.org/fact-tank/2019/12/16/u-s-lacks-mandated-paid-parental-leave/

MacMillan Uribe AL, et al. Exploring human resource managers' decision-making process for workplace breastfeeding-support benefits following the passage of the Affordable Care Act. *Matern Child Health J.* 2019;23(10):1348–1359.

Pesch MH, et al. Pediatricians advocating breastfeeding: let's start with supporting our fellow pediatricians first. *J Pediatr.* 2019;206:6–7.

Riaz S, Condon L. The experiences of breastfeeding mothers returning to work as hospital nurses in Pakistan: a qualitative study. *Women Birth.* 2019;32(2):e252–e258.

Rimes KA, et al. Maternity leave and exclusive breastfeeding. *Rev Saude Publica.* 2019;53:10.

Snyder K, et al. Workplace breastfeeding support varies by employment type: the service workplace disadvantage. *Breastfeed Med.* 2018;13(1):23–27.

Spencer BS, et al. African American women's breastfeeding experiences: cultural, personal, and political voices. *Qual Health Res.* 2015;25(7):974–987.

Tampah-Naah AM, et al. Maternal challenges of exclusive breastfeeding and complementary feeding in Ghana. *PLoS One.* 2019;14(5):e0215285.

U.S. Department of Health and Human Services, Office on Women's Health. Business case for breastfeeding. Page last updated: February 27, 2025. http://www.womenshealth.gov/breastfeeding/business-case-for-breastfeeding.html

U.S. Department of Labor. Employee Benefits Security Administration: Affordable Care Act Information for Workers and Families. April 8, 2025. https://www.dol.gov/agencies/ebsa/laws-and-regulations/laws/affordable-care-act/for-workers-and-families

World Alliance for Breastfeeding Action. End of year THANK YOU, and announcement of WBW 2015 slogan and theme. 2015. http://www.waba.org.my/

CHAPTER 26

Long-Term Maternal Conditions

The goal of lactation healthcare providers is to empower families to have positive nursing experiences. Chronic health conditions in either the parent or the infant have the potential to alter the normal course of nursing. Thus, some parents require special assistance. Any condition requiring medication raises the question of whether nursing is safe. Autoimmune disorders, obesity, or viruses may affect a parent's energy or otherwise impair the ability to nurse. Medical conditions or anatomical anomalies may affect fertility, impair milk production, or require special accommodations for nursing. Infectious disease may delay or place restrictions on nursing. Physical or neurological disabilities may create challenges with feedings. These parents will benefit from sensitive support and assistance with mitigating the effect their condition has on lactation. This chapter focuses on maternal/cis-female conditions and not medical conditions of nonbinary or trans parents. There may be some similarities, but research is lacking in this area.

KEY TERMS

Acetone
Acquired immune deficiency syndrome (AIDS)
Alactogenesis
Autoimmune disorder
Bariatric surgery
Cystic fibrosis
Cytomegalovirus (CMV)
Diabetes
Endometriosis
Epinephrine
Epstein-Barr
Exocrine system
Flash-heat method
Goiter
Hepatitis A
Hepatitis B
Hepatitis C
Herpes
Holder pasteurization
Human immunodeficiency virus (HIV)
Hypernatremia
Hypertension
Hyperthyroidism
Hypoplasia
Hypothyroidism
Infertility
Lactogenesis
Metabolic syndrome
Multipara
Obesity
Phenylalanine hydroxylase deficiency (PAH)
Phenylketonuria
Polycystic ovary syndrome (PCOS)
Postpartum thyroiditis
Pretoria pasteurization
Primipara
Prolactinoma
Raynaud's phenomenon
Rheumatoid arthritis
Scleroderma
Seroconversion
Sjögren's syndrome
Systemic lupus erythematosus
Thyroid disorder
Transplacental
Tuberculosis
Varicella zoster

Autoimmune Disorders

Autoimmune disorders (also called autoimmune diseases) affect about one in five people in the United States, and the incidence is emerging in countries that never had such diseases before. Autoimmune diseases occur when the immune system misfires and attacks the cells, tissues, or organs it normally protects. All autoimmune diseases have a genetic predisposition, and they tend to cluster in families. Environmental triggers such as diet, sun exposure, and a preceding infection may play a role in triggering the diseases in individuals with a genetic predisposition.

There are more than 80 autoimmune diseases, which clinicians consider to be a group of disorders (U.S. Department of Health and Human Services [USDHHS], 2021a). Some inherited genes are specific to a certain disease, whereas others predispose to autoimmunity in general. Autoimmune diseases share many common symptoms, and often an individual has more than one disease. The complex interplay of neurologic, psychological, and inflammation processes is related to the development of autoimmune and other chronic diseases.

Autoimmune diseases familiar to the public are multiple sclerosis, Graves' disease, **scleroderma**, Raynaud's phenomenon, inflammatory bowel disease, ulcerative colitis, Crohn's disease, **systemic lupus erythematosus**, Sjögren's syndrome, Type 1 **diabetes**, and **rheumatoid arthritis**. Fibromyalgia has gained recognition as a distinct clinical entity that often accompanies other autoimmune disorders. It exhibits a characteristic pattern of specific, intensely tender trigger points on the body. Allodynia, a condition of increased responsiveness to pain that is associated with fibromyalgia, causes perceived pain with even light touch. Chronic fatigue immune dysfunction syndrome is also linked to autoimmunity. Chronic fatigue and pain can affect coping abilities and mental outlook.

Women are three times more likely to be affected by an autoimmune disease than men (American Autoimmune Related Diseases Association, 2020). They are most vulnerable during their reproductive years, and the predominance among women may reflect the involvement of female hormones in the regulation of immune response. About 75% of diagnosed women are in their childbearing years. Many may have an undiagnosed autoimmune disease. Those who are afflicted often exhibit symptoms for several years before they are correctly diagnosed.

Proper diagnosis is one of the most difficult challenges related to autoimmune disease. You can suggest that parents with these symptoms learn the medical history of their immediate and extended family. You can also maintain a referral list of healthcare providers who have experience with autoimmune disease. One of the greatest challenges is obtaining a correct diagnosis. Many individuals seek a second, third, and fourth opinion over several years before they finally receive an appropriate diagnosis and treatment.

Pregnancy Implications

Some autoimmune diseases, such as multiple sclerosis, may improve during pregnancy. Others may worsen before or after childbirth. Some, including thyroid disorders, increase the risk of **infertility** and miscarriage (Dhillon-Smith et al., 2020). Individuals with lupus have about a 10% rate of miscarriage. They are also at higher risk for pregnancy complications including preeclampsia, HELPP syndrome (a life-threatening liver disorder thought to be a type of severe preeclampsia), intrauterine growth restriction (IUGR), and impaired kidney function, among others (Lupus Foundation of America, 2021). Some parents with lupus deliver preterm babies and will need lactation assistance to transition to full nursing.

Lactation Implications

Lactation is associated with remission or reduction of symptoms in some autoimmune diseases, including inflammatory bowel disease and multiple sclerosis (Alotiby, 2023). Human milk has protective factors that reduce the infant's risk of developing autoimmune disease, as discussed in **Chapter 9**. These include inflammatory bowel diseases such as Crohn's disease and ulcerative colitis, Type 1 (juvenile) diabetes, juvenile arthritis, multiple sclerosis, and celiac disease. Because of the genetic links in autoimmune diseases, parents with chronic medical conditions should be encouraged to nurse their children. Not nursing increases the risks of the child developing any of the scores of immune diseases.

Medications associated with autoimmune diseases should be individually considered in conjunction with a qualified healthcare provider. Most medications that treat lupus are compatible with nursing. These include corticosteroids (although there is some concern that these may affect milk production) and hydroxychloroquine or chloroquine, which are antimalarial medications. Some experts do not recommend methotrexate because of limited data on its safety (Hale & Krutsch, 2024). Lupus flares may be exaggerated postpartum and require close observation. Rheumatoid arthritis flares are also more common in the postpartum period, possibly because of hormone fluctuations. Although some medications to treat the disorder are incompatible during pregnancy, most are compatible with nursing (Bermas, 2024).

Endometriosis

Research suggests an association between abnormalities in the immune system and **endometriosis**, a chronic inflammatory disease in which endometrial cells and tissue migrate outside the uterus. It affects more than 10% of women of childbearing age and is a major cause of infertility and pelvic pain (Shigesi et al., 2019). Women with endometriosis have a two-fold increased risk of infertility compared with women without the condition. There is a genetic link associated with endometriosis (Joseph & Mahale, 2019). Endometriosis is also associated with environmental exposure to estrogen disrupter chemicals such as phthalates (Cai et al., 2019; Karwacka et al., 2019). **Chapter 11** discusses environmental contaminants and lactation.

Women with endometriosis have a higher incidence of autoimmune disorders than the general female population, including **hypothyroidism**, fibromyalgia, inflammatory bowel disease, celiac disease, asthma, and allergies (Shigesi et al., 2019). It is unclear which comes first, the endometriosis or the autoimmune condition, or whether they share the same pathophysiology. Because 41% of women with endometriosis have fertility problems, many women will become pregnant through assisted reproduction and then have problems with lactation (Sharma, 2021). A thorough medical history helps identify markers for lactation risk.

Sjögren's Syndrome

Sjögren's syndrome is an autoimmune disease that attacks secretory glands and impairs their ability to produce moisture. In most cases, the autoimmune response affects the tear ducts, salivary glands, and vagina (American College of Rheumatology, 2025). Sjögren's syndrome occurs mostly in women aged 40–60 years. There is no evidence that it affects the mammary glands. However, because the breast is a secretory organ, there is the possibility of a correlation despite minimal research on this topic (NHSinform, 2025). Sjögren's syndrome is associated with other disorders, including scleroderma and Raynaud's phenomenon (Retamozo et al., 2019).

Raynaud's Phenomenon

Raynaud's phenomenon is a neurovascular condition that is believed to affect about 3% of the general population (National Institute of Arthritis and Musculoskeletal and Skin Diseases [NIAMS], 2024). Primary Raynaud's has no known cause and secondary Raynaud's is related to another health condition. Primary Raynaud's usually appears between 15 and 25 years of age and is more common in women than men. It appears to occur more frequently in colder climates. This may be because people with the disorder have more Raynaud's attacks in colder climates. It is also more common in people with Scandinavian ancestry.

Pain in the extremities when exposed to cold is a marker for Raynaud's, which is a disorder of the small blood vessels in the skin. During a Raynaud's attack, restricted blood flow in the extremities causes numbness and a "pins-and-needles" sensation. Sometimes, dull pain and clumsiness occur. Skin color changes of the extremities follow a sequence of white (blanching or pallor) to blue (cyanotic) and then to red (rubor) as blood returns to the area. Raynaud's can also affect the nose and ears.

Cold is more apt to cause an attack when accompanied by physical or emotional stress. Sometimes stress alone causes vasoconstriction without exposure to cold. Injuries such as frostbite or surgery can cause Raynaud's phenomenon. Regular use of machinery such as chainsaws and vibrating drills can damage small blood vessels. Frequent typing and piano playing may worsen the condition. In addition to medical conditions, certain drugs can cause secondary Raynaud's, including some heart, blood, and migraine headache medications. Nicotine can also trigger symptoms (NIAMS, 2024). **Figure 26-1** presents conditions that may cause secondary Raynaud's.

Parents with Raynaud's may not be aware of it before pregnancy and may report never having symptoms before the baby's birth. A Raynaud's attack can affect a parent's dexterity and ability to relax during a feeding. Caution them that consuming caffeine, and nicotine via smoking or vaping, may worsen their symptoms by further constricting blood vessels.

Increasing intake of vitamin B_6 has helped in some instances. Vitamin B_6 passes readily into milk. Babies directly receiving excessive supplementary doses have experienced sedation, hypotonia, and respiratory distress. It is recommended that intake of vitamin B_6 not exceed 25 mg per day (Hale & Krutsch, 2024). There is no research to support the use of vitamin B_6 to treat Raynaud's phenomenon (Koschinski-Moller, 2021).

- Scleroderma—a thickening and hardening of the skin and other body tissues
- Systemic lupus erythematosus—a chronic inflammation of the skin and organ systems
- Rheumatoid arthritis—a chronic inflammation and swelling of tissue in the joints
- Blood flow reduction—problems that slow or stop blood flow in a vessel, such as inflammation and hardening of the arteries (arteriosclerosis)
- Nerve problems—problems that affect the nerves supplying the muscles
- Pulmonary hypertension—a condition in which pressure rises in the blood vessels of the lungs

Figure 26-1 Conditions that may cause secondary Raynaud's.

Data from U.S. Department of Health and Human Services (USDHHS), National Institute of Arthritis and Musculoskeletal and Skin Diseases (NIAMS). Raynaud's Phenomenon. May 2021. https://www.niams.nih.gov/health-topics/raynauds-phenomenon.

A Cochrane review found moderate-quality evidence that calcium channel blockers, such as nifedipine, may be minimally effective for treating primary Raynaud's. It appears that higher doses may be more effective than lower doses. Calcium channel blockers may reduce the frequency of primary Raynaud's phenomenon, although they may have little effect on severity (Klein-Weigel et al., 2021).

Raynaud's and Nipple Pain

A Raynaud's-like phenomenon can cause vasospasms of the nipple, as described in **Chapter 17**. Symptoms are a stinging, tingling, burning, painful sensation that persists after a feeding. The same triphasic color change occurs on the nipple as with the extremities (NIAMS, 2024). A poor latch can result in the baby compressing the nipple and causing a vasospasm. Sometimes, a parent may experience this kind of pain despite an effective latch. Some parents with nipple vasospasms report that the pain also occurs when they are exposed to cold.

Nipple vasospasm is severely painful and can lead to weaning if untreated. Your validation that the pain associated with secondary Raynaud's has a medical cause will be a relief. Refer parents to their healthcare provider for evaluation and treatment and provide current medical references if the provider is not familiar with nipple vasospasm related to lactation. As nursing rates increase, healthcare providers are becoming more familiar with Raynaud's phenomenon and treating appropriately. If a parent is on any of the medications associated with secondary Raynaud's, the provider may be able to adjust or change them. If vasospasms continue despite improving the baby's latch, other measures in **Figure 26-2** may provide relief.

- Seek treatment with medications, avoiding aggravating medications.
- Control stress and exercise regularly.
- Apply dry or moist heat immediately after nursing.
- Wear warm socks, gloves, hat, and scarf to protect the entire body from the cold.
- Avoid putting hands in cold water.
- Remove food from the refrigerator or freezer with gloves or potholders.
- Try to avoid cuts, bruises, and other injuries to the affected areas.
- Limit activities such as keyboarding, texting, sewing, or other detail work.
- Reduce or eliminate caffeine, nicotine, and other vasoconstrictors.
- Consider chiropractic, acupuncture, and/or biofeedback care.
- Consult a healthcare provider if questions or concerns develop.

Figure 26-2 Measures that may provide relief from secondary Raynaud's.

Data from U.S. Department of Health and Human Services (USDHHS), National Institute of Arthritis and Musculoskeletal and Skin Diseases (NIAMS). 2024.

Diabetes Mellitus

Worldwide, 422 million people have diabetes, with increases observed mostly in low- and middle-income countries (World Health Organization [WHO], 2023). People with diabetes may have difficulty conceiving because they can experience delayed menarche, menstrual abnormalities, and early menopause. Consistent glucose control is important for increasing fertility in these people (Kim et al., 2020; Thong et al., 2020). Quality prenatal high-risk care, including close monitoring of blood glucose levels and fetal size, enables many parents with diabetes to deliver healthy babies and meet their nursing goals.

Diabetes affects people of all ages and most forms are chronic (lifelong). All forms of diabetes are manageable with medications and/or lifestyle changes. Diabetes develops when pancreas production of insulin is minimal or absent, or when the body does not respond to the effects of insulin properly. In the absence of adequate insulin, glucose builds up in the bloodstream, causing high blood sugar (hyperglycemia). Diabetes is associated with other morbidities and causes of death (American Diabetes Association, 2020). An estimated 2 million annual deaths are directly caused by diabetes and kidney disease due to diabetes.

The high blood glucose levels in uncontrolled diabetes cause serious damage to nerves and blood vessels. Unable to metabolize carbohydrates for energy, the body burns fat as its energy source. When the fat metabolizes, increased amounts of ketones are formed. Ketones are acidic compounds that are removed from the body by the kidneys and excreted into urine. Surplus ketones can result in the kidneys being unable to remove them efficiently. The rapid buildup of ketones in the blood can result in metabolic acidosis or diabetic ketoacidosis, which can lead to coma and death.

Types of Diabetes

The three classifications of diabetes mellitus are insulin-dependent or type 1 diabetes, type 2 diabetes, and gestational diabetes mellitus (GDM). Impaired glucose tolerance (IGT) and impaired fasting glycemia (IFG) are intermediate conditions in the transition between normality and diabetes. People with IGT or IFG are at high risk of progressing to type 2 diabetes, although it is not inevitable (WHO, 2023).

Type 1 diabetes is an autoimmune disease with genetic risk factors that results in the inability of the pancreas to manufacture insulin. Type 1 diabetes is called *juvenile diabetes* because it appears primarily in children. It is also called *insulin-dependent diabetes* because individuals with type 1 diabetes must take insulin for the rest of their lives. Exclusive nursing for a prolonged period and delayed introduction of certain nutrients for babies may prevent the development of type 1 diabetes in the baby (Çiçekli & Durusoy, 2022). Type 2 diabetes is typically associated with dietary and lifestyle factors, including **obesity**. It can result from insulin resistance progressing to insulin dependence. Type 2 diabetes has many negative health effects, including an increased risk of cardiovascular disease.

Gestational diabetes occurs in 2% to 7% of pregnancies, usually within the second trimester. It occurs when placental hormones cause blood glucose levels to rise to higher-than-normal values but below the diagnostic threshold for diabetes. Thresholds differ from country to country. Gestational diabetes increases the risk for complications during pregnancy and at birth. Obesity, high blood pressure, and age are key risk factors for gestational diabetes. It can frequently be controlled by diet and moderate-intensity exercise. Sometimes oral medication or insulin is required.

Although gestational diabetes usually resolves after the birth, these women and their children are at increased risk of developing type 2 diabetes in the future. Nursing reduces this risk. Longer nursing duration reduces the risk more because longer-term nursing is associated with lower body mass, lower fasting glucose, lower triglycerides, and higher response to insulin (Ma et al., 2019). The prevalence of delayed onset of lactogenesis in parents with GDM is 35% (Wu et al., 2021). Being a primipara, having prepregnancy obesity, advanced age, and requiring insulin treatment for GDM are independent risk factors for delayed lactogenesis.

Babies of Diabetics

Before the adoption of insulin for diabetes, babies of gestational parents with diabetes often died, and the parent often died as well. Even with today's treatment, risks are still high for these parents with diabetes and their babies. The baby has twice the risk of serious injury at birth, triple the probability of cesarean delivery, and four times the rate of admission to a neonatal intensive care unit (NICU). The more poorly controlled the sugar levels are, the higher the risk of these outcomes (Centers for Disease Control and Prevention [CDC], 2024).

These babies are at risk for being large for gestational age (LGA) at birth and for being supplemented with formula because of hypoglycemia (low blood sugar) at birth. LGA babies are at higher risk for developing diabetes, and the early exposure to bovine proteins can be the triggering allergic event that impairs the body's ability to produce and use insulin (Güngör et al., 2019).

Prenatal Expression of Colostrum

Because of the increased risk of infant susceptibility to developing diabetes, many informed parents with diabetes do not want their babies to receive formula. Increasingly, expectant parents are taking steps to minimize the risk of formula supplementation. They may express colostrum prenatally, bring donor milk to the hospital, or request donor milk if the hospital offers it. With the prenatal provider's agreement that it is safe to do so, colostrum expression can begin after 37 weeks' gestation (Johnsen et al., 2021). A small amount of colostrum can be expressed, stored in syringes, and frozen. If the baby is due within a day or two, the colostrum can be refrigerated, not frozen. Some parents are not able to collect colostrum until after birth, especially first-time parents.

Approach clients with diabetes individually to identify their specific risk factors and needs. Help them tailor their care plan with their prenatal care provider before any colostrum expression to minimize preterm labor risk. Most parents view expressing colostrum prenatally as positive, enabling them to become familiar with milk expression and giving them a sense of security by having stored colostrum for use if needed after the birth. Using colostrum expressed prenatally significantly reduces formula supplementation in the hospital (Casey et al., 2019).

Nursing with Diabetes

Parents with diabetes face postpartum challenges of glycemic control and overall health, in addition to establishing nursing. Those who are active health consumers usually have a working knowledge of nutrition that will help them through the lactation period. Both the parent's and infant's blood sugar levels need careful monitoring because of the potential for low glucose following birth. Insulin needs drop dramatically after the delivery of the placenta. Frequent blood glucose tests in the first few days postpartum will help insulin-dependent parents determine their requirements. Insulin levels fluctuate erratically until lactation is established and fluctuate again when weaning occurs. Close monitoring is essential during these times.

Parents with insulin-dependent diabetes experience a delay in **lactogenesis** compared with those without diabetes. Diabetes may also be a risk factor for insufficient milk production. Nursing soon after birth, and frequently, is especially important to assist stage II lactogenesis. Parents with diabetes may worry about their health being affected by daily disruptions. Professional and peer lactation support can help reduce the risk of stress and ill health. Interdisciplinary management of nursing may include several healthcare providers, such as an obstetrician, a pediatrician, and an endocrinologist. A website for parents and health professionals on prepregnancy diabetes and lactation is being tested in Australia (Rasmussen et al., 2023).

Diabetes type can be a significant predictor of nursing initiation. Parents with complex medical pregnancies have lower odds of nursing intention and duration. Those with type 2 diabetes have lower intention to nurse than those with type 1 diabetes (Cordero et al., 2022) and higher levels of formula feeding at hospital discharge. Supportive hospital practices will increase the odds of any or exclusive nursing in medically complex pregnancies. People with diet-controlled diabetes have no nursing restrictions. Parents with insulin-dependent diabetes can nurse safely while continuing insulin therapy throughout lactation.

Diabetes increases the risk of yeast infections, both in the vaginal area and on the nipples. Moisture provides a breeding ground for fungus and can cause nipple pain. Keeping the nipples dry between feedings can help avoid this complication. If nipple pain fails to respond to the usual treatment, a yeast infection may be the cause (**Chapter 17** discusses thrush). Diabetes results in slow wound healing and neuropathy, which may affect the resolution of nipple pain. The delicate balance of diet, insulin, and exercise can be disturbed by an infection or by digestive or emotional upset. Reducing stress and removing milk regularly help avoid ductal narrowing and mastitis. If mastitis occurs, it will be important to monitor blood sugar closely and make necessary adjustments in the treatment regimen.

Diabetic Treatment During Lactation

Diabetes treatment is highly individual. Many people with diabetes feel they are at their healthiest and have better control over their diabetes during lactation than at any other time in their lives. Some parents may need to increase, rather than decrease, their dosage of insulin. Others may be able to decrease it significantly. Because of an altered hormone balance, parents with diabetes may experience improved glycemic control throughout lactation. Sugar is absorbed to produce the energy needed for milk production. Additionally, lactose is a component in the milk, and the activity of nursing expends more calories. This combination of factors often permits a higher caloric intake and lower insulin dosage.

During lactation, parents with diabetes generally require an increase in calories, carbohydrates, and protein. This varies with each individual, and precise dietary guidelines need to be part of the new regimen parents plan with their healthcare provider. If blood sugar climbs too high, **acetone** is released and transmitted to the baby through the milk. After several days of exposure to high acetone levels, the baby can develop an enlarged liver. An increase in carbohydrates, possibly accompanied by an increased insulin dosage, can control the risk of acetone migrating into the milk. Conversely, if blood sugar is too low, hypoglycemia may occur, releasing **epinephrine** and inhibiting letdown and milk production. Tight control of blood sugar levels helps prevent these extremes.

During any interruption in nursing, and especially during weaning, caloric intake and insulin dosage need to be adjusted to compensate for the decrease in the utilization of sugar for lactation. Whenever sugar is present in the urine, insulin dosage must increase gradually, and caloric intake must decrease to respond to the baby's feeding schedule. If the interruption is short-lived, a simple reduction in food intake may be sufficient, with no change in insulin dosage.

Insulin Resistance

Insulin resistance occurs when cells in the body do not respond as they should to insulin. The pancreas then makes more insulin to overcome increasing blood glucose levels. Over time, untreated chronic insulin resistance can lead to prediabetes and then type 2 diabetes. During pregnancy, insulin resistance ensures glucose for fetal growth. It can be accentuated by obesity, polycystic ovary syndrome (PCOS), and diabetes and may become severe (Kampmann et al., 2021).

Table 26-1 Symptoms of Metabolic Syndrome and Insulin Resistance

Symptoms of Metabolic Syndrome	Symptoms of Insulin Resistance Pertinent to Childbearing Parents
▪ High blood pressure ▪ Elevated blood glucose levels ▪ Elevated triglyceride levels ▪ Low levels of high-density-lipoprotein cholesterol ▪ Excess fat around the waist	▪ Excess weight gain ▪ Preexisting obesity ▪ Gestational diabetes ▪ High cholesterol ▪ Hypertension ▪ Acanthosis nigricans (dark skin in the armpits, groin and neck) ▪ Development of skin tags

Reproduced from the U.S. Department of Health and Human Services. The National Institute of Diabetes and Digestive and Kidney Diseases Health Information Center. Insulin Resistance and Prediabetes. May 2018. https://www.niddk.nih.gov/health-information/diabetes/overview/what-is-diabetes/prediabetes-insulin-resistance

Insulin resistance is the main feature in a cluster of symptoms in **metabolic syndrome**. Metabolic syndrome can lead to coronary artery disease, stroke, and type 2 diabetes. It is highly prevalent in higher-income countries and especially in the eastern Mediterranean region and the Americas (Noubiap et al., 2022). **Table 26-1** presents symptoms of metabolic syndrome and insulin resistance in childbearing parents.

Researchers believe metabolic syndrome may result from insulin resistance. The constant buildup of sugar in the blood sets the stage for disease later in life. Insulin resistance may also play a role in the poor nursing outcomes associated with obesity (Nommsen-Rivers et al., 2022). Some people with insulin resistance receive treatment with metformin, glitazones, and pioglitazones, which increase the body's sensitivity to insulin. Oral contraceptives may also be effective in increasing this sensitivity (Giraudo et al., 2023).

Obesity

Obesity is defined as having a body mass index (BMI) of 30 or greater. BMI is calculated from a person's weight and height and indicates body fatness and weight categories that may lead to health problems. Obesity adds to the global burden of chronic disease and disability. It is a major risk factor for cardiovascular disease, **hypertension**, stroke, cancer, and type 2 diabetes (WHO, 2021). The causes of obesity are multifaceted.

There is growing research interest in maternal obesity and childhood neurodevelopment, including maternal and fetal inflammation, the microbiome, and epigenetics (Tong & Kalish, 2021). Growing research indicates that some people have a genetic predisposition (genetic mutations) for weight gain. Modifiable factors influencing obesity include epigenetics, physical inactivity, insufficient sleep, excessive caloric intake, socioeconomic status, ethnicity, and psychological stress. The gut microbiome, certain medications, and endocrine disrupting chemicals in the environment are other factors associated with obesity (Masood & Moorthy, 2023).

Nursing and Obesity

The complex interplay between insulin, progesterone, and estrogen may cause delayed onset of lactogenesis II in parents who are obese. A blunted prolactin response may play a role in this, perhaps because of estrogen stored in adipose tissue (Diana et al., 2019). Obesity is associated with lower nursing rates and shorter duration. This may result from delayed lactogenesis and the physical difficulties of positioning, as well as bias within health systems (Achike & Akpinar-Elci, 2021). Parents with obesity are more likely to have a medically complex pregnancy and a cesarean delivery, further affecting lactation establishment.

Parents who are obese may have significant body image issues that make them reluctant to nurse or lead to early cessation. Body image concerns include dieting during pregnancy and the prenatal and postpartum physical changes that occur. Many parents who are obese have large breasts, which can create challenges with positioning and latch at feedings. The special aids for large breasts that nursing parents may need for positioning can make it more difficult to nurse discreetly in public. This might discourage some parents from nursing.

Weight bias and stigma from media, society, and healthcare professionals can impact a parent's decision to nurse. Well-meaning providers may not realize how offensive their language around weight loss sounds to their clients. The physical environment can also present a bias, such as too-small blood pressure cuffs, chairs, and gowns (Fruh et al., 2021).

Parents need positive professional support for nursing and to be validated as individuals, not merely as being obese. Referring to these clients as "parents with obesity" rather than "obese parents" recognizes the whole individual. Emotional and practical support from other nursing parents and a postpartum support group can increase your clients' confidence in their nursing experience. **Figure 26-3** provides tips to help with nursing.

- Place the breast on a pillow to take the weight off the baby.
- Place a small rolled blanket or washcloth under the breast to provide lift.
- Recline and place the baby prone on the chest (see Chapter 15 on laid-back/reclined nursing).
- Nurse in a side-lying position with the breast resting on the bed.
- Support the breast with a "sling"—a commercial sling attached to the bra or one fashioned by tying the corners of a baby blanket together.

Figure 26-3 Assisting large-breasted parents to nurse.

Health at Every Size (HAES) is an approach that addresses weight bias and stigma rather than focusing only on health outcomes. HAES promotes adopting a healthy lifestyle that includes body acceptance, intuitive eating, and physical activity for movement and health rather than for body shape (Hagen & Henningfield, 2023). You can support your clients with obesity by educating them as you would any other client and being mindful of the language you use when talking about their body and breasts. More information about the framework of HAES can be found at www.asdah.org.

One of the benefits of nursing is that it facilitates weight loss. Weight loss and maintenance appear to have a long-term association with having nursed. Parents with obesity who exclusively nurse for 4 months, with a duration of 12-plus months, retain less weight (an average of −8.0 kg) than those who do not nurse (Sharma, 2021). Cumulative weight gain between pregnancies can contribute to lifelong overweight, eventual obesity, and corresponding health problems (Rogozińska et al., 2019). Losing pregnancy weight is important to avoid the cumulative effect. There may also be a link between obesity, a high-fat diet during lactation, and infant programming for obesity (Larsen & Bode, 2021).

Bariatric (Weight-Loss) Surgery

As obesity levels soar, **bariatric surgery** has risen in popularity in affluent cultures. Rates in the United States rose from 13,000 procedures in 1998 to 270,089 in 2023 (American Society for Metabolic and Bariatric Surgery, 2025). Bariatric surgery limits either the amount of food a person can eat or the amount of food they can digest. The surgery carries major risks and complications, including infections, hernias, blood clots, and death. Moreover, without dramatic lifestyle and psychological and emotional changes, many individuals are at risk of regaining weight.

The risks of obesity are more compelling than the risk of surgery for many individuals. Bariatric surgery results in significant weight loss of 15% to 64%, depending on the type of surgery (Tamae Kakazu et al., 2020). It is an effective means of treating metabolic diseases such as diabetes (Aly et al., 2022). In a recent Italian study, individuals who had not achieved their goal weight within 2 years of the surgery were unlikely to achieve them. Those who lost their weight maintained their loss for an average of 4.8 years (Palumbo et al., 2023).

Bariatric surgery eligibility guidelines require that the individual be at least 80 pounds overweight. However, the procedure has become so popular that it is performed on people weighing less. Diabetes, heart disease, and sleep apnea are among the reasons for performing this surgery at lower weights. In some countries, those who may need it most cannot afford it. Adolescents are increasingly opting for bariatric surgery, with a five-fold increase in the number of adolescent bariatric procedures performed worldwide. The American Academy of Pediatrics (AAP) has issued guidelines for evaluating adolescents for these procedures (AAP, 2019).

Fertility and Pregnancy

Most women who have bariatric surgery are in their childbearing years. Pregnancy after bariatric surgery appears to reduce the risk of gestational diabetes and pregnancy-related hypertension, as well as reducing macrosomia in the infant. Pregnancy during a period of rapid weight loss is not recommended. These individuals should use some sort of contraception until their weight goal is achieved and maintained.

Because obesity lowers fertility rates, infertility is common in this population—as high as 41.9% in one study. Over 13% of women who have had bariatric surgery were also diagnosed with **polycystic ovary syndrome (PCOS)**. Bariatric surgery as a treatment option for women who are obese with PCOS and endometriosis is being studied.

Complications

Bariatric surgery risks major nutritional concerns post-surgery and parents will need to adhere to the dietary advice they receive in conjunction with their surgery. Nutritional needs are even greater during pregnancy. Gastric bypass surgery carries a greater risk both medically and nutritionally than the banding procedure, in which the stomach size is decreased. Complications such as severe anemia may result from nutritional deficiencies in iron, vitamin A, vitamin B_{12}, vitamin D, vitamin K, folate, and calcium. Thus, nutritional guidance and adherence are crucial (Shawe et al., 2019). Supplements can restore nutrition to adequate levels when taken consistently.

Infant of a gestational parent risk being born small-for-gestational-age (RóŻańska-Walędziak et al., 2020). Other complications include visual impairment from inadequate vitamin A; intracranial hemorrhage from inadequate vitamin K, and neurologic and developmental impairment from inadequate vitamin B_{12} (RóŻańska-Walędziak et al., 2023). These babies also have a higher risk of congenital abnormalities, IUGR, preterm birth, perinatal death, and admission to special care nurseries (Maslin et al., 2020; Shawe et al., 2019).

There is no consensus regarding vitamin and micronutrient supplementation while nursing. This makes it even more vital to obtain a parent's complete surgical history when a nursing baby exhibits any nutritional deficiencies, especially for those who had gastric bypass surgery, such as Roux-en-Y surgery (Akhter et al., 2019). A comprehensive overview of nutritional deficiencies can be found on the National Institute of Health website (Kamal et al., 2024).

Life After Bariatric Surgery

Parents who had bariatric surgery need to be referred to a nutritionist or dietitian. Nutritional supplementation is advised for life. Their nutritional status should be tested before conception, during pregnancy, and after delivery, with nutritional supplements targeted as needed. Testing should measure complete blood count, albumin, iron, folate, vitamin B_{12}, vitamin D, vitamin K, calcium, and phosphorus. The infants should also be evaluated and monitored for appropriate growth and adequacy of vitamin B_{12}, vitamin D, vitamin K, calcium, iron, and folate levels while they continue to nurse. Signs of problems for the baby include fussiness, poor weight gain, lethargy, and inadequate voiding or stooling. **Figure 26-4** identifies areas of key nutritional concern for a nursing parent who has undergone bariatric surgery.

Open-ended questions and thorough history taking will help you identify parents who have had bariatric surgery. Some parents may not mention gallbladder or bariatric surgery during a consultation, perhaps surmising that the history focuses only on surgery that affects the breast. A complete history is crucial to prevent babies of these parents from experiencing low weight gain, growth faltering, or neurologic damage from undernutrition. **Figure 26-5** presents information to gather about bariatric surgery when taking histories for parents and babies.

- Calories
- Vitamin B_{12}
- Vitamin K
- Folate
- Calcium
- Water-soluble vitamins, including vitamin D and vitamin C
- Iron
- Fat-soluble vitamins
- Protein
- Fat

Figure 26-4 Key nutritional concerns following bariatric surgery.

Data from Stefanski J. Breast-feeding after bariatric surgery. Today's Dietitian. 2006;8(1):47; Gadgil MD, et al. Laboratory Testing for and Diagnosis of Nutritional Deficiencies in Pregnancy Before and After Bariatric Surgery. Journal of Women's Health 2014;23(2):129-137.

Parent:

- When and what kind of surgery was performed
- Related surgeries such as plastic or breast surgery
- Complications from the procedure
- Parent's weight pattern
- Lab testing for nutritional deficiencies; frequency and results
- Current nutritionist/dietitian's recommendations
- Nutritional practices and supplements taken
- Recommendations from endocrinologist, obstetrician/gynecologist, or other provider

Baby:

- Any in utero and/or post-birth complications
- Weight and growth pattern
- Lab testing for nutritional deficiencies, frequency and results
- Amount and frequency of supplements used (if any), and type (e.g., parent's milk, donor milk, formula)
- Healthcare provider recommendations

Figure 26-5 Information to gather related to bariatric surgery.

Data from Kombol P. ILCA's inside track: a resource for breastfeeding mothers. Breastfeeding after weight loss surgery. J Hum Lact. 2008;24(3):341-342; Lamb M. Weight-loss surgery and breastfeeding. Clinical Lactation. 2011;2(3):17-21; Gadgil MD, et al. Laboratory Testing for and Diagnosis of Nutritional Deficiencies in Pregnancy Before and After Bariatric Surgery. Journal of Women's Health 2014;23(2):129-137.

Insufficient Milk Production

Insufficient milk production occurs when milk volume does not meet the nutritional needs of the infant. Primary insufficient milk is caused by medical conditions or anatomical issues in the parent. Parents with a history of infertility are at risk for primary insufficient milk production, though many parents who conceive by reproductive technology achieve ample milk production. Primary insufficient milk differs from a delay in lactogenesis that results from a cesarean delivery, hypertension, edema, hormonal birth control, diabetes, retained placenta, obesity, or a theca lutein cyst.

Secondary insufficient milk results from not thoroughly and regularly removing milk. Secondary causes are far more common than primary ones. Factors include timed or scheduled or infrequent feedings, pacifier use, medications, hormonal birth control, and herbs. Secondary lactation failure may also result from conditions that prevent adequate milk removal by the baby, such as preterm birth, ineffective latch or suck, and oral anomalies such as ankyloglossia. Impaired adrenocorticotropic hormone secretion may play a role as well. This hormone stimulates the production and release of cortisol, a stress hormone.

Prolactin and Insufficient Milk

Adequate milk production requires enough prolactin receptor cells in the breast. **Multiparas** are believed to have an increased number of prolactin receptors that bind with circulating prolactin. This may be reflected in or result in the lower serum levels of prolactin typically observed in multiparas. Despite the lower postpartum serum levels of prolactin, their babies take in significantly more milk than babies of **primiparas**.

Prolactin deficiency, or hyperprolactinemia, occurs when the anterior pituitary cells do not secrete prolactin, as measured by serum levels. This deficiency can occur with other anterior pituitary hormone defects or in isolation. It can be acquired or genetic. Some parents report a family history of **alactogenesis**, which is the absence of the onset of stage II lactogenesis, or minimal milk production.

Prolactin resistance is the inability of tissues to respond normally to prolactin. This condition may be caused by Sheehan's syndrome, smoking, retained placental fragments, **prolactinoma** (pituitary tumor), or hypothyroidism. Prolactin resistance may act much like insulin resistance, which suggests a possible genetic link (Moriwaki & Welt, 2021).

Prolactin deficiency or resistance may be an autoimmune condition that could benefit from dopamine agonists (Borba et al., 2019). A study using acupressure massage suggests that inflammation may inhibit prolactin release. It reported higher prolactin levels, reduced breast temperature, and significantly greater milk production by the third and fourth days postpartum (Lu et al., 2019). Researchers have found that a genetic deficiency in the pituitary gland results in low or absent prolactin function. This is associated with irregular menstrual cycles, gonadotropin imbalance, and infertility, as well as lactation (Blum et al., 2019).

Insufficient Glandular Tissue

When assessing parents with insufficient milk, pay careful attention to their breast development. Note the shape, symmetry, and vein prominence. Ask about breast growth, such as cup size changes during puberty and pregnancy. Ask about any changes after delivery and the sensation of fullness that accompanies the onset of full milk production. Palpate to determine the amount of glandular and fatty tissue and whether they are soft, flaccid, lumpy, or knotty. Environmental chemicals that are endocrine disruptors may also alter breast development (Kam et al., 2021). It is possible for a parent to experience insufficient glandular tissue with no associated risk factors (McGuire, 2019a).

Measure the space between the breasts to assess for **hypoplasia**. Spacing between the breasts (intramammary spacing) greater than 1.5 inches (3.81 cm) is a marker for insufficient milk (Kam et al., 2024). **Color Plates 5 to 8** compare normal and hypoplastic breasts. The lack of population-based studies makes it difficult to determine the worldwide prevalence of breast hypoplasia (Kam et al., 2023). Hypoplasia could be related to congenital syndromes such as Jeune and Poland syndromes.

Treatment for Low Milk Production

Medications such as metoclopramide and domperidone are commonly used as galactagogues to increase milk production. **Chapter 19** discusses these and other medications used as galactagogues. For parents with primary insufficient milk, insulin-sensitizing agents may help establish and maintain milk production. Metformin enhances insulin sensitivity in the liver and muscle, thus improving glycemic (sugar) control. Improved metabolic control with metformin may be associated with moderate weight loss. Other insulin-affecting medications with similar properties include glitazone, pioglitazone, and liraglutide. The field of gene therapies to address and resolve insufficient milk holds great promise.

Polycystic Ovary Syndrome (PCOS)

PCOS is a common endocrine disorder in about 18% of women in their childbearing years. It is associated with the accumulation of many incompletely developed ovarian follicles. The condition typically causes irregular menstrual cycles, scanty or absent menses, multiple small ovarian cysts (polycystic ovaries), mild to severe hirsutism (excessive hair), and infertility. Infertility in PCOS is related to anovulation (not ovulating). Many individuals who have this condition also develop diabetes with insulin resistance (USDHHS, Office on Women's Health, 2021b). PCOS carries lifelong health risks, and greater chances of developing life-threatening diseases (**Figure 26-6**).

PCOS and Obesity

PCOS may develop because of genetic and environmental factors, including obesity. Almost 50% of individuals with PCOS are obese. This can become a perpetual cycle because those with PCOS have higher rates of obesity, which increases PCOS symptoms. Weight loss is the first action suggested for parents with PCOS. PCOS can affect reproduction, metabolism, and psychological functions. Obesity concurrent with PCOS affects fertility through multiple factors. Some individuals with PCOS conceive spontaneously, whereas others require fertility assistance. Those who become pregnant can discuss with their healthcare provider whether the benefits of medication outweigh the risks during pregnancy. If PCOS medications are not used prenatally, parents may consider starting medication as soon as the baby is born.

- Impaired glucose tolerance, with more than 50% of individuals with PCOS experiencing type 2 diabetes or pre-diabetes before the age of 40
- Cardiovascular disease, with a 4 to 7 times higher incidence of heart attack than the same aged individuals without PCOS
- High blood pressure
- High levels of low-density-lipoprotein (bad) cholesterol and low levels of high-density-lipoprotein (good) cholesterol
- Endometrial cancer
- Sleep apnea
- Anxiety and depression

Figure 26-6 Conditions associated with a high risk of polycystic ovary syndrome (PCOS).

PCOS and Lactation

Parents with PCOS are often extremely motivated to nurse because of their difficulty conceiving. Nursing can help heal a fragile body image battered from infertility and repeated miscarriages. It is discouraging to struggle with infertility, achieve pregnancy through assisted reproductive technology, and then struggle to achieve full milk production. Faced with yet another challenge, these parents may decide to wean and need your sensitive validation of their choice.

It is difficult to predict lactation outcomes for parents with PCOS. One key marker is mammary growth during pregnancy. Parents with PCOS who have no breast growth during pregnancy seem to have more metabolic disturbance and impairment in milk production than those with PCOS who experience normal breast growth. Lowering insulin resistance may help to increase milk production. Treatment prenatally may improve pregnancy and health outcomes, as well as milk production. Cabergoline, an ergot alkaloid, is used to treat PCOS in pregnancy and may suppress lactation. Bromocriptine, also an ergot alkaloid, is used in fertility treatment to lower prolactin levels to conceive and can compromise milk production.

Insufficient milk may accompany a PCOS diagnosis or symptoms consistent with the syndrome (Kam et al., 2024). Parents with PCOS symptoms or insufficient milk will benefit from referral for a thorough physical and hormonal analysis. Some parents have observed an increase in milk production while using metformin, one of the medications used to treat the condition.

The relationship of hormonal disorders and insufficient milk production is an area of ongoing research. Parents with PCOS have higher androgen hormone levels, which are associated with negative nursing outcomes. Parents who fit these profiles and are using metformin or other medications can be encouraged to contact the Infant Risk Center, a university lactation research center (https://www.infantrisk.com) with the aim of helping advance knowledge and treatments for lactation difficulties.

Parents can maximize their nursing potential with skin-to-skin care and frequent feeding. They may also hyperstimulate milk production by hand expression and pumping after feedings. These parents will need close follow-up after hospital discharge, until lactogenesis II (secretory activation) occurs and they have normal milk production. Parents with PCOS may wish to plan ahead with their healthcare provider for possible supplementation.

Thyroid Disorders

The thyroid hormone plays a crucial role in heart and digestive function, metabolism, brain development, bone health, and muscle control. **Thyroid disorders** are common and relate to the reproductive cycle (Amino & Arata, 2020). Even slight hypothyroidism (low thyroid) can increase rates of miscarriage, fetal death, and cognitive deficits in babies. Excessive levels (**hyperthyroidism**) can affect heart rate and blood pressure and are a concern during pregnancy.

Some obstetric professionals recommend universal screening for thyroid disorders in pregnancy. Given the rising incidence of medical complexities during pregnancy, obstetric care providers will increasingly encounter clients with subclinical or overt symptoms of thyroid disorders (Stagnaro-Green et al., 2019). Because of hormonal fluctuations during pregnancy, close monitoring is important for expectant parents who have thyroid therapy. There is a link between untreated thyroid disorders and low milk production. Appropriate treatment may make a difference in establishing adequate milk production. Some parents with hyperthyroidism report ample milk production, whereas others have difficulty with letdown (Australian Breastfeeding Association [ABA], 2022).

Hypothyroidism

Hypothyroidism results from a deficiency in thyroid secretion. Symptoms include sluggishness, low blood pressure, dry skin, obesity, and sensitivity to cold. Replacement therapy with natural or synthetic hormone preparations can eliminate these effects. When thyroid supplementation is properly managed, parents can nurse with no risk to the baby's health. The supplementation they receive merely brings their thyroid levels to normal. Therefore, the amount of thyroid secretion the baby receives through the milk is equal to that of any other nursing parent. Thyroid supplement dose levels postpartum can likely be reduced to the prepregnancy level.

For a parent who is severely hypothyroid and receiving unusually high dosages of thyroid supplement, the additional thyroid hormone that passes to the baby through nursing can mask latent hypothyroidism in the baby. When weaning begins and the level of thyroid intake decreases, a baby with latent hypothyroidism could suffer neurologic damage. Newborn screening tests for congenital hypothyroidism.

Although hypothyroidism is linked to infertility, it is possible to conceive through assisted reproductive technologies. There is a link between untreated hypothyroidism and insufficient milk production (Kam et al., 2024). If a nursing parent has low milk production and a history or markers for a thyroid disorder, you might recommend thyroid testing.

Goiter

Adequate iodine intake is necessary for normal thyroid function. Even in countries with access to iodized salt, intake may be insufficient. Insufficient iodine can lead to a **goiter**, which is an enlargement of the thyroid gland, resulting in a thick-neck or double-chin appearance. An adequate concentration of iodine is needed in the milk for optimal neonatal thyroid hormone stores and to prevent impaired neurologic development. The iodine level in the milk responds quickly to the parent's increased intake, either by consuming iodine-rich foods or by taking supplements. A daily iodine intake of 150–250 μg for nursing parents is recommended (Delshad & Azizi, 2020; Jin et al., 2021; McGuire, 2019b).

Hyperthyroidism

Hyperthyroidism, present in less than 1% of pregnancies, is a condition in which the thyroid is overactive and produces too much thyroid hormone. Untreated hyperthyroidism is associated with infertility, recurring miscarriage, preeclampsia, IUGR, and postpartum hemorrhage (Stagnaro-Green et al., 2019). Thyroid storm, characterized by a rapid heartbeat, fever, and fainting,—is linked to maternal congestive heart failure (Sorah & Alderson, 2023). In animal studies, hyperthyroidism hindered prolactin release and was associated with impaired letdown and milk production (Pennacchio et al., 2017). The National Library of Medicine of the National Institutes of Health has useful resources for hyperthyroidism in the general population (Mathew et al., 2023) and in pregnancy (Sorah & Alderson, 2023).

Graves' disease is a form of hyperthyroidism in which pressure occurs on the eyes from supporting muscles, resulting in a staring, wide-eyed appearance. It accounts for 95% of hyperthyroidism cases during pregnancy (Sorah & Alderson, 2023). Graves' disease is associated with pernicious anemia, vitiligo, diabetes mellitus type 1, autoimmune adrenal insufficiency, systemic sclerosis, myasthenia gravis, Sjögren's syndrome, rheumatoid arthritis, and systemic lupus erythematosus (Wisse, 2022).

Diagnosis of Hyperthyroidism

Hyperthyroidism is diagnosed through blood tests that reveal abnormally high thyroid hormone levels and low levels of thyroid-stimulating hormone (TSH) produced by the pituitary gland. In rare cases, the pituitary gland produces excess amounts of TSH, thereby increasing levels of both TSH and thyroid hormones in the blood. Diagnostic scans using radiopharmaceutical contrast agents may require temporary or permanent weaning. The length of nursing cessation is contingent on the type of diagnostic test and imaging agent used. There are no restrictions for some materials, such as the contrast dyes frequently used for imaging (Hale & Krutsch, 2024). However, ^{131}iodine sodium iodide requires 8 days' abstention from nursing up to complete cessation, depending on the dosage. If it is used therapeutically to remove the thyroid gland, the period of abstaining from nursing could be much longer.

The U.S. Nuclear Regulatory Commission (USNRC) provides safety guidelines and detailed information on these radiological agents (USNRC, 2019). *Medications and Mothers' Milk* provides a summary of the most used agents and suggestions for protecting lactation (Hale & Krutsch, 2024). Milk can be expressed during brief cessation and saved by refrigerating or freezing. The radioisotopes break down in the expressed milk, just as they do in the body. The milk can be tested before use if there is concern about its safety.

Treatment of Hyperthyroidism

Three medications are commonly used for the treatment of hyperthyroidism. Methimazole is considered compatible with lactation. The active metabolite in carbimazole is methimazole so carbimazole is also compatible. Propylthiouracil has historically been recommended during lactation because only small amounts are secreted into the milk (Hale & Krutsch, 2024). Methimazole has fewer potential side effects during lactation compared with propylthiouracil. Low to moderate doses of methimazole are the preferred therapy (LactMed, 2024; Rind & Mariash, 2021).

Postpartum Thyroiditis

Postpartum thyroiditis causes thyroid function to fluctuate, resulting in either transient hyperthyroidism or hypothyroidism. Postpartum thyroiditis may be an immunologic flare that occurs after the immune suppression of pregnancy. This transient dysfunction usually resolves within a year after birth. Postpartum thyroiditis has been found in 5% of parents in the general population in the first year after birth (Rad & Deluxe, 2023). Fifty percent of parents with normal thyroid levels in the first trimester of pregnancy who test positive for thyroid autoantibodies develop postpartum thyroiditis (Peng & Pearce, 2022; Rad & Deluxe, 2023). Individuals with gestational diabetes and insulin-dependent diabetes have increased rates of this condition (Alexander et al., 2017). Permanent hypothyroidism results in 20% to 40% of women who experience postpartum thyroiditis (Rad & Deluxe, 2023). Parents with markers for hyperthyroidism or hypothyroidism should contact their healthcare provider for further evaluation and care.

Cystic Fibrosis

Cystic fibrosis (CF) is an inherited genetic disease that affects the **exocrine system**. An estimated 105,000 people have been diagnosed with CF across 94 countries, with close to 40,000 in the United States (Cystic Fibrosis Foundation, 2022). CF is significantly more prevalent in Caucasians. In most people, mucus, sweat, saliva, and digestive juices are thin and watery. The defective gene in CF makes these secretions thick and sticky, causing them to clog ducts and tubes throughout the body, including the pancreas and lungs. In addition to pulmonary complications, people with CF have an increased risk of diabetes.

Cystic Fibrosis and Pregnancy

Advances in research and medical treatments have extended the life span of people with CF. The median predicted survival age for individuals born in 2022 is 68.2 years. Medications have increased the fertility of people living with CF, although the incidence of subfertility (difficulty becoming pregnant) is 35% (Middleton et al., 2020). Many young adults with CF bear children after high-risk pregnancies. In 2022, 636 U.S. women with CF had pregnancies (Cystic Fibrosis Foundation, 2023). Childbearing does not appear to hasten the progression of the disease. Expectant parents with CF require support from a multidisciplinary team during pregnancy. There is often an increase in the frequency of clinical visits and possible hospitalization for some of these parent (Jain et al., 2022). Good pain relief during labor and birth is important (Middleton et al., 2020).

Cystic Fibrosis and Nursing

People with CF may have **hypernatremia** (too much salt in the blood), although human milk sodium levels are normal. During lactation, parents with CF can maintain their weight and support healthy infant growth. They will need nutritional support and medication management that is individualized to their specific needs (Jain et al., 2022). The disease may compromise the parent nutritionally. The caloric requirements of nursing may further compromise their nutritional status. Continual monitoring of nutrition is critical for nursing parents with CF.

Nursing parents report more illness-related visits and more flare-ups. A decrease in some areas of their quality of life may reflect the difficulty of balancing parenthood and self-care. As more data become available on nursing and the use of CF medications, these parents need individualized review by their health specialists. There are a variety of medication options for people with CF during pregnancy and postpartum. Ivacaftor is considered probably safe (Jain et al., 2022).

Parents with CF may be encouraged to learn that nursing enables them to get more rest than formula feeding. Urge them to rest when the baby naps, eat nutritiously, and keep their healthcare provider appointments to optimize their health. Helping a parent with CF nurse requires good communication with them and collaboration with their multidisciplinary healthcare team. Reflective listening may be an especially important skill. Mindfulness, awareness of your own feelings, and nurturing yourself will be important as you care for this vulnerable dyad.

Maternal Phenylketonuria

Globally, about 6% of infants are born with **phenylketonuria** (PKU) worldwide (Shoraka et al., 2020). The success of newborn screening for PKU, with resulting dietary management, has led to many babies with PKU growing to maturity and having children of their own. Healthcare providers thus now encounter maternal PKU, a situation with potential dangers for a developing fetus. PKU is an inherited error of metabolism caused by a deficiency in the amino acid enzyme phenylalanine hydroxylase. The disorder is termed **phenylalanine hydroxylase deficiency (PAH)**.

PKU Treatment

A special diet with phenylalanine-free proteins and other amino acid supplements has reduced mortality and morbidity in this population. The treatment regimen is complex, expensive, and challenging to maintain. Even with good compliance, people with PKU have higher risks of lifelong mood, anxiety, and attention-deficit disorders. Enzyme therapies, including the drug pegvaliase hold promise for enabling more dietary flexibility (Ashe et al., 2019). The manufacturer states that pegvaliase is not contraindicated during pregnancy and lactation, but there are scarce data available (Rohr et al., 2020). Neutral amino acids are also increasingly used. The drug sapropterin, a medication works in conjunction with dietary restrictions. It has promising outcomes for use during pregnancy. There are scarce data about sapropterin's safety during lactation. Research now focuses on the gut microbiome and gene therapies (Ashe et al., 2019).

PKU and Pregnancy

The toxic effects of elevated maternal phenylalanine on fetal development have added to recommendations that individuals with PKU follow treatment for life (Lichter-Konecki & Vockley, 2019). A special PKU diet is especially important during pregnancy. The phenylalanine overload resulting from a regular diet can affect fetal brain growth and formation. This damage occurs before birth, regardless of whether the baby inherits PKU. Results include intellectual disabilities, heart defects, microcephaly, brachygnathia (recessed mandible), IUGR, orofacial anomalies, and psychomotor deficiencies. These are classified as maternal PKU syndrome (Zeile et al., 2018).

Some people may not be aware that they had PKU as an infant. The phenylalanine overload during infancy may not have been high enough to cause the disease. However, it still could be high enough to cause brain damage in the developing fetus. Because the special diet may be discontinued as early as 5 years of age, they may not remember why they were on the diet at an early age. Lifelong adherence to the diet is recommended. Those who plan to begin a family should ask their parents about their medical history as an infant. Parents with PKU will benefit from anticipatory guidance on the importance of raising the child to know the familial history of the disorder, both in the parents and in the child. In many countries, infants are routinely screened for PKU and other metabolic conditions at about 48 hours after birth with parental consent.

Preconception counseling for individuals living with PKU will help in planning a healthy pregnancy. Parents with PKU can nurse. The theoretically slightly elevated phenylalanine levels in the milk can be safely metabolized by infants who do not have PKU. If parents take medication and nurse, you can refer them to the PKU MOMS subregistry or the Infant Risk Center to advance knowledge about PKU medications in lactation.

Infectious Diseases

Guidelines for safety while nursing are available for parents with chronic or acute infections (Meek & Noble). **Table 26-2** summarizes the most common diseases, with recommendations for nursing. Some are discussed in greater detail within this section. Timely referenced information and recommendations on infectious diseases and outbreaks are available from the CDC (https://www.cdc.gov), the AAP (https://www.aap.org), and the WHO (https://www.who.int). **Chapter 11** discusses medications and contraindications during lactation.

Tuberculosis

Tuberculosis (TB) is a bacterial disease that usually attacks the lungs, although it can attack other body parts as well. TB is among the top 10 causes of death. In 2020, 1.5 million people globally died from TB (WHO, 2022). It is the second-leading cause of death from a single infectious agent after COVID-19. Although more prevalent in underdeveloped regions, TB occurs in all countries. Pregnant individuals with HIV should be protected from TB which provides a route for maternal-to-child transmission of HIV.

Tuberculosis and Nursing

Nursing is safe with active TB with certain precautions. When the disease is discovered in the gestational parent before birth, treatment should begin immediately during pregnancy. Concentrations of first-line anti-TB drugs in human milk are low in the nursing newborn, making lactation compatible with the use of these medications. Because of the low concentration, the amount of drugs in the milk is not sufficient treatment for active or latent TB infection in a nursing infant. Thus, prophylactic treatment should start for the baby at birth. Nursing parents taking isoniazid should also take pyridoxine (vitamin B_6) supplementation to prevent or lessen some side effects (O'Connor & Brady, 2022).

When a parent's active TB is discovered after the baby is born, direct nursing recommendations vary among countries and the medical community. The CDC recommends that parents temporarily cease nursing but that the baby can receive expressed milk, provided there is no TB mastitis, which is a rare condition. Nursing may resume after the parent has been treated for 2 weeks and is determined to be no longer contagious (Meek & Noble, 2022a). If nursing is interrupted, milk expression every 2 to 4 hours will help establish and maintain milk production. The expressed milk may be fed to the baby. **Chapter 25** discusses milk production.

Breast Tuberculosis

Rarely, TB can occur within the breast. Breast TB constitutes less than 0.1% of known breast diseases (Galego et al., 2019). It is more common in young females and lactating parents. Breast TB presents 75% of the time as a hard lump. Pain and fever are the most common symptoms (Quaglio et al., 2019). Breast TB is easily confused with breast cancer or a breast abscess (Sinha & Rahul, 2019).

Timely diagnosis and treatment of breast TB are often delayed. The gold standard for diagnosis is the detection of *Mycobacterium tuberculosis* by acid-fast bacteria (AFB) Ziehl–Neelsen stain or the isolation of the organism from the lesion on culture (Quaglio et al., 2019). Parents with this disease should first be treated with antitubercular therapy before surgical treatment for resistant or residual masses.

The same nursing restrictions as those in pulmonary TB apply except that no expressed milk should be fed to the baby (Meek & Noble, 2022a). Asking open-ended questions and taking a thorough medical history help rule out all possibilities. Breast TB is an example of why it is important for nursing parents to be examined by their healthcare provider and not merely have multiple rounds of antibiotics called in to a pharmacy with the assumption that they have mastitis.

Hepatitis

Hepatitis is an inflammatory condition of the liver that is commonly caused by a viral infection. The seven known hepatitis viruses are labeled A, B, C, D, E, F, and G. Hepatitis A, E, and F viruses are transmitted through the ingestion of contaminated food or water. The B, C, D, and G viruses are transmitted mainly through blood or bodily fluids. Hepatitis A, B, and C are pertinent to maternal health and are discussed in this section.

Hepatitis A

Hepatitis A is a viral liver disease that is usually transmitted by ingesting food or water contaminated with the feces of an infected person. It can also be

Table 26-2 **Maternal Infections and Corresponding Nursing Management for Healthy Term Infants**

Infection/Disease	Continue Nursing	Conditions or Restrictions
Bacteria		
Mastitis	Yes	Complete full course of antibiotics.
Breast abscess	Yes	If there is obvious pus, pump and discard the milk from the infected side; continue nursing on the other side.
Active tuberculosis (TB)	Yes	Delay nursing until after 2 weeks of appropriate anti-TB therapy; provide TB prophylaxis for infant.
Urinary tract infection	Yes	None.
Bacterial infection	Yes	None.
Diarrhea	Yes	Practice good hand hygiene.
Parasites	Yes	None.
Malaria	Yes	None.
Fungi	Yes	None.
Candidal vaginitis (*Candida*)	Yes	Practice good hand hygiene.
Viruses		
Hepatitis A	Yes	Give immunoglobulin prophylaxis to the infant; practice good hand hygiene.
Hepatitis B	Yes	Prevent infant hepatitis B virus (HBV) infection with hepatitis B immune globulin (HBIG) at birth; immunize with HBV vaccine.
Hepatitis C	Yes	None.
Herpes (herpes simplex virus [HSV]-1, HSV-2)	Yes	Interrupt nursing and discard pumped milk until lesions heal (crusted); practice good hand hygiene.
Varicella zoster (chicken pox, shingles)	Yes	Give varicella zoster immune globulin (VZIG) for perinatal varicella zoster virus (VZV) occurrence; consider VZIG for postpartum occurrence.
Epstein–Barr	Yes	None.
Cytomegalovirus	Yes	None.
Enterovirus	Yes	Practice good hand hygiene.
Parvovirus	Yes	Continue nursing.
West Nile virus	Yes	Continue nursing.
Human T-lymphotropic virus (HTLV)-1, HTLV-2	No	Avoid direct nursing except in resource-limited countries.
HIV	Yes, with conditions	Continue nursing if viral suppression through antiretroviral (ART) is maintained during pregnancy, delivery, and postpartum. Avoid nursing where replacement feeding is considered acceptable, feasible, affordable, sustainable, and safe.

Data from Centers for Disease Control and Infection (CDC). Centers for Disease Control and Prevention (CDC). Contraindications to Breastfeeding or Feeding Expressed Breast Milk to Infants. 2023. https://www.cdc.gov/breastfeeding/breastfeeding-special-circumstances/contraindications-to-breastfeeding.html.

spread through close physical contact with an infectious person. People living in developing countries usually achieve immunity, and childhood infections are mild. Vaccines in countries with low rates of infection are recommended.

Hepatitis A symptoms can be mild to severe and include fever, fatigue, appetite loss, nausea and diarrhea, abdominal discomfort, dark-colored urine, and jaundice. Comfort measures include rest, nutrition, and fluid replacement. Antibodies have been detected in the parent's serum and milk. Parents with hepatitis A can nurse unless they become unwell or develop jaundice. In those cases, nursing may need to stop until they have recovered (National Library of Medicine, 2022).

Hepatitis B

An estimated 254 million people are infected with **hepatitis B** worldwide (WHO, 2024). Hepatitis B symptoms are like those of hepatitis A, with joint pain and clay-colored stools. The virus affects the liver and can result in chronic liver disease. It is spread by contact with the blood, semen, or other bodily fluids of an infected person and is mostly transmitted from the parent to the child during birth.

Hepatitis B viral DNA is detected in human milk and breast lesions, such as bleeding nipples. Although nursing might increase infant exposure, it is not a risk factor for transmission from the parent to the child (Meek & Noble, 2022a). Parents with the hepatitis B virus should take extra care with their nipples to avoid cracking and bleeding. There is no reason to delay nursing initiation.

The CDC recommends that infants born to hepatitis B–infected gestational parents receive hepatitis B immune globulin and the first dose of hepatitis B vaccine within 12 hours of birth, with the second and third doses at normal intervals. The baby should be tested between 9 and 18 months of age to verify that the vaccine worked and that the infant is not infected with hepatitis B through exposure to the parent's blood during birth (CDC, 2022b).

Hepatitis C

Worldwide, at least 50 million people have chronic **hepatitis C** infection (WHO, 2024), and no vaccine exists. The virus affects the liver and is spread through donated organs or contact with an infected person's blood. Symptoms are like those of hepatitis A and B, including joint pain and gray stools. Hepatitis C can be acute or chronic, leading to severe liver problems, including cirrhosis and cancer.

An estimated 1% to 2.5% of gestational parents are infected with hepatitis C, with a corresponding 5% risk for transmission from the parent to the infant during pregnancy or delivery (CDC, 2023a). Rates for blood-transmitted infections are higher in underdeveloped regions and among individuals with high-risk behaviors such as drug use involving needles and unprotected sex. Perinatal transmission risk can be lowered by avoiding fetal scalp electrodes, prolonged membrane rupture, and birth trauma when possible.

Like other viruses, hepatitis C virus RNA is present in human milk. However, nursing has not been proven to be a route for parent-to-infant transmission (Ruiz et al., 2019). The virus is transmitted through infected blood and not through human milk. Therefore, hepatitis C virus infection is not a contraindication to nursing. Recommended precautions include not nursing on a cracked or bleeding nipple and not using the milk from the affected side until the wound has healed (CDC, 2023b; Meek & Noble, 2022a). Antiviral therapies, including interferon, ribavirin, and directly acting antiviral agents, are compatible with nursing. Safety during lactation has not been established for newer drugs, including sofosbuvir and ledipasvir. They are therefore not recommended for nursing parents (Hale & Krutsch, 2024).

Herpes Viruses

Herpes is a viral infection that is contracted through direct contact with an active lesion or the bodily fluid of an infected person. Hundreds of herpes viruses have been identified. Eight of them manifest in humans, with varying degrees of severity and incidence. Herpes infections all have similar biologic behavior, are transmitted by a virus, and are highly contagious. They manifest themselves as skin lesions that begin as small red pimples, develop into fluid-filled blisters, and then dry up and heal. During the active phase, the blisters cause a burning, tingling, and itching sensation, often accompanied by fever and enlarged lymph nodes.

Exposure to active herpes lesions can be fatal to a neonate. All active lesions must be covered to prevent exposure. Nursing is acceptable if there are no herpetic lesions in the area or if active lesions on the breast are covered. If a lesion is present on the nipple or areola, nursing should be avoided. Expressed milk from that breast should not be fed to the infant until the lesion heals. Parents with a herpes lesion can express milk to maintain production on the affected side and discard the milk. The antiviral medications acyclovir, valaciclovir, and famciclovir can reduce herpes outbreaks. They are compatible with nursing and need to be started as soon as the tingling sensation signals the appearance of the vesicle(s).

Herpes Simplex

Herpes simplex 1 and 2 are the most common herpes viruses. Both viruses are contracted through close contact with an infected person whose skin is shedding the virus. The virus lies dormant in the nervous system and is asymptomatic until it becomes active. Common activating agents are fever; physical or emotional stress; lowered immunity, as with illness or pregnancy; exposure to sunlight; and certain foods or drugs. The infection can be present in the infant without any gestational parent history of herpes, usually presenting with upper and lower respiratory symptoms, a hoarse cry, and fever.

Herpes simplex 1 (cold sore or fever blister) usually appears as an open sore on the mouth and nose areas. Herpes simplex 2 (genitalis) is usually transmitted through sexual contact. It produces painful blisters on the skin and the moist lining of the sex organs. Exposure to herpes simplex viruses can be potentially fatal to the newborn. In addition to the other herpes simplex symptoms, herpes genitalis causes painful intercourse, urinary problems, and swelling in the groin area. Parents who experience their first genital herpes simplex virus infection in pregnancy are at the highest risk of transmitting the virus to the newborn.

Oral antiviral therapies are used to treat genital herpes in late pregnancy, usually with a prophylactic dose from 36 weeks' gestation to the birth of the baby. This has helped limit recurrence, the shedding of the virus at delivery, and the necessity of cesarean delivery. The effect of these drugs in helping prevent in utero infection is unclear. Neonates who contract the disease usually do so through direct contact with the infected tissue. A parent who has active lesions within 3 weeks of delivery should deliver by a cesarean section to ensure the baby's safety.

Varicella Zoster

Varicella zoster affects the central nervous system and causes chicken pox and shingles, which are highly contagious. Chicken pox is usually contracted by children, most commonly through direct contact or through droplets from the nose or mouth. Varicella zoster remains dormant in the body, and individuals infected with chicken pox are at risk for shingles later in life when the virus reactivates. Nearly one out of every three people in the United States will develop shingles in their lifetime (CDC, 2022c). As with any type of herpes, the infection is spread through contact with an active lesion. Parents contracting shingles need to practice diligent hygiene to avoid the risk of transmission to their baby. Active shingles on a breast appears in **Figure 26-7**.

Vaccination against chicken pox has lowered the incidence in the United States and other countries using the vaccine since the late 1990s. Adults who did not have chicken pox in childhood can prevent infection by receiving the vaccine before conception. The varicella vaccine is contraindicated during pregnancy. Individuals receiving the vaccine should make sure they are not pregnant prior to receiving it (Psarris et al., 2019).

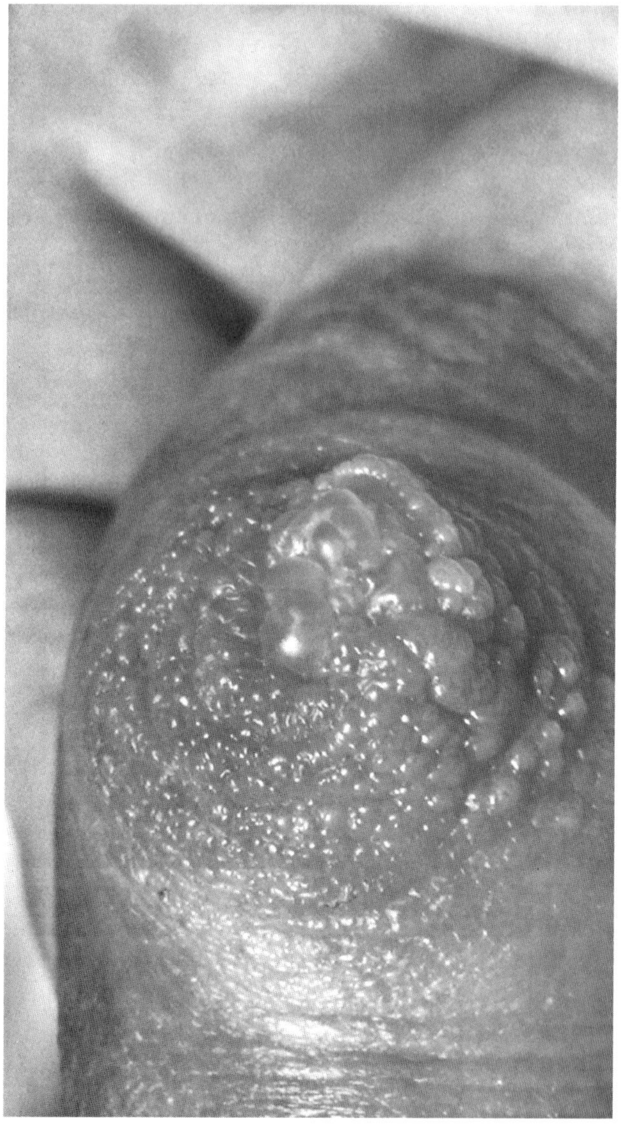

Figure 26-7 Active shingles (varicella zoster) on a breast.

Printed with permission of Shallon May-Rogers.

Contracting varicella during pregnancy carries risks for both the baby and the parent. If the parent has chicken pox at up to 20 weeks' gestation, congenital varicella syndrome may occur. The highest risk is between 7 and 20 weeks' gestation (Stanford Medicine, 2024). Congenital varicella syndrome consists of severe birth defects, including vision impairment, neurologic damage, and skin and limb deformities. A gestational parent may be treated with antiviral therapy, either alone or in combination with varicella zoster immunoglobulin. The parent and baby may remain together. Unless there are lesions on the breast, the baby may nurse (Blumental & Lepage, 2019; Meek & Noble).

When a chicken pox rash develops from 5 days before delivery up to 2 days after delivery, parents should receive varicella zoster immunoglobulin. This may not prevent infection but can reduce severity. When signs of chicken pox appear, the newborn can be treated with antiviral therapy. Nursing may continue when the baby has a chicken pox infection or exposure. Chicken pox or shingles contracted after delivery does not require isolation from the baby. If children at home have chicken pox and the parents do not test positive for antibodies, the newborn needs to receive the vaccine. The baby does not need to be isolated from siblings with chicken pox, regardless of having received varicella zoster immunoglobulin.

Epstein-Barr

Epstein-Barr is a virus that attacks the central nervous system and causes ongoing fatigue. Also called *infectious mononucleosis* (or "mono"), Epstein–Barr is acquired by most people in childhood and usually affects young adults up to age 35. It is known as the "kissing disease" because it is transmitted through human saliva. Epstein–Barr virus remains a lifelong dormant infection in some cells of the body's immune system. The virus is associated with the onset of autoimmune diseases, including lupus erythematosus, rheumatoid arthritis, and multiple sclerosis (Frappier, 2021). It is also associated with the development of cancers, including Hodgkin's disease and non-Hodgkin's lymphoma, nasopharyngeal carcinoma, and Burkitt lymphoma (CDC, 2020b; Houen & Trier, 2021).

Epstein–Barr virus is found in human milk (Francese et al., 2023). However, infection rates between nursed and formula-fed infants are similar, suggesting that nursing is not a primary source of infection. As with other viruses, human milk may confer passive immunity to the baby. Epstein–Barr infection in the parent does not contraindicate nursing. Because of the fatigue associated with Epstein–Barr, you can encourage parents to nurse lying down, nap or rest when the baby sleeps, and obtain as much household help as possible.

Cytomegalovirus

Cytomegalovirus (CMV) is a common virus for people of all ages. A healthy person's immune system usually prevents the virus from causing illness. CMV usually produces few symptoms and tends to reactivate intermittently without symptoms. Symptoms include fatigue, fever, swollen lymph glands, pneumonia, and liver or spleen defects. Nearly all adults are infected with CMV by the age of 50. CMV infection while pregnant results in congenital CMV infection in 1 out of every 200 infants. An estimated 40% to 50% of these infants may experience long-term health issues, including hearing and vision loss, intellectual disabilities, microcephaly, motor weakness, and seizures (CDC, 2020a, 2020b).

CMV can be shed in the bodily fluids of the infected person, including milk. There is not enough evidence to support withholding the parent's milk because of the risk of CMV infection (Meek & Noble, 2022a; Parker et al., 2021). Healthy, term infants can nurse even when the virus is shedding into the milk. Nursing babies may receive passive immunity to CMV through the milk. CMV in a gestational parent places preterm babies at a higher risk for becoming ill, however. The more preterm the infant is, the higher the risk, including below 32 weeks' gestational age and under 1000 g birth weight (Resch, 2022).

The greatest danger of CMV to infants is the possibility of **seroconversion** if a preterm or immunologically impaired infant of a seronegative gestational parent receives donor milk from a seropositive milk donor. Because the infant has not received **transplacental** antibodies, the infection could be serious. Although freezing may reduce the viral load of CMV in the milk, it does not change the risk of CMV sepsis-like syndrome (Meek & Noble, 2022a). Pasteurization destroys some of the milk's immunologic properties and can decrease the likelihood of CMV transmission. It provides donor recipients protection from CMV (Meek & Noble, 2022a). Pasteurization of donor milk is the standard for milk bank processing. **Chapter 22** discusses human milk banking.

Other Herpes Viruses

Three lesser-known herpes viruses also appear in humans. Human herpesvirus 6 (HHV6) presents as roseola infantum or exanthema subitum (rashes) and is usually self-limiting. Human herpesvirus 7 (HHV7) sheds in saliva and causes roseola; most children acquire it by age 3. Human herpesvirus 8 (HHV8) is a gamma herpes virus that appears to be spread through saliva and is commonly acquired in childhood. Human herpesvirus 8 (HHV8) is associated with Kaposi sarcoma, multicentric Castleman disease, and primary effusion lymphoma, diseases that most often occur in immunocompromised people. Malignancies associated with HHV8 are significantly higher in individuals living with HIV (Rewane & Tadi, 2023). Nursing has been found to be protective against HHV8 infection for children. A very low detected DNA load suggests that transmission of HHV8 via human milk is not likely (Francese et al., 2023).

Human T-Cell Lymphotropic Virus Type 1

The first human retrovirus to be discovered, human T-cell lymphotropic virus (HTLV), infects only T cells. The HTLV is in the same class of virus as the HIV/AIDS virus. Of the three subtypes HTLV-1, -2, and -3, HTLV-1 is the most prevalent and is highly oncogenic (having the potential to cause cancer) (Francese et al., 2023). HTLV is found in specific geographical areas, including Japan, the Caribbean, South and Central America, West Africa, and the southeastern United States. The virus affects at least 5 to 10 million people worldwide. Up to 10% of these people will progress to severe disease (Rosadas & Taylor, 2019).

HTLV infection usually develops without symptoms and can present years after exposure. It is transmitted through sex; blood exposure, including transfusions; and nursing. Transmission of the virus is primarily via human milk (Millen & Thoma-Kress, 2022). The disease is linked to adult T-cell leukemia/lymphoma, a rare and aggressive T-cell lymphoma, and myelopathy/tropical spastic paraparesis, a debilitating neurologic condition. HTLV can also lead to chronic health conditions, including uveitis, iritis, dermatitis, peripheral neuropathies, and arthritis (Tagaya et al., 2019).

Nursing for under 6 months (preferably no longer than 3 months as recommended in Japan) is not shown to increase the risk of parent–child HTLV-I infection transmission. However, nursing over 6 months significantly increases the risk (Rosadas & Taylor, 2022). Not nursing lowers the risk the most but must be weighed against the risks of unsafe formula feeding in low-resource areas. HTLV-1 is considered a contraindication to nursing (Meek & Noble, 2022a).

Human Immunodeficiency Virus

Human immunodeficiency virus (HIV) is a retrovirus that destroys the human immune system. It can lead to **acquired immune deficiency syndrome (AIDS)**, in which the body cannot fight off viral, bacterial, mycobacterial, and fungal pathogens. HIV is spread through sexual contact, bodily fluids, and intravenous drug use. HIV/AIDS is a major global health emergency that affects all regions of the world. It has caused millions of deaths and suffering for millions more. About 39 million people are living with HIV, and an estimated 1.7 million new infections occur annually. About 630,000 people died from AIDS-related conditions in 2022. HIV/AIDS especially affects children and birth parents. It is estimated that 4000 women between the ages of 15 and 24 are infected with HIV every week (UNAIDS, 2023).

When left untreated, HIV quickly leads to infection, disease, and death. No cure exists for HIV infection. Effective antiretroviral (ARV) drug therapy can slow the progression of the disease significantly and enable HIV-positive people to continue to lead productive lives. As of January 2022, 29.8 million people living with HIV were receiving antiretroviral therapy (ART) (UNAIDS, 2023). ART is recommended as a daily pre-exposure prophylaxis (called PrEP) for HIV-negative partners to prevent HIV infection (UNAIDS, 2023). ART is also used after exposure to prevent the development of HIV infection, especially in healthcare workers.

HIV and Nursing

Vertical transmission, or transmission from the birthing parent to the child, of HIV occurs from an HIV-positive parent to the baby during pregnancy, birth, or through nursing, especially mixed feeding (Prendergast et al., 2019). Rates of infection without any interventions are estimated at 15% to 45%. The effective use of ARV drug therapy significantly prevents infection if both the parent and child are treated during key stages (WHO, 2019). The WHO recommends ARV drug therapy to gestational parents and infants during pregnancy, birth, postpartum, and while nursing, as well as lifelong treatment for the parents.

WHO 2016 guidelines support HIV-positive parents to nurse for at least 12 months, with continued nursing for up to 24 months or longer (WHO, 2019; WHO & United Nations Children's Fund [UNICEF], 2016). ARV interventions for either the HIV-infected parent or the exposed infant significantly reduce the risk of postnatal transmission of HIV through nursing. The 2016 guidelines seek to balance HIV prevention with protection from other causes of child mortality (such as not nursing) and integrate HIV interventions into health services (WHO & UNICEF, 2016). Previous guidelines for industrialized countries had recommended that HIV-positive parents not nurse where replacement feeding is considered acceptable, feasible, affordable, sustainable, and safe.

Healthcare providers should inform HIV-positive parents that if their viral load is undetectable, the risk of transmitting HIV through nursing is less than 1% (CDC, 2023d, 2023e). HIV-positive parents from high-income regions who receive successful ART treatment are increasingly choosing to nurse their infants. Long-term studies are needed about the risks and benefits of various feeding modalities and the impact of not nursing on morbidity, mortality, and health (Moseholm & Weiss, 2020).

Human milk helps to prevent the oral transmission of HIV (Mangan et al., 2019). This may explain why exclusively nursed infants of HIV-positive parents have an 85% rate of noninfection. The milk is rich in oligosaccharides and glycoproteins, including tenascin, that broadly neutralize HIV by binding the virus. Other immune factors, such as lactoferrin and elafin, also play roles in neutralizing HIV in human milk (Morniroli et al., 2021).

Heat Treating the Milk

Human milk bank processing has demonstrated that heat treatment does not significantly alter milk's nutritional composition and is a far superior choice than easily contaminated infant formula. Heat treatment of expressed milk from parents known to be infected with HIV is an approach to safely provide human milk to exposed infants when direct nursing is not recommended.

Holder pasteurization, a low-temperature, long-time heating method (62.5°C for 30 minutes), is used in institutional human milk banking. It takes longer than the home heat treatment options of **Pretoria pasteurization** and the **flash-heat method** (**Figure 26-8**). These methods are an effective means of inactivating HIV in the milk. Most immunoglobulin activity in the milk survives the flash-heat method, suggesting that flash-heated milk is immunologically superior to infant formula (Capriati et al., 2019).

Pretoria Pasteurization:

- Place milk (between 50 and 150 ml) in a clean glass container and cover.
- Boil 450 ml water in a small pan of water and remove from the heat source.
- Place covered container upright in the pan of boiled water, cover the pan and leave for 20 minutes.
- Remove the container from the water, remove the cover, and cool to room temperature.

Flash-heat Pasteurization:

- Place milk (between 50 and 150 ml) into a clean uncovered glass container.
- Place the container upright in a small pan of water level about two finger widths above the level of the milk.
- Heat the water on a very hot fire or stove until it reaches a rolling boil.
- Remove the container from the water immediately and cool to room temperature.

Figure 26-8 Options for home pasteurization of human milk.

Modified from World Alliance for Breastfeeding Action (WABA). Understanding international policy on HIV and breastfeeding: a comprehensive resource. 2nd ed. 2018. https://waba.org.my/understanding-international-policy-on-hiv-and-breastfeeding/.

Zika and Ebola Viruses

Zika virus is spread mostly through the bite of an infected mosquito. The virus can be transmitted to the fetus during pregnancy and cause birth defects, including microcephaly. Despite limited research indicating that Zika viral material transfers into the milk, the baby can nurse. No parent-to-infant transmission through nursing or human milk intake was found in a systematic review, but more research is needed (Centeno-Tablante et al., 2021). There is no vaccine or medicine for Zika.

Ebola disease is caused by an infection with one of a group of viruses that are found primarily in sub-Saharan Africa. The Ebola virus is spread by close contact with an infected animal. Where a safe alternative is available, the baby should not nurse. When a parent has Ebola, the dyad should be separated. Nursing is not recommended during an active infection (CDC, 2020c; WHO, 2020). Nursing must be delayed until at least two consecutive tests 24 hours apart indicate no evidence of the virus.

Disabilities

One billion people, or 15% of the world's population, experience some form of disability, with a higher rate in underdeveloped regions (World Bank, 2023). With the resurgence of nursing and with increased fertility through assisted reproductive technology, more people with physical, neurologic, or other disabilities are bearing children. There are disparities in nursing outcomes for these parents (Brown et al., 2023). Barriers to nursing include lack of support, overall health related to the disability, little resource information, and difficulties with milk production or latch (Powell et al., 2018).

Physical Disabilities

It is important lactation caregivers gain understanding and be comfortable and confident in providing nursing support and care to parents with physical challenges. Practices that support nursing include the use of equipment and adaptations, breast pump use, physical help from other people with positioning and holding the baby, and peer support (Warkentin et al., 2021). Important aspects of care for people with disabilities are independence, staying in control, shared decision-making, and working with birthing care providers who are respectful of their autonomy (Blair et al., 2022).

People live with paralysis of varying degrees because of stroke, multiple sclerosis, spinal cord injury, traumatic brain injury, neurofibromatosis, cerebral palsy, or other causes. Parents with limited physical strength because of a muscular disease or injury can often nurse with help and adaptations. There is a lack of research for parents with these conditions.

In a recent case report, a parent experienced tetraplegia following a motor vehicle accident. Because of her previous experience of nursing her first child for 9 months, she was able to nurse her second baby for 3 months with assistance from care personnel, and nursing aids (Lee et al., 2019). Resources for parents with disabilities, including adaptive equipment, are available from nonprofit organizations (Christopher & Dana Reeve Foundation, 2021; Through the Looking Glass, 2020).

Neurologic Disabilities

Challenges for a parent with a history of seizures or a diagnosed seizure disorder, such as epilepsy, depend on the extent to which the disorder is controlled. Some people with seizure histories have symptoms preceding the seizure, from a few seconds to several minutes. For others, the seizure strikes with little warning. The safety of the infant is the primary concern. Parents can ensure there is a playpen nearby to quickly place the baby when they feel a seizure approaching. Support from pillows will provide a safe environment while nursing. A medical alert tag on the stroller when away from home will notify others if a seizure occurs.

Supporting Parents with Disabilities

New parents with disabilities want and need guidance, like any other new family. They may have cognitive and social needs as well as physical needs. A multidisciplinary and creative approach will help provide appropriate support for parents with disabilities to nurse their babies. Compile resources for local occupational and physical therapists who have experience or interest in helping parents achieve self-confidence and self-efficacy. Encourage parents to collaborate with their healthcare team to express their nursing needs and goals so that they will receive support. Recognizing the strengths and resiliencies of these parents will help healthcare providers focus on more than their physical limitations.

Summary

Parents with challenging circumstances involving their health often reach their nursing goals despite these obstacles. Some may need to change their goals to accommodate their special situation. Your assistance will be valuable to them as they navigate their unexpected parenting journey, including any necessary accommodations in nursing. You can help them recognize ways in which nursing and human milk helps meet the needs of their babies. Despite health conditions, parents can establish enriching and sound nursing practices that do not compromise their own health or that of the baby.

What You Learned—At a Glance

Conversation Starters with Parents

- What health conditions do you have that you think might affect nursing?
- What problems did you have with getting pregnant?
- What concerns do you have about nursing when you are sick?
- How will you manage feedings with your disability?

Special Health Conditions

- Autoimmune diseases such as chronic fatigue, Sjögren's syndrome, and Raynaud's phenomenon may affect nursing.
- There is a correlation between endometriosis, infertility, and autoimmune disorders.
- Insulin levels in nursing parents with diabetes may fluctuate erratically until lactation is established and again when weaning occurs.
- Individuals with diabetes are prone to yeast infections.

- Gestational diabetes places parents at higher risk for converting to type 2 diabetes.
- The cause of obesity is multifaceted. It may cause a delay in milk production because of an increase in surgical delivery, hormonal imbalances, and weight bias from healthcare professionals.
- Bariatric surgery for obesity carries lifelong nutritional implications.
- Primary insufficient milk may respond to metoclopramide, domperidone, or other medications.
- Decreasing insulin resistance may help increase milk production for those with PCOS.
- Properly managed thyroid supplementation is not a risk to an infant's health.
- Thyroid hormone in the milk can mask latent hypothyroidism in the baby.
- Nursing is safe with CF, with attention to special nutritional needs.

Infectious Diseases

- Nursing is safe with TB, with certain precautions and treatment.
- There is a low risk of transmitting hepatitis B or C to infants through nursing.
- Active herpes lesions must be covered to prevent infant exposure.
- Chicken pox contracted at delivery requires isolation from the newborn until the lesions heal; the milk can be given to the infant if there are no lesions on the breast.
- Nursing babies may receive passive immunity to CMV through human milk and transplacental antibodies.
- Very-low-birth-weight preterm babies are at risk for illness from CMV-positive milk.
- HIV-positive parents in industrialized nations may nurse if their viral loads are undetectable and they are taking anti-retroviral medications.
- With an undetectable viral load in the milk, the risk of transmitting HIV is less than 1%.
- HIV-positive parents in underdeveloped regions who receive antiviral therapy should nurse exclusively for 6 months and continue to nurse for up to 24 months.
- Mortality and morbidity rates for babies of HIV-positive gestational parents in underdeveloped regions are higher if the babies are not nursed.

Disabilities

- Increasing numbers of parents with disabilities are bearing children and nursing.
- Adaptive positioning and equipment for disabilities can accommodate nursing.
- The primary concern for parents with disabilities is the physical safety of the infant.
- Encourage a multidisciplinary approach for these families, and focus on their strengths and resiliencies, not solely on the disabilities.

References

Achike M, Akpinar-Elci M. The role of maternal prepregnancy body mass index in breastfeeding outcomes: a systematic review. *Breastfeed Med.* 2021;16(9):678–686.

Akhter Z, et al. Pregnancy after bariatric surgery and adverse perinatal outcomes: a systematic review and meta-analysis. *PLoS Med.* 2019;16(8):e1002866.

Alexander EK, et al. 2017 Guidelines of the American Thyroid Association for the diagnosis and management of thyroid disease during pregnancy and the postpartum. *Thyroid.* 2017;27(3): 315–389. Erratum in: Thyroid. 2017;27(9):1212.

Alotiby AA. The role of breastfeeding as a protective factor against the development of the immune-mediated disease: a systematic review. *Front Pediatr.* 2023;11:1–12.

Aly A, et al. Bariatric surgery: a call for greater access to coordinated surgical and specialist care in the public health system. *Med J Aust* 2022;217(5):228–231.

American Academy of Pediatrics, Section on Obesity, Section on Surgery; Armstrong SC, et al. Pediatric metabolic and bariatric surgery: evidence, barriers, and best practices. *Pediatrics.* 2019;144(6).

American Autoimmune Related Diseases Association, Inc. Women and autoimmunity. 2020. https://www.aarda.org/who-we-help/patients/women-and-autoimmunity/

American College of Rheumatology. Sjögren's syndrome. February, 2025. https://rheumatology.org/patients/sjogrens-disease

American Diabetes Association. The path to understanding diabetes starts here. 2020. https://www.diabetes.org/diabetes

American Society for Metabolic and Bariatric Surgery. Estimate of bariatric surgery numbers, 2011–2018. 2020. https://asmbs.org/resources/estimate-of-bariatric-surgery-numbers

Amino N, Arata N. Thyroid dysfunction following pregnancy and implications for breastfeeding. *Best Pract Res Clin Endocrinol Metab.* 2020;34(4):101438.

Ashe K, et al. Psychiatric and cognitive aspects of phenylketonuria: the limitations of diet and promise of new treatments. *Front Psychiatry.* 2019;10:561.

Australian Breastfeeding Association. Breastfeeding and thyroid disease. 2022. https://www.breastfeeding.asn.au/resources/breastfeeding-and-thyroid-disease

Bermas BL. Safety of rheumatic disease medication use during pregnancy and lactation. UpToDate. 2024. https://www.uptodate.com/contents/safety-of-rheumatic-disease-medication-use-during-pregnancy-and-lactation

Blair A, et al. Access to, and experiences of, maternity care for women with physical disabilities: a scoping review. *Midwifery*. 2022;107:103273.

Blum T, et al. Trpc5 deficiency causes hypoprolactinemia and altered function of oscillatory dopamine neurons in the arcuate nucleus. *Proc Natl Acad Sci USA*. 2019;116(30): 15236–15243.

Blumental S, Lepage P. Management of varicella in neonates and infants. *BMJ Paediatr Open*. 2019;3(1):e000433.

Borba VV, et al. Prolactin and autoimmunity: the hormone as an inflammatory cytokine. *Best Pract Res Clin Endocrinol Metab*. 2019;33(6):101324.

Brown HK, et al. Disability and in-hospital breastfeeding practices and supports in Ontario, Canada: a population-based study. *Lancet Public Health*. 2023;8(1):e47–e56.

Cai W, et al. Association between phthalate metabolites and risk of endometriosis: a meta-analysis. *Int J Environ Res Public Health*. 2019;16(19)3678.

Capriati T, et al. A modified holder pasteurization method for donor human milk: preliminary data. *Nutrients*. 2019;11(5):1139.

Casey JRR, et al. The effects of expressing antenatal colostrum in women with diabetes in pregnancy: a retrospective cohort study. *Aust N Z J Obstet Gynaecol*. 2019;59(6):811–818.

Centeno-Tablante E, et al. Update on the transmission of Zika virus through breast milk and breastfeeding: a systematic review of the evidence. *Viruses*. 2021;13(1):123.

Centers for Disease Control and Prevention. Cytomegalovirus (CMV) and congenital CMV infection. For healthcare providers. Reviewed August 18, 2020a. https://www.cdc.gov/cmv/clinical/

Centers for Disease Control and Prevention. Epstein-Barr virus and infectious mononucleosis. For healthcare providers. Reviewed 2020b. https://www.cdc.gov /epstein-barr/hcp.html

Centers for Disease Control and Prevention. Chickenpox (varicella). For healthcare professionals. October 21, 2022a. https://www.cdc.gov/chickenpox/hcp/index.html

Centers for Disease Control and Prevention. Hepatitis B questions and answers for health professionals. Reviewed March 30, 2022b. https://www.cdc.gov/hepatitis/hbv/hbvfaq.htm#overview

Centers for Disease Control and Prevention. Shingles (herpes zoster). For health care professionals. Reviewed February 3, 2022c. https://www.cdc.gov/shingles/hcp/index.html

Center for Disease Control and Prevention. CDC recommendations for hepatitis C testing among perinatally exposed infants and children—United States, 2023. Reviewed November 3, 2023a. https://www.cdc.gov/mmwr/volumes/72/rr/rr7204a1.htm

Centers for Disease Control and Prevention. Contraindications to breastfeeding or feeding expressed breast milk to infants. April 17, 2023b. https://www.cdc.gov /breastfeeding/breastfeeding-special-circumstances/Contraindications-to-breastfeeding.html

Centers for Disease Control and Prevention. Ebola virus disease. Mothers with confirmed or suspected Ebola virus disease (EVD) should not breastfeed their infants. Reviewed April 4, 2023c. https://www.cdc.gov/breastfeeding/breast feeding-special-circumstances/maternal-or-infant-illnesses/ebola.html

Centers for Disease Control and Prevention. HIV transmission. Reviewed February 2, 2023d. https://www.cdc.gov/breastfeeding/breastfeeding-special-circumstances/maternal-or-infant-illnesses/hiv.html

Centers for Disease Control and Prevention. How can I prevent transmitting HIV to my baby? Reviewed February 2, 2023e. https://www.cdc.gov/hiv/basics/hiv-prevention/mother-to-child.html

Centers for Disease Control and Prevention. Diabetes during pregnancy. May 2024. https://www.cdc.gov/maternal-infant-health/pregnancy-diabetes/index.html

Christopher & Dana Reeve Foundation. Parenting with paralysis. 2021. https://s3.amazonaws.com/reeve-assets-production/Parenting-Booklet-second-ed-online-8-27-21.pdf

Çiçekli İ, Durusoy R. Breastfeeding, nutrition and type 1 diabetes: a case-control study in Izmir, Turkey. *Int Breastfeed J*. 2022;27;17(1):42.

Cordero L, et al. Exclusive breastfeeding among women with type 1 and type 2 diabetes mellitus. *BMC Pregnancy Childbirth*. 2022;27;22(1):69.

Cystic Fibrosis Foundation. CF Foundation estimates increase in CF population. 2022. https://www.cff.org/news/2022-07/cf-foundation-estimates-increase-cf-population

Cystic Fibrosis Foundation. *Cystic Fibrosis Foundation Patient Registry 2022 Annual Data Report*. Bethesda, MD: Cystic Fibrosis Foundation; 2023.

Delshad H, Azizi F. Iodine nutrition in pregnant and breastfeeding women: sufficiency, deficiency, and supplementation. *Hormones (Athens)*. 2020;19(2):179–186.

Dhillon-Smith RK, et al. The prevalence of thyroid dysfunction and autoimmunity in women with history of miscarriage or subfertility. *J Clin Endocrinol*. 2020;105(8):2667–2677.

Diana A, et al. Breastmilk intake among exclusively breastfed Indonesian infants is negatively associated with maternal fat mass. *Eur J Clin Nutr*. 2019;73(8):1206–1208.

Francese R, et al. Viruses and human milk: transmission or protection? *Adv in Nutr*. 2023;14(6):1389–1415.

Frappier L. Epstein-Barr virus: current questions and challenges. *Tumour Virus Res*. 2021;12:200218.

Fruh SM, et al., Weight bias and stigma: impact on health. *Nurs Clin North Am*. 2021;56(4):479–493.

Hagen SJ, Henningfield MF. Health at Every Size pinciples: Clinician perspectives to limit weight stigma in medical care. *WMJ*. 2023;122(4):277–279.

Galego MA, et al. Tuberculosis of the breast: an uncommon presentation of an old disease. *BMJ Case Rep*. 2019;12(2):e227014. https://www.ncbi.nlm.nih.gov/books/NBK592383/

Giraudo F, et al. Effect on insulin sensitivity of combined oral hormonal contraceptives and progestin implant use in young women with T1D. *IPME Abstracts*. 2023;49:96.

Güngör D, et al. Infant milk-feeding practices and diabetes outcomes in offspring: a systematic review. *Am J Clin Nutr*. 2019;109(suppl 7):817S–837S.

Hale T, Krutsch K. *Hale's Medications & Mothers' Milk 2025–2026: A Manual of Lactational Pharmacology*. 21st ed. New York: Springer Publishing Company; 2024.

Houen G, Trier NH. Epstein-Barr virus and systemic autoimmune diseases. *Front Immunol*. 2021;11:587380.

Jain R, et al. Pregnancy in cystic fibrosis: review of the literature and expert recommendations. *J Cyst Fibros*. 2022;21:387–395.

Jin Y, et al. Use of iodine supplements by breastfeeding mothers is associated with better maternal and infant iodine status. *Biol Trace Elem Res*. 2021;199(8):2893–2903.

Johnsen M, et al. Antenatal breastmilk expression for women with diabetes in pregnancy—a feasibility study. *Int Breastfeed J.* 2021;16(1):56.

Joseph S, Mahale SD. Endometriosis Knowledgebase: a gene-based resource on endometriosis. *Database (Oxford).* 2019;2019: baz062.

Kam RL, et al. Modern, exogenous exposures associated with altered mammary gland development: a systematic review. *Early Hum Dev.* 2021;56:105342.

Kam RL, et al. Worldwide prevalence of breast hypoplasia in women: a systematic review. *Breastfeed Rev.* 2023;31(3):17–27.

Kam RL, et al. Breast hypoplasia markers among women who report insufficient milk production: a retrospective online survey. *PLoS One.* 2024;19(2):e0299642.

Kamal FA, et al. Nutritional deficiencies before and after bariatric surgery in low- and high-income countries: prevention and treatment. *Cureus.* 2024;16(2):e55062.

Kampmann U, et al. Extreme insulin resistance during pregnancy: a therapeutic challenge. *Endocrinol Diabetes Metab Case Rep.* 2021;20-0191.

Karwacka A, et al. Exposure to modern, widespread environmental endocrine disrupting chemicals and their effect on the reproductive potential of women: an overview of current epidemiological evidence. *Hum Fertil (Camb).* 2019;22(1): 2–25.

Kim C, et al. Infertility, gravidity, and risk of diabetes among high-risk women in the Diabetes Prevention Program Outcomes Study. *J Clin Endocrinol Metab.* 2020;105(3):e358–e367.

Klein-Weigel P, et al. Raynaud's phenomenon: a vascular acrosyndrome that requires long-term care. *Dtsch Arztebl Int.* 2021; 118:273–280.

Koschinski-Möller B. Raynaud's phenomenon in the breast nipple area. *Dtsch Arztebl Int.* 2021;118I(35–36):605.

LactMed. Methimazole. Drugs and Lactation Database. National Institute of Child Health and Human Development. Updated July 2024. https://www.ncbi.nlm.nih.gov/books/NBK501922/

Larsen JK, Bode L. Obesogenic programming effects during lactation: a narrative review and conceptual model focusing on underlying mechanisms and promising future research avenues. *Nutrients.* 2021;13(2):299.

Lee AHX, et al. Breastfeeding before and after spinal cord injury: a case report of a mother with C6 tetraplegia. *J Hum Lact.* 2019;35(4):742–747.

Lichter-Konecki U, Vockley J. Phenylketonuria: current treatments and future developments. *Drugs.* 2019;79(5):495–500.

Lu P, et al. Acupoint-tuina therapy promotes lactation in postpartum women with insufficient milk production who underwent caesarean sections. *Medicine (Baltimore).* 2019;98(35): e16456.

Lupus Foundation of America. Planning a pregnancy when you have lupus. June 27, 2021. https://www.lupus.org/resources/planning-a-pregnancy-when-you-have-lupus

Ma S, et al. Metabolic effects of breastfeed in women with prior gestational diabetes mellitus: a systematic review and meta-analysis. *Diabetes Metab Res Rev.* 2019;35(3):e3108.

Mangan RJ, et al. Determinants of tenascin-C and HIV-1 envelope binding and neutralization. *Mucosal Immunol.* 2019;12(4):1004–1012.

Maslin K, et al. Nutritional and perinatal outcomes of pregnant women with a history of bariatric surgery: a case series from a UK centre. *J Hum Nutr Diet.* 2020;33(3):386–395.

Masood B, Moorthy M. Causes of obesity: a review. *Clin Med (Lond).* 2023;23(4):284–291.

Mathew P, et al. Hyperthyroidism. In: *StatPearls.* Treasure Island, FL: StatPearls Publishing; 2023. https://www.ncbi.nlm.nih.gov/books/NBK537053/

McGuire E. Insufficient glandular tissue: a case report. *Breastfeed Rev.* 2019a;27(3):53–59.

McGuire E. Iodine, pregnancy and breastfeeding in Australia. *Breastfeed Rev.* 2019b;27(1):31–38.

Meek JY, Noble L. Section on Breastfeeding. Policy statement: breastfeeding and the use of human milk. *Pediatrics.* 2022a;150(1):e2022057988.

Middleton PG, et al. ERS/TSANZ Task Force statement on the management of reproduction and pregnancy in women with airways diseases. *Eur Respir J.* 2020;55(2):1901208.

Millen S, Thoma-Kress AL. Milk transmission of HTLV-1 and the need for innovative prevention strategies. *Front Med (Lausanne).* 2022;9:867147.

Moriwaki M, Welt CK. PRL Mutation causing alactogenesis: insights into prolactin structure and function relationships. *J Clin Endocrinol Metab.* 2021;106(8):e3021–e3026.

Morniroli D, et al. The antiviral properties of human milk: a multitude of defence tools from mother nature. *Nutrients.* 2021;13(2):694.

Moseholm E, Weis N. Women living with HIV in high-income settings and breastfeeding. *J Intern Med.* 2020;287(1):19–31.

National Institute of Arthritis and Musculoskeletal and Skin Disease. Raynaud's phenomenon. July 2024. https://www.niams.nih.gov/health-topics/raynauds-phenomenon

National Library of Medicine. Hepatitis A. In: *Mother to Baby Fact Sheets.* Brentwood, TN: Organization of Teratology Information Specialists; September 2022. https://www.ncbi.nlm.nih.gov/books/NBK582741/

NHSInform. Sjogren's syndrome. February 21, 2025. https://www.nhsinform.scot/illnesses-and-conditions/immune-system/sjogrens-syndrome/

Nommsen-Rivers LA, et al. Measures of maternal metabolic health as predictors of severely low milk production. *Breastfeed Medicine.* 2022;17(7):566–576.

Noubiap, JJ, et al. Geographic distribution of metabolic syndrome and its components in the general adult population: a meta-analysis of global data from 28 million individuals. *Diabetes Res. Clin. Pract.* 2022;188:109924.

O'Connor C, Brady MF. Isoniazid. In: *StatPearls.* Treasure Island, FL: StatPearls Publishing; 2022. https://www.ncbi.nlm.nih.gov/books/NBK557617/

Palumbo P, et al. Weight loss trend after bariatric surgery in a population of obese patients. *Clinical Nutrition ESPEN.* 2023;57:58–64.

Parker MG, et al. Section on Breastfeeding, Committee on Nutrition, Committee on Fetus and Newborn. Promoting human milk and breastfeeding for the very low birth weight infant. *Pediatrics.* 2021;148(5):e2021054272.

Peng CC, Pearce EN. An update on thyroid disorders in the postpartum period. *J Endocrinol Invest.* 2022;45(8):1497–1506.

Pennacchio GE, et al. Effect of hyperthyroidism on circulating prolactin and hypothalamic expression of tyrosine hydroxylase, prolactin signaling cascade members and estrogen and progesterone receptors during late pregnancy and lactation in the rat. *Mol Cell Endocrinol.* 2017;442:40–50.

Powell RM, et al. Breastfeeding among women with physical disabilities in the United States. *J Hum Lact.* 2018;34(2):253–261.

Prendergast AJ, et al. Transmission of CMV, HTLV-1, and HIV through breastmilk. *Lancet Child Adolesc Health.* 2019;3(4): 264–273.

Psarris A, et al. Immunizations during pregnancy: how, when and why. *Eur J Obstet Gynecol Reprod Biol.* 2019;240:29–35.

Quaglio G, et al. Breast tuberculosis in women: a systematic review. *Am J Trop Med Hyg.* 2019;101(1):12–21.

Rad NS, Deluxe L. Postpartum thyroiditis. In: *StatPearls*. Treasure Island, FL: StatPearls Publishing; 2023. https://www.ncbi.nlm.nih.gov/books/NBK557646/

Rasmussen B, et al. Development of a breastfeeding website for women with pre-pregnancy diabetes: a mixed-methods study. *Breastfeed Rev.* 2023:31(1):33–45.

Resch B. How to provide breast milk for the preterm infant and avoid symptomatic cytomegalovirus infection with possible long-term sequelae. *Life (Basel).* 2022;12(4):504.

Retamozo S, et al. Sjögren Big Data Consortium. Systemic manifestations of primary Sjögren's syndrome out of the ESSDAI classification: prevalence and clinical relevance in a large international, multi-ethnic cohort of patients. *Clin Exp Rheumatol.* 2019;37(suppl 118[3]):97–106.

Rewane A, Tadi P. Herpes virus type 8. In: *StatPearls*. Treasure Island, FL: StatPearls Publishing; 2023. https://www.ncbi.nlm.nih.gov/books/NBK556023/

Rind J, Mariash CN. Hyperthyroidism in pregnancy and lactation: a different paradigm? *J Endocr Soc.* 2021;5(4):bvab001.

Rogozińska E, et al. Gestational weight gain outside the Institute of Medicine recommendations and adverse pregnancy outcomes: analysis using individual participant data from randomised trials. *BMC Pregnancy Childbirth.* 2019;19(1):322.

Rohr F, et al. Discontinuation of pegvaliase therapy during maternal PKU pregnancy and postnatal breastfeeding: a case report. *Mol Genet Metab Rep.* 2020;22:100555.

Rosadas C, Taylor GP. Mother-to-child HTLV-1 transmission: unmet research needs. *Front Microbiol.* 2019;10:999.

Rosadas C, Taylor GP. Current interventions to prevent HTLV-1 mother-to-child transmission and their effectiveness: a systematic review and meta-analysis. *Microorganisms.* 2022;10(11):2227.

RóŻańska-Walędziak A, et al. The influence of bariatric surgery on pregnancy and perinatal outcomes—a case-control study. *J Clin Med.* 2020;9(5):1324.

RóŻańska-Walędziak A, et al. Nutritional implications of bariatric surgery on pregnancy management—a narrative review of the literature. *Medicina (Kaunas).* 2023;59(10):1864.

Ruiz L, et al. Unfolding the human milk microbiome landscape in the omics era. *Front Microbiol.* 2019;10:1378.

Sharma A. Endometriosis: diagnosis and management. *Best Practice Journal.* 2021:1–9. https://bpac.org.nz/2021/endometriosis.aspx

Shawe J, et al. Pregnancy after bariatric surgery: consensus recommendations for periconception, antenatal and postnatal care. *Obes Rev.* 2019;20(11):1507–1522.

Shigesi N, et al. The association between endometriosis and autoimmune diseases: a systematic review and meta-analysis. *Human Reproduction Update.* 2019;25(4):486–503.

Shoraka HR, et al. Global prevalence of classic phenylketonuria based on neonatal screening program data: systematic review and meta-analysis. *Clin Exp Pediatr.* 2020;63(2):34–43.

Sinha R, Rahul K. Breast tuberculosis. *Indian J Tuberc.* 2019;66(1):6–11.

Sorah K, Alderson TL. Hyperthyroidism in pregnancy. In: *StatPearls*. Treasure Island, FL: StatPearls Publishing; 2023. https://www.ncbi.nlm.nih.gov/books/NBK559203/

Stagnaro-Green A, et al. Universal screening for thyroid disease during pregnancy should be performed. *Best Pract Res Clin Endocrinol Metab.* 2019:101320.

Stanford Medicine. Chickenpox (varicella) and pregnancy. 2024. https://www.stanfordchildrens.org/en/topic/default?id=chickenpox-varicella-and-pregnancy-90-P02161

Tagaya Y, et al. 40 years of the human T-cell leukemia virus: past, present, and future. *F1000Res.* 2019;8:F1000 Faculty Rev-228.

Tamae Kakazu M, et al. Weight loss interventions as treatment of obesity hypoventilation syndrome: a systematic review. *Ann Am Thorac Soc.* 2020;17(4):492–502.

Thong EP, et al. Diabetes: a metabolic and reproductive disorder in women. *Lancet Diabetes Endocrinol.* 2020;8(2):134–149.

Through the Looking Glass. Serving families with disabilities since 1982. 2020. https://lookingglass.org/

Tong L, Kalish BT. The impact of maternal obesity on childhood neurodevelopment. *J Perinatol.* 2021;41:928–939.

UNAIDS. Global HIV & AIDS statistics—fact sheet. 2023. https://www.unaids.org/en/resources/fact-sheet

U.S. Department of Health and Human Services, Office on Women's Health. Autoimmune disease. February 22, 2021a. https://womenshealth.gov/a-z-topics/autoimmune-diseases

U.S. Department of Health and Human Services, Office on Women's Health. Polycystic ovary syndrome. February 22, 2021b. https://www.womenshealth.gov/a-z-topics/polycystic-ovary-syndrome

U.S. Nuclear Regulatory Commission. Consolidated guidance about materials licenses: program-specific guidance about medical use licenses, final report (NUREG-1556, 9, 3). September 2019. https://www.nrc.gov/reading-rm/doc-collections/nuregs/staff/sr1556/v9/

Warkentin T, et al. Breastfeeding positions and techniques used by Canadians with physical disabilities. *Disabil Health J.* 2021;14(4):101151.

Wisse B. Graves disease. MedLinePlus. U.S. Library of Medicine. National Institutes of Health. Reviewed February 1, 2022. http://www.nlm.nih.gov/medlineplus/ency/article/000358.htm

World Bank. Disability inclusion overview. 2023. https://www.worldbank.org/en/topic/disability

World Health Organization. HIV/AIDS. Updated November 15, 2019. https://www.who.int/en/news-room/fact-sheets/detail/hiv-aids

World Health Organization. Global hepatitis report 2024: action for access in low- and middle-income countries. Geneva: World Health Organization; 2024.

World Health Organization. Guidelines for the management of pregnant and breastfeeding women in the context of Ebola virus disease. February 2020. https://iris.who.int/bitstream/handle/10665/330851/9789240001381-eng.pdf?sequence=1

World Health Organization. Obesity and overweight. Updated June 2021. https://www.who.int/news-room/fact-sheets/detail/Obesity and overweight

World Health Organization. Global tuberculosis report 2021. 2.2 TB mortality. 2022. https://www.who.int/teams/global-tuberculosis-programme/tb-reports/global-tuberculosis-report-2021/disease-burden/mortality

World Health Organization. Diabetes. Fact sheet. April 5, 2023. https://www.who.int/news-room/fact-sheets/detail/diabetes

World Health Organization, United Nations Children's Fund. *Guideline: Updates on HIV and Infant Feeding: The Duration of Breastfeeding, and Support From Health Services to Improve Feeding Practices Among Mothers Living With HIV*. Geneva, Switzerland: World Health Organization; 2016. http://apps.who.int/iris/bitstream/handle/10665/246260/9789241549707-eng.pdf?sequence=1

Wu JL, et al., Gestational diabetes mellitus and risk of delayed onset of lactogenesis: a systematic review and meta-analysis. *Breastfeed Med.* 2021;16(5):385–392.

Zeile WL, et al. Maternal phenylketonuria syndrome: studies in mice suggest a potential approach to a continuing problem. *Pediatr Res. 2018*;83(4):889–896.

CHAPTER 27

Long-Term Infant Conditions

Providers of lactation care are likely to encounter infants whose physical condition is a factor in nursing. Parents of a baby born with a congenital disorder often progress through the classic cycle of grief, including denial, anger, rejection, and mourning for the loss of a "perfect" child. Circumstances may also cause parents to mourn the loss of an opportunity for a "normal" feeding experience. There is no set pattern or time progression for these emotions. You can be most helpful by being attentive and taking cues from the parents. Parents who do not reach acceptance during the typically brief time you spend with the family will need ongoing support.

KEY TERMS

Anomaly
Cleft lip
Cleft palate
Down syndrome
Duarte variant
Dysphagia
Eustachian tube
Galactosemia
Grommet
Hydrocephalus
Hypertension
Neurological impairment
Obturator
Otitis media
Palatal repair
Phenylalanine (Phe)
Phenylalanine hydroxylase deficiency (PAH)
Phenylketonuria (PKU)
Pierre Robin sequence
Sensory processing disorder (SPD)
Spina bifida

Congenital Conditions

Congenital conditions (also called birth defect) are structural or functional anomalies that occur during intrauterine life. They may be detected before birth, at birth, or in later infancy. Conditions vary in severity and may or may not affect life expectancy. When an infant is born with a health condition or neurological disorder, the effect on family members and their relationships depends on the type and severity of the disorder.

The available medical expertise and emotional support are factors in helping parents cope. Allow parents to work freely through their feelings until they reach a point of acceptance. Be sensitive in your support, recognizing that the term *birth defect* does not imply the infant is defective. When possible, refer to the infant's specific condition or use alternate terms, including *congenital disorder* or *congenital malformation* (World Health Organization [WHO], 2023).

The nutritional benefits derived from human milk are especially important to a compromised infant. Nursing or the use of human milk may help parents accept a challenging situation, confident that they are doing everything possible to comfort and nurture their baby. The bonding facilitated by nursing can lessen emotional stress and help the family through this difficult adjustment. At times, the infant's condition may prevent direct nursing or receiving human milk. Common infant conditions are presented here. If you encounter unusual infant conditions, turn to your multidisciplinary healthcare team and to your lactation colleagues. There is a global community of lactation professionals to help you in this interconnected age.

Heart Defects

Congenital heart defects are the most common birth defects in infants, occurring in up to 8% of live births worldwide (Wu et al., 2020). Defects can range from mild to severe, depending on their function and which parts of the heart are involved. Nutrition plays an especially important role for infants with cardiac anomalies, both before and after any surgery (Mangili et al., 2018). These infants are at increased risk for necrotizing enterocolitis (NEC), chylothorax, feeding difficulties, and slow growth (Davis & Spatz, 2019). There is also an increased risk of growth faltering, leading to a potential for cognitive delay, attention-deficit disorder, behavioral issues, and poor social and emotional development (Mangili et al., 2018).

Implications for Lactation

Many babies with cardiac issues are not able to nurse directly at first, often not until after surgery. Multidisciplinary healthcare provider support (including neonatologists, nurses, and surgical staff) is a key factor in a parent's decision to initiate and continue expressing milk. Lactation support is even more important when the diagnosis was not known before the birth and for parents who had not planned to nurse (Demirci et al., 2018). Parents will need timely instruction and support to begin milk expression as soon as possible. Human milk lowers the risks for NEC for babies with cardiac anomalies, (Cognata et al., 2019).

When the baby can nurse, staff education and active support for lactation are needed. The act of nursing improves the infant's coordination levels between sucking, breathing, and swallowing. If they are stable, immediate skin-to-skin contact helps these infants. Skin-to-skin contact while nursing also strengthens bonding in a stressful situation (Miranda et al., 2019). Feedings can be lengthy because of impaired cardiopulmonary function (Miranda et al., 2019). Babies with cardiac issues can expend more energy than their healthy counterparts, requiring more calories. Caregivers are often reluctant to encourage nursing because of uncertainty about how much milk the baby transfers. The use of prefeed/postfeed test weights in the neonatal intensive care unit (NICU) can be a helpful tool. Test weight use has been demonstrated to significantly increase the number of direct feeds and increase parental confidence (Gregory, 2018).

Infants with cardiac defects are at higher risk for **dysphagia**, a swallowing disorder that can cause coughing or choking and bringing food back up, sometimes through the nose. Dysphagia and oral feeding difficulties can lead to oral aversion. Infants exhibit more swallowing differences with bottle feedings than with nursing, with a higher risk for dysphagia (Souza et al., 2018). This risk lends even more support for direct feeding when possible. Feeding difficulties can persist with these infants long after they are discharged from the NICU. They may require continued nutritional support, including, at times, nasogastric (NG) tubes or percutaneous endoscopic gastronomy (PEG) tubes (Mangili et al., 2018).

A study of young adults who were born preterm and received human milk exclusively reported better cardiac function than for those who were exclusively formula fed. Thus, exclusive human milk feedings may improve cardiac function and reduce the risk of pulmonary **hypertension** in adulthood for infants born preterm (El-Khuffash et al., 2020).

Phenylketonuria

Phenylketonuria (PKU), also called **phenylalanine hydroxylase deficiency (PAH)**, is an autosomal-recessive genetic disorder. A metabolic block prevents the change of **phenylalanine (Phe)**, an amino acid, into tyrosine, a form the body can use. PKU occurs in approximately 1 in 24,000 live births in the United States and Europe, and 0.45 million individuals worldwide have PKU (Hillert et al., 2020). If PKU remains untreated, the body becomes overloaded with Phe, which results in central nervous system toxicity. Skin rashes, convulsions, cognitive impairment, and other problems can result.

The rate of debilitation depends on the degree of phenylalanine hydroxylase deficiency. Affected individuals with elevated Phe levels below 1200 μmol per L (20 mg per dL) have lowered risks for cognitive impairment, even with unrestricted diets. Individuals with higher elevated Phe levels, or classic PKU, are at risk for developing severe intellectual disability unless their diets are modified to low protein content (Hillert et al., 2020).

An infant with PKU appears healthy at birth, with diagnosis through a simple blood test that is part of standard newborn screening in most countries. With the universal screening of newborns, the most severe damage caused by PKU has been greatly reduced. Treatment initiated promptly during the first few weeks of life can avoid permanent damage. The infant requires stringent monitoring and a diet that restricts the level of Phe intake while providing a protein amount sufficient to allow appropriate growth. Continuing this diet regimen throughout the person's lifetime may help preserve normal cognitive function (Hillert et al., 2020). Maternal PKU is discussed in **Chapter 26.**

Implications for Lactation

Human milk is superior to any standard commercial infant formula for babies with PKU. It has a lower concentration of protein and a lower content of Phe—approximately 46 mg per 100 mL (Kalvala et al., 2023). The nursing infant's diet is adjusted for Phe based on weekly blood tests. After control is established, human milk, along with a supplement of Phe-free formula, meets the infant's requirements of low Phe.

Direct feeding and supplementation with a Phe-free formula provide good metabolic control and improve the growth and development of children with early diagnosis. Outcomes are better for infants who are fed human milk with appropriate supplementation than for formula-only infants. With support, these parents can successfully feed their babies human milk (Kalvala et al., 2023).

Low-Phe and Phe-free formulas are designed to be supplemented with cow's milk or a cow's milk–based formula. Consequently, vitamin and mineral supplements may be required to augment the nutrients present in human milk. If not, the addition of Phe-free formula to the infant's diet could result in a decrease in nutrient absorption. Additional fluid requirements may be minimal because of the lower solute load of human milk. Phe intake is difficult to determine precisely with direct nursing, making continued nursing a challenge. A recent scoping review of research noted there were no randomized controlled studies that compared infants fed human milk versus Phe-free formula (Kalvala et al., 2023).

Managing Lactation

Healthcare providers may interrupt nursing while they stabilize Phe levels and determine the infant's diet prescription. Milk expression can maintain production during this time. After control is established (with the level of Phe below 10 mg per dL) and the amount of Phe-free formula needed has been determined, human milk can be added to the infant's diet. The 2017 European Guidelines recommend alternating nursing with Phe-free formula (van Wegberg et al., 2017).

Some healthcare providers may recommend an alternative that allows continued nursing without interruption while control is being established, using one of two procedures. One method is to allow the infant to continue nursing and offer a Phe-free formula at each feeding. This requires maintaining a consistent daily intake of a prescribed volume of human milk and Phe-free formula. The other method is to substitute a Phe-free formula for one or two direct feedings per day and express milk at the missed feedings.

Historically, the management of PKU in infants involved the feeding of Phe-free formula along with nursing. The philosophy was to reduce milk intake by feeding the infant a prescribed amount of Phe-free formula prior to nursing (MacDonald et al., 2020). For the first 6 weeks of life, the infant's blood Phe levels and weights were monitored. However, a recent scoping review of the literature found no randomized controlled trial (RCT) studies to evaluate the effects of a nursing infant's milk ingestion compared to the low-Phe formula for the first 6 months. Therefore, the authors support the continuation of nursing for infants with PKU and advocate for additional studies (Kalvala et al., 2023).

Dietary Changes

PKU diagnosis is reconfirmed between 3 and 12 months of age, with a natural protein load calculated to provide a specific amount of Phe for 3 days. This is usually in the form of cow's milk or an evaporated milk formula. Parents who do not wish to interrupt nursing during this time can measure the Phe content of their milk to minimize error. Because dietary requirements change as an infant with PKU grows, parents can ask that the energy content of their milk be evaluated to determine whether a dietary adjustment is required. Guidelines for introducing solid foods are mostly the same as for any other infant. High-Phe foods such as eggs, meat, cheese, and cow's milk should be avoided.

Weaning a baby with PKU from nursing requires more structure than weaning other babies. To maintain a healthy balance, Phe intake must be monitored closely while replacing each dropped feeding with the appropriate amount of Phe-free or low-Phe formula or foods. Weaning may need to occur earlier than usual if healthcare providers have difficulty controlling the baby's Phe levels. When considering weaning, parents should designate a target date and estimate what the baby's weight will be to determine the requirements for Phe, protein, and energy at that time. They can then consult with a nutritionist specializing in PKU to calculate the amounts of Phe-free or low-Phe formula and other supplements needed.

Medication therapies for PKU continue to emerge. Sapropterin dihydrochloride could benefit individuals with PKU by lowering Phe or improving dietary Phe tolerance (MacDonald et al., 2020; Qu et al., 2019). Enzyme therapies, including pegvaliase and phenylalanine ammonia lyase, hold promise for reduced dietary restrictions (Ashe et al., 2019; Levy et al., 2018). These therapies may eventually enable parents whose babies have PKU to feed as they wish.

Counseling Implications

When unique circumstances place restrictions on nursing patterns, parents will benefit from support and advice on how to manage feedings and monitor their baby's intake. The baby's special care will require motivation, access to periodic blood checks, a support system, and a supportive medical team. Diligence in expressing milk when feedings are restricted will help to maintain production and prevent ductal narrowing and mastitis.

Periodic test weighing will track the amount of milk the baby consumes by measuring the amounts of Phe-free formula before nursing. Many healthcare professionals have learned more about using human milk with babies with PKU and work with families toward a positive outcome. One study reported that infants fed human milk with the appropriate Phe-free formula supplementation had significantly lower Phe levels and significantly higher weight gain than their formula-fed counterparts (Kose et al., 2018). You will need to stay informed on treatment strategies as new therapies for PKU are adopted for infants and children.

Galactosemia

Galactosemia is an inherited disease in which the liver enzyme that changes galactose to glucose is absent. Galactose is a simple sugar found in lactose, referred to as *milk sugar*. Screening for galactosemia is a routine test in newborn assessment. Diagnosis as early as possible can help prevent severe damage and even death (Welsink-Karssies et al., 2020). Galactosemia requires immediate and total weaning from all animal milks—including human milk—as well as other foods that contain galactose (Berry, 2021). The infant is placed on a special amino acid formula that is free of galactose.

Types of Galactosemia

There are three types of galactosemia, each caused by gene mutations and affecting different enzymes involved in breaking down galactose:

- Type I—classic galactosemia—is the most common and most severe form of the condition. It occurs in 1 in every 30,000 to 60,000 newborns. These infants soon develop feeding difficulties, lethargy, growth faltering, jaundice, liver damage, and bleeding. They can also develop bacterial infections and go into shock (American Liver Foundation, 2023).
- Type II—galactokinase deficiency—causes fewer medical problems, but affected infants develop cataracts. Occurrence ranges from 1 in 50,000 to 2,200,000 newborns (Ramani & Arya, 2023).
- Type III—galactose epimerase deficiency—can cause cataracts, delayed growth and development, intellectual disability, liver disease, and kidney problems. Symptoms range from mild to severe. The frequency of type III is very rare (Berry, 2021).

Duarte Variant

Although infants with galactosemia are generally unable to consume human milk, those with a form of classic galactosemia known as the **Duarte variant** are an exception. These infants have varying levels of enzyme activity, which allows them to ingest human milk. It is imperative for parents to consult with a specialist, such as a pediatric metabolic geneticist or endocrinologist, for ongoing guidance.

Dietary options with Duarte variant are either restricting dietary lactose and galactose for a year or so and then gradually introducing these items and testing for the individual's response or not restricting them at all (Fridovich-Keil et al., 2020). If the baby receives human milk, galactose levels need careful monitoring. Some nondairy formula may be needed; however, this is not always the case. Each infant needs to be assessed and followed individually.

Cleft Defects

A cleft is an opening in the upper lip or palate, or both, caused when these oral structures fail to fuse during the first trimester of pregnancy. Clefts can occur on one side of the mouth (unilateral) or both sides (bilateral). There can be a **cleft lip** only, a **cleft palate** only, or most commonly, a cleft of both the lip and the palate. A cleft in the palate results in an opening in the nasal cavity in the roof of the mouth. A cleft lip or cleft palate can affect the infant's ability to generate suction and obtain adequate nourishment.

An estimated 30% of clefts occur as part of other congenital anomalies, syndromes, and medical complications, including Pierre Robin sequence, Van der Woude syndrome, and 22q11 deletion syndrome (Academy of Breastfeeding Medicine [ABM], 2019; American Cleft Palate-Craniofacial Association, 2025). These require specialized medical care and often preclude nursing.

Rates of occurrence for a cleft defect vary, depending on the type of cleft. Clefts range from mild to severe and are among the most common birth defects. Worldwide, they range from 0.8 to 2.7 cases out of every 1000 live births (ABM, 2019). A combination of cleft lip and cleft palate occurs more frequently in people of Asian and Native American ancestry and least frequently in African Americans. When isolated and unaccompanied by another birth defect, the occurrence of babies born with clefts in the United States each year between 2010 and 2014 was approximately as follows (Mai et al., 2019):

- 1 in 1563 with cleft lip and palate
- 1 in 2807 with cleft lip only
- 1 in 1687 with cleft palate only

A child born with a cleft usually faces continuous treatment until adulthood. This may involve plastic surgery, orthodontics, management of ear fluid, and sometimes speech therapy. Each child's condition is unique, and treatment plans vary. Cleft palate treatment centers offer a comprehensive team approach to each child's needs. The child's prognosis and outcome are generally excellent unless the cleft is a part of a more serious syndrome.

Otitis media is common among children with cleft palates. It is thought that there is more chronic inflammation because of impaired formation and function of the **eustachian tubes** (Maina et al., 2022). The width of the cleft is associated with a higher incidence of acute otitis media (AOM) and otitis media with effusion (OME) before repair. Regardless of the width of the cleft palate, otitis media duration is a concern and requires long-term follow-up (Yoshitomi et al., 2022). The increased risk for otitis media appears unrelated to cleft repair and early treatment with feeding plates, called **grommets** or **obturators** (discussed later).

Parents' Reactions to a Cleft

Parents' reactions to their baby's condition are affected by the type of cleft. Predictably, the visibility of an unrepaired cleft lip, with or without a cleft palate, leads to an immediate emotional response. An isolated cleft palate is visible only when the infant cries and therefore elicits less emotional response. Avoid comments that might minimize the parents' concerns or deny their reactions. You can provide encouragement by commenting on how well they are doing in their parenting role and highlighting the baby's positive attributes.

Avoid suggesting that after surgery no one will know their child ever had a cleft. Despite tremendous surgical advances and remarkable results, traces of the cleft will exist. Although children with cleft defects can be affected by peer teasing, most children and adults with repaired cleft defects exhibit resilience and respond positively to family and therapeutic support (Stock et al., 2020).

Nursing Adjustments with a Cleft

As with all babies, human milk is the optimal food for babies with clefts. Nursing babies have fewer ear infections, and any milk that leaks into the nasal cavity is less irritating than infant formula. Both nutritive and nonnutritive sucking with nursing will aid in proper orofacial development and enhance bonding. The infant's birth order may affect nursing outcome. Multiparas, who typically establish initial milk production better than primiparas, may have an easier time nursing.

Feeding infants with clefts is often challenging and time-consuming, especially in the early weeks. Parents may feel discouraged or apprehensive about feeding their baby. A recent study of infants admitted to the NICU with a cleft lip and palate noted reduced odds of nursing at discharge (Tahmasebifard et al., 2023). Support will help parents overcome their fears and deal with obstacles.

The feeding assistance parents need depends on the type of cleft. In a study of babies with clefts (15% cleft lip, 29% cleft palate, 56% cleft lip and palate), only 5% of the babies nursed directly. Support identified by parents included lactation consultants, nurses, feeding therapists, and online support groups. Of these infants, 43% received expressed milk for 6 months or more (Madhoun et al., 2019). Only 29.5% of infants with cleft palates received human milk in one study. Of these, 76% received expressed milk, and 23% nursed directly (Gottschlich et al., 2018).

Although many parents find it difficult to transition to direct nursing, clinicians and parents should consider each baby's feeding strengths and limitations and never automatically dismiss that possibility. You can work with parents after surgical repair to help them and the baby learn to nurse nutritively. If the baby cannot achieve nutritive feeding, any nursing has value for comfort, oral development, and bonding. You can encourage parents to continue to provide their milk to minimize the child's risk of developing ear and respiratory infections.

Practical feeding suggestions from other families can offer insights into managing nursing with a cleft defect. Support groups can be helpful, and online resources offering parental support abound. Cleft teams include lactation and nutritional support members. A feeding protocol for infants with clefts is available from the ABM (2019). The immunological properties of human milk can be particularly valuable to these children because of the higher incidence of otitis media. Additionally, nursing offers these children improved speech development and aids in their visual development, as discussed in **Chapter 9**.

Nursing with a Cleft Lip

An isolated cleft lip presents no physiological impediment to nursing. The baby can usually nurse well and may be able to mold the open cleft around the breast tissue more easily than around a small rubber nipple. In many cases, the breast tissue fills the cleft to seal it off. Placing a thumb over the cleft while the baby nurses also improves the seal (**Figure 27-1**). This technique is sometimes called the "teacup" hold, with the parent compressing the areola skin together as one would hold a teacup handle. If the cleft in the lip is large, the nipple can be tipped to prevent the nipple from being pushed into the cleft (ABM, 2019). A syringe can also be used to feed an infant with a cleft palate when placed in a prone position (Genna, 2023). Parents benefit greatly from support and encouragement, despite the relative ease with which they may accomplish lactation.

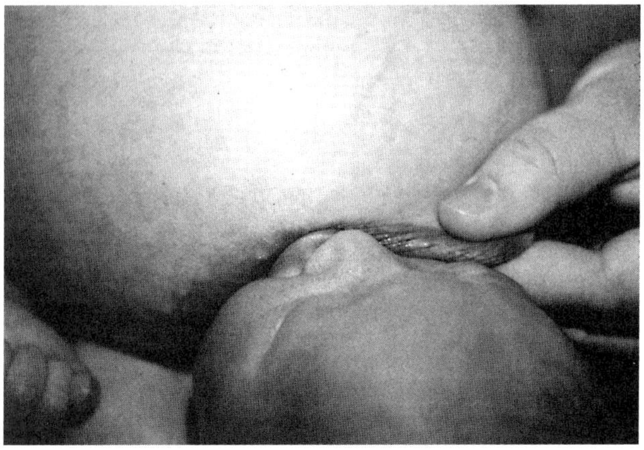

Figure 27-1 Using "teacup" hold to plug cleft lip.

Printed with permission of Kay Hoover.

Nursing with a Cleft Palate

A cleft palate poses a challenge to nursing. With a unilateral cleft palate, the nipple needs to enter the baby's mouth on the side of the cleft in such a way that the cheek on the side of the defect touches the breast. When the cleft is bilateral, the nipple should enter the baby's mouth at midline. Feeding in a position that keeps the baby's nose and throat higher than the breast can minimize milk leaking into the nasal cavity. The baby can straddle the parent's body while being held upright or in a side-sitting position.

Choking and milk leaking through the nose occur frequently in babies with cleft palates, regardless of feeding method. Although feeding can be time-consuming and frustrating, it often becomes easier after the first month. Milk expression maintains production, makes milk readily available at the beginning of a feeding, and removes milk that remains after a feeding. Skin-to-skin contact and initiating a feeding before the baby is completely awake will help encourage nursing. Short, frequent feedings avoid tiring the infant.

As an infant's tongue draws the nipple into their mouth, the tongue and palate create a vacuum to maintain the latch. The baby's gums compress the ducts to promote milk flow. With a cleft palate, the opening between the baby's mouth and nose prevents the baby from creating the vacuum needed for maintaining the latch. The baby uses shorter sucks with a faster rate of sucking and higher ratios of suck–swallow and generates a greater proportion of intraoral positive pressure (ABM, 2019). Babies with minor soft palate clefts are more likely to generate normal levels of suction and compression compared with their counterparts with larger clefts. Cupping the breast as the baby latches and continuing to support the breast will help the baby maintain a deep latch throughout the feeding.

Because a cleft palate prevents creating a vacuum in the oral cavity, the baby may very likely not be able to create the suction required in nursing. They may need expressed milk to supplement nursing. Specialty feeders, such as the Pigeon Cleft Palate Nurser, the Hazelbaker Feeder, and the Medela Special Needs (previously named Haberman) Feeder, are available. Parents will benefit from learning about the use of these alternative feeders. Squeezable bottles are reportedly easier to use than rigid feeding bottles. Alternative feeding methods prior to surgery can be beneficial. After surgery, feeding methods using suction reportedly yield more positive results (Dash et al., 2023). You can help each family find a feeding method that works best for them and their baby.

The parents will need to be attentive to their baby's weight pattern and monitor weight gain with weekly weight checks. A baby with a cleft palate needs a complete lactation assessment to determine their ability to transfer milk during nursing (after lactogenesis II has occurred). Pre- and post-feed weights should be used until the baby consistently transfers milk adequately. Counting voids and stools is an important marker for intake as well.

Milk transfer may be easiest at the beginning of a feeding when more milk is available. The baby's sucking may not feel particularly strong, especially if other children were nursed. These babies sometimes have difficulty extracting the hindmilk from the breast. Massaging the breasts before and during the feeding increases milk flow and makes it easier for the baby to transfer milk. A baby who is able to transfer milk from direct nursing needs to nurse on cue and with great frequency in the newborn period. Parents should aim for 8 to 12 feedings in 24 hours, initiating feedings if the baby fails to exhibit hunger cues.

Nursing with a Cleft Lip and Palate

If the baby has both a cleft lip and palate, the techniques discussed for a cleft palate apply. A more extensive cleft produces the most difficulty with feedings. Long-term use of a breast pump for expressing milk is likely to be even more necessary. Many parents pump exclusively and provide their milk through an alternative feeding method until the cleft palate is repaired. Nursing as often as possible enhances bonding and nipple stimulation for milk production. Nonnutritive nursing for comfort may aid in jaw development.

Nursing with a Submucosal Cleft Palate

A submucosal (also called a *submucous*) cleft palate results from abnormal soft palate muscle tissue. The gap between the disconnected muscles and the skin may appear as a bluish midline discoloration (**Figure 27-2**). The salivary glands may be involved as well, which can cause drooling. A bifid (forked) uvula, a short soft palate with muscle separation (furrow) in the midline, and a bony notch in the posterior of the hard palate are all markers for a submucosal cleft (Park et al., 2019). Because it is difficult to detect, a submucosal cleft of the soft palate can escape the newborn screening process.

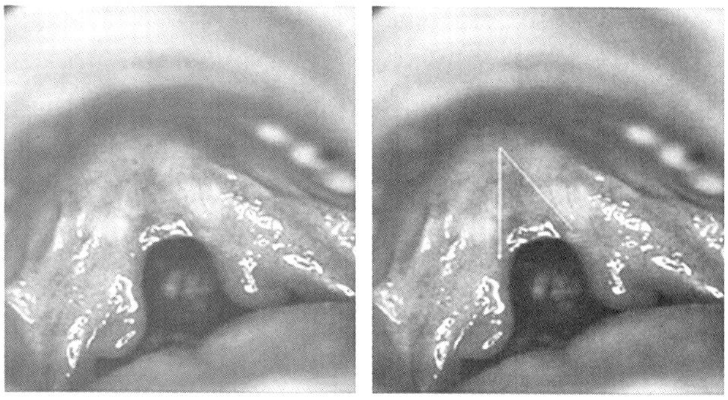

Figure 27-2 Submucosal cleft.

Printed with permission of Dr. Marie M. Tolarova.

Submucosal clefts occur in approximately 1 in 1200 live births because of genetic or environmental conditions. Sometimes, a submucosal cleft is discovered because of feeding difficulties or recurrent otitis media. Submucosal clefts diagnosed from a bifid uvula occur significantly earlier (19.5 months) than those found because of speech problems in toddlers (Jung et al., 2020). Speech problems, when they become evident, can include hypernasal speech (Ettinger et al., 2018). Early discovery and repair improve speech outcomes (Brosch et al., 2018). At times, the cleft eludes diagnosis until or throughout adulthood.

A submucosal cleft makes it difficult for the newborn to maintain sufficient vacuum to sustain a suck. An infant with feeding difficulties and the preceding symptoms needs referral for evaluation by an ear, nose, and throat specialist. A submucosal cleft can be a symptom of other more serious problems, such as velocardiofacial syndrome or chromosomal defects. DiGeorge syndrome, also called *22q11.2 deletion syndrome*, is a common genetic link (Solot et al., 2019). Surgical repairs may be performed (Ettinger et al., 2018; Solot et al., 2019).

Surgical Repair

Early cleft repair is associated with higher rates of nursing (Burianova et al., 2017). Surgical repair of a cleft lip is typically performed at about 3 months of age. Some surgical teams perform lip repair during the first few weeks postpartum. Repair of a cleft palate typically occurs at about 1 year. However, newer surgical techniques allow earlier **palatal repair** (Hammoudeh et al., 2017; Sakran et al., 2024). Palatal growth has historically determined the timing of the surgery. The goals for cleft palate repair have focused on anatomical closure of the palatal defect, improved speech, and minimizing disruption of maxillary growth.

Globally, there is variability in the technique utilized and timing of cleft palate repair, necessitating continued research (Naidu et al., 2022). Many families choose early palatal repair and may opt for surgery soon after birth. **Figure 27-3** (before surgery), **Figure 27-4** (immediately after surgery), and **Figure 27-5** (aged 11.5 years) illustrate a child with a unilateral cleft lip and palate who underwent palatal and lip repair at 11 days old. The baby transitioned to direct feeding by 6 weeks of age.

Research is needed to evaluate whether changes in surgical and anesthesia protocols will improve outcomes for children with clefts. In an attempt to minimize exposure to anesthesia, a single-stage repair of both cleft lip and palate may be done at 6 to 12 months of age. Studies indicate that dexmedetomidine may have protective neurological properties and enhance the effects of inhaled gases during anesthesia, but more research is needed (Fontanals et al., 2021).

Some healthcare providers permit infants to resume nursing immediately after surgery. Parents who are unable to nurse during this time can express milk and feed it to the baby through an alternative method. They can also freeze milk in preparation for the surgery. Because feeding difficulties primarily involve the palate, repair of a cleft lip usually does not alter nursing ability significantly. Nonetheless, lip repair provides an important psychological lift to parents.

Some cleft palate teams fit obturators (also known as *grommets*) over part of the cleft palate to assist in feeding (**Figure 27-6**). The baby still cannot create negative intraoral pressure, so assisted feeding is required (Hosseini et al., 2017). The use of nasal stents

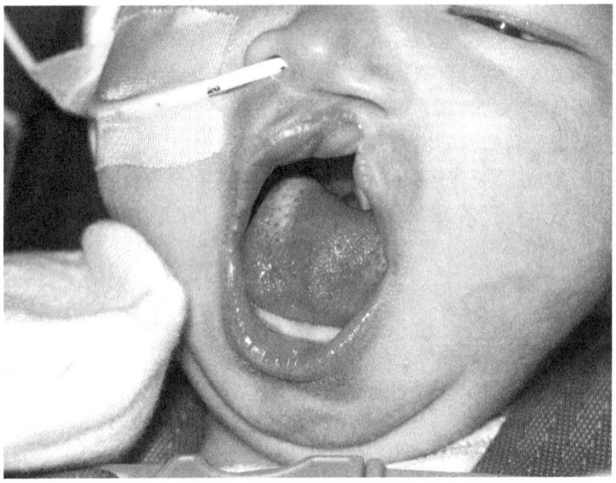

Figure 27-3 Cleft surgery repair—before surgery.

Printed with permission of Hollye Long.

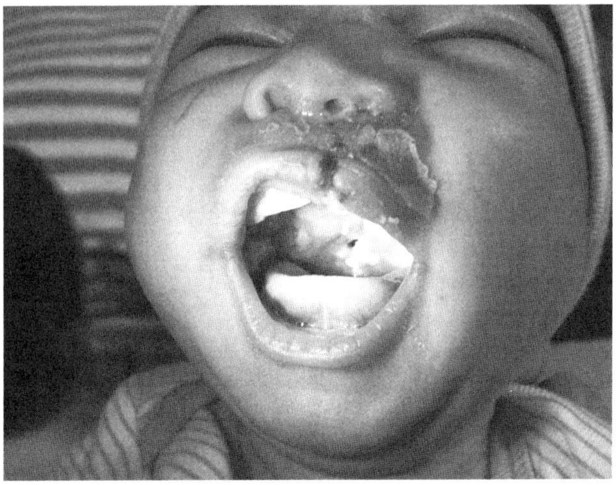

Figure 27-4 Cleft surgery repair—immediately after.

Printed with permission of Hollye Long.

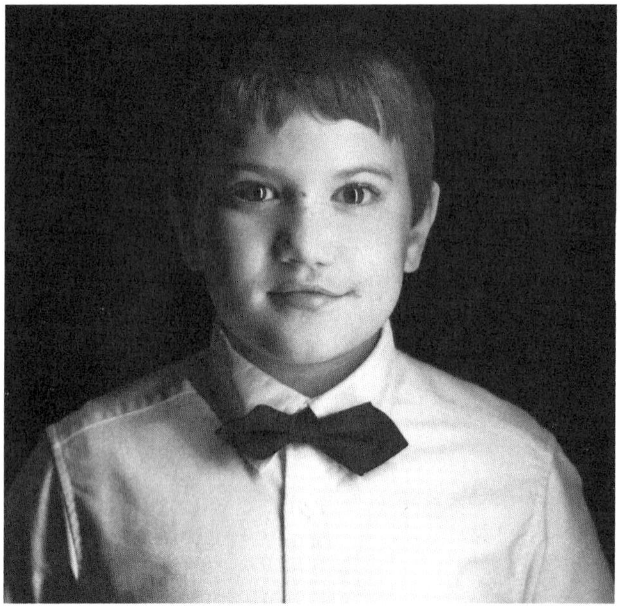

Figure 27-5 Cleft surgery repair—aged 11 years.

Printed with permission Hollye Long.

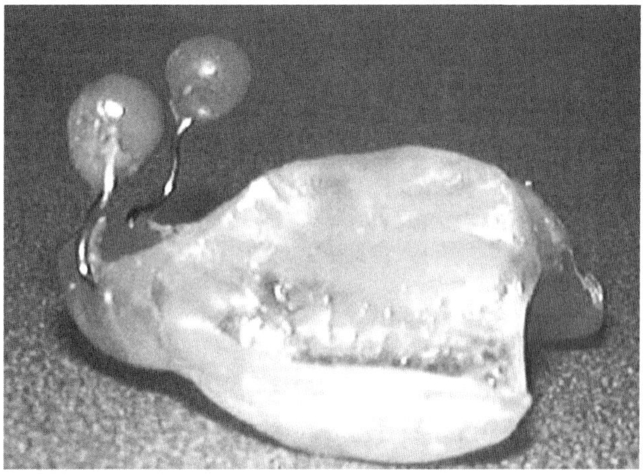

Figure 27-6 Obturator to bridge the gap in the cleft palate.

Printed with permission of Dr. Scott Franklin.

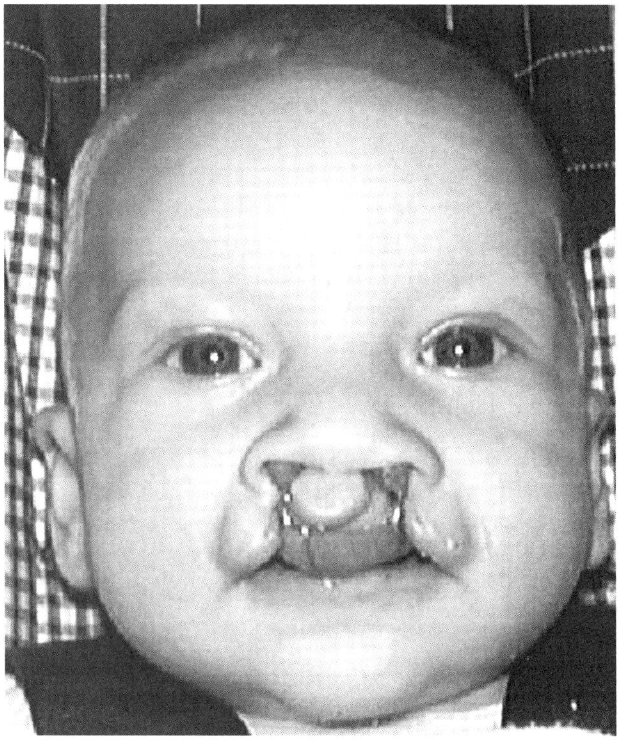

Figure 27-7 Nasal stent used in cleft surgery.
Printed with permission of Dr. Scott Franklin.

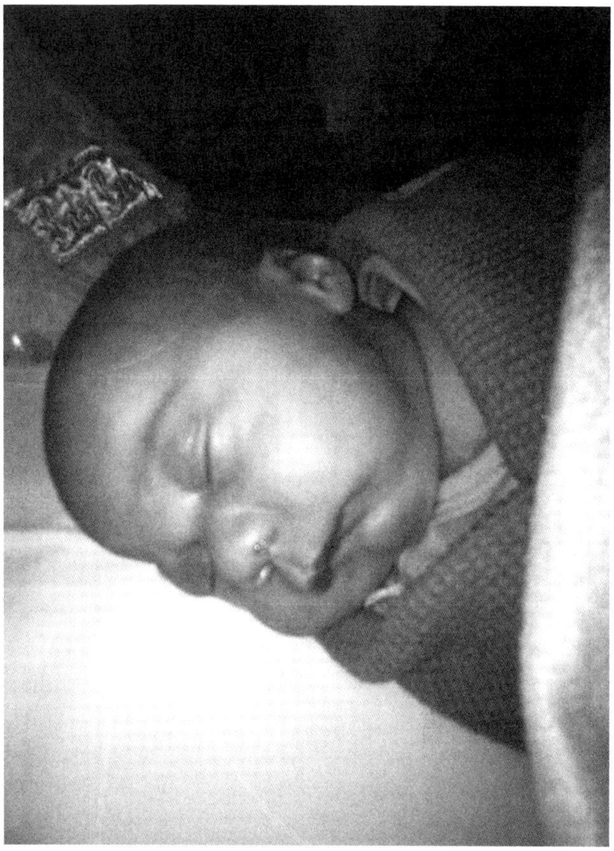

Figure 27-8 Infant with Pierre Robin sequence.
Courtesy of Pierre Robin Australia Inc.

helps minimize deformities and stretches the skin for repair, as illustrated in **Figure 27-7**. Obturators position the palate for repair and prevent dental arch collapse. Although some experts dispute its effectiveness for nursing, others assert that it enhances weight gain, facilitates nursing, and promotes early nutritional recovery (Muddasani et al., 2024).

Pierre Robin Sequence

Figure 27-8 illustrates an infant with **Pierre Robin sequence**, an **anomaly** characterized by micrognathia (a receding lower jaw). The condition is also characterized by displacement at the back of the tongue combined with a cleft palate and an absence of a gag reflex (Baxter & Shanks, 2023). Pierre Robin sequence, often shortened to "Robin sequence," was originally thought to be a specific disorder. It now refers to a grouping of clinical findings that may relate to other disorders—thus the name change from "syndrome" to "sequence" (Hurst, 2023).

Pierre Robin occurs in approximately 1 in every 8500 to 14,000 live births and appears equally in males and females (National Organization for Rare Disorders [NORD], 2018). It may be isolated and occur because of uterine growth restriction of the jaw, or it may be related to more than 45 different syndromes. Pierre Robin is associated with genetic disorders, most commonly Stickler syndrome, a connective tissue disorder that can cause blindness. Sometimes the baby's position in utero is the cause of the deformity. If uterine growth restriction is the cause, the jaw begins to develop after birth and usually catches up to normal by 4 to 6 years of age. If the condition is from a disorder, micrognathia continues and is a marker for other problems (NORD, 2018).

An infant with Pierre Robin can suffer severe respiratory distress and have difficulty maintaining an airway, particularly during the newborn period. This can lead to growth faltering, and some of these babies require endotracheal intubation and gavage feeding. The possible severity of airway obstruction and concerns about survival usually make direct nursing unlikely. Babies with Pierre Robin are prone sleep apnea so side sleeping is recommended (Kukkola & Kirjavainen, 2023).

Pierre Robin sequence occurs in varying degrees. An infant with a slight case may be able to nurse. An infant who cannot nurse initially can receive expressed milk. Babies with Pierre Robin are 15 times more likely to have poor feeding skills than babies without the syndrome (Dorise et al., 2019). After the infant gets through the crucial early stages of life and has developed sufficiently to maintain an airway without difficulty, the outcome is positive. The baby may be able to nurse at this time, depending on the caregiver's recommendations.

Support for the Parents

Understanding the emotions involved with cleft defects and staying current with treatments will help you provide reassurance and tactful, realistic information to parents. Parents report being overwhelmed with too much information during a time of initial emotional stress. It is especially important to limit the amount of information at one time, presenting it in gradual doses throughout the newborn period. Parents may benefit from the repetition of facts as they progress through the range of emotional reactions and become more receptive to explanations and suggestions. Support is crucial and extremely valuable (Stock et al., 2020), including support for bonding (Costa et al., 2019; Tsuchiya et al., 2019). Learning how to deal with the feelings of friends and family is also a concern.

You will benefit families by developing your understanding of, comfort with, and expertise in the treatment and outcomes for these babies and children. Parents need to know the signs and symptoms of illness, possible complications, expected difficulties in feeding, and information on deferring future treatment. Parents generally regard the craniofacial team with satisfaction. However, they often receive poor feeding advice from other caregivers who have low levels of knowledge and difficulty with cleft management. Resources and training are available globally through several organizations (March of Dimes, 2022; Operation Smiles, 2025; Smile Train, 2025).

Many new parents, especially those of first-born children with clefts, tend to attribute all behavior and feeding problems to the cleft. You can help them recognize behaviors that are largely part of the usual newborn pattern. Help them put the cleft in perspective and view their child as normal in other respects. Encourage them to become advocates for their child and to become comfortable with questioning and understanding all aspects of the child's treatment. It is important that you avoid evaluating or judging parents' feeding experience. The cleft palate feeding regimen can be trying, frustrating, and extremely time-consuming. Help parents recognize success in every effort.

Parents experience higher stress from infant feeding difficulties resulting from their child's congenital anomaly and not being able to nurse as they planned.

Table 27-1 Counseling Parents About Cleft Lip and Palate

- A cleft lip usually molds around the breast.
- Covering a cleft lip with a finger helps ensure good suction.
- With a unilateral cleft palate, the nipple enters on the side of the defect. The baby's cheek on the side of the defect should touch the breast.
- With a bilateral cleft palate, the nipple enters at midline. The baby's body can straddle the parent to nurse.
- A feeding plate (obturator) may be used to partially cover a cleft palate.
- Closely monitor weight gain, voids and stools, and frequency of feedings.
- Massaging the breasts before nursing will promote milk flow.
- Holding the breast in the baby's mouth provides additional support.
- Express milk after feedings and during surgical repair and feed the milk to the baby.
- Express milk after feedings to protect milk production.
- Feed the baby in an upright position to avoid choking or milk leaking from the baby's nose.
- If choking occurs, push the baby's chin to their chest to stop it. Resume the feeding when safe to do so.
- Use short, frequent feedings.
- Nurse when the baby is sleepy.
- If the baby can form a seal for latch, use of a tube-feeding device while nursing will encourage sucking.

Additional stressors include a lack of partner support, perceiving difficult infant dispositions, blame, anger, and concerns about the future (Boztepe et al., 2020).

Some parents are emotionally or physically unable to continue nursing for as long as they might have planned. It is important to recognize their disappointment, provide support and information about weaning, and remind them how the baby benefited from the nursing relationship and from their milk. Support groups across the globe give parents a unique, useful opportunity to relate to others who have dealt positively with the experience. **Table 27-1** presents counseling tips for parents about cleft defects.

Spina Bifida

Spina bifida is a neural tube defect present at birth that results in a gap in the bone that surrounds the spinal cord. Spina bifida occurs worldwide at an average of 1 case per 1000 births. Marked geographic variations occur, with the highest rates in Ireland

and Wales. France, Norway, Hungary, Czechoslovakia, Yugoslavia, and Japan have the lowest rates. The addition of adequate folic acid (400 µg per day) to the diet before conception has reduced spina bifida rates (Spina Bifida Association, 2025; U.S. National Institute of Neurological Disorders and Stroke [USNINDS], 2025b).

Most of these infants have weakness or paralysis below the spinal opening. Surgical repair may be unnecessary if the gap is small. When the gap is large enough to allow parts of the spinal cord to protrude, surgery may be required. Surgical repair usually occurs as soon as possible—within 24 to 48 hours after birth. The infant will be in the NICU after surgery, and parents will need help expressing, storing, and transporting their milk. There is little research on nursing infants with spina bifida. Barriers to nursing may be related to medical and surgical interventions, uninformed staff, or hospital routines (Hookway et al., 2021).

A baby with spina bifida can nurse as soon as it is allowed. A helper can carefully lift and carry the baby to the parent, support the baby with pillows, and make sure that positioning avoids pressure on the baby's spinal column. Feeding times will be brief until the baby has recovered from surgery. Longer feedings can begin as the baby grows stronger. The recovery process may take several weeks, during which time expressed milk can be provided. Parents may need feeding assistance and follow-up after the baby arrives home. Improved lactation outcomes result from prenatal education, informed staff, and a hospital dedicated to the value of human milk. Many infants go home on tube feedings and milk expression with hospital-grade breast pumps.

Despite the lack of research on lactation outcomes for babies with spina bifida, general lactation research confirms that nursing enhances parents' psychological adjustment. Because a diagnosis of spina bifida is often made during pregnancy, a prenatal consultation is an opportunity to discuss the importance of skin-to-skin contact, nursing, and remaining together (Church et al., 2020). Pillows, nipple shields, nursing supplementers, and bottles for nursing and providing their milk will help parents gain confidence in nursing. Be sure to remind parents that nursing and human milk can provide comfort and reduce pain during procedures (McPherson et al., 2020).

Down Syndrome

Down syndrome, also known as *trisomy 21*, is a chromosomal disorder in which the baby has an extra chromosome. Rates of occurrence vary geographically. In the United States, Down syndrome occurs in about 5700 babies per year (CDC, 2024a). Typical external signs include oval eyes that slant slightly upward, a protruding tongue that seems too large, abnormally shaped ears, a wide and flattened nose, and hypotonicity (low muscle tone). Other features include a short neck, white spots on the iris of the eye (called *Brushfield spots*), a deep transverse crease on the palm of the hand (Palmer crease), and a short stature (National Down Syndrome Society [NDSS], 2025) (**Figure 27-9**). Individuals with Down syndrome have a higher incidence of cardiac, neurological, and gastrointestinal health concerns as well as obesity (Magenis et al., 2022).

Typically, an infant with Down syndrome gains weight and grows in length more slowly than the average infant, regardless of feeding method. Special growth charts for children with Down syndrome reflect this (CDC, 2024b). Despite the slower growth and development, these children can usually pursue the same physical activities as other children. Immunological factors in human milk and easy digestibility make it especially beneficial to these babies. Children with Down syndrome may have a lower tendency toward obesity because of receiving human milk in infancy. **Chapter 10** discusses obesity in artificially fed infants.

Down syndrome is often diagnosed during pregnancy with confirmation by a blood test to determine the presence of extra material from chromosome. Because the test can take up to 2 weeks, families may experience a long waiting period of anxiety and grief. Providing lactation resources prenatally on establishing and protecting milk production will help parents understand that nursing their baby is possible. In one

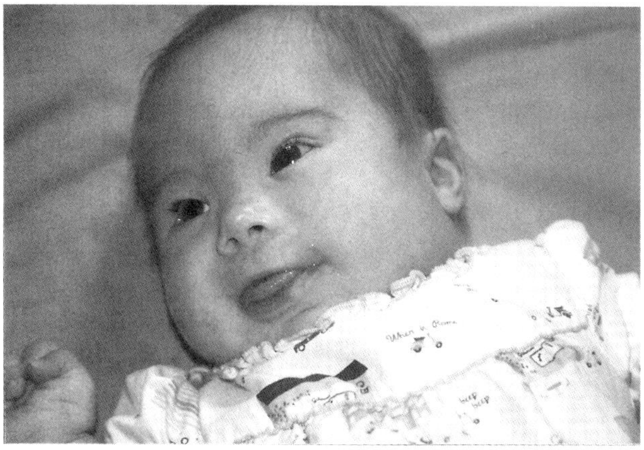

Figure 27-9 Infant with Down syndrome.

study, only 20% of families with a prenatal diagnosis received lactation information. Of the families in the study, 64% nursed for at least 6 weeks (Williams et al., 2022). Providing early education and continued support will encourage families to nurse their infants with Down syndrome.

Down syndrome does not cause initial feeding problems in all infants. Each infant needs evaluation on an individual basis. Mild cardiac complications allow nursing with little difficulty. Nursing may be contraindicated for a severe cardiac condition because of the activity required for direct feeding. In a study of feeding and swallowing difficulties, 55% of infants displayed some dysphagia, and 39% had severe dysphagia warranting feeding changes in the consistency of milk or formula or nonoral feeding (Stanley et al., 2019).

Most babies with Down syndrome are able to nurse directly. A systematic review revealed an exclusive nursing rate of 31.5% to 55.4%, with five studies reporting nursing for more than 6 months. Separation of the dyad, long hospital stays, sadness and fear, and low confidence were reasons cited for not nursing (Magenis et al., 2022). The average nursing duration is 7.7 weeks, compared to 23.4 weeks in healthy infants without Down syndrome (Coentro et al., 2020).

Lactation Management with Down Syndrome

Infants with Down syndrome often have hypotonia, which can cause a low intraoral vacuum. Hypotonia will cause the baby's head, arms, and legs to be loose and floppy. Difficulty rooting and sucking because of weak reflexes, sluggishness, and becoming easily fatigued at feedings can make it difficult for the baby to transfer milk sufficiently. Breast massage and milk expression to initiate letdown before nursing will facilitate milk transfer. Limited nutritive sucking and milk transfer can persist for several months because of delayed oromotor development. Nursing can help to strengthen oral muscles. Although extra feeding assistance and patience are needed in the early days, muscle tone will improve as the baby learns to nurse and exercises the facial muscles. Sucking and feeding improvement usually occur within a few months. The ABM's Clinical Protocol #16: Breastfeeding the Hypotonic Infant is an excellent resource for nursing a baby with Down syndrome (ABM, 2016).

Recommendations to support nursing in this population include early skin-to-skin contact and feeding initiation, feeding positions that provide head and chin support, working with tongue protrusion, therapeutic suck training, and milk expression. Parents can minimize the effort required from the baby during feedings by paying careful attention to signs of fatigue. Positioning that provides head and chin support will promote a deeper latch and improve the volume of milk transferred (Aguilar-Cordero et al., 2019). Any of the conventional nursing positions work well for an infant with Down syndrome. With the head and body well supported, the baby can reserve energy for nursing.

The baby's head should be slightly flexed but not drooped too far forward. A position that places the baby's throat slightly higher than the nipple prevents choking and gagging, especially in a laid-back position that allows the nipple to tilt upward. The side-lying position seems to work well for many of these babies, with the baby supported by several pillows and their head propped higher than the rest of the body. The side-sitting hold provides a greater ability to maintain latch. Using the Dancer hand position, illustrated in **Chapter 22**, can provide additional support.

When the baby latches, pressing down on the chin encourages a wide-open mouth. Parents can check that the bottom lip turns outward over the alveolar ridge. The typically flaccid, flat tongue may initially be unable to cup around the nipple and form a trough to carry the milk to the back of the throat. The parent can press down on the center of the tongue with their finger several times before each feeding to help the baby learn to shape the tongue appropriately.

Because the baby may be passive, parents may frequently need to observe and respond to subtle signs of wakefulness, such as lip and eye movements. The goal is to nurse for at least 10 to 12 minutes on each side every 2 to 3 hours. If the baby does not give cues, the parent will need to initiate feedings. A baby who has difficulty sucking can receive expressed milk after the feeding. Expressing milk after every feeding to ensure adequate stimulation for copious milk production and feeding the baby the expressed hindmilk will ensure that the baby's nutritional needs are met through the parent's milk.

Hydrocephalus

Hydrocephalus is an excessive accumulation of cerebrospinal fluid in the intracranial cavity. Also called hydrocephaly, the condition results from interference in the flow or absorption of fluid through the brain and the spinal canal. This causes the infant's head to enlarge as fluid increases. An estimated

10,000 people in the US and Canada are diagnosed with hydrocephalus every year (HCRN, 2024). It can be congenital or occur after birth.

Risk factors for hydrocephalus include consanguinity, maternal diabetes, pregnancy-induced hypertension, multiple gestation, oligohydramnios (low amniotic fluid), prenatal prescription drug and alcohol use, family history, and lack of prenatal care (Abebe et al., 2022). Hydrocephalus may also result from genetic abnormalities, developmental disorders (including spina bifida), meningitis, traumatic head injury, or subarachnoid hemorrhage (USNINDS, 2025a). In most cases, the baby has a high-pitched cry, muscle weakness, and neurological defects.

Hydrocephaly is primarily treated by surgical placement of a shunt or stent to drain the fluid. Endoscopic third ventriculostomy (ETV), a less invasive procedure, is increasingly used. The infant may need a feeding tube in the early days after surgery to ensure weight gain. Research on low-birth-weight preterm infants with severe neonatal brain injury found lower surgery rates for posthemorrhagic hydrocephalus (50% vs. 67%) after the use of human milk via nasal application. Nasal application of human milk transfers neurotrophins and stem cells to the brain. This research suggests that human milk may provide neuroprotection for preterm infants, reducing the rates of hydrocephalus that results from intracranial hemorrhage (Keller et al., 2019).

Nursing is possible with hydrocephaly, depending on the degree of **neurological impairment**. Human milk holds significant protection for these infants, including protection against shunt infection (Kalangu et al., 2020). If the infant is unable to directly nurse, the parent can pump and feed the baby expressed milk. These infants may have a weak or ineffective suck and tire easily. Adjustments in positioning and careful observation are important. The infant's head needs to be slightly above the nipple and well supported. Some parents find lying on their side with a pillow supporting the baby's head to be helpful. If pain occurs during feedings, the baby could develop a feeding aversion. Adjustment in feeding position should prevent pressure on the wound after surgery.

Neurological Impairment

Infants with neurological impairment can have varying degrees of mental deficiency and learning ability. The severity of impairment determines the degree to which an infant is able to nurse. An infant with severe impairment has an extremely poor attention span and cannot maintain concentration. Reflexes that were instinctive at birth may be forgotten. The baby requires continual reinforcement of instinctive reflexes as well as learned abilities.

Infants with neurological impairment may have hypotonia and hypertonia, resulting in non-rhythmic sucking skills. They often have a weak suck and weak reflexes for swallowing and gagging, and they often tire quickly when nursing (Children's Minnesota, 2024; Genna, 2023). They may overreact to stimuli, arching their body and biting when swallowing (tonic bite reflex). Ongoing assistance can help these infants accomplish effective latch and sucking for nursing.

Gentle organizing input before feeds, such as skin-to-skin contact, rhythmic rocking or swaying, and repetitive sounds (such as shushing), improves feeding. Positioning the baby's head level with the rest of their body can improve milk transfer. Nursing with the baby in an upright position and stroking downward under the chin will aid swallowing. If the baby arches their back, hold the baby with their flexed knees bent and the spine rounded. The use of swaddling and the Dancer hand position can also be useful (Children's Minnesota, 2024).

Babies who are born with a neurological impairment have a higher percentage of preterm births and may therefore require longer hospitalization than most babies. Generally, these parents need assistance and support to compensate for their babies' low muscle tone, as well as patience while the baby learns and relearns how to suck. They may need to manage separation from the baby, as well as the baby preferring bottle feeds because of sucking weakness. Depending on its severity, neurological impairment results in the infant rarely having a fully developed or strong suck and swallow reflex. Because milk transfer relies on a mature suck and swallow reflex, nursing is more challenging, and feedings take more time. The degree of difficulty depends on the severity of the impairment and parents' ability to cope with the emotional stress and practical aspects of nursing.

Short, frequent feedings may help compensate for the baby's difficulty in maintaining concentration and losing interest in nursing before transferring milk adequately. Because the baby may become frustrated waiting for milk to release, parents can express milk to initiate letdown before beginning feedings. For a baby who can maintain a latch and seal, a tube-feeding device may be useful while nursing. Babies with neurological defects need to be followed closely to ensure adequate intake, recognizing that supplementation with expressed milk may be necessary. When direct nursing is not possible, providing the

Table 27-2 Counseling Parents of an Infant with Neurological Impairment

Concern	Suggestions
Difficulty latching	■ Position the baby close to the nipple and adequately support their body. ■ Position the baby's lower lip outward from the bottom gum. ■ Press down the middle of the baby's tongue to create a groove for the nipple. ■ Use the Dancer hand position to provide support.
Difficulty sucking	■ Feed milk by a cup, dropper, spoon, bottle, or specialty feeding bottle (e.g., Pigeon, Special Needs, Hazelbaker).
Gagging or choking while nursing	■ Position the baby with their throat slightly above the nipple. ■ Stroke downward under the chin to aid swallowing.
Losing interest after several minutes of nursing	■ Pre-express milk to initiate letdown. ■ Express milk onto the nipple or into the corner of the baby's mouth. ■ Nurse more frequently, for shorter periods (e.g., 5 minutes) at a time. ■ Use a tube-feeding device while nursing to maintain milk flow and encourage sucking.
Unable to nurse effectively	■ Express milk and feed to the baby. ■ Hold baby skin to skin as often as possible. ■ Maximize close contact (e.g., wear baby in a sling if safe).

immunological protection of human milk is important for these children. **Table 27-2** presents counseling suggestions for neurological impairment.

Sensory Processing Disorder

Sensory integration is the process of the brain taking input from the five senses and forming a functional composite to comprehend the world around us. Failure of sensory integration to develop normally may result in problems in learning, development, or behavior. **Sensory processing disorder (SPD)** (previously called *sensory integration disorder*) is a pattern of dysfunction in individuals who have atypical responses to ordinary sensory stimulation. **Figure 27-10** presents risk factors in SPD.

- Birth weight of under 2200 g
- Under 36 weeks' gestational age
- Prenatal complications
- Maternal stress or illness
- Maternal use of medications or other drugs
- Birth complications, including operative deliveries
- Minority ethnicity
- Single parenthood
- Low socioeconomic status

Figure 27-10 Sensory processing disorder risk factors.

Modified from Star Institute. Sensory Spectrum Disorder. 2020. https://www.spdstar.org/basic/latest-research-findings#f2

One study found an increased risk of SPD in infants born preterm or via c-section. The disorder was found in 84% of preterm infants and 80% of infants born via c-section (Ptak et al., 2022). Another study of infants aged 4 to 24 months with siblings diagnosed with SPD suggests there may also be a genetic predisposition. The higher-risk infants exhibited more atypical physical characteristics. These included restricted movements and an asymmetrical tonic neck reflex that persisted beyond 6 months. The high-risk group also had lower sensory-seeking behaviors than the low-risk group. This suggests a possible reduced ability to explore the environment caused by subtle motor difficulties. These infants also had lower scores in language and cognition (Flanagan et al., 2019).

A baby who is hyporesponsive with low registration of sensory input, may fail to suck when nursing. A baby who is hyperresponsive may be hypertonic and easily overstimulated. When nursing, they might be overwhelmed by the repetitive stimuli and experience tactile input negatively. They might avoid latching and have an aversion to direct nursing. Excessive stimuli can make these infants irritable and difficult to calm (Freund-Azaria et al., 2023).

Special feeding strategies may help babies at both ends of the SPD spectrum transition to nursing more effectively. A hyporesponsive infant may respond to being held upright and finger feeding in that position, as well as gentle massage of the face, mouth, and palate. Strategies for the hyperresponsive baby include deeper pressure touch, swaddling, swinging the baby gently from head to toe in a blanket before feeding, and self-latch (Genna, 2023).

SPD is complex, and the baby will need multidisciplinary care, including an occupational or physical therapist. If you are able to attend the baby's evaluation or therapy, you can offer valuable insights from a feeding perspective and help parents advocate for continued nursing. An interdisciplinary approach benefits both these babies and their parents. Social media abounds with parents' firsthand accounts of children whose neurological impairment, autism, or other disorders first presented as feeding problems and the lack of healthcare support or validation encountered. A checklist for parents is available from the Sensory Processing Disorder Foundation (2024).

Support for Parents of Special Needs Infants

Parents of compromised infants may experience shock and grief at the birth of their "less-than-perfect baby." Nursing can help them form an attachment to their baby as they work through their emotions. These parents need a great deal of support and encouragement, and you are an important member of their support team. Reinforce their commitment to nursing and praise them for their diligence in coping with difficulties. Encourage parents and their partners to draw on each other for strength and support. Remind them of all the beneficial aspects of nursing for an infant with special needs. Maintain a list of specialists for easy referral. Also refer parents to a support group for families with challenged children. Such contact can help them deal with their grief and learn to celebrate their baby's uniqueness. **Chapter 24** discusses parental grief.

It is common for parents to experience negative feelings at times about their compromised baby. Their depression can be much more severe than postpartum depression, and these parents will need a great deal of support. You may be the only person with whom they can express their true feelings. They need to know that you are there for them. Provide lactation support with compassion, focusing on expressing empathy rather than trying to "fix" the problem. **Chapter 20** discusses postpartum depression.

Working with clients in emotional situations can put providers at risk for compassion fatigue. Compassion fatigue is secondary distress experienced by providers because of close contact with their clients' suffering. This differs from burnout, which is job dissatisfaction resulting from an uncontrollable and dissatisfying work environment (Kase et al., 2019). It is important to have the self-awareness to recognize when compassion fatigue is affecting your mental well-being and job performance.

Maintaining a positive attitude, flexibility, and critical thinking can lower the risk of compassion fatigue. Draw on support from those close to you and from your own support network. Engaging in mindfulness practices of self-care, accepting compassion from others, and remaining resilient through change can improve compassion satisfaction and overall mental and emotional well-being (Sist et al., 2022).

Summary

Having an infant with a health condition or neurological disorder poses challenges for parents. Some will reach their feeding goals despite these obstacles. Others may need to change their goals to accommodate their special situation. Your assistance will be valuable to them as they navigate their unexpected parenting journey, including any necessary feeding accommodations. You can help parents recognize ways in which nursing and providing expressed milk help meet their baby's needs. Despite health conditions, parents can establish enriching and sound feeding practices that do not compromise their baby's health. Nursing helps normalize the relationship between parents and a compromised baby and optimizes the baby's health through human milk.

What You Learned—At a Glance

Conversation Starters with Parents

- What health conditions does your baby have that you think might affect nursing?
- How are you managing feedings with your compromised baby?
- How are you and your partner emotionally handling having a compromised baby?
- What social support do you have to help you through this period?

Counseling Parents of a Compromised Infant

- Babies with cardiac issues may require more calories than healthy babies.
- Impaired cardiopulmonary function may increase the length of feedings.
- Test weights can improve direct nursing of babies with cardiac issues.

- Babies with cardiac issues are at higher risk for feeding difficulties, including dysphagia.
- Phe intake for an infant with PKU must be strictly monitored throughout lactation and structured weaning.
- A baby with PKU can receive Phe-free formula through a tube-feeding device while nursing.
- A baby with complete galactosemia cannot consume mammalian milk of any kind.
- A baby with the Duarte form of galactosemia may receive human milk with careful monitoring and a nondairy formula, such as one based on soy or amino acid.
- For a baby with a cleft lip, nursing may be easier than bottle feeding.
- Nursing with a cleft palate presents feeding challenges.
- Babies with Pierre Robin sequence can rarely nurse but benefit from receiving expressed milk.
- An infant with spina bifida may nurse depending on the level of impairment.

Neurological Impairment

- Ability to nurse will depend on the degree of impairment.
- The baby will require continual teaching and coaxing.
- Initiate feedings frequently in the absence of cues—at least every 2 hours—in the newborn period.
- Hold the baby upright with the nose and throat higher than the nipple.
- Hold the baby skin to skin frequently.
- Begin feedings before the baby is completely awake.
- Nurse for brief, frequent periods to avoid tiring the baby.
- Recognize signs of fatigue, cardiac complications, hypotonia, and difficulty rooting and sucking.
- Press down on the center of the tongue and use the Dancer hand position as needed.
- Express milk if the baby cannot nurse directly.

Special Health Needs

- Help parents deal with emotions and stages of grief for the loss of the "perfect" child.
- Avoid comments that minimize parents' concerns or deny their reactions.
- Give parents information in gradual doses during the newborn period.
- Help parents perceive their child as normal in other respects.
- Avoid judging parents' lactation decisions.
- Help with milk expression and provide follow-up care.
- Recognize symptoms of hyporesponsive and hyperresponsive babies
- Teach parents coping mechanisms and refer them to specialists.

References

Abebe MS, et al. Congenital hydrocephalus and associated risk factors: an institution-based case-control study, Dessie Town, North East Ethiopia. *Pediatric Health Med Ther.* 2022;13:175–182.

Academy of Breastfeeding Medicine. ABM clinical protocol #16: breastfeeding the hypotonic infant, revision 2016. *Breastfeed Med.* 2016;11(6):271–276.

Academy of Breastfeeding Medicine. ABM clinical protocol #17: guidelines for breastfeeding infants with cleft lip, cleft palate, or cleft lip and palate, revised 2019. *Breastfeed Med.* 2019;14(7):437–444.

Aguilar-Cordero MJ, et al. Assessment of the technique of breastfeeding in babies with Down syndrome. *Aquichan.* 2019;19(4).

American Cleft Palate-Craniofacial Association. Craniofacial conditions. 2025. https://acpacares.org/resource/craniofacial-conditions/

American Liver Foundation. Galactosemia. 2023. https://liverfoundation.org/liver-diseases/pediatric-liver-information-center/pediatric-liver-disease/galactosemia/

Ashe K, et al. Psychiatric and cognitive aspects of phenylketonuria: the limitations of diet and promise of new treatments. *Front Psychiatry.* 2019;10:561.

Baxter D, Shanks AL. Pierre Robin syndrome. In: *StatPearls.* Treasure Island, FL: StatPearls Publishing; August 7, 2023. https://www.ncbi.nlm.nih.gov/books/NBK562213/

Berry GT. Classic galactosemia and clinical variant galactosemia. In: Adam MP, Feldman J, Mirzaa GM, et al., eds. *GeneReviews.* Seattle, WA: University of Washington; March 11, 2021. https://www.ncbi.nlm.nih.gov/books/NBK1518/

Boztepe H, et al. Parenting stress in Turkish mothers of infants with cleft lip and/or palate. *Cleft Palate Craniofac J.* 2020;57(6):753–761.

Brosch S, et al. Submucous cleft palate and a congenitally short velum: effects of surgical intervention. *HNO.* 2018;66(8):598–604 [in German].

Burianova I, et al. Breastfeeding after early repair of cleft lip in newborns with cleft lip or cleft lip and palate in a Baby-Friendly designated hospital. *J Hum Lact.* 2017;33(3):504–508.

Centers for Disease Control and Prevention. Birth defects. Down syndrome. December 26, 2024a. https://www.cdc.gov/ncbddd/birthdefects/features/down-syndrome.html

Centers for Disease Control and Prevention. Growth charts for children with Down syndrome. May 16, 2024b. https://www.cdc.gov/birth-defects/hcp/down-syndrome-growth-charts/index.html

Children's Minnesota. Breastfeeding an infant with neurological problems. 2024. https://www.childrensmn.org/educationmaterials/childrensmn/article/15845/breastfeeding-an-infant-with-neurological-problems

Church PT, et al. Prenatal counseling: guidelines for the care of people with spina bifida. *J Pediatr Rehabil Med.* 2020;13(4):461–466.

Cognata A, et al. Human milk use in the preoperative period is associated with a lower risk for necrotizing enterocolitis in neonates with complex congenital heart disease. *J Pediatr.* 2019;215:11–16.e2.

Coentro VS, et al. Altered sucking dynamics in a breastfed infant with Down syndrome: a case report. *Int Breastfeed J.* 2020;15(1):71.

Costa B, et al. Satisfaction with health care in families following a diagnosis of cleft lip and/or palate in the United Kingdom. *Cleft Palate Craniofac J.* 2019;9:1055665619888318.

Dash M, et al. Feeding interventions among cleft lip/palate infants: a systematic review and meta-synthesis. *J Cleft Lip Palate Craniofac Anom.* 2023;10(1):14–25.

Davis JA, Spatz DL. Human milk and infants with congenital heart disease: a summary of current literature supporting the provision of human milk and breastfeeding. *Adv Neonatal Care.* 2019;19(3):212–218.

Demirci J, et al. Winging it: maternal perspectives and experiences of breastfeeding newborns with complex congenital surgical anomalies. *J Perinatol.* 2018;38(6):708–717.

Dorise B, et al. Feeding practices and growth of infants with Pierre Robin sequence. *Int J Pediatr Otorhinolaryngol.* 2019;118:11–14.

El-Khuffash A, et al. Preventing disease in the 21st century: early breast milk exposure and later cardiovascular health in premature infants. *Pediatr Res.* 2020;87(2):385–390.

Ettinger RK, et al. Timing of Furlow palatoplasty for patients with submucous cleft palate. *Cleft Palate Craniofac J.* 2018;55(3):430–436.

Flanagan JE, et al. Early identification of sensory processing difficulties in high-risk infants. *Am J Occup Ther.* 2019;73:7302205130.

Fontanals M, et al. Anesthetic considerations and complications of cleft palate repairs. What's new? *Curr Anesthesiol Rep.* 2021 Sep;11:257–264.

Freund-Azaria A, et al. Does infant sensory responsiveness explain exclusive breastfeeding 6 months after birth? A cohort prospective study. *Transl Pediatr.* 2023;12(6):1063–1075.

Fridovich-Keil JL, et al. Duarte variant galactosemia. In Adam MP, et al., eds. *GeneReviews.* Seattle, WA: University of Washington; June 25, 2020. https://www.ncbi.nlm.nih.gov/books /NBK258640/

Genna CW. *Supporting Sucking Skills in Breastfeeding Infants.* 4th ed. Burlington, MA: Jones and Bartlett Learning; 2023.

Gottschlich MM, et al. A retrospective study identifying breast milk feeding disparities in infants with cleft palate. *J Acad Nutr Diet.* 2018;118(11):2154–2161.

Gregory C. Use of test weights for breastfeeding infants with congenital heart disease in a cardiac transitional care unit: a best practice implementation project. *JBI Database System Rev Implement Rep.* 2018;16(11):2224–2245.

Hammoudeh JA, et al. Early cleft lip repair revisited: a safe and effective approach utilizing a multidisciplinary protocol. *Plast Reconstr Surg Glob Open.* 2017;5(6):e1340.

Hillert A, et al. (2020). The genetic landscape and epidemiology of phenylketonuria. *AJHG.* 107(2):234–250.

Hookway L, et al. The challenges of medically complex breastfed children and their families: a systematic review. *Matern Child Nutr.* 2021;17(4):e13182.

Hosseini HR, et al. Treatment outcomes of pre-surgical infant orthopedics in patients with non-syndromic cleft lip and/or palate: a systematic review and meta-analysis of randomized controlled trials. *PLoS One.* 2017;12(7):e0181768.

Hurst AC. Pierre Robin syndrome. December 31, 2023. http://www.nlm.nih.gov/medlineplus/ency/article/001607.htm

Hydrocephalus Clinical Research Network. Who we are. 2024. https://www.hcrn.org/

Jung SE, et al. Clinical interventions and speech outcomes for individuals with submucous cleft palate. *Arch Plast Surg.* 2020;47(6):542–550.

Kalangu KK, et al. Towards zero infection for ventriculoperitoneal shunt insertion in resource-limited settings: a multicenter prospective cohort study. *Childs Nerv Syst.* 2020;36:401–409.

Kalvala J, et al. Breast feeding in infants diagnosed with phenylketonuria (PKU): a scoping review. *BMJ Paediatr Open.* 2023;7(1):e002066.

Kase SM, et al. A cross-sectional pilot study of compassion fatigue, burnout, and compassion satisfaction in pediatric palliative care providers in the United States. *Palliat Support Care.* 2019;17(3):269–275.

Keller T, et al. Intranasal breast milk for premature infants with severe intraventricular hemorrhage-an observation. *Eur J Pediatr.* 2019;178(2):199–206.

Kose E, et al. The effects of breastfeeding in infants with phenylketonuria. *J Pediatr Nurs.* 2018;38:27–32.

Kukkola HL, Kirjavainen T. Obstructive sleep apnea is position dependent in young infants. *Pediatr Res.* 2023;93(5):1361–1367.

Levy HL, et al. Phenylalanine ammonia lyase (PAL): from discovery to enzyme substitution therapy for phenylketonuria. *Mol Genet Metab.* 2018;124(4):223–229.

MacDonald A, et al. PKU dietary handbook to accompany PKU guidelines. *Orphanet J Rare Dis.* 2020;15(1):171.

Madhoun LL, et al. Breast milk feeding practices and barriers and supports experienced by mother-infant dyads with cleft lip and /or palate. *Cleft Palate Craniofac J.* 2019;9:1055665619878972.

Magenis ML, et al. Down syndrome and breastfeeding: a systematic review. *J Intellect Disabil Res.* 2022;26(1):244–263.

Mai CT, et al & National Birth Defects Prevention Network. National population-based estimates for major birth defects, 2010–2014. *Birth Defects Res.* 2019;111(18):1420–1435.

Maina G, et al. Effectiveness of ventilation tube insertion for conductive hearing loss in children with chronic otitis media with effusion and non-syndromic cleft palate: a systematic review protocol. *JBI Evid Synth.* 2022;20(6):1560–1567.

Mangili G, et al. Feeding dysfunctions and failure to thrive in neonates with congenital heart diseases. *Pediatr Med Chir.* 2018;40(1).

March of Dimes. Cleft lip and cleft palate. 2022. https://www.marchofdimes.org/find-support/topics/birth/cleft-lip-and-cleft-palate

McPherson AC, et al. Nutrition, metabolic syndrome, and obesity: guidelines for the care of people with spina bifida. *J Pediatr Rehabil Med.* 2020;13(4):637–653.

Miranda VSG, et al. Cardiorespiratory parameters in infants cardiopathy: variations during feeding. *Codas.* 2019;31(2): e20180153.

Muddasani V, et al. The use of ultrasound-guided 3D-constructed obturator device in the management of cleft lip and palate: a case series. *Cureus.* 2024;16(7):e64948.

Naidu P, et al. Cleft palate repair: a history of techniques and variations. *PRS-GLOB OPEN.* 2022;10(3):e4019.

National Down Syndrome Society. About Down syndrome. 2025. https://ndss.org/about

National Organization for Rare Disorders. Pierre Robin sequence. 2018. https://rarediseases.org/rare-diseases/pierre -robin-sequence/

Operation Smiles. Strengthening the global health care workforce. 2025. https://www.operationsmile.org/global-health-equity/health-workforce-strengthening/

Park YH, et al. Treatment of velopharyngeal insufficiency in a patient with a submucous cleft palate using a speech aid: the more treatment options, the better the treatment results. *Maxillofac Plast Reconstr Surg.* 2019;41(1):19.

Ptak A, et al. The occurrence of the sensory processing disorder in children depending on the type and time of delivery: a pilot study. *Int J Environ Res Public Health.* 2022;19(11):6893.

Qu J, et al. Efficacy and safety of sapropterin dihydrochloride in patients with phenylketonuria: a meta-analysis of randomized controlled trials. *Br J Clin Pharmacol.* 2019;85(5): 893–899.

Ramani PK, Arya K. Galactokinase deficiency. In: *StatPearls.* Treasure Island, FL: StatPearls Publishing; 2023. https://www.ncbi.nlm.nih.gov/books/NBK560683/

Sakran KA, et al. Early cleft palate repair by a modified technique without relaxing incisions. *Cleft Palate Craniofac J.* 2024; 61(4):646–653.

Sensory Processing Disorder Foundation. Common sensory processing disorder behaviors – a checklist for all ages. 2024. https://www.spdfoundation.net/sensory-processing-disorder-checklist/

Sist L, et al. Self-care for nurses and midwives: findings from a scoping review. *Healthcare.* 2022:10(12):2473.

Smile Train. Training programs. 2025. https://www.smiletrain.org/medical-professionals/training-programs

Solot CB, et al. Speech-language disorders in 22q11.2 deletion syndrome: best practices for diagnosis and management. *Am J Speech Lang Pathol.* 2019;28(3):984–999.

Souza PC, et al. Findings of postoperative clinical assessment of swallowing in infants with congenital heart defect. *Codas.* 2018;30(1):e20170024.

Spina Bifida Association. Neural Tube Defects 2025. https://www.nichd.nih.gov/health/topics/factsheets/ntds

Stanley MA, et al. Clinical identification of feeding and swallowing disorders in 0-6 month old infants with Down syndrome. *Am J Med Genet A.* 2019;179(2):177–182.

Stock NM, et al. Promoting psychosocial adjustment in individuals born with cleft lip and/or palate and their families: current clinical practice in the United Kingdom. *Cleft Palate Craniofac J.* 2020;57(2):186–197.

Tahmasebifard N, et al. Early nutrition among infants admitted to the NICU with cleft lip and palate. *Cleft Palate Craniofac J.* 2023;60(3):299–305.

Tsuchiya S, et al. Association of cleft lip and palate on mother-to-infant bonding: a cross-sectional study in the Japan Environment and Children's Study (JECS). *BMC Pediatr.* 2019;19(1):505.

United Nations Children's Fund. Research on heart disease and health. 2019. https://www.unicef.org.uk/babyfriendly/news-and-research/baby-friendly-research/infant-health-research/infant-health-research-heart-disease-and-health/

U.S. National Institute of Neurological Disorders and Stroke. Hydrocephalus fact sheet. 2025a. https://www.ninds.nih.gov/Disorders/Patient-Caregiver-Education/Fact-Sheets/Hydrocephalus-Fact-Sheet

U.S. National Institute of Neurological Disorders and Stroke. Spina bifida. 2025b. https://www.ninds.nih.gov/health-information/disorders/spina-bifida?search-term=sspin%20bifida#toc-how-is-spina-bifida-diagnosed-and-treated-

van Wegberg AMJ, et al. The complete European guidelines on phenylketonuria: diagnosis and treatment. *Orphanet J Rare Dis.* 2017;12(1):162.

Welsink-Karssies MM, et al. Classical galactosemia: neuropsychological and psychosocial functioning beyond intellectual abilities. *Orphanet J Rare Dis.* 2020;15(1):42.

Williams GM, et al. Establishing breast feeding in infants with Down syndrome: the FADES cohort experience. *BMJ Paediatr Open.* 2022;6(1):e001547.

World Health Organization. Congenital disorders. February, 27, 2023. https://www.who.int/news-room/fact-sheets/detail/birth-defects

Wu W, et al. Incidence and mortality trend of congenital heart disease at the global, regional, and national level, 1990–2017. *Medicine (Baltimore).* 2020;99(23):e20593.

Yoshitomi A, et al. Relationship between cleft palate width and otitis media. *Laryngoscope Investig Otolaryngol.* 2022;7(6): 2126–2132.

PART 5

Professional Practice

CHAPTER 28

Professional Considerations

Lactation support providers are integral members of a nursing family's healthcare team. The members of the family's interdisciplinary healthcare team have varying degrees of knowledge and experience in basic lactation physiology and management, as well as counseling and communication skills. An **International Board Certified Lactation Consultant (IBCLC)** manages a full range of basic and specialized lactation care. Breastfeeding counselors provide peer support and refer to an IBCLC for complicated situations. Primary healthcare providers and other members of the healthcare team often learn more about lactation to fill gaps in their formal education. Lactation support providers are guided by professional practice documents that establish their scope of practice, required competencies, professional conduct, and legal parameters.

KEY TERMS

Certification
Code of professional conduct
Commission on Accreditation of Allied Health Education Programs (CAAHEP)
Continuing Education Recognition Points (CERPs)
Detailed Content Outline
Documentation Guidelines
Health Insurance Portability and Accountability Act (HIPAA)
Informed consent
International Board Certified Lactation Consultant (IBCLC)
International Board of Lactation Consultant Examiners (IBLCE)
Lactation Education Accreditation and Approval Review Committee (LEAARC)
Liability
Mentor
Professional burnout
Protected health information (PHI)
Role acquisition
Scope of practice
Standards of practice

Lactation Knowledge of the Healthcare Team

Practice-based interprofessional education helps health professionals learn teamwork skills and gain an understanding of the roles of others (Spaulding et al., 2021). Providers on the healthcare team need to be knowledgeable in lactation management and have the necessary skills and attitudes to provide meaningful advice and support to families. Hallmark traits of a capable practitioner are self-learning, self-efficacy, collaboration, creativity, and the ability to apply competencies to new tasks.

Lactation consultants are pivotal in helping other members of the healthcare team remain current with lactation skills and practices. When practitioners must refer routine situations to a lactation consultant for assistance, the families and staff can lose valuable time and delay resolution of a problem. Time constraints can make it difficult for busy health professionals to remain up to date with practical skills. Equipping healthcare providers with the necessary information and skills to aid and support nursing families can help minimize problems.

Filling Learning Gaps Among Team Members

The absence of adequate formal training in lactation accounts for much of the lack of tangible caregiver support. All healthcare members on the lactation team need to know how to support parents in a variety of situations during pregnancy, childbirth, and postpartum. An interdisciplinary approach to lactation education increases knowledge among healthcare professionals (Vilar-Compte et al., 2020). Sharing appropriate information across disciplines promotes a continuum of consistent, skilled care.

Interdisciplinary professional education improves student attitudes toward communication, shared problem-solving, and teamwork. It increases knowledge, skills, and behavior changes (Guraya & Barr, 2018; Teheux et al., 2021). Medical students report favorable attitudes toward interdisciplinary education throughout their medical training (Berger-Estilita et al., 2020). Consistent lactation education with hands-on interprofessional experiences should be taught across disciplines throughout undergraduate health courses, residency programs, and continuing education. Lactation information in medical textbooks needs updating and expansion as well (Radzyminski & Callister, 2015; Webber & Serowoky, 2017).

Professional Education of Team Members

Education during medical training and being surrounded by a culture in which nursing is the norm will enhance caregivers' lactation support and advice. During their professional education, learners should have opportunities to engage in all aspects of lactation, including teaching, research, advocacy, and professional development (Taylor & Bell, 2017). Curricula need to focus on improving students' lactation knowledge, attitudes, problem-solving, and support skills. Programs need to be evidence based, with consistent information and up-to-date best practices. Students need to acquire effective counseling and communication skills to feel confident supporting nursing families. They need to recognize cultural factors and social determinants that affect families.

Lactation education in medical curricula should include multidisciplinary and interprofessional application-based experiences, including didactic instruction, clinical practice, role playing, and skills labs (Chuisano & Anderson, 2020; Vilar-Compte et al., 2020). The American Academy of Pediatrics (AAP, 2023) and the American Academy of Family Physicians (AAFP, 2019) have lactation curricula for residents and continuing education, as well as lactation resources for practicing healthcare providers. Recently updated core competencies for interprofessional education of health professionals are a catalyst for improving team-based health care and enhancing health outcomes (Interprofessional Education Collaborative [IPEC], 2023).

A learning environment that coordinates early clinical learning opportunities, knowledge, skills, and judgment helps develop practice competency (Sahu et al., 2019). Structured and progressive learning supports cross-specialty demands in clinical practice (Liu et al., 2019). Providing opportunities to role-play situations in a receptive learning climate helps relieve anxiety and makes the anticipated situation less awkward when confronted with it in practice.

Virtual experiences offer opportunities to learn lactation management skills and increase confidence within a low-stress environment (Campbell et al., 2022; Grabowski et al., 2020; Sadovnikova et al., 2020; Webber et al., 2021; Weston & Zauche, 2021). Simulation can expose students to rare clinical scenarios and negate the need for real clients at clinical sites (Díaz et al., 2021; Sadovnikova et al., 2020; Weston & Zauche, 2021).

Continuing Education for Team Members

Teaching lactation management to hospital staff and other members of the lactation team is an ongoing process. Healthcare professionals inevitably experience uncertainty at various times in their clinical practice. Nurses who feel unprepared to help with lactation can develop confidence through learning by doing, open communication, and the growth of trust in colleagues (Newton et al., 2015). Teaching lactation management during the orientation of new nurses enhances their transition to professional practice.

The training of healthcare providers through the Baby-Friendly Hospital Initiative (BFHI) is an effective, low-cost strategy for raising awareness, providing consistent information, and ensuring appropriate lactation support. The Baby-Friendly model from the World Health Organization (WHO) and the United Nations Children's Fund (UNICEF) forms a framework for academic education, with elements aimed at specific professionals (Aryeetey & Dykes,

2018). Revision of Step 2 of the Ten Steps to Successful Breastfeeding requires that facilities "ensure that staff have sufficient knowledge, competence and skills to support breastfeeding." The focus on competency represents a shift from the length of training to a process that verifies staff competencies (Chapin et al., 2021).

Lactation consultants have a unique role in helping to fill the learning gaps among health professionals to enhance their competence and comfort in assisting with lactation. Team members need effective counseling and clinical skills, as well as an awareness of cultural and social factors related to infant feeding decisions (Campbell et al., 2022; Vanguri et al., 2021). Including a lactation consultant in teaching increases competency and affects lactation rates (Uzumcu et al., 2020).

In-service programs can be planned to meet the needs of both new and experienced staff to help achieve consistent lactation care. Inviting members of the healthcare team to attend continuing education sessions will contribute to consistency throughout the team. Nurses report significantly higher job satisfaction after collaboration with a multidisciplinary team (Baik & Zierler, 2019). Case-based learning, clinical simulations, practice, and feedback enable learners to process and apply information (Crowe et al., 2018; Hegland et al., 2017; Kurup et al., 2017; Tanis et al., 2019). Webinars and other forms of online learning increase the reach of educational offerings and provide opportunities for healthcare providers to learn on demand (Curran et al., 2019; Frisch et al., 2017). These and other techniques, such as seminars and short lactation updates at meetings or on bulletin boards, will help keep staff updated on current management practices.

World Breastfeeding Week and Month present timely occasions for lactation initiatives with motivational programs. A workshop or conference energizes people and generates enthusiasm for learning more about lactation. A bulletin board with monthly updates can include highlights of team members who have done something noteworthy related to lactation. Messages can be posted where people are likely to read them, such as in the breakroom, locker room, and restrooms.

Mentoring

Mentoring is effective in educating and supporting other healthcare providers to incorporate evidence into clinical practice. Work-based learning, with experiential teaching, is an effective means for staff to develop clinical skills and teamwork to deliver quality client care (Mianda & Voce, 2018). A skills-based team training approach, with high-frequency practice and mentoring, builds competency and confidence.

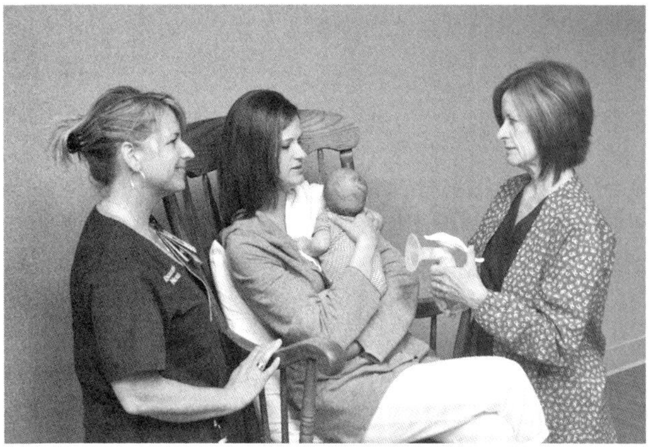

Figure 28-1 Staff member observes as the lactation consultant explains the use of a breast pump.

A lactation consultant is a valuable **mentor** for nurses and other caregivers as they acquire the knowledge and skills for assisting with nursing. Shadowing increases self-confidence and clinical skills among health professionals. A hospital staff member who asks for help in assisting at a feeding presents a teachable moment. Observing while a lactation consultant assists with the feeding will help increase their confidence in handling a similar situation in the future (**Figure 28-1**).

Preparing for the Lactation Profession

There are several modes of entry into the lactation consulting profession. Early in the profession, many entered from a background as a peer support counselor. With increased education requirements for **certification**, it is likely that most who enter the profession today will have some form of postsecondary degree. Many licensed healthcare providers add lactation consulting to their existing work in maternal and child health, including nursing, midwifery, dietetics, and healthcare provider practice. Some providers have advanced degrees in related fields, such as education, psychology, human development, public health, or another area that complements lactation consulting. Others have degrees in unrelated fields and change the direction of their careers after nursing their own children and wanting to help other families.

Formal Education

Preparation for the lactation profession begins with extensive education in all areas of lactation management and clinical practice, followed by formal certification through the **International Board of Lactation Consultant Examiners (IBLCE)**. The knowledge and skill base in the lactation field is broad and extensive. In the early years of the profession, many entrants to the field gained their knowledge through self-directed learning. As the profession evolves, formal education requirements have increased. Candidates for certification must demonstrate completion of education in the health sciences and lactation management, as well as clinical experience. The combination of health science subjects and the didactic and clinical instruction in lactation required for the profession constitutes 2 to 3 years of education.

Health Sciences

A foundation in health science enables lactation consultants to function as valued, respected members of the family's healthcare team. Certification candidates must demonstrate satisfactory completion of eight academic health science courses provided by an accredited institution of higher learning. These courses, typical preparation for allied health professionals, are described in the IBLCE *Health Sciences Education Guide*, with examples of typical course names and content (IBLCE, 2023a). Certification candidates must also complete six additional health science subjects through an institution of either higher learning or continuing education. **Table 28-1** lists the health science course and continuing education requirements for certification. Recognized health professionals will likely have completed the required courses through their professional education. Others will need to satisfy the requirements before applying for the certification examination.

Lactation Management

Lactation consultants need the competence to evaluate situations and apply appropriate knowledge, skills, and attitudes in both routine and nonroutine lactation management. Comprehensive lactation education is critical to the preparation of a competent clinician. A certification candidate must complete a minimum of 90 hours of lactation-specific education and 5 hours of education focused on communication skills. The candidate must confirm that the education covers the disciplines and chronological periods identified in the IBLCE **Detailed Content Outline** (IBLCE, 2023c), as described in **Table 28-2**. The education

Table 28-1 **Health Science Education for Lactation Consultants**

Equivalent of 1 semester of postsecondary higher education in:

- Biology
- Human anatomy
- Human physiology
- Infant and child growth and development
- Nutrition
- Psychology or counseling or communication skills
- Introduction to research
- Sociology, cultural sensitivity, or cultural anthropology

Continuing education in:

- Basic life support (e.g., cardiopulmonary resuscitation [CPR])
- Medical documentation
- Medical terminology
- Occupational safety, including security, for health professionals
- Professional ethics for health professionals (e.g., code of ethics)
- Universal safety precautions and infection control

Reproduced from International Board of Lactation Consultant Examiners. https://www.iblce.org. Printed with permission.

Table 28-2 **International Board of Lactation Consultant Examiners (IBLCE) Detailed Content Outline**

Disciplines	Chronological Periods
i. Development and Nutrition–Infant and Maternal	1. Prenatal
ii. Physiology and Endocrinology	2. Labor/birth (perinatal)
iii. Pathology—Infant and Maternal	3. Prematurity
iv. Pharmacology and Toxicology	4. 0–2 days
v. Psychology, Sociology, and Anthropology	5. 3–14 days
vi. Techniques	6. 15–28 days
vii. Clinical Skills	7. 1–3 months
A. Equipment and Technology	8. 4–6 months
B. Education and Communication	9. 7–12 months
C. Ethical and Legal Issues	10. Beyond 12 months
D. Research	11. General principles (including preconception)
E. Public Health and Advocacy	

Reproduced from International Board of Lactation Consultant Examiners. https://www.iblce.org. Printed with permission.

must be completed within 5 years immediately prior to exam application. Visit the IBLCE website for current requirements.

Certification candidates may complete the 95 hours of didactic education through conferences, workshops, or webinars. However, piecing education together in this manner does not guarantee the broad foundational knowledge and skills necessary for practicing as a competent clinician. Rigorous lactation education that provides a strong foundation is *critical* to establishing and maintaining a professional standard of care.

A certification requirement of a comprehensive lactation program would raise the standard of professional practice and provide a baseline of preparation for the lactation consulting profession. Aspiring lactation consultants are encouraged to seek a comprehensive course of study that prepares them not only for passing a minimal competency exam but also for acquiring the knowledge and skills to practice competently with nursing families. Lactation courses of varying lengths are available through on-site programs and distance learning.

The **Lactation Education Accreditation and Approval Review Committee (LEAARC)** established standards and a lactation curriculum to build educational consistency throughout the profession (LEAARC, 2018). LEAARC provides formal review and recognition of lactation courses. Links to courses endorsed by LEAARC are available on its website (LEAARC, 2025). LEAARC is a review committee for the **Commission on Accreditation of Allied Health Education Programs (CAAHEP)** for the accreditation of postsecondary lactation programs in universities and colleges (CAAHEP, 2025). Links to accredited programs are available on the CAAHEP website. Academic lactation programs are discussed later in the chapter.

Clinical Education

Clinical education is a significant component of the lactation consultant's formal preparation for the profession. A well-rounded lactation consultant needs clinical experience with different infant ages in the various settings that serve lactation families. This experience may be acquired in community support groups; health clinics; home visits; and maternity/infant care areas in hospitals, such as neonatal intensive care, labor and delivery, postpartum, and pediatric units. CAAHEP-accredited lactation programs provide the full range of clinical experience to students. LEAARC provides guidance for developing a clinical internship and for students seeking clinical experience (LEAARC, 2025).

Several resources are available to assist students in mapping their clinical instruction to obtain the necessary competencies. Clinical instructors and students alike use these resources to ensure balance when preparing for the profession.

- The Clinical Competencies for IBCLC Practice (IBLCE, 2018a) publication identifies specific experiences needed to prepare for the certification exam and work as a competent IBCLC.
- The LEAARC competency-based lactation curriculum covers all the IBLCE competencies. LEAARC also has a document for students to map their acquisition of clinical competencies (LEAARC, 2024).
- LEAARC's resource guide for establishing and maintaining a lactation clinical internship program includes a mapping document for clinical competencies.

Clinical practice, role playing, skills labs, and simulations are all effective methods for teaching clinical skills (Chuisano & Anderson, 2020; Weston & Zauche, 2021). Simulation-based experiences allowed continued clinical lactation education during the COVID-19 pandemic. The experience was positive for both interns and instructors. Simulation is a viable option for completing some of the required clinical hours. It can help standardize clinical education globally (Chamberlain et al., 2022).

Simulation exposes students to rare clinical scenarios and reduces the need for clinical sites. Learner outcomes from simulations are equal to or exceed outcomes from in-person clinical experiences (Díaz et al., 2021). Virtual clinical experiences increase learner confidence, remove the risk of working with real clients, and provide access to learners who live in remote areas (Campbell et al., 2022). Prebriefing and debriefing sessions help to round out virtual clinical experiences.

Ideally, a student acquires clinical skills through a formal internship under the guidance and coaching of an experienced clinical instructor who helps the student progress from novice to competent clinician. A structured program for supervised clinical experience provides opportunities for students to learn and practice skills in a variety of settings. This enables a novice clinician to progress toward expertise and an understanding of best practices in lactation care. Acquiring clinical experience outside a formal internship can be challenging. Hospitals do not typically allow a lactation consultant on staff to informally mentor students.

Aspiring lactation consultants who are nurses often obtain their clinical experience in the hospital where they are employed, documenting the hours they spend in lactation care. Nurses typically qualify for certification through the IBLCE Pathway 1. Pathway 2 (graduation from a CAAHEP-accredited postsecondary program) ensures a comprehensive program requiring that all competencies be acquired, supervised by an IBCLC clinical instructor qualified by education and experience. Pathway 3 requires that a student's clinical experience be acquired through a formal internship program supervised by an IBCLC with an approved mentorship plan. In the United States, limited access to clinical mentorships, as well as financial limitations, continue to hinder diversity among lactation professionals (Lima et al., 2024).

Academic Lactation Programs

Allied health professions typically require that students complete an integrated academic program of didactic and clinical preparation and then pass a certifying examination (CAAHEP, 2025). This required work can be incorporated into an academic certificate or degree program at a postsecondary institution. LEAARC assists colleges and universities in establishing academic lactation programs. As a review committee for CAAHEP, LEAARC reviews and recommends academic lactation programs for accreditation. Students who graduate from a CAAHEP-accredited lactation program qualify for the certification exam through Pathway 2.

As increasing numbers of academic programs emerge, wider availability of formal education will provide an avenue for young adults to prepare for the lactation consultant profession through postsecondary study, just as with other professions. Achieving consistency and quality among lactation education programs can lead to increased availability of accredited programs to prepare future members of the profession. With enough postsecondary programs available for aspiring lactation consultants, the profession can work toward the goal of requiring graduation from an academic program before certification. This raises the prominence of the IBCLC credential and the lactation consultant profession. The Pathway 2 programs are moving the profession toward that goal.

Certification

The IBLCE develops and administers the certification examination for lactation consultants. The IBLCE examination is recognized internationally as a measure of minimal competence in lactation consulting. It is administered in multiple languages and at numerous sites around the world. Since 1988, the IBLCE certification program has been continuously accredited by the National Commission for Certifying Agencies. Candidates who pass the exam are awarded the designation IBCLC.

Beginning in 2022, a newly formed IBCLC Commission manages initial certification and recertification, examination development, scoring, appeals, and ethics and discipline (IBCLC Commission, 2025). IBCLCs must provide evidence of basic life support education, 75 hours of **Continuing Education Recognition Points (CERPs)**, and 250 clinical practice hours every 5 years to maintain certification. They have the option to recertify by examination every 10 years and CERPs in alternate years. Those who wish to recertify by CERPs instead of exam must complete a Continuing Education (CE) Self-Assessment to identify areas that will require continuing education to maintain comprehensive knowledge and skills. Current requirements are available on the IBLCE website.

Acquiring the Role of Lactation Consultant

Moving into a new role is a dynamic process, especially when it involves a new career. New clinicians progress through their **role acquisition** at their own pace at each point in the process. The process of entering the lactation consulting profession is a time of personal growth as the learner acquires the skills, knowledge, and attitudes to provide quality assistance to families. Novices ultimately learn to adapt theory and book knowledge to each new situation and change their practices as researchers and practitioners discover and understand more about lactation. Many will model themselves after a mentor or other experienced colleague.

It is through exposure to a variety of practices that clinicians emerge with their own unique style and the ability to personalize their care. Remaining open to new practices and seeking new evidence-based information ensures continued growth in meeting the needs of parents and babies. The Dreyfus five-stage model of skill acquisition describes developmental stages beginning with novice and progressing through advanced beginner, competent, proficient, and expert (Dreyfus & Dreyfus, 1980). The model has been applied to the nursing profession (Benner, 2004). It describes the acquisition of the role of lactation consultant as well and is integrated into the discussion of the various stages that follow.

Novice Stage

The novice stage begins with the decision to enter the lactation consulting profession. Interest in the profession may derive from having enjoyed nursing, having received personal help from a lactation consultant, or a desire to expand a health profession role into helping families with nursing. A novice may have little or no experience and a limited understanding of the full range of the lactation profession. During this stage, they complete formal education in lactation management, acquire the necessary clinical skills, and become certified as an IBCLC.

As novices begin to apply their learning to clinical practice, their behaviors may be extremely limited, inflexible, and governed by rules. They match textbook learning with actual clinical cases and rely on standard care plans to guide them. They will continue to learn to recognize and assess signs and symptoms until they have experienced clinical problems such as mastitis, ankyloglossia, and low milk production in a range of clients.

Advanced Beginner Stage

A newly certified IBCLC will have functioned close to the level of a beginning lactation consultant in the final year of their clinical instruction. An increased level of professional responsibility at this stage heightens a sense of engagement with families and the ability to recognize various aspects of a situation. Although they might be eager to work independently, they may also welcome the security, support, and affirmation of a mentor. New practitioners pay close attention to the practice of colleagues. They tend to absorb information from colleagues as fact while actively seeking credible sources of information. They do not yet feel responsible for managing unfamiliar clinical situations. They typically focus on doing everything adequately while worrying about experiencing new situations and performing well without making mistakes.

Clinical care during this stage is guided by rules, protocols, care plans, and documents from professional organizations (described in the next section). It may be uncomfortable veering from a standard care plan to form decisions based on the needs of an individual parent and baby. For example, having learned about babies developing a preference for artificial nipples, a new practitioner may believe that a "good" lactation consultant does not use a nipple shield. Therefore, they may be reluctant to use one, even in circumstances in which it might be appropriate.

New practitioners feel vulnerable to criticism and have a heightened awareness of feedback on their own performance. Even an experienced provider may feel vulnerable taking on a new role as a lactation consultant. Curiosity, calmness, listening skills, responsiveness, humility, and accountability will help new practitioners grow and strengthen their proficiency as they mature as clinicians. At the same time, gaining self-awareness of their negative traits will help them learn compensatory skills and increase their effectiveness with families and colleagues.

Competent Stage

During the first and second years of practice, the development of skills and a grasp of clinical situations continue to evolve. The pace for gaining competence depends on the range of exposure to a variety of clinical experiences and numbers of nursing dyads. Learning from past experiences to develop forward-thinking—reflective learning—promotes learners' understanding of their core competencies and provides opportunities for personal critical reflection (Lane & Roberts, 2022). This reflection helps practitioners decide what is important based on previous experiences with other parents and babies. This stage is marked by excitement when performing well and remorse when performance is not as effective as it might have been because of missed relevant subtle signs and symptoms. These feelings act as a moral compass that continues to guide the practitioner's ethical and clinical learning.

At this stage, practitioners recognize that not everyone is a proficient or expert clinician. They identify conflicting advice among experts on many aspects of lactation care and may question overly generalized or broad advice. Rules, organizing, and planning begin to give way to perceiving the immediate demands of a situation. It becomes clear that there are many ways to approach situations. The practitioner is increasingly comfortable considering multiple approaches and weighing options as they tailor care to each dyad's needs and readiness.

Proficient Stage

The proficient practitioner has an enhanced ability to read situations and lets a situation guide their responses. They no longer believe they must have all the answers. Networking with other lactation consultants helps them mature in their role as they continue to learn the many ways to approach diverse aspects of lactation care. They can actively interpret the direction of changes in a situation and determine what can be ruled in and ruled out. When their grasp of a clinical situation is altered by changes or unexpected responses, they search for new understanding that leads to greater experiential clinical learning.

Reasoning, openness, and trust in what the practitioner observes and hears replace prediction, control, and confusion. When something unique or surprising occurs, they try to figure out why and how the situation is different. They continue to refine their comprehension of each situation and draw comparisons with past experiences and other parents and babies. They feel increasingly comfortable in many different circumstances. Interactions with parents are more spontaneous, with less fear of imperfection and a style that reflects their personality.

Expert Stage

An expert IBCLC understands the motives and whims of new parents and adjusts their teaching and guidance to complement their individual preferences. They use practical wisdom and integrate their grasp of situations with their responses. Intuition guides the practical assessment of situations and families' needs and wishes. Assessment of a situation becomes so linked with actions and outcomes that they are intuitively obvious. The practitioner fluidly responds to a situation even when the situation changes.

An expert IBCLC recognizes that parents are responsible for their choices. They are more accepting of parents who choose a path that may be less than optimal. Although they may seek opinions from others, they are quick to discard those that are incompatible with their personal approach. They look critically at research and adapt it to their clinical care. Clinical practice is guided by common sense, practical skills that reflect open-minded thinking, creativity, and thinking outside the box.

Professional Practice Documents

Lactation consultants work in concert with primary practitioners who care for families. They provide a level of care that facilitates continued health and wellness for the entire family, particularly in relation to lactation and early parenting. Several professional documents outline the behaviors that IBCLCs must follow.

Scope of Practice

The aim of a **scope of practice** is to protect the public by ensuring safe, competent, and evidence-based care. The Scope of Practice for IBCLCs (IBLCE, 2018b) affirms that lactation consultants have specialized knowledge and clinical expertise in lactation. It describes the activities for which lactation consultants are educated and in which they are authorized to engage. Lactation consultants have a duty to uphold the standards of the profession; to protect, promote, and support lactation; to provide competent services for families; to report truthfully and fully to primary healthcare providers and to the healthcare system; to preserve client confidence; and to act with reasonable diligence.

The lactation field in the United States contains a myriad of titles, credentials, certifications, educational backgrounds, and scopes of practice. This presents challenges to healthcare providers in making referrals, insurers in providing reimbursement for services, and policymakers when making recommendations. The various roles can also be unclear to families when seeking lactation support. Uniform identifiers have been suggested by several organizations to address this confusion. They all have similar categories of lactation consultant (IBCLC), lactation educator/counselor, and peer supporter. These titles distinguish between professional lactation care and the provision of lactation education and support (Strong et al., 2023).

Standards of Practice

Quality and service constitute the core of a profession's responsibility to the public. Lactation consultants are charged with providing quality care to the public and accepting responsibility for that care. **Standards of practice** describe what is considered best practice by a profession. The Standards of Practice for IBCLCs describe the tasks and skills an IBCLC should be able to perform (International Lactation Consultant Association [ILCA], 2013). Working within the appropriate scope of practice and demonstrating clinical competence, accountability, ethical practice, and legal responsibility are fundamental to maintaining professional standards.

Clinical Competencies

Anyone who provides health care is expected to demonstrate clinical competence. Lactation professionals must be clinically competent in their care of nursing families. The *Clinical Competencies for the Practice of IBCLCs* document encompasses the responsibilities and activities for an IBCLC's practice (IBLCE, 2018a). This document identifies competencies that enable IBCLCs to provide safe, competent, and evidence-based care. The LEAARC competency-based lactation curriculum complements the IBLCE competencies to ensure that lactation students learn these competencies during their precertification education.

Documentation Guidelines

Standard documentation ensures that a client's record is accurate, clear, and complete. The IBLCE **Documentation Guidelines** describe clinical documentation as the written, typed, or electronic record of information about a client or client group, which details the care provided (IBLCE, 2012). The record must communicate observations, assessments, the care plan, interventions, evaluations, outcome, and follow-up.

Documentation should be contemporaneous and recorded by the clinician with a date and signature. The record should be maintained securely in a way that protects client confidentiality. Documentation regarding client care has the potential to be admitted into legal proceedings, making their completeness and accuracy especially important.

Code of Professional Conduct

Members of the health profession are guided by a set of principles that outline the commitments and obligations to self, client, colleagues, society, and the profession. These principles set forth a **code of professional conduct** that protects the health, safety, and welfare of the public by establishing and enforcing qualifications of certification and issuing voluntary credentials to individuals who have attained those qualifications.

The *Code of Professional Conduct for IBCLCs*, governed and monitored by IBLCE, holds IBCLCs accountable for their practice (IBLCE, 2023b). It provides a framework for IBCLCs to carry out their essential duties and serves as a basis for decision-making. **Figure 28-2** presents the basic principles of the IBCLC *Code of Professional Conduct*.

1. Provide services that protect, promote, and support nursing.
2. Act with due diligence.
3. Preserve the confidentiality of clients.
4. Report accurately and completely to other members of the healthcare team.
5. Exercise independent judgment and avoid conflicts of interest.
6. Maintain personal integrity.
7. Uphold the professional standards expected of an IBCLC.
8. Comply with the IBLCE Disciplinary Procedures.

Figure 28-2 Principles of International Board Certified Lactation Consultant (IBCLC) *Code of Professional Conduct*.

Reproduced from International Board of Lactation Consultant Examiners. www.iblce.org. Printed with permission.

Ethical IBCLC Practice

Using evidence-based practices that are in the best interests of nursing families will help guide ethical practice. This requires remaining current through continuing education and skill development, as well as reading, understanding, and evaluating research. Recognizing and respecting that each family has its own personal beliefs and feeding goals will ensure appropriate care tailored to their needs.

Work within the profession's scope of practice to educate and guide parents and other family members in making their own decisions and collaborating on their care plan. Recognize that the use of lactation products is not always the solution of choice. Consider each situation appropriately and objectively within the context of all possible means of addressing a problem. Keep other members of the healthcare team informed of significant developments, especially when there is cause for concern. Treat all parents honestly, fairly, and equally. Always provide any promised follow-up care. If circumstances prevent the delivery of appropriate follow-up, document clearly that you made a good-faith effort. For example, if you promise to call a parent to learn how a care plan is working and you leave three or four messages with no response, or you send a text message, you have exercised due diligence. Document each contact with the date and time and indicate that you left a voice or electronic message asking them to call you if they need or desire further care.

Ethical Challenges

A variety of situations can raise the question of possible ethical implications or conflicts of interest. A framework for decision-making was proposed to help IBCLCs analyze and resolve such ethical dilemmas (Noel-Weiss et al., 2012). Avoiding a conflict of interest, or even the appearance of one, can sometimes be challenging. The potential for a conflict of interest exists for an IBCLC whose business includes the sale or rental of lactation equipment or products. It is also a risk for an IBCLC who works in a hospital as well as a private practice that relies on referrals. Including all available options when referring parents to sources for products or follow-up care can avoid the appearance of self-promotion. Another ethical challenge is considering a parent's experiences from a broad range of social, economic, and cultural contexts when suggesting interventions (Subramani et al., 2024).

A moral and ethical dilemma can also occur when a lactation consultant recognizes the need for a particular action and is not permitted to follow through because of organizational policies, provider orders, or other restrictions. Ethical practice intends that a lactation consultant does not undermine the primary caregiver's position. It is best to try to work within the parameters of a caregiver's advice as much as possible. When a disagreement occurs, it is important to discuss the discrepancy with the caregiver if possible and explain the evidence-based reasons for your position. If a family asks for recommendations for another healthcare provider, lactation consultant, or other allied healthcare practitioner, suggesting at least three names avoids the appearance of favoring one over another.

Much dialogue regarding ethics in lactation consultancy revolves around compliance with the *International Code of Marketing of Breast-milk Substitutes* (WHO, 1981). Other common themes are the use of alternative therapies, scope of practice, and legal aspects of practice. Ethical practice requires a clear understanding of biomedical ethics and, specifically, the unique ethical factors involved in lactation consulting. To promote professional ethics competency, IBLCE requires a minimum of 5 continuing education hours in ethics every 5 years to maintain certification. **Chapter 3** discusses ethics.

Legal Considerations

Lactation consultants must practice within the laws of the geopolitical region in which they live and must respect the family's rights to privacy and issues that are confidential in nature. To protect yourself legally, ensure that you are covered by liability insurance before practicing as a lactation consultant if such insurance is warranted in your geopolitical region. If you work for a hospital or government agency and perform only the duties within that scope of practice, your employer's liability insurance may provide sufficient coverage. However, many lactation consultants and other healthcare workers maintain liability insurance that will protect them in the employee role as well. Privately employed lactation consultants need to secure appropriate professional liability insurance.

Protecting Privacy and Confidentiality

Lactation consultants are ethically and legally obligated to respect and preserve a family's confidentiality and privacy. Practical safeguards prevent inadvertently disclosing identifying information. Speaking quietly and avoiding the use of client names when in public areas can guard against incidental disclosure. Privacy can be further protected by destroying research identifiers at the earliest opportunity and by isolating and locking file cabinets that contain client records.

Additional safeguards include encrypting **protected health information (PHI)** that is sent or maintained electronically, using secure electronic platforms for all electronic communication, and using strong passwords on all electronic devices. A confidentiality notice such as the one in **Figure 28-3** included in electronically transmitted reports ensures that the transmittal complies with privacy regulations. In the United States, the **Health Insurance Portability and Accountability Act (HIPAA)** requires that electronic platforms used for electronic health communication and records must be secure and HIPAA-compliant. Other countries have similar client privacy requirements.

Written consent to receive care and to share clinical information with other members of the healthcare team is standard practice. In a hospital, such consent usually occurs during admission. If you are the first point of contact, such as in private or clinic practice, it is important to obtain signed consent before initiating care. Consent is not required when sharing information anonymously with colleagues or in professional presentations if you avoid giving any clues about the client's identity.

Make a point to become familiar with client privacy regulations in your geopolitical region. In the United States, HIPAA prohibits the use or disclosure of a client's health information unless authorized by the client. However, in the case of suspected child neglect or abuse, the caregiver has authorization and a legal duty as a mandated reporter to report such instances to appropriate public health authorities. Many other countries have similar provisions. Anytime the

> The attached pages are my report of a recent lactation consultation. If you received this transmission in error, please respect the privacy of the people involved. Contact [your name, phone or fax number, or email address) to tell me I have sent it to the wrong recipient. Destroy the report you received by mistake.
>
> This report contains information that falls under the privacy sections of the Health Insurance Portability and Accountability Act of 1996. When you read it, you will see personal information and details about parents and infants. I have obtained consent from the family involved to transmit this report to their healthcare providers, as required by the International Board of Lactation Consultant Examiners Code of Professional Conduct and the International Lactation Consultant Association Standards of Practice.

Figure 28-3 Confidentiality notice to include with electronic communication.

Printed with permission of Elizabeth C. Brooks, JD, IBCLC.

potential health of a client or baby, or even that of a colleague, is at risk, an IBCLC has a duty to inform an appropriate person or authority. Secure electronic platforms and software programs designed for lactation practice that safeguard client privacy are available.

Client Relationships

Accepting a client creates certain contractual expectations and duties. Those duties exist regardless of whether clients pay for their services. Once a relationship is established, the caregiver has a duty to render the appropriate level of care unless the client authorizes their withdrawal. They have a duty to refer the client to another caregiver and not to abandon the client if they are unable to render appropriate care.

Establishing a Relationship

A client relationship is established whenever you and a parent have contact, whether in person, over the telephone, or via electronic communication. In some cases, you may create a client relationship simply through the act of making an appointment. When a parent arrives for a scheduled appointment, you are obligated to provide care or make alternate arrangements through referral to another competent practitioner. If your assessment reveals a problem that is beyond your competency, you must inform the parent of your concerns. Make sure parents understand the need for follow-up care and refer them to a competent practitioner when the problem is beyond your level of competency.

Voice and Electronic Contacts

A conversation by phone or teleconferencing platform can create a client relationship if you indicate acceptance or give comments that imply treatment. This is also the case with any form of electronic communication, including texts, social media responses, or emails. The content of a conversation determines whether it constitutes a relationship. You can avoid creating a client relationship through several measures. When a parent contacts you, first identify yourself and then ask their name and the purpose of the contact. If you determine that they need a referral, you can offer to make an appointment. If the parent declines, you can present options, such as going to the emergency department or contacting an appropriate caregiver or another lactation consultant. This avoids creating a client relationship if you do not give any comments that imply advice.

Where No Relationship Exists

Some interactions do not create a client relationship. A healthcare provider's request that you visit a client or review a client's record does not constitute a relationship. However, if the provider relies on you for lactation advice, and you are aware of this expectation, a relationship between you and the client is implied, and you are obligated to visit the client as soon as possible. In a hospital, generally, no relationship exists between you and clients after discharge. However, this usually does not apply if the client contacts you through the hospital (e.g., client portal or voice call).

Duration of a Relationship

When you have an established relationship with a client, you are legally required to continue care until the need for your services no longer exists, until the client withdraws from your care, or until you withdraw in a manner that does not constitute "abandonment" of the client. Performing services when needed avoids the potential of abandonment. When a healthcare provider asks you to evaluate a client, you can tell the client verbally, "I have been contacted by (name of provider) to evaluate you and your baby." Also, note this in the client's record. When you terminate the relationship, tell the client and write in the record, "I am signing off this case and will no longer follow this client. However, I will remain available if I am notified that additional consultations or assistance are required."

If you wish to withdraw from the relationship, you must give appropriate notice of your intentions, through either verbal, electronic, or written communication. You should state the status of the relationship, any need for follow-up care, and your intention to withdraw by a specific date that allows the client time to seek alternative care. You must indicate that you are available for emergencies until the stated date. In addition, you must state that the healthcare provider can obtain a copy of all records with the written permission of the client. A client's failure to pay for services they received does not justify your withdrawal without giving sufficient opportunity to obtain alternative care.

After providing notice of your intent to withdraw from a relationship with a client, you must refer the client to a competent replacement or to a specialist if the problem is outside a lactation consultant's competence or scope of practice. Substituting your services with those of another lactation consultant avoids abandonment. After securing written permission from the client, you can share case details with your replacement, both verbally and in writing. If a client fails to keep a follow-up appointment or to follow your advice, there are safeguards to ensure that the client understands the nature of the condition and the risks of failing to seek medical attention. Provide the client with an opportunity to visit you for counseling or care. Although you may share all this verbally with the client, you also need to follow it up in writing.

Informed Consent

Although **informed consent** may not always be a legal requirement, it is important to discuss specific topics with parents so that they are fully informed. Discuss the nature of a problem, the proposed treatment, and reasonable alternative treatments. Inform parents of the chance of success with the proposed treatment, as well as any inherent risks. Make sure they understand the consequences of failing to undergo treatment. You can explore alternative treatments and risks with colleagues to learn what they explain to their clients. Also consult current medical literature to document the frequency and severity of risks so that you can include this in your consent form.

Standard consent forms typically do not provide sufficient information about disclosures made to the client to establish that consent was adequately informed. Lactation consultants in a busy practice can ensure adequate legal protection by preparing information sheets for the courses of treatment. Both you and the client should sign the form, attesting that the client acknowledges receipt of the information. Generally, competent adults can give valid consent for infants. Therefore, a signed consent covers both the parent's and the infant's care. In addition to consent for treatment, you may want to include permission for photographs to be used for educational purposes. You can also upload photographs to the chart. Retain a copy of the signed consent for your files and provide a copy, either electronically or in print, to the client.

Record Retention

Client records provide a history of the dyad's health that is helpful to other care providers. Records help comply with statutes and other regulations, substantiate fees for third-party payment, and defend against professional negligence. In addition, client records (with identifiers removed) are a great source of research projects and are useful when preparing teaching presentations. Your geopolitical region defines how long you must retain records.

If you work in a healthcare provider's office, the state or province's medical practice act or licensing statutes may dictate the type of information to be included in a client's record. In the United States, these typically include a written or electronic record of a client's history, as well as examination and test results. To remain accredited, a hospital's records must contain identification data, client medical history, reports of relevant physical examinations, diagnostic and therapeutic orders, evidence of appropriate informed consent, clinical observations, reports of procedures and tests, and conclusions at the termination of hospitalization or evaluation of treatment.

Telephone calls, written and electronic correspondence, and appointments are all part of the official records. These demonstrate that you followed up on care or responded to a complaint in a timely fashion. They also demonstrate dates of appointments or a parent's failure to keep an appointment. Electronic medical records are commonplace in health care. **Chapter 2** discusses electronic medical recordkeeping, especially in a hospital setting.

Avoiding Liability

Becoming familiar with your local laws regulating the practice of health care will help you avoid placing yourself at risk for **liability**. Familiarize yourself with protocols in your practice setting and always perform within your scope of practice. Ensure that you are protected continuously by professional liability insurance. To safeguard against lawsuits, build positive relationships with clients and respect their autonomy. Avoid guaranteeing results or creating unrealistic expectations. Empower parents to make informed decisions rather than relying on you to direct their actions.

You can also minimize liability risk by recognizing when a case may be beyond your level of competence or when you may not have time to handle it. Document everything you do, as well as what you choose not to do, and why. Clients can request their records at any time, so avoid making negative notations in a record. Organize your workspace and keep necessary paperwork or electronic records accessible to make it convenient for timely documentation of what you do. Safeguard against lost records by ensuring that there are copies of all documentation. Cloud-based storage services provide long-term archiving of documents. In the United States, any cloud-based service must be HIPAA compliant.

Consulting a business attorney before opening a practice is a worthwhile investment. Incorporating a private practice may limit personal liability. Resources specific to starting and maintaining a lactation practice successfully include *Lactation Private Practice: From Start to Strong* (Frisbie, 2018a), *Paperless Private Practice for Lactation Consultants* (Frisbie, 2018b), and *Perspectives in Lactation: Is Private Practice for Me?* (Parkes, 2015).

Writing Expert Witness Reports

A seasoned lactation consultant or other healthcare professional may have occasion to provide expert court testimony where decisions concerning nursing infants and young children are made. A child protection case may involve an infant who was removed or is at risk of removal from their parent's care. In a criminal matter, a parent may be at risk for separation from the infant because the jail cannot accommodate keeping them together. In family law, the noncustodial parent may disagree with cosleeping, frequent feeding, or nursing beyond infancy. In one case, a parent discontinued nursing after being ordered to accommodate bottle feeding and overnight visits by the noncustodial parent (Feminist Legal Clinic, 2023).

A lactation consultant who has provided numerous expert reports in court shared tips for writing expert witness reports (Gribble, 2021):

- Begin with the report writer's qualifications and expertise, sources of information in the report, and a statement that everything considered relevant was included.
- Record the child's birth date, birth weight, current weight, relevant health information or medical conditions, and feeding history.
- Include relevant records or conversations with health professionals, experience expressing milk, or the infant's refusal of bottle feeds.
- Describe the importance of nursing with reference to relevant research, national and international recommendations, and the negative impact that cessation of nursing has on children.
- Personalize the information (e.g., "the parent has difficulty expressing milk," "the parent is following recommended lactation management," or "there is a family history of medical conditions that can be negatively affected by the cessation of nursing").
- Avoid overstating a case and ensure that there is evidence to back up every claim made.

If making recommendations, do not state that the child and parent must not be separated. Rather, recommend that the child's age and stage of development, their rights in relation to lactation, and the negative health impact of cessation of nursing be considered in the decision-making of the court. You might suggest that keeping the parent and child together, supervised, if necessary, until a decision is made would allow nursing to continue. If long separations are necessary, you could recommend accommodating milk expression and transport to the infant. In a criminal matter, the parent and baby might be placed in a unit that allows them to remain together. In family law, short visitation by the noncustodial parent or allowing the parent to be nearby may enable the infant to exclusively nurse.

Professional Growth

Remaining current in lactation practices and addressing personal challenges as a healthcare professional are important elements of a lactation consultant's continued growth. Opportunities abound for networking with others for collaboration, advice, and support. Continuing to learn about ways to enhance interactions with families will contribute to your personal growth as your competence and confidence continue to grow. Recognizing signs of potential burnout will help you achieve a comfortable balance and maintain your enthusiasm for working with families.

Continuing Education

Continuing education is an essential element of professional development that will help you remain current in your knowledge and clinical skills. Conferences, hands-on courses, seminars, webinars, and self-study modules assist healthcare professionals in meeting their personal education goals as well as fulfilling the requirements for maintaining licensure and certification. Employer support promotes continuing education, lifelong learning, and a culture conducive to learning (Chant & Westendorf, 2019; Rohan, 2017). Staff who continue their education develop clinical leadership and change-agent abilities (Ho et al., 2019).

Professional conferences provide valuable networking opportunities and cutting-edge education. National and regional professional organizations offer a variety of continuing education opportunities. Online networking opportunities are available through social media, including a myriad of Facebook groups and online lactation groups. Professional groups such as LinkedIn and Yammer allow professionals to share lactation information and seek answers to clinical questions. Becoming a member of your professional association, locally and internationally through ILCA, brings you in contact with other lactation professionals and provides access to a wealth of resources. ILCA membership includes a subscription to the *Journal of Human Lactation*, with new research and practice tips, case studies, and innovative approaches.

Maturing Through Experience

At times, working with nursing families may present discouraging experiences. Inevitably, something will occur that cannot be corrected or prevented. Such challenges can occur when parents experience medical complications or fail to follow through on advice. People in a parent's life may exert a negative influence that affects your assistance and the lactation outcome. Even your own approach with parents can create discouraging obstacles. At such times, it is helpful to express your frustrations or doubts to an understanding colleague.

Recognizing Limitations

Families and members of the healthcare team consider lactation consultants to be experts in lactation management. Being viewed as an expert can make it difficult to admit when we do not know something. It is important to acknowledge when you do not have all the answers and need to seek help from outside sources. Throughout your career, you may encounter an unusual situation, a medical question, or another circumstance that you cannot address adequately with your existing knowledge. Establishing professional resources helps you deliver complete and correct information. Developing collaborative relationships in areas that enhance your practice enables you to obtain assistance from others. Hospitals, healthcare providers, dietitians, pharmacies, medical libraries, service organizations, and universities are all valuable resources.

Cultivating contacts in related fields will help you provide families in your care with access to the information and services they need. A list of local referral resources may include physical therapists, occupational therapists, speech and language therapists, clinicians who treat oral structure anomalies, massage therapists, craniosacral therapists, acupuncturists, chiropractors, herbalists, and other specialists. In addition to establishing a network of personal resources, you can develop a reference library with current lactation texts and periodicals.

Discouraging Cases

There will invariably be parents who do not follow through on your advice and then experience what you consider to be negative results. Some of these outcomes may occur because of what you deem to be an inappropriate or ill-advised action. A parent may wean unexpectedly or earlier than you would consider optimal. Another may supplement with formula or introduce complementary foods at an early age. It is discouraging when lactation deteriorates because parents have not followed suggestions and advice. It is important to keep in mind that what parents do with your advice is their responsibility. They are accountable for the consequences of their actions; you are not. Your duty is to offer appropriate support and information. You must then step back and respect parents' autonomy and choices.

It is discouraging for both you and a highly motivated and determined parent who is unable to nurse for medical reasons. Other times, events may leave you feeling helpless, such as a baby dying or radical breast surgery that prevents lactation. These outcomes can affect you deeply when you have cultivated a caring relationship with a family. You may find it difficult to remove yourself emotionally from the situation, and need to work through your own grief.

Some discouraging situations involve people other than the parents in your care. Perhaps a parent's partner is unsupportive and resents your involvement. A member of the medical community may be unsupportive of your efforts or may consistently give incorrect lactation information. Although such situations can make it difficult to provide necessary help and advice, they offer opportunities as well. You can educate the partner or caregiver and try to determine the cause of the misinformation or lack of support. You can be open and frank about the partner's feelings and arrange follow-up contacts at times when the partner is not at home. You can provide medical research to share with the caregiver and encourage parents to share the positive aspects of their nursing. If parents ask you to recommend someone for a second opinion, providing several names will maintain your objectivity.

Personal Challenges

Our own personalities and communication styles can sometimes influence the way we approach parents. Each parent is unique, with their own personality, strengths, and limitations. Approaching parents with a focus on their individual needs ensures that you help them reach their goals. Examining your personal style and consciously working toward mitigating any weaknesses can help you overcome potential roadblocks in your communications. **Chapter 5** on communication and counseling and **Chapter 6** on consultations will assist you in avoiding barriers to your providing the assistance and support parents need.

Getting Overly Involved

Your influence on parents' behavior is limited, and your role is to encourage them to determine their own solutions. Parents can sometimes become overly dependent on a caregiver's assistance to the point that they fail to recognize and use their own resources. Encourage parents who rely on you too much to make their own decisions. Build their confidence and offer information with minimal guidance.

When problems are outside the realm of lactation, encourage parents to contact their healthcare provider, a mental health professional, a religious advisor, or other sources of advice and support. Parents need to understand that your services are restricted to lactation and related topics. If you are a licensed counselor or psychologist who has been counseling a parent in lactation and the nature of the contact changes, you need to renegotiate your relationship formally.

Counseling family members or close friends is discouraged. Emotional ties may cause you to have strong reactions to the choices they make. If lactation goes well, they may become overly dependent on you and fail to mature in their parenting as quickly as they might otherwise. If lactation does not go well, they may blame you regardless of the reason, thus harming your personal relationship. If you sense this may happen, it is wise to refer family members or friends to a colleague so that you may maintain your role as a loving family member or friend.

Discussing Your Nursing Experience

Parents often ask about their lactation consultant's personal nursing experience. Those who ask how long you nursed rarely really want to know that. More likely, they have a question about their own nursing. Capitalizing on your counseling skills can help you determine the real purpose of such a question. You might say, for example, "You're wondering how long to nurse your baby." It is important to keep the discussion focused on the parent. Discussing aspects of your life is unprofessional and diminishes the parent's experience. At times, it may be appropriate to give a short or humorous answer and immediately return the focus to the parent without elaborating on your personal experience.

Making Value Judgments

It may be challenging at times to remain objective and avoid the appearance of making value judgments. Your role is to empower parents as informed consumers by providing correct and appropriate information and advice. What parents do with that advice is their choice and their responsibility. Encourage parents to make decisions that fit into their lifestyle and then support their choices. Always leave room for parents to make a graceful exit if they seem uncomfortable with your suggestions. Clearly state, "You know best what you and your family can deal with at this time"—and mean it!

Interrupting

One of the greatest challenges in communication is allowing the other person to talk uninterrupted without interjecting your own comments. Effective listening involve the use of counseling skills to draw out parents and engage them in conversation. Resist the urge to interrupt or change the subject until an issue has been explored sufficiently. Such interruptions are common in many social and professional interactions, often requiring practice and careful attention to how you communicate.

Overwhelming Parents

Parents can feel overwhelmed by the amount of knowledge and skills they need for nursing, especially when it involves problem solving. Restricting the amount of information you give at any one time will avoid overloading parents with too much advice and information. Try to limit suggestions to two or three at a time. You can always follow up a contact with a telephone call, text, or email to determine if your plan worked. Clearly explain that there are more options and that if these suggestions do not work, you are available for further assistance.

Being Too Solution Oriented

Focusing too much on solutions runs the risk of failing to explore factors in a parent's life that may be significant to a situation. This risk is common in helping roles within the health profession, especially in a hospital setting, where staff time is limited. You can avoid missing important elements by listening carefully to feelings and concerns parents express. Engage in problem-solving only after you have gathered sufficient information and impressions. Observe their body language to gather impressions from what they are *not* saying. Allow parents time to define a situation and work toward solutions. Ensure that you respond to the parent's and baby's pace and that you do not rush to maintain your own schedule.

Failing to Follow Up

Routine follow-up in health care is an essential final component of every interaction. It confirms whether your advice has been helpful. Always follow through to learn if a situation has improved and to offer support. Make sure parents know how they may obtain help when they have questions or feel discouraged. If you plan to be away for an extended time, arrange for someone to provide assistance so that parents receive help when they need it. Remember that follow-up may involve referring families to community resources when it is apparent that you cannot resolve a problem.

Table 28-3 Signs of Emotional Burnout

Signs of Emotional Burnout	Physiological Reactions to Emotional Burnout
▪ Tunnel vision ▪ Loss of coping skills ▪ Lack of focus and concentration ▪ Inability to manage time ▪ Irrational behavior; a feeling of being on an "emotional roller coaster" ▪ Irritation; easily angered ▪ Tearful; crying for no reason ▪ Avoiding obligations and other avoidance behaviors ▪ Feeling that life is out of control	▪ Physical pain ▪ Weakness ▪ Fatigue ▪ Listlessness ▪ Depression ▪ Illness ▪ Becoming accident prone ▪ Insomnia or, conversely, sleeping excessively ▪ Anxiety ▪ Panic attacks

Avoiding Professional Burnout

Healthcare providers experience numerous pressures that place them at risk for stress and **professional burnout**. Almost everyone feels some degree of stress at work. Stress can result from excessive workloads, inefficient work processes, clerical burdens, work–home conflicts, lack of input or control with issues affecting their work lives, competing demands, and conflicting roles and relationships with colleagues and leadership (Hall et al., 2019; Tavella & Parker, 2020). How we cope with stress determines whether it leads to burnout. High levels of coping and optimism are associated with lower levels of burnout (Harolds, 2019a).

Stress that is not managed and controlled can lead to professional burnout, anxiety, and depression (Johnson et al., 2018). Burnout is most prevalent among people who work in service professions, and especially among healthcare providers (Rozario, 2019; Zarei et al., 2019). Females report higher levels of job strain than males (Jahnke et al., 2019; Riethof et al., 2019). Caregivers in maternal and infant health, and especially in lactation consulting, are predominantly female and are thus especially at risk for stress and burnout.

Personality is also a factor in burnout. Individuals who are prone to worry, irritability, and negative emotions are at higher risk for stress, compassion fatigue, and burnout (Kim et al., 2017). Those who are introverted and have low self-efficacy are also at risk for burnout.

Burnout is associated with emotional exhaustion, low work satisfaction, and depersonalization. Professional burnout and stress can cause suboptimal care, lower client satisfaction, reduced productivity, and high levels of absenteeism (West et al., 2018). There is a strong correlation between compassion fatigue and burnout (Zhang et al., 2018). Compassion fatigue is a form of burnout that is unique to professionals whose work involves caretaking or providing emotional support to others. Characterized by negative emotions and loss of empathy, compassion fatigue is a contributing factor in a client's satisfaction with their experience (Jilou et al., 2021; Klein et al., 2018; Xie et al., 2021). It is only by releasing tension that you can give compassionate care. **Table 28-3** describes signs of emotional burnout.

Work Environment

If you experience professional burnout, recognize that the problem you are experiencing is with your job and not with you. Healthy work environments are key to maximizing skills and performing optimally in the clinical arena (Brand et al., 2017; Slate et al., 2018). Job dissatisfaction can result from an imbalance between the effort you expend and the rewards you receive. Chronic work stress and unfavorable work conditions are associated with burnout and job dissatisfaction. It is not surprising that burnout has a direct effect on staff turnover (Kim & Kim, 2021; Tamata & Mohammadnezhad, 2023).

A healthy work environment will reduce the risk of staff burnout. The level of support from colleagues and superiors correlates with levels of job stress and burnout (Smith et al., 2018). Receiving cooperation and validation from colleagues can increase a sense of satisfaction in your work life. If a lack of cooperation and support from others creates work stress, you may need to use a new approach or find other avenues for garnering their support.

High job demands are a significant predictor of emotional exhaustion. Downsizing and lack of resources lead to constant psychological overtaxing, exhaustion, and cynicism. Health administrators can help avoid staff burnout by providing sufficient staffing and resources. Time constraints and staff shortages contribute to stress and can affect the quality of client care. Developing better time management skills often improves circumstances at work. An overwhelming workload may result from a lack of planning, prioritizing, or delegation skills. Measures to control these aspects of your job can prevent burnout and lead to increased job satisfaction and quality of care.

Job Satisfaction

Age, sufficient resources, meaningful work, and the impact of your efforts are significant predictors of job satisfaction. High levels of empowerment and the ability to influence a work situation reduce work-related stress and lower levels of burnout (Harolds, 2019a). Moving from higher levels of empowerment in a previous role to a less empowered position can correlate with a greater risk of burnout (de Las Heras-Rosas et al., 2021; Şenol Çelik et al., 2024). It is humbling to move from being an expert in a previous specialty to being a novice in a new role. Novice lactation consultants who had experienced high levels of empowerment in a related healthcare role may find it challenging as they move forward in acquiring expertise in their new role. Although acquiring the new role is desired, the life change can create anxiety (Dunbar et al., 2019).

Higher levels of job satisfaction are associated with positive coping strategies, self-confidence, optimism, and self-efficacy. Increasing general self-efficacy, reducing stress, and social support can alleviate job-related burnout (Yao et al., 2018). In addition, learning stress reduction techniques, developing interpersonal communication skills, and practicing mindfulness can decrease work-related anxiety (Green & Kinchen, 2021; Salvado et al., 2021; Tement et al., 2021). Empowerment, management support, and autonomy can decrease work stress and help to lower the risk of burnout (Burke et al., 2018; Hall et al., 2022; Moloney et al., 2020). Receiving support and encouragement from peers and being recognized for good performance increase job satisfaction and reduce the risk of burnout. Mentoring is a good tool for supporting the quality of job performance (Harolds, 2019b).

Delegating responsibilities helps you put your valuable time and energy into the most important functions. Training other staff to take calls and answer basic lactation questions gives them ownership and enables everyone to focus on priorities. Furthermore, empowering others to provide the first levels of lactation care helps minimize the types of problems that cause stress. If you are in private practice, consider asking a trusted colleague to take your referrals when you feel overwhelmed. You can record a message on your voice mail, send automatic responses to emails, and update your social media presence as appropriate to let families know you are unavailable.

High Expectations

Idealists who have high standards and believe they must do all the work themselves are at risk for burning out. High achievers who are full of enthusiasm and high expectations may fear falling short of self-imposed goals, resulting in disappointment and frustration. The need for perfection can reduce enthusiasm and tolerance and cause a loss of creativity and openness to change.

Failure to live up to our ideals increases the risk of burnout. Conflict between personal values and the values of the employer can create a feeling of powerlessness to change something we consider important. This can be magnified when combined with moral distress from knowing an ethically appropriate action and being unable to take that course. This can be especially taxing for lactation consultants whose employers violate the International Code by accepting gratuities from formula manufacturers and distributing formula discharge bags.

Balancing Work and Home

Factors in your life outside work can affect your satisfaction at work as well. It is often difficult for us to admit to our limitations and recognize that trying to be everything for everyone is unrealistic and impractical. When we attempt to do too many things, we cannot give our best to what is most important. We are in danger of emotional exhaustion and professional burnout anytime we fail to achieve a balance between professional responsibilities and personal needs (Fenwick et al., 2018; Lu et al., 2017). Work–life balance and self-care are key contributors to maintaining resilience (Bernuzzi et al., 2022; Cooper et al., 2020).

You cannot give the best of yourself when you feel stressed and stretched to the limit. Establishing personal boundaries and prioritizing the demands on your time help you achieve balance and reduce stress. Caring for nursing families often requires availability beyond a typical workday, sometimes 24 hours a day. Learn to limit commitments on your time and to say no when others ask more of you than you can give. Screen your calls, emails, and online queries when you feel unprepared to answer so that you may respond to messages at a more conducive time. Recapturing personal time to enjoy family, friends, and favorite activities helps you overcome burnout. Take the time to cultivate and nurture relationships with the important people in your life.

Make time for the most important person in your life—you! Plan special time to relax, pamper yourself, and enjoy activities that your busy schedule has not allowed. Use visualization and slow, deep breathing to relax and reclaim your strength and perspective. There are many online resources and mobile apps for incorporating mindfulness into your life. Your preferred means of physical exercise can also help rejuvenate you. Activities that you enjoy, such as massage, yoga, or manicures/pedicures are also ways to self-nurture and recharge. Maintaining perspective and finding humor in situations is especially important during times of stress. People with a sense of humor are healthier, happier people!

Renewing Enthusiasm

Learn how to recognize situations that make you feel uncomfortable, and work through them by discussing them with a colleague. Networking at conferences and meetings provides the opportunity for rejuvenation. Spending time with others in similar situations and learning new techniques can breathe new life into your job. Reading journals and technical information will expand your learning further. You can increase your professional support network by serving on committees and becoming active in your professional association.

If you enjoy community outreach, you might consider speaking to clinics, school health classes, nursing programs, and local organizations. If you enjoy writing, you could write an online blog, newsletter, or column on lactation for your local newspaper. You may also enjoy writing a column for a lactation or parenting website. If you enjoy education, you can teach lay counselors in the community or mentor lactation consultant interns. You can participate at the local, state, national, or global level in lactation protection and promotion efforts.

Undertaking a hobby or skill that has nothing to do with lactation can be rejuvenating. You might join a book club or pursue a new sport, exercise program, or musical instrument. Perhaps there are volunteer opportunities in your community. Nurturing your spirit helps you to be a well-rounded individual and not rely on your profession for your total sense of self. When you redefine your goals and relate them to your actions in this manner, you will be on your way toward developing a satisfying balance in your life. You will be able to continually reinvent yourself and bring a fresh, reinvigorated approach to the families in your care.

Summary

Members of the nursing dyad's lactation team must continually grow and thrive in the profession. Appropriate education and clinical experience prepare you to enter the lactation profession. Understanding the stages of acquiring your new role helps you anticipate each new challenge. Availing yourself of the networking and support from colleagues and your professional association enhances your effectiveness in working with families. Becoming certified and adhering to the profession's standards of practice and ethics ensures that you provide appropriate care. Recognizing your limitations and seeking assistance enables you to give your best effort to supporting and protecting lactation. Balancing your professional and personal lives helps you avoid burnout and maintain enthusiasm for helping nursing families.

What You Learned–At a Glance

Conversation Starters with Parents

- How well supported do you feel with your healthcare providers?
- How does your healthcare provider involve you in decision-making?
- How do you resolve conflicts with your healthcare provider?
- How effective is your healthcare team in meeting your needs?

Establishing Yourself in the Profession

- Acquire knowledge and skills through comprehensive lactation education and supervised clinical experience guided by the profession's clinical competencies.
- Acquire and maintain IBCLC certification.
- Work within your scope of practice.
- Evolve your skill level and confidence as you progress from a novice to an expert.
- Network with others to mature as a clinician.
- Reach out through social media, community presentations, and health fairs.
- Continue lifelong learning to remain current with clinical practice and research.

Legal Considerations

- Follow your *Code of Professional Conduct*.
- Ensure continuous coverage for professional liability insurance.
- Protect the privacy and confidentiality of clients and their families.
- Recognize what constitutes a client relationship and provide appropriate care.
- Ensure written informed consent before providing care.
- Retain client records appropriately.
- Build positive relationships with families.
- Avoid guaranteeing results or creating unrealistic expectations.
- Empower parents to make their own decisions and accept their choices.
- Work within the parameters of other caregivers' advice as much as possible.

Interdisciplinary Lactation Care

- Teach lactation care to all members of the health-care team to provide consistency.
- Launch a lactation initiative with a motivational program for the staff.
- Use creativity and humor to create a receptive learning climate.

Maturing Through Experience

- Learn how to deal with misinformation and lack of support.
- Accept your limitations.
- Avoid becoming overly involved or discussing your own lactation.
- Avoid making value judgments, interrupting, or overwhelming parents.
- Use counseling skills to avoid being too solution oriented.
- Provide appropriate and timely follow-up.
- Achieve a balance between professional responsibilities and personal needs.
- Recognize signs of burnout and learn how to manage and resolve it.
- Find new challenges and goals to renew your enthusiasm.

References

American Academy of Family Physicians. Breastfeeding support and resources toolkit. 2019. http://www.aafp.org/patient-care/public-health/breastfeeding/toolkit.html

American Academy of Pediatrics. Breastfeeding residency curriculum. 2023. https://www.aap.org/en/learning/breastfeeding-curriculum/

Aryeetey R, Dykes F. Global implications of the new WHO and UNICEF implementation guidance on the revised Baby-Friendly Hospital Initiative. *Matern Child Nutr.* 2018;14(3):e12637.

Baik D, Zierler B. RN job satisfaction and retention after an interprofessional team intervention. *West J Nurs Res.* 2019;41(4):615–630.

Benner P. Using the Dreyfus model of skill acquisition to describe and interpret skill acquisition and clinical judgment in nursing practice and education. *Bull Sci Technol Soc.* 2004; 24(3):188–199.

Berger-Estilita J, et al. Attitudes towards interprofessional education in the medical curriculum: a systematic review of the literature. *BMC Med Educ.* 2020;20(1):254.

Bernuzzi C, et al. The role of resilience in the work-life interface: a systematic review. *Work.* 2022;73(4):1147–1165.

Brand SL, et al. Whole-system approaches to improving the health and wellbeing of healthcare workers: a systematic review. *PLoS One.* 2017;12(12):e0188418.

Burke D, et al. Characteristics of nurse directors that contribute to registered nurse satisfaction. *J Nurs Adm.* 2018;48(10 suppl): S12–S18.

Campbell SH, et al. Educational resources and curriculum on lactation for health undergraduate students: a scoping review. *J Hum Lact.* 2022;38(1):89–99.

Chamberlain K, et al. Virtual lactation education in a pandemic. *J Hum Lact.* 2022;38(4):603–608.

Chant KJ, Westendorf DS. Nurse residency programs: key components for sustainability. *J Nurses Prof Dev.* 2019;35(4):185–192.

Chapin EM, et al. The paradigm shift in BFHI Step 2: from training to competency verification. *J Hum Lact.* 2021;37(3):532–538.

Chuisano SA, Anderson OS. Assessing application-based breastfeeding education for physicians and nurses: a scoping review. *J Hum Lact.* 2020;36(4):699–709.

Commission on Accreditation of Allied Health Education Programs. 2025. *About CAAHEP*. http://www.caahep.org

Cooper AL, et al. Nurse resilience: a concept analysis. *Int J Ment Health Nurs.* 2020;29(4):553–575.

Crowe S, et al. The impact of simulation-based education on nursing confidence, knowledge and patient outcomes on general medicine units. *Nurse Educ Pract.* 2018;29:70–75.

Curran V, et al. Adoption and use of mobile learning in continuing professional development by health and human services professionals. *J Contin Educ Health Prof.* 2019;39(2):76–85.

de Las Heras-Rosas C, et al. Organisational commitment in healthcare systems: a bibliometric analysis. *Int J Environ Res Public Health.* 2021;18(5):2271.

Díaz DA, et al. Comparison of clinical options: high-fidelity manikin-based and virtual simulation. *Nurse Educ.* 2021; 46(3):149–153.

Dreyfus SE, Dreyfus HO. *A Five-Stage Model of the Mental Activities Involved in Directed Skill Acquisition*. Berkeley, CA: University of California; 1980.

Dunbar G, et al. The transition from expert to novice and back to expert: ensuring competent and safe practice. *Clin Nurse Spec.* 2019;33(3):106–109.

Feminist Legal Clinic. In custody dispute, Va. judge orders breastfeeding mom to use bottle. 2023. https://feministlegal.org/in-custody-dispute-va-judge-orders-breastfeeding-mom-to-use-bottle-the-washington-post/#.ZGKMEk_MI7c

Fenwick J, et al. The emotional and professional wellbeing of Australian midwives: a comparison between those providing continuity of midwifery care and those not providing continuity. *Women Birth.* 2018;31(1):38–43.

Frisbie A. *Lactation Private Practice: From Start to Strong*. St. Petersburg, FL: Booklocker.com, Inc.; 2018a.

Frisbie A. *Paperless Private Practice for Lactation Consultants*. St. Petersburg, FL: Booklocker.com, Inc.; 2018b.

Frisch NC, et al. Expanding the reach of continuing educational offerings through a web-based virtual network: the experience of InspireNet. *Stud Health Technol Inform.* 2017;234:120–124.

Grabowski A, et al. Midwifery students better approximate their self-efficacy in clinical lactation after reflecting in and on their performance in the LactSim OSCE. *Adv Simul (Lond).* 2020;5:28.

Green AA, Kinchen EV. The effects of mindfulness meditation on stress and burnout in nurses. *J Holist Nurs.* 2021;39(4): 356–368.

Gribble KD. Writing expert reports for court in relation to breastfeeding infants and young children. *J Hum Lact.* 2021; 37(4):683–688.

Guraya SY, Barr H. The effectiveness of interprofessional education in healthcare: a systematic review and meta-analysis. *Kaohsiung J Med Sci.* 2018;34(3):160–165.

Hall LH, et al. Association of GP wellbeing and burnout with patient safety in UK primary care: a cross-sectional survey. *Br J Gen Pract.* 2019;69(684):e507–e514.

Hall VP, et al. The influence of leadership style and nurse empowerment on burnout. *Nurs Clin North Am.* 2022;57(1): 131–141.

Harolds JA. Quality and safety in health care, part L: positive psychology and burnout. *Clin Nucl Med.* 2019a;44(8):643–645.

Harolds JA. Quality and safety in health care, part XLIX: mentoring, coaching, and burnout. *Clin Nucl Med.* 2019b;44(7):566–567.

Hegland PA, et al. Simulation-based training for nurses: systematic review and meta-analysis. *Nurse Educ Today*. 2017;54:6–20.

Ho KH, et al. The technology implications of master's level education in the professionalization of nursing: a narrative inquiry. *J Adv Nurs.* 2019;75(9):1966–1975.

IBCLC Commission. 2025. About the IBCLC Commission. https://ibclc-commission.org/about/

International Board of Lactation Consultant Examiners. IBLCE documentation guidelines. 2012. https://ibclc-commission.org/wp- IBLCEcontent/uploads/2023/08/2012_February_28_DOC_documentation-guidelines_ENGLISH.pdf

International Board of Lactation Consultant Examiners. *Clinical Competencies for IBCLC Practice*. Falls Church, VA: International Board of Lactation Consultant Examiners; 2018a. https://ibclc-commission.org/ibclc-information/clinical-competencies-for-ibclcs/

International Board of Lactation Consultant Examiners. *Scope of Practice for International Board Certified Lactation Consultant Certificants*. Falls Church, VA: International Board of Lactation Consultant Examiners; 2018b. https://ibclc-commission.org/ibclc-information/scope-of-practice-for-ibclcs/

International Board of Lactation Consultant Examiners. Health sciences education guide. 2023a. https://ibclc-commission.org/ibclc-information/health-sciences-education-guide-2/

International Board of Lactation Consultant Examiners. *Code of Professional Conduct: International Board Certified Lactation Consultants*. Falls Church, VA: International Board of Lactation Consultant Examiners; 2023b. https://ibclc-commission.org/ibclc-information/code-of-professional-conduct-complaint-form/

International Board of Lactation Consultant Examiners. IBLCE detailed content outline. 2023c. https://ibclc-commission.org/ibclc-information/detailed-content-outline/

International Lactation Consultant Association. *Standards of Practice for Lactation Consultants*. 4th ed. Morrisville, NC: International Lactation Consultant Association; 2013.

Interprofessional Education Collaborative. IPEC core competencies for interprofessional collaborative practice revision, 2021–2023. 2023. https://www.ipecollaborative.org/

Jahnke SA, et al. The prevalence and health impacts of frequent work discrimination and harassment among women firefighters in the US Fire Service. *Biomed Res Int.* 2019;2019:6740207.

Jilou V, et al. Fatigue due to compassion in health professionals and coping strategies: a scoping review. *Rev Bras Enferm.* 2021;74(5):e20190628.

Johnson J, et al. Mental healthcare staff well-being and burnout: a narrative review of trends, causes, implications, and recommendations for future interventions. *Int J Ment Health Nurs.* 2018;27(1):20–32.

Kim H, Kim EG. A meta-analysis on predictors of turnover intention of hospital nurses in South Korea (2000–2020). *Nurs Open.* 2021;8(5):2406–2418.

Kim YH, et al. Influence of type D personality on job stress and job satisfaction in clinical nurses: the mediating effects of compassion fatigue, burnout, and compassion satisfaction. *J Adv Nurs.* 2017;73(4):905–916.

Klein CJ, et al. Quality of life and compassion satisfaction in clinicians: a pilot intervention study for reducing compassion fatigue. *Am J Hosp Palliat Care.* 2018;35(6):882–888.

Kurup V, et al. Role of in-situ simulation for training in healthcare: opportunities and challenges. *Curr Opin Anaesthesiol.* 2017;30(6):755–760.

Lactation Education Accreditation and Approval Review Committee. LEAARC Endorsed Courses. 2024. https://leaarc.org/endorse.html

Lactation Education Accreditation and Approval Review Committee. *Standards and Guidelines for the Accreditation of Lactation Consultant Education Programs.* Uxbridge, MA: Lactation Education Accreditation and Approval Review Committee; 2018.

Lactation Education Accreditation and Approval Review Committee. Who We Are. 2025. https://www.leaarc.org

Lane AS, Roberts C. Contextualised reflective competence: a new learning model promoting reflective practice for clinical training. *BMC Med Educ.* 2022;22(1):71.

Lima HK, et al. Assessing the landscape of lactation education: results of a pilot survey. *J Hum Lact.* 2024;40(2):276–285.

Liu YP, et al. Development of a nursing-specific Mini-CEX and evaluation of the core competencies of new nurses in postgraduate year training programs in Taiwan. *BMC Med Educ.* 2019;19(1):270.

Lu Y, et al. The relationship between job satisfaction, work stress, work-family conflict, and turnover intention among physicians in Guangdong, China: a cross-sectional study. *BMJ Open.* 2017;7(5):e014894.

Mianda S, Voce A. Developing and evaluating clinical leadership interventions for frontline healthcare providers: a review of the literature. *BMC Health Serv Res.* 2018;18(1):747.

Moloney W, et al. An integrative review of how healthcare organizations can support hospital nurses to thrive at work. *Int J Environ Res Public Health.* 2020;17(23):8757.

Newton JM, et al. A contemporary examination of workplace learning culture: an ethnomethodology study. *Nurse Educ Today.* 2015;35(1):91–96.

Noel-Weiss J, et al. Exploring how IBCLCs manage ethical dilemmas: a qualitative study. *BMC Med Ethics.* 2012;13:18.

Parkes K. *Perspectives in Lactation: Is Private Practice for Me?* Amarillo, TX: Praeclarus Press; 2015.

Radzyminski S, Callister LC. Health professionals' attitudes and beliefs about breastfeeding. *J Perinat Educ.* 2015;24(2):102–109.

Riethof N, et al. Burnout syndrome, mental splitting and depression in female health care professionals. *Med Sci Monit.* 2019;25:5237–5240.

Rohan AJ. Supporting nurses as lifelong learners. *Adv Neonatal Care.* 2017;17(4):235–236.

Rozario D. Burnout, resilience and moral injury: how the wicked problems of health care defy solutions, yet require innovative strategies in the modern era. *Can J Surg.* 2019;62(4):E6–E8.

Sadovnikova A, et al. Development and evaluation of a high-fidelity lactation simulation model for health professional breastfeeding education. *Int Breastfeed J.* 2020;15(1):8.

Sahu PK, et al. Best practices to impart clinical skills during preclinical years of medical curriculum. *J Educ Health Promot.* 2019;8:57.

Salvadó M, et al. Mindfulness-based interventions to reduce burnout in primary healthcare professionals: a systematic review and meta-analysis. *Healthcare (Basel).* 2021;9(10):1342.

Şenol Çelik S, et al. Structural and psychological empowerment and burnout among nurses: a systematic review and meta-analysis. *Int Nurs Rev.* 2024;71(1):189–201.

Slate KA, et al. Longitudinal study transformed onboarding nurse graduates. *J Nurses Prof Dev.* 2018;34(2):92–98.

Smith JG, et al. Association of the nurse work environment with nurse incivility in hospitals. *J Nurs Manag.* 2018;26(2):219–226.

Spaulding EM, et al. Interprofessional education and collaboration among healthcare students and professionals: a systematic review and call for action. *J Interprof Care.* 2021;35(4):612–621.

Strong G, et al. Speaking the same language: a call for standardized lactation terminology in the United States. *J Hum Lact.* 2023;39(1):121–131.

Subramani S, et al. Ethical issues in breastfeeding and lactation interventions: a scoping review. *J Hum Lact.* 2024;40(1):150–163.

Tamata AT, Mohammadnezhad M. A systematic review study on the factors affecting shortage of nursing workforce in the hospitals. *Nurs Open.* 2023;10(3):1247–1257.

Tanis SL, et al. Breastfeeding simulation with the standardized patient. *Nurs Women's Health.* 2019;23(2):141–147.

Tavella G, Parker G. A qualitative reexamination of the key features of burnout. *J Nerv Ment Dis.* 2020;208(6):452–458.

Taylor JS, Bell E. Medical education and leadership in breastfeeding medicine. *Breastfeed Med.* 2017;12(8):476–478.

Teheux L, et al. Intraprofessional workplace learning in postgraduate medical education: a scoping review. *BMC Med Educ.* 2021;21(1):479.

Tement S, et al. The impact of psychological interventions with elements of mindfulness (PIM) on empathy, well-being, and reduction of burnout in physicians: a systematic review. *Int J Environ Res Public Health.* 2021;18(21):11181.

Uzumcu Z, et al. Breastfeeding education in family medicine residencies: a 2019 CERA program directors survey. *Fam Med.* 2020;52(7):497–504.

Vanguri S, et al. ABM clinical protocol #14: breastfeeding-friendly physician's office—optimizing care for infants and children. *Breastfeed Med.* 2021;16(3):175–184.

Vilar-Compte M, et al. How much can Mexican healthcare providers learn about breastfeeding through a semi-virtual training? A propensity score matching analysis. *Int Breastfeed J.* 2020;15(1):59.

Webber E, et al. Using simulation to teach breastfeeding management skills and improve breastfeeding self-efficacy. *J Perinat Educ.* 2021;30(1):19–28.

Webber E, Serowoky M. Breastfeeding curricular content of family nurse practitioner programs. *J Pediatr Health Care.* 2017;31(2):189–195.

West CP, et al. Physician burnout: contributors, consequences and solutions. *J Intern Med.* 2018;283(6):516–529.

Weston J, Zauche LH. Comparison of virtual simulation to clinical practice for prelicensure nursing students in pediatrics. *Nurse Educ.* 2021;46(5):E95–E98.

World Health Organization. *International Code of Marketing of Breast-milk Substitutes.* Geneva, Switzerland: World Health Organization; 1981.

Xie W, et al. The prevalence of compassion satisfaction and compassion fatigue among nurses: a systematic review and meta-analysis. *Int J Nurs Stud.* 2021;120:103973.

Yao Y, et al. General self-efficacy modifies the effect of stress on burnout in nurses with different personality types. *BMC Health Serv Res.* 2018;18(1):667.

Zarei E, et al. Prevalence of burnout among primary health care staff and its predictors: a study in Iran. *Int J Environ Res Public Health.* 2019;16(12):2249.

Zhang YY, et al. Determinants of compassion satisfaction, compassion fatigue and burn out in nursing: a correlative meta-analysis. *Medicine (Baltimore).* 2018;97(26):e11086.

CHAPTER 29

Critical Reading and Review of Research

By studying this and other texts, you learn state-of-the-art information and many techniques to use in helping families with nursing. The ability to critically read and interpret scientific literature is a necessary skill to inform your practice and keep it current. This chapter provides background information on the processes of science used in scientific journal articles. It provides strategies for reading and analyzing research studies with discernment. These tools will be especially useful when the media reports on a study that sensationalizes a negative outcome or aspect of lactation. Positive studies also need to be scrutinized for bias, confounding variables, and causality links where there may be none. A "how-to" section on the structure and critical reading of scientific articles is aimed at readers who have little previous experience analyzing research. A mock article with commentary provides an opportunity to practice the techniques presented.

KEY TERMS

Abstract
Anchors
Assumptions
Average
Bell curve
Bias
Blind
Case-control study
Case studies
Chi-square
Cohen's Kappa
Cohort
Confidence intervals (CIs)
Confounding variables
Convenience
Correlation
Cronbach's alpha
Cross-sectional study
Dependent variable
Descriptive study
Dichotomous outcome
Distribution
Electronic publication (Epub)
Evidence-based practice
Evidence-informed practice
Experiment
Fabrication
Falsification
Generalize
Heterogeneity
Homogeneity
Hypothesis
Independent variable
Instruments
Internal validity
Likert scale
Logistic regression
Mean
Median
Meta-analysis
Nonprobability
Normal distribution
Null hypothesis
Observational study
Odds ratio
Open access
Operationalization
Outcome
Outliers
Output variables
Oximeter
P value
Peer review
Plagiarism
Population
Predictor variable
Probability
Prospective study
Qualitative study
Random assignment
Randomized clinical trial
Regression
Relationship
Reliability
Retrospective study
Review articles
Sample
Slope
Spurious
Statistical theory
Statistically significant
Systematic review
t-test
Validity
Variables
Variation

Evidence-Informed Versus Evidence-Based Practice

Healthcare practices rely largely on scientific research. This chapter addresses how to access and interpret scientific research and how to apply it appropriately to clinical care. Healthcare providers are generally favorable toward **evidence-based practices**. However, what does a clinician do when there is no scientific evidence to inform best practice? Scientific knowledge evolves over time, and there are not research trials to support all individual needs and concerns in health care.

Analyzing and applying multiple forms of evidence can be challenging, and inevitably, clinicians must rely on subjectivity. **Evidence-informed practice** is an approach to clinical care for situations where no evidence-based research trials or other scientific basis exists. The *evidence-based* model places evidence at the center, with input from the clinician's expertise, current best evidence, and client values and expectations. The *evidence-informed* model places clinical expertise at the core, with input from clinical circumstances, client preferences and actions, and current best evidence (Barreto et al., 2023; Faupel-Badger et al., 2022; Motani et al., 2019).

Evidence-informed health care ensures the most effective care combining the best available research evidence and management practices. The approach values clinician experience, intuition, and the clinical reasoning skills that come from working in a clinical specialty. An evidence-informed practice may be an emerging new practice that has no empirical evidence, has low risk for harm, is based on clinician expertise, and is acceptable to the client. As the practice becomes more established, it moves toward evidence-based practice as it demonstrates some evidence of benefit, low risk or no evidence of harm, and positive clinician and client experience. Evidence-informed practice is an essential component of best practice for an evolving profession such as lactation consulting.

Access to Scientific Journals

The internet provides easy access to scientific journals and research articles. Every major journal has a website with articles available online through free access, institutional or personal membership, or an individual fee basis. Articles usually appear online in advance of the print journal. When this is the case, the citation will include a notation such as "Epub 2019 June 20." For example: Togo A, et al. Repertoire of human breast and milk microbiota: a systematic review. *Future Microbiol.* 2019 May;14:623–641. doi:10.2217/fmb-2018-0317. Epub 2019 Apr 26. PubMed PMID: 31025880.

The "doi" number in the citation stands for "digital object identifier" and is an article identifier provided by the journal publisher. "Epub" stands for **electronic publication**. The "PubMed PMID" number is the identifying number for the article where it appears in PubMed, one of the databases for the National Center for Biotechnology Information (NCBI). NCBI provides access to extensive biomedical and genomic information, with tutorials for efficient use. PubMed has over 30 million citations for biomedical literature. It is easy to navigate and has a sophisticated search engine to list thousands of scholarly journal articles on a myriad of topics (NCBI, 2025).

EBSCO is a popular database company that requires a paid subscription. Most hospitals, schools, and libraries subscribe to this and other scientific/medical databases for use by employees, students, and patrons (EBSCO, 2025). The Directory of Open Access Journals (DOAJ) service provides **open access** to full-text, quality-controlled scientific and scholarly journals. DOAJ seeks to represent all subjects and languages and to prevent predatory journals from being listed in its database (DOAJ, 2025).

The Public Library of Science (PLOS) is another online publisher with a goal of immediate access to research (PLOS, 2025). The *International Breastfeeding Journal* (IBJ), an open-access lactation journal, covers all aspects of lactation, including original research, case studies, and editorials (IBJ, 2025). Accessible online journals, subject-specific preprint and Epub archives, and collections of learning components have increased the amount of information and the speed with which it is disseminated.

Types of Articles in Scientific Journals

Scientific journals contain many types of articles. Commonly, the first prose to appear is an editorial, and some journals print more than one. Editorials are interesting and often illuminating. The editor is a prominent person in the field whose knowledge is broad and whose perspective on how the field is changing is often insightful. Editorials are not studies, and they do not report on a particular study. Although they are not subjected to critical analysis, editorials do offer reasoned opinions from individuals who are usually experts in the field. The editorial may be a guest editorial or may be written by the editor or member of the editorial staff at the journal.

Case Studies

Many biomedical journals publish **case studies**—articles that report on one or more cases of a problem, diagnosis, or treatment. Case studies advance knowledge in a profession by enabling clinicians and novice researchers to share their work with the broader community. A case study often appears because there is interest in a particular topic. The diagnosis may be unusual, or the treatment may be risky, and it is therefore unlikely that any experiments will take place.

The absence of comparison subjects or comparison treatment prevents critical analysis. However, it is still important information to retain. For example, a case study may provide the only information available on the use of a particular drug during lactation. The case study may help guide an especially difficult decision in clinical practice. However, because of its limited nature, a case study cannot form the basis for generalizing to most nursing dyads.

Lactation case studies have features unique from many other professions. Rather than having a single case subject, the case usually includes a dyad and family, addressing physical and mental health domains over an extended period. An interdisciplinary team of healthcare providers is likely involved in caring for the dyad. The case study typically describes the course of infant feeding to explain an unusual situation or course of treatment.

Another example in lactation literature would be a case study on the use of a medication not often prescribed during lactation. Typically, the healthcare provider will describe the client's medical history and the circumstances leading to the medication's use. A description and discussion of the **outcomes** for the nursing dyad will then usually follow. Such a case study has a **sample** of one dyad.

Meta-Analyses

Meta-analysis is a research technique that pools the data and results of several studies to improve the strength of the conclusions. Meta-analyses usually focus on a specific aspect of treatments, tests, exposures, and associated outcomes. The question studied should be clearly stated in the article's title or **abstract**. Such articles usually contain the words *meta-analysis* or *meta-regression* in their titles or abstracts, making it easy to identify them. High-quality meta-analyses can reduce **bias**, provide adequate power to demonstrate real differences in outcomes, and help resolve the results of inconsistent studies (Hernandez et al., 2020).

Meta-analysis needs to account for differences in the data results (**heterogeneity**) to determine whether variations in treatment effects are attributable to more than chance fluctuations alone (Lin, 2020). Meta-regression merges meta-analytic and linear **regression** principles. It is a more sophisticated tool that is increasingly used to better determine outcome measures and covariate relationships (Xu & Doi, 2018). Because this type of study relies heavily on statistical **assumptions**, clinicians often need to judge quality and evaluate bias.

Review Articles

Review articles are written by one or more experts in the field who summarize and often critique the best and worst studies published on a topic. They do not combine the data and results as a meta-analysis does. The opinions of the experts play a role in the selection and the critical analysis of the articles to review. Little or no original data appear in a review article. A well-researched literature review can provide a critical analysis of the state of science about a specific topic. It should advance the field by creating new knowledge, not restating what is already known. A review article can identify the most recent information, important scientists in the field, and current controversies. These articles should contain the word *review* in the title or abstract. Including the word *review* in the database search will aid in finding this type of article.

A Cochrane review is a **systematic review** of primary research that explores the effects of interventions and diagnostic testing in health care and health policy (Cochrane Collaboration, 2025). Cochrane review topics are frequently updated. If methodology or a study within a review is found to be problematic, the review will be withdrawn and so noted. The reviews are published online by the Cochrane Collaboration, a nonprofit organization with collaborators from over 120 countries that does not accept commercial sponsorship.

Clinical Practice

Clinical practice articles often appear in journals for applied sciences such as nursing, dietetics, physical therapy, and medicine. Authors who have experience with a particular diagnosis, problem, deficit, or preventive technique share their accumulated wisdom with other clinicians. These articles offer valuable insights for clinical practice. *Clinical Lactation*, the journal of the U.S. Lactation Consultant Association (USLCA), is a lactation journal dedicated to clinical practice (USLCA, 2025).

Because clinical practice articles do not typically study a problem scientifically, there may be minimal presentation of data in graphs, tables, and figures. There also are no hypotheses or research questions. There typically will not be a control group, and the protocol may or may not be compared with another protocol. There may be summary information about how, for example, parents who followed a particular protocol coped with a particular problem. Although these articles are helpful, there is no substantive test of the authors' assertions. Therefore, clinical practice articles do not constitute the same quality of evidence as research does for changing care practices.

Longitudinal clinical lactation research studies encompass a period anywhere between pregnancy and weaning. The study needs to accommodate the infant's health and the parent's health, diet, body mass index, physical activity, and socioeconomic factors. It needs to consider the stage of lactation, milk composition, feeding patterns, frequency and exclusivity, and complementary and supplementary foods.

Online Surveys

Online platforms, email, and social media use surveys to rapidly gain large amounts of data on specific questions from targeted samples. With rigorous survey methodology, researchers can produce valid, robust, and meaningful data. Survey techniques are used frequently in lactation. The advantages of online surveys are speed, reach, ease, cost, flexibility, and automation. However, there is no interviewer to explore responses to open-ended questions and ask follow-up questions. Respondents also cannot seek clarification of unfamiliar or ambiguous terms. Furthermore, validity of responses can be skewed by over-representation of a particular viewpoint or respondents submitting duplicate responses, fraudulent information, or erroneous responses. Researchers must be cautious in claims based on their findings, and readers must carefully appraise research that is based on online surveys.

Research

Research articles put a long-held belief or new idea to a scientific test. Researchers subject themselves and their work to scientific investigation and the scrutiny of their peers. Because they take the risk that their colleagues may find their work wanting, it is important to approach the work of colleagues respectfully. Each article deserves careful attention, both for the growth of collective understanding about lactation and for the benefit of nursing families. Research articles follow a standardized structure.

Structure of a Scientific Article

Most scientific articles follow a format that provides a maximum amount of information in a limited amount of journal space. Well-written journal articles condense information effectively and demonstrate what the researchers did and why. Researchers explain the limitations of the study and provide justifiable conclusions from their work. With practice, you derive a clear sense of whether you agree with their conclusions, and you have clear reasons for your decisions. The growth of the science of lactation depends on this clear communication and on feedback given to researchers.

Nomenclature

Researchers are at the forefront of promoting lactation. The World Health Organization urges us to protect, promote, and support lactation. Lactation advocates generally fall into two distinct groups. The first group—researchers, editors, policymakers, and news media—*promotes* lactation impersonally. The second group—health professionals, counselors, educators, social media bloggers, and support groups—*protects and supports* lactation through personal interactions. Those who protect and support lactation have struggled with creating guilt and ill will if their messaging is too strong. With these role distinctions, the promoters can undertake a strong, risk-based approach, allowing those who protect and support lactation to use more neutral language with families.

The title of an article drives media headlines. If a study uses control and experimental groups, the title typically reflects the experimental group. Research comparing nursing to formula feeding often uses formula as the control group and nursing as the experimental group. A control group is the norm against which an experimental group is compared. The implication of nursing as the experimental group is that formula is the norm. Researchers are ethically required to present human milk as normal infant nutrition. Changing nursing to the control identifies formula as the **experiment** and places the focus on nursing, where it belongs. This presents challenges to policymakers and news media in managing any resulting controversy and potential shifts in public perception (Wiessinger, 2021).

Journal Identifiers

The abbreviated title of the journal often appears at the top of many scientific articles. For example, *Acta Paediatr* is the abbreviation for the journal *Acta Paediatrica*, a Scandinavian journal. Although the format for the name, volume number, pages, and year of publication varies from one journal to another, the format used by *Acta Paediatrica* illustrates the commonalities. This information is handy to have at the top of the first page of the article. Journals that do not have the journal name at the top usually put it at the end of the abstract or elsewhere on the first page.

Article Citation

Elements of this sample citation, "Almqvist-Tangen G, et al. Factors associated with discontinuation of breastfeeding before 1 month of age. *Acta Paediatr.* 2012;101(1):55–60" are as follows:

- *Acta Paediatr* is the journal's abbreviation, and it usually appears in italics.
- "2012" is the year of publication. In some journals, the year appears directly after the name of the journal.
- "101" is the volume of the journal. Most journals publish one volume every year; however, some publish two volumes per year.
- "(1)" is the issue number. When the issue number is included, it usually appears immediately after the volume in parentheses. Many journals publish an issue monthly. Some, like the *Journal of Human Lactation*, publish quarterly. Others, like *Lancet*, publish weekly. When locating an article or requesting one from a library, it is important to copy the numbers from the reference list carefully.
- "55–60" is the page range where the article is located. Most journals paginate continuously for 1 year. Volume 101 begins with page 1. If the first issue for that year ends at page 112, then the second issue begins at page 113, and so on. With continuous pagination, including the issue number is not necessary.

Predatory Journals

It can be difficult to discern legitimate scholarly journals from illegitimate or predatory journals. Predatory journals and publishers prioritize self-interest at the expense of scholarship. They use an exploitative business model with substandard quality control, deceptive publishing practices, and aggressive solicitation. They lack transparency and present false or misleading information. They do not use proper **peer review** to ensure scientific quality (Dinis-Oliveira, 2021; Gallent Torres, 2022; Mathew et al., 2022).

Predatory journals advertise aggressively for submissions and offer high acceptance rates. They vigorously invite researchers to publish via flattering and seemingly legitimate emails and charge authors fees for submission. Researchers diminish the quality of their work when their research is published in a predatory journal. Discerning clinicians need to critically examine the source of a research article to avoid illegitimate or predatory ones (JHL Editorial Team, 2020; Strong, 2019).

Title of the Article

A well-chosen title tells a lot about an article. In some journals, the title explains the main finding and may be two sentences long. This helps busy readers choose which articles are the highest priorities for their reading. The title of the sample citation tells you that the article studies reasons why parents discontinue nursing and that it studies babies younger than 1 month of age. A title identifying nursing as the control and formula feeding as the experiment may be "Formula Feeding Increases Risk of Sudden Infant Death Syndrome" rather than "Breastfeeding Reduces Sudden Infant Death Syndrome."

Authors

As you read research regularly, you begin to recognize the research interests of particular lactation scientists who publish several articles on aspects of a limited scope of conditions or problems. Often, you can acquire a good reference list on a single topic just by knowing a few researchers' names and noting the references in their articles. This will help in preparing a presentation or documenting the need for a practice change. When there are several authors, the citation will list the first author, followed by *et al.* The article will list all the authors, as in the illustration citation: Gerd Almqvist-Tangen, Stefan Bergman, Jovanna Dahlgren, Josefine Roswall, and Bernt Alm.

Abstract

Most journals ask authors to write a brief summary of (1) the reason they performed the study, (2) the main subjects and methods, (3) the findings, and (4) the conclusion. This constitutes the abstract, which is often the best guide for deciding whether an article is worth reading. Although the abstract may not answer all your questions about the study, it indicates what the authors considered most important. Each journal sets its own requirements for the length and format of the abstract. The abstract for the sample citation is as follows:

- **Background:** There is a slight decline in nursing initiation.
- **Aim:** Assess factors associated with discontinuation during the first 4 weeks.
- **Method:** Population-based longitudinal birth cohort study recruiting from 2007 to 2008 in southwestern Sweden with parent questionnaires and infants height, weight, head, and waist circumference.
- **Results:** 27% of parents had problems with pacifier use, smoking, sucking, staff support, and perceived poor weight gain.
- **Conclusion:** Support tailored to the parent's perspective can prevent problems.

Introduction

The authors usually begin with an explanation, in a few paragraphs, of why they studied the problem cited in the article. The introduction explains the clinical question that directed the researchers' study. This is typically where the **hypothesis** will be stated—an idea or explanation that has been observed, explored, and/or tested through an experimental process. There may also be clues as to why the authors made certain decisions, such as why they studied only infants younger than 6 weeks old or collected data only during a particular season.

In the introduction, the authors should declare funding sources and any potential conflicts of interest. Conflicts of interest include any outside factor that could influence the researchers' aims or study interpretation. Examples of conflicts that should be declared by authors are commercial grants, employment, speakership, or board membership in organizations related to the research topic, as well as researcher patents (Feldman & Mann, 2019). These declarations may appear at the end of the article instead.

Review of the Literature

The literature review explains the issues surrounding the problem studied and reviews past research. In some journals (e.g., the *New England Journal of Medicine*), the literature review is combined with the introduction. Nearly all articles discuss the research problem and past studies before they begin to explain the current research. The literature review narrows down the subject of interest. It cites previous studies and their findings and explains how the current study is different or better. Authors sometimes also explain weaknesses of past studies that their current study will correct.

Many funding sources will not support a study on a question that has received a great deal of previous research. Therefore, the researcher must either identify an aspect of the problem that was not covered or demonstrate that past research has not clarified an important point. Literature reviews could be very long, and journals usually want them to be limited to the most relevant studies. If you read such a review and do not find a study cited that you know is pertinent, space considerations could be the reason.

Methods

The goal of the methods section is to tell the reader how the scientists operationalized the hypotheses and questions that were studied. **Operationalization** is the process of strictly defining **variables** into factors that can be measured empirically and quantitatively. This section often begins with a description of subject recruitment. A member of the research team may have recruited subjects according to certain criteria (such as a previous preterm birth or giving birth to twins). Alternatively, subjects may have volunteered to be part of the study after learning about it through a childbirth class or an advertisement. Sometimes, the study relied on charts or other records, and the subjects were unaware of the study. Usually, journals require that authors state whether the study obtained approval from a human subjects review group and that the subjects gave informed consent.

Instruments

The methods section describes the tools (**instruments**) used to measure the outcome under study. The instrument may be, for example, a written questionnaire or survey, an electronic balance scale, a chemical test, a biopsy, or an ultrasound. The authors often explain the methods in much detail, including the way in which different measurement instruments led to the results.

For example, a milk sample collected early in a feeding will probably not have the same proportion of fat as a sample taken after milk was drained more fully. One study takes early milk samples and finds low vitamin A levels. The other study takes a sample after a complete feeding and finds higher vitamin A content. The difference might reflect the greater fat content in the complete feeding sample because vitamin A is fat soluble.

Definition of Terms

The methods section also defines the terms used in the study. When the authors say they included "nursing dyads," they need to define what they mean by *nursing* and by the term *dyads*. Do they mean exclusive nursing or partial nursing? Did they ask about the amount of any supplemental formula the baby consumed, or did they measure it? Is the dyad a biological pair, an adoptive pair, or a nonbinary pair?

Statistical Methods

Statistical methods usually appear in the methods section. The authors define the methods they used and why they chose them. They may explain that they applied more than one statistical test to the data to strengthen the conclusions. This can be the least familiar part of the article to read without a background in statistics. However, as you encounter statistical terminology, you can review tests online and self-tutor. You will quickly begin to find the same statistical tests applied frequently.

Results

Authors typically phrase their results carefully. The most important study results typically appear in graphs, tables, and charts. Tables often compare relevant characteristics between the experimental group and the control group. The title of the table or graph identifies its topic. A key below the table explains the statistical significance of the results. Tables helpfully summarize information about the subjects.

It may be tempting to read just the results because it seems like so much work to wade through the methods. However, reading only the results or the abstract of a study can limit the reader's understanding of both the general problem and the study's approach to it. Making the effort to understand the methods may prevent clinicians from inappropriately adopting a recommended change that is incompatible with best practice. The results of a study need to be considered in the context of the rest of the article so that the findings can be judged based on the specifics of that study.

Discussion

In the discussion, the authors explain their reason for conducting the study. They review the relevant literature, summarize the most important results, and suggest applications and further research. They also explain any weaknesses or problems with the project. Some of these explanations are in response to the comments of peer reviewers. These can be helpful to a reader who is unfamiliar with a particular area of research to think of alternative methods or interpretations. Although the earlier parts of the article are standard and prescribed by the journal, the discussion reveals more of the authors' thinking and creativity. By the time a study is ready for publication, the researchers have raised many questions in their minds, which they often explore in the discussion.

Conclusion

The concluding remarks are often provided as a separate section or may appear in the discussion section of the article. The authors restate the research topic and findings, mention additional questions spurred by the study, and advocate for additional research or actions if warranted.

References, Literature, and Bibliography

The final section identifies the articles cited in the literature review. It includes any article cited in the methods section if the authors used a method described in a separate article. Many journals permit the listing of additional articles related to the main topic. Online articles usually have hyperlinks to references, enabling readers to access other works concurrently as they read and evaluate the article.

Critical Reading of a Scientific Article

The process of critical reading results in various readers arriving at differing conclusions. Furthermore, if you reread an article later, you may assess its strengths and weaknesses differently from the first time you read it. This is where the fun lies in critical reading: in the challenge of the puzzles the science investigates.

Most studies are a mixture of well-done science and things that merit improvement. Honest investigators admit this in the discussion section. These imperfections reveal the nature of science. Science is a process, not a body of facts written in a textbook. Readers may become frustrated when they cannot clearly label a study as "good" or "bad." They may reject it entirely or they may apply every finding, blindly adopting the newest recommendation. The evidence for or against "truth" accumulates over time as a result of many imperfect studies. Clinicians who seek the best science to use in their practice realize they must keep reading and analyzing related research.

This discussion of critical reading suggests an order in which to read the parts of an article. For beginners, it might be helpful to use this standard approach early in the research process. A methodical approach helps the reader compare the strengths and weaknesses of a study in a defined way. This improves the ability to determine why studies differ in their findings and to clarify why a particular study may be unsatisfying. As you acquire more experience, you will create your own approach to reading and evaluating research. The following sections describe the steps of critical reading.

Step 1: Consider the Title

Scrutinizing the title will help determine what you expect the article will help present. Sometimes, a title may lead your thinking along one track, and the article turns out to be about a different facet than you were expecting. When you are aware of what you had expected, you can adjust more readily to what the authors actually meant.

Be alert to any bias in the wording of the title. For example, the health risks of infant formula feeding are not always accurately conveyed by the titles and abstracts of journal articles. A title that implies the "benefits" of nursing rather than the "risks" of not nursing may reflect bias.

What Do You Know About the Topic?

Your reading will be more critical if you identify your own knowledge before you begin. You may have chosen to read the article because of its importance for a problem that already interests you and that you have encountered several times in practice. Consider what you already know about the subject reflected in the title. Try to be specific in terms of what you know from other studies, textbooks, lectures, and experience. Taking time to review what you know helps you recognize any discrepancies between your knowledge and the author's claims. There may be legitimate reasons for those discrepancies. The scientists may have learned something new, for example.

How Would You Have Studied the Topic?

Consider how you would have studied the topic. For example, if the topic is nursing twins, where would you have obtained subjects? Would you want any specific age of twins? Would the gender of the babies be relevant? Would siblings affect the findings? If the twins were born before 35 weeks, could that complicate the causes of the problems you are studying? Do you need twins who were exclusively nursed?

Consider whether it is possible to conduct an experiment, or whether you can simply observe parents and babies who have made their own choices. Will it be easy to identify 20 or more twin sets that meet the criteria, or is the problem so unusual that the number of subjects will be limited? Does the problem occur in one ethnic or cultural group more than in other groups? If so, do you want to do a comparative study or focus more on only one group? The more questions you consider about how you would have done the study, the more readily you grasp the significance of the choices the researchers made.

What Will You Expect to Find?

Your brief review should suggest a short list of aspects you expect to find in the study. For example, you may expect the study to include both first-time nursing parents and experienced ones. Or you may expect it to include only preterm infants weighing over 2500 g. If the result turns out to be different from your expectations, you will be interested in the reasons. This may lead you to uncover a deficiency in the study.

Step 2: Read the Authors' Names

Noting author names is helpful, especially if you have read a previous work by the same author or authors and found the work to contain a problem. Are the shortcomings of the previous study corrected in this study? If the authors studied a previous problem in a way you thought was valuable, it will alert you to any changes in their methods or focus. If you never read work by these authors, noting their names gives you a reference point for future reading. As you develop familiarity with specific researchers, you will begin to discern their biases and gain more insight into your own biases and unfounded assumptions.

Step 3: Read the Abstract

Reading the abstract is the first point at which you confirm whether your assumptions about a study are correct. The abstract should describe the main characteristics of the subjects and methods. It will indicate whether the article is relevant to what you are studying. For example, if babies in a study on excessive crying are older than 6 months and you wanted information for 6-week-old infants, you may stop reading and seek a different article. If the article is about treating engorgement but does not mention the use of anti-inflammatory medications, reading the introduction and literature review may provide the rationale for the omission.

If the article reports a finding that contradicts what you know about the topic, it is not a reason to stop reading. Reading the abstract alerts you to the importance of specific aspects of the study that may justify the unexpected findings. The abstract may give you your first hint of the results the investigators believe warrant their recommendations. Knowing the direction in which the authors want to apply their findings prepares you to read for specific inclusions or exclusions in their work. Reading the abstract heightens your awareness of what the researchers believe is most important about their study.

Step 4: Study the Tables and Graphs

There are many kinds of tables, graphs, and charts. Their purposes range from summarizing information to clarifying complex patterns found in the data. Make a quick overview of the graphics to determine how many there are, their titles, and whether they are understandable. For each one, ask yourself why the authors chose to put the information in a summary form. Often, it is to save space because there is not enough space in many print journals for the authors to present their raw data (the actual numbers they collected or measured). They therefore summarize quantitative information in tables, graphs, and charts. Online journals may provide links to the study's raw data.

A table or graph may highlight an unusual aspect of the sample, method, or results. If a treatment produced a dramatic improvement in clients' conditions, for example, a graph may illustrate that most clearly. Graphs or tables that display results you consider minor while ignoring results that seem to be more important may suggest a possible bias. Consider whether the inferences or outcomes in the table data agree with the narrative. If they conflict and you cannot explain the difference in a plausible way, there may be a flaw in the article or an editorial error. When you read the results to decide whether the evidence supports the findings, you want to study the graphics closely. Critical analysis includes judging their clarity and consistency with the rest of the article.

Tables

Tables are often the simplest way to concisely capture a large amount of quantitative information. The most helpful tables have a title that reflects the main idea; the source of the data (e.g., from a survey or from client charts); and clear labels on each column and row, including the units of measurement and time (e.g., milliliters, kilograms, seconds, weeks, months). Some provide percentages of the total that each subgroup represents, as well as statistical test results.

Pay particular attention to whether the number of subjects reported in the tables is the same as that described in the narrative. The number of subjects who consented to participate initially is often greater than the number who participated in any particular aspect of the study. For example, the authors may have described their study to several childbirth preparation classes and obtained consent from 50 couples to observe the first feeding. What could happen to reduce that number? The researchers might have been out of town when two of the couples delivered. Perhaps another two parents were so tired after delivery that they refused to allow the researcher to observe them. Maybe three parents decided not to nurse. This reduces the sample size to 43 couples.

Therefore, if you read that 50 couples granted consent and that the total number of observations was 43, you might need to reread the part of the article that describes what happened to the other 7 couples. As long as the tables and text agree and there is an explanation of any apparent discrepancies, you can use the information in the tables to decide whether your clients are similar to the ones studied. You can also decide whether the tables and figures support the findings and reasoning claimed by the researchers.

Graphs

Graphs should have clear titles and labels and portray the data accurately. You need to study the scale of the graph carefully. In the graph in **Figure 29-1**, note that the scale goes from 0 to 20, so the height of the curved lines seems lower and less impressive than the height of the curves in the graph in **Figure 29-2**, in which the scale goes from 0 to 7. Either scale could be appropriate depending on the definition of the pain scale. However, the graphs create different reactions in the viewer. Because the **slope** or angle of the lines in Figure 29-1 is steeper than that of Figure 29-2, it appears that the change in pain was different from that illustrated in Figure 29-1. Actually, both reflect the same result. Although graphs can be helpful, they can also be misleading and require careful scrutiny.

Consider the source of the data in the graph. Suppose this study was one in which each parent was their own control, randomly assigned to treat one nipple and not the other. Suppose further that the authors claim that the treated nipple was sore for less total time than the untreated nipple. Although you might agree with that conclusion, you might wonder if it was a fair test. Perhaps some of the babies sucked more vigorously on the untreated nipple, causing it to be more painful than the treated nipple on day 1. This example is probably not what the authors would publish because it represents only one subject.

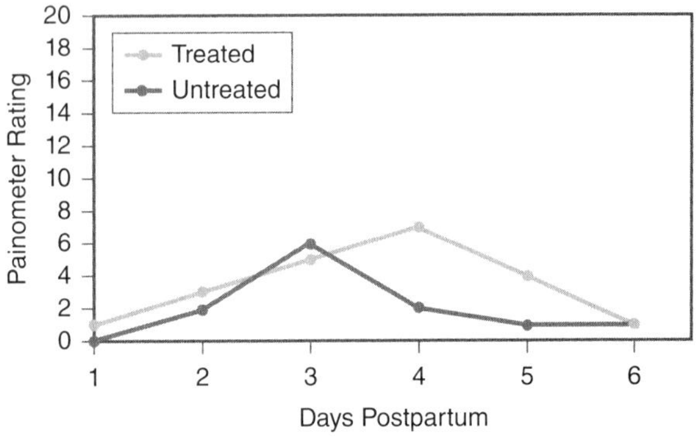

Figure 29-1 Changes in nipple soreness on a scale of 0 to 20.

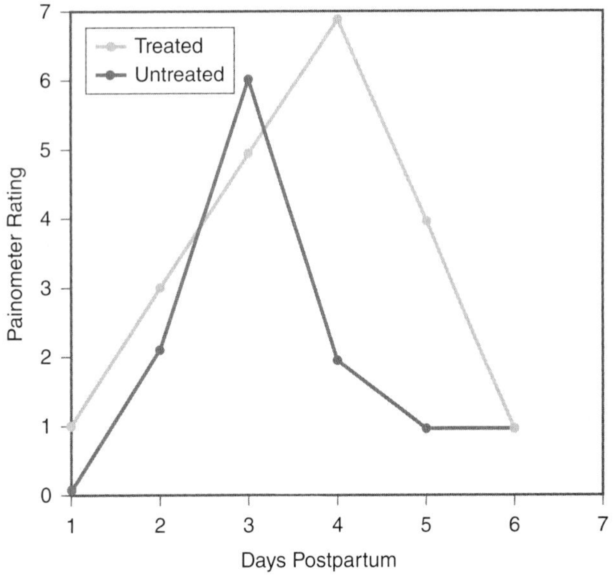

Figure 29-2 Changes in nipple soreness on a scale of 0 to 7.

Step 5: Read the Results

Read the results to get firmly in your mind what the authors claim to find. You need to understand their claims to read about their methods effectively. Pay particular attention to the subjects in the study and the relationships between variables. The first time you read the results section, determine whether the results are what the authors expected based on their theories and hypotheses. Before you read the article any further, get the results clear in your mind and consider whether those results were predicted.

Subjects

The subjects section of the article identifies the researchers' final sample. Perhaps they intended an equal proportion of first-time and experienced nursing parents. You then need to decide whether the sample was appropriate for the question they asked and whether the results are justified based on the kind of subjects they acquired.

Most researchers try to anticipate a certain number of study dropouts. However, sometimes more subjects drop out from one group than from the other. Consider whether their results could have been different if their original plan had worked. Dropouts can affect the results. Some leave the study because their problem resolves quickly and they no longer need the treatment. Some leave because they could not tolerate side effects of the treatment. Others drop out because the research process is a burden. Some families move before the study is completed.

Consider the implications of each reason that participants dropped out of the study. Would the findings have been different if the dropouts had remained in the study different? Suppose a study of parents who returned to employment at 6 weeks postpartum was trying to determine what factors made it likely that they would continue nursing to 12 weeks. One factor to study might be employer support. The researchers might enroll parents from the hospital who were planning to return to work at 6 weeks and continue nursing until at least 12 weeks. If a few subjects drop out because they expect a lack of support from their employer, the remaining subjects would disproportionately include more parents who expect support from their employers. It would then be likely that both those who continued and those who stopped expected support. This might lead the researchers to conclude that there was no difference between the two groups in terms of support. In reality, a higher proportion of those who expected no support simply left the study. The dropouts caused the study to experience **homogeneity** (similarity of data results) with respect to employer support, preventing detection of a difference in that factor.

Relationships

The investigators usually indicate that their study found a **relationship** between two or more variables. For example, they may have found a relationship between giving discharge packs containing formula to new parents and early discontinuation of nursing. The discharge packs are the **independent variable**, and the duration of nursing is the **dependent variable**. Consider all the logical steps needed to substantiate that finding.

Are the Data Consistent with the Claims?

In the discharge pack example, one result could be that more of the parents who received discharge packs needed to stop nursing earlier than did the parents who did not receive packs. The number of parents who stopped compared with those who continued must be significantly different in a statistical sense—**statistically significant**. It also needs to be convincingly different to you. Similarly, "early" weaning must be meaningfully different from "late" weaning.

Is There No Equal or Better Explanation?

In the discharge pack example, determine whether the data can rule out other possible competing explanations. Did more parents in the discharge pack group experience nipple pain? Was there a higher proportion of preterm infants? Were there more parents who intended to nurse for only 6 weeks or less? Ruling out these possible explanations makes it more likely that the discharge pack is the cause of the early weaning.

Does the Plausible Mechanism Link the Two Variables? In the discharge pack example, the mechanism for this causation might be that a discharge pack is a subtle message to the parent that the healthcare provider does not have confidence that they can make sufficient milk for the baby. The parent then doubts the adequacy of their milk production and weans early.

Step 6: Read the Methods

Reviewing the study's methods is the most important aspect of your critical reading because it determines whether the authors can justify their conclusions. The design of the study, the definitions of terms, the tools for measurement, and the statistical tests all contribute to your evaluation. When you have read and thought about the methods, recall the results. Do the study design, definitions, tools, and operations allow for the conclusions the researchers made? How could they have done the study differently to make you believe that the conclusions were more justified? What additional information about the methods would help you evaluate the findings more thoroughly?

Design of the Study

There are several shorthand ways of describing the design of a study to a scientific audience. When you recognize these basic study designs, you can understand the aspects of subject selection, data gathering, and comparisons that are drawn. You can also anticipate the kinds of conclusions warranted by the study's design. Some studies combine qualitative and quantitative data analysis techniques, garnering the strengths of both methods to provide a comprehensive understanding of a research problem or question. Such research collects and analyzes numerical data as well as qualitative data such as interviews, observations, or open-ended survey responses (Polit & Beck, 2022)

Observational Study. In an **observational study**, researchers study the effect of an intervention, risk, test, or treatment without trying to manipulate the research subjects. Observational studies may consist of prospective and retrospective **cohort** studies, case-control studies, or cross-sectional studies in which the researcher observes subjects and measures variables without assigning treatment (Riegelman, 2020).

An observational study can generally be completed quickly and inexpensively. It is often used because ethical or practical concerns prevent the researcher from conducting a traditional experiment. The lack of control and treatment groups makes it difficult to form inferences, and there is a risk of confounding variables and observer bias. Case study observational research offers a promising approach for researchers in healthcare settings who seek a more complete understanding of complex topics (Im et al., 2023). There is growing recognition of the value of using real-world evidence in decision-making (Baumfeld Andre et al., 2020).

Retrospective Study. A **retrospective study** (also called a *historical cohort study*) uses two comparison groups. The case subjects have the problem under examination, and the control subjects do not. Designing a study by first designating case subjects results in a design based on **output variables**. Output variables describe the subjects after follow-up or treatment. For example, the case subjects might be babies readmitted to the hospital with greater-than-expected weight loss during the first week of life. The control subjects would be babies without such weight loss, possibly found by a search of the charts in a pediatric practice. The purpose of such a comparison might be to determine whether there were any differences in the number of feedings or stools in the first 4 days of life or differences in the highest bilirubin level achieved that could be associated with the need for readmission. Such a retrospective study is a **case-control study**.

When the methods section declares that the design is retrospective, you expect to read a description of the groups chosen for comparison. You then want to know whether the groups were appropriate. Retrospective studies greatly depend on information recorded before researchers conducted the study. If a retrospective study concludes that babies who had stooled only once during their first 24 hours were at higher risk for readmission, you would want to know the accuracy of the recordkeeping of stools passed. In a retrospective study, the use of existing records may be all that is possible. The evidence gained from such a study may not be as strong as when the recordkeeping is more deliberate and planned.

Prospective Study. In a **prospective study**, subjects are sampled on the basis of input variables that are believed to influence the outcomes. The authors may have held staff education classes and designed new recordkeeping tools before data collection began. From the starting date forward, the staff would be asked to keep careful count of the number, color, and size of the stools on a certain cohort of babies designated as infants born from January 1 to June 30, 2019. If the number of stools related to the risk of readmission for weight loss, there would be greater confidence in this prospective study than in a retrospective one. The researchers ensured the accuracy of data collection before the study began.

Prospective studies may offer more complete information than a retrospective one. A disadvantage can be the length of time the cohort must be followed. However, longitudinal studies provide long-term insights. The U.S. Nurses' Health Study began in 1976 to investigate the long-term effects of oral contraceptives on women health. This is an example of a long-term prospective study evolved to investigate the risk factors for major chronic diseases in women and continues today (Nurses' Health Study, 2025).

Cross-Sectional Study. A **cross-sectional study** relies on recordkeeping or memory, much like a retrospective study does. However, researchers do not begin by identifying an affected group. Rather, they gather data from everyone at the same time. In a study about stooling and readmission rates in a cross-sectional design, for example, researchers might collect data at the time of all infants' 2-month visits. They would identify the affected group (readmitted infants) and compare the data about their stools, feedings, and bilirubin levels with the same information for the unaffected group. Cross-sectional studies are adequate for suggesting causative factors and relevant variables. The possibility that the data collection was too dependent on recall or missed too many possible subjects on the collection day or days limits confidence in the findings.

Descriptive Study. A **descriptive study** lists many relevant variables of a defined sample rather than comparing two groups. For example, a family practice office might want to know the characteristics of its childbearing families before designing a preconception class. The study might describe how many families in the previous year had borne a first child, how many had a second child, and how many nursed and for how long. Even though researchers gathered the information from one sample, they might publish their findings so that other family practices with similar types of families might benefit from the information. Descriptive studies require a thorough and careful description of the sample. Readers can then understand the similarities and differences between their groups of families and the one studied.

Qualitative Study. In a **qualitative study**, researchers observe subjects and events in a natural setting rather than establishing a control. They often study the meaning of an event or practice to the person experiencing it. Variables in a qualitative study are usually not measured in numbers, and differences between variables are not expressed numerically. Qualitative variables are often terms that the researcher believes change together, that is, category labels. For example, as "ethnic heritage" changes, so does the "critical support person." Qualitative research emphasizes getting a sense of the whole or comprehending the emergent properties of an experience instead of breaking down a phenomenon or experience into parts. Qualitative studies in lactation, for example, have described the feelings of parents who nursed a child for several years and the empowerment of low-income parents through nursing.

Experiments and Trials. In lactation research, it is less common to find studies designed as experiments. Problems that involve humans are difficult to conduct as experiments. However, researchers might study comparisons of equipment or differences between animals experimentally. The best information about a problem that involves humans comes from **randomized clinical trials**. Similar to experiments, these trials attempt to avoid bias in their comparisons. Treatment groups are as similar as possible at the beginning of the study, and great effort is made to identify any differences. Furthermore, the groups are treated the same in all ways except for the treatment itself. If the trial is **blind** as well, then knowledge of which treatment the client received remains secret until analysis of the data. This avoids the client's or clinician's assessment of the effectiveness of treatment being influenced by knowing to which treatment group the client belonged.

Suppose there was a new drug to eliminate mastitis caused by *Staphylococcus aureus*. To conduct a blind study, researchers disguise the new and old drugs, perhaps by using identical capsules, and administer them in the same manner. In that way, no one can distinguish one from the other. Only a system of codes detects the difference for later analysis. Both groups are otherwise healthy, first-time nursing parents of babies 2 to 6 months old. Therefore, the groups are as similar as possible. The severity of the mastitis is graded by strict criteria and by the same two clinicians for all subjects. Recommendations for other aspects of treatment (e.g., pain relief) are the same for all subjects. In a tightly controlled study like this, differences in cure rates between the two drugs are more likely to be attributable to the drugs than in a case-control or other less controlled study.

There are several reasons why more studies are not blinded, randomized trials. Ethical concerns preclude **random assignment** of people to potentially poorer treatments. For example, it would be unethical to assign one group of infants to be randomly nursed and another group to be artificially fed. It is also difficult to control many of the variables about people that result in comparison groups of humans who are different in many ways. In addition, large numbers of subjects are required when a trial attempts to study prevention of problems. Finally, precision in measuring "soft" outcomes—such as quality of bonding and attachment—is lower. Critical analysis of clinical trials involves judgments about the researchers having adequately identified and controlled important variables. Funding and recognition for researchers tend to be greater when their study outcomes are "harder" and more quantifiable.

Definitions

The authors should define key terms clearly enough for you to know who or what was included and excluded. Key concepts in the lactation field may include lactation, supplementation, multipara, infant, pain, treatment, and exercise. If the authors studied only multiparas, for example, all the possible differences in multiparas are variables. Did they have previous nursing experience, or did the authors assume they had nursed without asking? If the parents nursed previously, does it matter to the study's conclusions whether the previous experience was positive or negative? Is the age of the multiparas important? Is their experience coping with other stressful situations or child-rearing problems significant? Consider how the definition of multipara in the study might affect the results. Critically reading the definitions includes being able to state how a different or clearer definition could change the results or the interpretation of the results.

Tools (Instruments)

Research tools are the instruments, software, methodologies, and approaches researchers use to collect, analyze, and interpret data. Scales for weighing babies, survey questions, diet diaries, and pain ratings are examples of tools used in lactation studies. You may not be able to analyze a tool completely if you are not familiar with it. Still, you want to read the study because you may encounter similar tools in later reading. In addition, you will need to know how a defined term was measured to decide its applicability to your situation.

In better studies, the tools have undergone testing and measure the dependent variable consistently. The **reliability** of the measurement from one time to the next may be part of the reason the investigators chose to use this tool. Authors may assume some familiarity with the type of tool without explaining the general type in much detail. For example, they expect healthcare professionals to know what a **Likert scale**. Although they do not describe their Likert scale in detail, they should explain how it is different from others (whether it is a 5-point or a 7-point scale, for example). Likewise, they may expect an understanding of the use of a pulse **oximeter**, a device for measuring oxygen saturation levels and heart rate. They should specify whether the placement of the pulse oximeter was on a finger or a toe. Any details about the tool or its use should be described clearly so that you do not have serious questions about whether the quirks of the authors' method are more responsible for their results than the explanation for the results that they expound.

It is not necessary that the authors publish the entire tool in the article. Its length, developmental status, or potential profitability may prevent its publication. Examples or short versions of a survey's questions may help you decide whether the tone or complexity of the questions could have influenced the way subjects answered them. If you have serious concerns about the quality of the questions, you can contact the authors to request more information. Even if you agree with a study's conclusions, you may not want to use the study in a formal presentation until you have learned more about the tool so that you can adequately answer your audience's questions.

Operationalizing

Operationalizing identifies the specific research procedures used to gather data about concepts. The process allows researchers to clearly define and measure the variables they are studying. Suppose they are studying the change in pain after the application of a treatment. They should tell you how they define pain, which is often the subject's verbal or written report of the pain.

The tool for verbal reports of pain might be a 10-point scale in which the **anchors** (words used at specific points on the scale to describe what that number means) are "1 = no pain" and "10 = the worst pain you can imagine." You can then understand that the researchers operationalized the concept of "pain" by asking the subject to place a mark on the scale that best represented the level of pain before the treatment and again at a specified time afterward. Alternatively, they might have videotaped subjects before and after the treatment and watched for changes in facial expression.

Critical reading of a study's operationalization involves both its clarity and your judgment about its **validity**. The validity of a pain measure, for example, is often supported by expert review or by comparing the current pain tool with an older one and finding that the two agree. Although pain is difficult to measure because of its subjectivity, what is important is the person's determination of the amount of pain and whether that determination changes. A scale that reflects the changes is the operationalization of the pain. The construction of measurement scales is the subject of many research articles.

Statistics

A brief description of the main statistical approach used to evaluate the data is usually found in the methods section of the article. To some extent, the reader must rely on the peer-review process to catch any major problems in the statistics. The more you read lactation research, the more you become familiar with some of the common approaches used in certain research designs. Statistical tutoring and online learning options are available, many of them at no cost. This section describes common statistical ideas and tests.

Statistical Theory. Statistical theory is based on **probability**, a mathematical discipline that focuses on trying to precisely answer finely tuned questions about uncertain events. **Statistical theory** uses probability to answer real questions based on real data.

Sample size (the number of data points) is important. If there is an interesting trend (for example, if low-birth-weight babies tend to have lower IQ scores later in life), the larger the sample, the more likely the pattern in the data would convince us of the validity of what was observed. For example, in considering whether a coin is biased (i.e., tends to land heads more often than tails, or vice versa), you might flip the coin 100 times and record how often heads result from those 100 flips. Statistics would use the observed number of heads (the data) to determine if there is convincing evidence of a bias. If you observe only 37 heads in the 100 flips, a pattern that would happen less than 1% of the time if you were flipping a fair coin, you would conclude that the coin has some bias.

Study Frequency. Good studies aim for the largest sample size they can reasonably get. The statistical analysis tells the power of that sample size. Power relies on more than sample size. However, sample size is what researchers have the most control over, so they try to maximize it. For most purposes, researchers want a power of 0.80 (80%) or higher. If the power of a test is low, the reason for failing to find a significant difference between two groups could be that the sample selected was too small for a difference to occur, not that there is no real difference.

A power of 80% means that the data has an 80% probability of correctly rejecting the **null hypothesis**. The null hypothesis states that no statistical significance exists in a set of given observations, and therefore, the original study hypothesis, or alternative hypothesis, was not proven.

When you research nursing frequency at 10 days of age in your city, for example, you are studying a sample of the whole **population** of 10-day-old nursing babies (in the world, and maybe throughout human history). Your goal in studying the frequency in this sample may be to demontrate that the "normal" or "usual" or "**average**" frequency for all human babies at 10 days was *x*. You would then be trying to make a statement about the population by studying a sample of it. If your sample is large (500 subjects or more), the chance of an error in your estimate of *x* is far less than if your sample is only 20 subjects.

Statistical Tests. Statistical tests are tools that mathematically determine whether two sets of data are significantly different from each other. They help determine if there are relationships or differences between variables or groups in a data population. They provide a method to make quantitative decisions, testing the hypothesis about the significance of a particular sample. Each statistical test assumes certain things about the data. If those assumptions are not true, the test should not be used. Sometimes in the methods section, there is a brief statement about why a certain test was used and whether a particular assumption was met.

There are few hard-and-fast rules in statistical analysis. Statisticians may disagree about which test should be the first solution to try. They may question whether the assumption of a **normal distribution** of the data is true. A normal distribution describes much of the infinite data we could collect about the natural world. A normal distribution, plotted on a graph, resembles a **bell curve**. **Figure 29-3** illustrates a graph entitled "How much milk the 1-month-old infant takes at a single episode at the breast."

The left end of the graph identifies a few babies who take tiny amounts, perhaps when feedings are very frequent and short. The right end identifies a few babies who take a very large amount. Assuming that

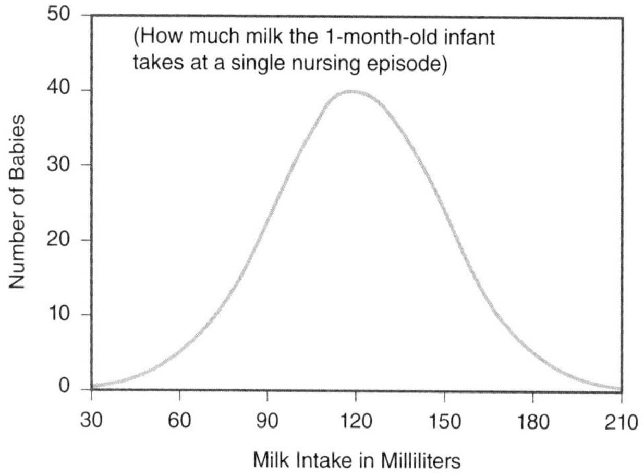

Figure 29-3 Centered bell curve.

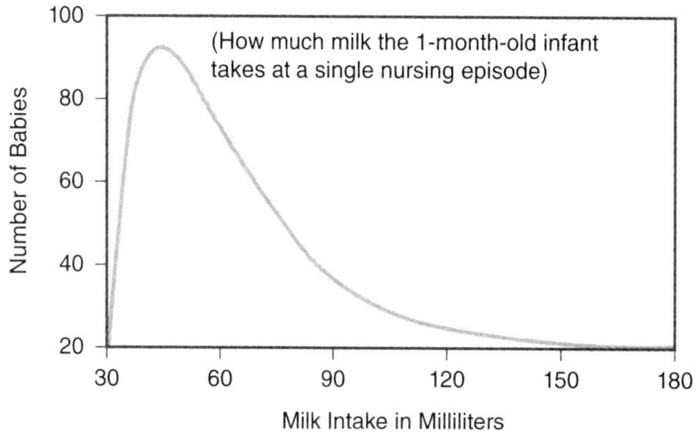

Figure 29-4 Unbalanced bell curve.

most babies take in about 120 mL, the center of the graph (the large hill or bell) represents what the bulk of babies do. Between the center and each extreme is a gradual slope.

Suppose the data on milk intake actually come from a distribution that resembles the graph in **Figure 29-4**. Here, the bulk (greatest number of values) of the data is at one extreme, not in the middle. The left side rises quickly, with a long slope on the right. Perhaps this is a group of preterm infants at 1 month of age whose intake tends to be less than that of full-term infants. A statistical test attempting to predict what happens in the bulk of this distribution by expecting it to be a normal distribution would be way off. The middle in this distribution is far to the left of where it would be with a normal distribution of the data. The data in **Figure 29-3** require a statistical test designed for this particular distribution. Researchers and statisticians need to carefully choose which tests to use and consider all the underlying assumptions, including the distribution of the data.

Statistical Significance. Statistical significance, or lack of significance, is determined by applying a statistical test to a result and calculating the probability of obtaining that result (or a more extreme result). The probability is reported as a **P value**. The P value measures the risk of rejecting a true null hypothesis. Most researchers want P values that are 0.05 or lower. Researchers want no more than a 5% or less chance of falsely stating that there is a real difference between two groups.

Confidence intervals (CIs) provide information about the statistical significance of a result. They represent the range within which a population's true value is expected to be found. A CI may measure the **median** (the middle point in a range of numbers) or the **mean** (the sum divided by the count). Usually, a 95% CI is reported. This describes the other possible results that are close to the one that came from the data and that are likely to contain the true population value. For example, if the mean (average) of weight gain from a study's sample was 200 g and the 95% CI was 185 to 215 g, it is likely that the population's true weight gain is somewhere between 185 and 215 g.

Large CIs (e.g., 50 to 350 g in this example) do not tell you very much. Nearly every weight gain falls somewhere in that interval, so you cannot tell the difference between a usual one and a more extreme one. Large CIs often occur with a small sample size. If you are comparing the weight gains in two different groups of infants and you expect them to be different, CIs should not overlap. So if the mean for group A (nursing) is 200 g (95% CI, 185–215 g) and the mean for group B (formula fed) is 220 g (95% CI, 205–235 g), the intervals share the values 205 to 215 g. These shared values mean that the real average weight gain could be the same for both groups. These CIs would not demonstrate a statistically significant difference between the two groups.

Common Statistical Tests and Terms. This section on common statistical tests and terms can help you understand some of the tests you are most likely to encounter. Tests range from determining whether two groups are significantly alike or different, the degrees of differences, and the relationship between variables to evaluating the reliability of an instrument.

Chi-Square. There are several slightly different versions of the **chi-square** test. It is typically used to determine whether the proportions in two groups are significantly different. You may want to determine, for example, whether the proportion of experienced nursing parents with mastitis is the same as the proportion of first-time nursing parents with mastitis. Large chi-square values usually lead to low, statistically significant P values.

Cohen's Kappa. The statistic **Cohen's Kappa** is used to demonstrate that two raters are in close agreement. It is calculated when two observers rate the same event on a scale. Values of 0.7 or higher are considered good.

Cronbach's Alpha. A researcher may use a **Cronbach's alpha** test to measures the internal consistency, or reliability, of an instrument. Values can range from 0.0 to 1.0. The closer they are to 1.0, the better the reliability.

Odds Ratio. Researchers use the **odds ratio** to compare the odds of something occurring in one group to the odds of it occurring in another group. For example, it is a way to compare the proportion of nursing babies who get otitis media with the proportion of formula-fed babies who get otitis media under similar conditions. If 2 of 10 nursing babies developed otitis media and 4 of 10 formula-fed babies developed otitis media, the ratio of those odds is 0.2/0.4 = 0.5. The odds of the nursing baby getting an ear infection were one-half the odds of the formula-fed baby.

An odds ratio would equal 1 if the odds for both groups are the same. CIs for odds ratios might be written like this: 0.5 (95% CI, 0.35–0.60). This means that the best estimate of the odds ratio could range from 0.35 to 0.60. Significant CIs for the odds ratio should not contain "1" (0.90–1.05, for example) because that would mean the odds ratio could be 1. This is another way of saying that the odds for the nursed baby were the same as the odds for the formula-fed baby. In studies comparing risks for nursed infants and formula-fed infants, we would expect to find that the formula-fed babies had higher risks.

Regression. Regression is a technique used to try to understand the relationship between variables. Simple regression relates one **predictor variable** (or independent variable) to one outcome variable (or dependent variable). Multiple regression relates several variables to one outcome variable. **Logistic regression** relates one or more variables to a **dichotomous outcome** variable (outcome measure in which there are only two possibilities). Regression may be used for a question such as "Do parent satisfaction, infant weight gain, and family support with the first nursed child relate to the decision to nurse or not nurse [dichotomous outcome] the next child?" Regression methods usually try to estimate how much change there is in the outcome variable for a one-unit change in the predictor variable. For example, "How much change occurs in infant crying time for each additional half hour of being carried in a baby sling?"

T-Test. Researchers use a **t-test** to determine if there is a significant difference between the means of two groups and to test a hypotheses about the mean of a sample. For example, you may want to know if the average weight loss of nursing newborns in hospital A is the same as the average weight loss for all nursing newborns in the country (where the national average is often considered a "norm" or "true" population value). A slightly different t-test could be used to compare the average weight loss of newborn babies in hospital A with that of newborn babies in hospital B.

Methodological Concerns in Lactation Research

The field of lactation has a unique set of concerns regarding research methodology. Because nursing involves two people, a study of a particular aspect of lactation can be affected by interactions between the nursing parent and baby. There are ethical issues related to intervening in the natural course of lactation. Methodology challenges include the following;

- Observing and measuring the process of feedings can disturb the natural process.
- Test weighing of infants may not be uniform. This can be resolved by careful instruction to the people who weigh the babies and by the use of electronic digital scales that are highly calibrated.
- It is difficult to equate the volume of expressed milk to the volume milk produced. Such volumes can be quite different unless good-quality pumps are used, pumping duration is adequate, milk lets down, and the study accounts for time of day.
- It is difficult to obtain a representative milk sample. Milk composition varies by length of time postpartum, time of day, proportion of milk drained, and gestation of the infant.
- A change in feeding method is one-directional, usually a change from nursing to formula feeding. For example, parents who began nursing may supplement or switch entirely to formula. Therefore, when studies encompass babies who have been formula-fed, some in the group may have nursed at some point and then formula-fed. This can make it difficult to interpret growth differences. It is difficult to study a switch from formula feeding to nursing because of the time-sensitive calibration of milk production. There may be ways to overcome this built-in direction, but the time-dependent nature of lactation may complicate interpretation.
- Studies of environmental contaminants often use human milk because it is easier to obtain than blood or other body tissue and because milk fats promote the accumulation of some chemicals in milk. However, the media may misunderstand the use of milk, implying that finding a pollutant in milk automatically means that feeding human milk is harmful. It also ignores the relevance of contaminants in other animal milks and plants.
- Studies of the effects of lactation on bone mineralization have sometimes been misunderstood because the time it takes to recover bone mass that was mobilized during lactation was longer than the length of the study.

Step 7: Read the Introduction and Literature Review

The introduction and literature review will help you understand some of the decisions the researchers made in light of the results they found and the methods they used. Most articles regarding lactation begin by citing expert bodies that recognize the superiority of human milk, followed by identifying a problem that prevents near-universal lactation. They might claim their study will address that problem, shed light on it, and help improve lactation rates.

Often, the authors explain and reference the theory underlying their approach to the problem and the hypothesis they want to test. Somewhere in this line of reasoning is the explicit or implicit statement of why the authors chose the problem to study. The literature review reveals how the authors' study is different from what has been done before and how their study is an improvement. If they have done a good job of this reasoning, they demonstrate that the problem is significant, that no one has adequately addressed it, and that their approach adds to the existing body of knowledge. Your experience and your reading of other articles and books will help you decide whether they have convinced you of this. The questions to consider are discussed in the following section.

Questions to Guide Your Literature Review

- Do you believe this is a significant problem? Have the authors explained why? If you were not very experienced in lactation, would their explanation be convincing?
- Are the summaries of the articles they cite accurate? If you know the studies, did they do a good job of stating the conclusions?

- If you know any of the studies, are they the appropriate ones to use? For example, if the new study is about excessive crying in fully nursing babies but the cited studies included partially nursing babies, what parts can legitimately be compared, and what parts must be different? Suppose the new study wants to use removal of dairy products from the parent's diet as a treatment. That could be a clear change in an exclusively nursing baby's diet. But in a baby who is also receiving supplements, a comparable change in diet would need to include removal of the formula. On the other hand, the older study may have found that firstborn infants suffered more excessive crying, and the new study might want to examine birth order. That aspect of both studies is more similar than exposure to cow's milk because birth order does not directly relate to cow's milk or the parent's diet.
- Did the authors omit any studies that you would have included? Are you aware of previous research about the problem that the authors left out? If it is an area of research with several previous studies, lack of space may be the reason. However, it may happen by design if the authors do not want to mention contrary studies, especially if the studies rejected what the authors wish to convey. Omitting relevant studies may also result from an inadequate literature search. Leaving out relevant studies can portray a misleading picture of the state of knowledge to those unfamiliar with the background information. Peer reviewers expect prospective authors to include the most important articles.
- Are the methods used in previous studies explained fully enough to judge whether the use or rejection of the studies in the new study is appropriate? For example, in a study of infection rates in children who attend day care versus those who do not attend day care, the literature review may describe the use of "written parental diaries" as the method. The authors may say that they propose to use the same method as previous studies—namely, having parents record weekly whether the child had fever, sore throat, and medical visits. Suppose they find that infection rates for children in day care are no different from those of stay-at-home children, despite previous studies finding a difference. In the older study, parents recorded symptoms on a daily basis and received biweekly reminders. That may explain why the older study found differences in rates, whereas the new study does not. You are searching for ways in which the current study is different from and similar to the older studies cited in the literature review. The authors should mention the differences and be clear about any aspects relevant to the current study.

Step 8: Read the Discussion

There is usually a link between the literature review and the discussion. The authors may explain the link at the beginning of the discussion section. They may offer an interpretation of the results that puts their findings into the context of other studies conducted on the same problem. Ask yourself whether the intentions the researchers declared based on their review of the current state of knowledge carried through to the methods and results. If they did something different from the studies cited earlier, ask whether it was an improvement. Consider whether the findings are as important as the authors claim and whether the state of knowledge about the problem is now more complete or clearer.

Speculation

The authors may stretch the interpretation of their findings into a more speculative understanding that links some aspects of the problem. As a critical reader, you can judge how plausible, realistic, and rational the link is. You do not know whether the link is correct, but you can consider whether it could exist and whether further suggestions by the authors along this line of reasoning are plausible.

An example of this is a study that found that peanut butter and jelly sandwiches correlate with higher milk production. Suppose the authors found evidence in the literature review that a chemical in peanuts caused an appetite increase in lab animals. They combined these two ideas to suggest that the reason peanut butter and jelly sandwiches are associated with higher milk production is that the sandwiches stimulate appetite in nursing parents who eat them. Although their research did not study the chemistry of peanuts or the overall calorie intake, they speculate that such a causal mechanism exists.

Suggestions for Further Research

Suggestions for further research provide a clear roadmap for studies to build upon previous work. These suggestions often arise from limitations the researchers identified in their study. Researchers may suggest that others carry on from their study to delve deeper into an aspect that time did not permit. They may suggest that a future study address a flaw in their research or test the speculations they made. They may suggest building on a particular finding of the research or filling gaps in the understanding of the problem that remain despite the knowledge gained from their study. Researchers may suggest examining a theory in another context, location, or culture. They may recommend taking the research in different directions or replicating the research results to draw further conclusions.

Flaws or Weaknesses

The authors may acknowledge some of the same flaws or weaknesses you detected in reading the article. Consider whether your assessment of the flaws (and their impact on your confidence in the results) is the same as that of the authors. If you believe the problems are more serious than the authors acknowledge, you want to read their justification as generously as you can. On the other hand, if the authors fail to note a flaw you uncovered, try to understand why. It could be that the goal or methods, as explained in the discussion, are different from your original understanding of them.

Step 9: Read the Results Again

Your first reading of the results section was to understand what the authors claimed to have found. Read the results again to decide whether you believe those claims were justified. You probably formed some judgments about this already, after reading the methods and discussion. Consider whether the authors convinced you that the data are consistent with the claims, there are no other equal or better explanations, and the mechanism links the variables.

Data Consistent with Claims

In deciding if the data are consistent with the claims, consider the example of the study testing the effect of discharge packs on the duration of lactation. If the study had 100 subjects (50 in the pack group and 50 in the nonpack group), and if 15 in the pack group weaned "early" but only 5 did in the nonpack group, is that a convincing difference to you? The difference would be statistically significant at $P = 0.05$. That is, there is only a 1 in 20 chance that a difference of 15 versus 5 (or a more extreme difference) occurred by chance. Therefore, statistically speaking, it is probable that the difference between the numbers of early weaners in the two groups is a real difference and not a chance occurrence. However, you could ask whether the difference is clinically important. Do 10 more "late" weaners out of 50 achieve enough additional health and relationship benefits to warrant discontinuing discharge packs?

This question is not just about statistics but also about values. Many healthcare providers probably consider this valid and important evidence against discharge packs. Skeptics, however, might argue, "If discharge packs are so bad, how did 35 of 50 parents go on to wean late in spite of them?" Considering answers to such questions helps you formulate responses you could use if you presented this study to skeptics.

Another Possible Explanation

Consider whether there is another possible explanation for the claimed relationship between variables. You need to scrutinize the numbers the authors present. Usually, you find that they have chosen appropriate ways to measure and summarize their data. Nevertheless, you may find that you have questions about their numbers that make you reluctant to agree with their conclusions.

Averages and Distribution Range

If the study found that parents who received discharge packs with formula nursed for 18 weeks and those who did not receive discharge packs nursed for 20 weeks, would you consider this to be an important difference? It could be a statistically significant difference between the groups, depending on the group sizes and the degree of **variation** in the averages. When an average (mean) is reported, you may want to know the **distribution** of each group's length of lactation. An average can be misleading if one subject (or a small number) has an extremely short or extremely long duration. **Figure 29-5** demonstrates the various ways a group could nurse for an average of 18 weeks.

Many parents in group 1 nursed for 18 weeks and four nursed for a shorter or longer time. The average in this distribution gives a good representation of the typical behavior in the group. The distribution range in group 1 is 25 − 11 weeks, for an average duration rate of 14 weeks. Group 2 included only one parent who nursed the "average" length of time and two parents whose duration was significantly different from the average (**outliers** with unusually small or large values for one of the variables being measured). The distribution range for group 2 is 50 – 2 weeks, for an average duration rate of 48 weeks. The distribution ranges in the two groups are dramatically different, as are the average duration rates of nursing.

Group 1	Group 2	Group 3
25 weeks	50 weeks	29 weeks
20 weeks	19 weeks	27 weeks
18 weeks	18 weeks	26 weeks
18 weeks	17 weeks	25 weeks
18 weeks	16 weeks	24 weeks
18 weeks	16 weeks	23 weeks
18 weeks	15 weeks	22 weeks
18 weeks	14 weeks	2 weeks
16 weeks	13 weeks	1 weeks
11 weeks	2 weeks	1 week
180 weeks	**180 weeks**	**180 weeks**

Figure 29-5 Ten subjects who nursed for an average of 18 weeks.

You might legitimately question whether the extremes in group 2 had much in common with the average. Specifically, you might wonder whether the parent who nursed for only 2 weeks had a difficult problem, such as a baby with ankyloglossia and a severe cardiac defect and would have nursed for only 2 weeks regardless of receiving a discharge pack. The results section may describe the reasons for weaning. If that information is absent or not collected, the authors cannot claim that discharge packs alone made a difference in the groups.

Closely examining the numbers to determine whether they are consistent with the claims may suggest a possible alternative explanation for the study's findings. A few parents may have had an extremely difficult problem that would have led to short duration of nursing, regardless of whether they received a pack. Excluding these factors from the calculation of duration might change the study's results. If the authors' data make you suspicious, you might ultimately be less willing to accept and apply the findings.

Also consider the other extreme in group 2. Suppose the parent who nursed for 50 weeks was in the group that received the discharge pack. You might ask, "If discharge packs are so bad, how did this parent manage to continue to nurse for so long?" Did the authors ask what the parents did with the packs. Did they use them? If yes, how old was the baby? Did they discard the formula? Authors rarely ask this question and presume that merely receiving a pack probably encourages formula use. The results would be stronger with data collected on the use of the packs, as well as any formula use among the group that did not receive the discharge pack.

Hidden Differences Between Groups

In group 3, there is quite a clear separation into two subgroups: one group nursed for 2 weeks or less, and the other group nursed for at least 22 weeks. Such a split might suggest the possibility of a major difference within the group. Perhaps subjects in the two subgroups received substantially different amounts of support. The subgroup who nursed longer may have had three or more support people, whereas the subgroup who nursed less may have had two or fewer support people. Although the entire group nursed for an average of 18 weeks, that average does not well represent the real story about the group. By trying to explain the duration of lactation using an average, the authors may have missed an alternative explanation for their findings related to differences in support.

Many studies randomly assign subjects to groups to avoid major hidden differences between groups (like the amount of support they received). The premise is that if subjects are assigned by chance to receive a discharge pack, differences other than receipt of a pack between groups will be approximately the same in both groups. Differences that could confuse the explanation of findings are called **confounding variables**. In randomized assignment to groups, each group has approximately the same number of multiparas, people with good support, people with inverted nipples, and so on. Therefore, all the reasons they could have stopped nursing early are the same in both groups except for receipt of a discharge pack. Random assignment allows researchers to conclude that the reason for weaning must be the single relevant difference between the groups—receipt of a discharge pack.

The best studies go even further to check whether random assignment worked. The authors report whether the groups were different at baseline in important ways. Consider whether they checked on the right things. For example, if you believe lack of support is important in early weaning, did the researchers check their groups to be sure that the average numbers of support people reported in the pack and nonpack groups were not statistically different? This checking for the differences and similarities achieved by random assignment is reported in the methods or results section. It is not possible to check for all differences. However, it is important to check for a few major ones. If you believe the researchers omitted something critical, you may be less likely to use the findings of the study.

Most articles related to the practice of helping parents with lactation do not have randomized groups.

Rather, they use a **convenience** (**nonprobability**) sample. Therefore, for a study about discharge packs, the sample might be the first 100 nursing parents after the starting date (in which parents 1–50 do not receive packs and parents 51–100 receive packs). Checking the basic similarity of groups is even more important in convenience samples than in randomized ones.

Plausible Mechanism for Relationship

In many studies, researchers hypothesize the mechanism and do not study it directly. This is especially true when the variables are not physiological but rather psychological or sociological. It may be challenging to determine if there is a plausible mechanism for the claimed relationship between variables. For example, sometimes authors address the reason lanolin seems to help heal nipple soreness in the literature review or in the discussion section. They usually do not address this in the results section unless they have studied the possible mechanism along with the relationship between variables. Along with testing whether lanolin led to faster healing, authors may have taken microscopic photos of cell changes in nipple skin to determine whether the differences in cell changes might explain healing differences.

Many mechanisms for important relationships between variables related to lactation are not straightforward. Demonstrating a plausible mechanism for how peer support compared with professional support leads to longer durations of nursing is not straightforward. Instead of dismissing research because of an inability to demonstrate mechanisms convincingly, most scientists and clinicians require plausibility and thoughtful consideration of mechanisms. In your critical reading, consider whether a mechanism is discussed and whether you judge that mechanism to be reasonable. If there is little consideration of how and why the variables are related as the study found them to be, you may be less likely to accept the study's findings.

Spurious Relationships

Sometimes, there is little discussion of mechanism because the mechanism is obvious. The greatest danger in the lack of a plausible mechanism is the acceptance of a **spurious** relationship. Spurious relationships between variables are those that seem statistically significant but have resulted from a **correlation** with no underlying meaning. Anytime a study finds a relationship for which the authors present no plausible mechanism, it could be spurious. This most often occurs when researchers notice a correlation in their data that was not the main relationship they were studying. In doing a variety of manipulations of the data, sometimes a relationship surfaces that is statistically significant. Although the authors may mention this "finding" in their article, it is not good science to claim it as a major result. Instead, they can consider the mechanisms and recommend further research.

Applying the Findings

After critically reading research with a discerning eye, a clinician must determine whether to apply the findings in their work. The process of critique presented in this chapter is structured around the parts of a scientific article because that is how most clinicians use it. However, some more general themes of the process of critical review are not determined solely through the article's sections. As a clinician who wants to decide whether to apply the results of a study to your work, you can ask yourself several questions.

What Was and Was Not Included?

Consider what the authors chose to include and exclude in their literature review, in their subjects, in the survey questions, and in the comparisons they made in data analysis. Did they adequately explain and justify their choices? Did their choices make the sample clients or study situation so different from your practice that you cannot justify using the results?

What Else Could Have Been Done?

Consider whether there is anything else the authors could have done in their research. Could they have included more subjects in the study? Could they have studied them for a longer period? Could there have been a more diverse ethnic base? Could they have included a control group? If you identify something, ask yourself why the authors might not have done that.

What Would Affect the Findings?

Consider whether any limiting factors might have affected the study's findings. For example, in a study examining intention to nurse, you may believe the authors should have included more low-income parents. That might have affected the finding that intending to nurse for more than 12 weeks is the best predictor of continuing to nurse for at least 6 weeks. You may reason that low-income parents must return to work by 6 weeks and that therefore, fewer plan to nurse past 6 weeks. For that reason, you might have chosen some other predictor variable to tell more about what enables them to continue to nurse to 6 weeks. In considering what the researchers might have done differently, you need to question how that might have changed the study's results.

Is There Publication Bias?

Bias in scientific research exists on multiple levels. Publication bias occurs when a study's publication is dependent on the results. A study is less likely to be published when the data do not reproduce previous results or when the results refute the researchers' initial hypothesis. These results are called *negative data* or *negative results*. This publishing dilemma exists throughout medical specialties (Gadde et al., 2018; Meyer et al., 2018; Scott et al., 2019).

Although getting papers with negative results published can be challenging, it is important that researchers publish them (Emborg, 2023). Negative results can add depth to a project and help to avoid publication bias. Studies that report positive or significant results or novel (new) ideas are more likely to be published. Outcomes that are statistically significant have higher odds of being fully reported.

The underpublishing of negative or non–statistically significant results is known in the publishing world as the "file drawer problem," in which such studies languish and never reach publication (Acar et al., 2018). This skewing can overestimate treatment effectiveness and increase unreliable decision-making (Mlinarić et al., 2017; Nair, 2019).

As awareness of publication bias has grown, researchers and analysts have begun taking steps to try to account for these flaws. One such step is to register a study ahead of time so that other scholars will know about the topic and hypothesis and can watch for the results, either positive or negative. A registry is available for clinical studies with human subjects through ClinicalTrials.gov, a global database provided by the U.S. National Library of Medicine (2019). Public awareness can reduce publication bias or at least make it more transparent (Elliott & Resnik, 2019).

Research Misconduct

Misconduct, fraud, and plagiarism are an increasing concern in academic research. There has been a 10-fold increase since 1975 in the number of scientific articles retracted because of fraud. **Fabrication** is described as the invention of data or cases, and **falsification** is the willful distortion of data or results. **Plagiarism** is the copying of ideas, data, or words without attribution.

In one review of retractions in medical and life science research papers 60% of the retractions were because of plagiarism, and 76% were because of image plagiarism (Stavale et al., 2019). The most common reasons for retracting a publication in obstetrics and gynecology are plagiarism and data falsification (Chambers et al., 2019). The nongovernmental organization Retraction Watch provides an online database of retracted studies, searchable by author, journal, and topic (Retraction Watch, 2024).

Industry-funded research is at risk for corruption when it lacks controls and accountability. Misconduct occurred in research about infant feeding with work conducted by Dr. Ranjit Chandra on allergies in infants and children (Newman, 2022). Chandra's claims that Nestlé Good Start formula could reduce infants' risk of developing allergies was cited for years in journals and textbooks until it was debunked.

It can be challenging to detect when errors or misconduct occur and to expose them. Witnesses to fraud or individuals suspecting fraud may be hesitant to report it because of fear of repercussions, retaliation, and being accused of complicity (Olesen et al., 2018). Institutions need to audit research, mandate reporting in cases of threat or harm, and protect whistleblowers from retaliation. There is also a need to standardize publication ethics training for researchers globally (Schroter et al., 2018).

Practicing Critical Reading

In this section you can practice reviewing an article using the process for critical reading presented earlier. Read the following mock article using steps 1 through 9 described in Critical Reading of a Scientific Article. Consider the questions presented in each section and answer them for yourself as you progress through the article. You may find it helpful to make notes about the strengths and flaws you find as you go through the review. After you complete your review, compare your ideas with those presented in the commentary that follows the mock article. You may find that you noted ideas not mentioned in the commentary. As long as you can justify them logically or by reference to other studies, your additional commentary is valuable.

Practice Article

Refusal to Nurse–Identifying Patterns

by Emma Halter and Makit Gogh
Journal of Intermittent Phenomena. 2021;13(2):110–114.

Abstract

A questionnaire was distributed to over 700 nursing parents in two suburban pediatric practices. Of this group, 200 reported having had experience with their babies rejecting nursing. There was a great deal of variation in reasons for the refusals—in measures tried, in other life events, and in parents' feelings. Stress and biting may be two types of events that precipitate refusals. Teaching parents about possible refusal in prenatal classes may help them realize they can overcome such discouraging events.

Introduction

Nursing parents often report[1,2] that their babies display a sudden lack of interest in nursing that persists long enough to cause concern about hunger and dehydration. The parents also experience engorgement. Refusing to nurse can lead to the introduction of formula, and weaning may follow soon after. For parents who intended to continue nursing longer, such unplanned weaning is emotionally difficult. Pediatric experts agree that continuing nursing for 6 months to 1 year is best for infant health.[3] Some scientists found that parents believe that the baby's rejection of nursing is related to the return of their menses[2] or to starting oral contraceptives.[4] There has been little attempt to study this phenomenon. As a first step, we collected data on nursing couplets in two private pediatric practices and identified any patterns. The study was approved by the Review Board of Busy Hospital, and subjects gave written informed consent.

Subjects and Methods

Participants were parents of currently nursing infants who were recruited by lactation consultants, nurses, and nurse practitioners in two large suburban group pediatric practices. From March 1, 2020, to May 31, 2020, all nursing parents whose babies had appointments for any reason were invited to complete a questionnaire while they waited to visit their providers. Those who needed help with child care to complete the survey received that help.

The questionnaire (**Figure 29-6**) was developed by the authors after reviewing books for parents and professionals that suggest causes and remedies for refusal to nurse. It was designed to be concise so that parents could finish it while they waited for their appointments (about 10 minutes to complete). Descriptive statistics were calculated for most responses. Correlations were determined for demographic characteristics and responses.

Results

During the 3-month period, the combined practices received 1032 nursing couplet visits. Because some couplets had multiple appointments, 955 couplets were offered a questionnaire. Of those, 780 agreed to complete the survey. For various reasons, only 600 questionnaires were complete enough to use. Of these, 400 had never had the problem of the baby rejecting nursing for 24 hours. **Table 29-1** presents the causes the remaining 200 parents identified for the rejection. Causes included newborn jaundice, medication, surgery, illness, separation, nipple pain, teething, and unknown. Newborn jaundice and teething were the most common causes, with 30 parents citing each as a cause. The refusals of interest were those that 70 parents marked as unknown reason, other reason, or preference for another food. Of course, because these parents were nursing at the time of the appointment, they had overcome the refusal. Many of the events that occurred near a refusal also occurred in couplets that never experienced refusal. The two strongest correlations, presented in **Table 29-2**, were an increase in family stress and biting. However, together these included only 15% of couplets who experienced refusal.

Discussion

Parents need lactation professionals who are aware of the potential for refusing to nurse and who can encourage them not to give up. That is probably the most important message of this study. Short periods of rejection are common. Determining a cause is extremely difficult. On the basis of this survey, we suggest educating parents in prenatal classes about possible refusals. Cautioning them against responding strongly to biting and emphasizing the

Your help with this questionnaire is greatly appreciated. We are trying to understand why some babies occasionally stop nursing for a few feeds. Please answer as fully as you can, and feel free to add any comments you would like.

1. Are you currently nursing?☐ Yes☐ No
2. How old is your nursing baby?______How old are you?______
3. Is this your first nursing baby?☐ Yes☐ No
   A. If yes, do you have other children?☐ Yes☐ No If yes, how many?______
   B. If no, how many other children have you nursed?______
4. With your currently nursing baby, if you have had any of the following problems at any time, please check:
   ☐Difficulty latching
   ☐Sore nipples
   ☐Teething
   ☐Engorgement
   ☐Breast infection
   ☐Ductal narrowing (plugged ducts)
   ☐Baby refused to nurse
   ☐Baby had a cold or stuffy nose that interfered with feeding
   ☐Biting
5. Since your baby was born, have you resumed your menstrual periods?☐ Yes☐ No
   A. If yes, how old was your baby when menstruation resumed?______
6. Please check any of the following birth control methods you have used since this baby was born and the age of the baby when you started using it:
   Method Age of baby when started use______
   ☐Condom (male or female)
   ☐Natural family planning
   ☐Lactational amenorrhea
   ☐Depo-Provera injection
   ☐Birth control pills
   ☐Intrauterine device (IUD)
   ☐Tubal ligation
7. Has your baby ever stopped nursing for at least 24 hours?☐ Yes☐ No

If no, you have finished this questionnaire. Thank you very much.

If yes, how old was your baby at the time?______

Please check all of the following that you feel apply to your situation, or write a brief description of why you think the baby stopped nursing:

☐Nursing stopped for at least 24 hours because:
☐Parent needed a medicine and was advised to temporarily stop nursing.
☐Parent and baby were separated by an unexpected event.
☐Baby had surgery.
☐Baby was too ill to nurse.
☐Baby was jaundiced.
☐Parent had sore nipples that needed rest.
☐Baby was teething.
☐Parent returned to work.
☐Baby had bitten parent and stopped nursing soon after.
☐Baby refused to nurse but would take other food.
☐Unknown. The reason for stopping was never clear.
☐Other: Please describe why you think your baby stopped nursing:

8. Please check all of the following that describe your feelings during the time your baby did not nurse:
   ☐Concerned baby was seaning.
   ☐Worried about hunger or dehydration.
   ☐Concerned about possible engorgement.
   ☐Relieved to have a short break.
   ☐Confused about what was happening.
   ☐Confused about the cause of the refusal to nurse.
   ☐Thought baby might be sick.
   ☐Other. Please describe:
9. Please check all of the following actions you tried to help resume nursing:
   ☐Kept trying to nurse in the usual ways.
   ☐Gave my baby time to feel better.
   ☐Called the lactation consultant, healthcare provider or counselor.
   ☐Talked to a family member or friend.
   ☐Nursed when my baby was sleepy.
   ☐Increased the amount of skin-to-skin contact.
   ☐Took a bath with my baby.
   ☐Used a sling or pack.
   ☐Tried to reduce the stress in my life.
   ☐Other. Please describe:

Thank you so much for your help. If you would like to learn the results of this study, please let us know at your next appointment.

Figure 29-6 Appendix A: Questionnaire for refusal to nurse.

importance of stress management may be the most specific strategies to emerge from these data, as presented in **Table 29-3**. There is no evidence that resuming menses or taking birth control pills, as suggested by others, is causal.

References

1. Complete D. Weaning from the breast. *Feed Babies J*. 2017; 11:335–339.
2. Empp A. Common concerns of nursing parents in a food assistance program. *Nutr Group Rep*. 2019;55:37–41.
3. Healthy World Alliance. Breastfeeding best for babies. *HWA*. 2019;56:123–125.
4. Wilgot E. Postpartum menstrual cycles. *Ann Fam*. 2018;33: 293–255.

Discussion of Practice Article

Title

The title of the article is, "Refusal to Nurse—Identifying Patterns." How will the authors define refusal to nurse? Although experienced nursing parents may

Table 29-1 Reasons for Stopping Nursing

Newborn jaundice	30
Medication use	10
Surgery	12
Illness of baby	20
Nipple pain	15
Separation of parent and baby	13
Teething	30
Unknown	70
Total couplets	200

Table 29-2 Correlations Between Unexplained Refusal to Nurse and Recent Events for Nursing Dyads

Event	Number of Dyads	*r* (Correlation)
Resuming menses within 1 week of strike (<3 months old)	5	0.21
Resuming menses	3	0.15
Starting birth control within same month	2	0.09
Increase in family stress	15	0.55
Biting	16	0.59

Table 29-3 Remedies Used to Overcome Refusal to Nurse

Remedy	Percentage of Parents Who Used It
Time and patience	83
Calling lactation professional	80
Nursing during sleep	50
Skin-to-skin soothing	55
Bathing together	30
Sling or pack	34
Trying to reduce stress	42

speak of this phenomenon as though everyone agrees on it, a clear definition is necessary to determine associated variables. What should be included and excluded? You might expect rejection by the baby for a certain length of time (more than one feeding) and for no obvious reason. Would it be reasonable to allow certain probable causes and disallow others?

What "patterns" do you consider based on the title? Do the authors intend to learn whether babies at a particular age are more likely to refuse to nurse? Will they study whether increased bottle use or separation often precede episodes? For parents who have nursed other children, is it likely that prior instances of refusal in the older child correlate with more refusals in the current nursing baby? Many patterns are possible, and you can compare the patterns you would like to be investigated with what the researchers chose.

What study design does the title suggest? Is this a trial to determine whether certain events cause or specific treatments cure refusal to nurse? Do you know of other studies of this phenomenon that have gained enough basic information to conduct such a trial? For this exercise, the topic of refusing to nurse was chosen because there is not much literature on it. Therefore, a descriptive study of some sort is more likely at this point in the development of knowledge.

If the authors intended to conduct a qualitative study, what kind of data might they collect? They might ask parents to tape-record the feelings they remember having and the effect on their confidence when the baby refused to nurse. Alternatively, they might try to include parents from many different cultures and compare the ways the parents describe the experience of refusal. If they do a quantitative study, they might try to find patterns by using correlation between variables as an outcome measure.

Authors' Names

Again, because this is a mock article, you will not find these authors' names in any database. However, for an actual article, if you wanted to know whether the authors had published on this topic previously, you could search an online database such as PubMed (https://www.pubmed.gov) or EBSCO (ebscohost.com) by author name. A simple internet search will easily yield an author's contact information and university or hospital affiliation as well. The author's body of work is usually included in the professional biography on the university's website. That can provide helpful background and additional studies or areas of expertise if you need more information.

Abstract

That 200 parents claim experience with their baby refusing to nurse might be surprising. This should start you thinking about the definition again. The definition may indicate that many more babies have refused to nurse than your experience suggests. Alternatively, it could be that this problem is more widespread than anyone realizes because no one has studied its prevalence before.

The source of subjects was two pediatric suburban practices. Will the authors provide more demographic data on income, education, race, ethnic heritage, and type of insurance? Will the results apply to parents in various ethnic and demographic groups? The authors used a questionnaire, which requires literacy. Did they determine whether any subjects had trouble reading English? Did they provide the questions in languages the parents use? Did the nature of the tool exclude parents with visual disabilities or language barriers? Why did the authors single out biting and stress as events to mention in the abstract? Were these especially strong findings or the only findings that parents can modify? What is their reasoning for suggesting that prenatal education might help?

Table 29-1: Reasons for Stopping Nursing. Note first that only 200 of the 900 mentioned in the abstract appear in this table. You will want to read why in the text. Are there reasons for refusing to nurse that you had thought of that are not on this list? The investigators should explain their reasons for these choices. Note that no descriptive statistics, such as percentages, or any tests of significance appear in this table.

Table 29-2: Unexplained Refusal and Recent Events. Why does the table focus on "unexplained" refusal to nurse, and how was that defined? Why do the events listed in this table differ from the "reasons" given in **Table 29-1**? Although the correlation statistic r is presented, no statistical significance is reported. None of the correlations is high ($r = 0.7$ or above) in many definitions. Do moderate correlations like 0.55 and 0.59 represent the most powerful of the possible variables associated with refusal to nurse? Has something been omitted from the study inadvertently? The text of the article should address these questions. The explanations may be too complex to include as footnotes to the table.

Table 29-3: Remedies. Did all the parents who completed the survey resume nursing after the refusal? If so, they do not represent parents whose babies weaned after the refusal. How would limiting the data collection to parents who overcame refusal to nurse limit the applicability of the findings? Are there other remedies that the authors should have included?

Results

Note that the parents targeted by the researchers were nursing at the time of the appointment. Apparently, parents who had stopped nursing after a refusal to nurse were not included. The strongest correlations between variables included in the questionnaire were those between refusal to nurse and biting and between refusal to nurse and stress. The descriptive data appear to support this claim, but there is no report of statistical tests. Consider whether the authors convincingly ruled out alternative explanations.

1. Do the investigators offer an analysis of whether parents who did not agree to participate were similar to or different from the parents who participated? This problem is similar to the "dropout" problem discussed in the Critical Reading section under Results. Some of these parents may be unable to read English. Without knowing more about the nonparticipants, it is difficult to know how to apply (**generalize**) the results.
2. Is the list of preceding events, such as medication use, surgery, and jaundice, in **Table 29-1** sufficiently explanatory to exclude them from the study? They are potentially confounding variables if the essence of refusing to nurse is that there is no "obvious" explanation. This is where definitions and the purpose of the investigation need to be clear to interpret the data properly.
3. Are there plausible mechanisms suggested or investigated for the relationships the authors found? Typically, the results section does not discuss the mechanism unless it was the focus of the study. In a descriptive study, it is important to consider how the relationships might work for the results to be taken seriously. Even if no strong evidence is available for a mechanism, if it does not violate known principles of physiology or human behavior, it is plausible. Both biting and stress could plausibly relate to refusing to nurse. As you read more of the article, you should be able to determine whether you believe the authors' explanations.

Methods

The design of this study is descriptive and cross-sectional. It takes a snapshot of the couplets in one area during a limited-time and contacts them only once. Thus, it illustrates a cross section of the population. It is also correlational; the researchers used a structured instrument to measure variables and then sought statistically significant relationships.

Was the definition of refusing to nurse clear and appropriate? From the questionnaire, you can determine that the definition was "stopped nursing for at least 24 hours." Knowledgeable professionals could disagree with this definition. Some might prefer a different time period or different wording. What is crucial is that the authors and parents mean the same thing when they use this definition.

If there were a big discrepancy in understanding the definition, the **internal validity** of the study would be in jeopardy. Because this is a new area of research, the investigators could have done a pilot study before this large study to be more certain about the meaning of this definition. In the pilot study they could have talked in more depth with parents about their experiences with refusing to nurse. They might have suggested different definitions until the parents and researchers agreed that they were identifying the same phenomenon. They could have asked lactation and child development experts for their opinions on the definition.

If you were to use this study to try to convince childbirth educators or pediatricians to address refusing to nurse, it would be important to discuss the topic as defined in this article and not to extend the findings to a looser or stricter definition. The choices listed in the questionnaire are not defined for parents, but most are probably reasonably clear. If you can think of multiple, significantly different interpretations for any of the phrases, you may have identified a less valuable part of the data.

Questionnaire

Review the questionnaire for whether it is designed to obtain unbiased information. You could ask many questions about the quality of this one. Even if reasonable people would disagree, it is important to think about some aspects of it. Here are just a few ideas about specific questions:

1. Item 1 does not ask whether the parent is nursing exclusively or partially. With a baby younger than 6 months of age, refusing to nurse could have been the cause of a switch to partial nursing. The investigators cannot determine such a switch from this question.
2. Questions such as item 3 about previous nursing experience often fail to ask whether the experience overall was positive or negative.
3. In item 4, it is not clear what information or relationship the investigators were seeking. It might have been useful to ask the age at which the parent experienced the problem to determine whether it was close in time to when the baby refused to nurse. It should probably have an "other" category in case the parent wants to list other problems they had. Among ones that might bear some relationship to refusing to nurse are those in which the baby has had some frustration in getting enough milk. These may include delayed lactogenesis, delayed or overactive milk ejection, nipples that needed reshaping, or bottle feeding that led to poor sucking.
4. In item 6, some of the contraceptive methods listed may not be familiar to all parents, but those who had used them would probably recognize them.
5. Item 7 does not allow for multiple instances of refusing to nurse. As a result, some parents may list multiple causes, intending them to refer to separate events. Often, researchers ask parents to indicate the most recent occurrence in their answer.
6. In item 8, the age of the baby greatly influences the parent's concern about refusing to nurse. With babies who are receiving complementary foods and other liquids, a 24-hour period of refusing to nurse may not be alarming. Therefore, it might be important to discuss the correlations separately for different age groups.

Subjects could be characterized by age, the number of children they have, the number of children they nursed, return of menses, use of contraception, and problems experienced. Other variables that might influence their experience and interpretation of refusing to nurse, such as ethnic group or planned duration of nursing, are not included. This often happens in descriptive studies. You will have to decide whether the information is useful to you even with some deficiencies.

Introduction and Literature Review

Because there is little research on this topic, the review is somewhat limited. Some authors seek what they believe is related research from other topics that cover the hypotheses they wish to highlight. For example, if they related refusing to nurse to stress in the parent, they might study other research on stress responses. These authors chose to seek patterns in a large number of couplets without a specific hypothesis. If you knew of articles they failed to include, you might judge their effort to be incomplete.

Discussion

If this is a representative cross section of nursing parents, the authors' statement that refusing to nurse is common is probably true. However, we are not certain what group this sample represents. We do know that it does not represent parents who weaned after their baby refused to nurse. Therefore, it can only be a piece of the puzzle. On the other hand, if refusing to nurse is common and most nursing parents handle it smoothly, then it would be important to understand how they coped in order to help others who may consider weaning as a result.

While the suggestion to educate parents about refusing to nurse is a good one, presenting it in a childbirth class may not be the best time. Similarly, although education about biting and stress is appropriate, we cannot expect them to resolve the problem of refusing to nurse on the basis of this study alone. Furthermore, although the authors claim to have found no evidence that resuming menses or taking birth control pills caused babies to refuse to nurse, this does not constitute the best evidence. A prospective study that queried parents about refusing to nurse beginning shortly after birth and that carefully recorded other possibly relevant variables on a regular basis would more likely detect a relationship.

Results Revisited

Depending on how convinced you are that this sample resembles your clients, you may want to initiate research yourself. At the very least, you could include questions about refusing to nurse in more of your routine follow-up calls. This study, like many descriptive studies, raises more questions than it answers. The moderate correlation of stress and biting with refusing to nurse (although the statistical significance is unknown) is consistent with the claim that these are two of the more common preceding events. The greatest failure of this study is its inability to rule out alternative explanations because of study design, a poorly characterized sample, and inadequate definitions. Although the authors discuss implications for practice, there could be a lot of disagreement on clinical implications because of the degree of uncertainty about so many possible confounders.

References

The references cited for the study appear to be relevant. Even though the parents in reference 2 may be a different sample than the ones in this study, the authors use that reference only to suggest what others have noted, which is appropriate.

Summary

Critically reading a scientific article is a skill that grows with experience and strengthens your practice as a lactation professional. Learning how to read and analyze research opens many doors for continued learning. Self-direction and self-education are hallmarks of the healthcare profession. As you mature in your clinical practice, be alert for opportunities to research and publish studies of your own. Opportunities may range from case studies to large prospective studies. You could have a great impact on the understanding of lactation!

What You Learned–At a Glance

Conversation Starters with Parents

- What sources do you use for information about nursing?
- What social media platforms do you visit regularly?
- What questions do you have about the scientific basis for information about nursing?
- What do you know about how commercialism affects nursing?

Types of Articles in Scientific Journals

- Editorials, although insightful, are not studies and are not critically reviewed.
- Scientific research is subject to weaknesses and fraud, making it important to read critically and question results.
- Case studies report on instances of a problem, diagnosis, or treatment and cannot be used to generalize.
- Meta-analyses combine data from several studies to test conclusions. Meta-regression is used to strengthen the validity of conclusions.
- Reviews are written by experts who analyze the best and worst studies and include little or no original data.
- Clinical practice articles report applications in real life.
- Research reports put a long-held belief or new idea to a scientific test.
- There are many open-access (free-use) journals and articles and an increase in predatory journals.

Structure of a Scientific Article

- Titles explain main findings and may be two sentences long.
- Authors tend to publish prolifically in a specific, narrow discipline.
- Many studies are funded, and some even published, by the pharmaceutical industry.
- Abstracts are brief summaries that explain a study.
- Introductions contain the study's purpose, parameters, and restraints.
- Literature reviews explain previous research.
- Methods describe how researchers operationalized the hypothesis; explain recruitment of subjects; describe the instruments and methods used to measure outcomes; and provide a definition of terms.
- Results are often displayed in graphs, tables, and charts that are peer reviewed for accuracy.
- Discussion reviews study reasons and other relevant literature, summarize results, and suggest applications and further research.
- References list the citations referred to in the article.

Beginning Critical Reading of an Article

- Consider the title of the article and what you know about the topic, how you would have studied it, and what you expect to find.
- Read the authors' names and the abstract.
- Identify terms and key concepts.
- Study the tables and graphs.
- Read the results for subjects, relationships, and data.

Methods for Justifying Conclusions

- Study design may be retrospective, case control, prospective, cross-sectional, survey, descriptive, qualitative, experiment, or trial.
- Tools (instruments) measure dependent variables consistently.
- Statistical theory is based on probability.
- Study frequency is based on samples of populations.
- Statistical tests include distributions, centered and unbalanced bell curves, CIs, chi-square, Cohen's Kappa, Cronbach's alpha, regression, and t-tests.
- The odds ratio is a summary of relative proportions in two different groups.

Finishing the Review

- Read the introduction and literature review, and consider significance and accuracy, appropriateness of studies cited, omissions, and thoroughness of explanations.
- Read the discussion and be alert for speculation, suggestions for further research, and flaws or weaknesses.
- Read the results again to check that the data are consistent with claims and that there is no other equal or better explanation.
- Be alert for spurious relationships.
- Determine what the researchers chose to include and exclude and why.
- Research any article or scientist that raises questions. Ties to industry may or may not be disclosed in the publication (although they should be).

References

Acar F, et al. Assessing robustness against potential publication bias in activation likelihood estimation (ALE) meta-analyses for fMRI. *PLoS One.* 2018;13(11):e0208177.

Barreto JOM, et al. Competency profiles for evidence-informed policy-making (EIPM): a rapid review. *Health Res Policy Syst.* 2023;21(1):16.

Baumfeld Andre E, et al. Trial designs using real-world data: the changing landscape of the regulatory approval process. *Pharmacoepidemiol Drug Saf.* 2020;29(10):1201–1212.

Chambers LM, et al. Plagiarism and data falsification are the most common reasons for retracted publications in obstetrics and gynaecology. *BJOG.* 2019;126(9):1134–1140.

Cochrane Collaboration. About us. 2025. https://www.cochrane.org/about-us

Dinis-Oliveira RJ. Predatory journals and meetings in forensic sciences: what every expert needs to know about this "parasitic" publishing model. *Forensic Sci Res.* 2021;6(4):303–309.

Directory of Open Access Journals. Find open access journals & articles. 2025. https://www.doaj.org

EBSCO Industries, Inc. Improving research around the world. 2025. https://www.ebsco.com

Elliott KC, Resnik DB. Making open science work for science and society. *Environ Health Perspect.* 2019;127(7):75002.

Emborg ME. Reframing the perception of outliers and negative data in translational research. *Brain Res Bull.* 2023;192: 203–207.

Faupel-Badger JM, et al. Advancing translational science education. *Clin Transl Sci.* 2022;15(11):2555–2566.

Feldman AM, Mann DL. Restoring public trust in scientific research by reducing conflicts of interest. *J Clin Invest.* 2019;129(10):3971-3973.

Gadde P, et al. Do dental research journals publish only positive results? A retrospective assessment of publication bias. *J Indian Soc Periodontol.* 2018;22(4):294–297.

Gallent Torres C. Editorial misconduct: the case of online predatory journals. *Heliyon.* 2022;8(3):e08999.

Hernandez AV, et al. Meta-analysis. *Chest.* 2020;158(1S):S97–S102.

Im D, et al. Qualitative research in healthcare: data analysis. *J Prev Med Public Health.* 2023;56(2):100–110.

International Breastfeeding Journal. Home. 2025. https://internationalbreastfeedingjournal.biomedcentral.com/

JHL Editorial Team. References from predatory publishers: policy statement for the *Journal of Human Lactation*. *J Hum Lact.* 2020;36(2):219–220.

Lin L. Comparison of four heterogeneity measures for meta-analysis. *J Eval Clin Pract.* 2020;26(1):376–384.

Mathew RP, et al. Predatory journals—the power of the predator versus the integrity of the honest. *Curr Probl Diagn Radiol.* 2022;51(5):740–746.

Meyer C, et al. Is publication bias present in gastroenterological research? An analysis of abstracts presented at an annual congress. *PeerJ.* 2018;6:e4995.

Mlinarić A, et al. Dealing with the positive publication bias: why you should really publish your negative results. *Biochem Med (Zagreb).* 2017;27(3):030201.

Motani P, et al. Lessons learned from Evidence-Informed Decision-Making in Nutrition & Health (EVIDENT) in Africa: a project evaluation. *Health Res Policy Syst.* 2019;17(1):12.

Nair AS. Publication bias—importance of studies with negative results! *Indian J Anaesth.* 2019;63(6):505–507.

National Center for Biotechnology Information. About NCBI. 2025. https://www.ncbi.nlm.nih.gov/home/about/

Newman M. Formula milk companies push allergy products despite flawed evidence. *BMJ.* 2022;376:o630.

Nurses' Health Study. Home. 2025. https://www.nurseshealthstudy.org/

Olesen AP, et al. In their own words: research misconduct from the perspective of researchers in Malaysian universities. *Sci Eng Ethics.* 2018;24(6):1755–1776.

Polit D, Beck C. *Essentials of Nursing Research: Appraising Evidence for Nursing Practice.* 10th ed. Philadelphia, PA: Lippincott Williams & Wilkins; 2022.

Public Library of Science. Open Science. 2025. https://plos.org/open-science/

Retraction Watch. Retraction watch database user guide. 2024. https://retractionwatch.com/retraction-watch-database-user-guide/

Riegelman RK. *Studying a Study and Testing a Test: Reading Evidence-Based Health Research.* 7th ed. Philadelphia, PA: Wolters Kluwer/Lippincott Williams & Wilkins; 2020.

Schroter S, et al. Biomedical authors' awareness of publication ethics: an international survey. *BMJ Open.* 2018;8(11):e021282.

Scott J, et al. An evaluation of publication bias in high-impact orthopaedic literature. *JB JS Open Access.* 2019;4(2):e0055.

Stavale R, et al. Research misconduct in health and life sciences research: a systematic review of retracted literature from Brazilian institutions. *PLoS One.* 2019;14(4):e0214272.

Strong G. Understanding quality in research: avoiding predatory journals. *J Hum Lact.* 2019;35(4):661–664.

U.S. Lactation Consultant Association. Clinical Lactation. 2025. uslca.org/clinical-lactation

U.S. National Library of Medicine. ClinicalTrials.gov. 2019. clinicaltrials.gov/ct2/home

Wiessinger D. Watch your step. *J Hum Lact.* 2021;37(3):464–468.

Xu C, Doi SAR. The robust error meta-regression method for dose-response meta-analysis. *Int J Evid Based Healthc.* 2018;16(3):138–144.

CHAPTER 30

Improving the Lactation Landscape

Promoting lactation presents unique challenges in societies where artificial feeding is perceived as the norm. Lactation promotion requires strong, confident leadership in changing the status quo in infant feeding. Seeking to understand other points of view and working for everyone's mutual benefit can help win support and arrive at creative solutions. Being an effective change agent requires assertiveness, persuasion, and an appreciation for the importance of giving recognition and praise. Understanding why others resist change helps resolve conflicts and identify common goals. This will help in defining problems and strategies for collaboration to overcome them and optimize health outcomes for families.

KEY TERMS

Assertiveness
Change agent
Personality types
Plan-Do-Study-Act (PDSA)
Social marketing
Transformational leadership

Strong Leadership

We inherently prefer to work with people we like. Human nature draws us to people who are cheerful, generous, and considerate of others. People who naturally exude these qualities find it easier to generate cooperation from those around them. Others may need to make a determined effort to present themselves in a manner that achieves positive results. Part of being an effective leader is instilling confidence in others. People respond well to a leader who is self-confident, assertive, and forthright.

Leadership Attributes

Effective leaders are approachable and inclusive. They are attentive, guard against snap judgments, and embrace change. The skills of a proficient leader include compassion, collaboration and participation, transparency, reflection, problem-solving, and accountability (Sullivan, 2017). Charisma, creativity, and innovation are common traits of an effective leader (Salau et al., 2018). Clinical leaders typically have values and beliefs that parallel their actions and interventions (Stanley & Stanley, 2018).

An effective problem-solver identifies problem areas, focuses on solutions, and prioritizes actions. When faced with questionable practices or unsupportive coworkers, a leader will try to learn the reasons for resistance to or lack of interest in what is proposed. Being attentive, with a goal of understanding what has led to a situation or the status quo, is an important first step to exploring appropriate solutions and garnering support for meaningful change.

The word *responsible* means that we are *able* to choose a *response*. It is not what happens to us but our *response* to what happens to us that determines the outcome. Although it is human nature to react immediately to events, there is always a gap between a stimulus and a response. The key to being effective is using that gap to choose an appropriate response. A spontaneous response is usually impulsive and based on feelings aroused by conditions. Such an impetuous reaction lacks forethought and may not lead to responsible action. A proactive leader helps others consider all elements of a proposed change before they choose their response.

Increasing Self-Confidence

Effective leaders do not allow fear of failure to undermine their self-confidence. When we do not produce the desired results, we need to change our approach. When we make a mistake or a wrong turn, we should acknowledge it, learn, and go on. Making mistakes is part of being a good leader and problem-solver. Leadership is a learning process that is strengthened as much by every failure as by every success. Responding to mistakes with purposeful insight is a sign of strength. Effective leaders help others recognize that every defeat is a step toward success.

Self-confidence is essential in actively facilitating change. How successful we view ourselves to be can determine the level of success we achieve. Focusing on our faults rather than on our strengths can prevent us from reaching our promotion goals. Increasing your creative confidence requires overcoming fear of the unknown, fear of being judged, fear of taking a first step, and fear of losing control. The principles outlined in this section will help you maintain perspective and increase your ability to act in a self-assured manner.

Much of our attitude involves the vocabulary we use in self-talk. If we continually expect to fail, we probably *will* fail! We can replace negative thoughts such as "I hope I don't . . ." with positive self-talk such as "I will . . ." (This is like parents who say they will *try* to nurse instead of that they *will* nurse.) We can convince ourselves how confident we are by saying to ourselves, "I am . . ." rather than "I wish I were . . ." or "I should be . . ." **Table 30-1** contains powerful statements to replace those that convey less affirmative messages. Positive and negative thinking are both learned habits. We can reprogram our minds to think positively by replacing negative thoughts with positive ones. Approach every situation with the belief that you will succeed. Focus on the best way to do the job right, and visualize yourself doing it!

Table 30-1 Powerful Language

Don't Say	Do Say
I have to . . .	I'll be glad to . . .
I'm no good at . . .	I'm getting better . . .
I failed . . .	Here's what I learned . . .
I'm going under . . .	I'm bouncing back . . .
This drives me crazy . . .	I can find a better way . . .
I can't do anything about it . . .	It's my responsibility to change . . .
We should have it ready by . . .	We will have it ready by . . .
Generally speaking, I tend to think . . .	I believe . . .
Do you have any questions?	What questions do you have?
It's not my fault. I couldn't help it.	I'm sorry. It was my responsibility.

Emotional Intelligence

A high level of emotional intelligence is required for problem-solving, interpersonal relations, stress management, and effective conflict management (Başoğul & Özgür, 2016). *Emotional intelligence* refers to the ability to identify and manage our emotions, as well as the emotions of others. It includes such attributes as self-awareness, self-understanding, impulse control, persistence, zeal, self-motivation, empathy, and tactfulness. You can improve your professional abilities by seeking to understand what others are trying to tell you, both verbally and nonverbally. Practice empathizing with others by imagining how you would feel in their circumstances. Consider how your emotions influence your decisions and behaviors (Gilar-Corbi et al., 2019).

Emotional intelligence in healthcare professionals positively affects caring behaviors. It can be influenced by age, experience, burnout, and job satisfaction (Nightingale et al., 2018). Higher emotional intelligence is correlated with increased leadership traits. As an individual's experience in health care grows, so, too, can emotional intelligence (Coskun et al., 2018). Emotionally intelligent leadership is important for providing high-quality health care (Carragher & Gormley, 2017). There is also a positive relationship between emotional competence and team members' attitudes about work. Emotionally intelligent leaders can improve behavior and teamwork (Coronado-Maldonado et al., 2023).

Increasing Assertiveness

High levels of **assertiveness** are characteristics of strong leaders and problem-solvers. Embracing assertive behavior as a strong asset increases our comfort and effectiveness when presenting ideas to others. Assertiveness is a learnable skill that can lower stress, reduce burnout, and improve competence (Kim, 2016; Yoshinaga et al., 2018). Being assertive involves recognizing a problem, suggesting a solution, identifying the behavior that is causing the problem, and expressing beliefs about the problem.

Lack of assertiveness and confidence is a barrier to leadership advancement for women in global health. Healthcare providers who assist with lactation are predominantly female. Women tend to be less assertive in self-promotion and more assertive when advocating for others. Women may worry that others will perceive their assertiveness negatively and interpret it as aggressive behavior. Reluctance to challenge healthcare practices may stem from a fear of conflict, stress, or reprisal. Assertiveness can lead to reframing confrontation to gain clarity instead of a means to engage in conflict.

Analyzing assertive behavior in others can increase our own assertiveness. Identify what it is about others that you admire. Observe what they say and how they say it, and decide which approaches and traits you want to emulate. You can then analyze your behavior and the ways you typically respond in situations that call for assertiveness. Do others pay attention when you have something important to say? Can you convince others of the merit of your information? Analyze times when you were assertive and times when you were not. Reflect on times when your actions were perceived as aggressive. Consider the language you used in each situation, including the nonverbal messages you conveyed. You might even document how you behaved in various situations, what worked, and what you could have done differently to be more effective.

You can practice assertiveness in everyday interactions with family, friends, coworkers, neighbors, and store clerks. Visualize yourself being assertive, and role-play situations with others. When you feel confident that you can approach an issue assertively, undertake an easy challenge first—one with a likelihood of success. If the results are not what you had planned, examine why it did not go the way you wanted, and reflect on what you can do differently. Keep a positive attitude and adjust your approach to the next challenge. Do not allow one setback to discourage you from continuing to work toward more assertive behavior.

Becoming a Change Agent

Being a **change agent** is key to reducing barriers to lactation and updating practices to support nursing families. A change agent is an individual who acts as a catalyst for change. Healthcare professionals are in an ideal position to plan and implement improvements in lactation promotion. Strong interprofessional healthcare teams develop ways of collaborating that enable leaders and followers to excel (Barry et al., 2021). Effective change agents possess leadership skills to command respect and the ability to navigate barriers and improve practices.

Transformational leadership helps facilitate the high-quality leadership and management needed for implementing change. The term *transformational leadership* refers to a leader's ability to inspire followers to change their expectations, perceptions, and motivations to work toward common goals. Transformational leaders work with a team to identify needed change, create a vision to guide the change, and initiate the change in tandem with the team. This approach encourages group collaboration and decision-making.

Recognizing the Need for Change

Recognizing the need to promote lactation correlates with society's perception of infant feeding. New parents receive continual messages that present infant formula and bottle feeding as the cultural norm for infants. Changing practices to support and promote lactation requires a cultural shift in the perception of infant feeding. Cultural beliefs evolve from the way people perceive their world. We cannot persuade others to change their perceptions and beliefs. Change must happen intrinsically from the inside out and at a pace that is comfortable for those who are undergoing the change. Creating high levels of trust and respect promotes open discussion and enhances beliefs that change is needed.

Figure 30-1 illustrates how two people can perceive the same image differently. One person readily recognizes an aristocratic young woman with a stylish hat. Another perceives a haggard older woman with a large nose, wearing a scarf. Neither perception is right or wrong. Each person simply perceives one image more readily than the other. In other words, one image stands out more clearly than the other and is recognized more easily. However, another more subtle image is also present and can be perceived with greater effort. Understanding this duality in perception sheds light on the challenge inherent in lactation promotion.

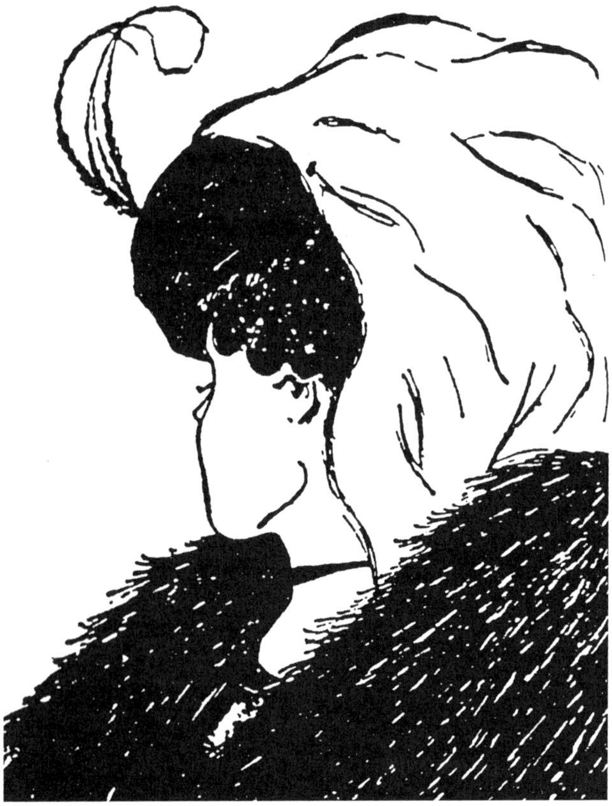

Figure 30-1 Both a young aristocratic lady and an older woman can be perceived in this illustration.

Reproduced from Hill, W. E. (William Ely), 1887-1962. Library of Congress Prints and Photographs Division Washington, D.C. 20540 USA. Retrieved from http://loc.gov/pictures/resource/ds.00175/

Assessing Readiness for Change

Organizations that value adaptability embrace change. Assessing readiness and increasing efforts to create individual, group, and organizational readiness for change will increase the likelihood of successful change. Employees' attitudes toward change are critical to successful implementation. Job satisfaction and organizational commitment are key elements in readiness for change. For employees to embrace a change, they must believe the change is needed, feel capable of implementing the change, and believe the change will benefit them. As the scale of change increases, employees may feel less positive about the process. Limiting the scope of the change may increase employee receptiveness.

The level of staff engagement strengthens the work climate for individual change readiness. Staff support will be greatest when changes feature their active input, and when changes are well founded and well communicated (Nilsen et al., 2019). People who participate in decisions feel empowered, with a sense of control and ownership of the change. Teamwork and participation in decision-making promote higher engagement and lower burnout (Hung & Chen, 2017). Implementing group-based interventions will help develop positive beliefs and collective readiness for change.

An organization that is receptive to change engages in efforts to identify, understand, accept, and internalize the emotions it arouses. Emotional turbulence is characteristic of strategic change. Leaders with the ability to manage emotionally turbulent situations develop mutual trust and respect to help people feel comfortable openly expressing themselves. High-quality communication increases acceptance, openness, and commitment. Failure to provide sufficient information, or providing poor-quality information, can create cynicism and rumors that may exaggerate the negative aspects of change. Handling a change effectively can avoid the risk of it being undermined or sabotaged.

Anticipating Resistance to Change

As common and inevitable as change is, people do not always welcome it. Understanding why others are resistant helps efforts to facilitate meaningful change. Resistance can be expressed in various ways. Individuals may be passively resistant by demonstrating either avoidance or a preference for what is consistent with their personal attitudes. Some may challenge the change, the source, or the tactics used. Others may selectively process aspects of the change that favor their original attitudes or behavior. Still others may assert their own views instead of challenging the change.

Recognizing that resistance is a natural part of the change process helps you capitalize on it and use it as a tool. Resistance can help identify weaknesses in the change strategies and plans. A low level of individual, group, or organizational readiness for change may present important insights for developing and improving the approach. Concerns from people with deep knowledge about the institution provides valuable insights and can lead to buy-in for the change.

Stages of Resistance to Change

Members of the team planning the change will vary in their level of acceptance or resistance. People who are most receptive will acknowledge that a problem exists and enthusiastically help to bring about the desired outcome. A more resistant person may argue that there is no problem and thus no need for change. Some members of the group may recognize the need for change but do not feel invested in it or doubt it will make a difference. Creating a safe place for everyone to discuss their reservations openly with the group will help members work through their reservations. Members need to move beyond their individual issues to focus on the group's efforts to plan and implement meaningful change.

The stages of resistance presented here are adapted from educational materials developed by SARAR International and published by World Neighbors in Action (Anand, 2005). Some possible arguments against lactation promotion appear with each stage. The stages are as follows:

1. *There is no problem.* I know human milk is good for babies, but infant formula is perfectly safe. It has fed babies for decades. Furthermore, parents have a right to choose how they want to feed their babies. They shouldn't be made to feel guilty if they choose to use formula.
2. *I recognize there is a problem, but it's not my responsibility.* I accept that nursing is superior to formula feeding. But I can't get involved. I don't have the time. Someone else will do it.
3. *I accept that we have a problem, but I doubt anyone's ability to change it.* Formula companies are too strong and influential, and our society does not see a problem.
4. *I accept there is a problem, but I'm afraid to get involved.* If I make too many waves, I might lose my job. I'm afraid of what others will think of me. I'm afraid of the time commitment.
5. *We believe we can do something about it, and I will begin to seek solutions.* We have a problem with infant feeding. I want to empower parents and help improve infant health. I will get involved, but I'm still unsure if we can make a difference.
6. *We know we can do it, and obstacles will not stop us.* I know I can make a difference. Working together, we can change things. Let's get started!
7. *We did it!* We finally have policies and procedures that promote lactation, and our staff is following the guidelines. We have returned control to parents and babies and are empowering parents to reach their feeding goals. Let's share our results with others!

Team members need to respect the process of change their colleagues undertake. Everyone enters the process at varying stages in their acceptance of an anticipated change. Each individual needs time and patience to progress at their own rate and cannot be expected to jump forward several stages at once. Many times, the greatest resister becomes one of the staunchest advocates when given the opportunity to progress through the necessary stages that lead to understanding and embracing a change. Some individuals may seem to slide backward during the period of change, depending on specific issues or information that surfaces. Some people never change their opinions or beliefs. Patience and flexibility are cornerstones to establishing consensus for moving forward with positive change.

Resistance to the Ten Steps to Successful Breastfeeding

The Ten Steps to Successful Breastfeeding are a guide to instituting changes in lactation policies and practices. By anticipating the reasons people resist these guidelines, you can select an approach to help resolve issues before they become obstacles. **Table 30-2** identifies examples of responses that may occur relative to each of the steps for lactation promotion.

Reasons for Resistance to Change

Understanding why someone resists the idea of change helps determine the most effective approach. Acceptance depends on the type of change and the amount of anxiety it elicits. Employees who trust management and identify with the organization tend to react positively toward change. Those who feel negatively tend to be ambivalent or resistant. Proposed changes in policies and practices will alter the way things have always been done. A change in routine can create tension and stress resulting from employee turnover, political battles, and a drain on money and time. Successfully motivating other people to accept change requires understanding their reasons for resistance.

Loss of Control. How people greet a change depends on the degree to which they feel they are in control of it. People who resist a change in routine may worry about losing their feeling of self-efficacy or power. Just as loss of control can lead to resistance, ownership typically leads to commitment. At every step in the process, it is important to recognize that change is exciting when it is done *by* us, and it is threatening when it is done *to* us. Increasing each person's involvement and participation and empowering them with legitimate choices promotes ownership.

Uncertainty. People who are unprepared mentally can feel threatened by a change, and their natural reaction is to resist. They may feel uncertain about where a proposed change will lead. Openly

Table 30-2 Responses to Arguments Against the Ten Steps to Successful Breastfeeding

Step 1	***(a) Comply fully with the International Code of Marketing of Breast-milk Substitutes and relevant World Health Assembly resolutions; (b) Have a written infant feeding policy that is routinely communicated to staff and parents; and (c) Establish ongoing monitoring and data-management systems.***
Stage of Resistance	**Argument**
There is no problem	We've had a policy for years. It's working well enough. We've been functioning well enough without a policy.
It's not my responsibility	I have too much to do already. I wouldn't know where to even begin writing a policy.
No one can do it	Even if we had a policy, no one would follow it. If parents aren't motivated to nurse, why bother?
I can't get involved	There are too many on the staff opposed to it. I wouldn't be able to get support from my supervisor.
Let's begin	I can explore policies in other hospitals. I can locate resources to help us with our policy.
We can do it	Let's bring people together from all departments to work on it. Let's survey our clients to learn how satisfied they are.
We did it!	We accomplished our goal! We have an infant feeding policy that promotes lactation and is routinely communicated to staff and parents.
Step 2	***Ensure that staff have sufficient knowledge, competence, and skills to support breastfeeding.***
Stage of Resistance	**Argument**
There is no problem	We have lactation consultants, so we don't need to train the rest of the staff. Our nurses know what they need to know about lactation.
It's not my responsibility	I don't have time to train everyone. I wouldn't know where to even begin with training.
No one can do it	The staff would never agree to extensive training. We don't have enough money or time to train the entire staff.
I can't get involved	Staff members would resent my suggestion that they need the training. I wouldn't be able to get support from my supervisor.
Let's begin	I can explore how other hospitals educate their staff. I will take an extensive course in lactation.
We can do it	Let's survey staff members to find out what they know about lactation. Let's form a committee with people from several departments.
We did it!	We accomplished our goal! Our staff are competent in supporting lactation.
Step 3	***Discuss the importance and management of breastfeeding with pregnant women and their families.***
Stage of Resistance	**Argument**
There is no problem	We give help and advice to parents when they are in the hospital. Teaching about lactation will create guilt in those who don't nurse.
It's not my responsibility	Parents learn what they need to know in their childbirth classes. It's the parents' responsibility to seek information.

No one can do it	We don't have the resources for prenatal teaching. Our clients want to formula feed.
I can't get involved	I don't have time to do prenatal teaching. I wouldn't be able to get support from my supervisor.
Let's begin	I can explore prenatal classes in other hospitals. I can make a questionnaire to screen parents with difficulties.
We can do it	Let's survey our clients to find out how satisfied they are. Let's explore what we can improve during labor and delivery.
We did it!	We accomplished our goal! Our staff helps expectant families understand the importance and management of lactation.
Step 4	***Facilitate immediate and uninterrupted skin-to-skin contact and support mothers to initiate breastfeeding as soon as possible after birth.***
Stage of Resistance	**Argument**
There is no problem	We start parents nursing as soon as they get to their room. Most babies are too sleepy to nurse right away.
It's not my responsibility	Relatives are excited to visit the baby. I'm too busy with postdelivery procedures.
No one can do it	The labor and delivery staff would never support such a policy. Babies get too cold nursing in the delivery room.
I can't get involved	The staff is getting tired of all my suggestions about lactation. I'm not very good at persuading people.
Let's begin	I can find someone in labor and delivery who will support the change. I can teach the staff about the importance of early initiation of nursing.
We can do it	Let's try it on a short-term basis and then evaluate it. We can find ways to keep babies warm in the delivery room.
We did it!	We accomplished our goal! Our staff helps parents initiate uninterrupted skin-to-skin contact and breastfeeding as soon as possible after birth.
Step 5	***Support mothers to initiate and maintain breastfeeding and manage common difficulties.***
Stage of Resistance	**Argument**
There is no problem	Nursing is a natural instinct; we don't need to teach it. There are plenty of support groups to help parents.
It's not my responsibility	I don't have time to help parents manage difficulties. I can't possibly visit every nursing parent.
No one can do it	We don't have enough staff to spend the time required for this. A lot of our staff don't believe in pushing lactation.
I can't get involved	I wouldn't get support from my supervisor for the time it would take. Staff won't spend so much time with nursing parents.
Let's begin	I can encourage staff to accompany me on rounds. I can propose telephone follow-up for nursing parents.
We can do it	Let's survey our clients about what would have helped them. Let's explore a program to mentor staff in lactation.
We did it!	We accomplished our goal! Our staff helps parents initiate and maintain nursing and manage common difficulties.

(continues)

Table 30-2 Responses to Arguments Against the Ten Steps to Successful Breastfeeding *(continued)*

Step 6	***Do not provide breastfed newborns any food or fluids other than breast milk, unless medically indicated.***
Stage of Resistance	**Argument**
There is no problem	We never do anything unless it is medically indicated. I am legally responsible for ensuring that the baby is not dehydrated.
It's not my responsibility	I can't influence hospital policies. Purchase of formula is an administrative decision, not mine.
No one can do it	The administration will never agree to begin purchasing formula. Formula companies will withdraw other funding if we make this change.
I can't get involved	I would not be able to get support from my supervisor. I won't be responsible for withholding fluids from a hypoglycemic baby.
Let's begin	I can explore how other hospitals have begun purchasing formula. I can teach staff the importance of exclusive nursing.
We can do it	Let's review the reasons we have been giving formula and water. Let's invite some parents in to discuss how they managed.
We did it!	We accomplished our goal! Our staff does not give nursing newborns any food or fluids other than human milk, unless medically indicated.
Step 7	***Enable mothers and their infants to remain together and to practice rooming-in 24 hours a day.***
Stage of Resistance	**Argument**
There is no problem	We have better security if babies are kept in the nursery. Babies could choke if they stay in the parents' rooms.
It's not my responsibility	Parents are tired after laboring and delivering. That is an administrative decision.
No one can do it	Nursery staff will lose their jobs if babies stay with their parents. Parents do not want to keep their babies in the room.
I can't get involved	I will never get support from the administration. The pediatric providers will not examine babies in the parents' rooms.
Let's begin	I can explore rooming-in policies at other hospitals. I can teach staff the importance of keeping babies and parents together.
We can do it	Let's invite pediatric providers to meet with the lactation committee. Let's record how much time babies spend away from their parents.
We did it!	We accomplished our goal! Our staff promotes 24-hour rooming-in for parents and their infants.
Step 8	***Support mothers to recognize and respond to their infants' cues for feeding.***
Stage of Resistance	**Argument**
There is no problem	It is more efficient to have scheduled feeding times. Babies need to get on a schedule as early as possible.
It's not my responsibility	I can teach the parents I visit, but I can't visit all of them. Parents will know when their baby wants to nurse.
No one can do it	Staff routines would be disrupted too much with unscheduled feedings. It would be too hard to monitor babies for hypoglycemia without a schedule.

I can't get involved	We have a lactation consultant who teaches parents. The logistics for unscheduled feedings would be too confusing.
Let's begin	I can teach staff the importance of the parent and baby setting the pace. I can help staff learn to recognize and teach feeding cues.
We can do it	Let's keep statistics to determine if schedules make a difference. Let's try it for 6 months and evaluate how it works.
We did it!	We accomplished our goal! Our staff teaches parents how to recognize and respond to their infants' feeding cues.
Step 9	***Counsel mothers on the use and risks of feeding bottles, teats and pacifiers.***
Stage of Resistance	**Argument**
There is no problem	We have to test sucking and swallowing with a bottle. Babies have strong sucking needs and pacifiers keep them calm.
It's not my responsibility	If parents want to use pacifiers, it is not my position to discourage them. Everyone uses pacifiers, so what's the big deal?
No one can do it	I'm the only one in the hospital who considers this to be a problem. Pacifiers and baby bottles are a part of our culture.
I can't get involved	The staff will think it takes too long to feed babies with a cup or spoon. There is nothing to document the use of cups for feeding babies.
Let's begin	I can teach staff about sucking preference and confusion. I can teach the staff how to cup feed a baby.
We can do it	Let's review why we use bottles. Let's teach parents to nurse rather than giving a pacifier.
We did it!	We accomplished our goal! Our staff counsels parents on the use and risks of feeding bottles, teats, and pacifiers.
Step 10	***Coordinate discharge so that parents and their infants have timely access to ongoing support and care.***
Stage of Resistance	**Argument**
There is no problem	We have the information at the desk if parents request it. Support groups make parents feel guilty if they wean early.
It's not my responsibility	Parents should seek help when they need it. Healthcare providers will refer parents for help if there is a problem.
No one can do it	We don't have enough resources to start a support group. Peer counselors do not always give sound advice and information.
I can't get involved	If I did this, I would have to do it on my own time. I don't have the resources to keep updating a referral list.
Let's begin	I can visit community support groups and foster a strong link. I can offer to train support counselors.
We can do it	Let's give a name and telephone number to nursing parents at discharge. Let's explore beginning an outpatient clinic and/or support group.
We did it!	We accomplished our goal! Our staff ensures that parents have timely access to ongoing support and care after discharge.

Adapted from World Health Organization. Ten Steps to Successful Breastfeeding. 2018. https://www.who.int/teams/nutrition-and-food-safety/food-and-nutrition-actions-in-health-systems/ten-steps-to-successful-breastfeeding?ua=1 sharing what is happening with everyone involved and providing sufficient groundwork or preparation can help to allay doubts and fears. Dividing a big change into several small steps over an extended period allows settling into one part of a change before experiencing the next step. Making sure everyone understands what will take place and when to expect more information helps to minimize uncertainty.

Difference. Routines will be different when change occurs, and some people want things to remain the same. With change, people must question familiar routines and habits. They must actively think about behaviors they had taken for granted and "reprogram" their daily routines. Conducting an inventory of current practices will help you keep what you are doing right and change only what needs to be adjusted. Minimizing the number of changes and leaving as many habits and routines as possible in place can help everyone find their comfort level.

Loss of Respect. Some people may believe that a proposed change implies that the old ways were wrong. They may feel embarrassed and self-conscious and fear seeming foolish because of past actions. Help everyone appreciate that their past actions were based on what was considered appropriate at the time. Practices evolve and change as new research and new knowledge become available. Praise others for their accomplishments under the old conditions and thank them for their willingness to evolve to meet present needs. Help them understand that you, too, have changed your practices, and encourage them to view the change positively.

Competence. Understandably, the prospect of change can cause concern about future competence. It is natural for people to worry about their ability to be effective with new practices. New ways often demand a new set of competencies, and they may wonder, "Can I do it?" or "*How* will I do it?" Equipping everyone with the necessary knowledge and skills for performing under the new rules is critical to success. Having access to experiential training, tools, techniques, and best practices will help others respond to the change (Aitkenhead et al., 2019; Visser et al., 2019). Positive reinforcement and ample opportunity to practice new skills without judgment through a formal mentorship or other supervised training allow others to observe and practice skills in a nonthreatening setting.

Disruption. A proposed change can be disruptive to some of the people involved. For example, it may interrupt plans or projects that others believe are more worthy. Meeting a deadline or attending a meeting may intrude on people's personal time. The time commitment required could interfere with days they are not scheduled to work or with planned family activities. Staff members may be required to go "above and beyond" their usual efforts, with more energy, time, and mental preoccupation devoted to the change. Validate these concerns and give support and recognition for the extra effort. Introduce changes with flexibility, and be sensitive to the effect the process has on those who must implement the change and operate in a new way.

Past Grievances. Sometimes unresolved grievances from the past can surface as you approach others with a proposed change. Undercurrents of professional jealousy or other resentments may obstruct efforts to achieve unity within the group. Perhaps someone had sought your support for a previous activity and was not satisfied with your response or your seeming lack of support. Perhaps a predecessor or colleague alienated staff with an offensive approach, and your motives are questioned. Teamwork requires leaving past grievances at the door so that everyone enters the process with equal status and an open mind. Remaining nonjudgmental and objective can help the team address past issues that could color attitudes so that everyone can focus on the present issues.

Real Threat. When a change occurs, the traditional way of doing things is replaced with new routines and a new set of expectations that challenge people to modify their practices. The process that took place may transform relationships among colleagues as well. Despite efforts at collaboration and unity, instituting a change may result in people needing to change their roles or lose status or power. For example, a proposed change to institute 24-hour rooming-in would alter staff routines and keep babies with their parents most of the time. Some staff will adapt to couplet care, while others may dislike the change enough to seek another role, resign, or retire. Everyone needs a supportive climate in which to let go of the past. Be sensitive to the loss of routines, comforts, traditions, rituals, and relationships. Avoid any pretense or false promises. Accept that a perceived threat is sometimes real. Some people may find the change too difficult or too disruptive to negotiate and thrive.

Conflict Management and Resolution

Introducing change inevitably creates a certain degree of conflict, which may surface as disagreement or discord. Conflict can be internal, between individuals, or between groups. It may arise because of opinion differences, competing goals, negative perceptions, poor communication, or unclear role expectations. Avoiding or ignoring conflict can lead to further conflict. Effective leaders embrace conflict as a natural part of the change process and manage it rationally and productively. *Conflict management* is an umbrella term for the way we identify and handle conflicts. It involves attempting to understand specific concerns and worries and recognizing an issue the way others perceive it.

Keeping an open mind and validating others' concerns and points of view can help resolve conflict. Conflict resolution is a form of negotiation, mediation, and diplomacy that reconciles opposing views while respecting and protecting the people involved. Conflict can be productive when it is brought out in the open to allow honest, frank, and positive relationships to develop among group members. It is through conflict that people learn to understand others and recognize the value of working together. Resolved conflict draws people closer together. In health care, effective conflict resolution can enhance team performance, lead to creative solutions, and improve client safety and outcomes.

Inevitably, conflicts will continue to surface as the process of change continues. It is better to address issues as they arise, no matter how minor they may seem. This fosters an environment in which honesty prevails and where neither side keeps an "account" of grievances against the other. People inherently work to satisfy their own personal needs, such as a need for money, power, self-actualization, or identity. They generally want others to accept them as they are and to like and appreciate them. Consequently, to resolve conflict, you must meet the other person's needs as well as your own.

Be Sensitive to Others

Sensitivity to another person's circumstances is important in all communication, and especially when a conflict occurs. Avoid confronting conflict in a public setting or in the presence of others who are uninvolved. Keep in mind that you are attempting to change behaviors, not people. Focusing on solutions rather than on individual problems will preserve solid relationships. Find ways for team members to work together through conflicts that stand in the way of reaching your goals. Because conflict involves both issues and feelings, it is important to get emotions out of the way before attempting to solve problems. When emotions surface, reflecting them back through active listening recognizes and validates them. This sets the stage for moving on to address problems and work toward solutions.

Coping with Difficult People

It is common for someone on your team to be regarded as difficult. You have tried everything in your arsenal to work with this person cooperatively. You have validated feelings and acknowledged concerns, and yet you continually meet with resistance. A change in approach may achieve more positive results. You cannot change the other person and you cannot directly change the way that person responds to you. What you *can* change is the way you relate to that person.

Finding a more effective way to communicate and present yourself can indirectly influence how the other person will respond:

- Be positive and avoid placing blame. Give recognition and praise for accomplishments.
- Write down exactly what you plan to say. This helps prepare for the interaction and helps release any underlying negativism before a confrontation. Role-playing the scenario may also help.
- Be aware of your body language. Face the person squarely, sit or stand erect, and lean forward to demonstrate a desire to interact in a meaningful way.
- Give your undivided attention and respond both verbally (e.g., "I understand . . ."; "I'm with you") and nonverbally (e.g., nodding, smiling, and maintaining eye contact).
- Recycle the other person's message to make sure you understood it correctly. After you have stated the message, pause for a response before continuing to speak.

Attention to the dynamics of meetings can help neutralize the efforts of a difficult person. Before the meeting, you can obtain input and support from others in the group. During the meeting, you can solicit reactions from allies by asking, for example, "How would you . . ."; "What do you think of . . ."; or "How many would agree?" Where you sit in a meeting can also reduce divisiveness. Sitting next to a difficult person minimizes the potential for conflict. It is difficult to spar with someone who is sitting immediately next to you. The various types of difficult people are presented in the next section.

The Aggressor. Some people are aggressive to the point of being hostile. They have a strong sense of what others should do and how they should do it, and they can be abrasive, abrupt, intimidating, and relentless. Their goal is to prove that you are wrong and they are right. An angry person cannot stay overtly angry for long if you remain calm. Be attentive and ready to answer quietly yet assertively. If they interrupt you, you can hold your ground by saying, "Let me finish." It is important not to allow an aggressor to seize control with negative energy.

The Saboteur. Someone may sabotage your efforts from behind the scenes. Although they avoid direct confrontation, they can be as divisive as one who confronts you openly. A saboteur may genuinely believe they are doing the right thing. They may frequently bring up irrelevant issues or question previous decisions. Never ignore a sniper! Left unchecked, this person can breed discontent and slowly undermine everyone's best efforts. Learn to recognize sabotage and minimize its effects. Address this person's behavior either privately or with a supervisor, as appropriate.

The Defeatist. A defeatist can infect others by dampening enthusiasm and undermining positive thinking. These people argue that "It won't work" or "It's no use" and refuse to buy into what the group is trying to accomplish. One way to challenge such people is to ask them for ideas on positive, realistic ways to solve problems. Take their complaints seriously and ask, "What's the worst possible scenario?" These people can bring strength to the group by identifying things that could go wrong. Put the matter back in their hands and engage them in considering solutions. Ask them to help identify tasks, processes, and people who may be affected by the proposed change. Engaging their talents in this way values their contributions to the process.

The Expert. People who consider themselves experts may appear pompous and arrogant. They can also be productive and talented when their participation is channeled appropriately. Avoid trying to assert yourself as the expert, and instead show that you respect their opinion and ask them to explain their point further. Be prepared and accurate in your interactions with these people. If their opinion is at odds with your recommendations, make sure that what you recommend is evidence-based and is supported by peer-reviewed research. You can ask politely for the same evidence for their recommendations as well. Asking them to research any new procedure or process helps invest them in the team and in the outcomes.

Achieving Unity

Identifying basic goals that everyone shares can establish common ground and help set the stage for debating strategies for moving forward. One common objective in lactation promotion is empowering new parents to achieve their goals. With that as a starting point, the group can begin to discuss strategies to accomplish this. You can then move on to determine how to meet on common ground with other related issues. Flexibility and compromise will help your team work through differences to achieve consensus on moving forward. Finding outcomes with mutual benefit sets a tone of cooperation and problem-solving and puts everyone on the same side instead of remaining adversarial.

An effective team builds on each person's strengths and compensates for weaknesses as it works toward achieving unity. An effective leader helps team members learn to sidestep negative energy and resist taking criticism personally. Communicating back and forth until the team reaches a solution that is mutually comfortable fosters trust and cooperation. Remaining open to new alternatives and compromises helps team members assume ownership of the proposed changes. As members increasingly feel ownership, they become more engaged, more invested, and ultimately, part of the solution.

Using Humor as a Tool for Change

Humor is an effective tool for reducing resistance and facilitating change. The comic relief of humor injected into a situation often presents a new perspective and leads to compromise. Humor fosters a positive climate and an energized work environment. A leader who maintains a good sense of humor improves relationships with team members, reduces power disparities, elevates work satisfaction and performance, and inspires innovation and creativity (Rosenberg et al., 2021). **Chapter 4** discusses the use of humor.

Beginning the Process of Change

Ultimately, people have very basic needs they want to meet through their work. Although priorities may vary, most people share many common desires. They want work that is interesting and challenging. They want appreciation for their efforts. They want to be involved in and important to the overall scheme. They want job security and reasonable pay. They want opportunities for career growth and advancement. Helping them meet these needs while instituting change reaps the support and cooperation necessary for success. Systematic preparation increases the ability to garner support for an anticipated change. Margaret Mead taught us, "Don't ever say one person can't change the world. It is the only thing that ever has."

Prepare Before Acting

Effectively initiating change will depend on how well you prepare before you approach others with your ideas. Evaluating current practices, identifying needed improvements, and gathering supporting research will lead to developing an action plan for implementing change. First consider which policies and procedures need to be changed. Before you approach anyone with your ideas, collect as much supporting data as possible for each change you have in mind. Such preparation before approaching others will be central to your success.

Evaluate Your Facility

Assess which of your present policies and practices follow current recommendations. It is important not to try to change everything all at once. First recognize the strengths of the organization by identifying what is right with the present system. Underscore with members of the group all the positive policies and practices that already provide good care for parents and babies. Many routines and practices can probably remain in place. Prepare a detailed rationale for any needed changes. Identify anticipated arguments and your possible responses to each one. Identify alternative approaches and methods in case you experience obstacles. This careful evaluation of your facility will prepare you to respond to obstacles and arguments as they arise.

Gather Data

After determining the changes that are needed, gather supporting research to support each proposed change. Identify the consequences of continuing to operate based on outdated policies and practices. Survey parents about the support they received in your hospital to learn what was good or bad and what could be improved. Document initiation rates and continuation rates at 2 weeks, 3 months, and 6 months. Compare your rates with those of other facilities in your community. Compare your facility's findings with national, state, provincial, or local statistics. Such data will validate the need for change and increase support from others. Continue to collect information throughout the change process, recording unanticipated outcomes or arguments that surfaced and any adjustments needed in your approach.

Managing Change

A thoughtful, strategic approach to a change initiative will increase long-term success. Many change management models are available online to guide organizations (Hart, 2023). The **Plan-Do-Study-Act (PDSA)** method is a commonly used tool in quality improvement (Agency for Healthcare Research and Quality, 2020; Institute for Healthcare Improvement [IHI], 2019). The approach provides a helpful structure for examining ways to promote lactation.

Step 1, Plan: Develop the Initiative

Initiating change and planning promotion efforts require strong teamwork. The first step in managing a change initiative is to form a team that will develop goals and measures and select the changes to implement.

Form a Team. In establishing your team, selecting team members with different points of view can provide valuable resources, insights, and perceptions. A variety of opinions and approaches enhances the team's knowledge and understanding. An effective team climate is one in which everyone feels equally empowered, safe, and comfortable when airing disagreements and concerns. Establishing the expectation that all members leave their credentials and personal agendas at the door helps to achieve this. An effective leader identifies the key issues and concerns and keeps everyone focused on topics rather than on personalities or job titles.

Attempting to understand an issue from another person's point of view enhances communication and garners support. Team members are more likely to be open to your ideas when you are genuinely open to their ideas. Listen until you can explain the other person's point of view as well as they can. Be open to allowing others' arguments and points of view to influence your thinking. The better you understand, the more you can appreciate alternative views and work toward creative solutions.

Creating mutual benefits for both sides of an issue helps everyone feel invested in and good about the outcome. If there appear to be losers on a particular issue, the team can seek ways for both sides to benefit so that there are only winners. When two opposing sides are unable to compromise, creative thinking can help identify whether an acceptable third alternative exists. An effective team works together to determine acceptable results and identify how to achieve those results.

In managing the team, it is important to designate tasks for a particular time and person. Effective leaders are comfortable delegating tasks to others and trusting them to do what is needed. Things may be done differently from how the leader would have done them—and perhaps even not done as well. However, relinquishing control to others and nurturing their growth are essential to developing a strong team. Such trust brings out the best in people and leads to enthusiastic and productive teamwork.

Set Aims. With your team in place, begin to identify areas for improvement, determine your initiative, and develop a plan. Knowing what you want the result to be will dictate how you plan to arrive there. Mapping it out with specific goals and visualizing it in your mind will help solidify a workable plan. The Code of Marketing of Breast-milk Substitutes (World Health Organization [WHO], 1981), the Ten Steps to Successful Breastfeeding (WHO, 1989), and the Global Strategy for Infant and Young Child Feeding (WHO & United Nations Children's Fund [UNICEF], 2003) provide research-based blueprints for lactation promotion. These seminal documents will help you identify current practices that can stay in place and guide the development of appropriate goals for changes in policies and protocols.

Establish Measures. The changes you wish to implement may involve behavior, attitudes, values, procedures, policies, or perhaps the entire structure. Establish specific short-term, intermediate, and long-term objectives, and then determine the metrics you will use to measure the outcome of each change. A goal of increasing lactation rates, for example, may have a short-term objective of increasing the rate to 58%, an intermediate objective of 68%, and a long-term objective of 75%. Reflect all these objectives in the timeline.

Select Changes. With objectives and metrics established, you are ready to identify needed changes and develop an action plan and strategies. For every change you wish to make, define the problem that makes that change necessary. For example, you may cite low initiation rates, high rates of engorgement, or large numbers of babies who have difficulty with latch. Determine the people who will be the most effective leaders in proposing and instituting the change. These are your change agents. Identify who the change will affect, and involve representatives from all affected areas in the process so that everyone has ownership of the change.

Try to anticipate all the issues involved in each individual objective, including the education required to empower the staff to implement the change. Consider how the change will be communicated and how it will affect people's levels of authority or power. Be mindful not to allow seemingly urgent matters to distract from important issues that need your attention. People often become so overly involved in what they perceive to be urgent that what is important receives little or no attention. What is urgent and what is important often are not the same. Focusing on what is important helps prevent the team's efforts from being diverted by distractions, crises, or obstacles. The team members can then prioritize important changes, develop a timeline, and stay committed to their goals.

Step 2, Do: Implement Your Plan

After you have defined the problems, goals, and strategies, you are ready to implement and test the planned changes. Major change cannot occur quickly. It could take many years for all changes to be fully implemented. Test a change or group of changes on a small scale to determine whether they created an improvement. If the results are positive, you can expand the tests and gradually incorporate larger and larger samples until you are confident that the changes can be adopted more widely.

In prioritizing changes, consider the anticipated level of difficulty in convincing others to support each one. Starting with a change that is likely to garner the most support gives you a greater chance of success. Changes that are least disruptive to routines or least controversial are likely to receive greater acceptance. For example, it may be much easier in a hospital setting with no lactation support to begin regular lactation rounds than to eliminate the practice of parents being given discharge bags from a formula company. Changes that improve client satisfaction are also positively received. Move slowly to issues perceived as more complicated or potentially problematic. At the same time, recognize that a change that seems easiest to you may not be the one that others favor.

Establishing a record of accomplishments with several of the easier changes prepares you for advancing to the more challenging ones. Leave the toughest hurdles until you have several of the less controversial and difficult changes in place. The success of introducing the earlier changes instills greater confidence in moving on to others. Additionally, after some of the changes are in place, people may be better able to recognize the larger picture and be more willing to support the tougher changes.

Step 3, Study: Analyze the Results

The team should evaluate both the positive and negative outcomes of each change and consider factors that might have contributed to the findings. A chart displayed in a team area or shared regularly at meetings can monitor the status of changes over time. Examining everyone's responses to the change will help identify any unanticipated problems that arise. Resolving problems immediately will maintain a high level of commitment among the staff. A willingness to risk failure and accepting failure in others is essential to successful change. Embracing disruptive innovation, along with all the unknowns that accompany it, helps create successful changes that guide an organization into the future (Luz et al., 2019; Marshall, 2019). Evaluating the outcomes associated with the change can help avoid jeopardizing long-term success.

Step 4, Act: Adjust the Process Based on the Results

Creating change requires continuous evaluation, improvement, and teamwork to achieve consistency. Repeating the PDSA cycle as you further refine your processes can help determine what action to take next. When a planned change works, you may be ready to implement it on a larger scale. If it does not achieve the desired results, define the failures, correct them, and refine the process in your next planning phase. If a plan does not work, it may be better suited for another time or environment. It may require overhauling the existing plan or developing a new one. Results generate momentum for changes until they are hardwired into the organization. When a change has become ingrained procedurally, you can standardize it and link it to the overall organizational structure. Customizable forms for facilitating organizational improvement are available online (IHI, 2019).

Capitalizing on Teamwork

The chances of success in creating change are greatest when change occurs through a multidisciplinary group of team members who share a common goal. The group needs to be large enough for a meeting to go on as planned when some members are absent. Careful attention to the makeup of members will increase team effectiveness. The personalities of team members will influence group dynamics. Attention to group dynamics and recognizing the efforts of everyone involved in the change process will increase success.

Team Makeup

All areas that will be affected by a change need to be represented on the change team. In a hospital, areas affected may include obstetrics, labor and delivery, postpartum care, neonatal intensive care, and pediatrics. A quality improvement representative is a valuable member of the team. U.S. hospitals accredited by The Joint Commission are required to have a process in place for quality improvement. In addition, consider other areas, such as housekeeping, management, home care, pharmacy, occupational therapy, and speech pathology. Bringing together a wide array of people to form an interdisciplinary team enables all those affected by the change to participate equally in the process.

Intercultural and interdisciplinary team diversity, when tactfully managed, increases the creative potential of teams (Tang, 2019). Respecting staff expertise and autonomy facilitates positive changes within the culture of an organization. Group dynamics will benefit from including people whom you have identified as allies, those you expect will resist, and those who seem to be neutral. Having such diversity in the group and getting buy-in from potential resistors helps avoid sabotage or the perception of one group being favored over another. People may be resistant not so much to change as to being controlled. Often, the greatest resistors become some of the most avid supporters after they understand the issues involved.

Types of Personalities

The variety of personal attributes and diversity with which people approach issues demonstrates the value of including the entire range of personalities in a group process. All personality types contribute positive traits to group dynamics and productivity. Personality types may vary among cultures, and it will help to capitalize on them when selecting team members. One theory identifies six basic personality types (Process

Communication Model, 2018). Taking the time to identify potential team members with each of these personalities will contribute positively to group dynamics:

- *Thinkers* welcome responsibility and are exceptional in detailed planning and organizing activities. They can structure their ideas logically and explain them quickly and comprehensively to others. They need a structured approach and want to be recognized for their contributions.
- *Persisters* perceive the world through the filter of their values, standards, and beliefs. People often admire their moral conduct and ethics. They are observant and willing to express their opinions and consider the opinions of others. They are extremely dedicated to their personal and professional development.
- *Harmonizers* are warm and compassionate and perceive the world through the filter of their feelings. They bring empathy and harmony into relationships and need to be recognized as a person. They respect people who recognize the importance of their emotions.
- *Rebels* are creative and can find solutions in situations when others perceive only problems. They are spontaneous, playful, and able to make boring tasks enjoyable. They are a source of positive energy and enthusiasm for others.
- *Imaginers* are introspective and think about all possible scenarios of different events. When talking to people, they do not give a lot of facts, preferring to analyze as many hypotheses and options as possible before reaching a conclusion.
- *Promoters* are charming and likeable. They are extremely resourceful and able to find solutions in every situation, as well as to rebound after a setback. They like to get to the point immediately. They need action and a dynamic environment to feel comfortable and alive.

Dynamics of a Team Meeting

Team functionality is dependent on compassionate, authentic leaders who help their teams thrive in the middle of complex situations (Shirey et al., 2019). The ultimate team goal is to find creative solutions that are mutually beneficial. The fact that not all members of the team share a common personal purpose should not prevent them from cooperating to reach group goals. Empowering team leadership will promote proactive behavior. The most proactive teams are those with higher levels of self-management and leaders who enhance the motivation, morale, and performance of team members.

It is important to learn as much as possible about the needs and concerns of each team member before proposing solutions. For group members to take ownership of a change, they need to be a part of designing it. The team leader should initially withhold their own goals to first learn the needs and goals of team members. In the process, the leader's agenda may change based on what others reflect. Knowing when to keep quiet, sit back, and let the discussion flow helps avoid the trap of beginning with a rigid preplanned agenda. After the leader states a position or proposal, they need to stop and let others respond.

Recognition and Praise

People like to be recognized for their efforts and respond favorably to positive feedback and expressions of gratitude. This is especially true when they believe they have made a special effort to help institute a change in practices. Creative incentives and rewards can encourage everyone's participation and compliance and create cooperation and goodwill. Examples of recognition include the following:

- Award a gift card for completing a learning module or attending an in-service program.
- Host a pizza party when a course is completed.
- Recognize a designated lactation supporter of the month.
- Publicize the lactation program and the hospital's commitment to lactation on the facility's website and social media accounts.
- Post a bulletin board with lactation updates, new policies, committee reports, and research summaries.
- Highlight changes in an electronic newsletter to community healthcare providers.

Lactation Promotion

There is a wide range of support for lactation promotion among the international healthcare community, governments, and organizations committed to protecting the health of infants and young children, as discussed in **Chapter 1**. Lactation promotion takes place at personal, institutional, political, and global levels. To advance lactation on a large scale requires multipronged interventions to overcome major policy, structural, and socioeconomic challenges (Hernández-Cordero & Pérez-Escamilla, 2022). Promotion strategies can target family, friends, health professionals, peer counselors, employers, and the communities in which parents live.

Lactation promotion is a form of **social marketing**, and effective marketing strategies increase awareness of lactation's importance. The relationship between social marketing and lactation is complex. Businesses use promotions to convert people's needs and wants into profitable company opportunities (Kotler & Armstrong, 2017). Social marketing applies the same principles for selling products to "selling" ideas, attitudes, and behaviors. In a health context, social marketing seeks to influence social behavior and benefit the target audience and society as a whole (Centers for Disease Control and Prevention [CDC], 2024).

Promotion campaigns create behavior change and implement research through coordination, monitoring, and evaluation. One such campaign, the Yale School of Public Health Becoming Breastfeeding Friendly (BBF), developed a toolbox that uses the analogy of interlocking gears working together to power an engine (Pérez-Escamilla et al., 2023). BBF has been implemented successfully in several countries with diverse socioeconomic, cultural, healthcare, and social systems. Each country focuses on the components where they have the greatest need. BBF can help guide the effective scaling up of lactation programs globally.

Promoting Lactation to Families

Lactation-friendly practices provide a framework within which families' needs can be met. Lactation promotion involves motivation, training, and coordination of the efforts of many people. Its success depends on the quality of education and support parents receive. Promotion needs to address a family's knowledge and skills gaps, misconceptions, and low self-confidence due to insufficient support (Samaniego et al., 2022). Education should include all family members whose opinions affect feeding decisions, especially partners (White et al., 2019). The intent to exclusively nurse in the first few weeks postpartum is more likely when the partner is perceived to prefer exclusive nursing (Wang et al., 2018).

Attitudes toward child care and parenting are pivotal in a family's infant feeding decision. Understanding these decisions can lead to new strategies for promoting and maintaining nursing. Promotion efforts for families need to encompass personal perceptions and societal norms. One study found that despite feeling positive about lactation, prospective parents viewed nursing as optional rather than the norm (Cha et al., 2021).

Reaching Families at Multiple Levels

Lactation promotion messages targeted at families need to reach them on multiple levels. A comprehensive approach places lactation promotion and advocacy within all aspects of their private and public lives. Mass media exposure is key to health promotion campaigns. Messages need to reach substantial proportions of the target audience frequently enough to be remembered. Promotion strategies need to consider parents' personal networks, including family, friends, work associates, schoolmates, media choices, and social networks. Creating supportive social media networks could help normalize nursing and reach young families more broadly across a diverse global online community (Galvão et al., 2021; Marcon et al., 2019). Websites, online videos, podcasts, apps, and e-mail are other electronic outlets for promotion to families.

Early Health Education

Knowledge, social influence, and exposure to nursing are significant in forming infant feeding attitudes, as discussed in **Chapter 3**. Normalizing nursing during adolescence and young adulthood helps develop favorable attitudes. Secondary schools are encouraged to incorporate age-appropriate information into textbooks and curricula at critical times in adolescent development. Including lactation promotion in school health curricula normalizes nursing and increases future intentions to nurse. Learning about lactation in school, with even a single interactive class, can positively affect lactation knowledge, attitudes, and intentions (Čatipović et al., 2018; Reyes et al., 2019). Teachers generally perceive school-based nursing positively (Moukarzel et al., 2019; Singletary et al., 2020).

Adolescents raised in an environment where lactation rates are low may never have witnessed a baby nursing. Exposing them to visual representations of nursing babies and introducing the topic to them with age-appropriate messages will reach them at a time when their own sexuality is emerging. Teaching classes at local schools provides an important community service and opportunities to answer questions for adolescents that may form the basis for later infant feeding decisions. **Figure 30-2** presents a sample teaching outline for a high school class.

Equity Factors in Lactation Promotion

Lactation promotion efforts can help mitigate inequities in health care, as discussed in **Chapter 3**. Limited

Opening discussion

- What have you heard about lactation? (address misconceptions and concerns)
- Were you nursed?
- Have you seen anyone nurse?
- Do you plan to nurse your children?

Paradigms of infant feeding

- Show illustrations that depict two possible interpretations (see Figure 30-1); relate to infant feeding practices
- Show images of animals nursing their young; relate to the normalcy of humans nursing

Changes in infant feeding practices

- Technological revolution and infant formula manufacturing
- World War II and women remaining in the workforce
- Return to nursing as prevailing infant feeding method

Why we need to return to nursing

- Health importance to babies, parents, family, society
- How nursing protects babies and parents

Show video that:

- Depicts parents nursing
- Shows how nursing works
- Puts nursing into the context of lifestyle

Closing discussion

- Reactions to video and seeing babies nursing
- Discuss how class may have altered previous answers

Figure 30-2 High school class on lactation.

access to skilled counseling, limited workplace support, gaps in legal provisions, weak monitoring and enforcement of the International Code, and limited maternity leave create structural barriers to lactation promotion (Samaniego et al., 2022). Dismantling inequities and inequalities in healthcare and lactation support needs to be at the forefront of promotional efforts.

Lactation disparities and inequities are prevalent among socioeconomic and racial groups (Jefferson, 2017). A social justice approach addresses gender, race, social, and cultural inequities and injustices that restrict access to opportunities and resources that influence lactation and health status (Smith, 2018). The Communities and Hospitals Advancing Maternity Practices (CHAMPS) promotes implementation of community- and hospital-based practices that address racial inequities in lactation (Burnham et al., 2022; Merewood et al., 2022). The concept of lactation equity requires both society and caregivers to advocate for all babies to be nursed regardless of status.

Culturally sensitive promotion strategies to address barriers to health equity are needed at every level to increase exclusive nursing and contribute to the health of all families. Lactation promotion needs to be geared toward low-income families, working parents, social networks, and the entire community. It needs to reflect historical and sociocultural factors for minority, indigenous, and other marginalized populations. Commitment, supportive policies, and comprehensive programs at the community level are factors in success.

Accommodations to circumstances are needed to reduce inequalities and support lactation. For example, prisons generally lack the structural conditions to accommodate lactation. Promotion efforts might include lactation rooms and trained staff in the facility or allowing in-home incarceration during the lactation period (Santos et al., 2022). Improving social and economic status will provide greater choice for all families regardless of race, class, or circumstance. Only when nursing represents a true choice for all families will it be truly equitable.

Cultural Factors in Lactation Promotion

Cultural norms can influence the types of marketing strategies to which families respond favorably. Promotion needs to reflect an understanding of a family's cultural heritage and respect deep-rooted cultural beliefs and traditions. Culturally sensitive interventions by community workers can make a big difference in helping families nurse exclusively. Teaching families about the importance of early and exclusive lactation, health education attendance, and support at birth helps reduce delayed initiation of lactation across diverse cultures and countries. **Chapter 3** discusses culture and lactation.

Health Factors in Lactation Promotion

In the early 2000s, lactation promotion began changing from a positive message of lactation's benefits to a risk-based message of the unfavorable consequences of *not* nursing. Idealization of nursing as "optimal" rather than normal may inadvertently reinforce a perception that formula feeding is the standard way of feeding babies. The deliberate marketing shift to health risks recognizes nursing as the norm for infant feeding and underscores its health imperative. Risk-based messages promote social and institutional change and encourage others in parents' lives to value nursing.

Framing promotion to identify the risks of not nursing does not mean that practitioners will refrain from recommending infant formula when it is needed.

Lactation professionals recognize when formula is medically indicated and help parents incorporate it into their feeding regimen. In addition, it is important to recognize that parents may perceive risks in choosing to nurse. Perceived barriers can be strong motivators in making decisions; thus, dispelling any misperceptions is an important element in promotion efforts.

Lactation promotion is especially critical among populations at high health risk. Nursing is the single most important preventive intervention against child mortality. Lack of awareness about lactation, lack of support from health workers, community cultural beliefs, and the unethical marketing of infant formula lead to under 40% of infants globally being exclusively nursed for 6 months (UNICEF, 2019b). The WHO estimates that about 820,000 child lives could be saved every year among children under 5 years if all children 0 to 23 months were optimally nursed (WHO, 2023). In addition, billions of dollars globally could be saved from unavoidable medical costs associated with maternal and infant illnesses and pediatric deaths from sudden infant death syndrome and necrotizing enterocolitis.

Promoting Lactation Within the Healthcare Profession

Hospitals and healthcare professionals are in the business of satisfying customer needs. In this regard, lactation promotion is no different from the marketing of any other health practice that improves the consumer's well-being. An institution adds value to its services by adopting a consumer-focused marketing strategy. Lactation promotion and support within health care need to be client centered and multidimensional. Melding and integrating the perspectives of multiple disciplines will help attain best practices for supporting and delivering consistent lactation care in healthcare settings.

Because most infant feeding decisions occur before delivery, antenatal lactation education and promotion are especially important. Hospitals and birthing centers offer numerous prenatal and postpartum opportunities for promoting lactation to families and caregivers. Continued ongoing lactation promotion and support in pediatric outpatient settings empower families' parenting self-efficacy and nursing throughout lactation (Meek, 2017; Thomas & Ware, 2019). The American Academy of Pediatrics (AAP) seeks to improve pediatricians' support of lactation by offering a lactation training curriculum and by helping pediatricians establish lactation-friendly practices (AAP, 2020).

Healthcare institutions can formalize their lactation support through written policies that protect nursing parents and support them throughout lactation. The Academy of Breastfeeding Breastfeeding-Friendly Physician's Office protocol optimizes care of infants and children (Vanguri et al., 2021). Examples of lactation-friendly policies are provided for pediatric practices (**Figure 30-3**) and obstetric practices

1. Develop or implement a current lactation protocol for use in your practice that is communicated to all staff. Provide copies to those who cover for you.
2. Arrange for all staff to attend inservices that teach the skills necessary to implement the protocol.
3. Inform all expectant parents about the benefits and management of lactation. Give written, noncommercial prenatal information on nursing, refer parents to lactation classes, and encourage partners to attend.
4. Help parents initiate and maintain lactation during hospital rounds. Perform newborn exams in the parent's room, showing parents how well-designed babies are for nursing.
5. If parent and baby are separated for medical reasons, confirm that an electric pump is available for expressing milk, and that milk is expressed at least 8 times in 24 hours. A prescription may be written for human milk, if necessary, to cover the cost of renting an electric pump.
6. Avoid the use of sterile water, glucose water, or formula for nursing newborn infants, unless medically indicated. Adequate amounts of milk are present at delivery in the form of colostrum.
7. Encourage parents to room-in 24 hours a day in the hospital. This protects the baby from disease in the nursery, provides opportunities for unrestricted contact and feeding, and encourages parents to become aware of their baby's needs and rhythms.
8. Advise parents to feed their infants on cue, 8 to 12 times each 24 hours. Teach behavioral feeding cues to avoid underfeeding or overhunger, with resulting infant behavioral disorganization.
9. Avoid the use of artificial nipples and pacifiers in newborn nursing infants. This approach decreases the incidence of nipple preference and its sequelae.
10. Have available on staff a lactation consultant or other healthcare provider whose responsibility can include prenatal teaching, hospital rounds, call-in times, and visits for lactation questions or problems. Or refer such situations to a lactation consultant in the community. Refer parents to support groups.

Figure 30-3 Ten steps to a Baby-Friendly Pediatric Practice.

Printed with permission of Marsha Walker.

1. Create and implement a lactation promotion and support policy for use in your practice that is communicated to all staff. Provide copies to those who cover for you.
2. Arrange for all staff to attend inservices that teach the skills necessary to implement the protocol.
3. Inform all expectant parents about the benefits and management of lactation. Give written, noncommercial information on lactation. Recommend that parents attend prenatal lactation classes that include partners. Refer parents to childbirth education classes.
4. Help parents initiate nursing within 1/2 hour of birth. Place and leave the infant on the parent's chest to promote prefeeding behaviors to initiate latch, suck, and organization of feedings.
5. If parent and baby are separated for medical reasons, confirm that an electric pump is available for expressing milk; that milk is expressed at least 8 times in 24 hours; that no nipple soreness, engorgement, or other problems arise from the use of the pump.
6. Avoid the use of sterile water, glucose water, or formula for nursing newborn infants, unless medically indicated. Adequate amounts of milk are present at delivery in the form of colostrum.
7. Encourage parents to room-in 24 hours a day to protect the baby from disease in the nursery, provide opportunities for unrestricted contact and feeding, and help parents learn their baby's needs and rhythms.
8. Advise parents to feed their infants on cue, 8 to 12 times each 24 hours. Teach behavioral feeding cues to avoid underfeeding or overhunger, with resulting infant behavioral disorganization.
9. Avoid the use of artificial nipples and pacifiers in newborn nursing infants. This approach decreases the incidence of nipple preference and its sequelae.
10. Have available on staff a lactation consultant or other healthcare provider whose responsibility can include prenatal teaching, hospital rounds, call-in times, and visits for lactation questions or problems. Or refer such situations to a lactation consultant in the community. Refer parents to support groups.

Figure 30-4 Ten steps to a Baby-Friendly Obstetric Practice.

(**Figure 30-4**). Coordinated care by a healthcare team from practices with these types of policies ensures optimal lactation support and care.

Hospital Promotion Efforts

Hospital practices vary considerably in their protection and support of lactation. Despite global promotion efforts, many hospitals provide marginal or no in-hospital lactation care. Conflicting advice, misconceptions, and inconsistencies between theory and practice affect the course of lactation. Parents need consistent technical assistance from caregivers who follow the health guidelines for optimal infant nutrition. Global strategies such as the Baby-Friendly Hospital Initiative (BFHI) BFHI (WHO & UNICEF, 2018) and the Global Strategy for Infant and Young Child Feeding (WHO & UNICEF, 2003) provide guidance for improving hospital practices with policies that are practical and action oriented. **Chapter 1** discusses the BFHI.

Hospital policies and practices that remove barriers during labor, delivery, recovery, and postpartum have a role in the duration of lactation. Pens, paper pads, coffee mugs, pamphlets, and other promotional items that display names and logos of formula manufacturers undermine lactation promotion efforts and send subliminal messages to staff and clients that formula is a healthy and desirable product. Removing such promotional items that detract from lactation is an important strategy.

The National Institute for Children's Health Quality (NICHQ) in the United States provides extensive training, quality improvements, and culture change to hospitals, states, and other organizations. Best Fed Beginnings, New York State Breastfeeding Quality Improvement in Hospitals, and the Texas Ten Step Star Achiever Breastfeeding Learning Collaborative are examples of initiatives that spread best practices among hospitals to support nursing families. Globally, organizations and health agencies that provide resources and models include the WHO and state/province health departments and ministries.

Caregiver Promotion

Health professionals are fundamental in lactation promotion. Lactation-friendly health care requires the genuine commitment of health professionals who work with young families. Healthcare providers need to recognize the influence they exert on clients. When they distribute infant formula or vouchers to parents, they place themselves in the position of advertising and promoting a product that compromises lactation. Healthcare professionals who support lactation can educate their peers and raise their awareness of parents' needs related to lactation.

Despite universal recognition of the health imperative of nursing, many providers fail to support families. A provider may acknowledge, for example, that sucking promotes milk production yet may advise formula supplements if a baby seems dissatisfied or hungry after nursing. Studies suggest that it is providers' culture and attitudes, not their knowledge, that most influence their efforts in lactation promotion and support (Holtzman & Usherwood, 2018). Education strategies that address attitudes and cultural factors may help to enhance their promotion and support of lactation.

UNICEF developed a pledge for physicians attesting to their commitment to protect, promote, and support lactation (Grant, 1994). Signing the pledge demonstrates a desire to support nursing families in their practices. The pledge was originally developed by UNICEF. In 2008, the World Alliance for Breastfeeding Action (WABA), in collaboration with the Academy of Breastfeeding Medicine (ABM), edited the pledge to address physicians specifically, presented in **Figure 30-5**. World Alliance for Breastfeeding Action (WABA). WABA/ABM Physician's Pledge to Promote, Protect and Support Breastfeeding, 2008. https://waba.org.my/v3/wp-content/uploads/2018/08/WABA-ABM-Physician-Pledge.pdf

Community Lactation Promotion

Opportunities for lactation promotion present themselves in many spheres of influence that affect parents' lives. Advocacy is needed to enact baby-friendly principles in communities throughout the world (Tomori et al., 2022). Promotion efforts should include advocating for adequate maternity leave and supportive workplace and childcare policies that enable parents to continue nursing (UNICEF, 2019a). Evidence-based advocacy generates the political will that drives legislation to release resources for workforce development and lactation programs in facilities and communities.

Governments and society have a responsibility to support lactation through policies and programs in the community. The complex and interrelated barriers across the social-ecological system require an integrated approach that goes beyond hospital birthing care and the health community. Education and promotional strategies toward improving lactation rates need to be targeted at the public, community organizations,

RECOGNIZING THAT breastfeeding plays an uniquely important role in health, development and survival of infants and young children and their mothers;

. . .optimally, breastfeeding is initiated within the immediate postpartum period with skin-to-skin placement, practised exclusively for 6 months, and continued for up to 2 years or more with appropriate complementary feeding;

. . .no substitute can provide the complex and dynamic balance of nutrients, antibodies, growth factors and living cells that make human milk the perfect food for human infants;

. . .women have the right to make their infant feeding decision based on complete and accurate information, and deserve to receive the skilled support of the medical community in achieving optimal breastfeeding;

. . .breastfeeding is an endangered natural resource that is needed to overcome the immune deficiencies of infancy and that requires my protection and support, and to provide adequate support, my skills must be maintained and up-to-date;

. . .my role as a physician is one of influence, authority, and trust, and that I wish above all else, to do no harm;

. . .the targets of the Innocenti Declarations are important to breastfeeding protection, promotion and support, and should be integrated into in my work and in my spheres of influence;

. . .both maternal and infant care, including medical intervention during pregnancy and L&D, should be carried out with consideration of the potential impact on breastfeeding;

. . .data on infant feeding practices must be part of normal health data collection and be monitored accordingly;

. . .current marketing practices - including free or low-cost distribution of human milk substitute supplies to hospitals or any other part of the health care system - create misunderstanding and asymmetry of information, and bias health workers and mothers concerning infant feeding choices;

. . .my government affirmed at the World Health Assembly in 1994 that the marketing and promotion of breast-milk substitutes should not be conducted anywhere in the health care system or by health care workers, and to promote, support and protect breastfeeding must be taken ***with urgency***; and,

. . .the promotion of health and prevention of morbidity and mortality are the duties and mandate of the responsible health care providers everywhere:

I, ______________________________ , hereby pledge to do my part to promote, protect and support optimal breastfeeding, to ensure that training of future physicians includes all evidence-based and necessary knowledge and skills, to provide leadership for the breastfeeding support team, and to work towards the four Innocenti Goals: to create multi-sectoral leadership, to ensure that facilities follow the Ten Steps, to support the WHO International Code of Marketing of Breast-milk Substitutes and end free or low-cost distribution of breastmilk substitutes in our health care systems, and to support paid maternity leave and workplace accommodation for breastfeeding mothers.

Figure 30-5 Physician's pledge to protect, promote, and support lactation.

The pledge was originally developed by UNICEF. In 2008, the World Alliance for Breastfeeding Action (WABA), in collaboration with the Academy of Breastfeeding Medicine (ABM) edited this pledge to address physicians specifically. Here is the link to WABA/ABM Physician Pledge http://waba.org.my/pdf/waba-abm-phy-pledge.pdf

employers, and others who can support young families. For example, the image of a parent feeding a baby in a toilet stall in **Figure 30-6** is part of an innovative social media campaign created by college students to highlight the inequity of shaming parents for nursing in public (When Nurture Calls, 2014).

Well-defined policies and strategies, financial resources, and strong political will are needed to deliver effective promotional efforts at the community level. Parents' beliefs and practices are strongly influenced by traditions within their culture and community. Therefore, a strategy for promoting early and exclusive nursing needs to incorporate traditional beliefs and practices into modern messages on lactation (Bazzano et al., 2017; Karim et al., 2019; Thow et al., 2017). A social and cultural change of the whole community toward lactation increases rates. Community-based promotion can raise public awareness and increase support for lactation within the community (Anderson et al., 2017; Lambert et al., 2018). One community-based program partnered with local hospitals to increase lactation awareness and improve support through an ongoing multilevel approach (Leruth et al., 2017).

Efforts to create a lactation-friendly community can begin by developing local criteria with political and social leaders in the community who are committed to the initiative. Components can include lactation training for local health workers and referral sources for families to receive additional care. In addition, support can be established in the community to assist parents in making informed choices. A community-wide peer support system and removal of practices, distributors, shops, and services that violate the International Code of Marketing of Breast-milk Substitutes will further this community effort.

Parents' groups in the community are encouraged to commit resources and time to lactation promotion. Artists can portray the beauty and power of lactation through paintings, photographs, poems, and plays. The media can present lactation as a natural part of our culture. Coordinated community efforts to return lactation to the cultural norm will empower parents to nurture their babies in the manner that nature intended. Long-term strategies for community promotion are described in **Figure 30-7**.

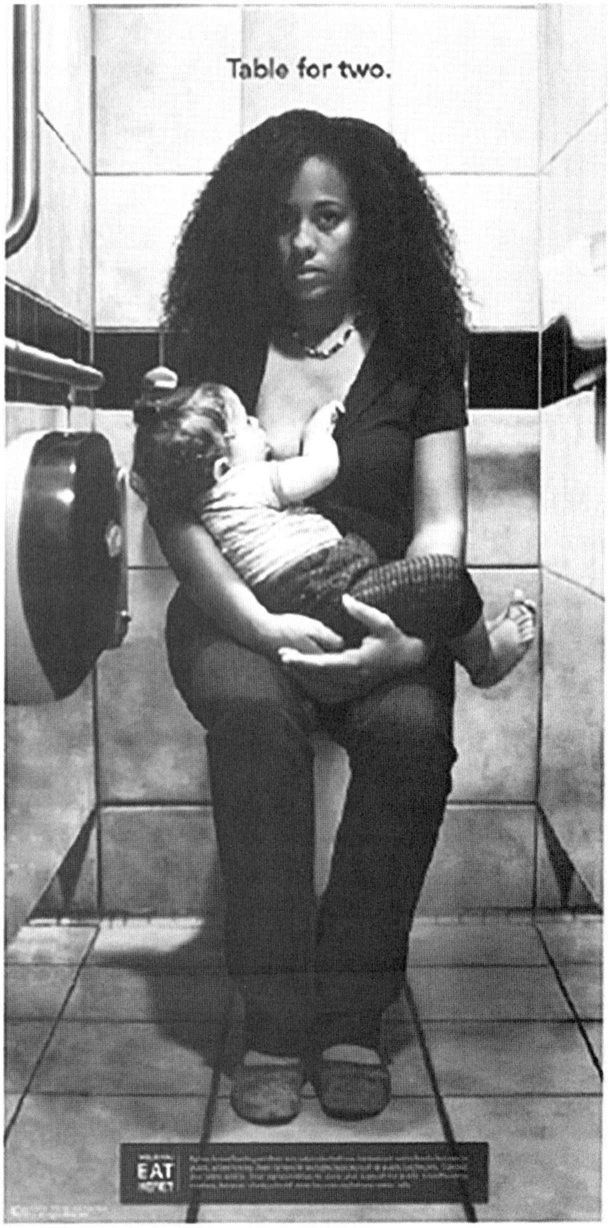

Figure 30-6 When nurture calls.

© When Nurture Calls

- Ensure that maternity centers practice all of the Ten Steps to Successful Breastfeeding.
- Take action to implement fully all articles of the International Code of Marketing of Breastmilk Substitutes and its subsequent World Health Assembly (WHA) resolutions.
- Enact and enforce legislation to protect the rights of nursing employees.
- Educate communities to value parents' contributions to the health of their children and thus the health of the community and the world.
- Encourage institutions to ensure convenient antenatal care, respect from caregivers, good obstetrical services, and patient-focused delivery procedures.
- Provide counseling and clinical services for lactation and birth spacing.
- Enlist community, health, religious, and political leaders to promote the primary healthcare principles of preventive health education and empowerment of families.

Figure 30-7 Long-term strategies for community promotion of nursing.

Data from the Department of Child and Adolescent Health and Development (CAH), World Health Organization. *Community-Based Strategies for Breastfeeding Promotion and Support in Developing Countries*. 2003. Geneva, Switzerland.

Summary

Demonstrating effective leadership and helping others embrace change can help return lactation to the cultural norm and ensure every child's basic human right to be nursed. Lactation-friendly health care creates a family-friendly environment. International and community initiatives can guide and support the promotion of optimal nutrition for infants and young children. The success of lactation promotion results from countless small changes enacted one person at a time, hospital by hospital, and country by country. It requires the combined efforts of lactation professionals and all other members of the healthcare profession and lactation support community, as well as the most important people involved—nursing families!

What You Learned–At a Glance

Conversation Starters with Parents

- What hospital practices made it difficult for you to nurse your baby?
- How did your hospital solicit your feedback on the nursing support you received?
- How supported do you feel in your cultural traditions related to nursing?
- How do your healthcare providers promote lactation?

Strong Leadership

- Build on your personal attributes, emotional intelligence, and assertiveness.
- Assess the need and readiness for change, and plan for resistance.
- Allow individuals to progress at their own pace in the change process.
- Recognize reasons for resistance to change.
- Recognize the needs of others, identify common goals, neutralize negativity and divisiveness, and use humor to diffuse resistance.

Initiating Planned Change

- Gather data and evaluate your facility.
- Form a committee represented by affected areas and diverse personality types.
- Identify needed changes and develop objectives and measures to evaluate achievement of your goals.
- Prioritize changes and build on improvements slowly.
- Analyze the results from implementing changes and make necessary adjustments.
- Give recognition and praise for everyone's efforts.

Lactation Promotion to Families

- Reach families at multiple levels with education, support, and advocacy.
- Address family lifestyles and social and economic status.
- Reflect an understanding of cultural heritage, traditions, and acculturation.
- Address health factors with risk-based messages to promote change.

Lactation Promotion Within the Healthcare Profession

- Insufficient staffing, lack of continuity, ineffective guidelines, and lack of commitment interfere with lactation promotion.
- Despite global promotion, many parents receive marginal or no in-hospital lactation care.
- Promotion strategies need to remove barriers in labor, delivery, and postpartum care.
- The BFHI and Global Strategy for Infant and Young Child Feeding provide guidelines for creating changes in facilities.
- Education needs to address the attitudes and culture of healthcare professionals.
- Community promotion reaches organizations, employers, and the public with policies, strategies, resources, and political will.

References

Agency for Healthcare Research and Quality. Plan-Do-Study-Act (PDSA) directions and examples. Health literacy universal precautions toolkit, 2nd edition. 2020. https://www.ahrq.gov/health-literacy/quality-resources/tools/literacy-toolkit/healthlittoolkit2-tool2b.html

Aitkenhead S, et al. How the Leading Change, Adding Value framework enables nursing, midwifery and care staff to transform practice. *Br J Nurs.* 2019;28(18):1210–1212.

American Academy of Pediatrics. The breastfeeding curriculum. 2020. https://www.aap.org/en-us/advocacy-and-policy

/aap-health-initiatives/Breastfeeding/Pages/Breastfeeding-Curriculum.aspx

Anand RK. *Transforming Health Colleagues into Breastfeeding Advocates. WABA Activity Sheet No. 3*. Penang, Malaysia: World Alliance for Breastfeeding Action; February 7, 2005. https://www.waba.org.my/resources/activitysheet/acsh3.htm

Anderson J, et al. Brookings supports breastfeeding: using public deliberation as a community-engaged approach to dissemination of research. *Transl Behav Med*. 2017;7(4):783–792.

Barry ES, et al. Leadership and followership in military interprofessional health care teams. *Mil Med*. 2021;186(suppl 3):7–15.

Başoğul C, Özgür G. Role of emotional intelligence in conflict management strategies of nurses. *Asian Nurs Res (Korean Soc Nurs Sci)*. 2016;10(3):228–233.

Bazzano AN, et al. Qualitative studies of infant and young child feeding in lower-income countries: a systematic review and synthesis of dietary patterns. *Nutrients*. 2017;9(10).

Burnham L, et al. Mississippi CHAMPS: decreasing racial inequities in breastfeeding. *Pediatrics*. 2022;149(2):e2020030502.

Carragher J, Gormley K. Leadership and emotional intelligence in nursing and midwifery education and practice: a discussion paper. *J Adv Nurs*. 2017;73(1):85–96.

Čatipović M, et al. Breastfeeding intention and knowledge in secondary-school students. *Acta Clin Croat*. 2018;57(4):658–668.

Centers for Disease Control and Prevention. Gateway to health communication & social marketing practice. October 16, 2024. https://www.cdc.gov/health-communication/php/communication-resources/index.html

Cha E, et al. Client-centered breastfeeding-promotion strategies: Q methodology. *Int J Environ Res Public Health*. 2021;18(6):2955.

Coronado-Maldonado I, et al. Emotional intelligence, leadership, and work teams: a hybrid literature review. *Heliyon*. 2023;9(10):e20356.

Coskun O, et al. Emotional intelligence and leadership traits among family physicians. *Postgrad Med*. 2018;130(7):644–649.

Galvão DMPG, et al. Use of new technologies and promotion of breastfeeding: integrative literature review. *Rev Paul Pediatr*. 2021;40:e2020234.

Gilar-Corbi R, et al. Can emotional intelligence be improved? A randomized experimental study of a business-oriented EI training program for senior managers. *PLoS One*. 2019;14(10):e0224254.

Grant JP. *Physician's Pledge to Protect, Promote and Support Breastfeeding*. New York: UNICEF; 1994.

Hart J. Top 10 change management models: a comprehensive overview. The Knowledge Academy. June 1, 2023. https://www.theknowledgeacademy.com/blog/change-management-models/

Hernández-Cordero S, Pérez-Escamilla R. What will it take to increase breastfeeding? *Matern Child Nutr*. 2022;18(suppl 3):e13371.

Holtzman O, Usherwood T. Australian general practitioners' knowledge, attitudes and practices towards breastfeeding. *PLoS One*. 2018;13(2):e0191854.

Hung D, Chen PH. Ready for change? The role of physician and staff engagement, burnout, and workplace attributes. *J Ambul Care Manage*. 2017;40(2):150–157.

Institute for Healthcare Improvement. How to Improve: Model for Improvement. 2019. https://www.ihi.org/resources/how-improve-model-improvement

Jefferson UT. Breastfeeding exposure, attitudes, and intentions of African American and Caucasian college students. *J Hum Lact*. 2017;33(1):149–156.

Karim F, et al. Prevalence and determinants of initiation of breastfeeding within one hour of birth: an analysis of the Bangladesh Demographic and Health Survey, 2014. *PLoS One*. 2019;14(7):e0220224.

Kim M. Development and effects of assertiveness training applying Dongsasub training for nursing students in clinical practice. *J Korean Acad Nurs*. 2016;46(4):490–500.

Kotler P, Armstrong G. *Principles of Marketing*. 17th ed. Harlow, UK: Pearson Education Ltd.; 2017.

Lambert AW, et al. Community-based breastfeeding support with the Tiger Babies breastfeeding support tent. *Nurs Women's Health*. 2018;22(2):138–147.

Leruth C, et al. A multilevel approach to breastfeeding promotion: using healthy start to deliver individual support and drive collective impact. *Matern Child Health J*. 2017;21(suppl 1):4–10.

Luz S, et al. Characteristics and behaviours of formal versus informal nurse champions and their relationship to innovation success. *J Adv Nurs*. 2019;75(1):85–95.

Marcon AR, et al. Protecting, promoting, and supporting breastfeeding on Instagram. *Matern Child Nutr*. 2019;15(1):e12658.

Marshall DR. Unleashing the power of nurse innovators. *J Nurs Adm*. 2019;49(2):55–56.

Meek JY. How to establish a breastfeeding-friendly pediatric office. *AAP News*. April 17, 2017. https://publications.aap.org/aapnews/news/11076/How-to-establish-a-breastfeeding-friendly?autologincheck=redirected

Merewood A, et al. Assessing the impact of a statewide effort to improve breastfeeding rates: a RE-AIM evaluation of CHAMPS in Mississippi. *Matern Child Nutr*. 2022;18(3):e13370.

Moukarzel S, et al. Getting schooled: teachers' views on school-based breastfeeding education in Lebanon. *Int Breastfeed J*. 2019;14:3.

Nightingale S, et al. The impact of emotional intelligence in health care professionals on caring behaviour towards patients in clinical and long-term care settings: findings from an integrative review. *Int J Nurs Stud*. 2018;80:106–117.

Nilsen P, et al. Implementation of change in health care in Sweden: a qualitative study of professionals' change responses. *Implement Sci*. 2019;14(1):51.

Pérez-Escamilla R, et al. Gearing to success with national breastfeeding programmes: the Becoming Breastfeeding Friendly (BBF) initiative experience. *Matern Child Nutr*. 2023;19(suppl 1):e13339.

Process Communication Model. Personality types. 2018. https://processcommunicationmodel.com/six-personality-types/

Reyes C, et al. Investigating the effectiveness of school-based breastfeeding education on breastfeeding knowledge, attitudes and intentions of adolescent females. *Midwifery*. 2019;70:64–70.

Rosenberg C, et al. Humor in workplace leadership: a systematic search scoping review. *Front Psychol*. 2021;12:610795.

Salau O, et al. Integrated datasets on transformational leadership attributes and employee engagement: the moderating role of job satisfaction in the fast moving consumer goods (FMCG) industry. *Data Brief*. 2018;19:2329–2335.

Samaniego JAR, et al. Implementation and effectiveness of policies adopted to enable breastfeeding in the Philippines are limited by structural and individual barriers. *Int J Environ Res Public Health*. 2022;19(17):10938.

Santos MVD, et al. Promotion, protection and support for breastfeeding in prisons: a scoping review. *Cien Saude Colet.* 2022;27(7):2689–2702.

Shirey MR, et al. Integration of authentic leadership lens for building high performing interprofessional collaborative practice teams. *Nurs Adm Q.* 2019;43(2):101–112.

Singletary N, et al. Exploring North Carolina family and consumer sciences teachers' attitudes towards breastfeeding and infant feeding education practices. *J Hum Lact.* 2020;36(4):766–775.

Smith PH. Social justice at the core of breastfeeding protection, promotion and support: a conceptualization. *J Hum Lact.* 2018;34(2):220–225.

Stanley D, Stanley K. Clinical leadership and nursing explored: a literature search. *J Clin Nurs.* 2018;27(9–10):1730–1743.

Sullivan EJ. *Effective Leadership and Management in Nursing.* 9th ed. Upper Saddle River, NJ: Prentice Hall; 2017.

Tang M. Fostering creativity in intercultural and interdisciplinary teams: the VICTORY model. *Front Psychol.* 2019;10:2020.

Thomas J, Ware JL. Top 10 ways busy pediatricians can support breastfeeding. *AAP News.* October 24, 2019. https://publications.aap.org/aapnews/news/14432/Top-10-ways-busy-pediatricians-can-support

Thow AM, et al. Opportunities for strengthening infant and young child feeding policies in South Asia: insights from the SAIFRN policy analysis project. *BMC Public Health.* 2017;17(suppl 2):404.

Tomori C, et al. What works to protect, promote and support breastfeeding on a large scale: a review of reviews. *Matern Child Nutr.* 2022;18(suppl 3):e13344.

United Nations Children's Fund. Breastfeeding and family-friendly policies. July 2019a. https://www.unicef.org/sites/default/files/2019-07/UNICEF-Breastfeeding-Family-Friendly%20Policies-2019.pdf

United Nations Children's Fund. *The State of the World's Children 2019. Growing Well in a Changing World. Children, Food and Nutrition.* New York: UNICEF; 2019b. https://www.unicef.org/reports/state-of-worlds-children-2019

Vanguri S, et al. ABM clinical protocol #14: breastfeeding-friendly physician's office-optimizing care for infants and children. *Breastfeed Med.* 2021;16(3):175–184.

Visser GHA, et al. Framework for safe delivery: a call to action. *Int J Gynaecol Obstet.* 2019;146(1):1–2.

Wang S, et al. When fathers are perceived to share in the maternal decision to breastfeed: outcomes from the Infant Feeding Practices Study II. *Matern Child Health J.* 2018;22(11):1676–1684.

When Nurture Calls. May 6, 2014. https://www.behance.net/gallery/16685319/When-Nurture-Calls-Campaign

White B, et al. Gamifying breastfeeding for fathers: process evaluation of the Milk Man mobile app. *JMIR Pediatr Parent.* 2019;2(1):e12157.

World Health Organization. *The International Code of Marketing of Breast-milk Substitutes.* Geneva, Switzerland: World Health Organization; 1981. https://www.who.int/publications/i/item/9241541601

World Health Organization. *Protecting, Promoting, and Supporting Breastfeeding: A Joint WHO/UNICEF Statement.* Geneva, Switzerland: World Health Organization; 1989.

World Health Organization. Infant and young child feeding. 2023. https://www.who.int/news-room/fact-sheets/detail/infant-and-young-child-feeding

World Health Organization, United Nations Children's Fund. *Global Strategy for Infant and Young Child Feeding.* Geneva, Switzerland: World Health Organization; 2003. https://www.who.int/publications/i/item/9241562218

World Health Organization, United Nations Children's Fund. Protecting, promoting, and supporting breastfeeding in facilities providing maternity and newborn services: the revised Baby-Friendly Hospital Initiative 2018 implementation guidance. Geneva, Switzerland: World Health Organization; 2018. https://www.who.int/publications/i/item/9789241513807

Yoshinaga N, et al. Is modified brief assertiveness training for nurses effective? A single-group study with long-term follow-up. *J Nurs Manag.* 2018;26(1):59–65.

Glossary

A

ABO incompatibility Blood type incompatibility between a birth parent and baby that causes the parent to produce antibodies that destroy the infant's red blood cells, leading to rapid development of jaundice.

Abstract In research, a summary of a scientific article that describes the purpose, scope, results, and conclusions about a study or topic.

Acculturation Integration into a new culture.

Acetone A ketone (chemical) formed when the body uses fat instead of glucose sugar for energy. Usually a sign that cells lack insulin or cannot effectively use available insulin.

Acinus Any small saclike structure, such as one found in a gland. Also called *alveolus*.

Acquired immune deficiency syndrome (AIDS) Disease of the human immune system caused by infection with the human immunodeficiency virus (HIV). Transmitted by contact with bodily fluids, including blood and semen.

Acrocyanosis Bluish tinge of the hands and feet.

Acrodermatitis enteropathica A rare long-term disease of infants. Symptoms are blisters on the skin and mucous membranes, hair loss, diarrhea, and growth faltering.

Active immunity Long-term immunity that protects the body from new infection; gained from the production of antibodies.

Active listening A counseling technique that paraphrases a message and reflects it back to the sender.

Acute bilirubin encephalopathy (ABE) Acute manifestations of neurological damage caused by excessive bilirubin in the first weeks after birth.

Adiponectin Cell-signaling proteins secreted by fat tissue.

Adipose tissue Tissue made of fat cells arranged in lobes.

Adrenal hormones Hormones produced in the adrenal glands, including estrogen, progesterone, steroids, cortisol, and cortisone and chemicals such as adrenalin, norepinephrine, and dopamine.

Adverse childhood experiences (ACE) Potentially traumatic events that occur in childhood such as violence, abuse, or neglect.

Affirmation Validating concerns, showing acceptance, and praising actions or attempts.

Alactogenesis Absence of the onset of stage II lactogenesis (secretory activation).

Albumin A protein made by the liver.

Allergen A foreign substance that can cause an allergic response in the body.

Alpha-lactalbumin Protein in the whey portion of human milk that assists with the synthesis of lactose. Bactericide against *Streptococcus pneumoniaes*.

Alternate feeding method Infant feeding method other than direct nursing, including spoon, cup, syringe, paladai, supplemental tube or nursing system, and bottle.

Alternate massage Technique that compresses the breast when the baby pauses during a feeding. Used to encourage sucking and increase milk production. Also called *breast compression*.

Alternative hunches Intuitive attempts to continue problem-solving after testing an original hunch.

Alveolar ridge The bony ridge of the jaw that contains the tooth sockets. Also called the *gumline*.

Alveoli Tiny glands in the breast that produce milk.

Amastia Rare condition in which breast tissue and the nipple-areolar complex fail to develop.

Amazia The presence of the nipple-areolar complex with no underlying glandular tissue.

Amenorrhea The absence of the monthly flow of blood and discharge of mucous tissues from the uterus through the vagina (menstruation).

Amino acids The basic building blocks that make up proteins in the body; the end products of protein digestion.

Amphetamines Stimulant drugs with street names such as ecstasy, harmony, and love that quickly migrate from the bloodstream into the milk.

Amylase An enzyme that aids the breakdown of starch in digestion.

Analgesia Absence of the sensation of pain because of an interruption in the nervous system pathway through the use of analgesics that relieve pain without loss of consciousness.

Anchor In research, a word or phrase used at the numerical end points of a written scale to describe the extremes of feeling or thought measured by the scale.

Anemia A decrease in red cells in the blood, in hemoglobin, or in total volume, reducing the blood's ability to carry oxygen. It occurs in about half of all pregnancies.

Anesthesia Partial or complete loss of sensation with or without memory loss because of disease, injury, or administration of an anesthetic agent, usually by injection or inhalation.

Ankyloglossia Tight lingual frenulum. A defect in which the membrane under the tongue is too short, limiting movement of the tongue. Also known as *tongue tie*.

Anomaly Change from what is regarded as normal; an inherited problem with growth of a structure.

Anovulatory Failure of the ovaries to produce, mature, or release eggs.

Anoxia Lack of oxygen.

Antibacterial Agent that destroys bacteria or suppresses their growth or ability to reproduce.

Antibodies A protein substance that is developed in response to and interacts specifically with an antigen to form the basis of immunity.

Antibody response Process by which proteins produced in the blood become attached to antigens on infectious organisms' antibodies to render them harmless or cause them to be destroyed.

Anticipatory guidance A counseling technique that provides encouragement, help, and guidance to prevent or minimize problems.

Anticipatory stage The first of four stages in role acquisition which includes collecting information and beginning to learn about a new role.

Antigen A substance foreign to the body, often a protein.

Antimicrobial Preventing or destroying the development of microorganisms.

Antiparasite Substance that protects against an organism that lives in or on another organism (its host) and benefits by deriving nutrients at the host's expense.

Antiviral An agent that kills a virus or suppresses its ability to replicate, inhibiting its capability to multiply and reproduce.

Apgar Newborn test performed at 1 minute of life and again at 5 and 10 minutes measuring heart rate, respiratory effort, muscle tone, reflex irritability, and color with each receiving a score of 0, 1, or 2.

Apnea Failure to breathe.

Approach behaviors Signals the baby sends to indicate a willingness to interact, such as tongue extension, bringing their hand to their mouth, or rooting.

Appropriate for gestational age (AGA) Born at the appropriate size for the number of weeks of gestation. When full term, the baby is heavier than 2500 grams (about 5.5 lb) and lighter than 4000 grams (about 8.75 lb).

Arachidonic acid Polyunsaturated fatty acid that has anti-inflammatory properties and can act as a vasodilator.

Areola The dark, circular area surrounding the nipple.

Assertiveness Self-assurance and confidence without being aggressive.

Assessment In healthcare, an evaluation of an individual that includes physical examination and medical history.

Assisted reproductive technology (ART) Reproductive technology to achieve pregnancy by artificial or partially artificial means, primarily in infertility treatments.

Assisted vaginal delivery (or operative vaginal delivery) (AVD or OVD) Vaginal delivery of a baby with the help of forceps or a vacuum device.

Assumption In statistics, a condition that must be true of the data for the statistical test to be used accurately.

Asymmetrical latch A latch with more of the breast below the nipple in the baby's mouth.

Asymmetry Disparity in size or shape.

Athelia The complete absence of the nipple-areolar complex, although there is underlying tissue.

Atopic dermatitis Allergic tendency (possibly inherited) to rash or inflammation of the skin.

Atresia Absence of a normal body opening.

Atrophy Loss of size of a part of the body because of disease or other influences. A natural occurrence in the final stage of lactation (involution).

Attending A counseling technique that involves listening and observing in a noninterfering manner.

Attentive listening A skill that involves being fully engaged and actively focusing on a speaker's words and message.

Autocrine control Local control within a gland. In lactation, a secretory product from one type of cell influences the activity of the same type of cell, suggesting that milk that is left in the gland acts to inhibit the production of more milk.

Autoimmune disorder Disorder in which the body's immune system attacks and destroys its healthy tissues. More than 80 types of autoimmune disorders exist, and females are more frequently affected than males.

Autonomic nerves Nerves that can function independently without outside influence.

Average In research, the sum of the values (in the group being averaged) divided by the number of members of the group.

Average baby Baby who is generally quiet, alert, and listening while awake; nurses between 8 and 12 times per day; and sleeps from 12 to 20 hours per day.

Avoidance behaviors Signals the baby sends to indicate an unwillingness to interact, such as frowning, wrinkling their brow, squinting, closing their eyes, or clenching their fists.

Axilla Pyramid-shaped space forming the underside of the shoulder between the upper part of the arm and the side of the chest. Also called *armpit*.

B

Baby blues Mild depression felt for several weeks after birth, frequently appearing around the third day postpartum. There may be bouts of tearfulness and sadness mingled with happiness and excitement. It is more common with a first baby.

Baby-Friendly Community Initiative (BFCI) An extension of the Baby-Friendly Hospital Initiative (BFHI) that provides continued lactation support to communities upon facility discharge after birth with a comprehensive support system through support groups.

Baby-Friendly Hospital Initiative (BFHI) Health initiative of the World Health Organization (WHO) and United Nations Children's Fund (UNICEF) launched in 1991 to protect, promote, and support lactation.

Baby training Feeding and putting infants to sleep at specific times, including feeding on a schedule. Emphasizes infants going to sleep on their own without nursing, rocking, bottles, or pacifiers.

Bactericidal Having the ability to destroy bacteria.

Bacteriostatic Having the ability to restrain the development of bacteria.

Bariatric surgery Weight loss surgery to limit either the amount of food consumed or the amount of food digested.

Barrier methods Contraception with physical or chemical barriers to prevent fertilization, including sponge and diaphragm, and male and female condoms.

Basal Referring to the fundamental or basic, as in the lowest body temperature or lowest prolactin level.

Basal metabolic rate Rate at which the body uses energy when at rest to perform body functions.

Baseline The starting value(s) before applying a treatment or test.

Bauer crawling reflex Reflex in which pressure on the soles of the feet elicits spontaneous crawling efforts and extension of the baby's head.

Bell curve The shape of the normal distribution on a graph, resembling the shape of a bell.

Bias In scientific studies, the tendency of a sample to misrepresent the whole population because the sample does not reflect the total target population studied. In statistics, the tendency to consistently overestimate or underestimate a true value.

Bifurcated or bifid Splitting into two branches or parts.

Bili-bed Fluorescent light to treat jaundice, with light rays emitting from a flat pad under the baby in an open bassinet.

Bili-blanket/bili-wrap Fluorescent fiber-optic wrap to treat jaundice, in which a flat light paddle is placed on the baby's back so that the baby can be held and fed during treatment.

Bili-light Fluorescent light to treat jaundice with light rays shining from an overhead light; the infant's eyes must be shielded by a patch.

Bilirubin A by-product of the breakdown of the hemoglobin portion of red blood cells.

Bioavailability The amount of a nutrient, drug, or other substance that is active in the tissues.

Biological nurturing See *laid-back nursing*.

Bisphenol A (BPA) An organic compound with two phenol functional groups thought to be hazardous to health.

Blind In research, a characteristic of a study in which the treatment is kept secret from the person receiving it and, often, from those giving the treatment as well.

Blood and lymph systems The blood, heart, and blood vessels form the circulatory system. The lymphatic system (lymph, lymph nodes, and lymph vessels) supports the circulatory system by draining excess fluids and proteins from tissues back into the bloodstream, thereby preventing tissue swelling.

Blood glucose The main simple sugar in blood that provides energy to all cells in the body.

Blood incompatibility Blood type incompatibility between a birth parent and baby that causes the parent to produce antibodies that destroy the infant's red blood cells, leading to rapid development of jaundice.

Body language Nonverbal messages sent by body position and gestures.

Body length An indicator of appropriate growth. At 1 year of age, a baby's length is typically about 1½ times the body length at birth.

Body mass index (BMI) A measure of the body that considers a person's weight and height to gauge total body fat in adults.

Bolus A round mass of food or liquid ready to be swallowed; a dose of a substance given intravenously.

Bonding Interaction between parents and their infant to form a unique, lasting relationship.

Bovine immunoglobulin G (IgG) Immunoglobulin specific to cow's milk, which can cause abdominal discomfort and excessive crying in the infant because of its high levels or long half-life.

Bradycardia A condition in which the heart contracts steadily but at a rate below normal.

Breast abscess A pocket of pus inside the breast, most commonly occurring during lactation.

Breast compression See *Alternate massage*.

Breast massage Manual massage to facilitate letdown and milk expression.

Breast pump A device to mechanically remove milk, which may be manual, battery, or electric.

Breastfeeding-associated jaundice Neonatal jaundice caused by mismanagement of lactation. Also called *lack-of-breastfeeding jaundice* and *suboptimal intake jaundice*.

Breastfeeding Report Card Report from the Centers for Disease Control and Prevention showing the extent to which infants are nursed in each U.S. state.

Breastmilk jaundice A rare type of neonatal jaundice caused by a factor in the milk, appearing between the fourth and seventh day of life. Also called *late-onset jaundice*.

Bristol Breastfeeding Assessment Tool (BBAT) A lactation assessment tool that facilitates accurate, rapid appraisal to target advice to parents acquiring early nursing skills and for those experiencing problems with an older baby.

Buccal frenula Folds of mucous membranes connecting buccal mucosa to alveolar mucosa.

Buccal pads A fat pad over the main cheek muscle that is evident in full-term infants and not fully developed in preterm infants. Also called a *sucking pad.*

Buprenorphine Partial micro-opioid receptor agonist and a kappa-opioid receptor antagonist drug used instead of methadone to treat opiate dependency.

C

Caffeine Component in coffee, tea, cola, chocolate, and some medications that can cause excessive crying in sensitive infants.

Calcium Dietary mineral that gives bones their rigidity and teeth their hardness.

Calming techniques Techniques to help soothe a fussy baby.

Calories Units of energy a food or beverage provides.

Candida albicans A tiny, common yeastlike fungus in the mouth, digestive tract, and vagina and on the skin of healthy persons.

Candidiasis A yeastlike fungal infection commonly afflicting the vagina that produces a thick vaginal discharge. Can be transmitted to the baby at birth and cause candidiasis in the baby's mouth and digestive tract, which appears as white patches or ulcers. May also occur on the nipples.

Cannabis (marijuana) Plant containing tetrahydrocannabinol (THC), an ingredient with narcotic and psychoactive effects. Believed to lower or inhibit prolactin levels and possibly affect milk production.

Capillaries Tiny blood vessels in the circulatory system that link the arteries and the veins.

Caput succedaneum A collection of fluid between a newborn's scalp and skull formed from pressure of the cervix on the infant's head during labor. The swelling begins to recede soon after birth.

Carbohydrates Sugars and starch in food that provide energy and play key roles in the immune system.

Care plan Documentation that describes a problem, options for solving it, and plans for follow-up.

Carpal tunnel syndrome Progressive condition caused by compression of a key nerve in the wrist resulting in numbness and pain; may interfere with comfortable positioning for feedings.

Case-control study Research that compares cases (people with the problem studied) with controls (similar people without the problem studied).

Case studies Studies describing one or several instances of a diagnosis, problem, or situation that arose in practice.

Casein Component of the proteins in milk.

Categorical data In research, data that can be classified but not quantified, such as the survey responses "very satisfied," "satisfied," "unsatisfied," and "very unsatisfied."

Celiac disease Autoimmune disorder in which ingestion of gluten leads to damage in the small intestine.

Centers for Disease Control and Prevention (CDC) An agency of the U.S. Public Health Service established in 1973 to protect public health through the prevention and control of diseases and other preventable health conditions and to respond to public health emergencies.

Cephalhematoma (also spelled *cephalohematoma*) Swelling from blood pooled under the scalp. It may begin in a baby during labor and may slowly become larger in the first few days after birth. It may result from trauma, often from forceps or vacuum extraction.

Change agent Someone who promotes organizational transformation by focusing, educating, and modeling effectiveness, improvement, and development.

Chiropractic care Care that emphasizes diagnosis, treatment, and prevention of mechanical disorders of the musculoskeletal system, especially the spine, theorizing that these disorders affect general health via the nervous system.

Chi-square In research, a statistical test to determine if there is a significant association between categorical variables.

C-hold Technique to help with latch with the free hand cupping the breast to form the letter *C* and the thumb on top and fingers curved below, well behind the areola.

Cholecystokinin (CCK) A gastrointestinal hormone released during sucking that enhances digestion, sedation, and a feeling of satiation and well-being.

Cisgender Personal identity and gender that corresponds with the sex assigned at birth.

Clavicle Long, curved horizontal bone above the first rib, forming the front portion of the shoulder. Also called the *collarbone.*

Cleft lip Upper lip with one or more clefts (splits) resulting from the failure of the upper jaw and nasal areas to fuse in the embryo.

Cleft palate A complete or partial opening through the hard and soft palates into the nasal area at birth. It is often linked to a cleft in the upper lip.

Clustered feeding Period of almost constant wakefulness and nursing, generally in the early evening. Also referred to as *bunched feedings.*

Clutch hold See *Side-sitting hold.*

Cocaine Illicit drug that stimulates the central nervous system and causes irritability, jitteriness, tremors, increased heart and respiratory rates, and convulsions or seizures in the infant.

Code of Professional Conduct A set of International Board of Lactation Consultant Examiners (IBLCE) principles that provides guidance in professional practice and conduct.

Cognitive learning Learning that involves perception and judgment.

Cohen's kappa In research, a statistical test to measure concordance for dichotomous data, with kappa values of 0.7 or higher generally considered evidence of excellent agreement.

Cohort In research, a group studied together because of a characteristic or experience they have in common.

Cohort study Observational research that follows a group of participants with a characteristic or experience in common over a period of time, examining how certain factors affect health outcomes.

Colicky behavior Extreme fussiness that is characterized by a baby's piercing cry, severe abdominal discomfort, and inability to be comforted. Now called *excessive crying*.

Colostrum Milk secreted during pregnancy, after childbirth, and before the onset of mature milk.

Combined spinal–epidural (CSE) A regional technique that combines rapid onset of a spinal anesthesia with epidural anesthesia and analgesia that remains in place to provide long-lasting relief.

Commission on Accreditation of Allied Health Education Programs (CAAHEP) Agency that accredits academic lactation programs in postsecondary institutions.

Complementary feeding Adding new foods to the growing nursing infant's diet to meet the energy and nutrient needs that are not met by human milk alone.

Complete protein complement An incomplete protein food combined with other incomplete protein foods to fill in the missing nutrients.

Complex carbohydrates Carbohydrates that contain important vitamins and minerals, take longer to digest than simple carbohydrates, and do not stimulate a craving for more food. Foods in this category include vegetables; fruits; and whole-grain cereals, rice, breads, and crackers.

Confidence intervals (CIs) In statistics, the range within which a population's true value is expected to be found.

Conformity Attitude or behavior that occurs in response to pressure toward a social norm.

Confounding variables In research, a characteristic, attribute, or experience of people in a study that could confuse the interpretation of the study's results.

Conjugation The process by which the liver converts bilirubin into a form that can be broken down and passed into the intestine for excretion.

Connective tissue Fibrous tissue that supports and contains the fatty tissue and the milk-producing and milk-transporting tissues in the mammary gland.

Constipation Condition in which feces are molded and firm to the touch, appearing like pellets or marbles.

Consumer responsibilities The responsibility of consumers to become informed and manage outcomes, as in their health and the health of their children.

Consumer rights The right to information that will enable one to grow as an informed consumer.

Continuing Education Recognition Points (CERPs) Required professional education for International Board Certified Lactation Consultants (IBCLCs) to maintain their credential.

Contraception Use of a technique or device to prevent pregnancy.

Control In research, the group of individuals in a study to whom the treatment was not given (in an experiment) or who do not have the problem of interest (in a case-control study). The amount or type of regulation of study conditions the researchers can exercise.

Convenience In research, a type of sample selected by the researcher that is not random or carefully defined but rather readily accessible.

Coombs' test Test that measures the presence of antibodies to red blood cells in the blood.

Cooper's ligaments Ligaments that run vertically through the mammary gland and attach the deep layer of subcutaneous tissue to the dermis of the skin.

Core Curriculum for Interdisciplinary Lactation Care Text that identifies core knowledge for the lactation profession.

Correlation In research, shown to be associated by a specific statistical test.

Cosleeping Practice in which the infant sleeps with the parents.

COVID-19 A coronaviral disease that became a global pandemic, with resulting safety concerns for nursing newborns and families.

Cow's milk The milk of bovines (cows) and the most used substance in artificial infant formula.

Cow's milk protein allergy Response by the infant's immune system to bovine milk and products containing bovine milk proteins.

Cradle cap (seborrheic dermatitis) Thick, scaly dandruff mostly found on the newborn's scalp and sometimes on the face, ears, neck, or diaper area. Also known as *seborrheic dermatitis*.

Cradle hold Sitting position with the baby's body across the parent's abdomen and the baby's head resting in the crook of the arm, supporting the baby's body with the opposite hand.

Craniosacral Referring to the skull, spine, and sacrum; gentle manipulation to reduce pain and tension.

Cronbach's alpha In research, a test to determine whether items on a scale or tool are internally consistent or whether they measure the same concept in a similar way.

Cross-cradle hold The same holding technique as the dominant hand hold but used for the less dominant hand as well. See *Dominant hand hold*.

Cross-nursing Nursing another parent's baby.

Cross-sectional study Research that examines a question at one point in time (such as surveys of a neighborhood all collected within the same week).

Cultural humility An ongoing process of self-exploration and self-critique combined with a willingness to honor the beliefs, customs, and values of others and accept them for who they are.

Culture The environment that surrounds us and influences our beliefs and attitudes.

Cup feeding Alternate feeding method in which the baby is fed with a cup.

Cystic fibrosis An inherited condition in which the cells that produce mucus, sweat, and digestive juices do not function correctly, causing thick, sticky secretions that obstruct the lungs and other organs.

Cytokines A family of growth factors secreted primarily from leukocytes that stimulate humoral and cellular immune responses, as well as the activation of phagocytic cells.

Cytomegalovirus (CMV) A usually benign herpes virus that can lead to severe systemic damage in preterm infants and people with suppressed immune systems.

D

Dancer hand position Position that begins in the C-hold position, bringing the hand forward to support the breast with three fingers and bending the index finger to gently hold the baby's cheek on one side, with the thumb holding the other cheek. A technique to help the baby's tongue form correctly for nursing and provide stability for the baby to stay latched. Originated by Sarah Danner and Ed Cerutti.

Dehydration Large loss of water from the body tissues.

Demographics Variables that describe basic characteristics of subjects, such as age, gender, place of residence, income, education, and ethnicity.

Dependent variable In research, the aspect or characteristic of test subjects, or of their experience, that a researcher is trying to understand or explain. In a study of the effect of calories on weight gain, for example, weight gain is the dependent variable.

Dermis The layer of skin immediately below the outer layer (epidermis) that contains blood and lymph vessels, nerves and nerve endings, glands, and hair follicles.

Descriptive study In research, usually a study that explores a phenomenon by describing it in detail rather than trying to control any aspects of it.

Detailed Content Outline An International Board of Lactation Consultant Examiners (IBLCE) document that identifies the clinical skills topics and chronological periods required for certification.

Detoxify Speed up the removal of harmful substances from the body.

Diabetes A disorder of carbohydrate metabolism resulting from inadequate secretion or utilization of insulin.

Diabetic mastopathy The presence of a benign tumor-like breast mass in individuals with insulin-dependent diabetes mellitus.

Diaper rash Small, reddened, pimple-like rash in the diaper area that responds to frequent diaper changes, careful washing, air drying, and over-the-counter ointments or creams.

Diarrhea Feces that are looser than normal, very watery, and may be greenish and very foul-smelling.

Dichlorodiphenyldichloroethylene (DDE) Main breakdown product of dichlorodiphenyltrichloroethane (DDT).

Dichlorodiphenyltrichloroethane (DDT) Pesticide used in farming and banned in most countries because of potential harm to humans.

Dichotomous outcome An outcome measure in which there are only two possibilities, such as yes/no or true/false.

Dietary reference intake (DRI) System of nutrition recommendations from the Institute of Medicine (IOM) of the U.S. National Academy of Sciences.

Digital baby weight scale A device to weigh babies that is designed for measurement accuracy.

Digital technique Use of a finger to assess an infant's oral structure or to perform suck assessment and/or training.

Disorganized suck Temporary sucking difficulty due to illness, preterm birth, medications, a delay in the first feeding, a neuromotor dysfunction, variations in oral anatomy, or nipple preference from the use of an artificial nipple.

Disparity Inequality in access to power and opportunities based on gender, gender identity and expression, sexual orientation, class, language, race, color, culture, ethnicity, nationality, marital status, geography, immigration, generation, religion, ability, size, or age.

Distribution In research, the way the values of a variable (independent or dependent) range; how many values are small, medium, and large. Often, this is shown graphically.

Documentation Guidelines An International Board of Lactation Consultant Examiners (IBLCE) document that provides suggestions for clinical recordkeeping for the lactation professional.

Dominant culture Specific behaviors, rituals, values, and social customs that constitute a societal norm.

Dominant hand hold Position with the baby's head supported in the dominant hand and the baby's body supported with the forearm. The baby can nurse on the nearest side, and then the arm can move the baby across to the opposite side.

Donor milk Human milk that is expressed and donated to a human milk bank to be given to another baby.

Dopamine A hormone made in the adrenal gland that acts as a prolactin inhibitor.

Doula An experienced caregiver who helps parents immediately before, during, and/or after delivery.

Down syndrome A disorder in which the baby is born with an extra chromosome, also known as *trisomy 21*.

Duarte's variant Variation of galactosemia, in which the infant can consume human milk (either totally or partially) with careful monitoring of galactose levels.

Duct system A system of ducts and ductules through which milk flows from the alveoli out to the nipple pores.

Ductal narrowing Compressed duct that restricts milk flow when the surrounding tissue is inflamed or swollen. Previously referred to as *blocked duct* or *plugged duct*.

Ductule Small duct that drains milk from the alveoli into larger ducts that terminate in the nipple.

Dyad Two individuals who form one unit, each dependent on the other, such as a nursing dyad of parent and baby.

Dysfunctional suck Sucking anomaly that requires a referral to a physical, occupational, or speech therapist with specialization in infant disorders.

Dysphagia A disorder that causes difficulty swallowing and possibly coughing or choking and bringing food back up, sometimes through the nose. It can lead to oral aversion.

Dysphoric milk-ejection reflex A physiological condition that causes intense negative feelings when the milk lets down.

E

Eclampsia A hypertensive disease during pregnancy with multisystem involvement and possible coma and convulsive seizures. A severe complication of preeclampsia that occurs in the second half of pregnancy and is characterized by hypertension and protein in the urine, and possible coma and convulsive seizures.

Eczema Swelling of the outer layer of skin that may be itchy and red, have small blisters, and weep.

Edema A local or generalized condition in which body tissues contain excessive fluid.

Edinburgh Postnatal Depression Scale (EPDS) Scale for rating the degree of postpartum depression.

Electronic communication Communication through computer, phone, voice mail, text messaging, email, or social media.

Electronic health record A comprehensive patient history maintained electronically and designed to share information across providers, hospitals, and regions.

Electronic medical record Standard medical and clinical data gathered by a healthcare provider and maintained electronically.

Electronic publication (Epub) The publishing of original works online before or in lieu of print.

Empathetic listening A counseling technique of listening with the intent to understand emotionally and intellectually.

Empowerment The act of promoting or influencing self-actualization. The process of becoming stronger and more confident.

Endocrine Pertaining to a gland that secretes directly into the bloodstream.

Endometriosis Condition in which the tissue (endometrium) normally lining the uterus grows outside the uterus, frequently causing pain and infertility.

Engorgement Swelling or congestion of body tissues; overfullness.

Engrossment Parents interacting with their infants.

Enteral Within or by way of the intestines.

Environmental contaminant Impurity in human milk that results from contamination of the environment by such chemicals as dichlorodiphenyltrichloroethane (DDT), polybrominated biphenyl (PBB), and polychlorinated biphenyl (PCB) that then enter the food chain and are consumed.

Enzyme A protein that speeds up or causes chemical reactions in living matter.

Epidermal growth factor Growth factor in human milk that stimulates cell growth, proliferation, and differentiation.

Epidermis The outer layers of the skin made up of an outer, dead portion and a deeper, living portion. Epidermal cells gradually move outward to the skin surface, changing as they go, until they become flakes.

Epidural analgesia Agent injected into the epidural space of the spinal cord to create loss of feeling in the body from the injection site down.

Epidural anesthesia Agent injected into the epidural space of the spinal cord to create total loss of feeling in the body from the uterus down. Used for cesarean delivery.

Epigenetics Study of the epigenome, the cellular layer that sits on top of the genome, and the mechanisms that turn genes "on" or "off."

Epiglottis The cartilage-like structure that overhangs the trachea like a lid and closes during swallowing to prevent food from entering the trachea.

Epinephrine A hormone secreted by the adrenal gland in response to stress or fear that increases heart rate, opens airways, and is part of the "fight-or-flight" reaction. Also known as *adrenaline*.

Episiotomy A surgical incision to enlarge the vaginal opening during childbirth.

Epithelium The tissue that covers the internal and external surfaces of the body.

Epstein pearls Small protein-filled harmless cysts that look like tiny white bumps on the gumlines or palate.

Epstein–Barr A herpes virus spread through bodily fluids, especially saliva. Symptoms include fatigue; fever; and swollen lymph nodes, liver, and spleen. The virus can cause infectious mononucleosis, also known as the "kissing disease."

Erythema toxicum Pink to red macular (raised) area in newborns with a yellow or white center. It has no apparent significance and requires no treatment.

Estrogen The hormone that stimulates growth of the reproductive organs, including alveoli and ducts in the mammary gland.

Eustachian tube Tube lined with mucous membrane that joins the nose–throat cavity (nasopharynx) and the inner ear (tympanic cavity).

Evert Protrude outward.

Evidence-based practice Practice based largely on scientific research.

Evidence-informed practice Practice where no evidence-based research trials or other scientific basis exists that combines the clinician's knowledge and expertise, the patient's needs and preferences, and clinical circumstances with the best available evidence from research.

Exchange transfusion Medical procedure that replaces blood with donated blood or plasma.

Exclusive nursing Infant feeding with no drinks or foods other than human milk; no pacifiers or artificial nipples; no limits on feeding frequency or duration; and ensuring at least 8 to 12 feedings in 24 hours, including night feedings.

Exclusively pump Remove milk from the breast to feed the baby rather than directly nursing.

Exocrine gland Type of gland that releases substances through ducts onto body surfaces or into body cavities.

Exocrine system System of exocrine glands, including sweat, mammary, and salivary glands.

Exogenous Derived from outside the body.

Experiment Research in which the scientist selects a sample and applies a treatment or action to part of the sample to measure the differences between treated and untreated parts.

Extremely low birth weight (ELBW) Born weighing under 2 lb, 3 oz (1000 g).

F

Fabrication In research, the presentation of fake data or results as true research.

Failure to thrive (FTT) Term that was replaced by growth faltering to better capture the symptoms of inadequate nutrition in infants. See *Growth faltering*.

Falsification In research, exclusion or manipulation of research data or materials to achieve a desired result, not a true outcome.

Fat necrosis A lump of dead or damaged tissue after breast surgery, radiation, or another trauma.

Fat-soluble vitamins Vitamins A, D, E, and K.

Fatty tissue Body tissue containing stored fat that serves as a source of energy and cushions and insulates vital organs; component of the breast.

Feedback inhibitor of lactation (FIL) A term previously used to describe human whey protein that regulates milk production by inhibiting milk synthesis when milk remains in the breast.

Fiber-optic blanket See *Bili-blanket/bili-wrap*.

Fibroblast growth factor Hormone that controls a wide range of biological functions and regulates cellular proliferation, survival, migration, and differentiation.

Fibrocystic breast A common type of benign condition that causes lumpiness in the breast.

Finger feeding A feeding method in which the baby sucks on a finger with a 5-, 6-, or 8-French oral gastric tube that leads to the liquid placed along the fat pad of the finger, extending a few centimeters beyond the tip of the finger. See also *Tube feeding*.

Fistula An abnormal passage from an internal organ to the body surface or between two internal organs.

Flange The portion of a breast pump that is placed against the breast to form suction.

Flanged Extending outward, flaring, as in the baby's upper and lower lips curled outward when latched.

Flash-heat method Milk treatment in which a container is placed into a pan of water, heated to a rolling boil, and then removed.

Flat nipple A nipple that remains flat when compressed, neither everting nor inverting.

Flatulence Excessive gas in the stomach and abdomen, causing pain.

Flexion A state of being bent or curved.

Flora Bacteria, fungi, and other microorganisms normally occurring on or in the body.

Fluoride A compound added to water supplies or toothpaste or ingested as a supplement to reduce tooth decay.

Fontanel A space between the bones of an infant's skull covered by tough membranes.

Food intolerance An adverse reaction to specific foods, which occurs in about 10% of the population and may be chronic and progress to severe illness.

Food sensitivity In lactation, an infant's reaction to something in the parent's diet.

Football hold See *Side-sitting hold*.

Forceps Instrument to help a difficult childbirth, to quickly deliver a baby with breathing problems, or to shorten normal labor. The blades of the forceps are put into the vagina one at a time and applied to opposite sides of the baby's head, with the baby's head held firmly between the blades.

Foremilk The high lactose milk that is present at the beginning of a feeding.

Formal stage The second of four stages in role acquisition, a time in which the role is viewed more personally.

Frenotomy A procedure to release a tight frenulum by clipping or laser cautery. Also called *frenectomy* or *frenulotomy*.

Frenuloplasty A procedure to release a tight frenulum that involves deep cutting and stitches. Also called *frenoplasty*.

Fussy baby A baby who is consistently fretful, crying, or unsettled for no discernible reason.

G

Galactagogue (also spelled *galactogogue*) Food, drink, medication, or herb that is believed to increase milk production.

Galactocele A cyst caused by the blockage of a milk duct that contains a thick, creamy, milk-like substance and may be discharged from the nipple when compressed.

Galactopoiesis Stage III lactogenesis, which marks the establishment and maintenance of mature milk.

Galactorrhea Secretion and release of milk unrelated to childbirth or lactation; excessive or inappropriate milk production. Also called *spontaneous lactation*.

Galactose A simple sugar produced by the breakdown of lactose (milk sugar).

Galactosemia An inherited disorder caused by lack of an enzyme that prevents the body from breaking down galactose, causing it to build up to toxic levels in the blood.

Gastroenteritis Inflammation of the stomach and intestines that can cause nausea, vomiting, diarrhea, and cramps.

Gastroesophageal reflux (GER) A backflow of acidic contents of the stomach into the esophagus that produces burning pain, often resulting from failure of the lower esophageal sphincter to close.

Gastroesophageal reflux disease (GERD) Medical diagnosis of gastroesophageal reflux associated with persistent symptoms or complications, including esophagitis, low weight gain, growth faltering, and respiratory disorders.

Gastrostomy Gavage feeding in which a tube is placed through the skin directly into the stomach.

Gavage feeding A feeding method in which a tube is passed through the nose, mouth, or skin into the stomach.

Gender assignment The classification at birth as either male or female based on the inspection of the external genitalia or other indicators.

Gender dysphoria Distress experienced when a person's gender identity differs from the sex assigned at birth.

Gender expression The way a person publicly expresses their gender.

Gender identity A person's innate sense of their gender.

Gene expression Process by which information encoded in a gene is used to synthesize products such as RNA or proteins.

Generalize In research, extending the results of a study beyond the people studied to include a larger group who are more or less like them.

Genetically modified (engineered) food Foods derived from bioengineered modified organisms that have had changes introduced into their DNA using various methods of genetic engineering.

Gestational age The age of a fetus or a newborn, usually stated in weeks, dating from the first day of the last menses.

Gestational ovarian theca lutein cyst A cyst filled with clear, straw-colored fluid that develops in the ovary when an egg is not impregnated, shrinks, and is shed during menstruation.

Ghrelin A peptide hormone that signals hunger to the brain, often called the "hunger hormone."

Glandular tissue Functional part of the breast that produces and transports milk.

Global Data Bank on Infant and Young Child Feeding Pooling of information by the World Health Organization from national and regional surveys and studies focusing on the prevalence and duration of nursing and complementary feeding practices.

Global Strategy for Infant and Young Child Feeding World Health Organization (WHO) and United Nations Children's Fund (UNICEF) strategy released in 2003 to address appropriate, evidence-based feeding practices for infants and young children that are essential for attaining and maintaining proper nutrition and health.

Glucuronic acid An agent that conjugates bilirubin in the liver.

Glycan A polysaccharide or oligosaccharide.

Goiter Enlarged thyroid gland, resulting in a thick-looking neck or double-chin appearance.

Gonadotropins Protein hormones secreted by the pituitary that stimulate the activity of the gonads.

Grommet See *Obturator*.

Growth factor A naturally occurring substance capable of stimulating cellular growth, proliferation, healing, and cellular differentiation.

Growth faltering Term that replaced the term failure to thrive to better capture the symptoms of malnutrition in infants, adding aspects of infant behavior and motor development to weight parameters.

Gut closure Closure of open junctions in cells of the infant's immature gut, which protects the infant from the risk of necrotizing enterocolitis, diarrheal disease, and allergies.

H

Half-life The time needed for a drug's level in the bloodstream to decline to one-half of its beginning level.

Hard palate Thin horizontal bony plate in the roof of the mouth, in line with the end of the upper alveolar ridge.

Head circumference Measurement of a head around its largest area, from above the eyebrows and ears and around the back of the head.

Health consumerism Exerting control as a responsible decision-maker concerning health care.

Health disparities Inequalities in health when members of certain population groups do not have the same health status as other groups.

Health equity The opportunity for all people to attain their full health potential.

Health inequities Health disadvantages that are modifiable, associated with social disadvantage, and considered ethically unfair.

Health Insurance Portability and Accountability Act (HIPAA) U.S. regulations to protect patient privacy in health care.

Healthy People 2030 Science-based, 10-year national objectives for improving the health of all Americans.

Hematocrit A measure of the number of red cells in blood, stated as a percentage of total blood volume.

Hemoglobin The portion of the red blood cell that transports oxygen to all parts of the body.

Hemolysis The destruction of red blood cells, leading to the release of hemoglobin into the bloodstream.

Hemorrhagic disease Disease of the newborn caused by a lack of vitamin K.

Hepatitis A Liver inflammation caused by the hepatitis A virus, which is transmitted by infected food and water, with symptoms of fatigue, fever, liver enlargement, and jaundice.

Hepatitis B A liver infection caused by the hepatitis B virus, which is transmitted by bodily fluids. May be acute (malaise, fever, jaundice) or chronic (asymptomatic) and may lead to scarring of the liver (cirrhosis) or liver cancer.

Hepatitis C A usually asymptomatic chronic liver infection caused by the hepatitis C virus, which is transmitted by blood transfusions, hemodialysis, and needle sticks. May lead to scarring of the liver (cirrhosis) or liver cancer. Considered the most serious hepatitis infection because of the lack of symptoms until years later.

Heroin Highly addictive drug of abuse that converts to morphine when it enters the body.

Herpes A family of eight viruses that infect humans with varying degrees of severity: herpes simplex 1, herpes simplex 2, herpes varicella, herpes zoster, Epstein–Barr, cytomegalovirus, and herpes simplex 7 and 8.

Heterogeneity In research, variability among studies in a systematic review that may be clinical, methodological, or statistical.

High-risk infant An infant born at risk because of a medical condition or social situation.

Hindmilk The high-fat milk resulting from the letdown reflex, which forces milk from the alveoli and washes fat from the walls of the ducts.

Hirschsprung's disease A congenital condition in which muscles in the infant's intestines lack proper nerve cells and the stool does not pass easily beyond that point. These infants frequently have large, bloated abdomens from the collection of stool and gas.

History In health care, information relevant to the health of the parent and infant, both past and present, including significant illnesses, disorders, and surgeries.

Holder pasteurization Heat treating liquid at either 56°C or 62.5°C (132.8°F or 144.5°F).

Homogeneity The state of being all the same. In studies hypothesizing that two groups are different in important ways, finding sameness between them invalidates the results.

Hospital privileges Permission granted to a healthcare provider to practice at a healthcare facility.

Human immunodeficiency virus (HIV) Virus that attacks and weakens the body's immune system, thus allowing opportunistic viruses, bacteria, parasites, and fungi to cause illness and death.

Human milk bank A service to collect, screen, process, and distribute donated milk to meet the medical needs of individuals for whom it is prescribed.

Human milk fortifier (HMF) Nutrients added to expressed milk to enhance the growth and nutrient balances of VLBW infants and ELBW infants.

Humoral factors Factors such as antimicrobial immunoglobulin antibodies and multiple proteins that are transported by the circulatory system.

Hunch Using intuition to develop a hypothesis.

Hunger cues A progression of signs that indicate an infant's desire to feed, beginning with body wriggling and rapid eye movement (REM), followed by mouthing movements, passing their hand(s) over their head, and bringing a hand to their mouth. Also referred to as *feeding cues.*

Hydatid disease Parasitic infection that can mimic a galactocele.

Hydration Water balance within the body.

Hydrocephalus An increase in abnormal cerebrospinal fluid within the cranial cavity that can lead to skull enlargement (especially the forehead) and brain atrophy.

Hyperalimentation The administration of nutrients by intravenous feeding, especially to individuals such as preterm infants who cannot ingest food through the alimentary tract.

Hyperbilirubinemia A condition characterized by excessive bilirubin in the blood, which causes yellow coloring of the tissues, membranes, and secretions. Also referred to as *jaundice.*

Hypernatremia Overconcentration of sodium in the blood, caused by excess loss of water and electrolytes resulting from diarrhea, excessive sweating, or inadequate water intake.

Hyperprolactinemia A condition characterized by elevated prolactin levels in the blood.

Hypertension High blood pressure persistently exceeding 140/90, often without external symptoms.

Hyperthyroidism A condition in which the thyroid gland produces too much thyroid hormone, causing weight loss, hair loss, nervousness, increased heart rate, and moodiness. Frequently caused by Graves' disease, an autoimmune disorder.

Hypertonic A condition characterized by abnormally high tension or tone, especially of the muscles.

Hypocalcemia A condition characterized by inadequate calcium in the blood.

Hypoglycemia A condition characterized by low blood glucose levels.

Hypopituitarism See *Sheehan's syndrome.*

Hypoplasia A condition characterized by an incomplete or underdeveloped organ or tissue, usually the result of a decrease in the number of cells.

Hypothalamus The portion of the brain forming the floor and part of the side wall of the third ventricle; it triggers the release of hormones.

Hypothesis In research, an expected relationship between two variables expressed before a study and around which the study is designed.

Hypothyroidism A deficiency of thyroid secretions causing low metabolism.

Hypotonic A condition characterized by abnormally low tension or tone, especially of the muscles.

Hypoxia Insufficient oxygen in the cells, characterized by rapid heartbeat, high blood pressure, contraction of blood vessels, dizziness, and mental confusion.

I

Iatrogenic Induced inadvertently by a medical practitioner, treatment, or diagnostic procedure.

Idiopathic granulomatous mastitis (IGM) A benign condition that causes long periods of significant inflammation of the breast and overlying skin.

Immunoglobulin Group of five distinct antibodies in the serum and external secretions of the body that provide immunity; includes immunoglobulin (Ig)A, IgD, IgE, IgG, and IgM.

Immunoglobulin A (IgA) The immunoglobulin that has the highest concentration in colostrum and human milk and is the most biologically active; it is available only through human milk.

Immunological Providing immunity to disease by stimulating antigens.

Implants Devices or tissues placed inside or on the surface of the body, as in breast implants.

Implicit bias Having attitudes towards people or associating stereotypes with them without conscious knowledge.

Independent variable The aspect of research subjects or their experience that may explain or predict the result or outcome. In a study of the effect of calories on weight gain, for example, calories are the independent variable.

Inducing lactation Stimulating milk production in individuals who have not gone through pregnancy.

Induction A method of artificially or prematurely stimulating labor.

Infant acne Skin condition resembling adolescent acne that appears on the newborn's face, primarily the nose, forehead, and cheeks. It usually starts at about 2 weeks of age, disappears at 8 to 10 weeks, and is believed to result from sebaceous gland stimulation by maternal or infant hormones.

Infant Breastfeeding Assessment Tool (IBFAT) Tool that assesses infant behavior during a feeding.

Infant states Six states of infant sleep and wakefulness: deep sleep, light sleep, drowsy, quiet and alert, active and alert, and crying.

Infertility Failure to conceive after 12 months of unprotected intercourse.

Informal stage The third of four stages in role acquisition, marked by modifying, blending, and individualizing one's role.

Informed consent Consent to care based on sufficient information.

Inhibited letdown Failure of milk to let down because of a weak suck, ineffective latch, fatigue, anxiety, fear, or pain.

Injectables Artificial hormonal preparations administered by a deep intramuscular injection and slowly absorbed into the bloodstream, providing sufficient levels of contraceptive hormone for 1 to 3 months, depending on the type of contraceptive used.

Innervation The distribution or supply of nerve fibers or nerve impulses to a part of the body.

Innocenti Declaration Declaration to promote, protect, and support lactation, produced and adopted by policymakers from the World Health Organization (WHO) and United Nations Children's Fund (UNICEF) at the Spedale degli Innocenti in Florence, Italy, in 1990.

Institutional bias Discriminatory policies and practices within an organization against groups of people.

Instruments In research, measurement tools to aid in subject, client, or patient evaluation, such as scales, indexes, questionnaires, interviews, and informal observations. In statistics, instruments are mathematical formulas used to estimate causal effects.

Insufficient glandular tissue A condition of arrested development in which the breasts remain below the normal size, also called *hypoplasia.*

Insulin-like growth factor Proteins with high sequence similarity to insulin, part of a complex system that cells use to communicate with their physiologic environment.

Intercostal nerves Any of 11 nerves on each side of which is an anterior division of a thoracic nerve lying between a pair of adjacent ribs.

Internal validity In research, the assurance that extraneous variables are not responsible for observed results.

International Board Certified Lactation Consultant (IBCLC) A healthcare professional who specializes in the clinical management of lactation and is certified by the International Board of Lactation Consultant Examiners.

International Board of Lactation Consultant Examiners (IBLCE) A nonprofit corporation established in 1985 to develop and administer certification for lactation consultants.

***International Classification of Diseases* (ICD-11) codes** The eleventh revision of the coding system created by the World Health Organization that is used to code various medical records, including diseases, symptoms, abnormal findings, and external causes of injury.

International Code of Marketing of Breast-milk Substitutes (the International Code) A set of resolutions developed in 1979 by the World Health Organization (WHO) and the United Nations Children's Fund (UNICEF) that regulates the marketing and distribution of any fluid intended to replace human milk, devices used to feed such fluids, and the role of healthcare workers who advise on infant feeding.

International Lactation Consultant Association (ILCA) The professional association for lactation consultants founded in 1985 for health professionals who specialize in promoting, protecting, and supporting lactation.

Intimate partner violence (IPV) Physical, sexual, or psychological harm by a current or former partner.

Intraductal papilloma Benign tumor within a duct that is often associated with a spontaneous bloody discharge.

Intralipids Lipids given with total parenteral nutrition.

Intramuscular (IM) Referring to the inside of a muscle, such as an injection into a muscle to administer medicine.

Intrauterine device (IUD) A contraceptive copper or hormonal device placed into the uterus to prevent a fertilized egg from implanting.

Intrauterine growth restriction (IUGR) Condition in which the fetal weight is estimated to be below the 10th percentile for its gestational age.

Intravenous Referring to the inside of a vein, such as with a tube inserted into a vein to provide nutrients or medication directly into the bloodstream.

Intubation Medical procedure in which a tube passes into a body opening, such as with a breathing tube through the mouth or nose or into the trachea to provide an airway for anesthetic gas or oxygen.

Inverted nipple Nipple that retracts when compressed.

Involution A normal process marked by decreasing size of an organ, such as in involution of the uterus after birth or the involution of the breast after weaning.

Iron Mineral required in red cell formation, with greater amounts needed during pregnancy to support the growing fetus and placenta and to increase red cell mass.

J

Jaundice See *Hyperbilirubinemia*.

K

Kangaroo care See *Skin-to-skin care*.

Keratin The tough surface layer of dead skin developed in response to pressure.

Kernicterus Chronic and permanent brain damage caused by excessive bilirubin depositing in the brain tissues.

Kilocalorie (kcal) Unit of heat equal to the amount of heat required to raise the temperature of 1 kilogram of water by 1 degree at 1 atmospheric pressure. Used by nutritionists to characterize the energy-producing potential in food.

L

Labial frenum A membranous band of tissue that connects the upper lip to the upper alveolar ridge (gumline). Also called the *maxillary*, *upper*, or *superior frenum*.

Lactase An enzyme that increases the conversion rate of milk sugar (lactose) to glucose and galactose, carbohydrates needed by the body for energy.

Lactase deficiency (lactase nonpersistence) Digestive disorder characterized by the body's inability to produce enough lactase, an enzyme needed to break down lactose.

Lactation Education Accreditation and Approval Review Committee (LEAARC) Organization that established and maintains standards in lactation consultant education, recognizes lactation courses, and recommends academic lactation programs for accreditation through the Commission on Accreditation of Allied Health Education Programs (CAAHEP).

Lactational amenorrhea method (LAM) Contraception method that relies on three conditions: menses have not yet returned, the baby nurses around the clock without other foods, and the baby is younger than 6 months.

Lactiferous sinus Former description of the ducts beneath the areola, now considered to be a temporary dilation during letdown as milk passes through the ducts.

Lactobacillus bifidus Organism in the intestinal tract of nursing infants that discourages the colonization of bacteria.

Lactocyte Specialized epithelial cells in the mammary gland responsible for synthesizing and secreting milk.

Lactoengineering Process of separating milk components to fortify human milk to meet the needs of very low-birth-weight and extremely low-birth-weight infants.

Lactoferrin An iron-binding protein that increases absorption of iron.

Lactogenesis The phases during which milk production and secretion are established.

Lactogenesis I Initiation of milk synthesis.

Lactogenesis II Copious milk production.

Lactogenesis III Establishment of mature milk production; also called *galactopoiesis*.

Lactose The type of sugar present in human milk. Also called *milk sugar*.

Lactose intolerance A disorder resulting in the inability to digest milk sugar (lactose) because of lactase deficiency.

Lactose overload Excessive lactose intake in the infant, which may produce green, frothy, loose, and frequent stools; poor weight gain; bloated abdomen; and large amounts of gas.

Laid-back nursing A nursing position where gravity and primitive neonatal reflexes allow the baby to find and latch onto the nipple. The parent lies on their back with the baby placed tummy down on the chest. Also called *prone position, posture feeding, and biological nurturing*.

Large for gestational age (LGA) Infant designation determined by size and weight at birth being in the top 10% of the growth rate appropriate for gestational age.

Larynx Part of the air passage connecting the throat with the windpipe (trachea) that leads toward the lungs; rises and is closed off by the epiglottis during swallowing.

Latch The infant grasping the nipple and surrounding tissue to form a seal and generate negative pressure to begin sucking.

LATCH Acronym for a system to assess the infant's ability to latch and evaluate audible swallowing as a determinant of milk intake: **L**atch, **A**udible swallow, **T**ype of nipple, **C**omfort, and **H**old.

Late-preterm (LPT) Born between the gestational ages of 34 weeks and 0/7 days through 36 weeks and 6/7 days (formerly called near term).

Leaky gut syndrome A condition in which the intestinal lining becomes inflamed, thin, and porous, allowing incompletely digested proteins to cross into the bloodstream.

Learning climate The prevailing influence or set of conditions characterizing the setting in which learning takes place.

Learning style Manner in which an individual acquires and processes information in learning situations, including styles such as visual, auditory, kinesthetic, and reading/writing.

Leptin A peptide hormone in human milk that regulates energy intake and expenditure, including appetite and metabolism.

Lesbian, gay, bisexual, transgender, queer, questioning, plus (LGBTQ+) Term used in the United States to describe non-cisgender sexual orientation or gender identity that includes lesbian, gay, bisexual, transgender, queer or questioning, and other identities that fall outside these categories.

Letdown Milk ejection triggered by nipple stimulation or as a conditioned reflex.

Leukocytes Cells in human milk that fight infection.

Liability Obligation to provide care meeting the standard of practice for a profession.

Likert scale A measurement scale for attitude or opinion that uses fixed-choice response formats to measure levels of agreement or disagreement with the statement. Pronounced "lick-ert".

Liminality A transitional stage between a previous cultural norm and a return to culturally normal status.

Lingual frenulum A fold of mucous membrane under the center portion of the tongue.

Lipase A digestive system enzyme that increases the breakdown of fats (lipids).

Lipids Group of naturally occurring molecules that includes fats, waxes, sterols, fat-soluble vitamins (such as vitamins A, D, E, and K), monoglycerides, diglycerides, triglycerides, phospholipids, and others.

Lobule A small lobe, a cluster of 10 to 100 alveoli.

Lochia Discharge that is composed of blood, mucus, and tissue caused by the gradual renewal of reproductive structures after childbirth. Its color transforms from red to pink and then to white in about 2 to 4 weeks.

Logistic regression In research, a statistical technique for studying relationships between variables that can be used when the dependent (outcome) variable is dichotomous (only two possibilities).

Long-chain polyunsaturated fatty acid Fatty acid that promotes optimal neural and visual development.

Low birth weight (LBW) Born weighing less than 5 lb, 8 oz (2500 g) at birth.

Luteinizing hormone A hormone produced by the anterior lobe of the pituitary gland that regulated the menstrual cycle in females.

Lymph A thin, clear, slightly yellow fluid in the lymphatic system that is about 95% water with a few red blood cells and variable numbers of white blood cells.

Lymph nodes Small, rounded masses that filter lymph fluids and trap bacteria and cast-off cell parts to arrest the spread of infection.

Lymphatic system Complex network of capillaries, thin vessels, valves, ducts, nodes, and organs that absorb excess blood fluids from the tissue spaces and return them to the heart.

Lymphocyte A lymph cell or white blood cell.

Lysozyme An enzyme with antiseptic actions that destroys some foreign organisms.

M

Macroglossia Abnormal enlargement of the tongue.

Macrophages White blood cells that can surround and digest foreign substances in the body.

Macular Of, relating to, or characterized by a spot or spots; raised.

Malignancy The state or presence of a malignant (cancerous) tumor.

Malnutrition Inadequate nutrition from improper diet, regardless of the number of calories consumed.

Mammary gland Exocrine gland (organ) that functions independently to extract materials from the blood and convert them into milk.

Mammary ridge The line extending from the armpit to the inner thigh of the fetus; sometimes the site of an extra (supernumerary) nipple. Also called the *milk line.*

Mammogenesis Stage during which the breast develops to a functioning state.

Manual expression Removal of milk from the breast by manual manipulation. Also called *hand expression.*

Masseter muscle The muscle that closes the mouth; the principal muscle in chewing.

Mastitis Swelling and redness of breast tissue that often causes pain and warmth, and can lead to fever and chills. Also called *breast infection.*

Mastitis spectrum A spectrum of conditions causing inflammation of the mammary gland because of ductal inflammation and edema in the supporting tissue. It can lead to inflammatory mastitis and, if not treated, acute bacterial mastitis.

Maternity Practices in Infant Nutrition and Care (mPINC) A survey conducted about every 2 years by the U.S. Centers for Disease Control and Prevention that assesses maternity care practices and provides feedback to U.S. hospitals, enabling them to make improvements that better support lactation.

Mature milk Composition of human milk after 7 to 10 days postpartum.

Maxillary frenum See *Labial frenum.*

Mean In research, the average of an array of numbers.

Meconium The first stool of a newborn that is greenish black to dark brown, with a tarry consistency.

Median The middle point in a range of numbers.

Menses Uterine blood and cellular debris discharged during menstruation.

Mentor Experienced person who provides expertise to help less experienced individuals advance their careers, enhance their education, and build their networks. Term used in lactation for helping students acquire clinical skills.

Meta-analysis In research, a method of putting together the results of many studies and reanalyzing them as if they had all been parts of one big study.

Metabolic Referring to metabolism, the sum of all chemical processes in the body as they relate to the movement of nutrients in the blood after digestion.

Metabolic syndrome Cluster of diseases that includes obesity, hypertension, cardiovascular disease, and diabetes.

Methicillin-resistant *Staphylococcus aureus* (MRSA) Any strain of *S. aureus* bacteria that is resistant to a large group of antibiotics, including penicillins and cephalosporins.

Microaggression Subtle behavior directed at a member of a marginalized group that has a negative, derogatory effect.

Microbiome Aggregate of microorganisms that reside on the surface and in deep layers of skin, in the saliva and oral mucosa, in the conjunctiva, and in the gastrointestinal tract.

Micrognathia A condition in which the lower jaw is smaller than usual, potentially causing problems with feeding and breathing.

Milia Very small "whiteheads" that are keratin deposits within the dermis. Also called *infant acne.*

Milk banking See *Human milk bank.*

Milk bleb/blister A blocked nipple pore.

Milk-ejection reflex (MER) A reflex stimulated by sucking and mediated by oxytocin in which milk flows from the alveoli into the milk ducts.

Milk/plasma ratio The quantity of a drug or its metabolite in human milk in relation to its quantity in the parent's plasma or blood.

Milk-producing tissue Glands (alveoli) in which milk synthesis takes place.

Milk sharing Informal sharing of human milk.

Milk stasis Buildup of milk in the breast, usually from ineffective or infrequent removal.

Milk synthesis The process of making human milk by joining together several elements.

Milk transfer Transfer of milk to the baby through nursing.

Milk-transporting tissue System of ductules, secondary ducts, and nipple pores through which milk travels to the baby.

Minerals Nutrients and vitamins that the body needs to work properly.

Minimal nursing Nursing one to three times a day, with complementary or supplementary feedings providing the remaining nourishment. Typical scenario for gradual weaning.

Mixed message A communication or impression that is indistinct or confused.

Modified side-sitting hold Nursing position with the baby on the parent's side with the top of the baby's head toward the middle of the parent's chest and the feet facing away.

Molding Asymmetrical appearance of the baby's head after birth caused by the overlapping of skull bones.

Monosaccharide The simplest form of carbohydrate.

Montgomery glands Small raised areas around the nipple that enlarge during pregnancy and lactation and secrete a fluid that lubricates the nipple.

Morbidity The condition of suffering from an illness or abnormal condition or quality.

Moro reflex A normal newborn reflex caused by a sudden loud noise, resulting in drawing up of the legs, an embracing position of the arms, and usually a short cry.

Mortality The number of deaths in a population.

Mother–Baby Assessment (MBA) A tool to evaluate the progress of feedings by observing signaling, positioning, fixing, milk transfer, and ending.

Motility Capable of motion.

Motivational interviewing A client-centered counseling technique that draws out the client's reasons for change rather than just giving information about change.

Mottling A white and reddish coloration of the skin on the baby's trunk and extremities. Also called *cutis marmorata.*

Mucin A glycoprotein in human milk, saliva, bile, salivary glands, skin, connective tissues, tendon, and cartilage.

Multipara Having given live birth to more than one child.

Myelin A fatty substance in the coverings of various nerve fibers that gives the normally gray fibers a white, creamy color.

Myers-Briggs Type Indicators Personality type, strengths, and preferences identified in a self-report inventory to study the influence of personality on how individuals obtain and process information and how they make decisions.

Myoepithelial cells Smooth muscle layers that enclose the alveoli and ducts of the mammary gland.

N

Naloxone A pure opioid antagonist that reverses the effects of opioids, especially with overdoses. Trade name: Narcan.

Naltrexone Opioid receptor antagonist used primarily in the management of alcohol dependence and opioid dependence. Trade names: Revia, Depade.

Nasogastric (NG) Gavage feeding with a tube passing through the nose into the stomach.

Nasopharynx Part of the throat behind the nose, reaching from the back of the nasal opening to the soft palate.

Natal tooth A tooth that is present at the time of birth.

Natural family planning A birth control method based on abstaining from sexual intercourse during the time of ovulation.

Necrotizing enterocolitis (NEC) Inflammation of the intestines and especially of the human ileum that results in tissue death.

Neo-BFHI An initiative published in 2015 with recommendations for improving lactation support for preterm and ill infants.

Neonatal abstinence syndrome (NAS) A group of problems that occur in a newborn exposed to addictive opiate drugs in utero.

Neonatal intensive care unit (NICU) An intensive care unit in a hospital for preterm and ill newborn infants. Also called a *special care unit* or *special care nursery.*

Neonatal tooth A tooth that erupts within 30 days from birth.

Neonate A newborn infant up to 6 weeks of age.

Nerves Fibers or bundles of fibers that transmit impulses of sensation to the brain or spinal cord and transmit impulses from these to the muscles and organs.

Neural tube defect A condition in which congenital defects (such as anencephaly and spina bifida) result from incomplete closure of a neural tube early in embryonic development.

Neurological impairment Limited or impaired capacity of the nervous system with difficulties in areas such as memory and cognitive functioning.

Neuromotor dysfunction Impaired or abnormal functioning of the brain and motor function.

Neurotransmitter Chemical released from a nerve terminal that changes or results in the sending of nerve signals across spaces separating nerve fibers.

Neutrophil A type of white blood cell; a granulocyte containing enzymes that digest microorganisms.

New Ballard Scale (NBS) Gestational assessment tool that evaluates the tone of the infant's total body, wrist, biceps muscle, knee joint, shoulder girdle, and pelvic girdle.

Nil per os (NPO) Latin term that translates to "nothing by mouth."

Nipple, common A nipple that protrudes slightly when at rest and becomes erect when stimulated.

Nipple correction Technique to evert a nipple to improve infant latch.

Nipple, cracked A nipple with a crack or fissure lengthwise or crosswise along it.

Nipple, flat A nipple with a very short shank that does not become erect in response to stimulation.

Nipple, inverted A nipple that remains retracted, both when at rest and on stimulation.

Nipple, inverted appearing A nipple that appears inverted but becomes erect when stimulated.

Nipple, retracted A nipple that appears graspable but retracts on stimulation.

Nipple everter Device for everting the nipple.

Nipple pores Openings on the end of the nipple through which milk flows.

Nipple preference A baby's preference for an artificial nipple over the parent's nipple, resulting from sucking alternately on both, which requires two different mechanisms.

Nipple shield An artificial nipple used over the nipple during nursing.

Nonbinary Having a gender identity that cannot be described as exclusively male or female.

Nonnutritive sucking (NNS) Fluttery, non-drawing sucks, with alternating sucking bursts and resting.

Nonprobability In research, a type of sampling other than random, such as convenience sampling.

Normal distribution In research, the dispersal of data from measuring many natural phenomena; a common assumption in statistical tests.

Normal fullness Increased amounts of blood and lymph necessary for milk production that cause the breasts to become fuller, heavier, and slightly tender; not to be confused with engorgement.

Normal newborn jaundice Mildly elevated bilirubin levels in a healthy newborn from normal red blood cell breakdown that typically appears between the second and fifth days of life and resolves quickly. Also called *physiologic jaundice of the newborn.*

Nosocomial Hospital acquired, as in a nosocomial infection.

Nucleotides Compounds derived from nucleic acid and secreted by mammary epithelial cells that play key roles in the function and growth of the gastrointestinal and immune systems.

Null hypothesis In research, a condition where no statistical significance exists in a set of given observations, and therefore, the original study hypothesis, or alternative hypothesis, was not proven.

Nursing strike Nursing abstinence; a baby's rejection of nursing.

Nursing supplementer A device for supplemental feeding while nursing via a small tube placed from the end of the nipple to a container of milk, which may be a commercial system (bottle or collection bag), a standard bottle, a bag, or a syringe.

Nutrient A substance or ingredient, released by digestion and then absorbed, that promotes growth, provides energy, and maintains life.

Nutritive sucking (NS) An organized continuous sequence of long drawing sucks that produces a regular flow of milk.

O

Obesity A body mass index (BMI) of 30 or greater.

Obestatin A peptide hormone in human milk that increases appetite.

Observational study A type of study in which a researcher observes and documents participants' behaviors without influencing or interfering with the behavior.

Obturator A feeding plate placed over a cleft palate to aid in feeding the baby. Also called *grommet.*

Odds ratio In research, a descriptive measure of the association between two variables, with the odds of one group in the numerator and the odds of another group in the denominator. If the odds are greater in the numerator, the odds ratio is greater than 1.

Office on Women's Health The department that coordinates women's health–related activities across the U.S. Department of Health and Human Services Health Resources and Services Administration (HRSA).

Olfactory sense The ability to perceive and distinguish odors.

Oligosaccharide A carbohydrate in human milk that discourages the growth of pathogens in the intestinal tract.

1,000 Days Partnership that promotes targeted action and investment to improve nutrition for parents and children in the 1000 days between pregnancy and the child's second birthday.

Open access Research journal articles distributed online, free of cost or other access barriers.

Open-ended question A form of question that cannot be answered by "yes" or "no," often beginning with *who, what, when, where, why, how, how much,* and *how often.*

Operationalization The process of defining the concepts to be studied in terms of measurable variables and relationships, including choosing instruments or tools.

Operative vaginal delivery (OVD) Delivery with the use of forceps or a vacuum device to assist in transitioning the fetus to extrauterine life.

Oral aversion Reluctance, avoidance, or fear of accepting sensation in or around the mouth, including nursing or bottle feeding. May be caused by intubation, tube feedings, and other invasive procedures.

Oral structure Parts of the mouth that include the lips, vestibule (the area between the teeth, lips, and cheeks), mouth cavity, gums, teeth, hard and soft palate, tongue, and salivary glands.

Orbicularis oris muscle Circular muscle surrounding the mouth that closes the lips.

Orogastric (OG) Gavage feeding with a tube passing through the mouth to the stomach.

Otitis media Swelling or infection of the middle ear, a common disease of childhood that is less frequent in nursing babies.

Outcome The results of any treatment or action. In research, the outcome is usually the same as the dependent variable.

Outliers In research, unusually small or large values for one of the variables being measured. Outliers can distort an average. Researchers often try to offer explanations for why a few values are so different from most others.

Output variables In research, variables that represent the outcome or the result that is being measured or predicted in a given analysis or model. If a sample is selected based on an "effect" of jaundice, for example, babies would be studied only if they are jaundiced. Jaundice would be the output variable that divides babies into two comparison groups.

Over-the-counter medication Drugs that can be purchased without a prescription.

Oximeter A small clip-on instrument that noninvasively estimates the oxygen saturation of blood.

Oxytocin Hormone that stimulates the smooth muscles to contract, specifically those surrounding the alveoli in the breast (causing the release of milk) and those in the uterus (causing uterine contractions). A synthetic form is Pitocin.

P

P value In research, the level of marginal significance within a statistical hypothesis test, with P representing the probability of the occurrence of a given event. Used to provide the smallest level of significance at which a null hypothesis is rejected.

Paced feeding Bottle-feeding method that allows babies to suck, swallow, and breathe as they would during nursing.

Paget's disease Rare form of breast cancer that appears on the nipple and areola. Usually there will also be one or more tumors inside the same breast.

Paladai Cup-feeding device used to feed babies in India and other countries.

Palatal repair Surgery to repair a cleft palate.

Palate The roof of the mouth. The hard portion in the front is called the *hard palate*. The soft portion in the back is called the *soft palate*.

Palmar grasp A primitive newborn reflex that curls the fingers when the palm of the hand is tickled.

Paradigm shift A change from one way of thinking to another, typically new, idea.

Parenchyma Functional parts of an organ. In the breast, it includes alveoli and lactiferous ducts.

Parenteral Nongastrointestinal, intravenous.

Parent-led weaning Weaning initiated by the nursing parent without cues from the baby. Also called *mother-led weaning*.

Passive immunity Immunity from antibodies carried through the placenta to the fetus or through human milk.

Passive listening A type of listening, such as attending.

Pathogen Any microorganism that can cause a disease.

Pathologic jaundice Jaundice that results from such conditions as infections in the blood or liver, diseases of the liver, obstructions in the gastrointestinal system, and interference with the binding of the bilirubin in the bloodstream.

Patient Protection and Affordable Care Act U.S. government 2010 Patient Protection and Affordable Care Act, which requires most employers to provide reasonable break time and a private place for nonexempt employees to express milk.

Patient-controlled epidural anesthesia (PCEA) A programmed infusion pump that delivers boluses of anesthetic solution on demand from the wearer.

Peer review A process conducted by scientific journals in which an article submitted for publication is read and approved by several scientists with relevant knowledge. They are peers of the authors, and they can suggest improvements or reject the article.

Peptide A molecule chain of two or more amino acids.

Percutaneous endoscopic gastrostomy (PEG) tube A feeding tube placed through the skin directly into the stomach for delivery of nutrition.

Perineum The approximate boundary of the pelvic outlet that passes to the urogenital ducts and rectum. Also the area between the anus and the posterior part of the external genitalia.

Periosteum A fiberlike covering of the bones with nerves and blood vessels that supply the bones.

Peristalsis The wavelike, rhythmic contraction of smooth muscle. Movement of the infant's tongue in compressing breast tissue against the hard palate to receive milk.

Persistent organic pollutants (POPs) Organic compounds that are resistant to environmental degradation through chemical, biological, and photolytic processes.

Personal stage The final of four stages in role acquisition. The time in which one's style evolves to be consistent with one's personality.

Phagocyte A cell that can engulf particles such as bacteria, other microorganisms, aged red blood cells, and foreign matter.

Phencyclidine hydrochloride (PCP) Recreational dissociative drug, also known as Angel Dust, that is stored in fat tissue and excreted slowly from the body.

Phenylalanine An amino acid in food protein that can accumulate to dangerous levels in a baby with phenylketonuria. Abbreviated as Phe.

Phenylalanine hydroxylase deficiency (PAH) Genetic intolerance to the essential amino acid phenylalanine (Phe), with a range of severity in disorders, including phenylketonuria (PKU).

Phenylketonuria (PKU) A hereditary disease that, if not treated early, can cause brain injury or severe impairment in intellectual ability in the baby.

Philtrum The midline space between the upper lip and the nose.

Phototherapy Use of a bili-light to treat infantile jaundice.

Phthalates Estrogen-mimicking compounds found in various plastics that infants can be exposed to by artificial feeding.

Physiologic jaundice See *Normal newborn jaundice*.

Phytoestrogens Estrogen in a plant, such as the phytoestrogen in cabbage (used to treat engorgement).

Pierre Robin sequence A newborn condition of an unusually small jaw combined with a cleft palate, downward displacement of the tongue, and absence of a gag reflex.

Pilot study In research, a small trial run of a study to test processes or instruments planned for use in the main study so that problems can be worked out.

Pincer grasp Use of the thumb and forefinger to pick up objects, usually occurring at about 8 to 9 months of age.

Pinch test A test for inverted nipples, performed by gently compressing the nipple between the thumb and forefinger and observing the degree of protrusion that results.

Pitocin A synthetic form of oxytocin.

Pituitary A small, rounded body at the base of the brain that secretes hormones. The anterior pituitary secretes prolactin; the posterior pituitary secretes oxytocin.

Placenta The spongy structure that grows on the wall of the uterus during pregnancy to nourish the baby.

Placenta accreta Condition in which the placenta grows too deeply into the uterine wall.

Placenta previa Condition in which the placenta lies very low in the uterus and covers all or part of the cervix.

Placental retention Retention of placental fragments after birth, which can cause hormones to remain at pregnancy levels and inhibit lactation.

Placid baby Baby who nurses as few as four to six times in 24 hours, sleeps as much as 18 to 20 hours per day, and is usually quietly alert and tranquil when awake.

Plagiarism Use of another person's ideas or work and claiming it as one's own.

Plan-Do-Study-Act (PDSA) A method to guide the process of change and test whether a change produces the intended improvement.

Plugged duct See *Ductal narrowing*, a more accurate description for blockage in a milk duct.

Pneumothorax Collection of air or gas in the chest causing the lung to collapse.

Polybrominated diphenyl ethers (PBDEs) Chemicals used in computer plastics, foam cushions, textiles, and other products that accumulate in animals and people.

Polycystic ovary syndrome (PCOS) A variable disorder marked by amenorrhea, excessive hair, obesity, infertility, and ovarian enlargement; usually initiated by an elevated level of luteinizing hormone, androgen, or estrogen that results in an abnormal cycle of gonadotropin release by the pituitary gland. Also called *polycystic ovarian disease*, *polycystic ovarian syndrome*, and *Stein-Leventhal syndrome*.

Polymastia Accessory breasts.

Polysaccharides Class of carbohydrates, such as starch and cellulose, consisting of several monosaccharides joined by glycosidic bonds.

Polythelia Condition in which there are one or more supernumerary nipples along the mammary ridge.

Pooled milk Donor milk that is pooled and heat treated to ensure the absence of HIV, hepatitis, and other viruses and bacteria.

Poor weight gain Gaining weight at a slower rate than other children of the same age and sex, the most obvious symptom being smaller size.

Population The whole group of people who have some characteristic(s) under study, of which the sample actually studied is just a part.

Postpartum depression A mild to moderate mood disorder that lasts from 1 to 6 weeks postpartum, characterized by mood changes, sleep disturbances, and fatigue. It may include the inability to cope with life, feeling no attachment to the baby, worrying that something is not "right," and occasional thoughts of suicide.

Postpartum psychosis A mental health emergency that can lead to a loss of control, rational thought, and social functioning. It may include overwhelming confusion, hallucinations, and attempts at self-harm or harming the child.

Postpartum thyroiditis Inflammation of the thyroid within a year after giving birth. Hyperthyroidism, hypothyroidism, or one after the other may occur.

Postterm Born after 42 weeks' gestation.

Posttraumatic stress disorder (PTSD) Persistent mental and emotional stress resulting from injury or psychological shock.

Posture feeding See *Laid-back nursing*.

Power In research, the degree of mathematical likelihood that a given sample size and test will find a difference between comparison groups when there really is a difference.

ppm Parts per million.

Prebiotics Nondigestible food ingredients that stimulate the growth or activity of bacteria in the digestive system that are beneficial to the health of the body.

Predictor variable Independent variable that is believed to influence the result.

Pretending A type of listening that gives a noncommittal response, trying to be polite and not focusing attention to the speaker.

Preterm Born before 37 weeks' gestation.

Pretoria pasteurization Pasteurization method in which the container of milk is placed into water already heated from 56°C to 62°C in an aluminum pot for about 15 minutes.

Primary group Group, such as a family, in which an individual forms close, personal, and enduring relationships.

Primipara An individual who has completed one pregnancy.

Primitive neonatal reflexes (PNRs) Innate adaptive newborn responses; automatic movements controlled by the brainstem that integrate over time as the brain matures.

Probability In research, the likelihood of something happening, calculated by dividing the number of times an event occurs by the total number of trials conducted.

Probes Directing the conversation to pinpoint issues and feelings that need to be expressed openly.

Probiotics Dietary supplements of live microorganisms thought to be beneficial to the body's health; lactic acid bacteria and bifidobacteria are the most common types of microbes used as probiotics.

Professional burnout Feelings of exhaustion, dissatisfaction, and reduced professional ability resulting from stress linked to work.

Progesterone The hormone responsible for the development of the placenta and mammary glands.

Projectile vomiting Violent expulsion of the contents of the stomach with enough force to send it over 1 foot.

Prolactin The hormone that stimulates breast development and production of milk during pregnancy and lactation.

Prolactin inhibitory factor (PIF) A factor produced in and released from the hypothalamus that prohibits the release of prolactin.

Prolactin receptor cells Sites within the alveolar cells that are receptors for prolactin. Frequent nursing in the early postpartum period is thought to lay down more receptor sites, enabling greater milk production for the duration of lactation.

Prolactinoma A benign pituitary tumor that secretes prolactin.

Prone Position of the body when lying face downward. An infant sleeping position to avoid.

Propylthiouracil Medication to treat hyperthyroidism and Graves' disease by lowering the amount of thyroid hormone to normal levels.

Prospective study In research, a study that collects data as events happen rather than from old records or memory.

Prostaglandin One of several strong hormonelike fatty acids that act in small amounts on certain organs.

Protected health information (PHI) A person's private medical information, including history, prognosis, and treatment, which is protected under privacy regulations such as Health Insurance Portability and Accountability Act (HIPAA) regulation in the United States.

Protecting, Promoting, and Supporting Breastfeeding A joint World Health Organization (WHO) and United Nations Children's Fund (UNICEF) statement issued in 1989 to increase awareness of the critical role that health services play in promoting lactation.

Protein Large biological molecules, or macromolecules, consisting of one or more long chains of amino acid residues. A complete protein food contains all the essential amino acids. An incomplete protein food lacks essential amino acids and must be combined with other incomplete protein foods that fill in the missing nutrients.

Pyloric stenosis A congenital bowel obstruction in infants in which the outflow valve of the stomach does not open enough to permit stomach contents to pass through. It is most common in firstborn White male infants and is characterized by projectile vomiting.

Q

Qualitative study Research that gathers participants' perceptions, experiences, and behavior. Statistical analysis is not typically used, and changes in practice are not often recommended, except at a conceptual level. Often, such studies lead to further studies.

R

Random assignment A technique that distributes research participants across different groups, such as treatment and control groups, to eliminate bias and ensure fairness. Examples are a coin flip or a random number chart.

Randomized clinical trial An experiment or experiment-like type of research in which the scientist controls many aspects of the study. Subjects are randomly assigned to their groups. Potential confounders are measured, and analysis is planned before data collection.

Rapid eye movement (REM) Stage of sleep characterized by quick, random eye movements.

Range In research, the number that results from subtracting the lowest from the highest value in the data.

Raynaud's phenomenon Sporadic attacks of interruptions in blood flow to the extremities (fingers, toes, ears, and nose), resulting in tingling, numbness, burning, and pain. Nipple vasospasms can mimic Raynaud's.

Rebirthing Simulation of the birth experience in which the baby is placed on the abdomen in a bath of warm water and allowed to latch on their own; also called *remedial co-bathing*.

Reciprocity The capacity to engage in social exchange.

Recurrent mastitis Breast infection that occurs more than one time during a single lactation.

Reflective listening See *Active listening*.

Reflexes Involuntary and nearly instantaneous movements in response to a stimulus.

Regression In research, a statistical method for estimating how variables are related in a study.

Relactation Resumption of lactation beyond the immediate postpartum period.

Relationship In research, the connections between two or more variables that can be measured and analyzed. Connections can be spurious, correlated, or causal.

Reliability In research, the property possessed by good-quality measurement tools that ensures they measure a concept or characteristic the same way each time.

Remedial co-bathing See *Rebirthing*.

Reproductive coercion A form of domestic violence in which partner behavior is used to maintain power, control, and domination in the relationship by controlling pregnancy outcomes, including forced pregnancy or termination.

Resistin Protein peptide in human milk secreted by fat cells that may control growth rate in utero and aid in the baby's metabolic development.

Respiratory distress syndrome (RDS) A common condition of preterm infants that is characterized by delayed onset of respiration and low Apgar score; caused by the lungs not being fully developed.

Respiratory syncytial virus (RSV) Multistrain virus that causes severe respiratory disease, including bronchitis and pneumonia, in infants and children.

Retinoids A class of chemical compounds that are related chemically to vitamin A.

Retrospective study In research, a study in which a result is identified in a group of subjects, and then the past experiences of those subjects are examined to see what might have led to the result.

Reverse-cycle nursing A feeding pattern used during regular separations, with the baby nursing when the dyad is together.

Reverse pressure softening Massage method to help soften the areola caused by edema to aid the baby in latching.

Review articles In research, articles in which one or more experts summarize and often critique the best and worst studies published on a topic, with little or no original data included.

Rh incompatibility Blood incompatibility between a birth parent and baby when the parent is Rh negative and the baby is Rh positive.

Rheumatoid arthritis An autoimmune disorder that can cause joint pain and damage throughout the body, usually on both sides of the body.

Rickets Condition caused by lack of vitamin D, calcium, and phosphorus; marked by abnormal bone growth.

Role acquisition Stages of acquiring new roles in life, either personally (e.g., parent) or professionally (e.g., lactation consultant). Characterized by anticipatory, formal, informal, and personal stages.

Rooming-in Nursing parent and baby sharing the same hospital room, beginning as soon as possible after birth.

Rooting reflex An automatic oral action exhibited by healthy newborns to help them find and latch onto a nipple to begin feeding. A newborn's natural instinct to turn their head toward a stimulation and make sucking motions when touched on the cheek.

Rotavirus Class of viruses that cause diarrheal illness and lead to hospitalization.

S

Sample In research, the group of people or subjects who are selected to participate in a study.

Sarcoidosis A multisystemic disease that may involve breast parenchyma and can be confused with benign or malignant tumors.

Scleroderma A rare condition in which skin and connective tissues harden and contract; may be isolated or systemic.

Scope of practice The duties and responsibilities that healthcare professionals are allowed to undertake based on their professional license and legal regulations. The activities in which International Board Certified Lactation Consultants (IBCLCs) are authorized to engage to protect the public by ensuring safe, competent, and evidence-based care.

Searching response Newborn bobbing and bouncing behavior demonstrated when searching for the nipple.

Sebaceous Fatty, oily, or greasy, usually referring to the skin's oil-secreting glands or to their secretions.

Secondary groups Social groups in which relationships are relatively impersonal (e.g., school, work, religious, and recreational groups).

Secretory activation Stage II lactogenesis, signifying copious milk secretion.

Secretory differentiation Stage I lactogenesis; the beginning of the third trimester of pregnancy.

Selective listening Form of listening that hears only certain parts of what is said.

Self-efficacy One's belief in the ability to perform well.

Sensory input A message, perception, or awareness the mind receives while processing information.

Sensory processing disorder (SPD) A condition in which the brain has trouble receiving and responding to information that comes in through the senses.

Sepsis A serious condition in which the body responds improperly to an infection.

Seroconversion The production of specific antibodies against specific antigens. A change from a seronegative to a seropositive condition.

Sexual abuse A continuum of unwanted sexual activity that ranges from coercion to contact abuse (unwanted kissing, touching, or fondling) to rape.

Sheehan's syndrome A condition that occurs when severe blood loss during childbirth causes long-term damage to the pituitary gland. Also called *hypopituitarism*.

Side-lying position A nursing position in which the parent lies on one side with the baby alongside, facing them.

Side-sitting hold A nursing position with the baby held along the parent's side with their feet toward the back; also known as the *football* or *clutch hold*.

Simple carbohydrate The simplest type of sugar that causes a sudden rise in blood sugar level after ingestion, followed by a rapid drop and a craving for more food. When consumed in the absence of nutritional foods, simple carbohydrate foods may cause fatigue, dizziness, nervousness, or headache.

Sjögren's syndrome An autoimmune disorder that causes dry eyes and mouth; frequently concurrent with rheumatoid arthritis and lupus.

Skin-to-skin care Technique in which the baby is held in skin-to-skin contact upright and prone against the chest, wearing only a diaper, with the parent and baby wrapped together to maintain body temperature. Preferably used immediately after birth, to facilitate infant transition to extrauterine life and nursing.

Sleep training Term used for a parenting approach that encourages babies to fall asleep by themselves and to sleep for long stretches; includes scheduling feedings and allowing the baby to cry.

Slope In research, the slope of a line on a graph, used in regression analysis to understand the relationship between two or more variables. The slope shows how much the dependent variable changes when the independent variable increases.

Slow weight gain Growth in which a baby gains weight steadily, although slowly, and stays on a particular growth curve.

Small for gestational age (SGA) Classification for a newborn in the bottom 10% of growth rate in size and weight considered appropriate for gestational age. Infant whose growth was retarded and who was delivered before 37 weeks (preterm) or after 42 weeks (postterm).

SMART goals An acronym for goals that stands for Specific, Measurable, Achievable, Realistic, and Timely.

Social determinants Conditions in the environment in which people are born, live, learn, work, play, worship, and age.

Social marketing The use of marketing techniques to influence people's behavior to help individuals choose strategies that best fit their readiness for action and their resources.

Social toxicant Mood-changing substance, such as tobacco, coffee, tea, alcohol, marijuana, and other social drugs.

Soft palate Soft tissue behind the hard palate in the roof of the mouth, in line with the end of the upper alveolar ridge.

Soporific Sleep-inducing agent (e.g., warm milk).

Sphincter A circular band of muscle fibers that narrows a passage or closes a natural opening in the body.

Spina bifida A neural tube defect present at birth that results in a gap in the bone that surrounds the spinal cord.

Spinal anesthesia A form of regional anesthesia involving injection of a local anesthetic into the cerebrospinal fluid (CSF), generally through a fine needle, usually 3.5 inches (9 cm) long.

Split-brain theory Theory that the brain's hemispheres process information differently, with the left hemisphere handling language and analytical tasks and the right hemisphere processing spatial and emotional elements.

Spontaneous lactation See *Galactorrhea*.

Spurious Not being what it purports to be. The relationship between two variables when statistical significance is found, but the significance is caused by a third variable that is hidden or unclear.

Standards of practice Stated measures or levels of quality that serve as models for the conduct and evaluation of practice.

Standing orders Documented standard orders for patient care in stipulated clinical situations.

Statistical theory Mathematical ideas about probability and infinite cases that underlie the applied tests commonly used by researchers.

Statistically significant In research, description of an outcome that did not happen by chance, with an underlying relationship that caused the event.

Structural bias Cultural values in a society that are ingrained in daily life.

Subclinical mastitis (SCM) Low-grade, asymptomatic inflammation of mammary tissue.

Sublingual Under the tongue.

Submucosal cleft A palatal cleft that is covered by skin and may not be discovered until feeding difficulties or speech problems occur.

Sucking pattern Pattern of an infant's nutritive and nonnutritive sucking.

Sudden infant death syndrome (SIDS) The sudden death of a child of less than 1 year of age, in which the death remains unexplained after a thorough autopsy and detailed death scene investigation. SIDS is a subgroup of sudden unexplained infant death (SUID).

Sudden unexplained infant death (SUID) A broad term that encompasses sudden infant death syndrome (SIDS) and includes all unexpected infant deaths prior to investigation.

Superbill Itemized form used by healthcare providers to reflect rendered services.

Supernumerary nipple Extra nipple, other than the one normally found on each breast, which may be present along the milk lines. Also called *polythelia* and *accessory nipple*.

Supine Lying flat on the back.

Supplementary feeding Additional feeding given to the infant in place of or after nursing, which may be human milk or infant formula. Also called *topping off* the infant.

Supportive and sustaining tissue Tissues between the milk-producing and milk-transporting tissues, including nerves, fatty tissue, connective tissue, and the blood and lymph systems.

Suppressor peptides Inhibiting peptides in human milk that cause a cessation of milk secretion during milk stasis and engorgement.

Swaddling Wrapping the baby, confining their arms and legs to inhibit the startle reflex and provide a feeling of warmth and security.

Systematic review In research, a review that uses repeatable methods to find, select, and synthesize all available evidence.

Systemic bias Prejudice, bigotry, or unfairness directed toward individuals of an oppressed or marginalized group.

Systemic lupus erythematosus An inflammatory autoimmune disorder affecting the joints, skin, kidneys, blood cells, brain, heart, and lungs. Symptoms may include joint pain, fatigue, and a characteristic "butterfly" rash on the cheeks and bridge of the nose.

T

Tail of Spence Breast tissue that extends into the axilla.

Tandem nursing Nursing more than one child of different ages.

Technology-mediated support Support provided through telephone, texting, videoconferencing, and other tools and applications.

Ten Steps to Successful Breastfeeding Steps formed by the World Health Organization (WHO) and United Nations Children's Fund (UNICEF) to promote sound lactation practices and policies worldwide.

Tertiary The third level of sophistication of development, as in a specialized, highly technical tertiary-level healthcare facility.

The Joint Commission An independent, not-for-profit organization that evaluates and accredits healthcare organizations in the United States.

Thelarche Onset of secondary breast development, usually occurring at the beginning of puberty.

Third-party reimbursement Reimbursement to the healthcare provider in which the provider bills the insurance company and the insurance company reimburses the provider.

Thrush See *Candidiasis*.

Thyroid disorder Abnormal thyroid function; either low (hypothyroid), high (hyperthyroid), or inflamed (thyroiditis).

Tonic neck reflex A primitive infant reflex present until 3 or 4 months of age that prevents the baby from rolling over until adequate neurological and motor development occurs. Lying on their back, the infant extends their arm and leg on the side of the body opposite to the direction the head is turned. Also referred to as the *fencer position*.

Total parenteral nutrition (TPN) Intravenous nutrition that bypasses the digestive system.

Transcutaneous bilirubin (TcB) measurement system Noninvasive handheld device held over the baby's skin to indicate the bilirubin level.

Transdermal patch A contraceptive skin patch that emits hormones (progestin or combined progestin and estrogen) that are absorbed through the skin to prevent ovulation and pregnancy.

Transformational leadership Leadership that inspires followers to change their expectations, perceptions, and motivations to work toward common goals.

Transforming growth factor β Protein that controls proliferation, cellular differentiation, and other functions in most cells.

Transient nipple soreness Temporary nipple soreness in the first week postpartum as the nipples become accustomed to the infant's sucking.

Transitional milk Milk that is present at stage II lactogenesis, around the second or third day postpartum, when blood flow increases and copious milk secretion begins. The milk that is between colostrum and mature milk.

Transplacental Across or through the placenta.

Trauma-informed care An approach that recognizes the widespread impact of trauma and focuses on safety, trust, collaboration, empowerment, and cultural sensitivity. Assuming that an individual is more likely than not to have a history of trauma and acknowledging the role trauma has in their lives.

Trophic Promoting cellular growth, differentiation, and survival, especially related to nutrition, as in "trophic feeds."

Trough Channel through which the milk travels; formed in the center of the infant's tongue during sucking.

t-test In research, a test to decide between two contradictory hypotheses about the mean of a sample.

Tubal ligation A sterilization process in which the fallopian tubes are surgically cut, blocked, or sealed off to prevent conception from occurring.

Tuberculosis A highly infectious bacterial disease, primarily concentrated in the lungs, spread by tiny droplets released into the air by coughing and sneezing.

Tuberculosis mastitis An extremely rare form of tuberculosis that often mimics breast carcinoma. It usually occurs on the Indian subcontinent and Africa.

Turgor Normal strength and tension of the skin caused by outward pressure of the cells and the fluid that surrounds them.

U

Unconjugated In jaundice, bilirubin that is not bound to albumin and circulates freely in the bloodstream. It can migrate toward tissues with high fat content, including the brain and nervous system.

United Nations Children's Fund (UNICEF) An agency of the United Nations, established in 1946 and charged with protecting the lives and health of children.

U.S. Department of Agriculture (USDA) The government agency that oversees the Special Supplemental Food Program for Women, Infants, and Children, referred to as *WIC*.

U.S. Surgeon General's Call to Action to Support Breastfeeding U.S. call to action listing concrete steps that can be taken at multiple levels throughout the country to reduce barriers to lactation.

V

Vaccine Weakened or dead microorganism given to a person to produce antibodies against the virus.

Vacuum extraction Vaginal delivery of the infant assisted by a machine that applies suction to the infant's head.

Vaginal ring A soft, flexible ring worn inside the vagina as a contraceptive method. The ring emits hormones (progestin or a combination of progestin and estrogen) to prevent pregnancy.

Validity A property of research methods that conveys how well they capture or measure the phenomenon or concept under study.

Vancomycin-resistant *Enterococcus* (VRE) Group of bacterial species of the genus *Enterococcus* that is resistant to the antibiotic vancomycin.

Vancomycin-resistant *Staphylococcus aureus* (VRSA) Strain of *S. aureus* that is resistant to the glycopeptide antibiotic vancomycin.

Variable In research, a characteristic or effect of either the hypothesized "causes" or "outcomes" under study. If feeding is a partial cause of jaundice, the number and amount of feedings, and the possible bilirubin levels are variables.

Variation In statistics, the measure of how much data points differ from each other and from the mean. It is expected that most phenomena are not the same when measured over time or when measured in different individuals. The variation in the number of times each day that a baby wants to nurse and the variation in the number of feedings between different babies on the same day are both examples.

Varicella zoster A herpes virus that affects the central nervous system and causes chicken pox and shingles.

Vasospasm Sharp and often persistent contraction of a blood vessel, reducing blood flow. Observed in nursing as nipple vasospasm. See *Raynaud's phenomenon*.

Vegan Diet that excludes meat, eggs, dairy products, and all other animal-derived ingredients.

Vegetarian Diet that excludes red meat, poultry, seafood, and the flesh of any other animal.

Ventral On the abdomen.

Vernix The creamy protective coating on the newborn.

Very low birth weight (VLBW) Infant born weighing less than 3 lb, 5 oz (1500 g).

Vicarious trauma Secondary trauma that is triggered by exposure to another person's traumatic experiences.

Virus A tiny organism that grows only in the cells of another organism.

Vitamin D Vitamin found in foods and supplements that is essential for the absorption of calcium and the prevention of rickets in children. The body manufactures vitamin D under the influence of sunlight.

Vitamin K Vitamin essential for blood clotting.

Vitamins Any of various organic substances that are essential in small quantities for normal growth and metabolism.

Voice tone Pitch level, rate of speech, and volume when speaking.

Voiding Urination.

Vulnerable population People who are socioeconomically disadvantaged, such as racial or ethnic minorities, uninsured and underinsured individuals, homeless individuals, imprisoned individuals, immigrants, and those in the LGBTQ+ community.

W

Warmline A telephone line that is answered electronically and asks the caller to leave a message for a return call.

Water-soluble vitamins Vitamins that are absorbed into the bloodstream during digestion and need to be taken regularly through diet. They include Vitamin C and the B-complex vitamins.

Wet nursing Nursing an infant other than one's own.

Whey The watery part of milk that remains after the formation of curds.

Witch's milk Milk secreted by the newborn's breasts that disappears shortly after birth.

World Health Assembly (WHA) Decision-making body of the World Health Organization (WHO) composed of health ministers from its 194 member states.

World Health Organization (WHO) An agency of the United Nations that plans and coordinates global health care and assists member nations to combat disease and train healthcare workers.

Y

Yeast infection See *Candidiasis*.

Z

Zuska-Atkin's disease A rare and often painful disorder characterized by milk duct fistulas and recurrent abscesses located within and around the nipple.

Index

Note: Page numbers followed by *f* and *t* indicate materials in figures and tables, respectively.

D

G

H

I

J

K

L

M

N

O

Q

R

S

T

U

V

W

Y

Z

Notes

Notes

Notes

Notes

Notes

Notes

Notes

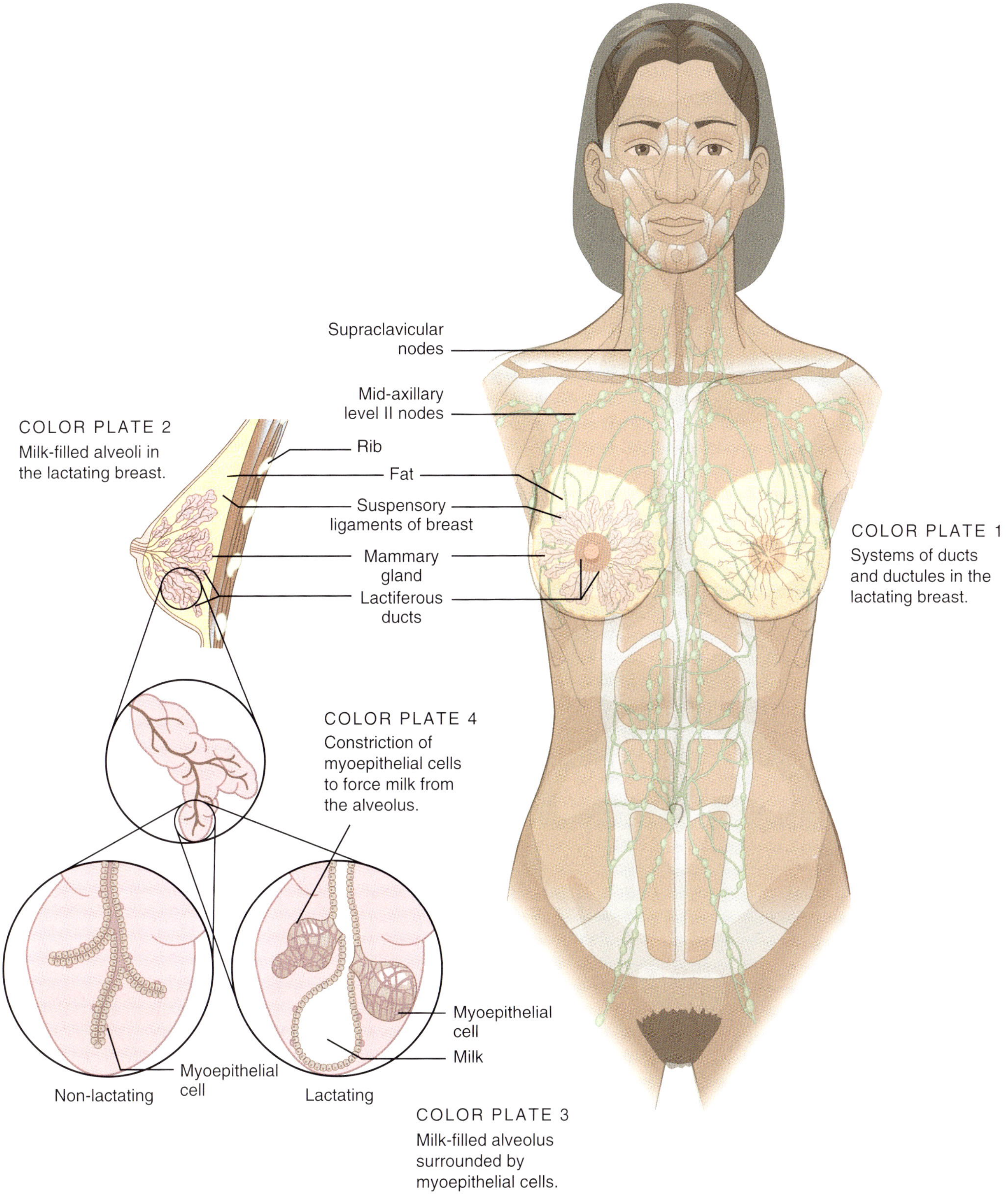

Color Plate 1-4 (1) System of ducts and ductules in the lactating breast. (2) Milk-filled alveoli in the lactating breast. (3) Milk-filled alveolus surrounded by myoepithelial cells (4) Constriction of myoepithelial cells to force milk from the alveolus.

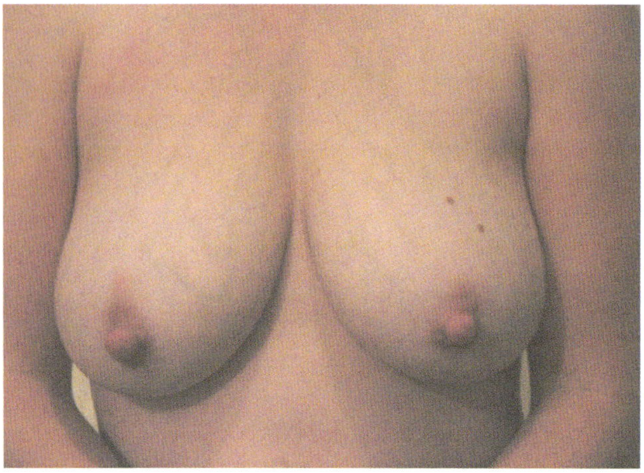

Color Plate 5 Type 1: Rounded breast with normal lower medial and lateral quadrants.

Printed with permission of Anna Swisher.

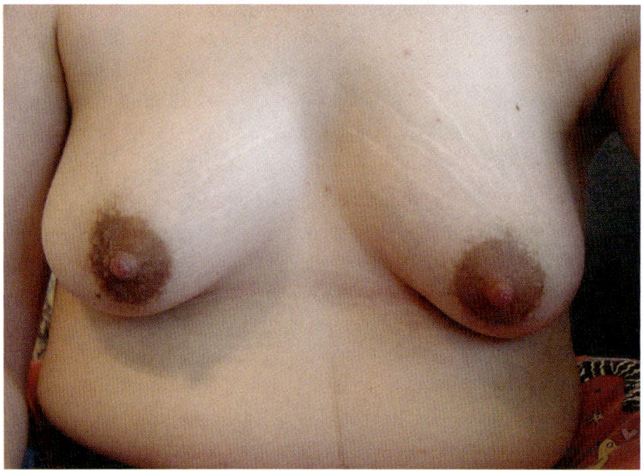

Color Plate 6 Type 2: Hypoplasia of the lower medial quadrant.

Printed with permission of Anna Swisher.

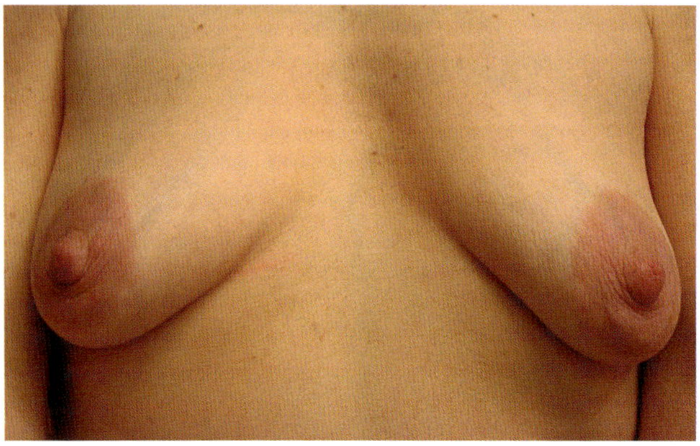

Color Plate 7 Type 3: Hypoplasia of the lower medial and lateral quadrants.

Printed with permission of Anna Swisher.

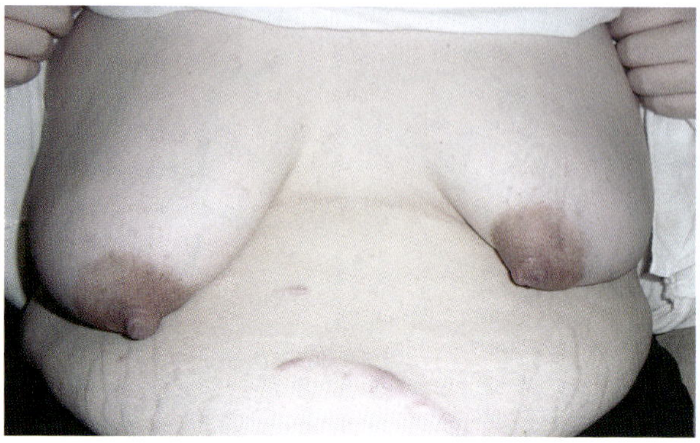

Color Plate 8 Type 4: Severe constrictions with minimal breast base; areolae may be very bulbous.

Printed with permission of Anna Swisher.

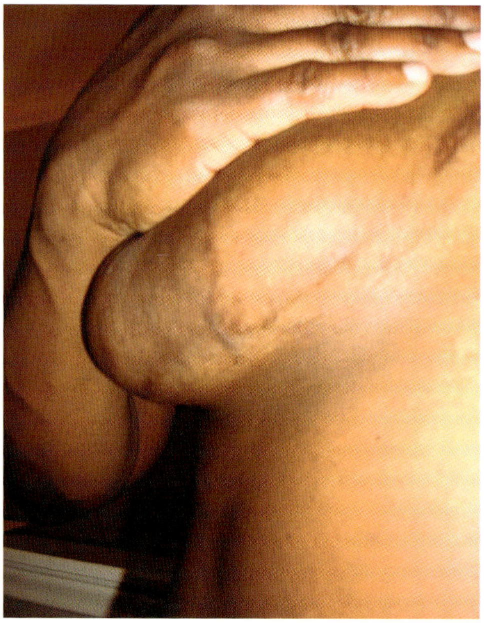

Color Plate 9 Scars from breast surgery can be a marker for severed ducts.

Printed with permission of Anna Swisher.

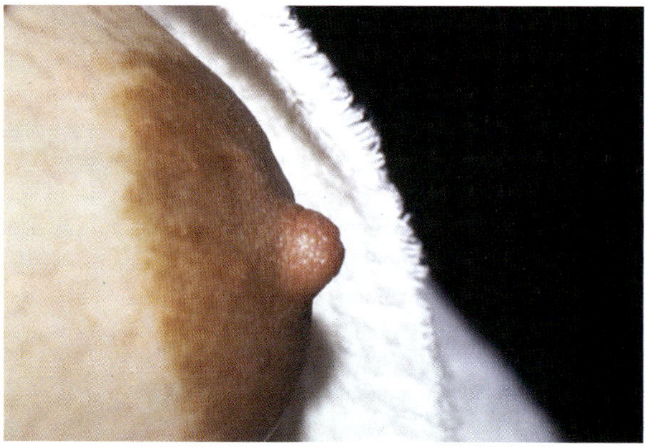

Color Plate 10 Nipple appears normal.

Printed with permission of Kay Hoover.

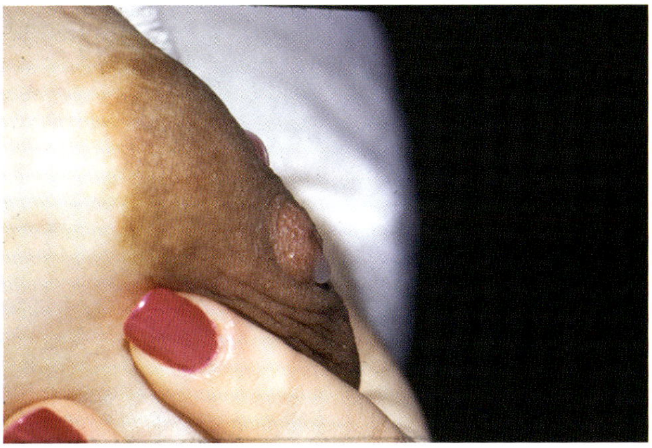

Color Plate 11 Nipple from Color Plate 10 inverts when stimulated.

Printed with permission of Kay Hoover.

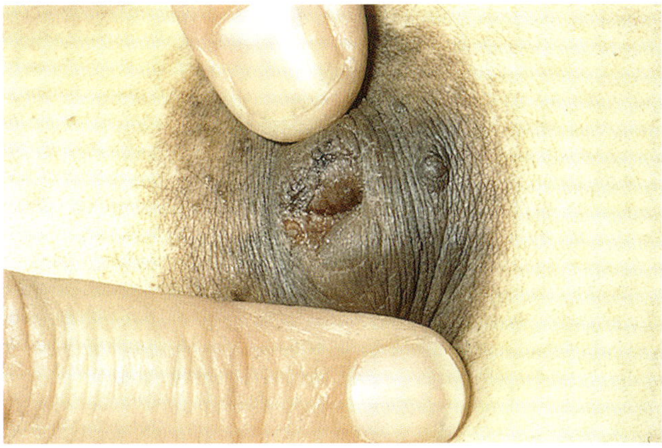

Color Plate 12 Nipple appears dimpled.

Printed with permission of Jan Riordan.

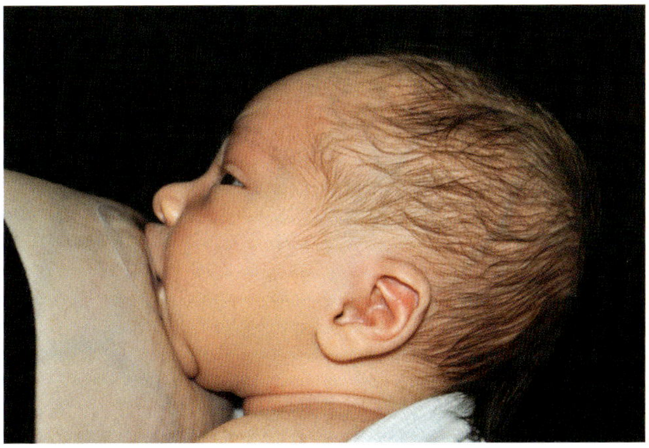

Color Plate 13 Baby latching onto the breast with the aid of a nipple shield.

Printed with permission of Anna Swisher.

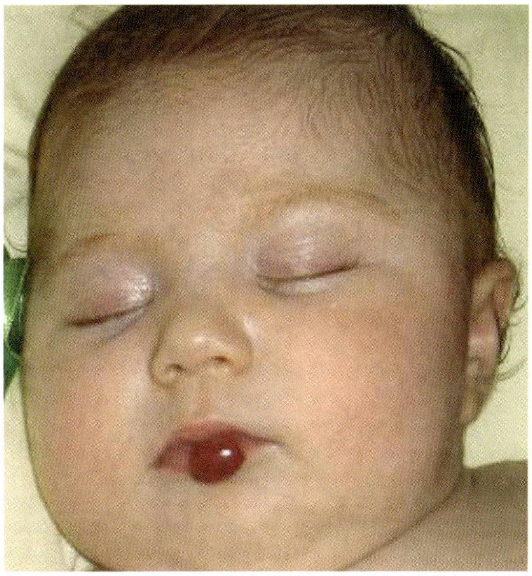

Color Plate 14 Hemangioma on infant lip.

Courtesy of Megha Tollefson. Infantile Hemangiomas: An Update, Mayo Clinic, September 29, 2014.

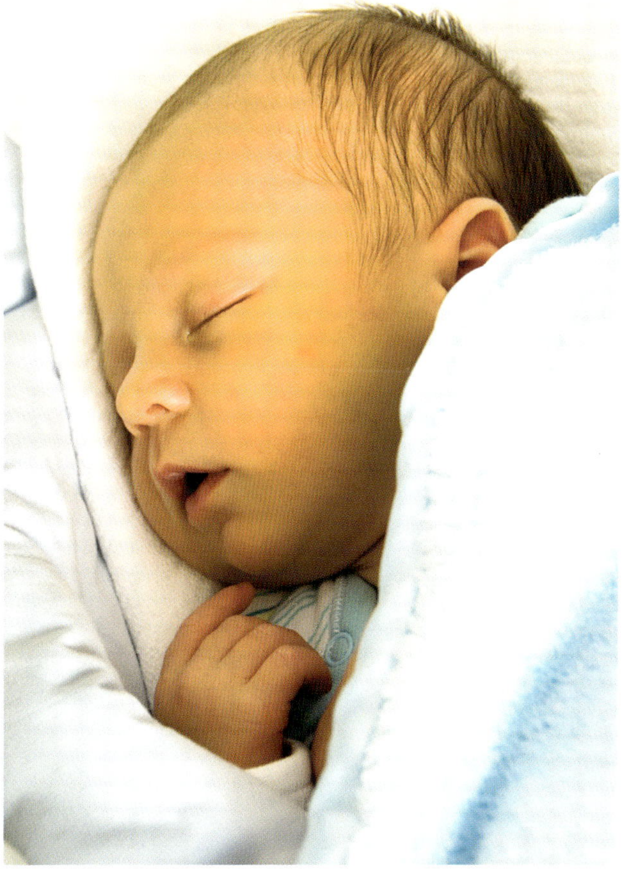

Color Plate 15 Hyperbilirubinemia.

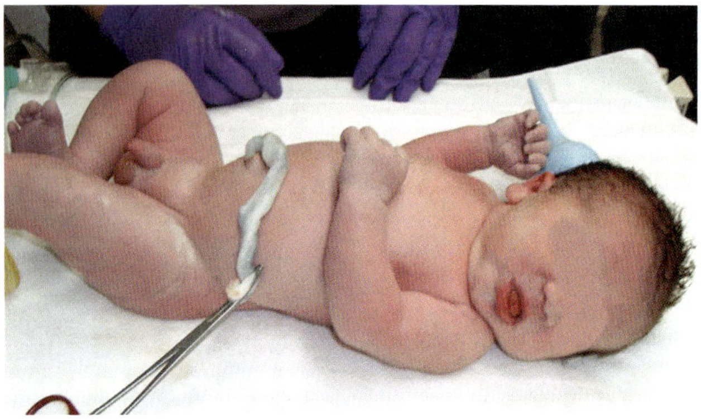

Color Plate 16 Acrocyanosis.

Printed with permission of Dr. Charlie Goldberg.

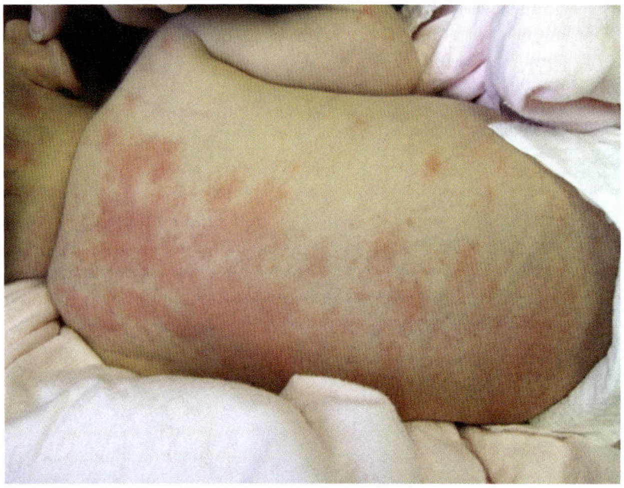

Color Plate 17 Erythema toxicum.

Printed with permission of Dr. Jeffrey Hull.

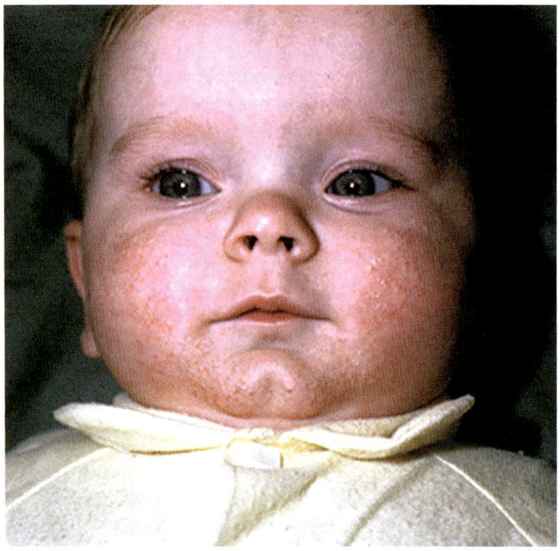

Color Plate 18 Infant acne.

Printed with permission of Dr. Kenneth Greer.

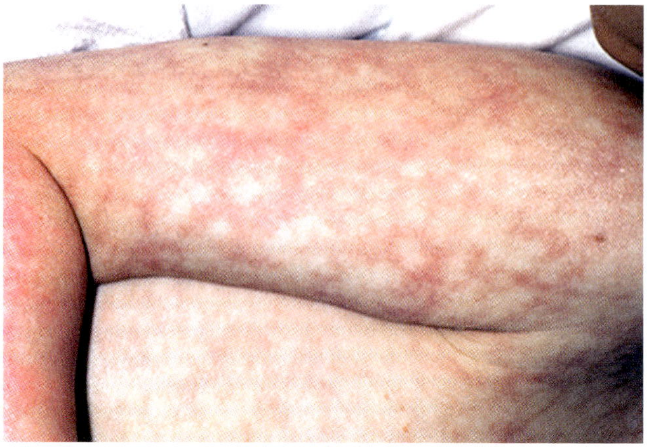

Color Plate 19 Mottling.

Printed with permission of Dr. Kenneth Greer.

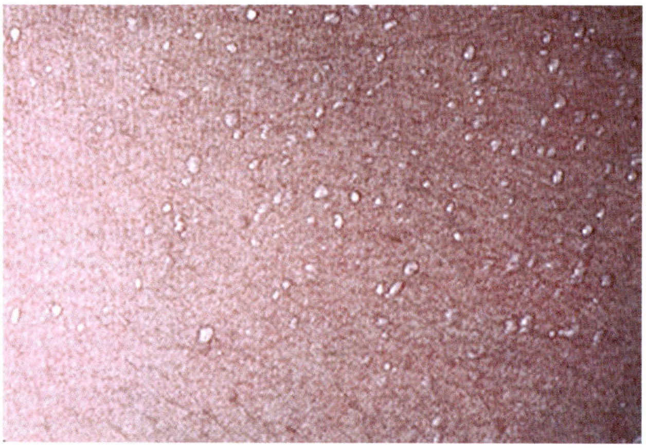

Color Plate 20 Milia.

Printed with permission of Dr. Kenneth Greer.

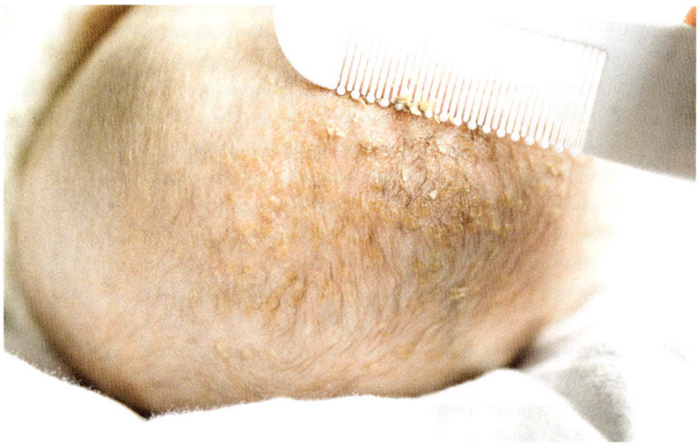

Color Plate 21 Cradle cap.

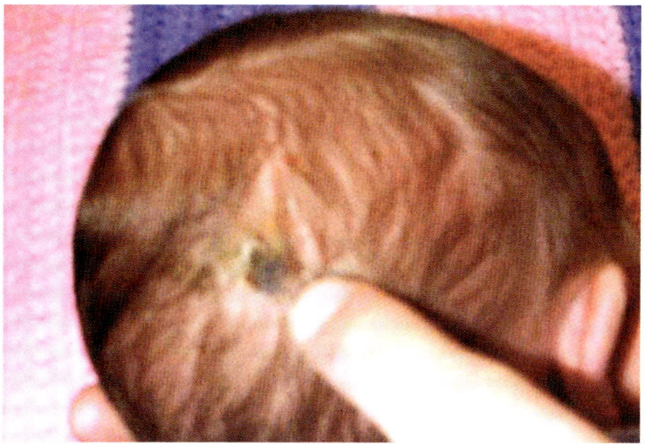

Color Plate 22 Baby with a cephalhematoma on his head.

Printed with permission of Anna Swisher.

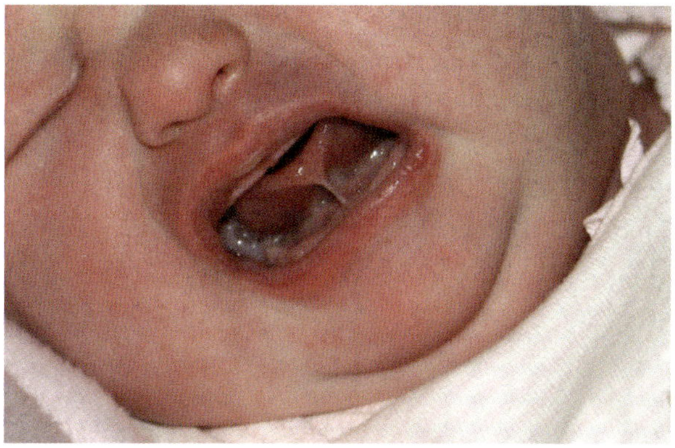

Color Plate 23 A tight frenulum.

Printed with permission of Anna Swisher.

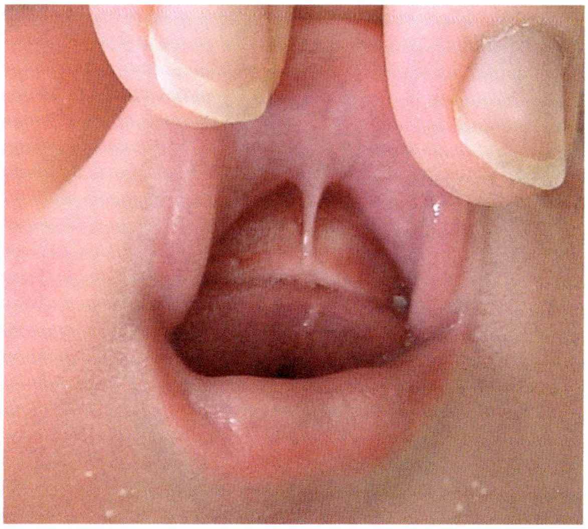

Color Plate 24 A tight frenum.

Printed with permission of Anna Swisher.

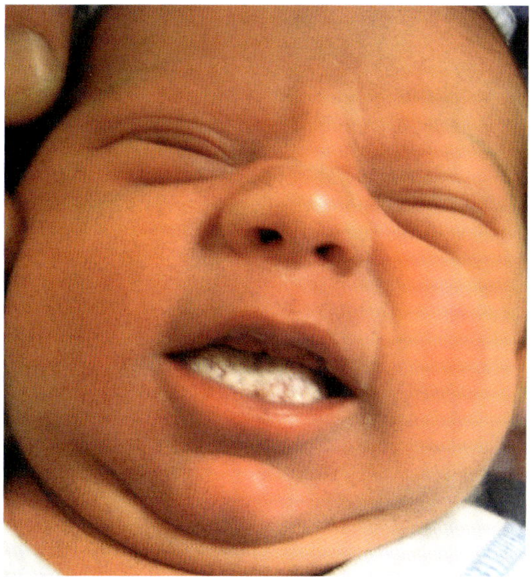

Color Plate 25 Baby with thrush in his mouth.

Printed with permission of James Heilman, MD, and Wikipedia.

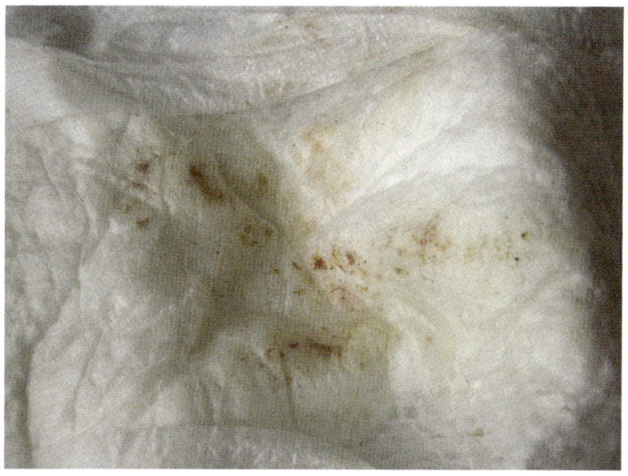

Color Plate 26 Urate crystals in a diaper.

Printed with permission of Judith Lauwers.

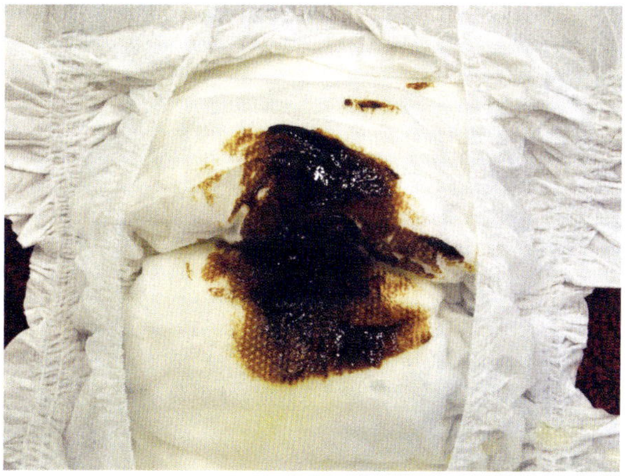

Color Plate 27 Meconium.

Printed with permission of Anna Swisher.

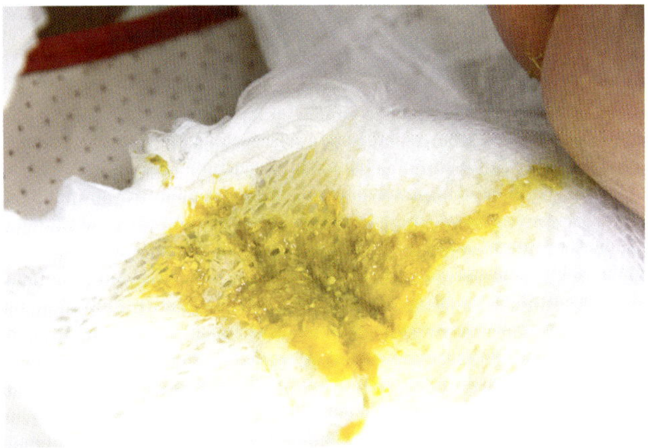

Color Plate 28 Breastmilk stool.

Photo by Every Mother, Inc.

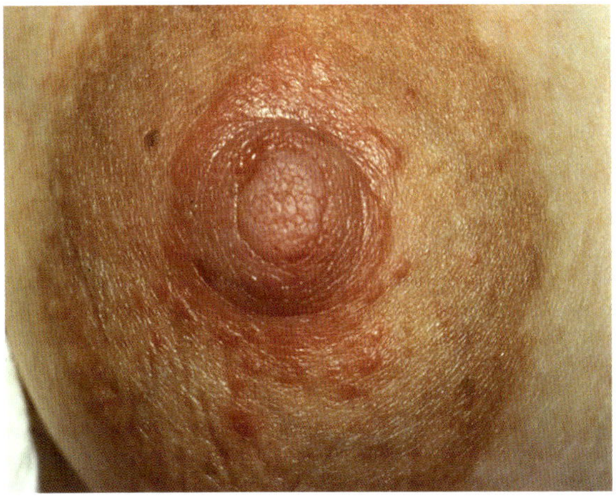

Color Plate 29 Thrush on the nipple.

Printed with permission of S.J. Parker.

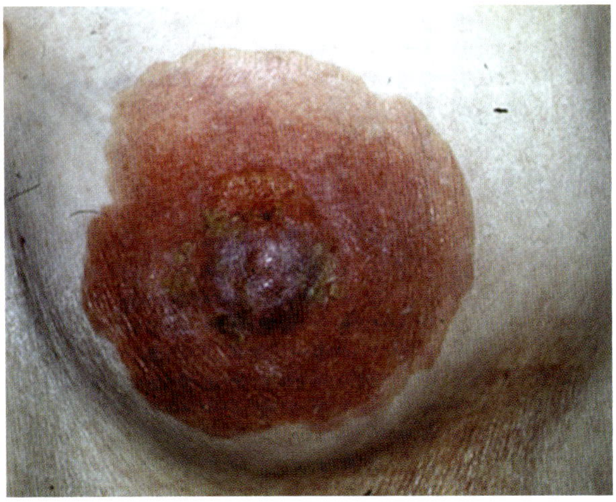

Color Plate 30 Paget's disease on the nipple.

Printed with permission of S.J. Parker.

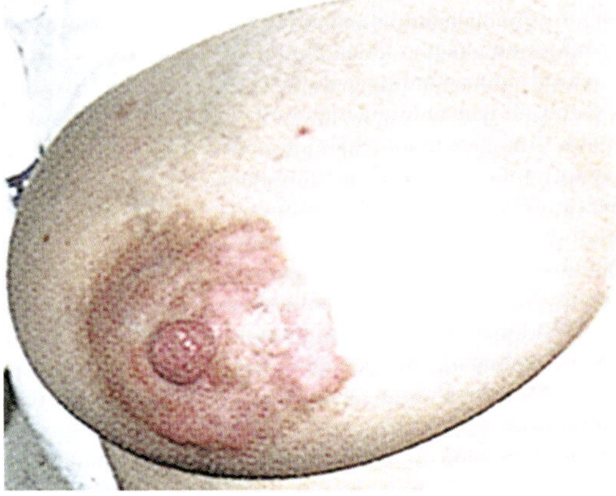

Color Plate 31 Psoriasis on the nipple.

Printed with permission of Karen Foard.

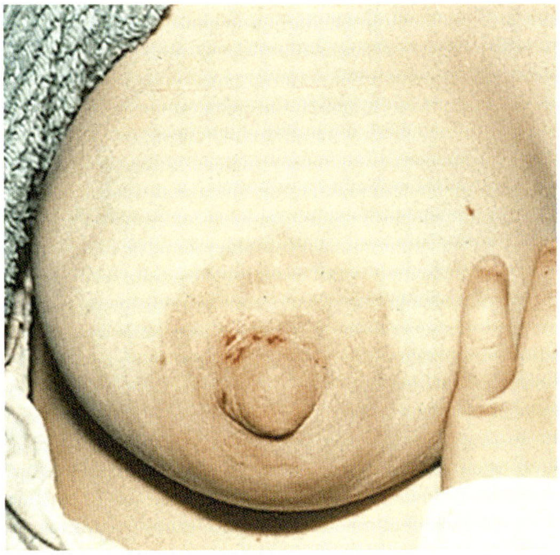

Color Plate 32 Herpes on the nipple.

Printed with permission of Chele Marmet.

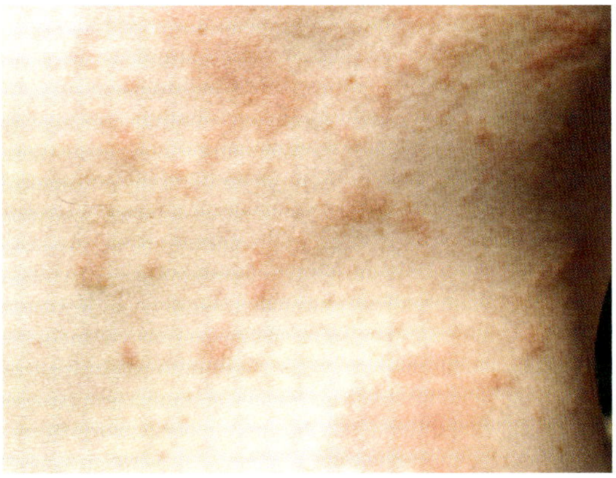

Color Plate 33 Poison ivy on the breast.

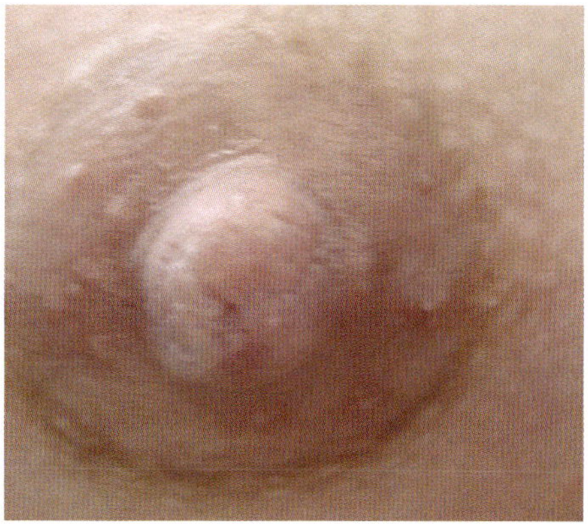

Color Plate 34 Stage I nipple trauma described in Table 17-3.

Printed with permission of Anna Swisher.

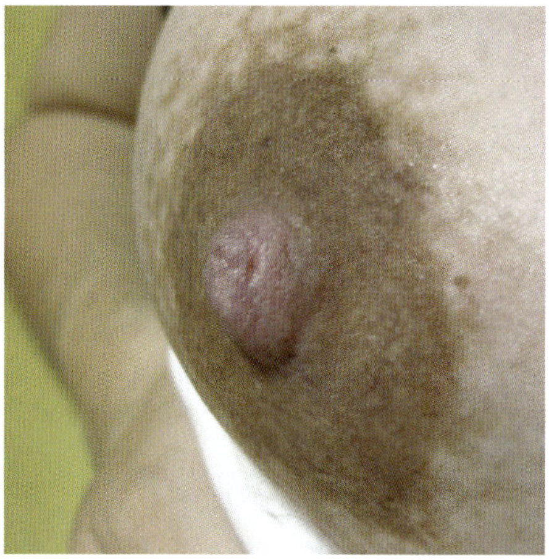

Color Plate 35 Stage II nipple trauma described in Table 17-3.

Printed with permission of Anna Swisher.

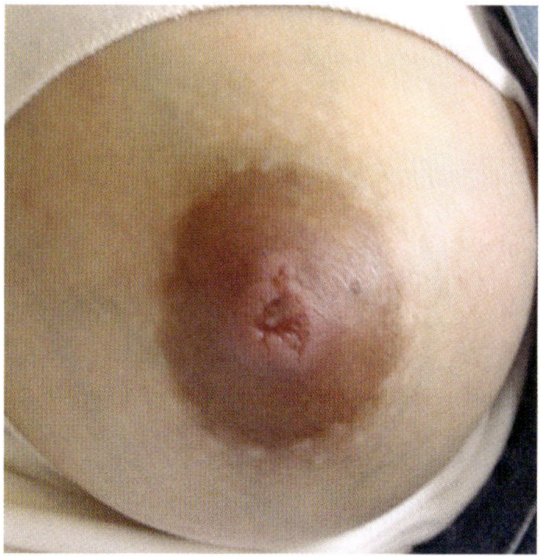

Color Plate 36 Stage III nipple trauma described in Table 17-3.

Printed with permission of Anna Swisher.

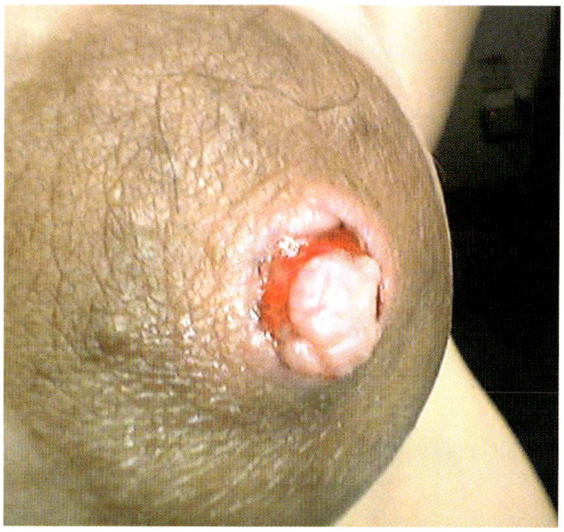

Color Plate 37 Stage IV nipple trauma described in Table 17-3.

Printed with Permission of Linda Hill.

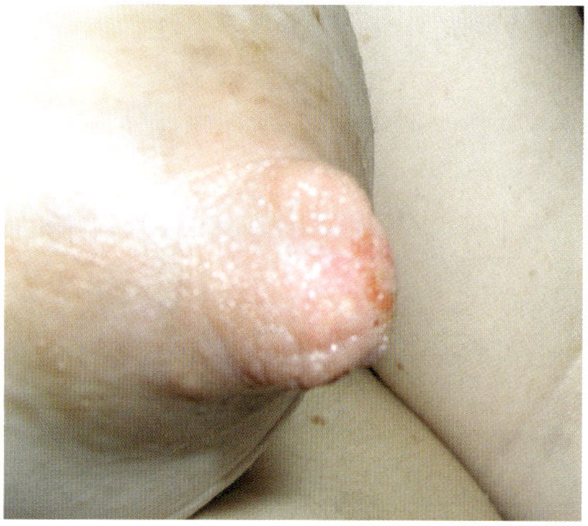

Color Plate 38 Cracked nipple.

Printed with permission of Catherine Watson Genna, BS, IBCLC.

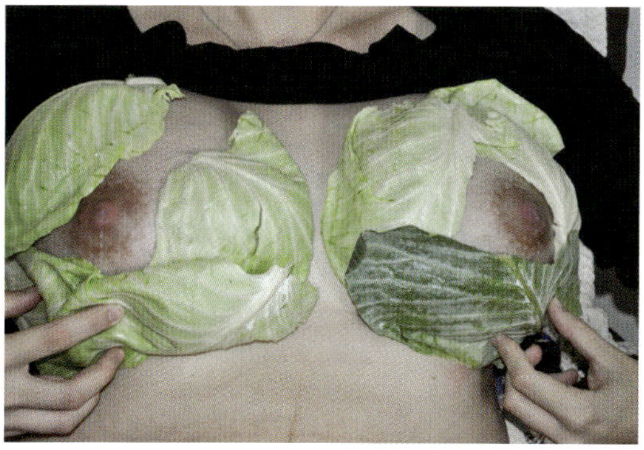

Color Plate 39 Mother with cabbage on her breasts to relieve engorgement.

Printed with permission of Anna Swisher.

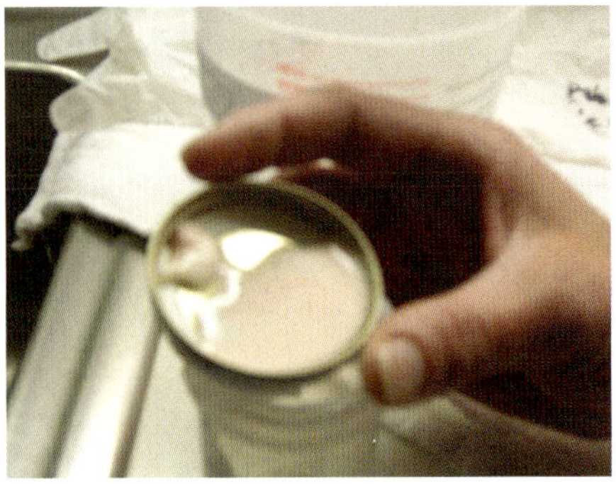

Color Plate 40 Lump in milk released from a breast infection.

Printed with permission of Judith Lauwers.

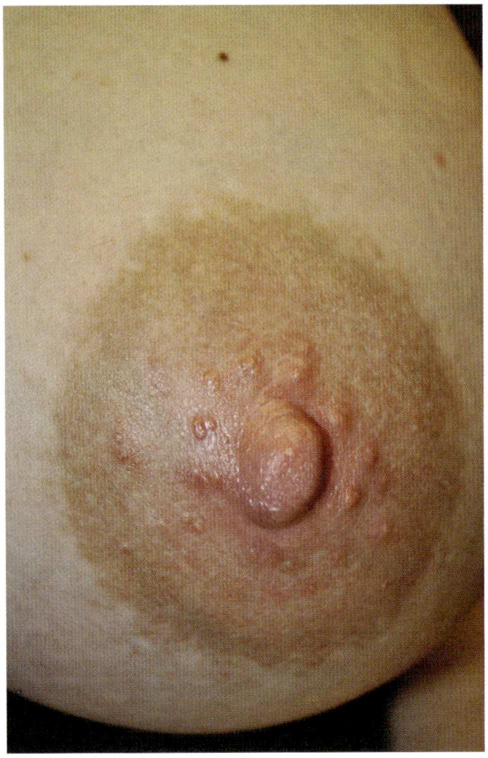

Color Plate 41 Milk blister on the nipple.

Printed with permission of Anna Swisher.

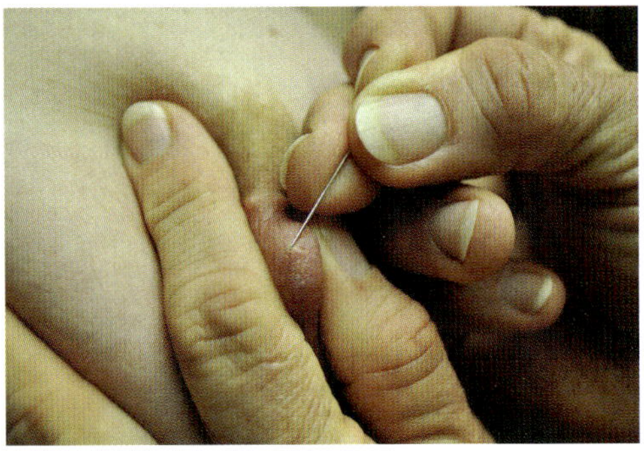

Color Plate 42 Opening a blister or bleb with a sterile needle.

Printed with permission of Anna Swisher.

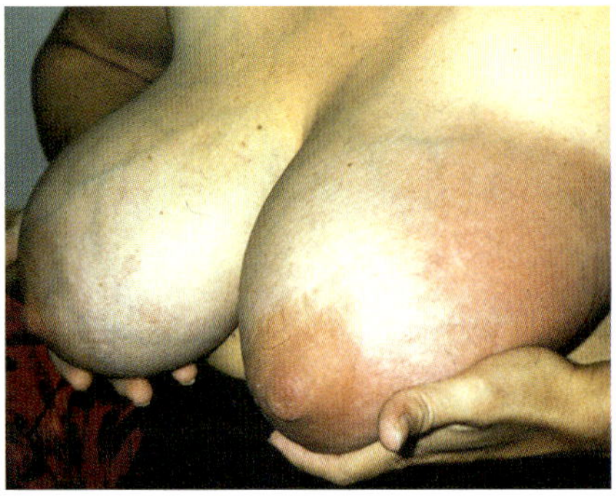

Color Plate 43 Mother with mastitis.

Printed with permission of Sarah Coulter Danner.

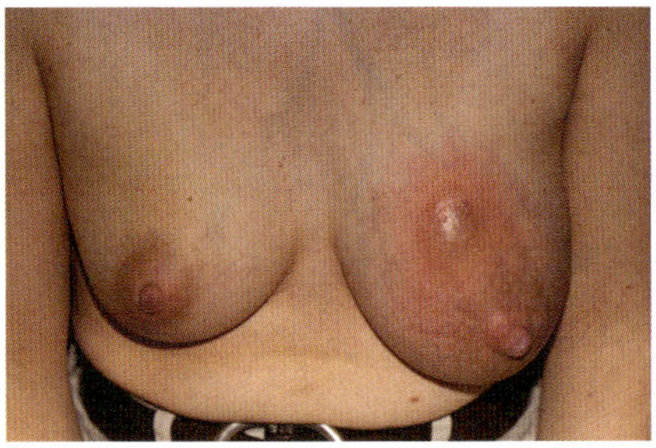

Color Plate 44 Breast abscess before surgery.

Printed with permission of Kay Hoover and Barbara Wilson-Clay.

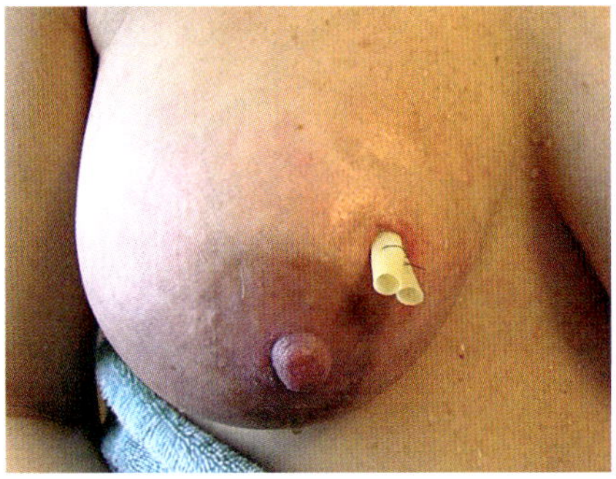

Color Plate 45 Breast abscess after surgery.

Printed with permission of Kay Hoover and Barbara Wilson-Clay.

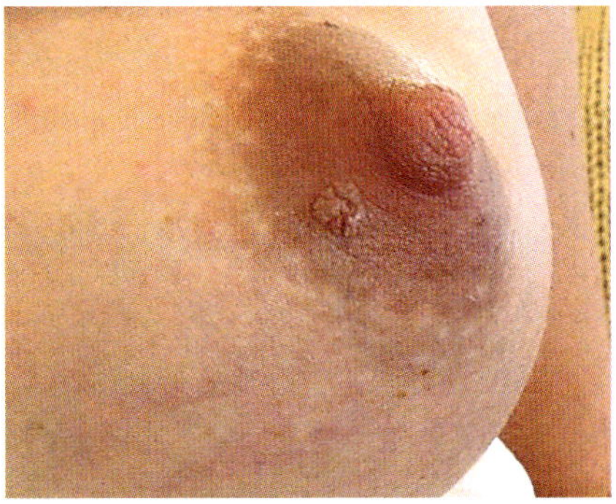

Color Plate 46 Scar on breast (bottom left) from childhood injury.

Printed with permission of Anna Swisher.